MEDICAL RADIOLOGY

Diagnostic Imaging

Springer-Verlag Berlin Heidelberg GmbH

Ph. Demaerel (Ed.)

Recent Advances in Diagnostic Neuroradiology

With Contributions by

A. Abanou · E. Achten · D. Balériaux · F. Barkhof · L. Bellinger · E. Bergers · P. Brys
J. Byrne · E. A. Cabanis · F. Calabro · A. G. Clifton · Ph. David · Ph. Demaerel
J. M. Donovan Post · V. Dousset · M. Droessaert · Z. Fan · P. Flamen · D. Gambarelli
N. Girard · P. D. Griffiths · M. Grisoli · S. Halpin · A. J. Holz · M. D. Hourihan
M.-T. Iba-Zizen · A. Jackson · R. H. Jäger · O. Jansen · M. Jidal · J. R. Jinkins · Z. Liu
F. Maes · K. Miszkiel · W. Mukonoweshuro · T. P. Naidich · P. M. Parizel · Z. Patay
C. Raybaud · F. Rio · M. Ryan · M. Savoiardo · P. D. Schellinger · E. Sklar · S. Sunaert
W. Taylor · L. van den Hauwe · D. Vandermeulen · J. W. Van Goethem · P. Van Hecke
K. Van Leemput · A. D. Waldman · G. Wilms · L. Xiong · I. Yousry · T. A. Yousry · Q. Zeng

Series Editor's Foreword by

A. L. Baert

With 367 Figures in 925 Separate Illustrations, 34 in Color and 18 Tables

Springer

Philippe Demaerel, MD, PhD
Professor, Department of Radiology
University Hospitals K.U.L.
Herestraat 49
3000 Leuven
Belgium

Medical Radiology · Diagnostic Imaging and Radiation Oncology
Continuation of
Handbuch der medizinischen Radiologie
Encyclopedia of Medical Radiology

ISBN 978-3-642-63003-3 ISBN 978-3-642-56662-2 (eBook)
DOI 10.1007/978-3-642-56662-2

Library of Congress Cataloging-in-Publication Data
Recent advances in diagnostic neuroradiology / P. Demaerel (ed.); with contributions by E. Achten ... [et al.]; foreword by A. L. Baert.
p.; cm. -- (Medical Radiology)
Includes bibliographical references and index.

1. Brain--Imaging. 2. Spinal cord--Imaging. 3. Spine--Imaging. I. Demaerel, P. (Philippe), 1963- II. Series.
[DNLM: 1. Neuroradiography--methods. 2. Nervous System Diseases--diagnosis. WL 141 R295 200]
RC386.6.D52 R43 2000
616.8'04754--dc21 00-020834

Originally published by Springer-Verlag Berlin Heidelberg New York in 2001
Softcover reprint of the hardcover 1st edition 2001

Cover-Design and Typesetting: Verlagsservice Teichmann, 69256 Mauer

SPIN: 107 188 33 21/3130 – 5 4 3 2 1 0

To my wonderful wife
INGELE

and our sons
RIK, VICTOR and PHILIP GEORG

Foreword

The tremendous progress in the radiological management of patients suffering from neurological disorders which has been achieved during recent years is now widely recognized by all neuroscientists as well as by the large medical community.

In no other radiological subdiscipline is the impact of the new sectional imaging modalities, especially MRI, on clinical practice so evident and so massive as in the neuroradiological field. The editors of this series are convinced that, notwithstanding the availability of numerous excellent textbooks on modern neuroradiology, this volume still will be able to fill some niches in the rapidly evolving and large neuroradiological imaging database.

I am extremely grateful for the highly professional engagement and the enthusiasm of Prof. P. Demaerel during the preparation of this book. He was not only able to engage a select group of outstanding internationally recognized neuroradiologists and to perform the necessary editorial work on the different topics, but also to contribute excellent chapters from his own hand. I congratulate him and all co-authors on this superb performance. I am convinced that this volume, like so many others in the Medical Radiology diagnostic series, will meet the great success it certainly deserves with clinicians, neuroradiologists and all other professionals daily engaged in the neurosciences.

Leuven

ALBERT L. BAERT

Preface

Several excellent textbooks exist on diagnostic adult or pediatric neuroradiology, and the purpose here was certainly not to provide another overview of neuroimaging. Rather, this volume was conceived as an addendum to the existing references on neuroradiology; the topics selected are those where significant progress has been achieved in the past 2–3 years.

Techniques and clinical applications in MR imaging are evolving so rapidly that the challenge of keeping up with the innovations is enormous. Instead of devoting a section to the physics of MR imaging, we opted for six topics that are usually barely treated in the standard textbooks. These include management, quantitative MR imaging and neuroanatomy. Other chapters deal with progress in sequence design, contrast media and spectroscopy.

The sections on the brain and the spine each begin with an introductory chapter. Three topics are discussed in both sections: trauma, tumors, and post-therapeutic imaging. Four chapters are devoted to vascular disease of the brain, including the role of MR angiography. The imaging approach to a series of clinical entities is discussed in more detail than in the standard textbooks: epilepsy, multiple sclerosis, degenerative disease, AIDS and neurofibromatosis. There is a chapter on imaging in ophthalmology and one on the imaging of endocrine diseases. Three topics were chosen in the field of pediatric neuroradiology. In the section on the spine there are also chapters on infections and lymphoproliferative diseases.

There is certainly some overlap of material, which has the advantage that chapters can be read individually. One of the express goals was to offer relatively short contributions to inform the interested reader rapidly on recent advances in the given field.

I wish to thank the more than 50 contributors for their tremendous efforts to make this book possible. We hope that this volume will provide a state-of-the-art selection of topics in the field of diagnostic neuroradiology and that it will further expand the expertise of the reader.

Leuven

Philippe Demaerel

Contents

Techniques in Neuroradiology

1 Management in Neuroradiology

Paul M. Parizel

CONTENTS

1.1 Introduction

The term 'management' has many definitions. In the clinical sense, management of a disease or a patient is thought of as the whole system of care and treatment. In the business world, management is usually defined as the executive function of planning, organizing, coordinating, directing, controlling and supervising a business. This implies a judicious use of means to accomplish an end, directed by art or craft (Webster's Third New International Dictionary 1986).

In this time and age, where cost containment is an essential element in all health care systems, neuroradiology, like other specialties, has come under intense scrutiny to reexamine resource management and to pursue additional efficiencies. One of the methods of achieving this goal is by applying the concept of 'total quality management', which should reduce costs while improving both efficiency and quality of care. Management rules and guidelines, which apply to the business world (profit organizations), are not, however, immediately transferable to medical departments, which are, in most European countries, non-profit organizations. As a reminder, a summary of the different types of organizational structures is provided in Table 1.1.

Table 1.1. Types of organizational structures

	Private	Public
Profit	e.g. companies	e.g. state enterprises (postal services, national railway system)
Non-profit	e.g. unions, charitable institutions, cultural organizations	e.g. city hospitals, government institutions (ministry of health), schools

In the present chapter, I will not address the highly political and controversial question of whether neuroradiology should exist as an independent department, or whether it should function as a section in a radiology department, or as a unit in a larger neurosciences clinical division. To avoid controversy, throughout this chapter, I will use the hybrid term 'neuroradiology department/section'.

1.2 Characteristics of a Neuroradiology Department/Section

The functioning of a (neuro)radiology department/section is governed by distinctive characteristics which are intrinsic to the so-called services sector:

P.M. Parizel, MD, PhD
Department of Radiology, University of Antwerp, Wilrijkstraat 10, 2650 Edegem, Belgium

- Intangibility. The concept of intangibility implies that the perception by the customer of the service provided is not directly linked to objectively measurable criteria of performance. A neuroradiology unit has two types of customers: the *referring physician* and the *patient*. The referring physician is, to a large extent, able to appreciate the quality of the diagnosis or interventional procedure provided, but his/her behaviour will also be influenced by other aspects of the production process: ease of scheduling, waiting list, speed of the reporting, etc. Conversely, our other type of customer, namely the patient, is usually not in a position to judge the quality of the care provided by the neuroradiologist (appropriateness of the examination, correctness of the diagnosis, quality of the treatment, etc.). The patient's judgement will often rely on subsidiary functions: was it difficult to get an appointment and was there a waiting list? Was the time schedule for the appointment respected? Were the people friendly? Did the report reach the referring physician in time? Was the department clean and modern? etc.
- Inseparability: the service cannot be separated from the person(s) of the provider(s) of the service, i.e. the neuroradiologist(s). This characteristic also limits the scale of operation. One interventional neuroradiologist can treat only so many patients. Moreover, though great care is given to the education and training of neuroradiologists, the skilled expertise provided in a department is inseparable from the qualification and experience of the individual performing the procedures. Managers of departments or hospitals tend to disregard this principle and think in terms of interchangeability of people or 'full time equivalents'. Successful management of a neuroradiology department/section implies respect for the strengths and prowess of each individual.
- Heterogeneity: it is impossible to standardize output among several providers of presumably the same service. All neuroradiological procedures are not of the same quality, and it is often difficult to judge the quality of the service provided. For example, even for a relatively straightforward 'product' such as a radiological report, there are no objective standards to judge the quality or completeness. In light of these problems of standardization and quality evaluation, an important challenge in managing a neuroradiology section, or any enterprise of the same kind, is to ensure consistent and high-quality performance.
- Fluctuating demand: by definition, medical demand fluctuates considerably. Ideally, a department should be structured so that it can adequately meet peak demands, without having too much overcapacity. There are only two possible solutions: (1) level the demand; (2) adaptable production capacity. An electronic scheduling system can be of great value in levelling demand, and in avoiding great fluctuations. Adaptability of the production capacity is more difficult to achieve. The practice of hiring mobile CT or MRI scanners has not gained wide acceptance in Europe.

It is important to keep in mind that the level of quality is remembered long after the illness is forgotten. Therefore, total quality management systems should be integrated in neuroradiology to improve efficiency and quality.

1.3 Task Definition of a Neuroradiology Department/Section

Good management presupposes a clear and unambiguous definition of the goals and priorities for neuroradiologists within the organizational structure in which they are employed (independent neuroradiology department versus neuroradiology section as part of the radiology department; university or teaching hospital setting versus large community hospital; etc.). In the following paragraphs, I have attempted to itemize the tasks of a neuroradiologist.

1.3.1 Patient Care

Patient care is, by any standard, and regardless of the type of practice, our *core business activity*. Neuroradiologists are trained to devote the best of their energies and creative skills towards *the practice of diagnostic and interventional radiology*. Generally, neuroradiologists are highly regarded for their professional skills and level of expertise, not only by their fellow radiologists, but also by their clinical colleagues in the fields of neurosurgery, neurology, ENT, ophthalmology, psychiatry, orthopedics, etc. Recognition by peers has been one of the driving forces in the development of neuroradiology as a specialty in its own right.

1.3.2 Educational Activities

Educational activities (teaching at undergraduate, graduate and postgraduate level) constitute an essential part of radiology in academic centres and teaching hospitals. These activities are time-consuming and tend to reduce the efficiency of patient throughput. Nevertheless they are mandatory for the continued survival of neuroradiological skills and knowledge. Economic pressures tend to reduce the time and personnel available for teaching activities. It should be made clear to hospital administrators, that if a radiology department wants to maintain a position of leadership in training students, residents, fellows, visiting radiologists, etc., this will cost time and more staff will need to be hired.

1.3.3 Scientific Research

Scientific research is highly desirable for neuroradiologists to keep abreast of the rapid developments in their field. Again, though many hospitals or universities encourage their staff members to adopt a high scientific profile (published papers, abstracts at meetings, etc.), they are reluctant to provide the necessary staffing or organizational framework for these activities. Management systems should address this issue. If the organization wants to maintain a scientific profile and presence on an international level, it will need to create a framework and provide personnel to achieve this goal.

1.3.4 Interdisciplinary Communication and Cooperation

Neuroradiology has traditionally had strong ties with neurosurgery. Historically, neuroradiological procedures such as air encephalography were first practised by neurosurgeons. Over the past decades, the symbiotic relationship with neurosurgeons has proved to be durable and mutually beneficial. A similarly advantageous affinity has developed over the past decade with ENT surgeons, who are increasingly relying on imaging techniques for the diagnosis, staging and interventional radiology management of certain diseases. Conversely, the interdisciplinary relationship between neuroradiology and neurology has been more strained. The introduction of cross-sectional imaging techniques such as computed tomography (CT) in the 1970s and magnetic resonance imaging (MRI) in the 1980s has given rise to turf battles in many hospitals. In some countries, neurologists perform a substantial percentage of CT and MR scans of the brain, and, to a much lesser extent, of the spine. Neuroradiologists have not always been successful in managing these conflicts of interest. The introduction of a total quality management system in the hospital should be viewed as a unique opportunity to resolve these turf battles, to the benefit of the patient, and of efficient work flow.

1.3.5 Interprofessional Communication and Cooperation

In many, if not most, departments, neuroradiologists have tended to neglect the administration, organization and communication aspects of their activities. Relations with hospital managers are often strained. Neuroradiology is often singled out as an example of technologically advanced high-cost medicine. Moreover, the diagnostic or therapeutic yield of many neuroradiology procedures is less visible than of many other specialties.

1.4 Management in Neuroradiology: Needs and Opportunities

Economic pressures are impacting all facets of the health care system. Radiology departments, and even more so neuroradiology departments/sections, are under close scrutiny by government planners, hospital managers and financial officers, because they are perceived as being capital-intensive and because of their high-tech aura. In many hospitals, they have become primary targets for cost control. Neuroradiology is particularly visible and vulnerable to cost controllers because of the high purchase and maintenance price of instruments and the need for continuous system upgrades (Margulis et al. 1994). The need to keep up with the rapid pace of scientific and technological developments may lead to a spiralling increase of health care expenditures (Hillman et al. 1994a; Hillman 1994b).

These developments are driving the need for greater efficiency and for changes in the organizational fabric of a neuroradiology department/section. Changes involve not only patient-care related issues, but also all of the other aspects pertaining to the daily activities in neuroradiology. It is my opinion that the introduction of a total quality management (TQM) system should be regarded as a golden opportunity to restructure a neuroradiology unit and to clearly redefine the goals and ambitions of all parties concerned.

TQM changes the production and distribution processes and the relationship between suppliers and patients in a hospital. In the area of science, TQM aims to provide a more structured approach to research activities within the department. The same holds true for teaching and education tasks. The successful functioning of a TQM system requires tools to monitor the performance of the neuroradiology department/section, such as: quality assessment, information support systems, bench marking, information support systems, real-time control, etc. Bench marking is the first step towards improving productivity because it creates a baseline for assessing progress and it enables a department/section to compare itself with other institutions; cost, quality and service should also be included in the bench marking process.

1.5 Guidelines Towards Efficient Management

Within the limited scope of this chapter, it is of course impossible to review the entire management process for a neuroradiology department/section. In the following paragraphs, I will focus on a few items, which I consider important in the efficient management of a unit.

1.5.1 People Management

Neuroradiologists should be encouraged to become more involved in managerial responsibilities and to play an advisory role on quality issues. *Decentralized decision making* is an important tool to help individuals gain control over their immediate work environment. Protocol driven approaches for certain diseases and clinical questions can save time. Therefore, the development of algorithm based strategies by neuroradiologists for CT and MR examinations saves time and streamlines the patient flow.

Highly unusual in academic or community hospitals, but very effective as a management tool, is the introduction of *incentives*, based on results achieved by individuals or sections. This requires an unequivocal definition of the goals to be achieved: patient care, scientific activities (papers published, abstracts accepted, grant money generated), educational activities, management, contacts with other departments, etc. Good management should strive to create a caring work environment, and to develop a skilled professional staff with a high level of integrity.

Cost containment should not initially be performed on expenditures for auxiliary personnel (receptionists, secretaries, etc.), who are the interface of the neuroradiology department/section with the customers (referring physicians and patients). In the 'services sector', cutting costs by reducing ancillary personnel may cause a negative spiral which is sometimes referred to as the 'strategic management trap' (Fig. 1.1).

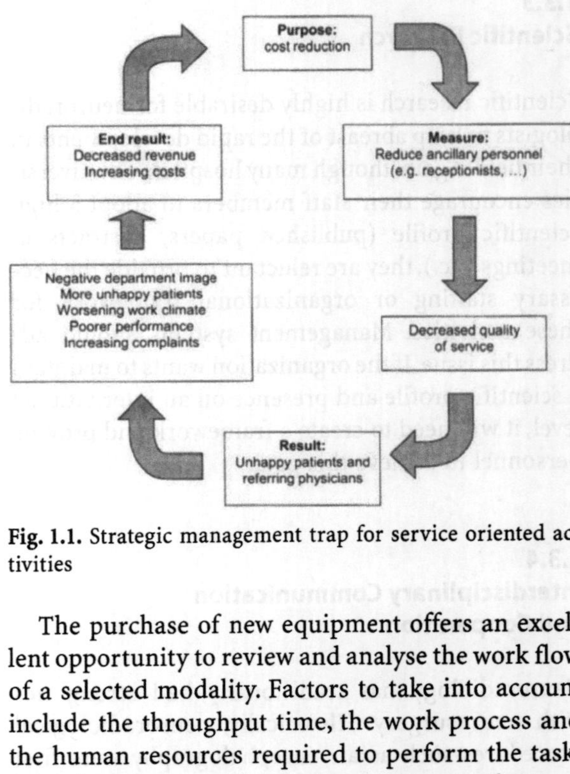

Fig. 1.1. Strategic management trap for service oriented activities

The purchase of new equipment offers an excellent opportunity to review and analyse the work flow of a selected modality. Factors to take into account include the throughput time, the work process and the human resources required to perform the task. Many hospitals spend very large amounts of money on new equipment, without operations analysis or staff training.

1.5.2 Patient Scheduling

In today's world of integrated hospital and radiology information systems (HIS and RIS), a centralized electronic scheduling system for patients should be used. Access to the scheduler should be achievable simultaneously from multiple hospital domains and units (ambulatory care services, patient wards, physician offices, etc.) as well as within the radiology domain. Figure 1.2 provides an example of a scheduling work flow. The electronic appointment book automatically suggests scheduled time slots, based on patient availability and clinical pathways. An electronic scheduling system can prevent resource overbooking, procedure-procedure interaction, and inappropriately utilized resources. Separate schedules can be maintained for inpatients and outpatients.

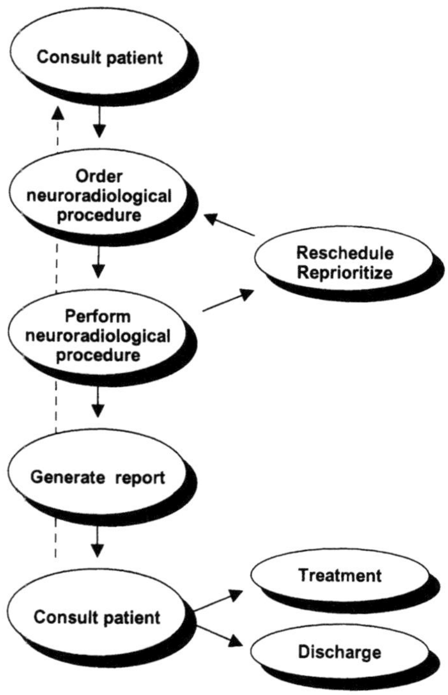

Fig. 1.2. Neuroradiology scheduling workflow

Ultimately, the electronic appointment book reduces the number of phone calls required to coordinate schedules across several units, and ensures that the patient is available at the required time. Moreover, the scheduler can automatically confirm appointments by notifying the referring physician either through e-mail, letter or fax. This system is efficient and saves time for the administrative staff.

1.5.3 Patient Waiting Areas

Theoretically, use of a centralized electronic scheduling system reduces waiting times and ensures an efficient patient flow for neuroradiology procedures. Nevertheless, when the patient has to wait (e.g. due to intervening emergency procedures, technical malfunction, etc.), it is important to inform patients while they wait, by giving them literature, or providing a video. Separate waiting areas for different image acquisition modalities are useful to regulate patient flows, and to avoid misunderstandings. The days of the central waiting area are over.

1.5.4 Image Processing and Management

It is self-evident that neuroradiology, as well as other imaging divisions, will evolve towards a filmless, electronic image management and viewing paradigm. Even today, a very substantial amount of routine neuroradiologic images are generated in digital format: CT, MRI, angiography. It is therefore natural that neuroradiology departments/sections should be among the first to adopt picture archiving and communications systems (PACS), since such an important part of their image output is already in digital format. Nevertheless, it should be emphasized that PACS is not a toy for radiologists, but a tool for the hospital and the medical community as a whole. Therefore the expenditures for a PACS system should not be billed to the (neuro)radiology department/section, but should be evenly distributed over the hospital. The ultimate goal is for a PACS system to be hospitalwide, including all imaging modalities online. Workstations must be able to display past with current images, together with providing access to the patient's clinical history. Though PACS requires considerable investments, part of the money can be recuperated in storage space, increased efficiency, decreased need for archiving personnel in the file room, decreased film expenditures, etc.

1.5.5 Reporting

Neuroradiologists can and should make good use of the opportunities provided by the rapid developments in computer technology to improve reporting systems. Integration of data from different sources can help the decision-making process and allows closer collaboration with other disciplines. With PACS, immediate comparison with previous examinations is possible without the need for actual transport of hard copy films.

Digital reporting is gaining increased acceptance. The challenge is to create reports simply, easily, quickly and inexpensively. Immediate reporting, also known as real-time reporting, is the digital equivalent of what used to be called 'wet reading' in the old days. It implies that images are imported as soon as they are generated and accepted as appropriate. From a managerial point of view, it is important to remember that immediate reporting presupposes a sufficient number of skilled radiologists to provide a continuous service. In teaching hospitals, the 'film-reading sessions' with medical students, residents and fellows will need to be redefined. In most European centres, on-line reporting is not a realistic option because departments are generally understaffed.

The information of the radiology report needs to be integrated into the electronic patient record. It can be entered into RIS by transcription (relatively slow, labour intensive and therefore expensive) or by speech recognition. Though at present only a few departments are using speech recognition software to generate reports, tremendous technological advances show great promise in this area, and it is likely that speech recognition will become the standard in a few years time.

Neuroradiology lends itself well to 'structured reporting', with a controlled vocabulary and predefined format. Structured reporting allows standardization of data collection and consistent interpretation of these data. This has opened the way to measure outcomes analysis.

It should be understood that these changes will ultimately generate more work for the radiologist, but the quality of diagnosis and of reporting will be enhanced.

1.6 Conclusion

Quality in neuroradiology can only be achieved when there is a commitment and a will from the top management of the hospital to wholeheartedly support this goal. There are three key elements to the successful management of a neuroradiology department/section of the 21st century:

1. High-quality and state-of-the-art image acquisition equipment (neuroangiography suite, magnetic resonance imaging unit(s), computed tomography, interventional room, etc.) is a prerequisite for high standards of care. The practice of neuroradiology is changing rapidly, and a judicious investment policy is required.
2. A strategic plan to implement ongoing advances in image processing (digital radiology, PACS) and reporting will ultimately save costs and generate a higher standard of care. Seamless integration of image acquisition modalities with viewing and reporting devices is the key to successful data management.
3. Most important, however, is the human resources management for medical and paramedical personnel. All too often, superbly equipped hospitals and departments have been unable to build and hold together a team of dedicated and skilled professional staff through lack of long-term vision in people management. Administrative and managerial support systems should help department or section heads to improve their team-building skills. This is even more important in academic or university centres, where the financial rewards are lower than in private hospitals.

Many members of the medical profession experience an almost visceral reaction of aversion and negation whenever the term 'management' is mentioned. Yet, efficient management of a busy neuroradiology department streamlines the work flow and can help physicians to spend more time providing medical care to their patients. Given the efforts to reduce healthcare costs in general, and the cost of diagnostic and interventional neuroradiological procedures in particular, neuroradiologists should fully support the drive towards quality management in order to increase efficiency and care standards for our patients. The increasing complexities of a modern neuroradiology department/section enhance the need for efficient management. In this context, it is also wise to remember the words of Prof. Alexander Margulis: "High imaging technology retains similarity to the most ancient one: fire. It is an excellent servant, but a terrible master when it escapes control" (Margulis et al. 1994).

References

Hillman BJ (1994a) Outcomes for research and cost-effectiveness analysis for diagnostic imaging. Radiology 193:307–310

Hillman BJ (1994b) New imaging technology and cost containment. AJR 162:503–506

Margulis AR, Kucharzyk J, Hetts SW, Werne AM (1994) High imaging technology and health care expenditures. Eur Radiol 4:1–3

Webster's Third New International Dictionary (1986) Merriam-Webster Inc. Publishers, Springfield, Massachusetts, USA

2 Progress in Neuroanatomy

TAREK A. YOUSRY, INDRA YOUSRY, THOMAS P. NAIDICH

CONTENTS

2.1 Introduction

Anatomy is the basis of radiology and a major pillar of neuroradiology, neurology and neurosurgery. Technical advances in neuroimaging – especially magnetic resonance imaging (MRI) – now enable us to visualize, in vivo, details of the brain that were difficult to assess just a few years ago. These advances provide the finer anatomic display of gyri, sulci, cranial nuclei and cranial nerves required to complement concurrent advances in neurosurgery and neurofunctional imaging.

T.A. YOUSRY, MD; I. YOUSRY, MD
Abteilung für Neuroradiologie, Klinikum Grosshadern, Marchioninistrasse 15, 81366 München, Germany
T.P. NAIDICH, MD, FACR
Professor of Radiology, Director of Neuroradiology, The Mount Sinai Medical Center, One Gustave L. Levy Place, Department of Radiology, Box 1234, New York, NY 10029-6574, USA

2.2 Technical Considerations

2.2.1 The Cortex

Three-dimensional (3D) T1-weighted sequences such as MPRAGE (magnetization prepared rapid acquisition gradient echo) or SPGR (spoiled gradient recalled acquisition in the steady state) have made it possible to acquire a 3D data set with a slice thickness of 1 mm in one plane and to reformat the data to display any structure in any required plane with equal resolution. The 3D format and the reduced slice thickness have also permitted reconstruction of images of the brain surface of good quality (Figs. 2.1a, 2.2a). An impression of the cortical surface can also be obtained using the technique described by KATADA (1990). Combining the latter technique with venous MRA can give precise information as to the relationships between gyri and cortical veins (TSUCHIYA et al. 1999).

With current techniques at field strengths of 0.1–1.5 T, it is not yet possible to characterize the cytoarchitectonic or myelogenic features of the cortex. With more powerful magnets of 3.0 T or more, however, it is already possible to visualize the lines of Genari in the primary visual field (V1), and it should become possible to see other intracortical features in the near future.

2.2.2 The Cranial Nerves

Visualization of the cranial nerves was significantly improved by the use of sequences that give a cisternographic effect, for example, the 3D CISS (three-dimensional Fourier transformation constructive interference in steady-state) sequence. In these images the image contrast depends on the ratio of T2 to T1. Since this ratio approaches unity in cerebrospinal fluid (CSF), but is much lower in nerve tissue, the 3D

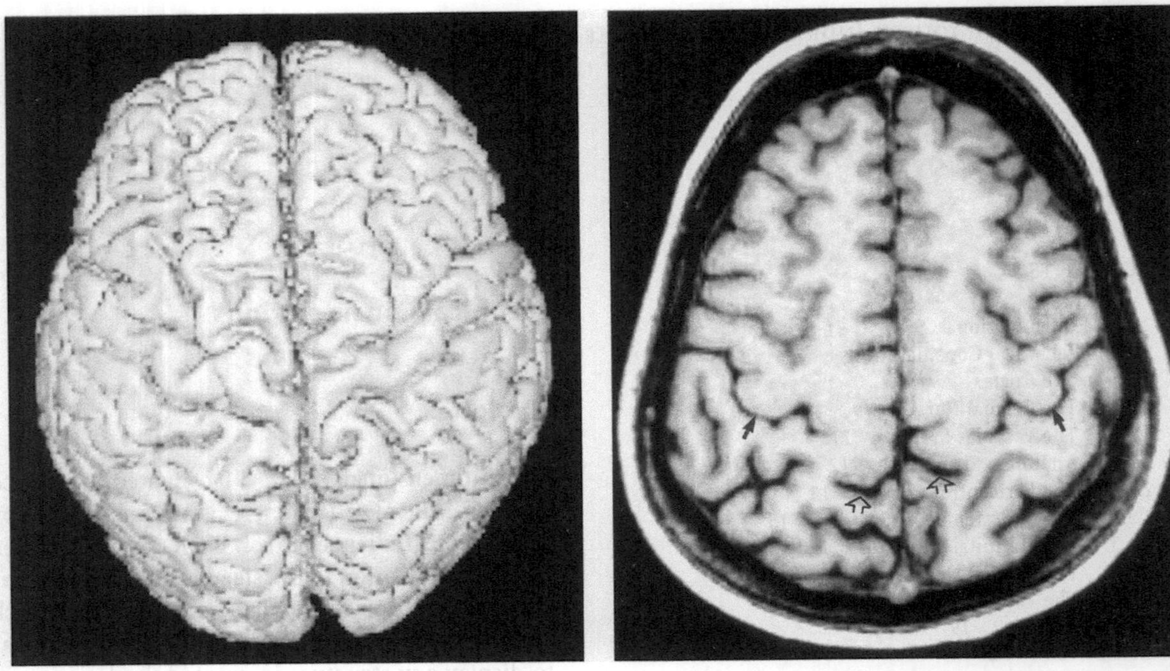

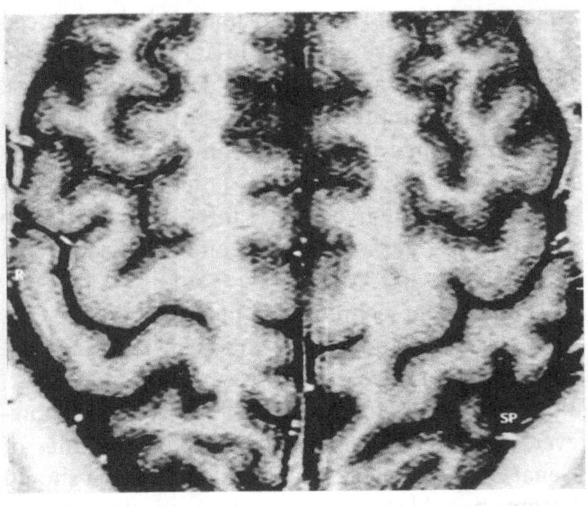

Fig. 2.1a–c. Pericentral region. Axial landmarks. Convexity surface rendering from a 3D data set acquired as a sagittal plane T1 w MPRAGE sequence (**a**). In the axial plane (**b** T1w MPRAGE sequence, **c** T1w inversion recovery sequence) the W-shaped knob of the precentral gyrus is easily identified (*arrows in* **b**). Furthermore, the pars marginalis of the cingulate sulcus of both hemispheres appears as a horizontal bracket (*open arrows in* **b**). The medial end of the central sulcus enters the pars bracket immediately anteriorly. The full sagittal dimension of the precentral gyrus is thicker than that of the postcentral gyrus (**b,c**). The cortex of the precentral gyrus is thicker than cortex of the postcentral gyrus (**c**)

CISS sequence achieves high CSF/nerve contrast and fine display of the intracisternal segments of the cranial nerves. These techniques have improved the assessment of cranial nerves. In addition, the 3D CISS sequence visualizes other intracisternal structures such as arteries and veins, permitting us to assess possible neurovascular compressions. Other studies have shown that 3D FSE (fast spin echo) sequences can yield similar results.

A newly developed ultra-long echo train length (ETL) 3D FSE and half-Fourier technique, performed in less than 3 min, is almost comparable to the conventional 3D-FSE images, performed in 15 min, for depicting anatomic details and pathologic findings. Implementation of the ultra-long ETL and half-Fourier 3D-FSE imaging technique enables acquisition of inner ear MR studies in a vastly reduced time, with high spatial resolution, without significant penalty (Naganawa et al. 1998). 3D FSE sequences have made possible 3D reconstruction of the endolymphatic and perilymphatic labyrinth of the inner ear (Hans et al. 1999).

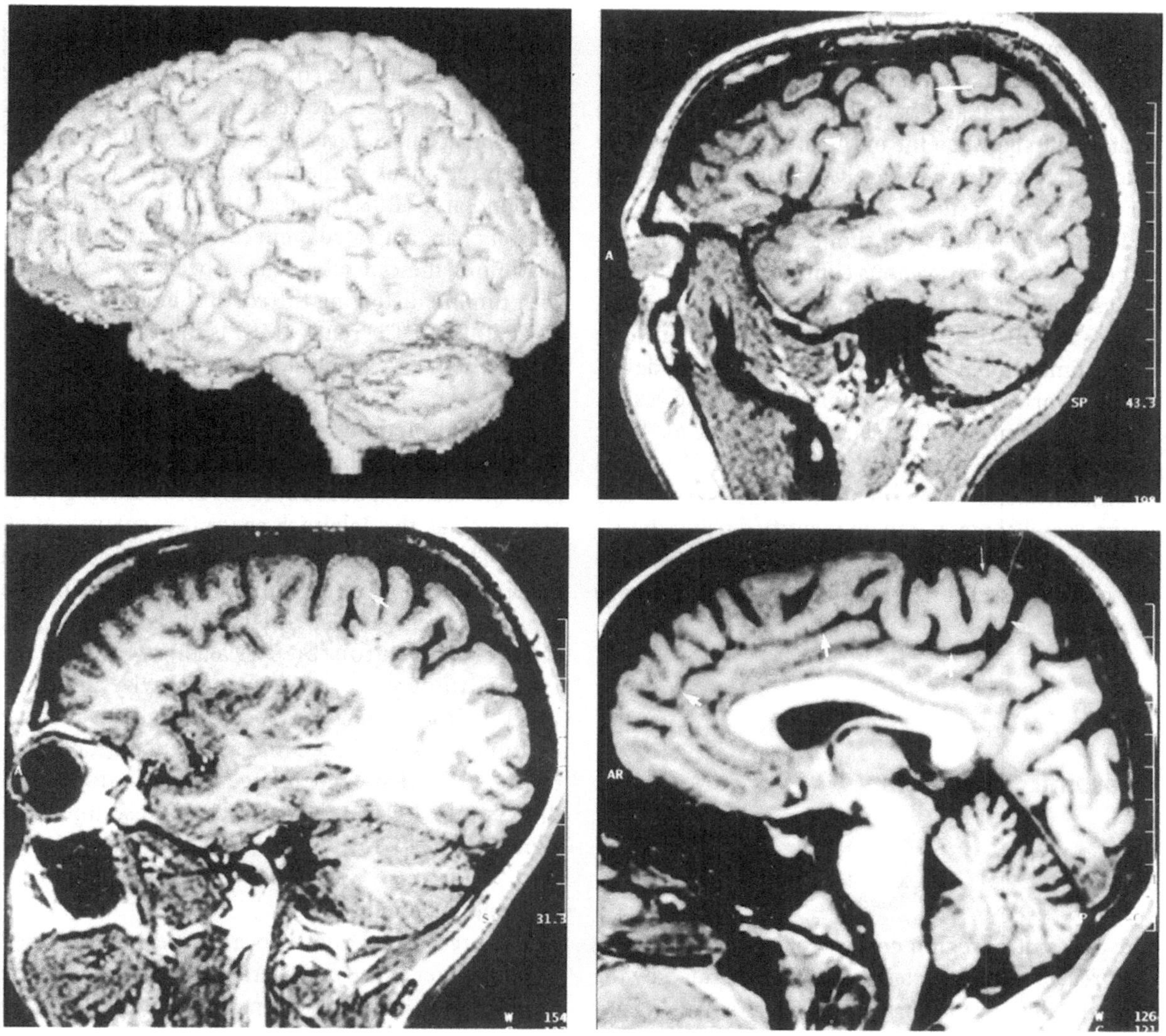

a b c d

Fig. 2.2a–d. Pericentral region. Sagittal landmarks (T1w MPRAGE sequence). **a** Left lateral convexity surface rendering from a 3D data set acquired as a sagittal plane T1 w MPRAGE sequence. Anterior is the reader's left. **b** In the sagittal plane the anterior horizontal (*long thin arrow*) and anterior ascending (*short thin arrow*) rami of the sylvian fissure are first identified on the lateral sections, and used to identify the M shape of the inferior frontal gyrus. Posterior to this gyrus, in order, lie the precentral sulcus (*short arrow*), the subcallosal gyrus, the central sulcus (*long arrow*) and the postcentral gyrus. **c** At the level of the insula, the posteriorly directed hook (*arrow*) of the motor hand area defines the precentral gyrus. **d** The cingulate sulcus and its ramus marginalis (*arrows*) are first identified. The central sulcus (*thin arrow*) lies immediately anterior to the ramus marginalis and is oriented such that it curves posteriorly, to course nearly perpendicular to the ramus marginalis

2.2.3 The Vascular System

Two major techniques for MR angiography (MRA) are used to evaluate the vascular system: time of flight (TOF) MRA and phase contrast (PC) MRA. In comparison to digital subtraction angiography (DSA), it has been shown that MR angiography with maximum pixel intensity projection images has a sensitivity of 87% and a specificity of 88%. MR angiography source images have a sensitivity of 89% and a specificity of 63% in depicting the presence of a vessel segment of the circle of Willis. The positive predictive value of an arterial segment with a diameter of at least 1 mm was 99%. An arterial segment shown to have a diameter of at least 1 mm on the MR source image is almost always present and patent in vivo (Stock et al. 1996). The advantage of the TOF technique over the PC technique is that the TOF images also display the adjacent cerebral structures on the source images. The source images are of special interest for anatomical studies, because they combine cortical and vascular anatomy, so that the relationship between the brain and its vessels can be studied in vivo, non-invasively. This is especially true for the arterial system.

For the venous system similar results can be obtained by using intravenous contrast media with the TOF sequence, the MPRAGE sequence or the SPGR sequence (BRAUN et al. 1996a,b). Furthermore, three-dimensional imaging methods were developed to portray vascular anatomy, displaying vessels extracted from 3D data sets (BULLITT et al. 1997; GLOGER et al. 1994a–c).

Finally, it should be mentioned that vessels and nerve-vessel contacts can be identified using the 3D CISS sequence by following a vessel's course from the parent vessel to the area of supply or drainage (YOUSRY et al. 1999).

2.3 Anatomic Structures

2.3.1 The Pericentral Cortex

The pericentral region consists of two parallel gyri, the precentral and postcentral gyri, separated by the central sulcus. Superiorly, the central sulcus nearly always reaches the cerebral margin and may extend onto the medial interhemispheric surface of the brain. In this location, the precentral and postcentral gyri fuse to each other to form the paracentral lobule around the upper of the central sulcus. Inferiorly, the central sulcus rarely reaches the sylvian fissure. Instead, the precentral and postcentral gyri fuse together to form the subcentral gyrus between the inferior end of the central sulcus and the sylvian fissure. Functional and anatomical MRI have both been used to define significant regions along the precentral gyrus (primary motor cortex) and the postcentral gyrus (primary sensory cortex).

Functional Methods. Using functional MRI (fMRI) it can be shown that the motor hand area is located at the middle genu of the central sulcus in a portion of the precentral gyrus that displays a characteristic omega or epsilon shaped "knob" or "knuckle" (YOUSRY et al. 1995; NAIDICH and BRIGHTBILL 1996a). Using MEG (magnetoencephalography) it is possible to identify the postcentral gyrus reliably (SOBEL et al. 1993). Using PET (positron emission tomography), it can be shown that the cortical representation of the sensory hand area is located along the anterior bank of the postcentral gyrus at a characteristic curve of the central sulcus immediately posterior to the motor hand area (RUMEAU et al. 1994). Further, the detection of an "activated" vein can assist in the identification of the central sulcus, especially in patients with tumors distorting the cortical anatomy (YOUSRY et al. 1999). Currently fMRI is increasingly being used to define the central region preoperatively.

Anatomical Methods. CT has shown that the profound normal variability of the cortical anatomy can limit the use of standard systems for localizing anatomy, such as the Talairach space (STEINMETZ et al. 1989). Therefore, specific signs have been developed to help to identify the individual portions of the pericentral region more directly (YOUSRY et al. 1995; NAIDICH and BRIGHTBILL 1996a,b; IWASAKI et al. 1991; NAIDICH et al. 1995). The sensitivity and specificity of these signs has been evaluated and the multiple signs combined into a system for localizing the central sulcus and related gyri (NAIDICH and BRIGHTBILL 1996a). The newest and most important signs are briefly reviewed:

1. Axial plane images

a) The precentral knob: A focal, posteriorly directed protrusion of the precentral gyrus designated the precentral knob has been shown by fMRI to be the site of the hand motor area. This focal motor region is seen on axial CT and MRI images as inverted omega (90%) or as a horizontal epsilon (10%) in all cases (Fig. 2.1). This sign has a high interrater reproducibility (Yousry et al. 1997a) as well as a high "applicability" (Naidich and Brightbill 1996a).

b) The pars bracket sign: In axial plane CT and MRI, the pars marginalis of the cingulate sulcus of the left and the right cerebral hemispheres appear together as a horizontal bracket. The medial end of the central sulcus enters the pars bracket immediately anterior to the pars marginalis in 94%–96% of cases (Fig. 2.1), whereas the postcentral sulcus enters the pars bracket in only 3%. Thus, the relationship of a sulcus to the pars bracket permits accurate identification of the central sulcus, hence the term "bracket sign". This sign is also characterized by a high applicability (Naidich and Brightbill 1996a,b).

c) Thickness of pre- and postcentral gyri: Several studies have shown that the full sagittal dimension of the precentral gyrus is thicker than that of the postcentral gyrus (Fig. 2.1) (Naidich and Brightbill 1996a; Naidich et al. 1995). Further, the thickness of the *cortex* of the precentral gyrus is also greater than that of the postcentral gyrus (Meyer et al. 1996). Using T1 weighted turbo inversion recovery sequences the mean cortical thicknesses of the anterior (PrG) and posterior (PoG) banks of the central sulcus were found to be 2.70 and 1.76 mm for both hemispheres with a mean cortical thickness ratio of 1.54 (Fig. 2.1c) (Meyer et al. 1996). The difference in cortical thickness is based on and explained by cytoarchitectonic studies (Naidich and Brightbill 1996a; Brodmann 1909; von Economo and Koskinas 1925).
These three signs are the most important and most reliable for attempting to localize the central sulcus in the axial plane (Naidich and Brightbill 1996a).

2. Sagittal plane images
Other signs have been developed to identify pericentral structures in the sagittal plane:
a) Lateral sagittal plane. The "M" shape of the inferior frontal gyrus. The anterior horizontal and anterior ascending rami of the sylvian fissure extend upward into the inferior frontal gyrus, giving it the shape of a letter "M". The first vertical line of the "M" represents the pars orbitalis. The middle "v" of the "M" represents the pars triangularis. The posterior vertical line of the "M" represents the pars opercularis of the inferior frontal gyrus. Identification of the "M" provides the starting point for subsequent, sequential identification of the precentral sulcus, precentral gyrus, central sulcus and postcentral gyrus (Fig. 2.2) (Naidich et al. 1995; Steinmetz et al. 1990; Naidich et al. 1997).
b) Middle sagittal plane: The precentral knob. The posteriorly directed expansion of the precentral gyrus at the hand motor area may be identified at the level of the insula as a posteriorly directed hook which defines the position of the precentral gyrus, the central sulcus and the postcentral gyrus in 92% of cases (Fig. 2.2) (Yousry TA et al. 1997a).
c) Medial sagittal plane: The pars marginalis. The cingulate sulcus is followed posteriorly and then superiorly to identify the pars marginalis at the cerebral margin. The central sulcus lies millimeters anterior to the pars marginalis. Characteristically the central sulcus curves posteriorly and is oriented such that it curves downward and posteriorly to course nearly perpendicular to the pars marginalis (Fig. 2.2) (Naidich and Brightbill 1996a).
As in the axial plane, all these signs should be combined and handled as one system to localize the central region and the adjacent frontal and parietal areas (Naidich and Brightbill 1996a).
c) Neonatal imaging
In infants under the age of 3 months, the immature state of the myelination provides an additional sign for identifying the pericentral structures. At term the white matter of the precentral and postcentral gyri is more mature than the surrounding white matter. As a result it shows readily identifiable high signal intensity on T1-weighted images and low signal intensity on T2-weighted sequences (Yoshiura et al. 1998). This difference in intensity is a reliable sign for identifying the pericentral region. It is speculated that this difference in signal intensity reflects more advanced development of the nerve cells, oligodendroglial cells, synaptic density, and dentride formation, which may cause decreased interstitial water and increased lipid content of the membranes within the cortex (Korogi et al. 1996a).

2.3.2 The Supratemporal Surface

The transverse temporal gyrus of Heschl (synonym: Heschl's gyrus, HG) is the primary auditory cortex (A1) of the brain. It courses anterolaterally over the superior surface of the temporal lobe from the posterior border of the insula medially to the convexity surface of the temporal lobe laterally. It divides the superior surface of the temporal lobe into an anterior *planum polare* and a posterior *planum temporale*. The size of the planum temporale exhibits substantial bilateral asymmetry. The planum temporale appears to be significantly larger in the dominant hemisphere, and reflects dominant language processing (Flechsig 1908; Geshwind and Levitsky 1968; von Economo and Horn 1930; Steinmetz et al. 1991; Witelson and Pallie 1973). The morphometric characteristics and asymmetries of the planum temporale have been studied extensively in disorders such as dyslexia (Leonard et al. 1993; Galaburda et al. 1985; Hynd et al. 1990) and schizophrenia (Petty et al. 1995; Kulynych et al. 1995), with conflicting results as to the presence and extent of asymmetry of the planum temporale in these conditions.

Heschl's gyrus corresponds to Brodmann area 41 (BRODMAN 1909). Usually, only a restricted posteromedial portion of Heschl's gyrus can be considered the true site of A1 (LIEGEOIS-CHAUVEL et al. 1991). A second Heschl's gyrus may be present posterior and parallel to the first and may occasionally be functionally included in A1 (LIEGEOIS-CHAUVEL et al. 1995). Controversy persists as to the number of Heschl's gyri seen in association with hemispheric asymmetry. Some authors claim that one Heschl's gyrus is usually found in the left hemisphere, whereas 2 Heschl's gyri are usually found in the right hemispheres. Other recent studies have shown no hemispheric asymmetries in the number of Heschl's gyri. Using fMRI, activation related to white noise stimulation was found to be confined to the posterior aspect of the superior temporal gyrus, centered on Heschl's gyrus. Pure tone discrimination was localized to Heschl's gyrus (BINDER et al. 1994). High tones activated the medial part of Heschl's gyrus, whereas low tones activated the lateral parts of Heschl's gyrus (STRAINER et al. 1997). Speech activation was located in the posterior part of the superior temporal gyrus and was associated with significantly more widespread activation than were noise stimuli (BINDER et al. 1994).

Using MRI, a system was developed to accurately identify Heschl's gyrus in the axial, sagittal and coronal planes. In the *sagittal plane* just lateral to the insula the characteristic shape of Heschl's gyrus can easily be identified directly on the supratemporal surface without need for additional landmarks. Depending on the number of Heschl's gyri present, Heschl's gyrus may assume the form of a single "omega", a "mushroom" (VON ECONOMO and HORN 1930), a "heart" (VON ECONOMO and HORN 1930), or a double Ω (Fig. 2.3a) (YOUSRY TA et al. 1997b). In the *coronal plane,* perpendicular to the bicommissural plane, the section on which Heschl's gyrus is identified best is characterized by the tent-like shape formed by the convergence of the two fornices, and the presence of the VIIIth cranial nerves (Fig. 2.3b) (YOUSRY TA et al. 1997b). In the *axial plane,* the slice which best reveals Heschl's gyrus is the section which displays the adhesio interthalamica (massa intermedia of the thalamus) (Fig. 2.3c) (YOUSRY TA et al. 1997b).

2.3.3 The Occipital Lobe

The occipital lobe is important for the many visual areas (V1–V3) it contains. The primary visual area (V1) is located in the striate cortex. Most of the striate cortex extends along the calcarine sulcus (KOROGI et al. 1996b). However, the actual extent of the striate cortex within the calcarine sulcus is variable. Approximately 30% of the striate cortex may be exposed on the medial surface posteriorly. In other cases nearly all of the striate cortex lies hidden within the calcarine sulcus, extends into the parieto-occipital sulcus and/or lies on the tentorial surface of the occipital lobe (KOROGI et al. 1996b). The precise course of the calcarine sulcus also varies. Typically, the sulcus runs obliquely, first extending anterosuperiorly from the occipital pole partway toward the parieto-occipital sulcus and then further anteroinferiorly to its junction with the parieto-occipital sulcus (Fig. 2.4). KOROGI et al. classified the degree of continuity of the calcarine sulcus into three groups. In the first group (50%) the sulcus was found to be continuous without major branches. In the second group (26%), the calcarine sulcus gave off major branches. In the third group (24%), the calcarine sulcus showed significant disruptions (KOROGI et al. 1996b). In the coronal plane, the positions of the two calcarine sulci and the two parieto-occipital sulci were found to be symmetric in only 60% of cases. A significantly low position of one calcarine sulcus was found in 24%, whereas a unilateral V-shaped arrangement of the calcarine and the parieto-occipital sulcus was encountered in 16% (KOROGI et al. 1996b). The vertical separation between the two calcarine sulci in the coronal plane was found to be more than 10 mm in 12% of cases (KOROGI et al. 1996b). The exact position and symmetry of the calcarine and parieto-occipital sulci may also be influenced by the magnitude of any occipital petalia. These variations necessarily complicate the identification of the calcarine sulcus, and are therefore important to be known.

2.3.4 *The Cranial Nerves*

The visualization of the cisternal segments of the cranial nerves is determined, in part, by the specific anatomy of each cranial nerve: e.g., the nerve's diameter, the course of the nerve, and the volume of surrounding cerebrospinal fluid (CSF). Nerves with small diameters are difficult to visualize using conventional sequences.

Studies of the cranial nerves have mainly been performed using T1-weighted sequences (CAILLET et al. 1990; SUZUKI et al. 1989; FUERXER et al. 1997; PARRAVANO et al. 1993; MAJOIE et al. 1997; MARTIN

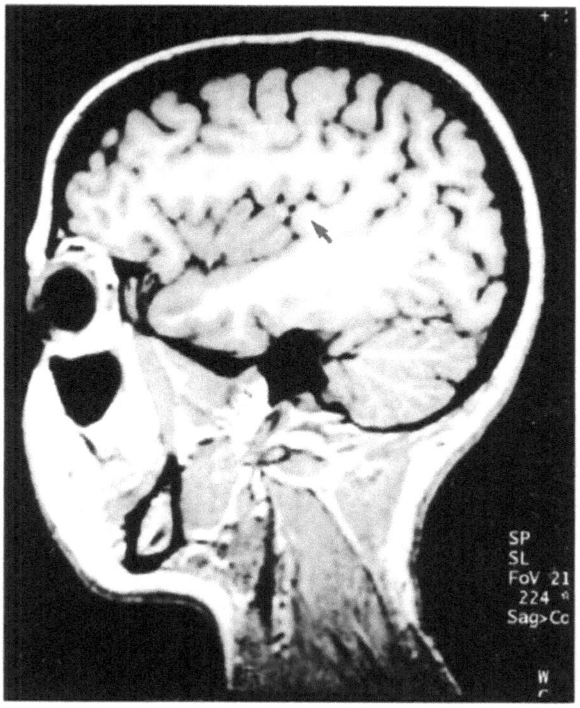

a

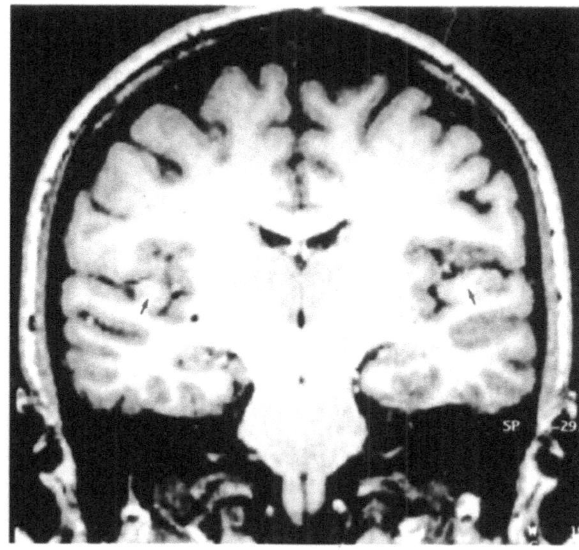

b

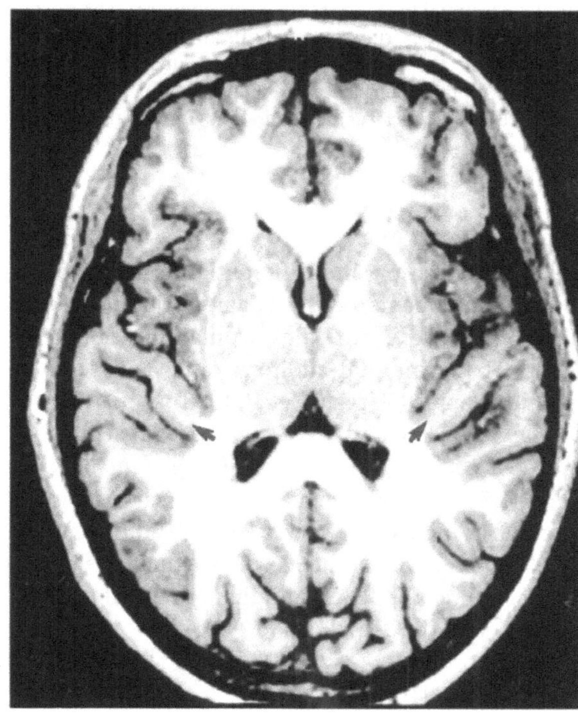
c

Fig. 2.3a–c. Heschl's gyrus. Landmarks in three planes (T1w MPRAGE sequence). **a** In the *sagittal plane* just lateral to the insula, the *shape* of HG (*arrow*) is so characteristic that it can easily be identified directly on the supratemporal surface without need for additional landmarks. Depending on the presence and extent of any intermediate sulcus, HG may appear Ω-shaped, on medial sections of the temporal lobe and insula. **b** In a *coronal plane* perpendicular on the bicommissural plane, the section on which HG (*arrows*) is identified best is characterized by (1) a tent-like shape formed as the two fornices converge to join with each other and (2) the presence of the VIIIth cranial nerves. **c** In the *axial plane* HG (*arrows*) is identified by its temporal location and its characteristic anterolateral course on the section on which the adhesio interthalamica can be identified

et al. 1992). Although routine spin echo T2-weighted sequences have not been systematically evaluated, they are thought to be inferior to T1-weighted sequences (Caillet et al. 1990). However, T2-weighted sequences are important because of their high sensitivity in detecting vascular or inflammatory pathologies affecting the brainstem and/or the cranial nerve nuclei and root entry zones. FLAIR (fluid attenuated inversion recovery) sequences, which null the signal of CSF routinely, enable visualization of some nerves, such as cranial nerve III.

Casselman et al. (1993) introduced the 3D CISS sequence for imaging the inner ear and the cerebellopontine angle. This steady-state refocused gradient-echo sequence is flow compensated (Deimling and Laub 1989) and can therefore be used to image small structures surrounded by CSF, with high contrast and resolution. These images are similar to those obtained from cisternography performed by intrathecal administration of contrast media. Casselman et al. (1993) showed that the combination of high contrast and high spatial resolution allowed de-

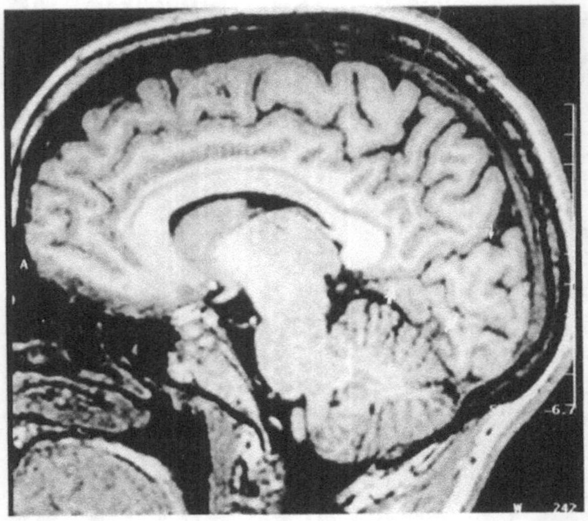

Fig. 2.4. Occipital lobe (T1w MPRAGE sequence). The calcarine sulcus (*arrows*) runs obliquely in an anterosuperior direction from the occipital pole to its junction with the parieto-occipital sulcus (*thin arrow*) to form the anterior calcarine sulcus. The calcarine sulci show a gradual posterior declination

tailed visualization and differentiation of the individual components of the facial-vestibulocochlear nerve complex in the fluid-containing compartments of the internal auditory canal and cerebellopontine angle (Yousry I et al. 1998).

The 3D CISS and T2 weighted-FSE sequences proved especially good for identifying cranial nerves I and II. The 3D CISS sequence was clearly superior for identifying cranial nerves III, V, VII, VIII and the IX–XI complex. Only the 3D CISS sequence showed cranial nerves IV, VI, XII and the individual components of VIII (Yousry I et al. 1998).

A) The Trigeminal Nerve(V)

The trigeminal nerve and its ganglion are easily identified on MRI (Fig. 2.5) (Yousry I et al. 1998). T1-weighted contrast enhanced sequences demonstrate a thin rim of peripheral enhancement along the anterior and superior aspects of Meckel's cave and a thin rim of curvilinear enhancement between the medial surface of the cave and the cavernous portion of the internal carotid artery (Fig. 2.5). This rim of enhancement represents the dural layers that define Meckel's cave (Downs et al. 1996). The remaining contents of Meckel's cave are isointense with CSF. The trigeminal ganglion shows two patterns of enhancement. (1) In the first, MRI shows a discrete, semilunar, enhancing structure within the inferolateral aspect of Meckel's

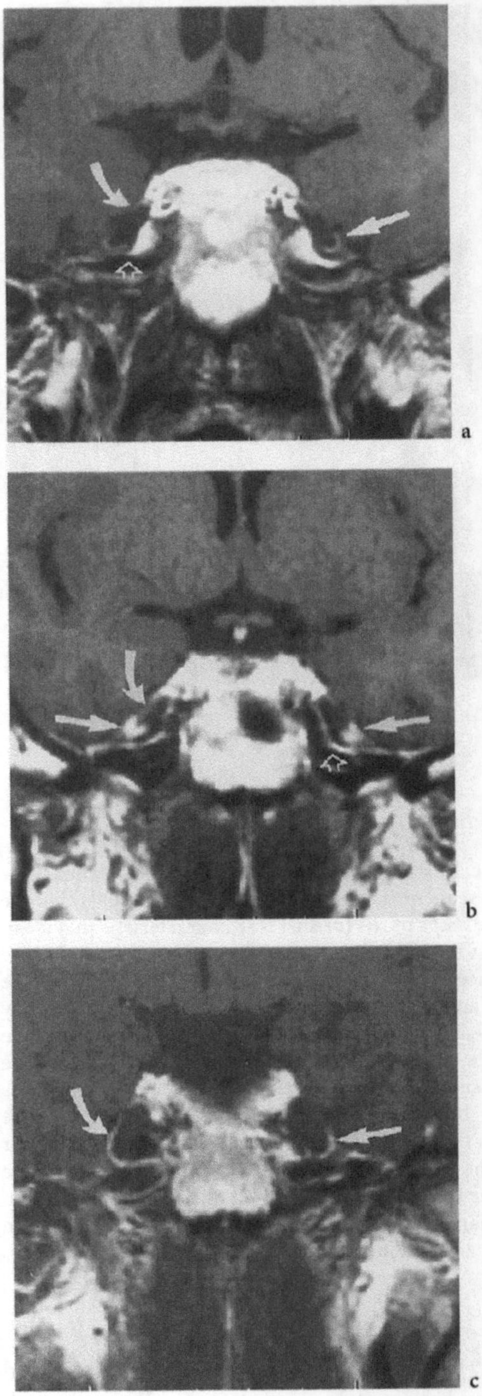

Fig. 2.5a–c. Meckel's cave (contrast enhanced T1w sequence) (from Downs DM et al. with permission). **a** T1w MR image shows enhancement of the thin trigeminal ganglion (*straight white arrow*). The internal carotid artery (*open arrow*) and the lateral wall of Meckel's cave (*curved arrow*) are also shown. **b** The trigeminal ganglia enhance (*straight arrows*). They are thicker and more nodular than in **a**. **c** The thin, enhancing trigeminal ganglion (*straight arrow*), located inferolaterally, blends with the dura (*curved arrow*)

cave. The convex margin of this structure is always oriented inferolaterally. Its contour may vary from thin and regular to thick and nodular. The actual enhancement may vary from linear superomedial extensions into the cave from the semilunar structure, through a separate linear band oriented along the long axis of the cave anterolaterally, to a separate round focus of enhancement within the cave. (2) In the second (12%), no distinct enhancing structure can be seen within the cave. Instead, a thickened semilunar area of enhancement blends with the inferolateral dura and is thought to represent the ganglion. Both enhancement patterns are probably related to the lack of a blood-brain barrier in the region of the trigeminal ganglion, and therefore both have to be considered normal (Downs et al. 1996).

b) The Abducens Nerve (VI)

Since abducens nerve palsy is the most common isolated ocular nerve palsy (Rosenberg 1991), extensive efforts have been made to identify cranial nerve VI (Yousry I et al. 1999; Casselman and Dehaene 1998; Mamata et al. 1998; Ohtsuka et al. 1996; Depper et al. 1993). To date it has proven to be nearly impossible to identify VI reliably and regularly by standard radiological techniques, including conventional MRI. The main difficulties are the nerve's oblique anterosuperolateral course from the brainstem to Dorello's canal and its small cross-sectional area of 0.43–1.85 mm^2 (Lang et al. 1974).

The radicular fibers of VI derive from a nucleus situated in the pons, immediately beneath the floor of the fourth ventricle, opposite the median eminence. The nucleus, together with the facial nerve fibers that course around it, form a recognizable "facial colliculus" on the posterior surface of the brainstem (i.e., floor of the fourth ventricle) (Fig. 2.6). The facial colliculus can be recognized by its shape, which is helpful in localizing central lesions affecting the nucleus of VI. More recently, cranial nerve VI can be reliably identified in its cisternal and in its petroclival course by using the 3D CISS sequence. The root exit zone (REZ) of VI is usually located in the pontomedullary sulcus (94%). In 6% the REZ lies superior to the pontomedullary sulcus (Fig. 2.6). The abducens nerve is surrounded by a sheath that may consist of arachnoid tissue (93%) and/or dura (21%). The arachnoid-dural sheath follows the nerve into the cavernous sinus, where it becomes thinner and disappears. CSF within the sheath can surround VI for a variable distance. On occasion, a CSF-filled evagination of the arachnoid can be detected on MRI in the region where VI exits the prepontine cistern. In the majority of cases the evagination corresponds to Dorello's canal, which can be identified regularly (94%) (Fig. 2.6) (Yousry I et al. 1999).

The identification of VI is facilitated by the use of anatomic landmarks such as Dorello's canal (in all planes) and the facial colliculus (in the transverse plane only). That cisternal structure which enters Dorello's canal must be cranial nerve VI. It should be noted that it is often easier to identify Dorello's canal first and then follow VI back to the pontomedullary sulcus. The search for VI in the axial plane can be facilitated by starting on those sections on which the facial colliculus is identified (Yousry I et al. 1999).

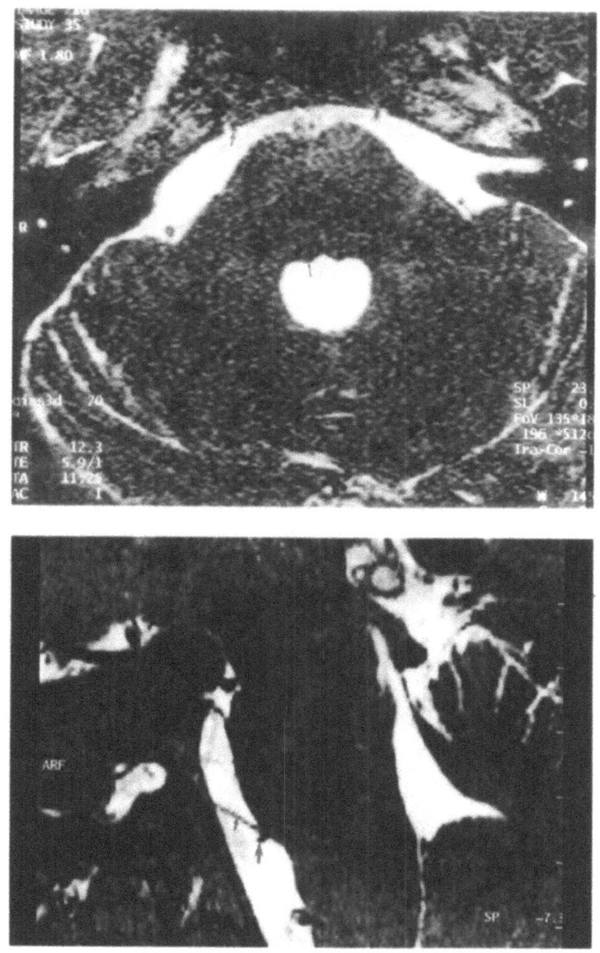

Fig. 2.6a,b. Cranial nerve VI (3D CISS sequence). The facial colliculus – the site of the VI nucleus– is readily identified on the posterior surface of the brainstem (floor of the fourth ventricle) (**a** *thin arrow*). The cisternal course of VI (*short arrow*) starts at the pontomedullary sulcus and continues superolaterally until it reaches the dural porus (**b**). At the porus, an evagination of CSF corresponding to Dorello's canal is easily identified (**a** *short arrow*). The neurovascular relationship is appreciated in the sagittal plane (**b**). In this patient the AICA (*arrow*) passes inferior to VI

c) The Facial and the Vestibulocochlear Nerve (VII and VIII)

MRI studies of the internal auditory canal now demonstrate that the facial, cochlear, superior vestibular, and inferior vestibular nerves show characteristic configurations that differ identifiably in different portions of their course from the brainstem to their termination. Cadaveric studies and MR studies in vivo have also revealed clear variations in the anatomy and relationships of the facial and vestibulocochlear nerves (Kim et al. 1998; Dailiana et al. 1997).

Near the brainstem, VII usually lies anterior to VIII (67%), but may lie anterosuperior or anteroinferior (23%) to VIII. At this location, VIII is approximately rectangular in cross-section in 83%, crescentic in 16%, and round in 2%. The cochlear nerve represents the most inferior part of VIII (Fig. 2.7) (Kim et al. 1998).

In the midcistern, VII is located anterior to a shallow groove in VIII (64%). In 5% of cases, VIII changes from its rectangular shape (near the brainstem) to a curved shape. This change is independent of any earlier or later division of VIII (Fig. 2.7).

At the porus acousticus, VIII occupies the posterior portion of the canal and has not yet fasciculated into its three terminal portions. Instead, the cochlear and superior vestibular nerves can be identified as rounded enlargements of the nerve complex. The inferior vestibular nerve appears as a shallow region or as a small round structure situated between the cochlear nerve and the superior vestibular nerve. Ninety-five percent of the vestibulocochlear nerves are curved and crescent shaped; 5% appear rectangular. Where VIII curves at the porus acousticus, the cochlear and vestibular portions of VIII occupy the anteroinferior and posterosuperior portions of the canal, respectively. In 90% the inferior vestibular nerve can be identified as a small, round, or oval structure inferior to the superior vestibular nerve, with some fibers connecting to the cochlear nerve (Fig. 2.7) (Kim et al. 1998).

In the Mid Internal Acoustic Canal. In the midportion of the internal auditory canal (IAC), cranial nerve VII occupies the anterosuperior portion of the canal (Fig. 2.7).

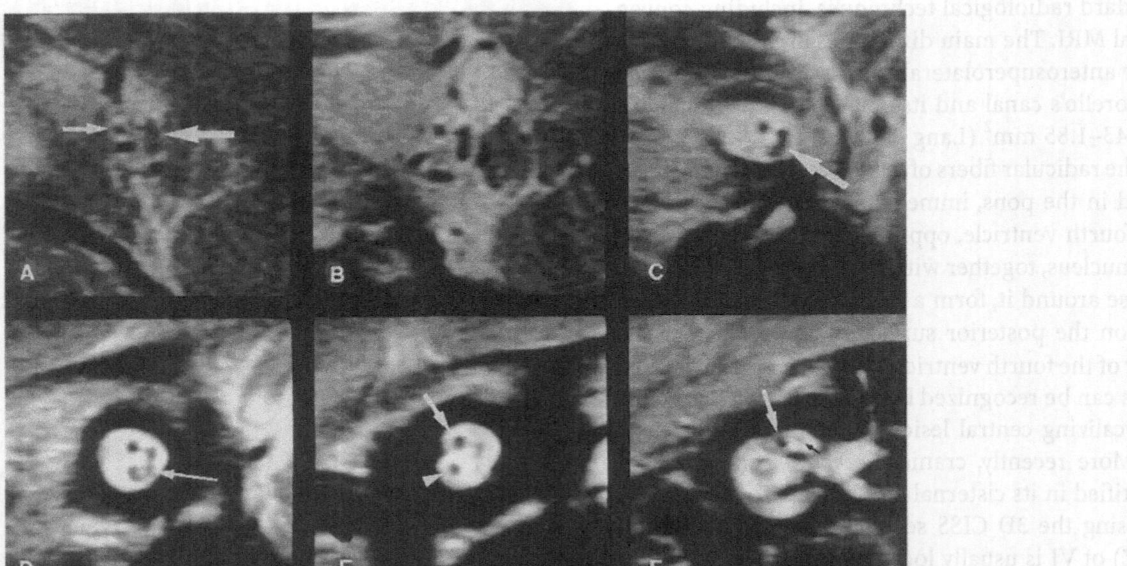

Fig. 2.7A–F. Cranial nerves VII-VIII (T2w FSE sequence) (from Kim H.-S. et al. with permission). **a** Near the brainstem, the cross section of VIII (*large arrow*) is rectangular. VII is located anterior to the superior portion of VIII. **b** In the midportion between the brainstem and porus acusticus, VII and VIII have a similar shape and relationship. **c** At the porus acusticus, VIII has changed to a curved shape. **d** In the midportion of the IAC, VIII divides into the superior vestibular, inferior vestibular, and cochlear nerves. The inferior vestibular nerve (*arrow*) is oval, with a connecting portion between the superior vestibular and cochlear nerves. **e** In the lateral portion of the IAC, the facial (*arrow*) and the cochlear nerves (*arrowhead*) are similar in size. The inferior vestibular nerve is the smallest one. **f** VII (*white arrow*) and the superior vestibular nerve (*black arrow*) above the transverse crest are seen in the most lateral portion of the canal

In the Lateral Internal Acoustic Canal. The cochlear and vestibular nerves usually separate from each other about 3–4 mm from the lateral end of the internal auditory canal. The vestibular nerve divides into the inferior and superior vestibular nerves 1–2 mm from the falciform crest. Near the transverse crest, the superior and inferior vestibulocochlear nerves are completely separated, and the facial and cochlear nerves move farther anterosuperiorly and anteroinferiorly, respectively. The cross sections of the facial, cochlear, and superior vestibular nerves are round. Small fibers connect the superior and inferior vestibular nerves as well as the cochlear and inferior vestibular nerves. Most of the inferior vestibular nerves are irregularly shaped, with connecting fibers to the cochlear and superior vestibular nerves. The cochlear nerve is the largest segment of VIII in 88%. The superior vestibular nerve is larger than the inferior vestibular nerve in 81%. The facial and cochlear nerves are of similar size in 36%. When right and left sides are compared, the relative sizes of the four nerves are symmetrical in 70% (Kim et al. 1998).

Thus, the facial nerve remains superior and anterior to the vestibulocochlear nerve or its branches and maintains its tubular shape throughout its course in the canal. VIII occupies the posterior inferior portion of the canal, with a shape that changes along its course from rectangular (at the brainstem), to tubular (at the entrance of the canal), to crescent-shaped (in the canal) before it divides into individual nerves (Rubinstein et al. 1996).

Using a high-resolution T1-weighted sequence (prototype three-dimensional Fourier transform gradient-echo that permits a very short echo time: 4.2 ms), the facial nerve can be visualized within the parotid gland (72%) by identifying VII in the stylomastoid foramen and then following the nerve inferiorly on sequential sections through the parotid gland. Curved reformations help to confirm the identity of the nerve (Dailiana et al. 1997).

2.3.5 The Vascular System

2.3.5.1 Arteries

Using the TOF sequence it is possible to identify easily all the arteries of the circle of Willis. In addition, it is also possible to display small vessels, such as the length of the anterior choroidal artery from its origin to its entrance into the choroid plexus of the temporal horn. The relation of this vessel to the posterior communicating artery, the uncus, parahippocampal gyrus and the choroid fissure can be easily assessed (Fig. 2.8) (Wiesman et al. 1999).

The relationship between small arteries of the posterior fossa and the cranial nerves is often better visualized when using sequences such as the 3D CISS sequence. A detailed assessment of the neurovascular relationship of VI was made possible by using the 3D CISS sequence. Noninvasively, it was shown that the AICA passes inferior to VI in 63.8% and superior to it in 29.8% (Fig. 2.6). In 6.4% the relationship between the blood vessel and nerve could not determined, because they appeared to merge into one structure. This appearance could represent penetration of the nerve by the blood vessel (Naidich et al. 1976) or, in rare instances, duplication or fenestration of the artery, with VI passing through the arterial branches (Yousry I et al. 1999).

It is not always possible to differentiate between arteries and nerves on the MR images. In general, however, differences in the signal intensity, the course of the depicted structures, their topography and the pattern of affluents and confluents make it possible to differentiate between arteries and nerves (Braun et al. 1996a,b; Yousry I et al. 1999).

2.3.5.2 Veins

Cortical vessels are of special importance for planning the operative approach to cerebral lesions such

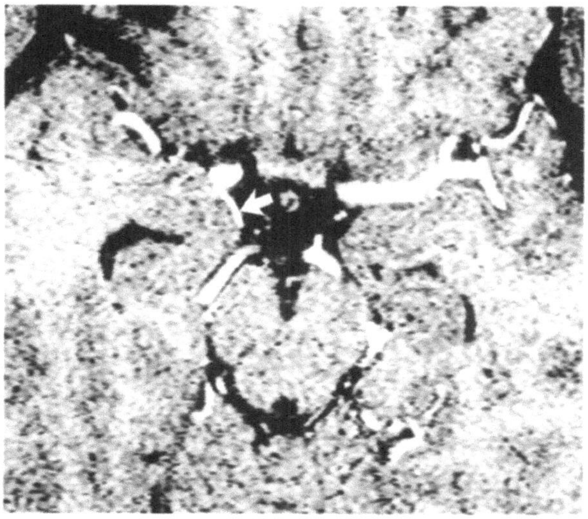

Fig. 2.8. Anterior choroidal artery. The anterior choroidal (*arrow*) artery is identified at its origin, along its course around the uncus (MRA TOF sequence)

as tumors. Combining surface anatomy scanning using HASTE sequences with PC venograms, permits an accurate visualization of the relationships of the cortical surface and its cortical veins (Tsuchiya et al. 1999).

Using contrast enhanced T1-weighted SPGR images it is also possible to identify the superficial venous structures of the brainstem (Braun et al. 1996b). The venous system is organized into a lattice of vertical and transverse collecting channels. The veins lie deep to the overlying arteries, close to the surface of the brainstem, and delineate the contour of the brainstem more precisely. Therefore the veins may usually be distinguished from the arteries.

The superior petrosal vein represents one of the major longitudinal ascending anastomoses on the lateral aspect of the brainstem (Fig. 2.9). This vein can be accurately identified by MRI in 95% (Braun et al. 1996b). When the superior petrosal vein is absent, the more anteriorly located longitudinal pontine veins drain the petrosal venous territory instead. The superior petrosal vein is located in the posterior and lateral portion of the cerebello-pontine cistern, posterior to the VIIIth cranial nerve and adjacent to the flocculus. Among the veins that drain the superior petrosal vein, the vein of the lateral recess of the 4th ventricle can always be identified (Braun et al. 1996a). The superior cerebellar hemi-

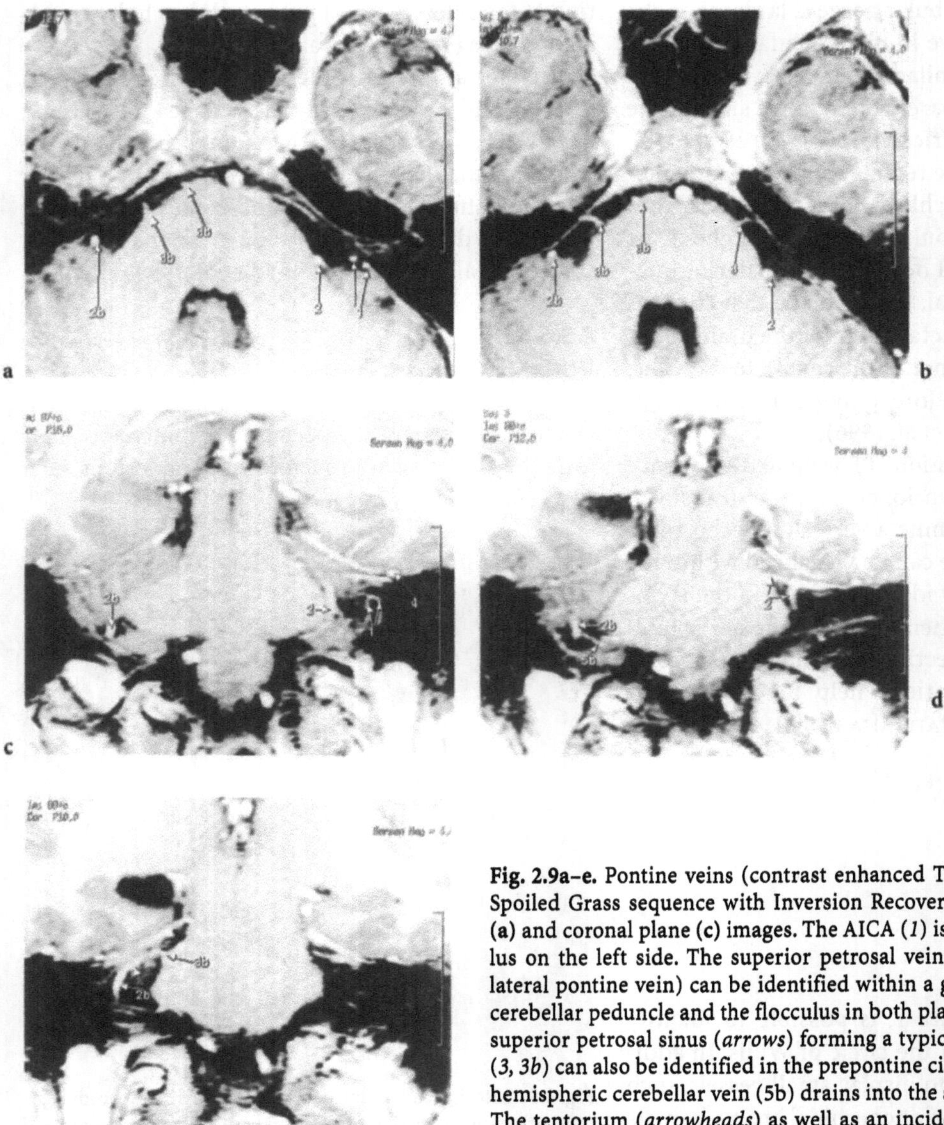

Fig. 2.9a–e. Pontine veins (contrast enhanced T1w 3D Gradient Echo Fast Spoiled Grass sequence with Inversion Recovery Preparation). Transverse (**a**) and coronal plane (**c**) images. The AICA (*1*) is identified near the flocculus on the left side. The superior petrosal vein (*2, 2b*; also known as the lateral pontine vein) can be identified within a groove between the middle cerebellar peduncle and the flocculus in both planes (**a–e**). It drains into the superior petrosal sinus (*arrows*) forming a typical hook (**d**). Bridging veins (*3, 3b*) can also be identified in the prepontine cistern (**a,b**). The right lateral hemispheric cerebellar vein (5b) drains into the superior petrosal vein (*2b*). The tentorium (*arrowheads*) as well as an incidental arachnoid cyst in the right lateral fissure are also identified. (Courtesy M. Braun)

spheric vein can only be identified in 52%. The anastomosis with the lateral mesencephalic vein is visualized in 72.5% (Braun et al. 1996b). Lateral to the trigeminal nerve the superior petrosal vein bends laterally into the superior petrosal sinus forming a characteristic hook in 76% (Fig. 2.9). The superficial pontine veins form a thin network covering the anterior and lateral aspect of the pons. This network is formed by longitudinal and transverse veins. The former can be identified in 72.5% in the axial plane, the latter - although functionally dominant - in only 56.2% (Braun et al. 1996b).

References

Binder JR, Rao SM, Hammeke TA et al. (1994) Functional magnetic resonance imaging of human auditory cortex. Ann Neurol 35: 662–672

Braun M, Bracard S, Anxionnat R, Roland J, Picard L (1996a) The veins of the medulla oblongata: MRI cross-sectional anatomy. Surg Radiol Anat 18: 201–207

Braun M, Bracard S, Huot J-C, Roland J, Picard L (1996b) Pontine veins. MRI cross-sectional anatomy. Surg Radiol Anat 18: 315–321

Brodmann K (1909) Vergleichende Lokalisationslehre der Grosshirnrinde. Verlag von Johann Ambrosius Barth, Leipzig

Bullitt E, Liu A, Aylward S, Soltys M, Rosenman J, Pizer SM (1997) Methods for displaying intracerebral vascular anatomy. AJNR Am J Neuroradiol 18: 417–420

Caillet H, Delvalle A, Doyon D et al. (1990) Visibility of cranial nerves at MRI. J Neuroradiol 17: 289–301

Casselman JW, Dehaene I (1998) Imaging of the IIIrd, IVth, and VIth cranial nerves. Neuro-Ophthalmology 19: 63–68

Casselman JW, Kuhweide R, Deimling M, Ampe W, Dehaene I, Meeus L (1993) Constructive interference in steady state-3DFT MR imaging of the inner ear and cerebellopontine angle. AJNR Am J Neuroradiol 14: 47–57

Dailiana T, Chakeres D, Schmalbrock P, Williams P, Aletras A (1997) High-resolution MR of the intraparotid facial nerve and parotid duct. AJNR Am J Neuroradiol 18: 165–172

Deimling M, Laub GA (1989) Constructive interference in steady state for motion sensitivity reduction. SMRM. Berkeley: Book of Abstracts of the Society of Magnetic Resonance in Medicine, p 642

Depper MH, Truwit CL, Dreisbach JN, Kelly WM (1993) Isolated abducens nerve palsy: MR imaging findings. AJR Am J Roentgenol 160: 837–841

Downs DM, Damiano TR, Rubinstein D (1996) Gasserian ganglion: appearance on contrast-enhanced MR. AJNR Am J Neuroradiol 17: 237–241

Flechsig P (1908) Bemerkungen über die Hörsphäre des menschlichen Gehirns. Neurologisches Centralblatt 27: 2–7

Fuerxer F, Carlier R, Iffenecker C, Schaison G, Doyon D (1997) L'imagerie par résonance magnétique des voies olfactives dans le syndrome de Kallmann de Morsier. J Neuroradiol 23: 223–230

Galaburda AM, Sherman GF, Rosen GD, Aboitiz F, Geschwind N (1985) Developmental dyslexia: four consecutive patients with cortical anomalies. Ann Neurol 18: 222–233

Geshwind N, Levitsky W (1968) Human brain: left-right asymmetries in temporal speech region. Science 161: 186–187

Gloger S, Gloger A, Vogt H, Kretschmann HJ (1994a) Computer-assisted 3D reconstruction of the terminal branches of the cerebral arteries. I. Anterior cerebral artery. *Neuroradiology* 36: 173–180

Gloger S, Gloger A, Vogt H, Kretschmann HJ (1994b) Computer-assisted 3D reconstruction of the terminal branches of the cerebral arteries. II. Middle cerebral artery. Neuroradiology 36: 181–187

Gloger S, Gloger A, Vogt H, Kretschmann HJ (1994c) Computer-assisted 3D reconstruction of the terminal branches of the cerebral arteries. III. Posterior cerebral artery and circle of Willis. Neuroradiology 36: 251–257

Hans P, Grant AJ, Laitt RD, Ramsden RT, Kassner A, Jackson A (1999) Comparison of three-dimensional visualization techniques for depicting the scala vestibuli and scala tympani of the cochlea by using high-resolution MR imaging. AJNR Am J Neuroradiol 20: 1197–1206

Hynd GW, Semrud-Clikeman M, Lorys AR, Novey ES, Eliopulos D (1990) Brain morphology in developmental dyslexia and attention deficit disorder/hyperactivity. Arch Neurol 47: 919–926

Iwasaki S, Nakagawa H, Fukusumu A et al. (1991) Identification of pre- and postcentral gyri on CT and MR images on the basis of the medullary pattern of cerebral white matter. Radiology 179: 207–213

Katada K (1990) MR imaging of brain surface structures: surface anatomy scanning (SAS). Neuroradiology 32: 439–448

Kim H-S, Kim D-I, Chung I-H, Lee W-S, Kim K-Y (1998) Vestibulocochlear nerves in the subarachnoid space and internal auditory canal. AJNR Am J Neuroradiol 19: 1155–1161

Korogi Y, Takahashi M, Sumi M et al. (1996a) MR signal intensity of the perirolandic cortex in the neonate and infant. Neuroradiology 38: 578–584

Korogi Y, Takahashi M, Okuda T et al. (1996b) MR topography of the striate cortex: correlation with anatomic sections. Int J Neuroradiol 2: 534–540

Kulynych JJ, Vladar K, Fantie BD, Jones DW, Weinberger DR (1995) Normal asymmetry of the planum temporale in patients with schizophrenia. Three-dimensional cortical morphometry with MRI. Br J Psychiatry 166: 742–749

Lang J (1974) Eintritt und Verlauf der Hirnnerven (III, IV, VI) "im" Sinus cavernosus. Anat Entwickl-Gesch 145: 87–99

Leonard CM, Voeller KK, Lombardino LJ et al.(1993) Anomalous cerebral structure in dyslexia revealed with magnetic resonance imaging. Arch Neurol 50: 461–469

Liegeois-Chauvel C, Laguitton V, Badier JM, Schwartz D, Chauvel P (1995) [Cortical mechanisms of auditive perception in man: contribution of cerebral potentials and evoked magnetic fields by auditive stimulations]. Rev Neurol 151: 495–504

Liegeois-Chauvel C, Musolino A, Chauvel P (1991) Localization of the primary auditory area in man. Brain 114: 139–151

Majoie CBLM, Hulsmans F-JH, Verbeeten B Jr et al. (1997) Trigeminal neuralgia: comparison of two MR imaging techniques in the demonstration of neurovascular contact. Radiology 204: 455–460

Mamata Y, Muro I, Matsumae M et al. (1998) Magnetic reso-

nance cisternography for visualization of intracranial fine structures. J Neurosurg 88: 670–678
Martin N, Le Bras F, Krief O, Chedid G, Marsault C, Nahum H (1992) Anatomie IRM in vivo du paquet acoustico-facial. J Neuroradiol 19: 88–97
Meyer JR, Roychowdhury S, Russell EJ, Callahan C, Gitelman D, Mesulam MM (1996) Location of the central sulcus via cortical thickness of the precentral and postcentral gyri on MR. AJNR Am J Neuroradiol 17: 1699–1706
Naganawa S, Itoh T, Fukatsu H et al. (1998) Three-dimensional fast spin-echo MR of the inner ear: ultra-long echo train length and half-Fourier technique. AJNR Am J Neuroradiol 19: 739–741
Naidich TP, Brightbill TC (1996a) Systems for localizing fronto-parietal gyri and sulci on axial CT and MRI. Int J Neuroradiol 2: 313–338
Naidich TP, Brightbill TC (1996b) The pars marginalis. Part I: A "bracket" sign for the central sulcus in axial plane CT and MRI. Int J Neuroradiol 2: 3–19
Naidich TP, Kricheff II, George AE, Lin JP (1976) The normal anterior inferior cerebellar artery. Radiology 119: 355–373
Naidich TP, Valavanis AG, Kubik S (1995) Anatomic relationships along the low-middle convexity. Part I: Normal specimens and magnetic resonance imaging. Neurosurgery 36: 517–532
Naidich TP, Valavanis AG, Kubik S, Taber KH, Yasargil MG (1997) Anatomic relationships along the low-middle convexity. Part II: Lesion localization. Int J Neuroradiol 3: 393–409
Ohtsuka K, Sone A, Igarashi Y, Akiba H, Sakata M (1996) Vascular compressive abducens nerve palsy disclosed by magnetic resonance imaging. Am J Ophthalmol 122: 416–419
Parravano JG, Toledo A, Kucharczyk W (1993) Dimensions of the optic nerves, chiasm, and tracts: MR quantitative comparison between patients with optic atrophy and normals. J Comput Assist Tomogr 17: 688–690
Petty RG, Barta PE, Pearlson GD et al. (1995) Reversal of asymmetry of the planum temporale in schizophrenia. Am J Psychiatry 152: 715–721
Rosenberg RN (1991) Comprehensive neurology. Raven Press, New York
Rubinstein D, Sandberg EJ, Cajade-Law AG (1996) Anatomy of the facial and vestibulocochlear nerves in the internal auditory canal. AJNR Am J Neuroradiol 17: 1099–1105
Rumeau C, Tzourio N, Murayama N et al. (1994) Location of hand function in the sensorimotor cortex: MR and functional correlation. AJNR Am J Neuroradiol 15: 567–572
Sobel DF, Gallen CC, Schwartz BJ et al. (1993) Locating the central sulcus: comparison of MR anatomic and magnetoencephalographic functional methods. AJNR Am J Neuroradiol 14: 915–925
Steinmetz H, Ebeling U, Huang YX, Kahn T (1990) Sulcus topography of the parietal opercular region: an anatomic and MR study. Brain Lang 38: 515–533
Steinmetz H, Furst G, Freund HJ (1989) Cerebral cortical localization: application and validation of the proportional grid system in MR imaging. J Comput Assist Tomogr 13: 10–19
Steinmetz H, Volkmann J, Jäncke L, Freund HJ (1991) Anatomical left-right asymmetry of language-related temporal cortex is different in left- and right handers. Ann Neurol 29: 315–319
Stock KW, Wetzel S, Kirsch E, Bongartz G, Steinbrich W, Radue EW (1996) Anatomic evaluation of the circle of Willis: MR angiography versus intraarterial digital subtraction angiography. AJNR Am J Neuroradiol 17: 1495–1499
Strainer JC, Ulmer JL, Yetkin FZ, Haughton VM, Daniels DL, Millen SJ (1997) Functional MR of the primary auditory cortex: an analysis of pure tone activation and tone discrimination. AJNR Am J Neuroradiol 18: 601–610
Suzuki M, Takashima T, Kadoya M, Takahashi S, Miyayama S, Taira S (1989) MR imaging of olfactory bulbs and tracts. AJNR Am J Neuroradiol 10: 955–957
Tsuchiya K, Hachiya J, Hiyama T, Maehara T (1999) A new MRI technique for demonstrating the surface of the brain together with the cortical veins. Neuroradiology 41: 425–427
von Economo C, Horn L (1930) Über Windungsrelief, Maße und Rindenarchitektonik der Supratemporalfläche, ihre individuellen und ihre Seitenunterschiede. Z Neurol Psychiatrie 130: 678–757
von Economo C, Koskinas GN (1925) Die Cytoarchitektonik der Hirnrinde des erwachsenen Menschen. Verlag von Julius Springer, Wien Berlin
Wiesman M, Yousry I, Seloos K, Camelio S, Yousry TA (1999) Identification of the anterior choroid artery using 3D-TOF source and 3DFT-CISS MR images. 11th European Congress of Neurosurgery, EANS. Copenhagen, Denmark, p 77
Witelson SF, Pallie W (1973) Left hemisphere specialization for language in the newborn. Neuroanatomical evidence of asymmetry. Brain 96: 641–646
Yoshiura T, Iwanaga S, Yamada K et al. (1998) Perirolandic cortex in infants: signal intensity on MR images as a landmark of the sensorimotor cortex. Radiology 207: 385–388
Yousry I, Camelio S, Wiesmann M, Yousry TA (1998) Improved visualization of the cranial nerves: a comparative study between TSE and 3 DFT-CISS sequences. Symposium Neuroradiologicum. Philadelphia
Yousry I, Camelio S, Wiesmann M, et al. (1999) Detailed magnetic resonance imaging anatomy of the cisternal segment of the abducent nerve: Dorello's canal and neurovascular relationships and landmarks. J Neurosurg 91: 276–283
Yousry TA, Schmid UD, Alkadhi H et al. (1997a) Localization of the motor hand area to a knob on the precentral gyrus. A new landmark. Brain 120: 141–157
Yousry TA, Fesl G, Büttner A, Noachter S, Schmid UD (1997b) Heschl's gyrus: anatomic description and methods of identification in MRI. Int J Neuroradiol 3: 2–12
Yousry T, Schmidt D, Alkadhi H, Winkler P, Schmid U, Peraud A (1995) New anatomic landmark for the identification of the precentral gyrus: validation and characterization. Radiology 197(P): 373

3 Technical Progress in Neuroradiology and Its Application

ALAN JACKSON

CONTENTS

3.1 Introduction

The discovery of X-rays by Wilhelm Roentgen on 8 November 1895 marked the birth of imaging as a clinical speciality. Within 6 months X-ray systems were in clinical use in hospitals across Europe and the United States (ABRAHAMS 1986). Throughout the following century other new imaging technologies such as ultrasound, CT and MRI repeatedly demonstrated their ability to revolutionise clinical practice in all areas of medicine.

The introduction of new imaging technologies follows a typical pattern. First tentative reports lead to a flurry of research activity, gradual definition of possible clinical benefits and eventual introduction into clinical practice. As technologies have become more complex this development cycle has progressively become longer. The suggestion that magnetic gradients could be used to encode position dependent information from NMR was made by LAUTERBUR in 1973. Despite the unprecedented research and development activity that ensued, clinical MRI systems were not available for almost a decade (SCHENK and LEUE 1996). In view of this, logic suggests that the next revolution in imaging is almost undoubtedly already in development and that, given sufficient insight, we should be able to predict the new tools we may be using in 10 or 20 years time. Several potential candidate technologies do suggest themselves. Electron spin magnetic resonance offers the possibility of examining atoms with unpaired electrons, potentially providing a tool for imaging of free radicals and transitional metals (BERTINI and DRAGO 1980; WEIL et al. 1994). Electrical impedance tomography continues to improve and offers the possibility of continuous cerebral imaging of blood flow at low cost (MORUCCI and RIGAUD 1996; KORZHENEVSKII et al. 1997). Synchrotron radiation with accurately defined wavelength and high amplitudes offers the potential for imaging systems based on X-ray diffraction and molecular specific absorptionometry. Nanotechnology developments offer a massive potential for invasive diagnostic and therapeutic devices. In fact, although this is a seductive exercise the next revolution in imaging will probably be as unexpected as previous ones.

Following the introduction of new technologies into clinical use, further development and extension of their functionality is inevitable. This evolution of existing technologies is continuous and is easier to predict than the development of new concepts since it is driven by clinical need and limited only by engineering capability. Major changes are already occurring in the practice of neuroradiology, which will provide impetus for the development of new technologies. The most important of these are the increasing demands for physiological data and image quantification and the growth of image guided surgery and interventional neuroradiology. Equally important is the change in working practice that is occurring as a result of the increasing power and availability of computing technology. It is safe to predict that PACS systems will become the norm in clinical departments. Radiological workstations can be expected to evolve into far more sophisticated tools. Tele-

A. JACKSON, PhD, MB, ChB, MRCP, FRCR
Imaging Science and Biomedical Engineering, Medical School, University of Manchester, Oxford Road, Manchester, M13 9PT, UK

conferencing, image analysis, 3D data display and voice recognition software are already commercially available. New functionality including automated image annotation, report interpretation, semi-automated anatomical segmentation, automated access to reference texts, identification and display of exemplar cases and formal decision support systems are all currently being developed. The integration of computer based systems via web technology will also impact on neuroradiology at many levels from day to day clinical practice through to training and continuing medical education.

The rest of this chapter will attempt to illustrate the technological developments that will impact on the practice of neuroradiology in the near future. The sheer scope of these makes it impossible to be comprehensive. Some major developments will occur which are not discussed, some developments are addressed in other chapters and some of the technologies described here may be surpassed or fail to fulfil their expectations.

3.2 Advances in MR imaging

Recent advances in MRI technology have largely arisen as a direct consequence of the increasing interest in various forms of functional imaging. Dynamic imaging methods require rapid image acquisition and high spatial resolution, which are dependent on rapid gradient switching. Techniques such as diffusion imaging also require high gradient amplitudes, which are dependent on amplifier performance and gradient coil design. In response to these demands all high end clinical imaging systems are now available with high performance gradient subsystems, typically capable of achieving peak gradient strengths in excess of 20 mT/m with switching times of 200 μs or less. Such systems can perform single shot echo planar imaging with imaging matrices of 64 or even 128. Although these systems were primarily intended for functional imaging studies, they considerably expand the capabilities of MRI in standard clinical practice.

3.3 Clinical Uses of Fast Imaging Techniques

Fast imaging methods such as fast spin echo (FSE) are increasingly used in routine clinical examinations to increase patient throughput. The widespread availability of fast spin echo has produced a viable alternative to standard spin echo techniques for T2 weighted brain and spine imaging, with significant savings in scan times. Fast spin echo image acquisition trains have also allowed routine clinical use of the inherently slow inversion recovery imaging sequences including short tau inversion recovery (STIR) and fluid attenuated inversion recovery (FLAIR). The fast inversion recovery technique can be modified to obtain exquisite grey/white matter contrast and use of a 3D fast spin echo acquisition allows whole brain volume imaging with thin slices (3–5 mm) in under 4 min (Fig. 3.1). The STIR sequence suppresses fat signal using a 180° RF pulse to invert the longitudinal magnetisation as an initial excitation pulse. Image acquisitions are then performed with the inversion time (TI) equivalent to the null point for fat (approximately 0.69+T1 at 1.5 Tesla) (Bydder and Young 1985). The STIR sequence is relatively robust to problems with magnetic field homogeneity and allows lengthening of the TE in comparison to standard spin echo sequences which provides increased contrast effects from T1 recovery and T2 decay (Fig. 3.2). The combination of STIR with fast spin echo techniques has largely overcome the problems of increased imaging time which are incurred by the long TRs required by conventional

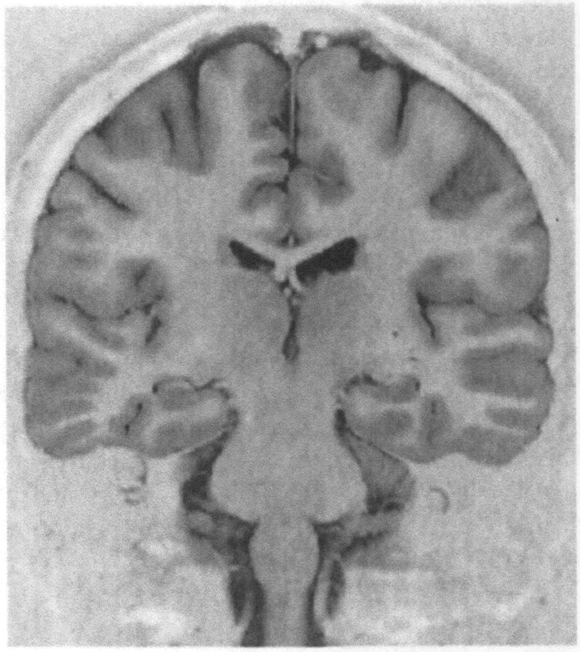

Fig. 3.1. Inversion recovery fast spin echo image of a normal brain. The slice thickness is 3 mm and image acquisition of the entire brain was performed in approximately 4 min

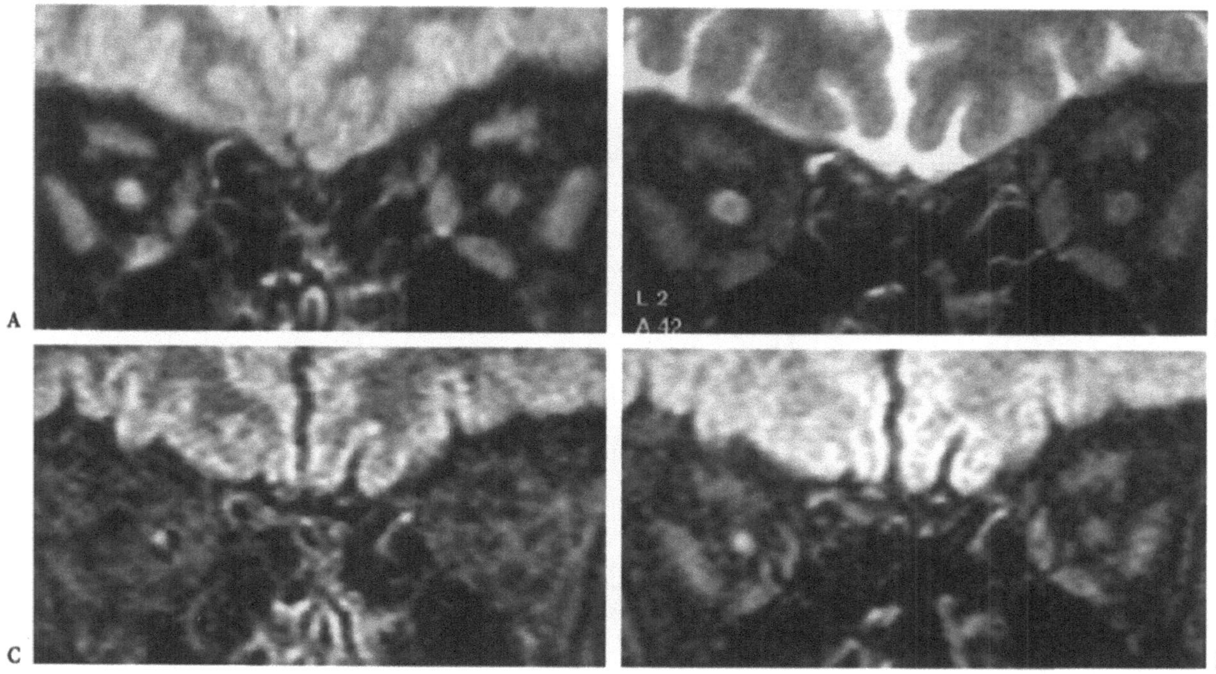

Fig. 3.2A–D. Images of a patient with right-sided optic neuritis. **A** STIR image shows good quality fat suppression and high signal from the optic nerve and surrounding CSF. **B** SPIR fat suppression again shows good quality fat suppression, and heavy T2 weighting allows differentiation between the optic nerve and surrounding CSF. Comparison of the signal within the nerve to normal white matter in the frontal lobe is difficult due to partial volume artefact with surrounding CSF. **C** DAIR image shows suppression of both CSF and fat. High signal in the right optic nerve is clearly visible. There is, however, some chemical shift effect making the optic nerve appear eccentrically placed within the optic nerve sheath. **D** SPIR/FLAIR image shows good quality suppression of CSF and fat. The right optic nerve is clearly seen to be of high signal towards the normal nerve and can be directly compared to the white matter in the frontal lobe

STIR sequences. The FLAIR sequence uses the same approach to suppress the signal from free fluid by elongation of the TI to approximately 2600 ms at 1.5 Tesla (De Coene et al. 1992). The combination of the FLAIR sequence with fast spin echo collection is often called fast-FLAIR and has become a standard sequence for brain imaging in many centres. In addition to improving the demonstration of lesions adjacent to CSF the fast-FLAIR sequence reduces the dynamic range of the images and allows the use of long TE values producing very heavy T2 weighting (Fig. 3.3). The limitations of the STIR sequence led to the development of fat suppression techniques based on the use of frequency specific selective partial inversion recovery (SPIR) pulse sequences (Oh et al. 1988; Tien 1992). These techniques are heavily dependent on the homogeneity of the main field and are highly sensitive to the presence of paramagnetic disturbances. Nonetheless, the improvements in magnet technology and particularly the introduction of iterative active shimming protocols allow the use of frequency specific fat suppression, even over large fields of view, on all commercial high field systems. In these sequences the inversion pulse inverts only the fat magnetisation while leaving water resonances undisturbed. This technique will not suppress areas of T1 shortening due to contrast enhancement allowing its use in combination with postcontrast T1 weighted acquisitions (Fig. 3.4). The SPIR technique is compatible with a wide range of sequences allowing the acquisition of T1 and T2 weighted images. It also differentiates fat from tissues with T1 values similar to that of fat and does not alter the contrast between normal non-fatty tissues.

The use of fast inversion recovery and frequency-specific tissue suppression techniques has also led to the development of hybrid sequences capable of suppressing signal from two tissues. These sequences use either a combination of two inversion recovery preparation pulses (dual attenuation inversion recovery, DAIR) or combine SPIR fat suppression with a fast-FLAIR sequence (SPIR-FLAIR). The SPIR-FLAIR sequence was developed to allow a highly T2 weighted sequence to be used in the orbit to examine the optic nerve whilst suppressing signal from both orbital fat and perineural CSF (Fig. 3.2) (Jackson et al. 1998). The DAIR sequence can also be used in this way (Fig. 3.2) but offers some additional flexibility

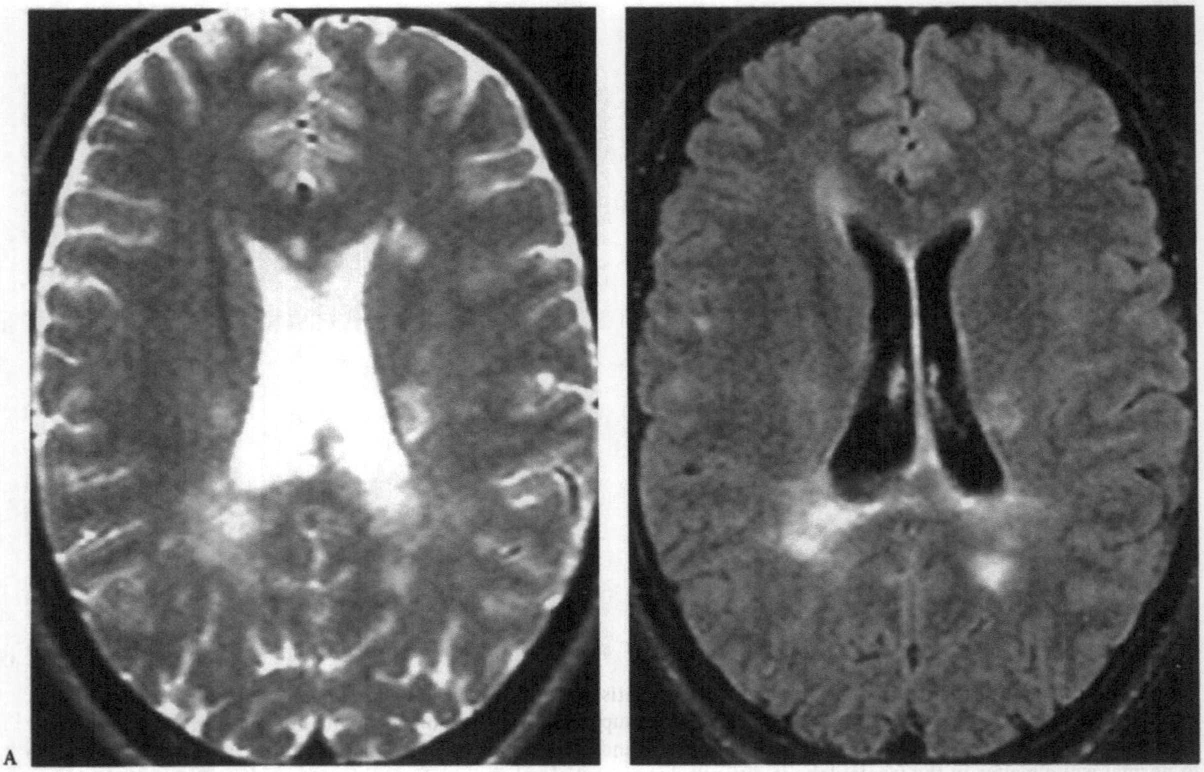

Fig. 3.3A,B. Images of a patient with multiple sclerosis. A T2 weighted conventional spin echo sequence shows high signal lesions within the brain and adjacent to the CSF. B Fast spin echo FLAIR image at the same level shows demyelination with far higher conspicuity than conventional T2 weighted images. Slice thickness was 3 mm and the entire brain was imaged in under 4 min

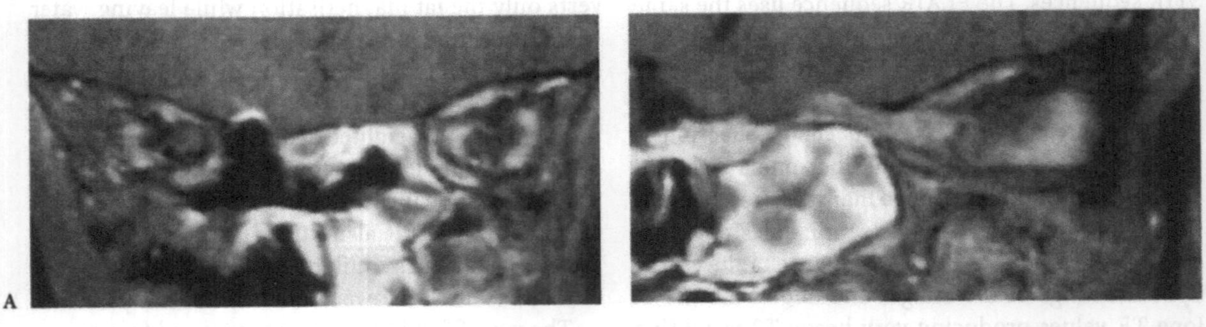

Fig. 3.4A,B. Images of an optic nerve sheath meningioma extending through the optic canal. Both images are postcontrast T1 weighted volume acquisitions using a SPIR fat suppression prepulse. A Enhancing nerve sheath tumour is clearly seen in the left orbit. B Parasagittal oblique section shows the anteroposterior extent of the tumour clearly delineated from orbital fat

since it can be used to suppress signal from any combination of tissues. This approach has been used to develop methods for "gray matter only" and "white matter only" images by suppressing signal from CSF and either white or grey matter respectively. Although these techniques currently have no clear clinical role, they may simplify the quantitative analysis of grey matter disorders and could improve the delineation between normal and pathological tissues.

The widespread availability of fast spin echo also allows the use of high spatial resolution imaging techniques with large matrices and thin slices. The combination of FSE with volume acquisitions provides a powerful combination for the production of high spatial resolution data sets with high signal to noise ratios (Fig. 3.5). Constructive interference in steady state (CISS) 3D Fourier transform MRI provides an alternative technique for the production of

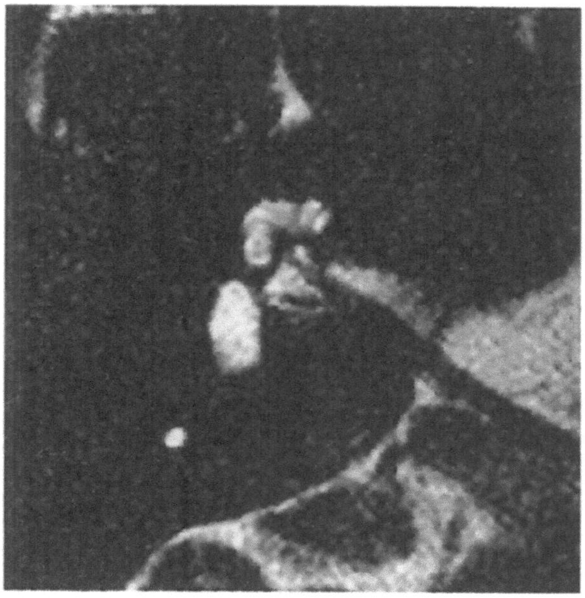

Fig. 3.5. Image of the cochlea and vestibule in a normal volunteer. The image is a fast spin echoT2 weighted volume acquisition with an in-plane and through plane resolution of 0.5 mm

similar high resolution T2 weighted images. The ability of these sequences to produce very high resolution heavily T2 weighted images has been widely used for the imaging of the basal cisterns and of the vestibulocochlear system (Fig. 3.5). These data sets provide exquisite anatomical detail and lend themselves to the use of three-dimensional visualisation techniques to provide images which can be viewed at the workstation and anatomically realistic 3D models (Figs. 3.6, 3.7) (Jackson et al. 1998; Shigematsu et al. 1998).

Echo planar imaging (EPI) techniques are also beginning to make an impact on clinical scanning protocols in a number of areas. Although single

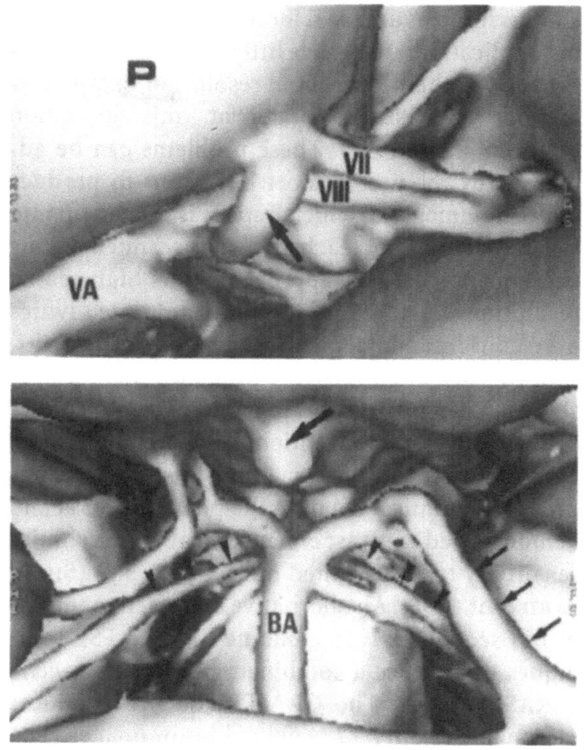

Fig. 3.7A,B. Three-dimensional isosurface renderings of the basal systems using a CISS 3D Fourier transform image acquisition. **A** Anterior to posterior virtual endoscopic view from a viewpoint within the chiasmatic system shows the infundibulum (*arrow*), basilar artery (*BA*), and ocular motor nerves (*arrowheads*) between the posterior cerebral and superior cerebellar arteries. Well-developed posterior communicating artery (*small arrows*) is seen. **B** Anterior to posterior virtual endoscopic view of the left cerebellopontine angle clearly shows the spatial relationship between the nerves (*VII, VIII*) and the PICA (*arrow*) (*VA* vertebral artery, *P* pons). (Images taken from Shigematsu et al. 1998)

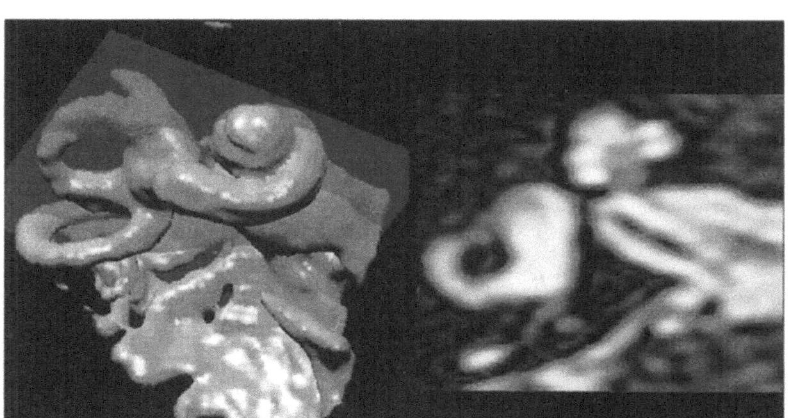

Fig. 3.6. Isosurface rendering of the vestibular cochlea system in a normal volunteer. The left-hand image demonstrates the isosurface render clearly showing the cochlea, basal turn and semicircular canals. A plane is projected through the 3D reconstruction and the primary image data from that plane is represented on the right

shot techniques are ideal for many functional imaging applications, they have little use in a clinical setting due to their low spatial resolution, spatial distortion and severe water/fat misregistration (OZDOBA et al. 1997). These problems can be addressed by the use of short EPI trains to produce multishot images in which k space is broken up into several sections and each section is scanned during subsequent TRs. This approach allows high spatial resolution whilst retaining significant time savings over conventional sequences. The use of a multishot EPI inversion recovery sequence was recently shown to demonstrate brain pathology with similar conspicuities to conventional T2 weighted spin echo sequences. At the same time this sequence improved anatomical detail in the posterior fossa and demonstrated contrast enhancement with a similar sensitivity to T1 weighted images (Fig. 3.8) (SHEPPARD et al. 1998). An alternative approach to the use of EPI sequences is to combine EPI and FSE techniques to produce a combined gradient-spin-echo (GRASE) image. The GRASE sequence produces reasonable quality T2 weighted brain images (Fig. 3.9) and is ideal to exclude major pathology or for use in uncooperative patients; however, several studies have found it has a markedly diminished sensitivity for detecting small lesions (FELLNER et al. 1995; PATEL et al. 1995a).

The fast spin echo, echo planar and GRASE sequences can all be used for the acquisition of single shot images in which an entire k space data set is collected within a single TR. As would be expected these imaging techniques whilst fast suffer from significant image degradation and are unsuited for routine brain or spine imaging (OZDOBA et al. 1997). However, both single shot FSE and GRASE suffer far less from image distortion than single shot EPI and have been suggested as possible imaging methods in uncooperative or claustrophobic patients. The combination of half-Fourier acquisition and single-shot turbo spin-echo (HASTE) offers a very rapid imaging technique with good spatial resolution that may also be used in these circumstances (SUGAHARA et al. 1997; GREENSPAN et al. 1998). In diagnostic practice all these methods remain suboptimal and must be used with caution. However, single shot FSE, GRASE and HASTE all provide promising techniques for real time image guidance (Fig. 3.10) and for dynamic imaging techniques designed to assess movement.

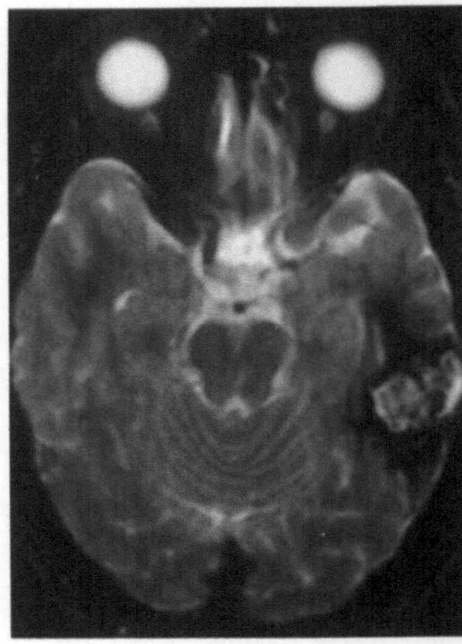

Fig. 3.9. Benign tumour of the temporal lobe demonstrated on GRASE images. Image thickness is 5 mm and acquisition of images through the whole brain was performed in under 2 min

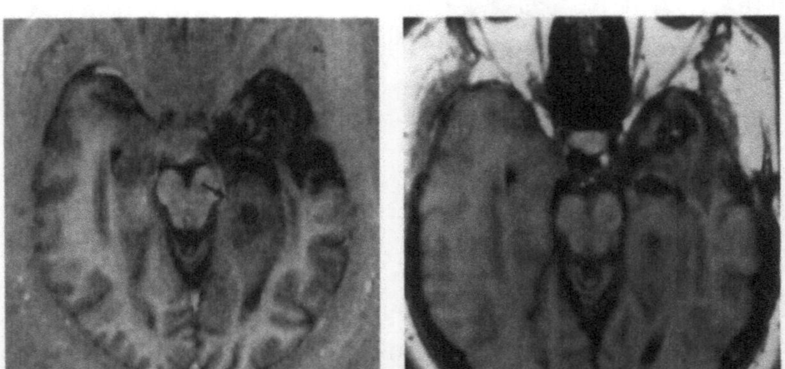

Fig. 3.8A,B. Unenhancing recurrent tumour nodule within the medial left temporal lobe demonstrated by (A) an inversion recovery echo planar acquisition and for comparison (B) a conventional non-contrast T1 weighted spin echo image. (Images are taken from Sheppard et al. 1998)

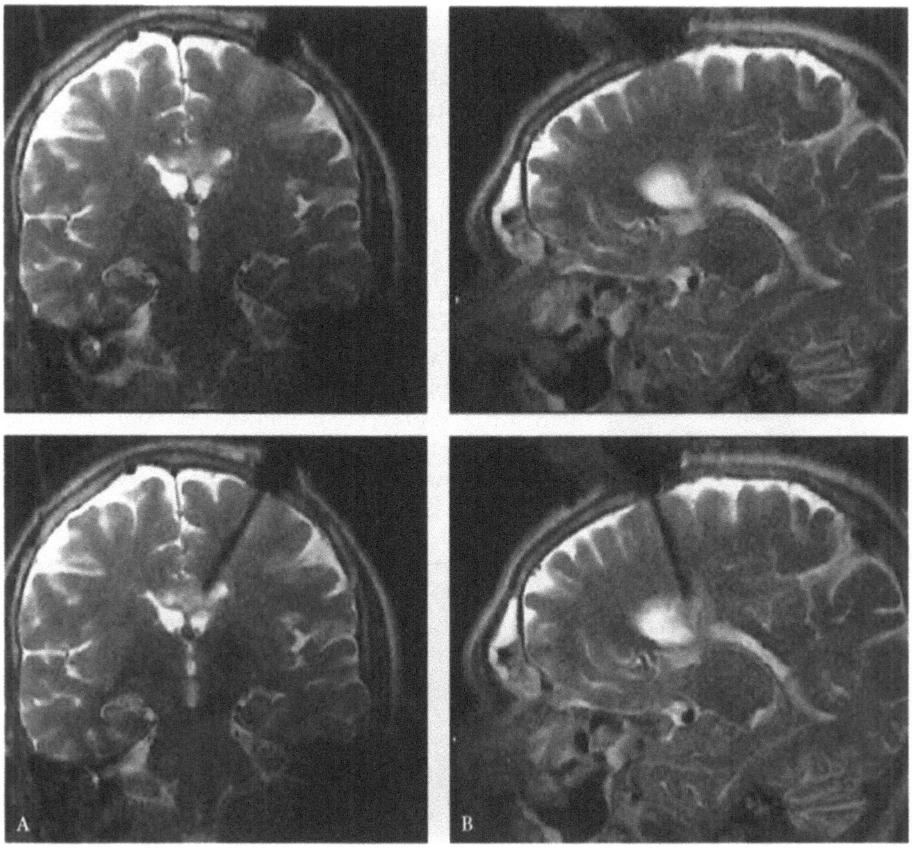

Fig. 3.10. A,B Primary glioma of the corpus callosum demonstrated on T2 weighted HASTE images. **C,D** HASTE images acquired during frameless image-guided biopsy of the lesion. Note the needle track. (Images courtesy of Philips Medical Systems)

3.4 Magnetic Resonance Angiography

The availability of improved specification MR scanners has also produced changes in the practice of magnetic resonance angiography. In "time of flight" angiography (TOF), phase dispersal due to turbulent non-laminar flow can lead to artefactual signal loss and misrepresentation of vascular anatomy. The use of very short TE values and of volume acquisitions and larger imaging matrices to ensure small voxel size significantly reduces phase dispersion (GRAVES 1997). The second main problem with TOF techniques is the gradual loss of longitudinal magnetisation, which occurs as a vessel penetrates into the imaging volume. The maximum slice thickness is limited because of this saturation effect and the optimal flip angle is a compromise between adequate background tissue suppression and preservation of signal in moving spins. Background tissue suppression can be improved by use of an off-resonance magnetisation transfer pulse to saturate protons in the bound water of the brain parenchyma and so enhance contrast between arteries and brain. The variation in arterial signal due to loss of longitudinal magnetisation can be reduced by use of a TONE (Tilted Optimised Nonsaturating Excitation) sequence which uses a variable flip-angle to decrease spin saturation as the vessel traverses an imaging volume (Fig. 3.11). The flip angle is set lower at the entry side and gradually increased as it approaches the exit side, increasing signal intensity in the distal arteries. An alternative approach is the MOTSA (multiple overlapping thin slab acquisition) which uses multiple thin slabs to minimise saturation effects. This approach combines the increased sensitivity to slow flow of a thin slice 2D acquisition with the 3D features of smaller voxel size (less phase dispersion) and the potential for 3D reconstruction.

An alternative approach to cerebral MRA is to depict the vessel lumen itself by enhancing the signal void created by flowing protons. This renders the vessel black in contrast to the surrounding stationary tissue. This technique is called "black blood" or "dark blood" angiography (EDELMAN et al. 1990). The availability of 3D T2 weighted fast spin echo and GRASE sequences has led to a re-evaluation of the black blood technique with sever-

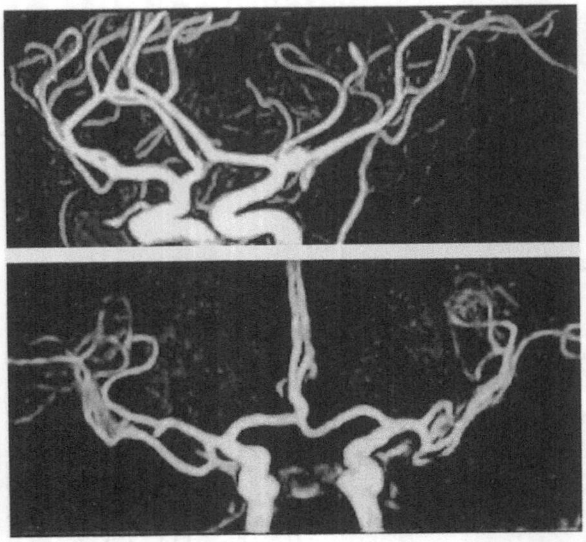

Fig. 3.11. Time of flight (TOF) angiogram in the circle of Willis in a normal volunteer. Images demonstrate the use of TONE to maintain signal intensity in vessels as blood penetrates into the imaging block

al advantages over conventional TOF. One advantage is that signal loss due to turbulence, which would cause image degradation on TOF images, contributes to the desired signal void. A second advantage is the ability of black blood to separate vessels from surrounding haematoma, which is not possible with the TOF technique (Fig. 3.12). Black blood also produces more accurate 3D visualisations of aneurysm morphology than TOF angiography due to the high signal contrast that occurs at the vessel boundary and the insensitivity of the technique to turbulent flow (Fig. 3.13). Black blood images have found an application in the extracranial carotid vessels but can be problematic in the intracranial circulation because of the intimate relationship of the internal carotid artery to the skull base. The signal void produced by bone is difficult to differentiate from the signal void produced from flowing blood so that aneurysms of the distal internal carotid may be impossible to visualise with the black blood technique (Naganawa et al. 1997).

A more recent development also resulting from the access to rapid imaging methods is the use of contrast subtraction angiography. Rapid acquisition of T1 weighted images before and during passage of a contrast bolus allows the production of high signal to noise subtraction angiograms (Fig. 3.14). This technique is of particular benefit in the extracranial vessels where it is able to produce high-resolution 3D angiograms of the entire extracranial vasculature. These subtraction angiograms do not suffer from dephasing effects in areas of rapid or turbulent flow and will reliably demonstrate short segment stenoses and confidently differentiate them from occlusive lesions (Sardanelli et al. 1999). The subtraction technique is highly dependent on the acquisition of the contrast image occurring during the peak arterial contrast bolus, which also serves to reduce distracting venous filling. Although this can be attempted by manual timing of the contrast injection, this technique is unreliable and unsatisfactory. The use of various automatic scan-triggering techniques has therefore become standard. The presence of the contrast bolus entering the neck is detected by measuring the change in signal intensity in a rapid image acquisition, which then

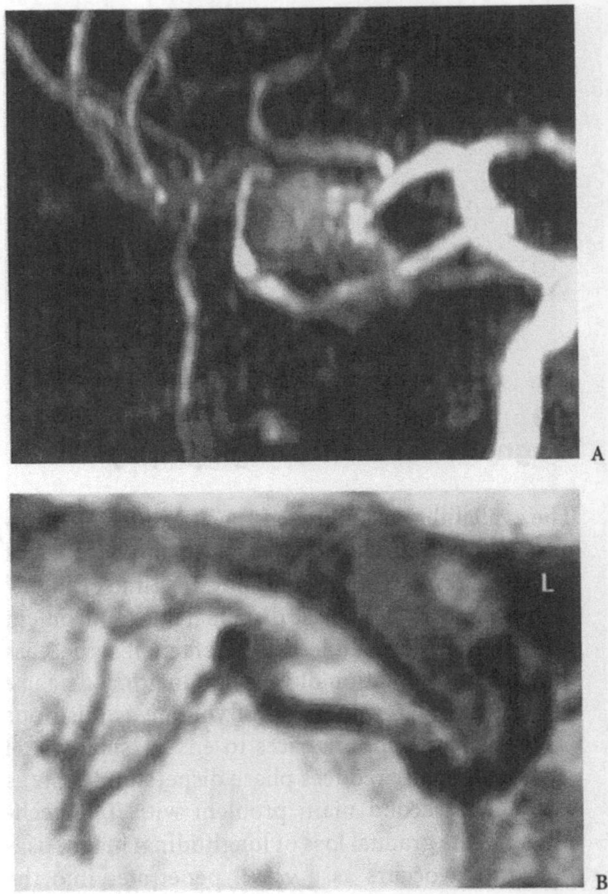

Fig. 3.12A,B. Small bifurcation aneurysm of the right middle cerebral artery with surrounding haematoma. A Maximum intensity projection of TOF angiogram shows loss of detail around the middle cerebral artery bifurcation due to high signal haematoma. The aneurysm cannot be seen. B Black blood angiogram clearly shows the outline of the aneurysm and its relationship to the surrounding vessels. The haematoma is not evident

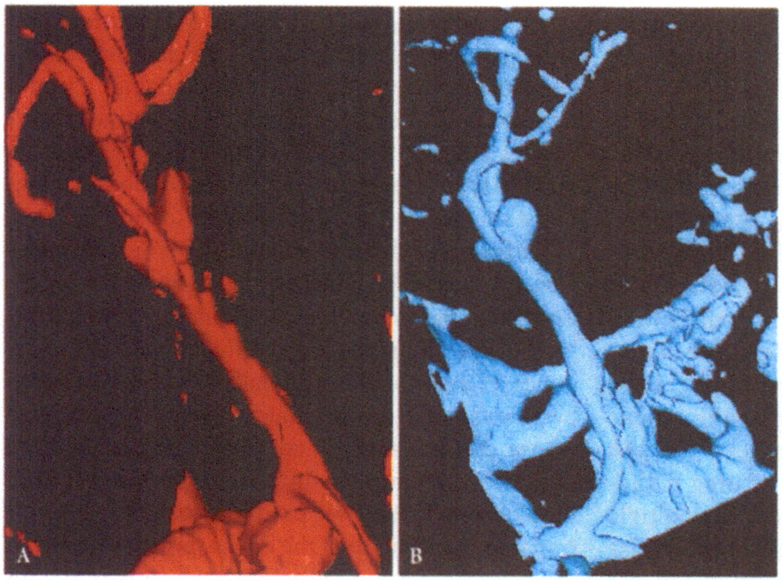

Fig. 3.13A,B. Aneurysm of the bifurcation of the middle cerebral artery. **A** Time of flight angiogram with isosurface rendering demonstrates distortion of the aneurysm which appears to be "cone shaped". **B** shows 3D rendering from black blood angiography which more clearly shows the rounded bilobed nature of the aneurysm

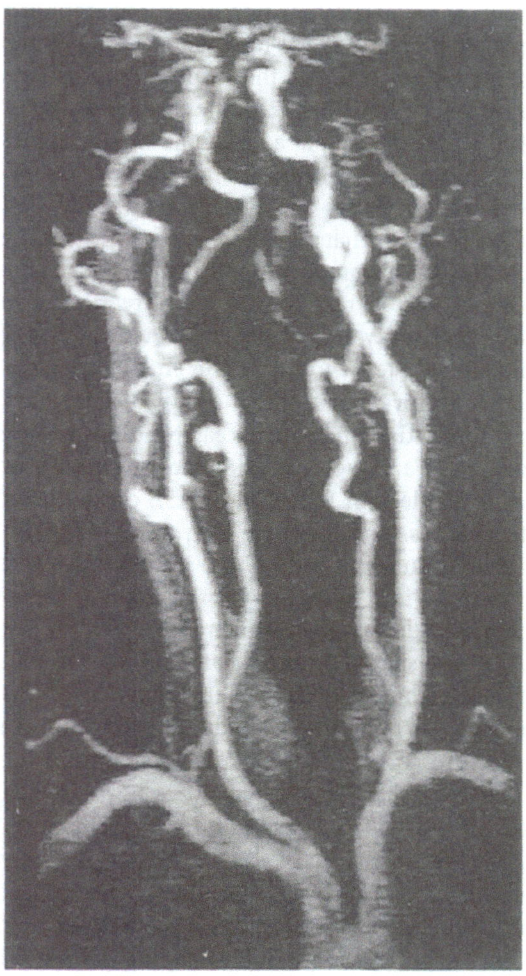

Fig. 3.14. Contrast subtraction MRA of the extracranial vessels demonstrating an occlusion of the right internal carotid artery

triggers the scan itself. These bolus-tracking packages are now becoming available on all commercial MRI systems (Foo et al. 1997).

The clinical applications of intra- and extracranial MR angiography are discussed in Chaps. 12 and 13.

3.5 Magnetisation Transfer and Diffusion Weighted Imaging

The use of new MR contrast mechanisms is also beginning to have a profound effect on clinical practice in neuroradiology. Of these the most notable are magnetisation transfer (MT) and diffusion weighted imaging. Both these techniques can be used to detect abnormalities beyond the resolution of conventional MR images. Magnetisation transfer contrast results from the presence of two separate pools of protons within tissue: bound immobile protons associated with macromolecules such as myelin and free mobile protons associated with free water. Pulsed MT imaging is achieved by application of an off-resonance radio frequency before the pulse sequence to preferentially saturate protons in the bound pool, which then transfer magnetisation to mobile protons in the free water. The change in net signal intensity depends on the strength of the saturation pulses and on the structure of the macromolecular matrix. The amount of magnetisation transferred can be represented as the magnetisation transfer ratio (MTR). Decreases in MTR have been demonstrated in areas of demyelination, inflammation, Wallerian degeneration and in human and experimental brain tumours (Ikezaki et al. 1997). The measurement of MTR appears to be unaffected by tissue anisotropy and is increasingly used as a method of quantifying abnormalities in isotropic white matter tracts affected by inflammatory and ischaemic disease. Despite this the exact clinical benefits of MT imaging remain unclear. The MT ratio is thought to reflect the structural integrity of tissues with an important contribution from myelin and axons. In multiple sclerosis decreases in MTR appear maximal during the acute enhancing phase, slowly recovering as the lesions mature (Hanyu et al. 1998). This suggests that MT imaging may provide a tool for elucidating pathophysiology and monitoring treatment in multiple sclerosis. In tumours MTR has been shown to improve the accuracy of tumour classification and was superior to other conventional sequences in the classification of intra-axial tumours allowing differentiation between low-grade astrocytomas, haemangioblastomas and craniopharyngiomas (Kurki et al. 1995). Kato et al. demonstrated regional decreases in MTR in pyramidal tract in patients with amyotrophic lateral sclerosis which were sufficiently specific to aid diagnosis (Fig. 3.15) (Kato et al. 1997). Taylor-Robinson et al. (1995) demonstrated a correlation between globus pallidus MT contrast and blood ammonia levels ($P<0.05$), which also correlated to the severity of hepatic encephalopathy in patients with liver dysfunction. These disparate observations suggest that MTR images may become an increasingly important feature of diagnostic imaging strategies in a number of brain diseases.

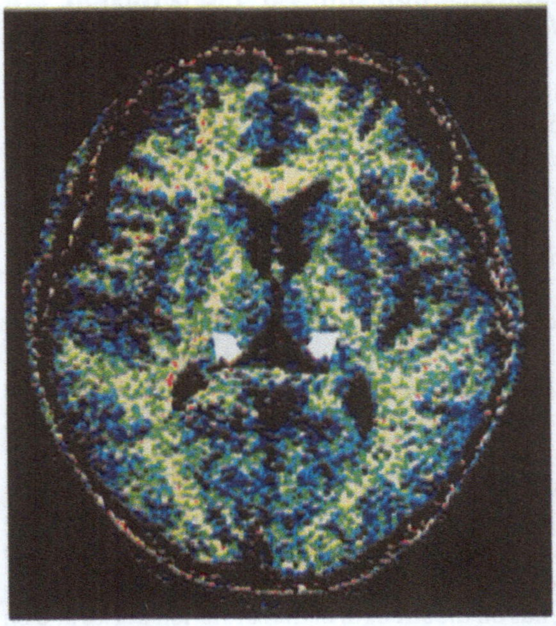

Fig. 3.15. Magnetisation transfer ratio image of the internal capsule in a patient with amyotrophic lateral sclerosis. Note the focal decreases in MTR in the position of the pyramidal tract (*arrows*). (Image from Kato and Matsamura 1997)

Diffusion weighted imaging (DWI) sequences have been available for many years but it is only recently that the technique has become widely clinically available. In principle the diffusion technique depends on motion related signal loss which is induced by the use of large matched de-phasing gradients whose effects cancel if no motion is present. The presence of Brownian diffusion of protons within the sample will however produce signal loss proportional to the strength of the dephasing gradients and the degree of proton diffusion that occurs in the interval between the application of the two gradients. Repeated imaging using increasing diffusion gradient strengths allows calculation of the apparent diffusional coefficient (ADC) for each pixel. Since the gradients are directional the ADC measurements represent vectors which are classically acquired along the three principal axes of the main magnet bore. As interest in diffusional anisotropy has increased more workers are now measuring the full diffusion tensor, which requires measurements in six directions to allow precise quantification of the true diffusional vector magnitude and direction. The clinical practicality of DWI depends on the ability of the imaging sequence to correct for small physiological patient movements, which occur during image acquisition. Patient movements can be minimised by rapid imaging and most diffusion sequences are now based on single shot EPI, FSE, GRASE or multishot EPI techniques. Because of the long scan times, DWI images are also sensitive to phase shifts, which vary from view to view. To correct for this many DWI sequences use a double echo sequence in which the fast echo carries spatial information and the second "navigator" echo has no spatial encoding. Variations in the phase of the navigator induced by motion are then used to correct phase errors occurring in the fast imaging echo. These navigator echo corrected images show significant reduction in movement related phase echo and make clinical DWI realistically achievable (Mori and van Zijl 1998). The clinical role of DWI is already well defined in some areas and continues to grow as more stable imaging techniques become widely available. The largest application of DWI is likely to be in the investigation of cerebral ischaemia. In both clinical studies and animal models

DWI demonstrates a rapid fall in ADC with a gradual return to normal followed by an increase in ADC over baseline values (Schlaug et al. 1997). In acute stroke, demonstration of decreased ADC (Fig. 3.16) may be the only imaging abnormality whilst T2 remains normal (Geijer et al. 1999; Gonzalez et al. 1999). In the late phase of stroke, areas of increased ADC allow confident identification of lesions which are at least several days old and corresponds to cellular breakdown and with loss of diffusional barriers (Fitzek et al. 1998). The identification of an area of T2 abnormality with ADC values around normal may indicate either cellular recovery or progressive cellular necrosis. In these cases DWI alone is not sufficient to predict outcome and evidence of the perfusional status of the tissue must be sought. This combination of DWI and perfusion imaging, often known as the "brain attack" protocol, offers considerable promise for the assessment of acute stroke, for treatment planning and for the assessment of new therapeutic strategies (Lovblad et al. 1997; Barber et al. 1998; Berry et al. 1998; Read et al. 1998). The imaging approach of stroke is discussed in Chap. 10. Other clinical uses for DWI are less well defined. The ability to measure regional anisotropy has led several groups to examine the potential utility of DWI in white matter development and white matter disease. In the newborn the AC of white matter is considerably greater than in adults and there is a close correlation with gestational age with ADC dropping as gestational age increases. Measurements of diffusional anisotropy do not show a similar correlation and it has been suggested that ADC measures reflect brain water content whilst diffusional anisotropy gives information concerning brain microstructure (Neil et al. 1998). This conclusion is supported by observations in multiple sclerosis where diffusion tensor imaging identifies significantly altered water diffusion properties in the normal-appearing white matter of patients compared with control subjects (Fig. 3.17), and can distinguish between lesion types. The highest diffusion is seen in destructive (T1 hypointense) lesions, whereas the greatest change in anisotropy is found in inflammatory (gadolinium-enhancing) lesions (Werring et al. 1999b). DWI has also been used to visualise the degree and distribution of white matter tract lesions in a variety of disease states including trauma, tumours and stroke (Werring et al. 1998a; Nakada et al. 1999; Werring et al. 1999a). DWI also has several potential applications in cerebral tumours. The use of DWI in patients with epidermoid tumours of the posterior fossa allows confident demonstration of the tumour, which can be isointense on conventional MR sequences. The DWI characteristics of cerebral abscess have also been suggested to be of diagnostic use with abscesses showing high signal on DWI images compared to benign brain tumour, which appeared hypointense (Kim et al. 1998). More excitingly the changes in ADC observed after tumour therapy in both humans and animal models appear to correlate closely with the histological changes taking place within the tumour (Chenevert et al. 1997; Sugahara et al. 1999). In an animal model of brain tumour diffusion displayed a strong treatment effect and increased by 55% 6–8 days following treatment, and before tumour regression (Chenevert et al. 1997). Diffusion and relaxation times returned to pre-treatment levels by 12 days after treatment. Histological examination showed that the observed increase in diffusion reflected an increase of extracellular space following

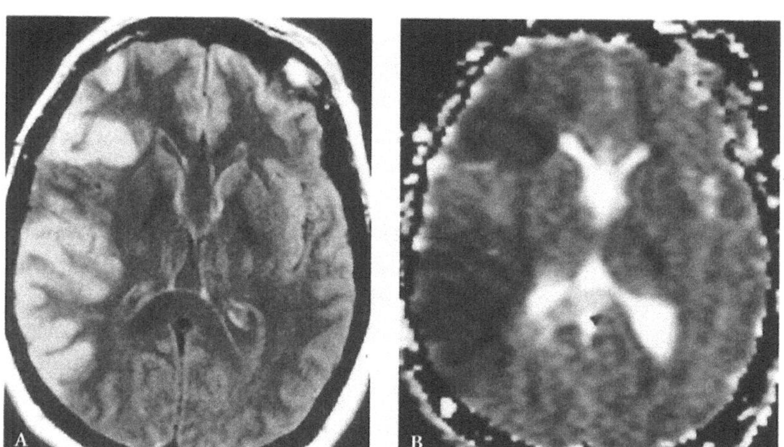

Fig. 3.16A,B. Right-sided middle cerebral artery stroke imaged 3 h after onset. **A** T2 weighted fast FLAIR image demonstrates extensive signal abnormality in the distribution of the middle cerebral artery. **B** Apparent diffusional coefficient image calculated from fast spin echo navigator echo corrected primary images using three gradient values. The image shows extensive areas of decreased ADC in a distribution of the stroke

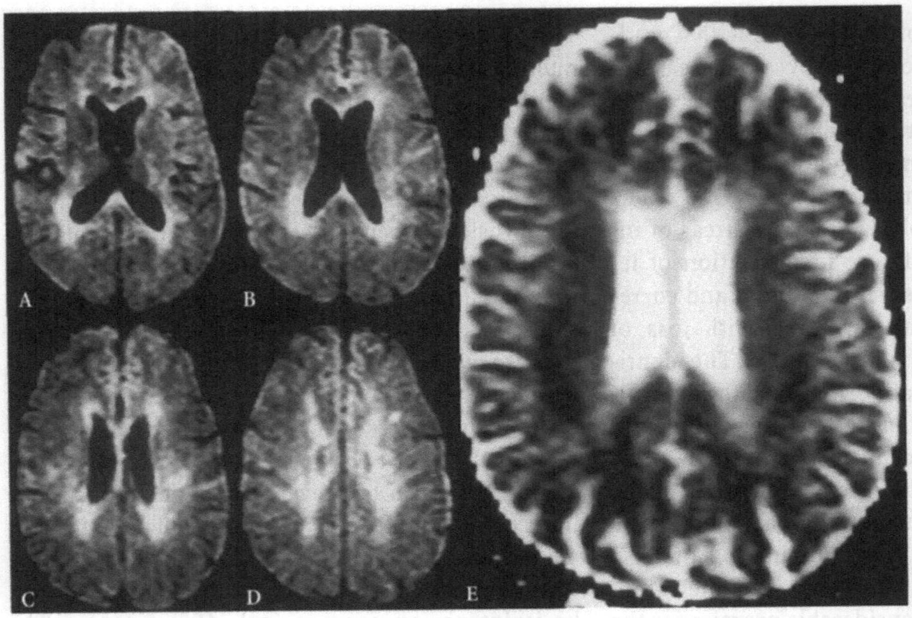

Fig. 3.17A–E. Diffusion-weighted images in a patient with multiple sclerosis. Images A–D show the primary images acquired with a combination of diffusion and T2 weighting. Note the extensive periventricular high signal abnormality. E Apparent diffusional coefficient image calculated using the data in image B together with two other diffusion-weighted images at the same level. Note the high diffusional coefficient in CSF and the areas of high diffusional coefficient lesions in the immediate periventricular region. Comparing the image

treatment. Furthermore, the subsequent apparent diffusion coefficient decrease was a result of repopulation of the space by viable tumour cells at a rate dependent on the surviving tumour cell fraction and recurrent tumour doubling time. These results suggest that diffusion measurements are sensitive to therapy induced changes in cellular structure and may provide an early non-invasive indicator of treatment efficacy.

3.6 Dynamic MR Imaging Techniques

The ability of modern MRI systems for rapid image acquisition enables the design of studies based on temporal variations in signal intensity. These include the blood oxygen level dependent (BOLD) functional MR technique, which detects small inherent signal changes in the brain resulting from regional changes in blood flow and techniques for the measurement of cerebral perfusion parameters based on the signal changes resulting from contrast agent passage and uptake.

3.6.1 Functional Imaging

The BOLD technique depends on small changes in signal intensity which occur on T2* weighted images when local cerebral activation occurs. Neuronal activation causes an increase in local blood flow which outstrips the increased cerebral oxygen requirements so that the local concentration of deoxyhaemoglobin falls. Since deoxyhaemoglobin is a paramagnetic compound, this causes a rise in signal intensity which occurs some seconds after the onset of neuronal activation and persists for the duration of the task. The amplitude of this signal change is small, usually less than 8%, and often much smaller, which makes the identification of true activation related signal change difficult. In order to facilitate this the commonest functional imaging paradigm follows a "boxcar" design with alternating periods of activation and rest. This experimental design allow the use of cross-correlation statistics to identify true activations despite poor signal to noise characteristics in the original images. Unfortunately the use of a boxcar paradigm is restrictive and the need to use all the image data renders the technique exquisitely sensitive to motion artefact, which may present as failure to detect activation or, more worryingly, as spurious activation. These motion-related artefacts can be reduced by the use of rigid body co-registration algorithms and data re-sampling prior to calculation of the cross-correlation coefficient. However, this is time consuming and will not correct for large movements. The limitations of the boxcar experimental design have led to the increased use of event related fMRI. This technique records MR signal at fixed time periods after stimulus presentation which allows the identification of BOLD responses to transient single stimuli and allows far more flexibility in the design of the experimental paradigm. These fMRI methodologies are largely employed in research studies of brain function; however, they are also being increasingly used to identify eloquent cortical areas in surgical planning (Fig. 3.18).

3.6.2
Perfusion Imaging

Despite the importance of cerebral perfusion measurements in diagnostic neuroradiology, no ideal clinically acceptable technique exists. The gold standard technique for measurement of regional cerebral blood flow is to use PET in combination with a short lived isotope such as oxygen-15 water. However, this is very costly and more suitable to research applications than clinical use. ^{99m}Tc HMPAO SPECT scanning is clinically acceptable and of considerable value in the diagnosis of many disorders such as the dementing diseases. Unfortunately SPECT is of relatively low resolution and does not produce quantitative images of CBF but qualitative images of marker distribution, which reflect perfusion, local atrophy and neuronal metabolic activity. The introduction of spiral CT has led to a resurgence of interest in the Xe inhalation technique, which is discussed more fully later in this chapter.

MR techniques for the measurement of cerebral perfusion have been based on either dynamic imaging of contrast bolus passage or identification of protons flowing into an imaging volume by spin tagging techniques. The dynamic contrast enhanced technique for MR perfusion imaging uses a dynamic imaging acquisition of the first passage of an intravenously injected contrast bolus through the brain (Rosen et al. 1990). Either T1 or T2 weighted images may be collected; however, most studies use T2* weighted sequences since paramagnetic effects increase the signal change in areas of low vascularity. Images must be collected with a temporal resolution of approximately 2 s or less in order to allow accurate analysis of the contrast bolus. The passage of contrast causes a transient drop in signal intensity which can be used to calculate the rate of change of T2* (ΔR2), which is linearly proportional to contrast concentration. The contrast concentration time course in each voxel can then be analysed to generate vascular parameters, which describe the blood flow pattern in the

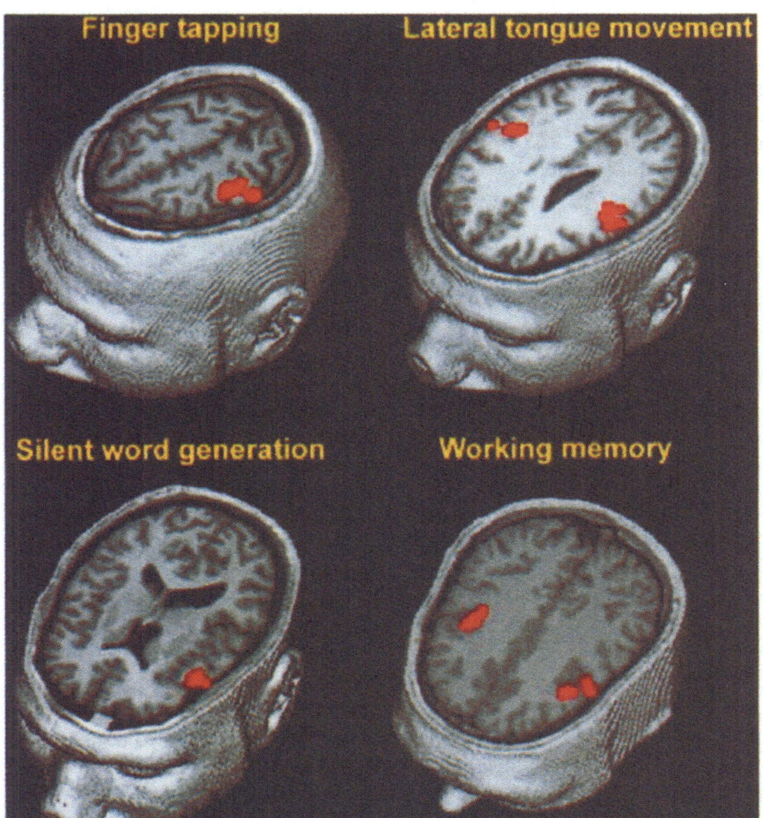

Fig. 3.18. Three-dimensional renderings of functional imaging using the BOLD technique in a normal volunteer to demonstrate areas of eloquent cortex

voxel. In order to remove the effects of contrast recirculation the analysis is commonly performed by fitting a gamma variate curve to the contrast concentration time course data (Fig. 3.19). This data can be used to calculate the relative cerebral blood volume (rCBV), which is proportional to the area under the curve, the mean transit time (MTT), which is equal to the width of the curve and the contrast arrival time (T0) and time to peak contrast concentration (TTP). The relative cerebral blood flow (rCBF) is calculated by dividing the rCBV by the MTT (Fig. 3.20). The measurement of rCBF obtained in this way is a relative one and direct comparisons between patients are not possible. This results in part from the non-linearity of the CBV measurements which are produced from T2* weighted images but mainly from variations in the MTT measurement due to bolus dispersal. In order to address this problem accurate measurements of the arterial input function can be simultaneously acquired and used to deconvolute the time course data to reduce the effects of bolus dispersion. This deconvolution step allows estimation of true blood flow and supports the use of the technique for clinical measurements (Rempp et al. 1994). An alternative technique is to assess contrast bolus volume by measurement of venous contrast concentrations; this technique is more stable, technically simpler and produces excellent agreement with other "gold standard" methods for the measurement of CBF (Hagen et al. 1999). Of equal importance is the ability of the technique to demonstrate contrast arrival time parameters T0 and TTP. The presence of compensatory small vessel dilatation in response to local falls in cerebral perfusion pressure gives rise to significant regional prolongation of TTP and T0. These changes reflect the degree of regional autoregulation and are highly sensitive indicators of brain at risk of infarction (Fig. 3.21). The technique is valuable in the investigation of extracranial carotid disease and of cerebral arteritides. It also is increasingly being applied in other disease states such as neoplasia and the neurodegenerative disorders (Fig. 3.22) (Sandson et al. 1996; Kluytmans et al. 1997; Kassner et al. 1999).

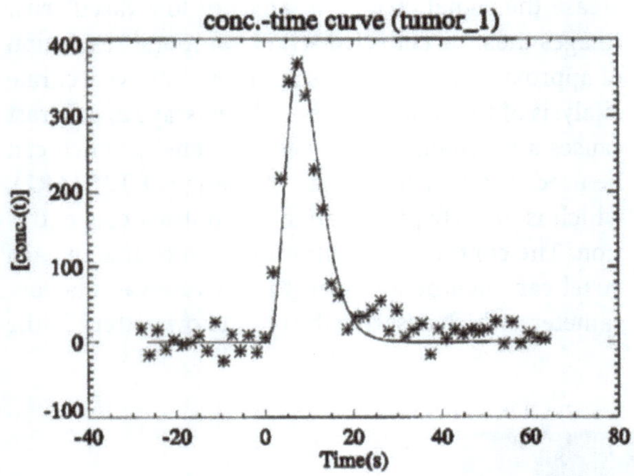

Fig. 3.19. Shows the change in contrast concentration against time in a single voxel from a malignant brain tumour. Data points are fitted to a gamma variat curve shown as *a dotted line* which is then used to calculate haemodynamic variables

Several techniques for cerebral perfusion imaging have been described which avoid the need for intrave-

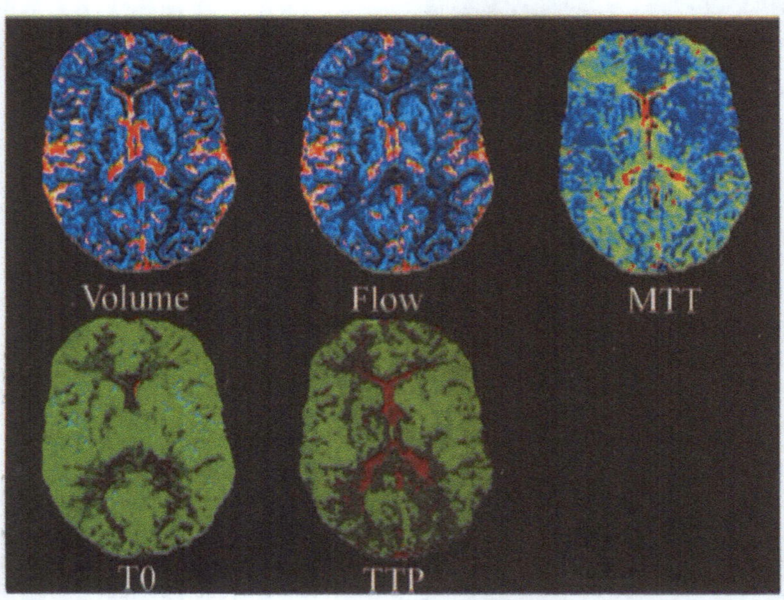

Fig. 3.20. Parametric imaging of perfusion-related haemodynamic variables calculated from dynamic susceptibility contrast enhanced MRI. Images show relative cerebral blood volume (*top left*), relative cerebral blood flow (*top middle*), mean transit time (*top right*), time to contrast arrival (*bottom left*), and time to peak contrast concentration (*bottom right*). The distribution of cerebral blood volume and cerebral blood flow follows clear anatomical demarcations. Mean transit time, T0 and TTP maps all show slight prolongation in the anterior and posterior cerebral watersheds

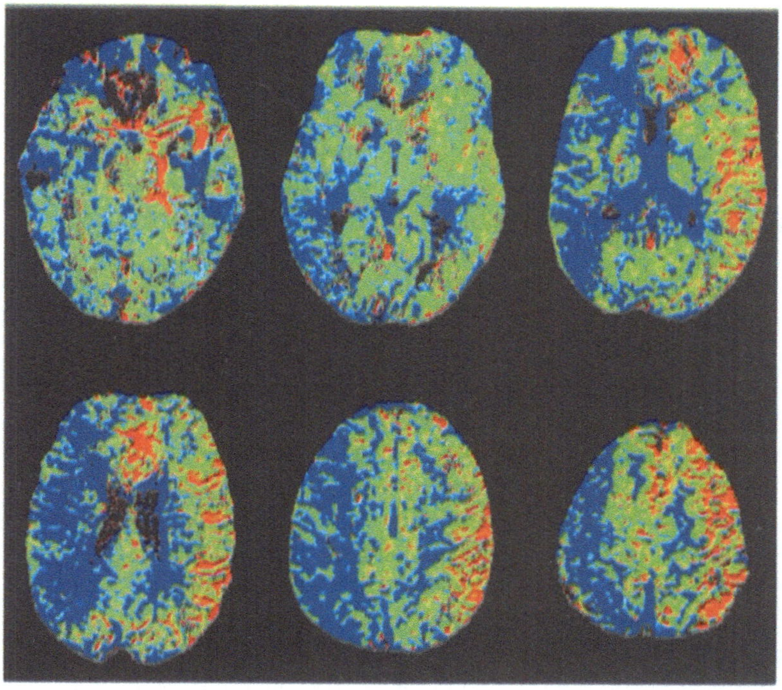

Fig. 3.21. Time to peak concentration maps from dynamic susceptibility contrast enhanced imaging in a patient with severe right-sided carotid stenosis. The images show marked asymmetry with prolongation of TTP in the distribution of the right middle cerebral artery and its watershed zones. The changes are most marked in the areas of the watershed and deep white matter

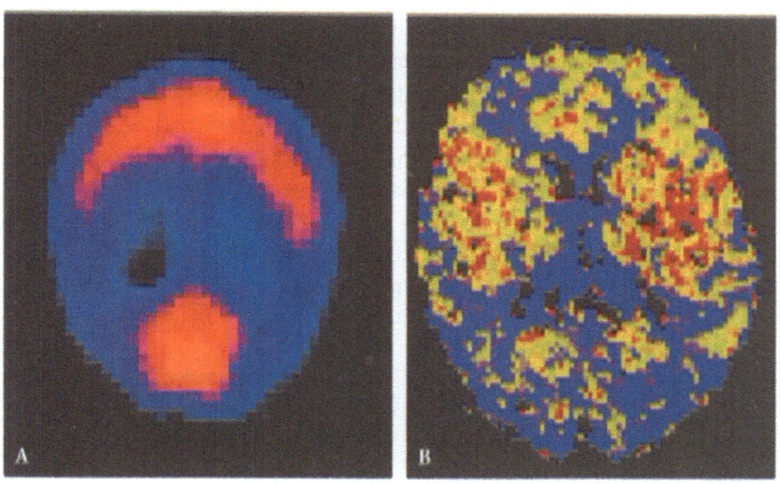

Fig. 3.22A,B. Images from a patient with Alzheimer's disease. **A** Tc HMPAO SPECT image in the axial plane demonstrates bilateral parietal areas of underperfusion. **B** TTP map from dynamic susceptibility contrast enhanced imaging sequence demonstrates corresponding areas of prolonged TTP in the posterior parietal and occipital cortices

nous contrast injections. These techniques use pulsed labelling of arterial spins by a radio frequency inversion pulse and use images acquired with and without labelling to measure regional perfusion. The techniques are complicated by loss of the spin tag due to the relatively short T1 of the inflowing blood compared to the rate passage of blood through the brain. Thus, although arterial tagging in the neck is theoretically optimal from a biological standpoint and works well in small animals, it is extremely difficult to implement in humans. The alternative approaches of labelling spins immediately adjacent to the imaging plane have their own problems regarding direction of inflow, selection of optimal inflow times and inadvertent labelling of venous inflow. This has given rise to a number of alternative approaches to spin labelling which include echo-planar MR imaging with alternating radio frequency (EPISTAR), flow sensitive alternating inversion recovery (FAIR), uninverted FAIR (UNFAIR), and quantitative imaging of perfusion using single subtraction (QUIPPS). A review of these techniques and their problems has been published by Patel et al. (1995b). Despite the technical problems and the extremely small signal changes seen after spin tagging these techniques appear promising as a method of quantitative perfusion imaging.

3.6.3 MR Imaging of Angiogenesis

The time course of tissue enhancement has long been of interest in many disease states, particularly in the diagnosis and classification of tumours. In recent years it has been increasingly appreciated that tumour growth is dependent on the growth of new blood vessels, known as angiogenesis, which is stimulated by the release of growth factors from the tumour cells. Many growth factors have been identified but vasoactive endothelial growth factor (VEGF) has been most strongly associated with tumour blood vessel development. VEGF increases the permeability of existing capillary membranes allowing easier diffusion of metabolites into and out of the tumour and stimulates the proliferation of the blood vessel lining cells and growth of new vessels. The elucidation of this angiogenic cascade has led to a new therapeutic approach to cancer with the development of "anti VEGF" therapies. The development of these therapies has led to increased interest in the imaging of angiogenesis both for diagnosis and for treatment planning and monitoring.

The features of angiogenic tissue, which can be examined by MRI, include increased vascular density, disorganisation of vascular anatomy, variability in vessel size and increased permeability of endothelium due to VEGF activity. The measurement of vascular density can be estimated using the first pass analysis of rCBV described above (Fig. 3.23). Vascular disorganisation and variability in vessel size can be estimated by examination of the late "re-circulation phase" of the first pass bolus or by comparison of the contrast related signal change on T2 and T2* weighted images. These later methods have been very recently described and require clinical validation; however, they theoretically appear to offer powerful techniques for the localisation of angiogenic tissue.

Since VEGF activity is associated with marked increase in endothelial permeability, one alternative approach to the imaging of angiogenesis is to quantify the permeability of vascular endothelia (Dvorak et al. 1995; Amoroso et al. 1997; Brasch et al. 1997). The VEGF mediated increase in endothelial permeability correlates to malignant behaviour in a variety of tumour types (Goldman et al. 1993; Jensen 1998) and has been implicated in the formation of peritumoural edema and tumour cysts (Criscuolo 1993; Provias et al. 1996). The presence of high endothelial permeability in tumours has also been implicated in the generation of haematogenous metastases and in the viability of these metastases in other tissues (Zetter 1998). Imaging studies to measure endothelial permeability rely on the accurate measurement of marker concentrations in the blood stream and in the tumour over time. These measurements can then be combined with a pharmacokinetic model of marker distribution to calculate a transfer constant related to permeability. Several appropriate pharmacokinetic models have been described of distribution (Larsson et al. 1990; Brix et al. 1991; Tofts and Kermode 1991; Tofts et al.

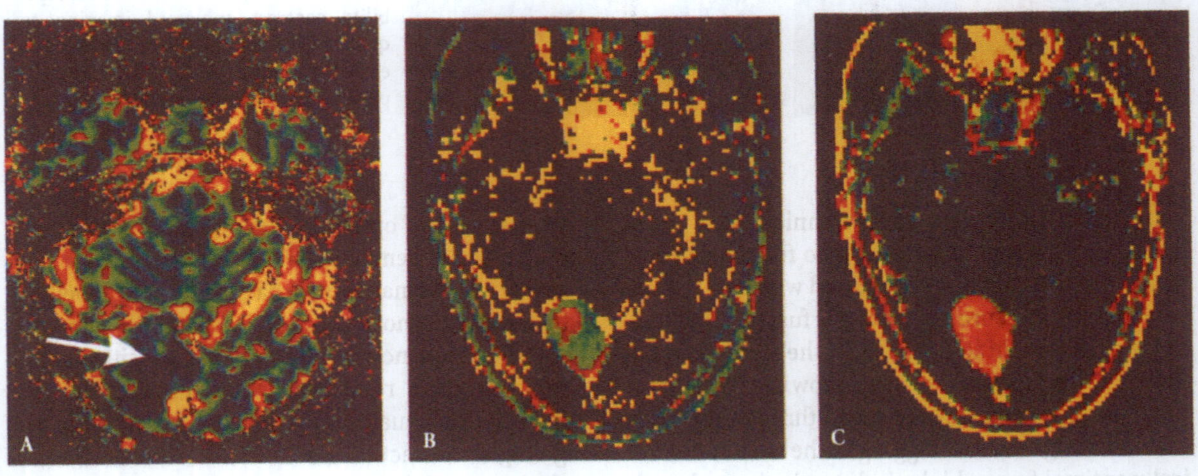

Fig. 3.23A–C. Parametric images in a patient with a low-grade tentorial meningioma. **A** Cerebral blood volume map calculated from T2 weighted dynamic susceptibility contrast enhanced imaging shows a very low cerebral blood volume within the tumour itself (*arrow*). **B** Map of endothelial surface area permeability product (*K*) shows an area of moderately high permeability (*red*) in the centre of a tumour which has intermediate permeability (*green*). **C** Contrast distribution space (*VL* shows high contrast distribution space suggesting a large extracellular fraction within the tumour

1995). The most commonly used model was described by BRIX et al. (1991) and calculates a transfer constant (*k12*) for passage of contrast between the blood stream and the tumour interstitium which is related to vascular permeability. The model described by TOFTS et al. (1995) represents a more comprehensive approach which aims to calculate a true absolute value for endothelial permeability surface area product (*k*). The rationale behind this more complex and methodologically demanding approach is to produce a measurement which is independent of variables, such as receive gain, contrast dosage, patient cardiovascular status, etc. This makes the Tofts model attractive for monitoring changes of tumour vasculature during treatment and determining the surrogate end points for treatment in longitudinal comparison and multicentre trials. The Tofts model estimates two independent variables: the surface area endothelial permeability product (*k*) and the contrast distribution volume (*vl*), which corresponds to the size of the extracellular space (Fig. 3.23). Values of *k* are highly reproducible and are independent of the scanner type; they show close correlation with aggressive behaviour of tumours across many tumour types (Fig. 3.24).

3.7 Interventional MR

The use of MRI for image guidance in both conventional and frameless stereotaxic surgery is continuing to grow. Dedicated MRI systems for interventional procedures are available from several manufacturers. One approach to this type of system has been the production of "open" magnets, effectively splitting the hardware component of the magnet itself into two physical moieties to allow access for the surgeon in the main field. This places restrictions on the magnet design so that these systems tend to be of low field strength with restricted gradient performance compared to current diagnostic machines. An alternative approach is to combine conventional MR systems with X-ray screening and ultrasound to allow multimodality control of operative procedures (Fig. 3.25). This approach allows real time control of surgical procedures, which can then be supplemented by functional imaging to identify eloquent cortex or spectroscopic imaging to identify optimal sites for tumour biopsy (Fig. 3.26).

3.8 Advances in CT Technology

The widespread availability of spiral CT systems has resulted in a number of concurrent developments related to the improvement in image acquisition speed. The combination of fast spiral CT and image reconstruction from partial acquisition has made real time CT fluoroscopy possible and these systems are now commercially available. CT fluoroscopy is invaluable for procedures such as spinal biopsy and for a wide range of non-neuro applications. Fast spiral acquisition also allows the use of CT for contrast angiography using the same approach described for MR. Acquisition of a series of 1-mm slices over approximately 1 min during contrast bolus passage

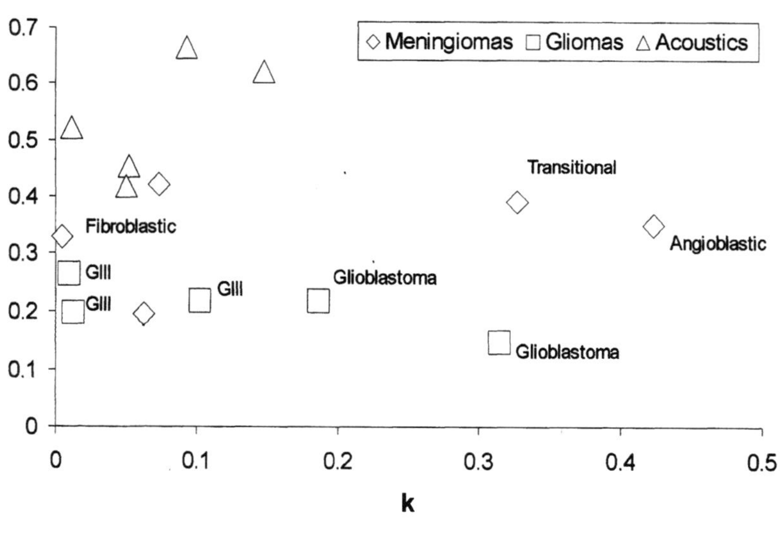

Fig. 3.24. A plot of endothelial surface area permeability product (*K*) against contrast distribution space (*VL*) in 15 patients with cerebral tumours. Patients with acoustic neuroma show high values of *VL* in keeping with the known histological characteristics of the tumour. High values of *K* (>0.15) as seen only in patients with glioblastoma and aggressive meningiomas

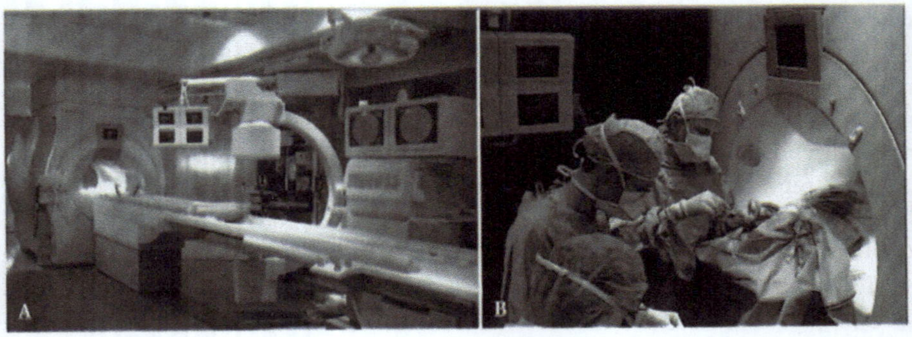

Fig. 3.25. A Interventional magnetic resonance imaging suite. The system consists of a 1.5-Tesla imaging unit connected by continuous table to a C-arm digital subtraction angiography unit seen in the centre of the image. Angiographic and MR images can be displayed simultaneously and synchronised. **B** Operative areas are provided at both ends of the magnet bore; this figure shows two surgeons performing a frameless image-guided brain biopsy using the surgical operating space at the far end of the magnet bore. (Images courtesy of Philips Medical Systems)

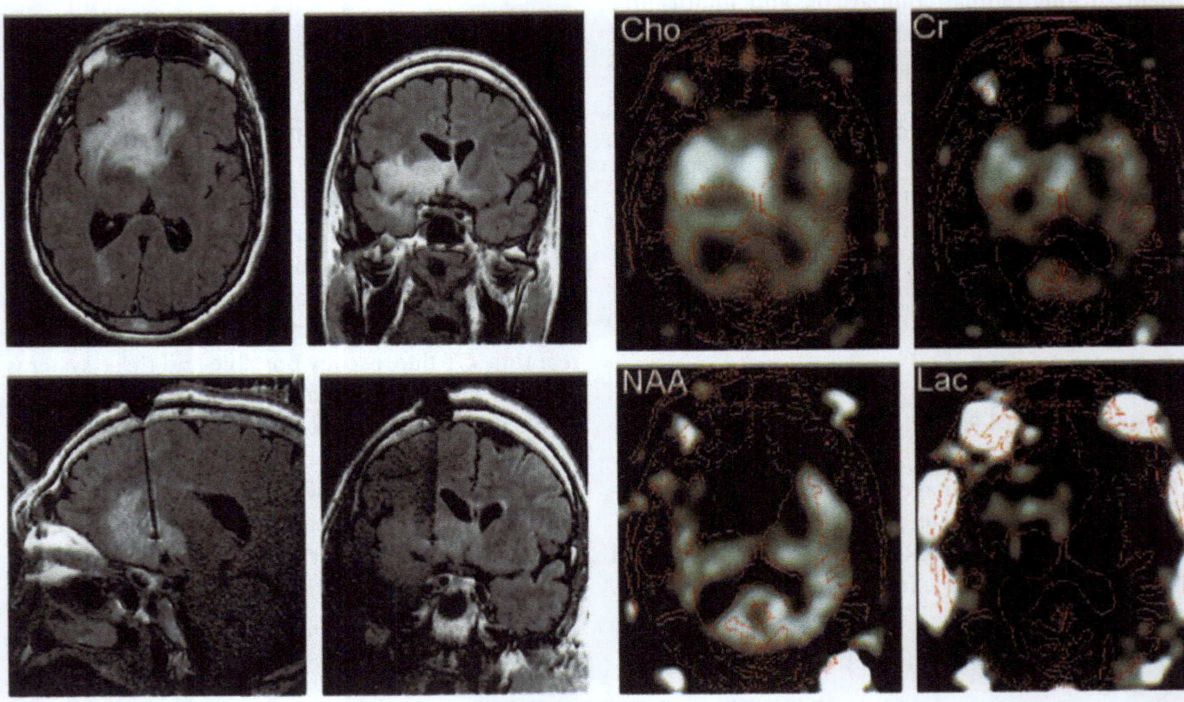

Fig. 3.26A–C. Interventional procedure on a patient with a primary cerebral glioma. Images *at the top left* are postcontrast HASTE T1 weighted images demonstrating the enhancing mass lesion in the base of the brain. The outline of the tumour from the axial images is then overlayed on spectroscopic imaging shown in **B. B** Tumour area shows the high central area with high choline concentration lying in the posterior half of the enhancing mass. **c** Image-guided stereotaxic biopsy of the identified site. The needle can be seen to lie in the posterior half of the central area of the tumour. (Images courtesy of Philips Medical Systems)

provides excellent detail of arterial anatomy, which can be improved by subtraction of matching non-contrast images (Imakita et al. 1998). This technique has been used for screening for intracranial aneurysms, evaluating subarachnoid haemorrhage (Fig. 3.27), planning surgical therapy and pre-embolic assessment of AVMs (Tanaka et al. 1997). Rapid imaging of contrast bolus passage can also be used to measure CBV, CBF and MTT using image-processing techniques identical to those described for MRI. The use of CT for dynamic contrast perfusion imaging has advantages in terms of absolute flow quantification but suffers from limited tissue coverage due to the high temporal resolution required for this technique. The introduction of "multislice" CT systems will overcome many of these restrictions so that

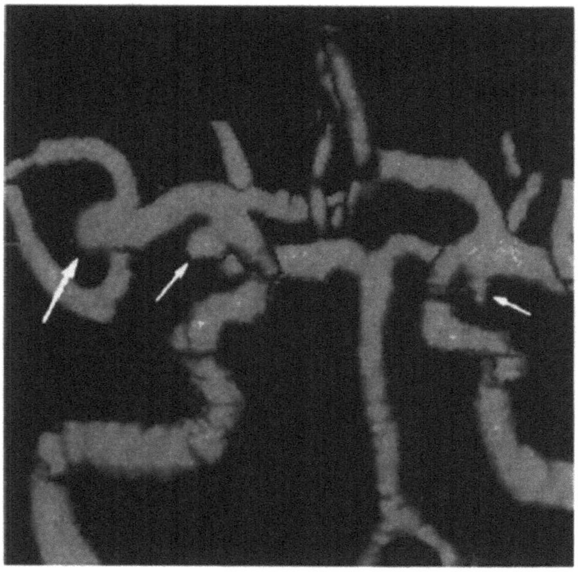

Fig. 3.27. Three-dimensional isosurface render of a subtraction CT angiogram showing right MCA bifurcation (*arrow*) and bilateral ICA-anterior choroidal artery aneurysms (*short arrows*). (Image from Imakita et al. 1998)

dynamic CT perfusion imaging may become an attractive clinical option. Use of a simpler analytical approach allows calculation of accurate CBV measures from whole brain, which may be sufficient for identification of reperfusion in acute stroke but appears limited for other uses (Hunter et al. 1998). A more promising technique for cerebral perfusion imaging is the use of inhaled xenon as a contrast agent. Subjects inhale xenon gas, which is freely diffusible from vasculature into brain parenchyma. At steady state, concentrations of Xe in the tissue reflect regional perfusion allowing calculation of absolute blood flow. The technique allows whole head imaging, and problems with sedation due to the anaesthetic action of Xe are minimised by rapid spiral CT data collection. Although the technique involves ionising radiation, it provides highly accurate quantitative measurements and has been validated in several experimental and clinical studies (Hagen et al. 1999).

3.9 Advances in Angiography and Image Processing

The availability of increased computing power and the growth of effective local and international networking is also producing significant changes in practice. Over the past 10 years there has been a rapid increase in availability of 3D visualisation tools for clinical use and some techniques, particularly maximum intensity projection rendering (MIP), are already considered an essential part of investigations such as MRA and CTA (Figs. 3.11, 3.27). With the increase in imaging hardware performance, MR and CT data sets are now of sufficiently high spatial resolution and quality to allow the use of more sophisticated visualisation algorithms. Techniques such as isosurface rendering are now available on most commercial clinical image analysis systems and have been applied to a wide range of clinical investigations including vascular imaging (Figs. 3.6, 3.7, 3.13, 3.27). As these techniques become more sophisticated they are able to combine 3D data sets from different modalities and are likely to perform an increasing role in routine clinical work. Figure 3.28 shows a series of MRA images of a patient with a posterior communicating artery aneurysm. The standard MIP image (Fig. 3.28A) is of poor quality and is inadequate for full pretreatment assessment of the aneurysm for coiling or clipping. An isosurface rendering of the same data set (Fig. 3.28B) provides excellent detail of the aneurysm neck and of the branch vessel arising from it. The 3D isosurface model can be interactively rotated in real time to allow selection of the optimal view for aneurysm coiling, if this is appropriate, and a pseudo-DSA image can be calculated from the MRA data (Fig. 3.28C). These pseudo-DSA projections show the view likely to be obtained at angiography and allow selection of the optimal projections for intervention prior to the angiography. Coregistration of T2 weighted FSE volume scans allows identification of blood clot within the aneurysm, which can then be incorporated into the 3D model (Fig. 3.28D) showing a much larger, partially thrombosed, aneurysm which was not appreciated from the TOF data alone. The ability to generate 3D data for planning of neuroradiological interventional procedures is extremely valuable since the placement of embolic materials or coils can easily be misjudged when working with 2D angiographic projections. This problem has been addressed by the development of 3D rotational angiography systems, which acquire multiple images during contrast injection whilst rotating the C-arm of the intensifier through an arc around the patient's head (Fig. 3.29). These rotational views allow the anatomy to be viewed as a movie loop providing depth information to the operator at the time of angiogram. These rotational images can then be used to calculate a true 3D data set, which can be isosurface rendered and interactively rotated on a computer workstation (Fig. 3.29). This

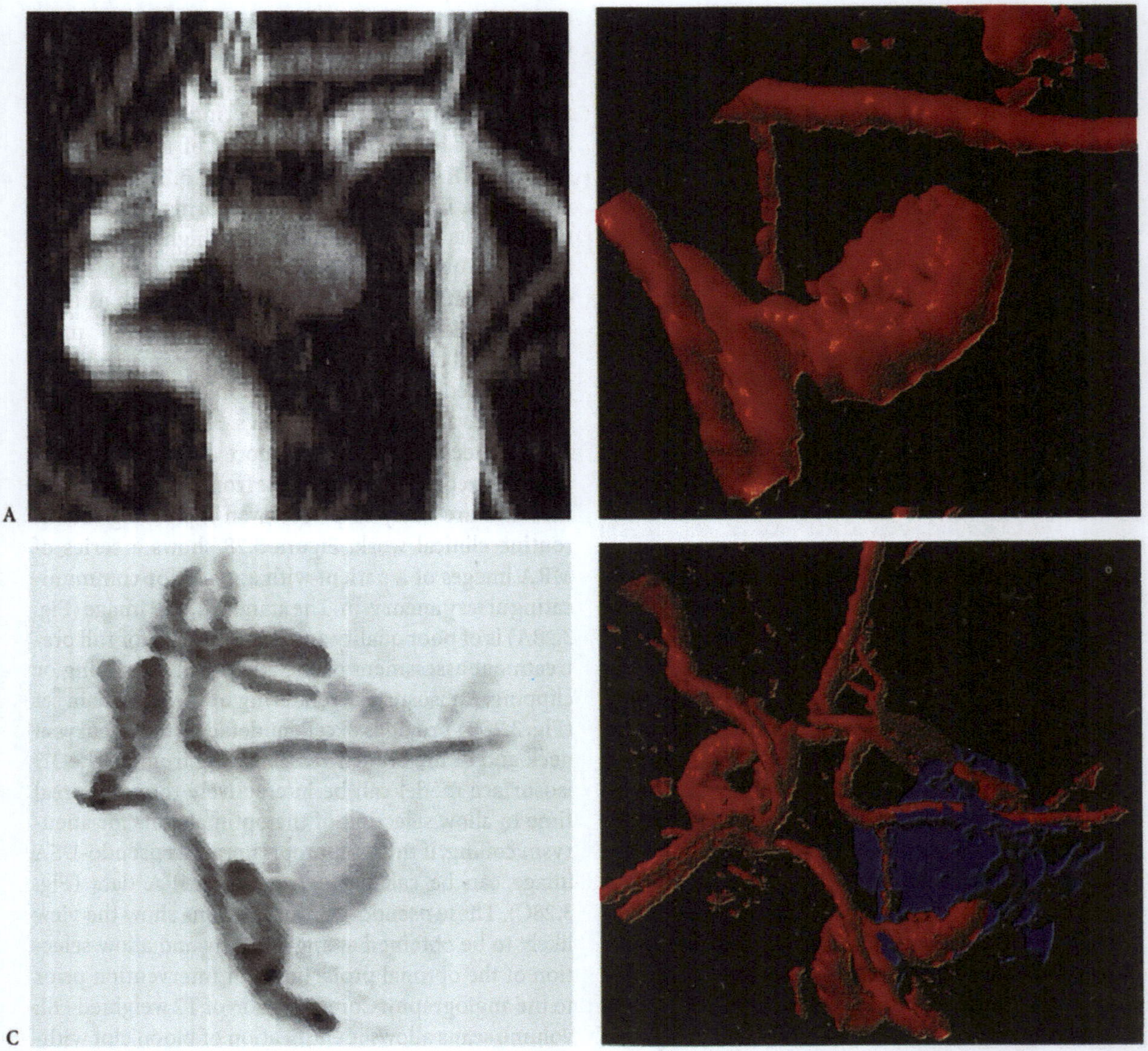

Fig. 3.28A–D. Images from a patient with a left-sided posterior cerebral artery aneurysm. **A** Maximum intensity projection of a time of flight angiogram shows a large aneurysm and displacement of the overlying posterior cerebral artery. The neck of the vessel is poorly seen. **B** Isosurface rendering from the same time of flight data set clearly shows the neck and the branch vessel arising from it. **C** "Pseudo-DSA" view derived from time of flight angiographic data. This view has been selected to demonstrate the optimal view of the neck available on angiography. **D** Isosurface render of coregistered time of flight angiography and T2 weighted volume acquisitions. This image demonstrates the vascular anatomy and the origin of the aneurysm derived from the time of flight angiogram *in red* together with the large intra-aneurysmal haematoma identified from the T2 volume data set *in blue*

allows detailed 3D analysis of vascular anatomy using data acquired from a single angiographic run and guarantees that the optimal angiographic projection can always be identified.

Improvements in computing power are also increasing the role of image postprocessing in clinical practice. The combination of high spatial resolution volume imaging from both CT and MR with automated image coregistration techniques allows the production of subtraction images (Fig. 3.30). These methods are of considerable value in improving the demonstration of contrast-related changes, assessing cerebral atrophy and identifying areas of tumour growth. Automated segmentation techniques for the identification of normal and pathological tissues and for automated measurements of tumour volumes and growth rates are increasingly reported and will soon become commercially available (Fig. 3.31). The role of

A

B

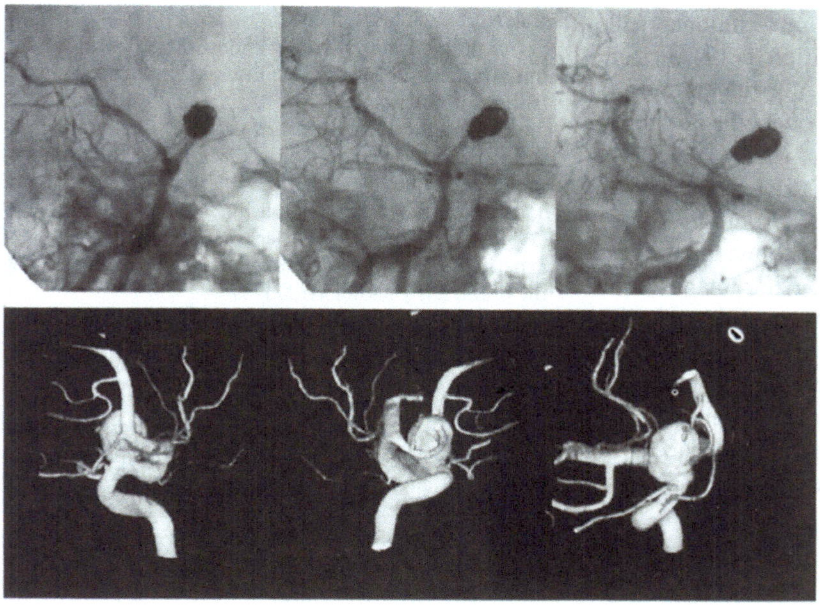

Fig. 3.29A,B. Images from two patients with intracerebral aneurysms. **A** *Top row* demonstrates a series of subtraction angiography images from a rotational dynamic run in a patient with an anterior communicating artery aneurysm which has been coiled using GDC detachable coils. **B** *The bottom row* of images demonstrate 3D reconstructions generated from rotational angiographic data in another patient with a large ICA termination aneurysm. The isosurface 3D rendered models can be rotated real time to gain a clear understanding of the 3D anatomy. (Image courtesy of Philips Medical Systems)

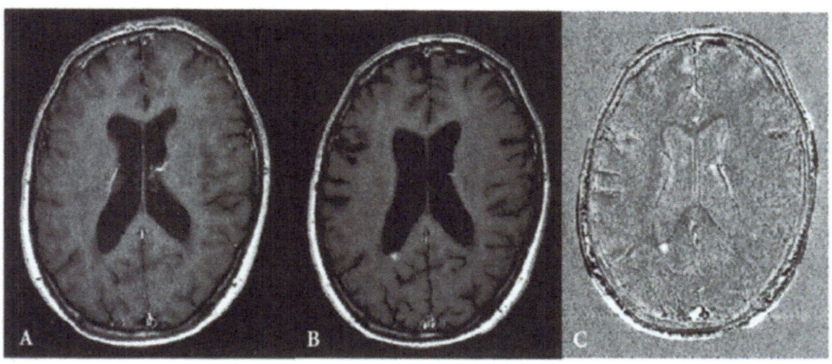

Fig. 3.30A–C. Images from a patient with multiple sclerosis showing an acute enhancing plaque at the anterior horn of the right lateral ventricle. **A** Unenhanced T1 weighted image. **B** Contrast enhanced T1 weighted image. **C** Subtraction imaging following coregistration of the imaging volume. Note the increased conspicuity of the enhancing lesion

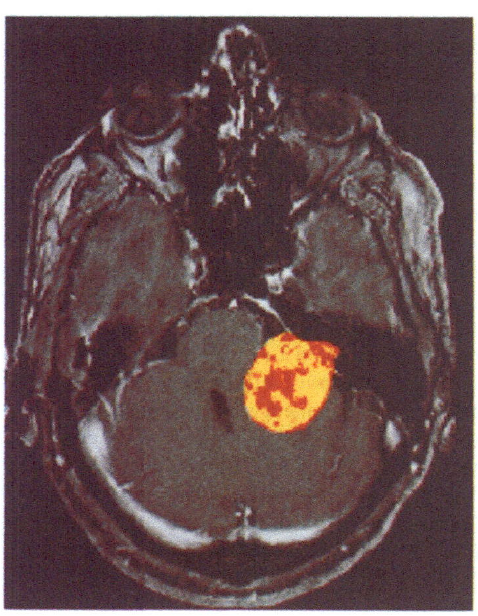

Fig. 3.31. Automatic identification of tumour pixels in a patient with a large acoustic neuroma. The probability of individual pixels belonging to the acoustic neuroma was calculated using matched pre- and postcontrast T1 weighted images. This probability map was then used to calculate a tumour probability map based on the assumption that the tumour would be a single large mass lesion. These combinations of imaging techniques have allowed accurate demonstration of the tumour and measurement of its size

these algorithmic and visualisation techniques will continue to require clinical definition, but it is clear that their role will grow significantly. Integration of image analysis and PACS systems offers the potential for automated image comparison, which is already technically feasible and which is restricted only by the cost of the computing systems. One solution to the cost implications of complex algorithmic analysis is the increasing use of web technology for image management and analysis. As the software tools available for the web become more sophisticated it is likely that the infrastructure of many departments will change to a distributed high bandwidth image management network with centralised high powered, multiprocessor, servers dedicated to image management and analysis.

References

Abrahams H (1986) Radiology. In: Walton J, Beeson P, Scott R (eds) The Oxford companion to medicine. Oxford University Press, Oxford, pp 1193–1198

Amoroso A, Del Porto F, Di Monaco C, Manfredini P, Afeltra A (1997) Vascular endothelial growth factor: a key mediator of neoangiogenesis. A review. Eur Rev Med Pharmacol Sci 1: 17–25

Barber PA, Darby DG, Desmond PM et al. (1998) Prediction of stroke outcome with echoplanar perfusion- and diffusion- weighted MRI. Neurology 51: 418–426

Berry I, Ranjeva JP, Duthil P, Manelfe C (1998) Diffusion and perfusion MRI, measurements of acute stroke events and outcome: present practice and future hope. Cerebrovasc Dis 8(S2): 8–16

Bertini I, Drago RS (1980) ESR and NMR of paramagnetic species in biological and related systems. Kluwer

Brasch R, Pham C, Shames D et al. (1997) Assessing tumor angiogenesis using macromolecular MR imaging contrast media. J Magn Reson Imaging 7: 68–74

Brix G, Semmler W, Port R et al. (1991) Pharmacokinetic parameters in CNS Gd-DTPA enhanced MR imaging. J Comput Assist Tomogr 15: 621–628

Bydder GM, Young IR (1985) MR imaging: clinical use of the inversion recovery sequence. J Comput Assist Tomogr 9: 659–675

Chenevert TL, McKeever PE, Ross BD (1997) Monitoring early response of experimental brain tumors to therapy using diffusion magnetic resonance imaging. Clin Cancer Res 3: 1457–1466

Criscuolo GR (1993) The genesis of peritumoral vasogenic brain edema and tumor cysts: a hypothetical role for tumor-derived vascular permeability factor. Yale J Biol Med 66: 277–314

De Coene B, Hajnal JV, Gatehouse P et al. (1992) MR of the brain using fluid-attenuated inversion recovery (FLAIR) pulse sequences. AJNR 13: 1555–1564

Dvorak HF, Brown LF, Detmar M, Dvorak AM (1995) Vascular permeability factor/vascular endothelial growth factor, microvascular hyperpermeability, and angiogenesis. Am J Pathol 146: 1029–1039

Edelman R, Mattle H, Wallner B et al. (1990) Extracranial carotid arteries: evaluation with "black blood" MR angiography. Radiology 177: 45–50

Fellner F, Schmitt R, Trenkler J, Fellner C, Bohm-Jurkovic H (1995) Turbo gradient-spin-echo (GRASE): first clinical experiences with a fast T2-weighted sequence in MRI of the brain. Eur J Radiol 19: 171–176

Fitzek C, Tintera J, Muller-Forell W et al. (1998) Differentiation of recent and old cerebral infarcts by diffusion-weighted MRI. Neuroradiology 40: 778–782

Foo TK, Saranathan M, Prince MR, Chenevert TL (1997) Automated detection of bolus arrival and initiation of data acquisition in fast, three-dimensional, gadolinium-enhanced MR angiography. Radiology 203: 275–280

Geijer B, Brockstedt S, Lindgren A, Stahlberg F, Norrving B, Holtas S (1999) Radiological diagnosis of acute stroke. Comparison of conventional MR imaging, echo-planar diffusion-weighted imaging, and spin-echo diffusion-weighted imaging. Acta Radiol 40: 255–262

Goldman CK, Kim J, Wong WL, King V, Brock T, Gillespie GY (1993) Epidermal growth factor stimulates vascular endothelial growth factor production by human malignant glioma cells: a model of glioblastoma multiforme pathophysiology. Mol Biol Cell 4: 121–133

Gonzalez RG, Schaefer PW, Buonanno FS et al. (1999) Diffusion-weighted MR imaging: diagnostic accuracy in patients imaged within 6 hours of stroke symptom onset. Radiology 210: 155–162

Graves M (1997) Magnetic resonance angiography Review Article. BJR 70: 6–28

Greenspan SL, Mathews VP, Caldemeyer KS, Patel MR (1998) FLAIR and HASTE imaging in neurologic diseases [published erratum appears in Magn Reson Imaging Clin North Am 1998 May; 6(2): x]. Magn Reson Imaging Clin North Am 6: 53–65

Hagen T, Bertyla K, Piepgrass U (1999) Correlation of regional cerebral blood flow measurements by stable xenon CT and perfusion MRI. J Comput Assist Tomogr 23: 257–264

Hanyu H, Imon Y, Sakurai H et al. (1998) Diffusion-weighted magnetic resonance and magnetization transfer imaging in the assessment of ischemic human stroke. Intern Med 37: 360–365

Hunter G, Hamberg L, Ponzo J et al. (1998) Assessment of cerebral perfusion and arterial anatomy in hyperacute stroke with three-dimensional functional CT: early clinical results. AJNR 19: 29–37

Ikezaki K, Takahashi M, Koga H et al. (1997) Apparent diffusion coefficient (ADC) and magnetization transfer contrast (MTC) mapping of experimental brain tumor. Acta Neurochir Suppl (Wien) 70: 170–172

Imakita S, Onishi Y, Hashimoto T et al. (1998) Subtraction CT angiography with controlled orbital helical scanning for detection of intracranial aneurysms. AJNR 19: 291–295

Jackson A, Sheppard S, Laitt R, Kassner A, Moriarty D (1998) Optic neuritis: MR imaging with combined fat- and water-suppression techniques. Radiology 206: 57–63

Jensen RL (1998) Growth factor-mediated angiogenesis in the malignant progression of glial tumors: a review. Surg Neurol 49: 189–196

Kassner A, Jackson A, Hofmann A et al. (1999) Dynamic contrast susceptibility imaging demonstrates regional abnormalities of time-to-peak contrast concentration in Alzheimer's disease. Proceedings 7th nnual meeting of the Society for Magnetic Resonance in Medicine, Philadelphia, May 1999, p 1527

Kato Y, Matsamura K, Kinosada Y, Narita Y, Kuzuhara S, Nakagawa T (1997) Detection of pyramidal tract lesions in amyotrophic lateral sclerosis with magnetisation transfer measurements. AJNR 18: 1541–1547

Kim YJ, Chang KH, Song IC et al. (1998) Brain abscess and necrotic or cystic brain tumor: discrimination with signal intensity on diffusion-weighted MR imaging." Am J Roentgenol 171: 1487–1490

Kluytmans M, van de Grood J, Klijn C, Folkers P, Mali W, Viergeven M (1997) Dynamic susceptibility contrast MR perfusion imaging in unilateral symptomatic internal carotid artery occlusion. Proceedings of the ISMRM

Korzhenevskii A, Kornienko V, Kul'tiasov MY, Kul'tiasov Y, Cherepenin V (1997) Electrical impedance computerized tomograph for medical applications. Instruments and Experimental Techniques 40: 415–421

Kurki T, Lundbom N, Valtonen S (1995) Tissue characterisation of intracranial tumours: the value of magnetisation transfer and conventional MRI. Neuroradiology 37: 515–521

Larsson H, Stubgaard M, Frederiksen J, Jensen M, Henriksen O, Paulson O (1990) Quantitation of blood-brain carrier defect by magnetic resonance imaging and gadolinium-DTPA in patients with multiple sclerosis and brain tumors. Mag Reson Med 16: 117–131

Lauterbur P (1973) Image formation by induced local interactions: examples employing nuclear magnetic resonance. Nature 242: 190–191

Lovblad KO, Baird AE, Schlaug G et al. (1997) Ischemic lesion volumes in acute stroke by diffusion-weighted magnetic resonance imaging correlate with clinical outcome. Ann Neurol 42: 164–170

Mori S, van Zijl PC (1998) A motion correction scheme by twin-echo navigation for diffusion-weighted magnetic resonance imaging with multiple RF echo acquisition. Magn Reson Med 40: 511–516

Morucci J, Rigaud B (1996) Bioelectrical impedance techniques in medicine. Part III: Impedance imaging. Crit Rev Biomed Eng 24: 655–677

Naganawa S, Ito T, Shimada H et al. (1997) Cerebral black blood MR angiography with the interleaved multi-slab three-dimensional fast spin echo sequence. Radiat Med 15: 385–388

Nakada T, Nakayama N, Fujii Y, Kwee IL (1999) Clinical application of three-dimensional anisotropy contrast magnetic resonance axonography. Technical note. J Neurosurg 90: 791–795

Neil JJ, Shiran SI, McKinstry RC et al. (1998) Normal brain in human newborns: apparent diffusion coefficient and diffusion anisotropy measured by using diffusion tensor MR imaging. Radiology 209: 57–66

Oh CH, Hilal SK, Cho ZH (1988) Selective partial inversion recovery (SPIR) in steady state for selective saturation magnetic resonance imaging (MRI). In: Book of abstracts Society of Magnetic Resonance in Medicine Seventh annual meeting

Ozdoba C, Remonda L, Heid O, Lovblad K, Schroth G (1997) High resolution echo-planar imaging of the brain: is it suitable for routine clinical imaging? Neuroradiology 39: 833–840

Patel MR, Klufas RA, Shapiro AW (1995a) MR imaging of diseases of the brain: comparison of GRASE and conventional spin-echo T2-weighted pulse sequences. Am J Roentgenol 165: 963–966

Patel MR, Siewert B, Warach S, Edelman RR (1995b) Diffusion and perfusion imaging techniques. Magn Reson Imaging Clin North Am 3: 425–438

Provias J, Claffey K, Guha A (1996) Expression of vascular permeability factor/vascular endothelial growth factor (VPF/VEGF) in meningiomas and associated peritumoral edema (Meeting abstract). Proceedings Annual Meeting Am Assoc Cancer Res 37: A1018

Read SJ, Jackson GD, Abbott DF et al. (1998) Experience with diffusion-weighted imaging in an acute stroke unit. Cerebrovasc Dis 8: 135–143

Rempp KA, Brix G, Wenz F, Becker CR, Guckel F, Lorenz WJ (1994) Quantification of regional cerebral blood flow and volume with dynamic susceptibility contrast-enhanced MR imaging. Radiology 193: 637–641

Rosen BR, Belliveau JW, Vevea JM, Brady TJ (1990) Perfusion imaging with NMR contrast agents. Magn Reson Med 14: 249–265

Sandson TA, O'Connor M, Sperling RA, Edelman RR, Warach S (1996) Noninvasive perfusion MRI in Alzheimer's disease: a preliminary report. Neurology 47: 1339–1342

Sardanelli F, Zandrino F, Parodi RC, De Caro G (1999) MR angiography of internal carotid arteries: breath-hold Gd-enhanced 3D fast imaging with steady-state precession versus unenhanced 2D and 3D time-of-flight techniques. J Comput Assist Tomogr 23: 208–215

Schenk J, Leue W (1996) Instrumentation: magnets coils and hardware. In: Atlas S (ed) Magnetic resonance imaging of the brain and spine. Lippincott-Raven, Philadelphia, pp 1–27

Schlaug G, Siewert B, Benfield A, Edelman RR, Warach S (1997) Time course of the apparent diffusion coefficient (ADC) abnormality in human stroke. Neurology 49: 113–119

Sheppard S, Davis P, Kater G, Peterson J (1998) Inversion recovery echo-planar MR in adult brain neoplasia. AJNR 19: 267–273

Shigematsu Y, Korogi Y, Hirai T et al. (1998) Virtual MRI endoscopy of the intracranial cerebrospinal fluid spaces. Neuroradiology 40: 644–650

Sugahara T, Korogi Y, Hirai T et al. (1997) Comparison of HASTE and segmented-HASTE sequences with a T2-weighted fast spin-echo sequence in the screening evaluation of the brain. Am J Roentgenol 169: 1401–1410

Sugahara T, Korogi Y, Kochi M et al. (1999) Usefulness of diffusion-weighted MRI with echo-planar technique in the evaluation of cellularity in gliomas. J Magn Reson Imaging 9: 53–60

Tanaka H, Numaguchi Y, Konno S, Shrier DA, Shibata DK, Patel U (1997) Initial experience with helical CT and 3D reconstruction in therapeutic planning of cerebral AVMs: comparison with 3D time of flight MRA and digital subtraction angiography. J Comput Assist Tomogr 21: 811–817

Taylor-Robinson SD, Oatridge A, Hajnal JV, Burroughs AK, McIntyre N, deSouza NM (1995) MR imaging of the basal ganglia in chronic liver disease: correlation of T1-weighted and magnetisation transfer contrast measurements with liver dysfunction and neuropsychiatric status. Metab Brain Dis 10: 175–188

Tien RD (1992) Fat-suppression MR imaging in neuroradiology: techniques and clinical application. Am J Roentgenol 158: 369–379
Tofts P, Berkowitz B, Schnall M (1995) Quantitative analysis of dynamic Gd-DTPA enhancement in breast tumours using a permeability model. Magn Reson Med 33: 564–568
Tofts PS, Kermode AG (1991) Measurement of the blood brain barrier permeability and leakage space using dynamic MR imaging: fundamental concepts. Magn Reson Med 17: 357–367
Weil J, Bolton J, Wertz J (1994) Electron paramagnetic resonance. Wiley Interscience
Werring DJ, Clark CA, Barker GJ et al. (1998) The structural and functional mechanisms of motor recovery: complementary use of diffusion tensor and functional magnetic resonance imaging in a traumatic injury of the internal capsule. J Neurol Neurosurg Psychiatry 65: 863–869
Werring DJ, Clark CA, Barker GJ, Thompson AJ, Miller DH (1999a) Diffusion tensor imaging of lesions and normal-appearing white matter in multiple sclerosis. Neurology 52: 1626–1632
Werring DJ, Clark CA, Parker GJ, Miller DH, Thompson AJ, Barker GJ (1999b) A direct demonstration of both structure and function in the visual system: combining diffusion tensor imaging with functional magnetic resonance imaging. Neuroimage 9: 352--361
Zetter BR (1998) Angiogenesis and tumor metastasis. Ann Rev Med 49: 407–424

4 Quantitative MR Imaging

Dirk Vandermeulen, Frederik Maes, Koen Van Leemput

CONTENTS

4.1 Introduction

MR imaging is superior to other imaging techniques for studying diseases of the nervous system due to its high spatial resolution and the inherent high soft tissue contrast. Conventional MR imaging based diagnosis is mostly based on cross-sectional views on analog films, resulting in subjective and descriptive or qualitative results. The digital character of MR, however, offers the opportunity to extract additional quantitative and objective information on organ shape and function for diagnosis and therapy support. Clinical requirements for extracting such information have grown considerably in neurological applications. Image based brain analysis is no longer limited to absolute measurements of volumes and distances, but also includes changes over time and intersubject differences, requiring even more accurate quantification of more objects (not only the total brain but also substructures) with more complex shapes. In multiple sclerosis, for instance, measurements are not restricted to total lesion load, but also include white matter changes and lesion evolution over time, time of lesion onset and disappearance, and spatial distribution of lesions. In schizophrenia, subtle volumetric and morphological differences between matched populations of schizophrenics and normal controls, such as of the hippocampus and of left versus right hemisphere asymmetry, have to be quantified to differentiate between normal variation and abnormal brain development. In epilepsy surgery planning, subtle malformations of the cortex need to be detected in high-resolution MR imaging by comparison with a matched control group.

However, accurate quantitative analysis of structural and physiological parameters from medical images is usually a very difficult problem due to limitations intrinsic to the image acquisition process itself, such as poor contrast, limited resolution, partial volume effects, noise, intensity inhomogeneities and artifacts. Improving the reliability of image measurements thus requires robust and well-validated algorithms for automated computer-based image analysis. These include: image enhancement and restoration to improve the discrimination of relevant features in the image and to suppress the influence of image noise and artifacts; image segmentation to define and delineate the structures of interest in the image; and image registration and fusion to integrate multiple images of the same scene in a single representation and to track changes over time and image visualization to support qualitative and quantitative analysis of the images in three dimensions.

In this chapter we will concentrate on image segmentation and image registration algorithms. We give an overview of the algorithmic state-of-the-art, provide pointers to the relevant literature and show how these algorithms can be applied in MR-based analysis of disease patterns occurring in multiple sclerosis, schizophrenia and epilepsy.

D. Vandermeulen, PhD; F. Maes, PhD; K. Van Leemput, MSc
Medical Image Computing, ESAT-PSI and Radiology, Faculties of Engineering and Medicine, Kardinaal Mercierlaan 94, Heverlee, 3001 Leuven, Belgium

4.2 Image Segmentation

Medical image segmentation refers to the process of assigning anatomical labels to pixels in 2D images or voxels in 3D images. The objects that need to be segmented in the different applications are very diverse. First, normal appearing anatomical structures such as the ventricles, basal ganglia, etc., can be delineated for the purpose of comparing a group of patients to a matched control group (schizophrenics vs. normals, e.g.). Second, in many applications, the segmentation and quantification of pathological structures such as tumors and lesions is required, as lesion volume and shape and their change over time contain important quantitative information for diagnosis and treatment feedback.

Methods for image segmentation can be classified according to the amount of a priori model knowledge that is implemented: (1) manual delineation, (2) low-level segmentation, (3) model-based segmentation and (4) interactive segmentation.

4.2.1 Manual Delineation

Pure manual delineation is the basic segmentation program offered on most medical workstations. Manual delineation may be most suited for quick experiments or measurements on a limited number of cases, which otherwise would require important modifications to existing software. However, manual delineation of objects in 3D medical images by a trained expert is often tedious, time consuming and highly subjective because of ambiguity in the images. For instance, the outline of the object of interest may not be entirely visible in the image, such that the observer has to rely on prior knowledge when inferring invisible contours. Moreover, the perceived location of the boundary in the image displayed on a computer screen is sensitive to the setting of the intensity window when studying the image (Semelka et al. 1990) and on screen calibration parameters (Pizer and ter Haar Romeny 1991). Interpretation of the images by a human observer therefore suffers from large interobserver and intraobserver variability, which introduces uncertainty into the quantitative measurements extracted from the images and decreases the significance of the clinical findings derived from these measurements.

The variability of image measurements may be reduced and the efficiency of the measurement procedure increased by automating the measurements using computer vision methods. Computer vision strategies for computer-aided segmentation can be classified as either low-level or model-based.

4.2.2 Low-level Segmentation Methods

Low-level segmentation methods, such as intensity thresholding, edge detection, region growing, region merging and morphological operations, rely entirely on image operators that analyze the intensity, texture or shape locally in each voxel in the image. When the contrast between the object and its background is sufficiently high, it suffices to specify a threshold on the original image intensity values. Edge detection techniques find the boundary between an object and its background by looking for pixels with high intensity gradients, which may be combined into closed contours by edge tracking and grouping (Ogniewicz et al. 1993). Region growing combines neighboring pixels with similar local characteristics, starting from a seed pixel or by analysis of the intensity or its gradients (Griffin et al. 1992; Eberly and Pizer 1994) in a local neighborhood around each pixel. The dual approaches of edge detection and region growing may be combined in a single strategy that simultaneously looks for intensity similarity within a region and discontinuity at its boundary (Pavlidis and Liow 1990; Haddon and Boyce 1990; Chu and Aggarwal 1993).

4.2.3 Model-based Segmentation

Model-based methods incorporate knowledge about the global shape of the object to be segmented or its semantic context and relationship to other objects in the scene. These approaches usually involve some kind of optimization to find the instance of the model that best fits the image data, such as fitting contours to object boundaries or intensity models to image regions. Physics based deformable contour models (Terzopoulos 1987) model the boundary in 2D or surface in 3D of the object to be segmented as an elastic membrane that deforms under the influence of external image derived forces (which attract the membrane to object edges, e.g.) and internal elasticity constraints such as boundary continuity and smoothness (Kass et al. 1988). Models may also be learned from a training set of segmented examples to model average shape and normal variability (COOTES et al. 1994). An extensive survey of the use of deformable contours in medical image analysis has recently been compiled by MCINERNEY and TERZOPOULOS (1996).

Alternatively, image segmentation may be formulated as fitting appropriate intensity models to the data, such as mixtures of Gaussian distributions (WELLS et al. 1996a) while preserving object boundary discontinuities. However, since brain and non-brain tissues often show spectral overlap in MR images, these methods when applied to images of the brain generally require some postprocessing in order to improve the segmentations. Furthermore, the presence of a spatially smoothly varying intensity inhomogeneity or bias field (SIMMONS et al. 1994) in MR images complicates matters. Although not always visible for a human observer, such a bias field can cause serious misclassifications when intensity-based segmentation techniques are used (Fig. 4.1).

WELLS et al. (1996a) used the idea that in order to make a good classification the bias field must be known, but estimation of that bias field is helped by a good classification. This leads to an iterative method, interleaving classification with bias correction. Their algorithm requires that the user manually selects representative points for each of the classes considered. However, such user interaction is time consuming and yields subjective, irreproducible segmentation results. Furthermore, pixels that are not trained can cause serious bias estimation errors. This typically occurs in regions surrounding the brain, which consist of several different types of tissues.

VAN LEEMPUT et al. (1999a, 1999b) extended this algorithm by including a third step estimating the class-conditional distribution parameters (typically means and variances of normal distributions describing the expected intensities per tissue or structure). It turns out that, in this procedure, classes consisting of different tissues do not interfere with the bias estimation (Fig. 4.2). Furthermore, a digital brain atlas in the form of a priori probability maps for the location of the tissue classes is used to initialize the algorithm. As a result, this method yields a fully automatic classification of brain tissues and simultaneously corrects for the MR bias field.

A particular problem related to the finite resolution of MRI data is the partial volume (PV) effect.

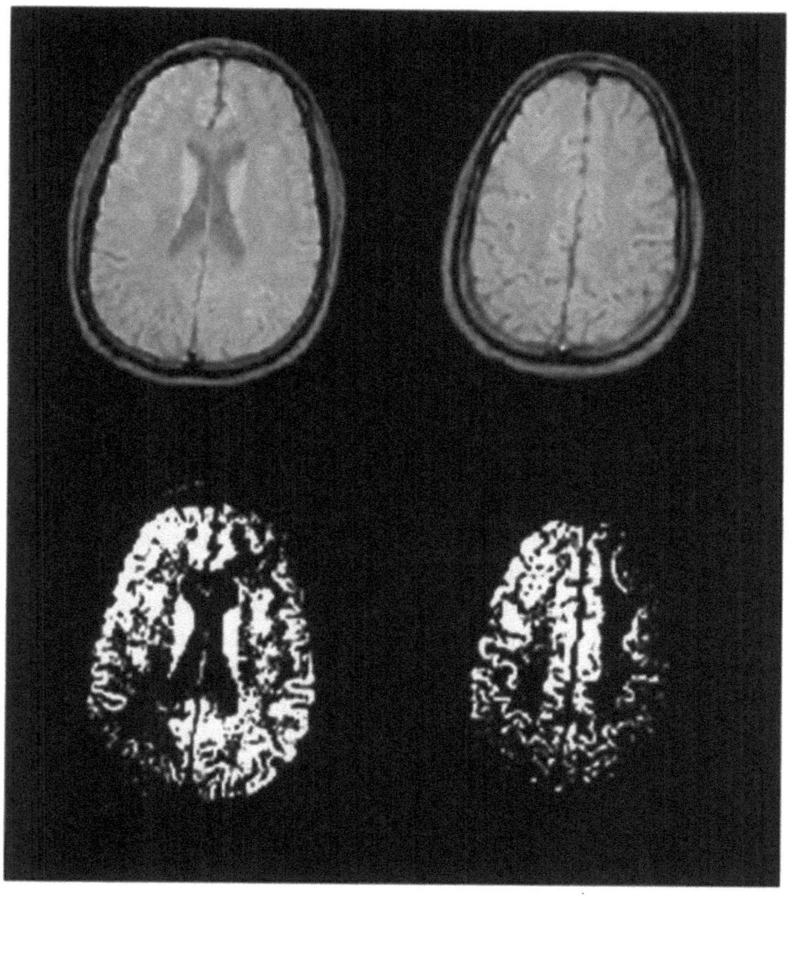

Fig. 4.1. *Top* Two MRI slices shown with conventional display window. *Bottom* Same images with very narrow window indicating the bias present in the data

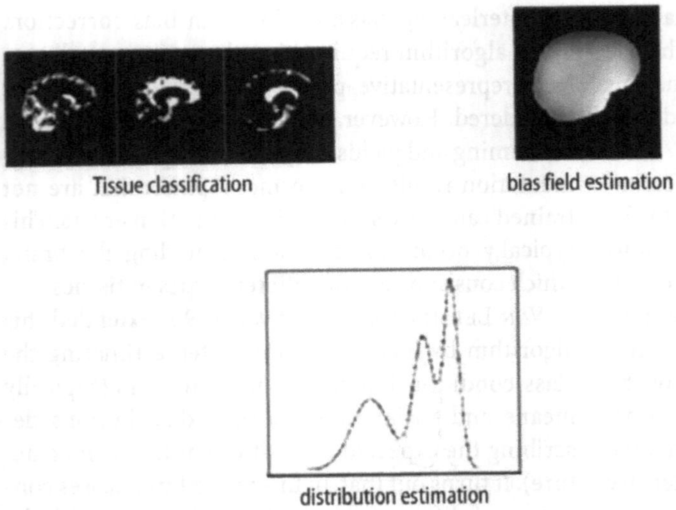

Fig. 4.2. Iterative procedure for brain tissue classification including bias field correction and class-conditional distribution parameter estimation as developed by Van Leemput et al. (1999a, 1999b)

Whereas the traditional model assumes that each voxel in the image belongs to only one single class, voxels that lie on the border between different tissue types violate this assumption. In reality, these voxels are really a mixture of tissues and every segmentation method that tries to assign them exclusively to one class is condemned to fail. The problem is especially important in images of the brain since the interface between gray and white matter is highly complex, which results in a non-negligible percentage of PV voxels compared to the volume of pure tissue voxels. Misclassification of this thin interface therefore gives immediate rise to considerable segmentation errors. Ideally, the model should be adjusted so as to model a mixture of tissue types in each voxel rather than a single tissue type only. Choi et al. (1991) introduced the concept of so-called mixels (mixed pixels), but they had to introduce heuristics in order to arrive at a workable solution. More recently, Laidlaw et al. (1998) applied the intensity distribution of partial volume mixtures of two tissues derived by Santago and Gage (1995) to the segmentation problem. However, the time figures they sketch are far too high for the method to be practically useful. Further research is therefore needed.

4.2.4 Interactive Segmentation

Although low-level segmentation techniques are popular because of their simplicity and speed, their application to medical images is usually limited to high contrast objects. Model-based approaches are more robust as these methods can cope with uncertainty in locally computed image features by propagating evidence gathered from neighboring locations. However, model-based approaches are computationally expensive if the number of degrees of freedom of the model is large, such that in practical applications models are necessarily simple. Moreover, the anatomical and medical knowledge the human expert relies on when detecting and delineating pathological structures is difficult to make explicit in a complete and unambiguous way. Hence, while fully automated model-based segmentation algorithms have been developed for certain specific applications, complete automation does not seem feasible for quantification of pathology in general.

Recently new strategies have been presented (Griffin et al. 1994; Vincken et al. 1997; Beard et al. 1994; Maes et al. 1995) for semi-automated segmentation that aim to combine the advantages of higher efficiency and lower subjectivity of automated algorithms with the ability of the human observer to rely on application specific expert knowledge. The segmentation is essentially performed interactively by the expert user, but is facilitated and accelerated by the use of computer methods. Instead of trying to solve the entire segmentation problem automatically, these methods are designed to provide powerful and intelligent assistance to the clinical user. This intelligence is based on the idea that the segmentation is facilitated if the image can be partitioned in primitive regions such that all pixels of the same region belong to the same object. Ideally, only one such region should correspond to each object, but in practice such a partitioning will be an oversegmentation of the image (there will be more regions than objects). If such a partitioning is available, the segmentation problem is reduced to selecting those regions in the partitioning that belong to the object of interest. The segmentation does not need to consider individual pixels, but can proceed at the level of primitive entities at a larger scale by treating all pixels that belong to the same region as one single entity. This drastically reduces the number of segmentation decisions to be made, which increases robustness and efficiency while decreasing variability. Selecting the regions that make up the object of interest may be done automatically when prior knowledge about the scene or appropriate object models are available. Instead, a hierarchy of merged primitive regions is computed automatically and used as input for subsequent interactive computer-aided segmentation of the object of interest (Fig. 4.3).

The first type of interaction consists of the user dragging the mouse pointer over the object in the screen, whereby all regions hit by the mouse are selected and displayed in the image. With these tools the user thus effectively "paints" the object in the image on the screen (Fig. 4.4).

Alternatively, the user may specify a region of interest around the object to be segmented or indicate points in the image that do or do not belong to the object of interest. The algorithm then searches for the largest combination of primitive regions that satisfies these constraints, which can be adjusted interactively by the user if needed (Fig. 4.5).

Because of the underlying hierarchical primitive region representation, these methods are able to automatically compute the boundary of the object of interest from just a few user specified clues. Because the user does not need to accurately indicate the object's outline manually, these methods are more efficient than totally manual delineation and because the boundary is computed from the image intensities directly, they are also much less subject to observer variability. Moreover, they are not targeted at a specific application, but are designed to have large applicability for a variety of different objects in a variety of images, offering the clinical user a single tool that enables him to quickly segment objects with different appearance in the image without limiting restrictions regarding image contrast or imaging modality.

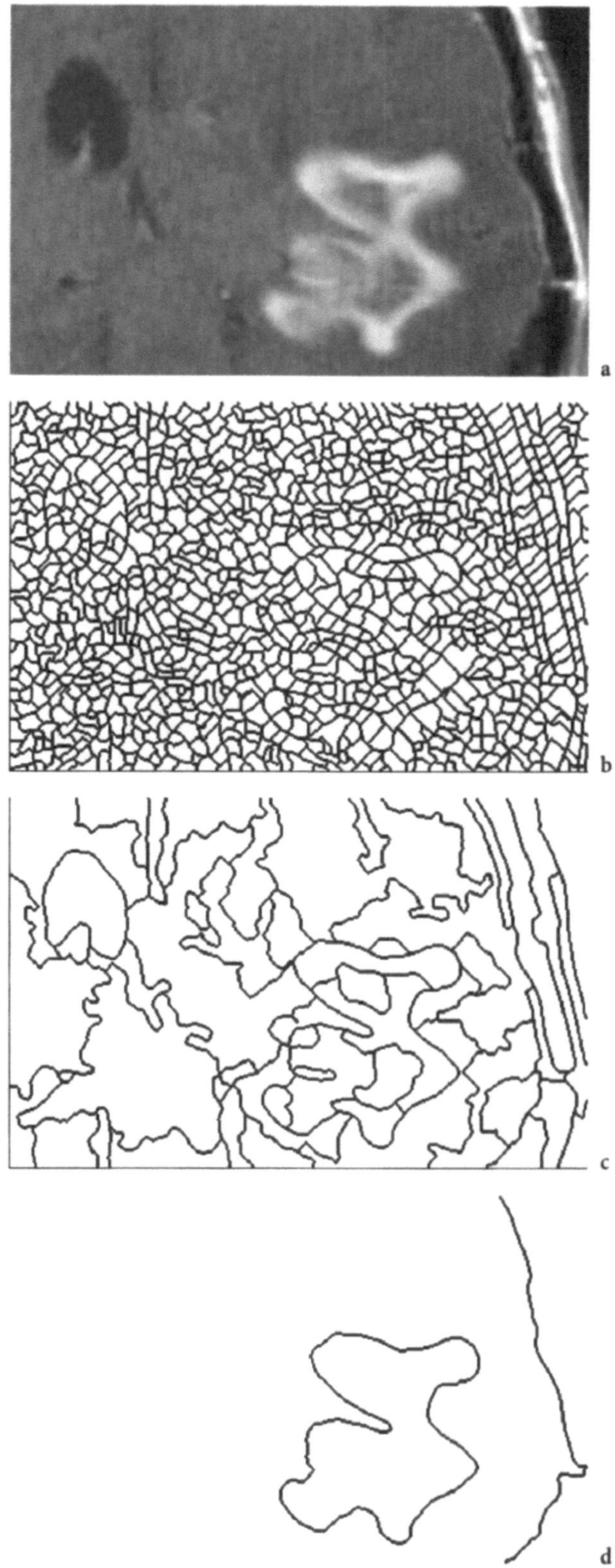

Fig. 4.3a–d. Interactive segmentation. Original axial MR image of a brain tumour (**a**). Image (**a**) subdivided in elementary homogenous regions. Regions are iteratively and automatically merged into larger regions based on intensity homogeneity criteria (**c**,**d**)

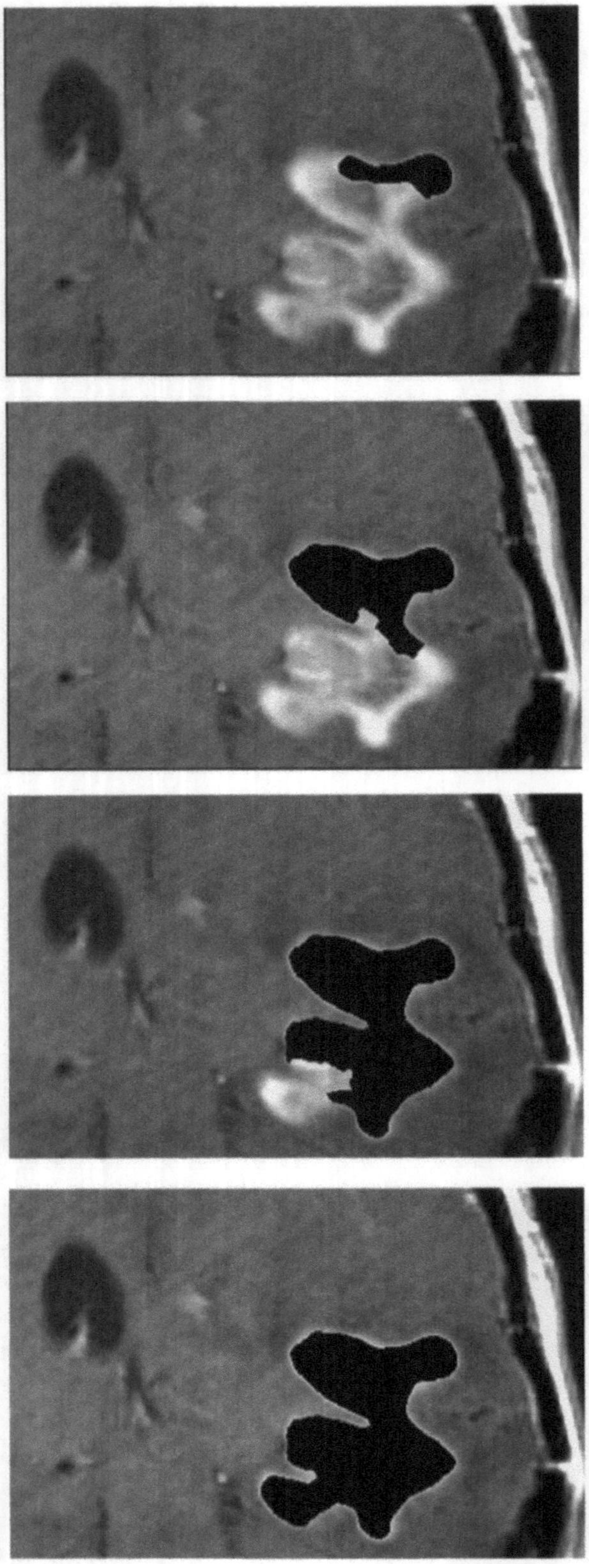

Fig. 4.4a–d. Interactive segmentation ("paint brush") of Fig. 4.3a. The four subfigures display subsequent user interactions: User selects the regions that belong to the object of interest by dragging the mouse pointer over it

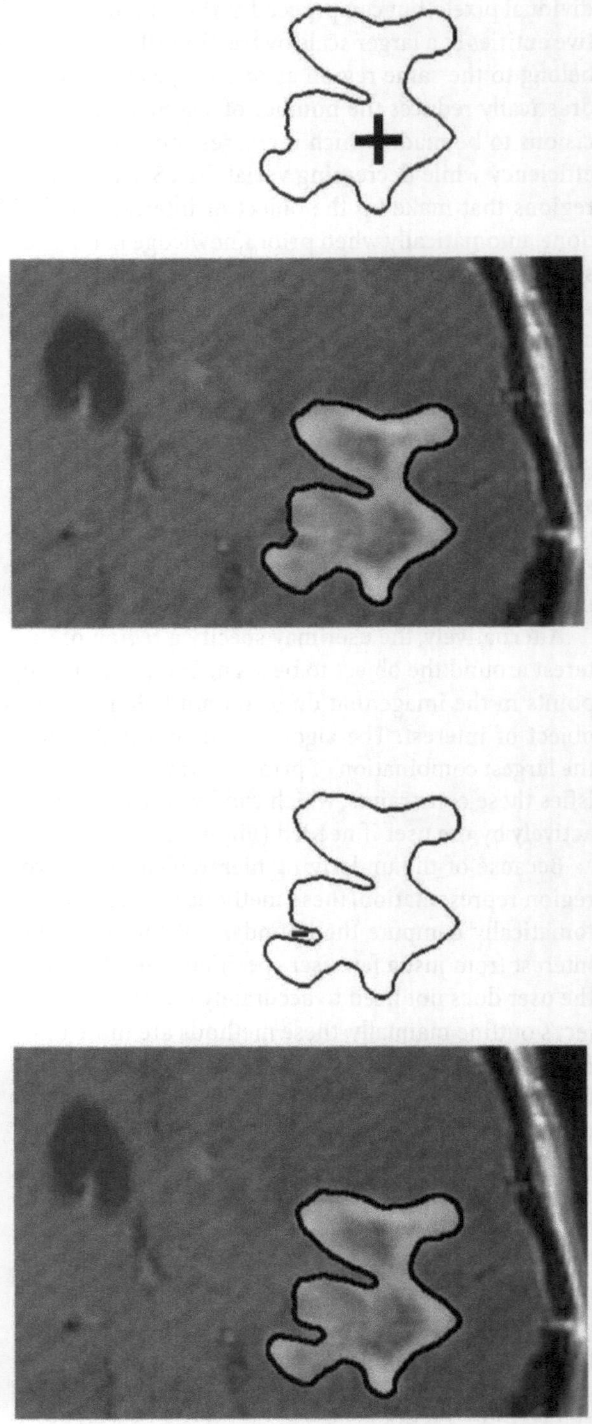

Fig. 4.5a–d. Interactive segmentation ("point and click") of Fig 4.3a. Alternatively the user can click points inside (labeled as +) and points outside (labeled as –) (**a**). In this case the border of the rectangular region of interest is labeled as outside points. The user may refine the contour by specifying additional points (**c**). The largest region matching these consists in immediately shown to the user (**b,d**)

4.3 Image Registration

Medical decisions in diagnosis, therapy planning and therapy follow-up often rely on information extracted from 3D radiological images obtained using a variety of imaging modalities, such as CT, MR or PET. Because these modalities are based on different physical principles, they often offer complementary information to the clinician. In many applications the clinician therefore benefits from integrated visualization and analysis of multimodal images, which may be acquired at the same or at different time points. In stereotactic MRI-based neurosurgery planning for biopsies or functional interventions, additional vascular information is provided by MRA. For brain function analysis, functional information obtained from PET or fMRI images is combined with anatomical information provided by MR imaging. Quantification of brain morphometric changes over time in schizophrenia or of lesion evolution in MS requires analysis of multispectral (PD, T1, T2, etc.) MR images acquired at different time points.

Retrospective registration of 3D medical images for clinical applications is not a trivial problem, due to the sometimes large differences in patient positioning in the scanner, the different image content and resolution of the images, the possible presence of modality specific image degradations and artifacts and pathology induced distortions. Moreover, patient related changes over time may have occurred between both acquisitions, for instance because of a surgical intervention.

In many clinical settings, 3D images are still displayed with a light box as a sequence of 2D cross-sectional slices printed on radiographic films. When interpreting multiple images jointly, the clinician mentally has to construct a picture of the 3D geometric relationship between the different sets of slices, relying on application specific medical and radiological expert knowledge to interpret the geometrical clues provided by anatomical landmarks visible in each of the images separately. It is clear that when one wants to exploit the benefits of digital imaging and medical image processing for quantitative analysis of multimodal images, computer methods have to be applied to the registration problem. The registration may be done manually by the user tuning the registration parameters assisted by visualization software that supplies visual feedback of the quality of the registration (Pietrzyk et al. 1994). While such a subjective approach may be sufficient to support clinical decisions in some applications, a more objective and mathematically formal registration procedure is needed when higher accuracy is required, as for instance in neurosurgery, or if clear anatomical references are missing or uncertain in one of the images. Automated retrospective registration of 3D multimodal images is therefore a fundamental task in medical image processing.

4.3.1 Rigid Registration

While in some applications it is important to recover local non-rigid deformations, many intrapatient studies involve only the estimation of an affine geometric transformation, assuming that the registration transformation can be adequately modeled as the combination of 3D translation and rotation and possibly 3D scaling and skew. The rigid body assumption is well satisfied inside the skull in 3D scans of the head if scanner miscalibration, geometric distortion of the images and patient related changes, for instance due to interscanning operations, can be neglected.

An overview and classification of registration techniques has recently been compiled by Maintz and Viergever (1998). Following their terminology, registration procedures can be classified according to problem statement, registration paradigm and optimization procedure. The problem statement includes criteria such as the object or region of interest, the modalities involved, dimensionality of the data both spatially and in time, intra- versus inter-subject or atlas registration, and the nature of the transformation to be recovered. The registration paradigm involves the image features and the correspondence criterion used to compute the registration. The optimization procedure includes the search strategy and the degree of interaction required.

Registration methods can be classified according to the registration paradigm as being either extrinsic, i.e., making use of external objects or markers introduced in the imaged space specifically for registration purposes (e.g., pasted onto the skin or screwed into the cranium), or intrinsic, i.e., based on the image information generated by the object under study itself (e.g., anatomical landmarks). Intrinsic methods can be classified as either point based, surface based or voxel based. External marker based registration is usually very accurate, but cannot be applied retrospectively. Point based methods rely on manually indicated anatomical landmarks or automatically computed geometrically salient points. Although very versatile, these methods are labor-intensive if user interaction is required and their accuracy depends on the accurate localization of a sufficient number of corresponding landmarks in all modalities. Surface based registration requires delineation of corresponding surfaces in each of the images separately. But surface segmentation algorithms are generally highly data and application dependent and surfaces are not easily identified in functional modalities such as PET.

Voxel based registration methods optimize a functional measuring of the similarity of all geometrically corresponding voxel pairs for some feature (e.g., intensity). The main advantage of voxel similarity based (VSB) methods is that feature calculation is straightforward or even absent when only gray values are used, such that the accuracy of these methods is not limited by segmentation errors as in point or surface based methods. By extending the features from points to surfaces to all voxels in the image, knowledge of point-to-point correspondence is traded for a larger set of samples that is accounted for by the similarity measure.

For intramodality registration multiple VSB methods have been proposed that optimize some global measure of the absolute difference between image intensities of corresponding voxels within overlapping parts or in a region of interest. These criteria all rely on the assumption that the intensities of the two images are linearly correlated, which is generally not satisfied in the case of intermodality registration.

Maes et al. (1997) and Wells et al. (1996b), inspired by the work of Woods et al. (1993), recognized the information theoretic nature of the registration problem and proposed, independently of each other, to use the much more general notion of mutual information or relative entropy as a non-linear generalization of cross-correlation. Mutual information (MI) is a basic concept from information theory, measuring the statistical dependence between two random variables or the amount of information that one variable contains about the other. The MI registration criterion states that the mutual information of the image intensity values of corresponding voxel pairs is maximal if the images are geometrically aligned. Because no assumptions are made regarding the nature of the relationship between the image intensities in both modalities, maximization of mutual information is a very general and powerful criterion that can be applied automatically without prior segmentation on a large variety of applications.

This idea has soon attracted a lot of interest from the research community. West et al. (1997) compared multiple retrospective rigid image registration algorithms with each other and with a gold standard (defined by rigidly attached reference markers) on MR imaging, CT and PET images of the brain. In these experiments, the algorithms based on mutual information (or related concepts) turned out to be the most versatile, robust and accurate.

4.3.2 Non-rigid Registration

Rigid registration methods apply global and rigid transformations, which are useful when rigid body assumptions are likely to hold. However, they cannot account for non-rigid morphological variability between and within subjects. For applications where this variability matters, e.g., segmentation of brain structures by matching an individual brain to a labeled brain template, also called brain warping, non-rigid matching must be used. Other applications include: registration of intraoperative imaging data with preoperative images that deliver intraoperative guidance, and tracking changes over time in pathological structures during treatment (radiotherapy, drug treatment). A very recent exhaustive compilation on non-rigid registration in the context of brain warping was presented by Toga (1999).

Similar to the rigid registration algorithms, non-rigid registration strategies can be categorized according to the registration paradigm. For obvious reasons, all of the proposed algorithms for non-rigid registration are intrinsic.

Point based non-rigid registration methods rely on manually indicated anatomical landmarks or automatically computed geometrically salient points (high local curvature, e.g.) and use the well-established armamentarium of thin-plate splines (Bookstein 1991) to interpolate the deformation between the landmarks (Meyer et al. 1997).

For brain imaging, lines corresponding to anatomical features such as sulcal, gyral or ventricular curves can be automatically extracted using local curvature based criteria and can be matched in reference and target data sets (Subsol 1999).

Readily identifiable anatomical surfaces such as the cortical and ventricular surfaces have been used for surface based warping (Davatzikos 1996). Each of the surfaces is parameterized and matched with their counterparts in the corresponding scan and their correspondences guide the volumetric transformation or warping from one brain to the other. While determining correspondence, higher-level structural and anatomical information is used to ensure the biological validity (Thompson and Toga 1996).

Hybrid methods, combining voxel similarity measures (cf. below) and either lines or surfaces, have been proposed in matching cortical regions (Collins et al. 1996; Thompson and Toga 1996).

The more traditional non-rigid voxel-similarity-based registration algorithms use gray-value correlation or functions thereof like normalized correlation (Collins et al. (1994) or sum-of-squared-differences (Christensen et al. 1996; Woods et al. 1998) as a measure of similarity between a reference scan and the corresponding voxels in the target scan. More recent procedures use optic-flow based schemes (Thirion 1998) and mutual information based similarity criteria (Kim et al. 1997). Each of these procedures estimates a deformation vector at each voxel such that the similarity criterion is optimized. Since many such solutions exist that may be anatomically infeasible, additional restrictions are imposed on the resulting transformation. These transformations need to contain enough degrees of freedom to model expected local variations while needing to interpolate the transformation calculated at a sparse subset of the image voxels. For instance, one can model the whole image grid as an elastic, viscoelastic or fluid continuous medium. The registration then consists in minimizing a cost function evaluated at each image voxel that measures simultaneously the intensity similarity between the target image and the currently deformed reference image and the amount of deformation between the reference image and its currently deformed version. The main drawback of this and similar procedures is their high computational complexity requiring powerful, even parallel, computers. By building approximate models of these physical continuum mechanics models, Thirion (1998) succeeded in generating an algorithm that behaves almost similarly while running orders of magnitude faster (warping one 3D brain MR image of 256×256×128 voxels to a similarly sized image requires about 30–60 min on a state-of-the-art single processor computer). As a result, studies involving many large data sets can now be performed without necessitating excessively powerful machines.

Dawant et al. (1998), for instance, used this algorithm for automated atlas-based segmentation of internal brain structures and found that, for large scale structures such as the brain or the cerebellum, the resulting contours are virtually indistinguishable from outlines drawn by an experienced radiologist (Fig. 4.6).

A recent evolution in non-rigid registration involves the incorporation of statistical expectations about the deformations. By defining probability distributions on the space of deformation transformations applied to the reference template, statistical parameters of these distributions can be estimated from a database to determine the magnitude and directional biases of deformation (Thompson and Toga 1996). The calculated statistics allow abnormal pathological deviations to be detected as well as to detect the characteristic features discriminating two different populations (e.g., schizophrenics vs. normal controls).

4.4 Selected Applications in Brain Morphometry

Brain morphometry studies techniques for measurement of the size and shape of the brain and its parts. Morphometry used to depend mainly on postmortem dissection, but since the advent of non-invasive MR imaging, large volumes of data are becoming available from normal as well as abnormal individuals in vivo. Furthermore, the study of growth and time evolution of diseases (tumour staging, etc.) becomes possible by analysis of images acquired at different times.

The basic requirements for improved morphometry are similar in the different applications. Measurement of size is hampered by the difficulties of detecting and localizing the boundaries of structures in images (segmentation), particularly in three dimensions. Improved registration techniques are needed for matching whole images, or representations of specific anatomical objects, obtained at different times or with different imaging modalities or in different individuals.

4.4.1 Multiple Sclerosis

The role of MRI in assessing the progression of multiple sclerosis (MS) and in monitoring the effect of a drug therapy is of increasing importance. This is caused by the higher sensitivity and objectivity of an

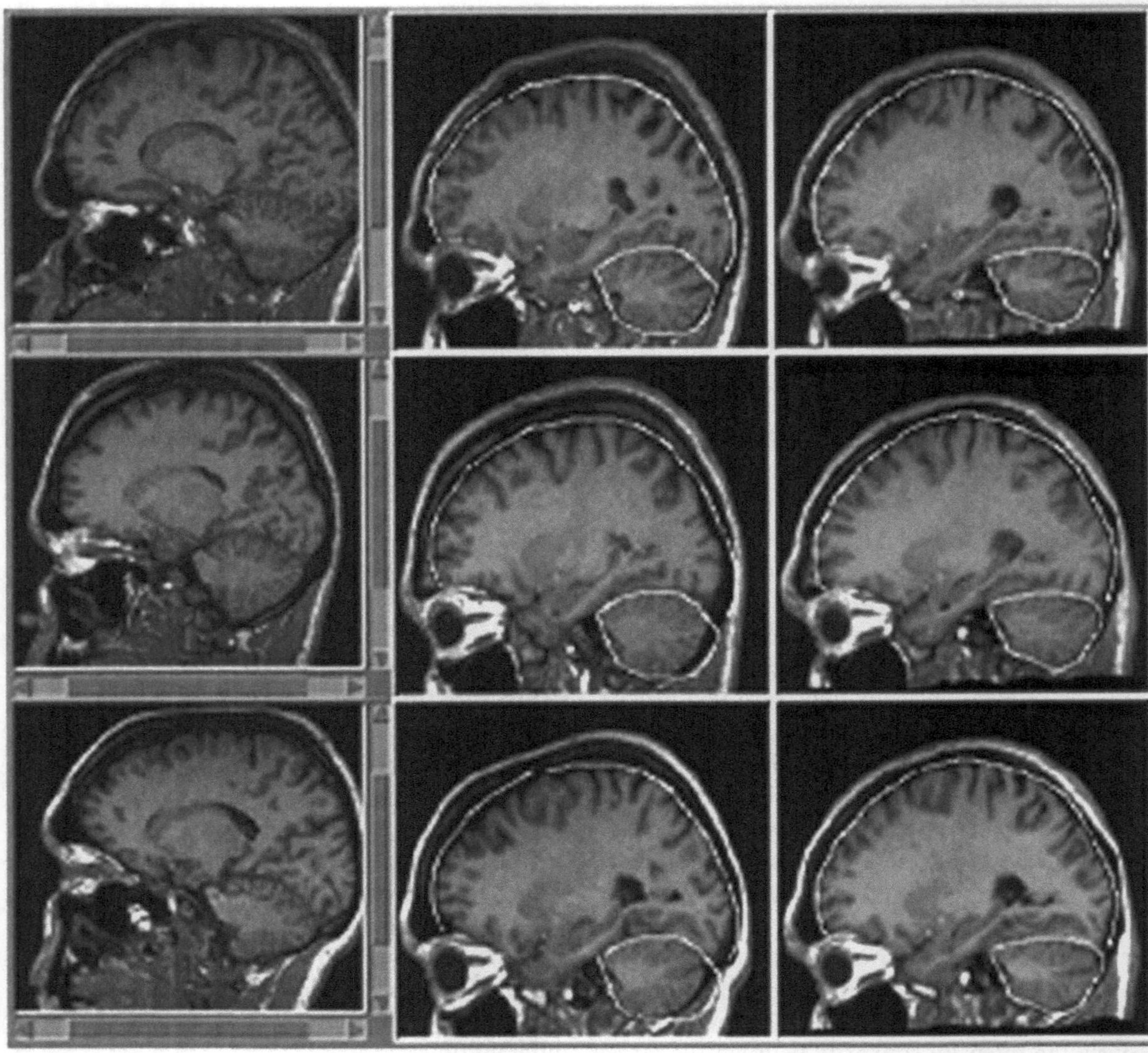

Fig. 4.6. Automated atlas-based segmentation. Surface contours delineated in a reference or template MR image are warped to a target study using the non-rigid transformation calculated by the algorithm (Dawant et al. (1998). Original sagittal slices of 3 individuals (left). Atlas warping after affine registration (middle). Atlas warping after non-rigid registration (right)

MR-based surrogate index compared to traditional clinical disability scales (Evans et al. 1997), in combination with the widespread availability of MR imaging. In clinical trials, manual analysis of the MR images by human experts is too time-consuming because of the large amounts of data involved. Furthermore, the inter- and intraobserver variability associated with manual delineations complicates the analysis of the results. Finally, it is not clear how a human rater combines information obtained from the different channels when multispectral MR data are examined. Therefore, considerable efforts have been made by the medical imaging community to come up with fast automated methods that produce more objective and reproducible results (Zijdenbos et al. 1994; Johnston et al. 1996; Udupa et al. 1997). However, most of these techniques still require some human interaction and/or ad hoc processing steps, which can make the results not fully objective. Zijdenbos et al. (1998) proposed and validated a fully automated pipeline for MS lesion segmentation from T1-, T2- and PD-weighted images. However, they used a fixed classifier that must be retrained in cases where different scanner types or pulse sequences produce contrast variations.

Van Leemput et al. (1999c) present a fully automated technique for segmenting MS lesions from T1-, T2-, and PD-weighted MR images that automatically retrains the classifier. More specifically, a model-based iterative algorithm is used that simultaneously corrects for MR field inhomogeneities, estimates tissue class distribution parameters, and

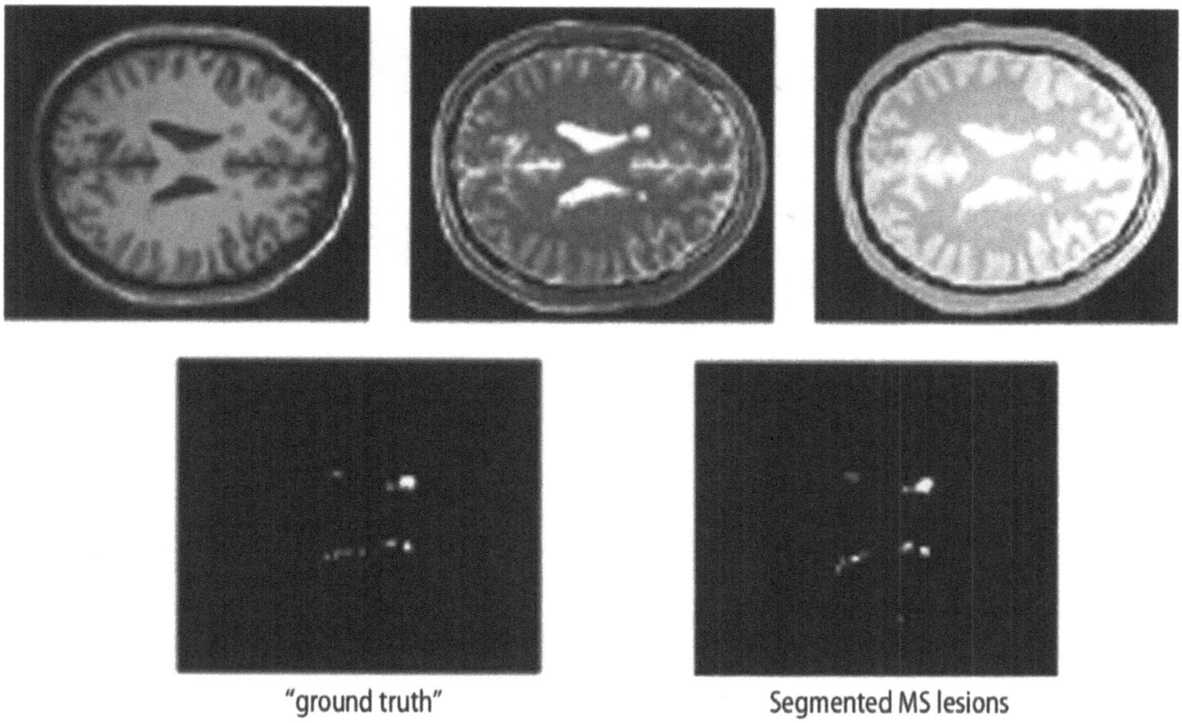

Fig. 4.7. Qualitative example of the performance of the automated algorithm of Van Leemput et al. (1999c) for MS lesion segmentation on simulated MR images with MS lesions. *Top row* T1-, T2- and PD-weighted images. *Bottom row from left to right* Lesion ground truth and final segmentation map

classifies the image voxels. The method is fully automated by mapping each image to a digital brain atlas that contains spatially varying prior probabilities for gray matter, white matter and CSF. The MS lesions are detected as voxels that are not well explained statistically by the model. Furthermore, since almost 95% of the MS lesions are located inside white matter, this information can be added to the model by restraining their search within the prior spatial probability map of white matter. In order to give a qualitative impression of the performance of the algorithm, it was applied to simulated MR images that were generated by the BrainWeb MR simulator (Cocosco et al. 1997).[1] These consist of T1-, T2- and PD-weighted images in which also MS lesions are present. In order to achieve as realistic conditions as possible, images with a typical 3% noise level and a severe MR bias field of 40% were used. These images are depicted [fig:brainweb] along with the ground truth for the MS lesions and the final automatically detected lesions (Fig. 4.7).

The performance of the algorithm was also evaluated by comparing its results with tracings by trained human experts as part of the BIOMORPH project.[2] The method was validated by comparing the total lesion load (TLL) of automatically detected lesions on 20 scans with those detected by a human expert. As pointed out by Evans et al. (1997), the most important requirement for an automated method is that its measurements change in response to a treatment in a manner proportionate to manual measurements. Van Leemput et al. (1999c) therefore performed a linear regression analysis, rather than attempting to show that the TLL of the automated method does not differ significantly from that of the manual segmentations. Regression analysis shows that the automatic segmentations indeed change proportionately to the manual segmentations. Overall, very careful qualitative inspection of the segmentations did not reveal consistent failings in any of the methods. MS lesion segmentation is challenging for human observers and automated methods alike. Disagreement over boundary placement of specific lesions typically contributes only a small fraction of the total error. More important is disagreement over

[1] Available at http://www.bic.mni.mcgill.ca/brainweb/

[2] Development and Validation of Techniques for Brain Morphometry (BIOMORPH). EU-Biomed Project No. 95-0845. Partners in the BIOMORPH project are: University of Kent at Canterbury, Kent, UK; ETH, Zurich, Switzerland; University of Oxford, Oxford, UK; INRIA, Nice, France; Katholieke Universiteit Leuven, Leuven, Belgium.

whether or not a lesion was present in a certain locality (object identification). There is no true gold standard available for evaluating methods, and correct identification of MS lesions remains a major challenge for human observers and automated methods alike.

Multiple sclerosis is a progressive disease that requires a study of lesion evolution over time. In contrast to the previous approaches that analyze the images in a static way, a number of methods were recently proposed that analyze MS lesions in the spatiotemporal (3D and time) domain, consisting of a whole time series of mutually coregistered 3D MR images (Guttman et al. 1994).

In order for this time-series analysis to be carried out, the data needs to be preprocessed: the within image intensity inhomogeneity and between image intensity scaling needs to be corrected and all data sets for a single individual need to be coregistered (Fig. 4.8).

In Gerig et al. (1998), time series analysis proceeds as follows: for each voxel along the time-axis, features [such as standard deviation, first derivative of time signal, maximum and minimum gradient (corresponding to increase and decrease of brightness), etc.] are calculated followed by a non-linear fuzzy combination of these features. The resulting segmentation is shown in Fig. 4.9. Only dynamically changing lesions are segmented, while static lesions are suppressed. Additional attributes can be calculated that contain information about the time of maximum increase and the time of maximum decrease of brightness, thus expressing the lifetime of pixels of a single lesion. The "time-map" further yields information about the correlation of different lesions with respect to the dynamic time change.

Since this method studies intensity changes over time, it is very sensitive to errors in the temporal

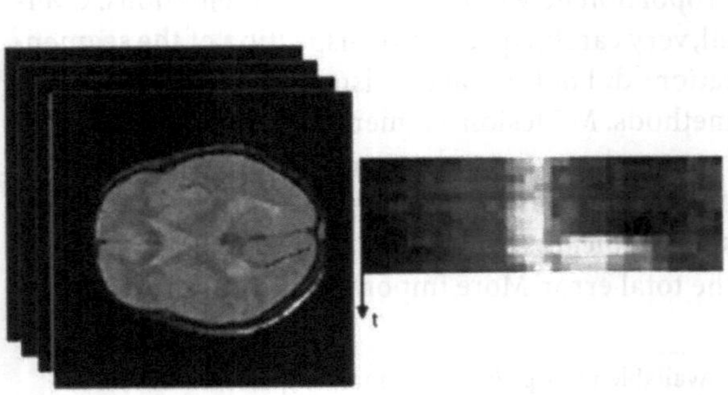

Fig. 4.8. Temporal analysis of MS lesions. The time series of MR images is mutually coregistered and intensities are normalized. *The figure on the right shows* a 1D cross-section (*horizontal axis*) tracked over time (*vertical axis*). This profile corresponds to the *black line in the image on the left*

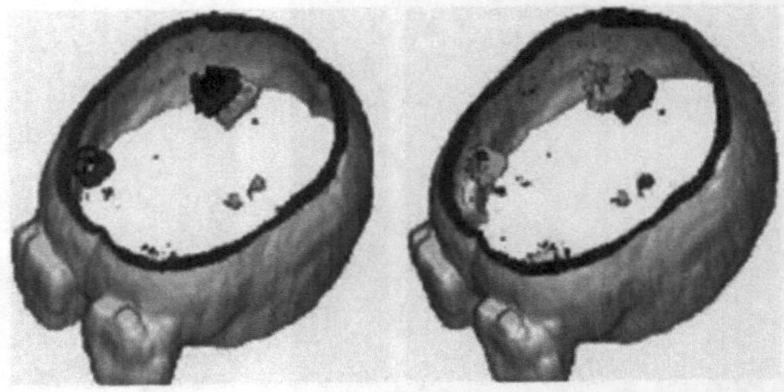

Fig. 4.9. Three-dimensional display of MS lesions segmented by the spatiotemporal procedure of Gerig et al. (1998). *The gray code* corresponds to the time of appearance (*left*) and disappearance (*right*)

coregistration. When the registration is inaccurate, it is hard to distinguish evolving lesions from edges of misaligned anatomical structures (cortex, ventricles, etc.). Furthermore there is no direct relationship between the amplitude of lesion evolution (shrinkage or expansion) and temporal variation of intensity. Finally, spatial correlation between neighboring voxels is not taken into account.

In contrast, Rey et al. (1999) and Thirion and Calmon (1999) present a method based on the calculation of the apparent motion between two images. Each pair of consecutive 3D images is first rigidly aligned. Then, a non-rigid deformation or displacement field is calculated representing an estimate of the apparent motion. By calculating scalar vector operators (such as the Jacobian, measuring locally shrinking or expanding regions), changing lesions can thus be detected. A nice property of this operator is its invariance with respect to any rigid misalignment. Figure 4.10 shows a result of such a spatiotemporal analysis calculated by retaining only the significantly changing regions.

4.4.2 Schizophrenia

Several studies have reported morphological differences in the brains of schizophrenic patients when compared to normal controls (DeLisi et al. 1995), such as enlargement of the cerebral ventricles, changes in corpus callosal area, reduction in temporal cortex as well as more widespread subtle cortical decline, and decreased or reversed cerebral asymmetries. These findings suggest the presence of structural brain pathology in schizophrenia. Some hypotheses have been proposed about schizophrenia as a syndrome of anomalies in normal brain develop-

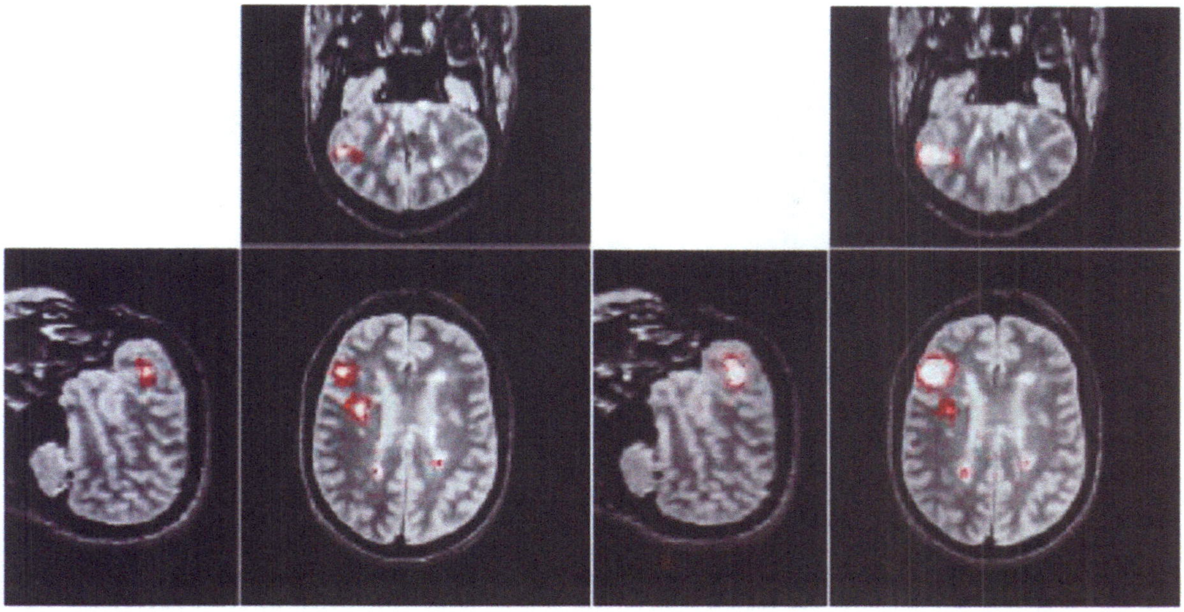

Fig. 4.10. Segmentation of evolving MS lesions based on the procedure of Rey et al. (1999)

ment (Crow et al. 1989) whose origin may be genetically determined. Characterization of the morphological processes in schizophrenia may lead to new pharmacological treatments, aimed at prevention and cure rather than suppression of symptoms. There is in addition a particular focus on asymmetry as the defining characteristic of the human brain and the correlate of language. Techniques are required for describing and quantifying cerebral asymmetries to determine where these are located, how variable they are between individuals and how the distribution in individuals with schizophrenia differs from that in the general population.

Prima et al. (1998) developed a method that allows the automatic extraction of the brain symmetry plane from MR data. A disymmetry map is then computed by mirroring each image w.r.t. this symmetry plane and calculating the non-rigid deformation between the original images and its mirrored copy (Fig. 4.11). Finally, by non-rigidly registering or warping the images of different subjects to a reference image, it is possible to compute a mean disymmetry map that includes statistical estimates of variability.

In Maes et al. (1999), a method is presented for quantifying cerebral gray and white matter asymmetry from MR images. The method consists of bias field correction, tissue segmentation and atlas-based separation of left and right hemispheres and relies on state-of-the-art algorithms for rigid and non-rigid image registration and intensity-based voxel classification (Van Leemput et al. 1999a, 1999b). Because all steps in the procedure are completely automated and do not require interactive intervention or user specified parameters, the results are highly reproducible and consistent. White and gray matter are segmented after bias correction by the intensity-based tissue classification algorithm of Van Leemput et al. (1999b). Separation of the computed white and gray matter probability maps into left and right halves is achieved by non-rigid registration of the study image to a template MR image in which left and right hemispheres have been carefully segmented.[1]

The delineations of left and right hemispheres in the template image were transformed into binary label images, which were subsequently edited by morphological operations to match the brain envelope rather than the individual gyri and sulci to be more robust against differences in local cortical topology. The template image is matched to the study image by a combination of affine (Maes et al. 1997) and locally non-rigid transformations (Thirion 1998). The resulting deformation field is then applied to the label images, such that matched outlines of left and

[1] This image and the segmentations were retrieved from the Internet Brain Segmentation Repository (IBSR) available at http://neuro-www.mgh.harvard.edu/cma/ibsr. Maintained by Andrew Worth at the Center for Morphometric Analysis, Massachusetts General Hospital, Charlestown, MA, USA.

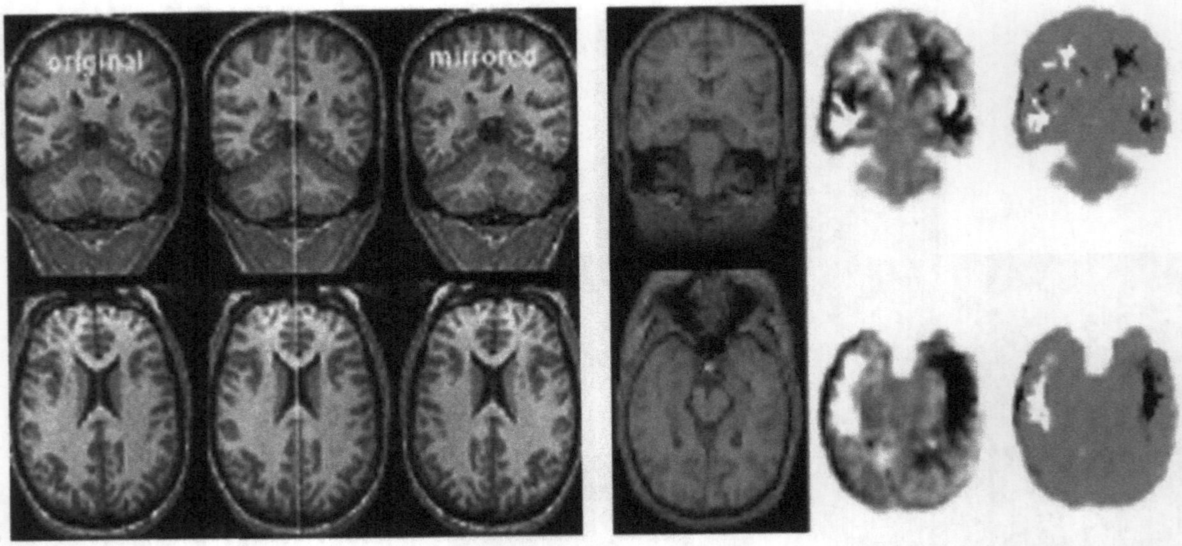

a b

Fig. 4.11a,b. A symmetry map over a population of normal male controls calculated by the procedure of PRIMA et al. (1998). First each image is mirrowed w.r.t. its mid-sagittal plane (a). The original image is non-rigidly warped to its mirrowed copy. Regions of local expansion or contraction are then calculated from the deformation field. The results are shown after additional warping of individual MR scans to a standard MR scan (b). *Bright areas* correspond to regions larger than its counterpart. *Dark regions represent regions that are smaller*

right hemispheres are obtained. These are used to separate left and right halves in the original gray and white matter segmentations and, at the same time, to remove non-relevant structures such as the cerebellum and brain stem. Finally, volumes for gray and white matter for each half of the brain separately are computed by integrating the corresponding probability maps within the brain regions of interest defined by the matched template image. Figure 4.12 illustrates that the gray and white matter segmentation maps obtained from the original images are correctly split into separate maps for left and right hemispheres by non-rigid registration with the labeled template image.

Various authors have presented alternative techniques to separate the brain hemispheres by the so-called mid-sagittal plane, defined as the plane that best fits the interhemispheric fissure of the brain (MARAIS et al. 1996) or as the plane that maximizes similarity between the image and its reflection relative to this plane (LIU et al. 1998; PRIMA et al. 1998). The advantage of the approach of MAES et al. of intensity-driven non-rigid registration to a labeled template image is that it does not assume the boundary between both hemispheres to be planar.

4.4.3 Epilepsy

Epilepsy is the most frequent serious primary neurological illness. Around 30% of epilepsy patients have epileptic seizures that are not controlled with medication. Epilepsy surgery is by far the most effective treatment for these patients with refractory partial epilepsy and is also the cheapest option besides vagus nerve stimulation and administration of antiepileptic drugs.

The aim of any presurgical evaluation in epilepsy surgery is to delineate the epileptogenic zone as accurately as possible. The epileptogenic zone is that part of the brain that has to be removed surgically in order to render the patient seizure free. Once the epileptogenic lesion is defined and the indication for surgery is made, the data of the different imaging techniques are transferred to a neuronavigation system (image guided neurosurgery or frameless stereotaxy), to enable the surgeon to resect exactly that part of the brain where the epileptogenic zone is located. This is all the more important when the lesion is located in or near functionally important cerebral cortex.

With the conventional investigation methods, the epileptic lesion and epileptogenic zone cannot always be defined accurately enough to proceed to a surgical intervention. This is often the case when visual inspection of high resolution MR images does

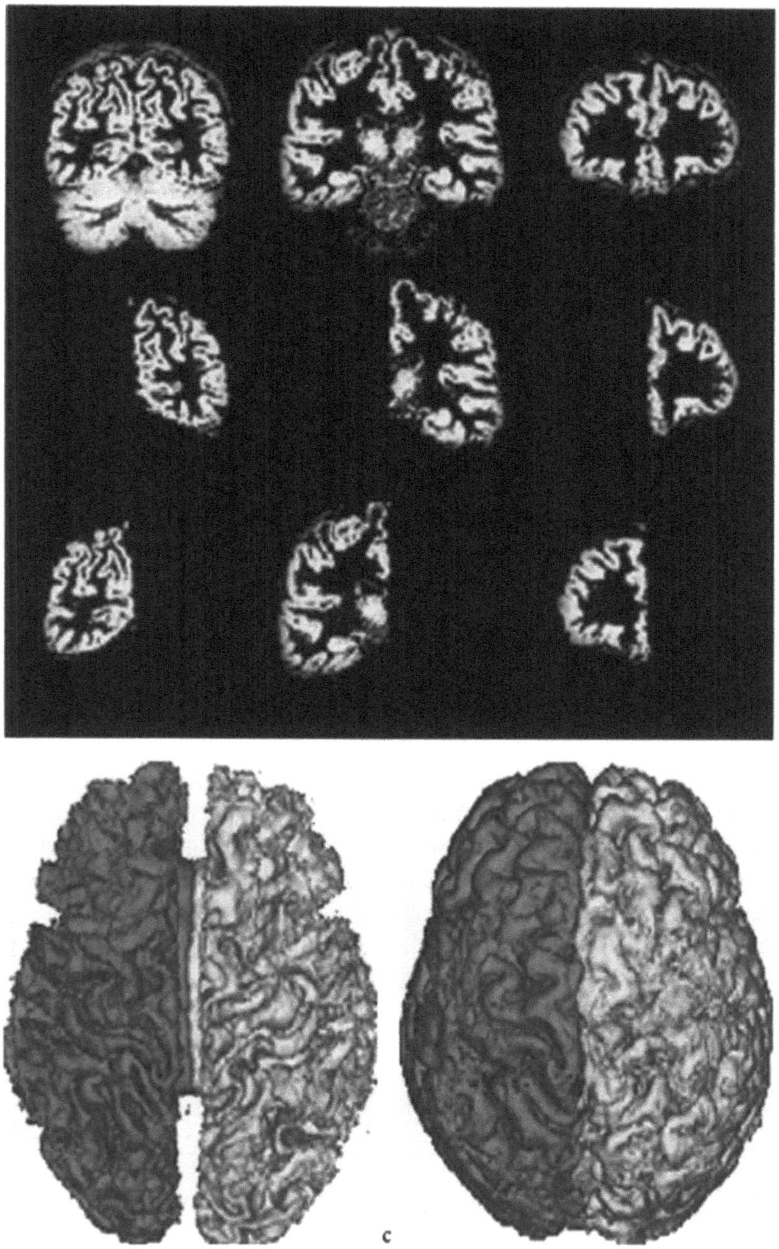

Fig. 4.12a–c. Left-right hemisphere gray matter and white matter separation according to the method of Maes et al. (1999) on high quality high resolution data, consisting of a single sagittal T1-weighted image (Siemens Vision 1.5 T scanner, 3D MPRAGE, 256×256 matrix, 1.25 mm slice thickness, 128 slices, FOV = 256 mm, TR = 11.4 ms, TE = 4.4 ms) with good contrast between gray matter, white matter and the tissues surrounding the brain. Coronal sections through the gray matter segmentation map before (*top row*) and after left-right and cerebrum-cerebellum separation (**a**). A 3D-entering of the segmental white (**b**) and gray (**c**) matter is shown

not show a lesion. The underlying pathological lesion in these cases most often is a form of malformation of cortical development (MCD). MCDs are a frequent cause of epilepsy. MR features of MCD include cortical thickening, blurring of the gray-white matter transition, and white matter hyperintensity (Chan et al. 1998). Sisodiya et al. (1995) described a semi-interactive technique to segment gray matter on 3D MR images in order to better detect abnormalities in cortical thickness. They reported subtle MCD that was not detected on visual inspection of the images. Manual segmentation of the gray matter, however, is time consuming and difficult to implement in a clinical context. Free et al. (1998) used a voxel-by-voxel comparison of automatically segmented gray matter to compare structural MR imaging of the brains of control subjects with those of patients with epilepsy. First, each 3D MR image is automatically segmented into gray matter, white matter and CSF, resulting in an image representing the individual spatial distribution of GM, called the GMDM. Next, each GMDM image is transformed, using an affine spatial transformation to a normalized reference space (Talairach), to remove differences in patient positioning (translation, rotation) and size differences (scaling). Subsequently, individual GM-

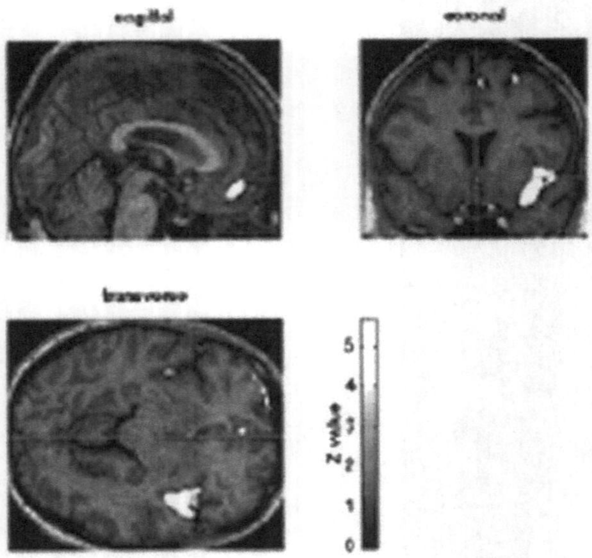

Fig. 4.13. Result of the statistical voxel-by-voxel analysis for abnormal gray matter density in epilepsy patients. The three orthogonal views show projections of clusters of significantly abnormal gray matter voxels in a 3D MR image of a single epileptic patient

DMs of patients are compared to those of control subjects. Statistically significant deviations in GM-DMs are analyzed on a voxel-by-voxel basis and correlated with other clinical patient data (Fig. 4.13).

The resulting analysis identified MCD and abnormalities beyond the visualized lesion in individual patients with MCD. Moreover, Sisodiya et al. (1997) reported that patients with hippocampal sclerosis (HS) in combination with subtle MCD, detected with their semi-interactive segmentation technique, had a worse prognosis after surgery compared with patients with HS who did not have these MCD, probably because the epileptogenic zone is too extensive to be removed completely.

4.5 Conclusion

In this chapter we have given an overview of algorithmic developments in MR image segmentation and registration. Segmentation and registration are essential components of many quantitative MR image analysis tasks.

In image segmentation, we have indicated two major strategies that are actively being investigated: on the one hand, the completely automatic procedures which are typically tailored to specific applications and are often used for large scale studies where the investment in development of automatic image analysis algorithms is smaller than the effort otherwise needed in manual interaction; and, on the other hand, the interactive segmentation methods, which try to combine the computational power of machines with the intelligent interaction of a human expert. This strategy is optimal in small scale studies where incorporation of domain specific knowledge into the algorithm would be too cumbersome or even impossible.

In image registration, we have stressed the success of intensity or voxel similarity based methods, in particular those based on information theoretic concepts, in rigid registration of brain images. No major advances are to be expected in this area. Non-rigid registration, on the other hand, is still an open problem and an active research area with no single satisfactory general solution, yet. In the context of brain warping, the major obstacle that remains, besides reduction in computational complexity, is a clear, understandable model of feasible deformations mapping one brain to another brain or a template. Here the continuum mechanics models need to be combined with more specific knowledge about brain development. This combination will require some knowledge engineering, extracting the information stored in medical textbooks and converting it into manageable computer algorithms.

Acknowledgements. The authors wish to acknowledge input from the scientific collaborators in the BIOMORPH project [Development and Validation of Techniques for Brain Morphometry (BIOMORPH). EU-Biomed Project No. 95–0845]. Partners in the BIOMORPH project are: University of Kent at Canterbury (UKC), Kent, UK; ETH, Zurich, Switzerland; University of Oxford, Oxford, UK; INRIA, Nice, France; Katholieke Universiteit Leuven (KUL), Leuven, Belgium. Clinical input was provided in particular by ACF Colchester (UKC), L. DeLisi (Stony Brook, NY, USA), T. Crow (Oxford) and W. Van Paesschen (KUL).

References

Beard D, Eberly D, Emminger B et al (1994) Interacting with image hierarchies for fast and accurate object segmentation. In: Proc SPIE Medical Imaging 1994: Image Processing, vol 2167, pp 10–17

Bookstein F (1991) Morphometric tools for landmark data. Cambridge University Press

Chan S, Chin SS, Nordli DR et al. (1998) Prospective magnetic resonance imaging identification of focal cortical dysplasia, including the non-balloon cell subtype. Ann Neurol 44: 749–757

Choi HS, Haynor DR, Kim Y (1991) Partial volume tissue classification of multi-channel magnetic resonance images – a mixel model. IEEE Trans Med Imaging 10: 395–407

Christensen G, Rabbitt RD, Miller MI (1996) Deformable templates using large deformation kinematics. IEEE Trans Image Processing 5: 1435–1447

Chu CC, Aggarwal JK (1993) The integration of image segmentation maps using region and edge information. IEEE Trans Pattern Analysis and Machine Intelligence 15: 1241–1252

Cocosco CA, Kollokian V, Kwan RKS et al. (1997) BrainWeb: online interface to a 3D MRI simulated brain database. Neuroimage 5(4) part 2/4: S425

Collins DL, Neelin P, Peters TM et al. (1994) Automatic three-dimensional intersubject registration of MR volumetric data into standardized Talairach space. J Comput Assist Tomogr 18: 192–205

Collins DL, Le Goualher G, Venugopal R et al. (1996) Cortical Constraints for non-linear cortical registration. In: Hoehne KH, Kikinis R (eds) Visualization in biomedical computing. Lecture notes in computer science, Springer Verlag, vol 1131, pp 307–316

Cootes T, Hill A, Taylor C et al. (1994) The use of active shape models for locating structures in medical images. Image and Vision Computing 12: 355–366

Crow TJ, Ball J, Bloom SR et al. (1989) Schizophrenia as an anomaly of development of cerebral asymmetry. Arch Gen Psychiatry 46: 1145–1150

Davatzikos C (1996) Spatial normalisation of three-dimensional brain images using deformable models. J Comput Assist Tomogr 20: 656–665

Dawant BM, Thirion JP, Maes F et al. (1998) Automatic 3D segmentation of internal structures of the head in MR images using a combination of similarity and free-form transformations. In: Hanson KM (ed) Proc SPIE Medical Imaging 1998: Image Processing, vol 3338, pp 1528–1539

DeLisi LE, Tew W, Xie SH et al. (1995) A prospective follow-up study of brain morphology and cognition in first-epsiode schizophrenic patients: preliminary findings. Biol Psychiatry 38: 349–360

Eberly D, Pizer SM (1994) Ridge flow models for image segmentation. In: Proc SPIE Medical Imaging 1994: Image Processing, vol 2167, pp 54–64

Evans AC, Frank JA, Antel J et al. (1997) The role of MRI in clinical trials of multiple sclerosis: comparison of image processing techniques. Ann Neurol 41: 125–132

Free SL, Woermann FG, Duncan JS (1998) Voxel-by-voxel comparison of automatically segmented grey matter: a rater-independent comparison of structural MRI in patients with epilepsy. Epilepsia 39 (Suppl.6): 98 (Abstract)

Gerig G, Welti D, Guttman C et al. (1998) Exploring the discrimation power of the time domain for segmentation and characterization of lesions in serial MR data. In: Wells WM, Colchester A, Delp S (eds) Proc. of the 1st international conference on medical image computing and computer-assisted intervention, MICCAI '98. Lecture notes in computer science, Springer Verlag, vol 1496, pp 469–480

Griffin LD, Colchester ACF, Robinson GP (1992) Scale and segmentation of grey-level images using maximum gradient paths. Image and Vision Computing 10: 389–402

Griffin LD, Colchester ACF, Roll SA, Studholme CS (1994) Hierarchical segmentation satifying constraints. In: Proc British Machine Vision Conference, BMVC '94, pp 135–144

Guttman CRG, Ahn SS, Hsu LE et al. (1994). The evolution of multiple sclerosis Lesions on Serial MRI. Am J Neuroradiol 16: 1481–1491

Haddon JF, Boyce JF (1990) Image segmentation by unifying region and boundary information. IEEE Trans on Pattern Analysis and Machine Intelligence 12: 929–948

Johnston B, Atkins MS, Mackiewich B et al. (1996) Segmentation of multiple sclerosis lesions in intensity corrected multispectral MRI. IEEE Trans Med Imaging 15: 154–169

Kass M, Witkin A, Terzopoulos D (1988) Snakes: active contour models. Int J Comput Vision 1: 321–331

Kim B, Boes JL, Frey KA et al. (1997) Mutual information for automated unwarping of rat brain autoradiographs. Neuroimage 5: 31–40

Laidlaw DH, Fleischer KW, Barr AH (1998) Partial-volume bayesian classification of material mixtures in MR volume data using voxel histograms. IEEE Trans Med Imaging 17: 74–86

Liu Y, Collins RT, Rothfus WE (1998) Automatic bilateral symmetry (midsagittal) plane extraction from pathological 3D neuroradiological images. In: Hanson KM (ed) Proceedings SPIE Medical Imaging 1998: Image Processing, vol 3338, pp 1528–1539

Maes F, Collignon A, Vandermeulen D et al. (1997) Multimodality image registration by maximization of mutual information. IEEE Trans Med Imaging 16: 187–198

Maes F, Vandermeulen D, Suetens P, Marchal G (1995) Computer-aided interactive object delineation using an intelligent paintbrush technique. Proceedings 1st International conference on computer vision, virtual reality and robotics in medicine, CVRMED '95, Lectures notes in computer science, Springer, vol. 905, pp 77–83

Maes F, Van Leemput K, DeLisi LE et al. (1999) Quantification of cerebral grey and white matter asymmetry from MRI. In: Proceedings of medical image computing and computer-assisted intervention – MICCAI '99. In press.

Maintz JBA, Viergever MA (1998) A survey of medical image registration. Med Image Anal 2: 1–36

Marais P, Guillemaud R, Sakuma M et al. (1996) Visualising cerebral asymmetry. In: Hoehne KH, Kikinis R (eds) Proceedings visualization in biomedical computing. Lecture notes in computer science, Springer Verlag, vol 1131, pp 411–416

McInerney T, Terzopulos D (1996) Deformable models in medical image analysis: a survey. Med Image Anal 1: 91–108

Meyer C, Boes J, Kim B et al. (1997) Demonstration of accuracy and clinical versatility of mutual information for automatic multimodality image fusion using affine and thin plate spline warped geometric deformations. Med Image Anal 1: 195–206

Ogniewicz R, Vehkomäki T, Székely G (1993) Extraction of closed boundaries from fragmented edge maps using shape-oriented grouping procedures. In: Lemke HU, Inamura K, Jaffe CC, Felix R (eds) Proceedings Computer assisted radiology, Springer Verlag, pp 334–340

Pavlidis T, Liow YT (1990) Integrating region growing and edge detection. IEEE Trans on Pattern Analysis and Machine Intelligence 12: 225–233

Pietrzyk U, Herholz K, Fink G et al. (1994) An interactive technique for three-dimensional image registration: validation for PET, SPECT, MRI and CT brain studies. J Nucl Med 35: 2011–2018
Pizer SM, ter Haar Romeny BM (1991) Fundamental properties of medical image perception. J Dig Imaging 4: 1–20
Prima S, Thirion JP, Subsol G et al. (1998) Automatic analysis of normal brain dissymmetry of males and females in MR images. In: Wells WM, Colchester A, Delp S (eds) Proceedings of the 1st International conference on medical image computing and computer-assisted intervention – MICCAI '98. Lecture notes in computer science, Springer Verlag, vol 1496, pp 770–779
Rey D, Subsol G, Delingette H et al. (1999) Automatic detection and segmentation of evolving processes in 3D medical images: application to multiple sclerosis. In: Kuba A, Samal M, Todd-Pokropek (eds) Proceedings Information processing in medical imaging. Lecture notes in computer science, Springer Verlag, vol 1613, pp 154–167
Santago P, Gage HD (1995) Statistical models of partial volume effect. IEEE Trans Image Proc 4: 1531–1540
Semelka RC, Tomei E, Wagner S et al. (1990) Normal left ventricular dimensions and function: Interstudy reproducibility of measurements with cine MR imaging. Radiology 174: 763–768
Simmons A, Tofts PS, Barker GJ et al. (1994) Sources of intensity nonuniformity in spin echo images at 1.5 T. Magn Reson Med 32: 121–128
Sisodiya SM, Free SL, Stevens JM et al. (1995) Widespread cerebral structural changes in patients with cortical dysgenesis and epilepsy. Brain 118: 1039–1050
Sisodiya SM, Moran N, Free SL et al. (1997) Correlation of widespread preoperative magnetic resonance imaging changes with unsuccessful surgery for hippocampal sclerosis. Ann Neurol 41: 490–496
Studholme C, Hill DLG, Hawkes DJ (1996) Automated 3-D registration of MR and CT images of the head. Med Image Anal 1: 163–175
Subsol G (1999) Crest-lines for curvature-based warping, In: Toga AW (ed) Brain warping. Academic Press, pp 241–262
Terzopoulos D, Platt J, Barr A et al. (1987) Elastically deformable models. Computer Graphics 21: 205–214
Thirion JP (1998) Image matching as a diffusion process: an analogy with Maxwell's demons. Med Image Anal 2: 243–260
Thirion JP, Calmon G (1999) Deformation analysis to detect and quantify active lesions in 3D medical image sequences. IEEE Trans Med Imaging 18: 429–441
Thompson PM, Toga AW (1996) High-resolution random-mesh algorithms for creating a probabilistic three-dimensional surface atlas of the human brain. Neuroimage 3: 19–34
Toga AW (1999) Brain warping. Academic Press
Udupa JK, Wei L, Samarasekera S et al. (1997) Multiple sclerosis lesion quantification using fuzzy – connectedness principles. IEEE Trans Med Imaging 16: 598–609
Van Leemput K, Maes F, Vandermeulen D et al. (1999a). Automated model-based bias field correction of MR images of the brain. IEEE Trans Med Imaging. Accepted for publication.
Van Leemput K, Maes F, Vandermeulen D et al. (1999b). Automated model-based tissue classification of MR images of the brain. IEEE Trans Med Imaging. Accepted for publication.
Van Leemput K, Maes F, Bello F et al. (1999c) Automated segmentation of MS lesions from multi-channel MR images. In: Proceedings of medical image computing and computer-assisted intervention – MICCAI '99. In press.
Vincken KL, Koster ASE, Viergever MA (1997) Probabilistic multiscale image segmentation. IEEE Trans Pattern Analysis and Machine Intelligence 19: 109–120
Wells WM, Grimson WEL, Kikinis R et al. (1996a) Adaptive segmentation of MRI data. IEEE Trans Med Imaging 15: 429–442
Wells WM, Viola P, Atsumi H et al. (1996b) Multi-modal volume registration by maximization of mutual information. Med Image Anal 1: 35–51
West J, Fitzpatrick JM, Wang MY et al. (1997) Comparison and evaluation of retrospective intermodality brain image registration techniques. J Comput Assist Tomogr 21: 554–566
Woods RP, Grafton ST, Watson JDG et al. (1998) Automated image registration II: Intersubject validation of linear and non-linear models. J Comput Assist Tomogr 22: 155–165
Woods RP, Mazziotta JC, Cherry SR (1993) MRI-PET registration with automated algorithm. J Comput Assist Tomogr 17: 536–546
Zijdenbos AP, Dawant BM, Margolin RA et al. (1994) Morphometric analysis of white matter lesions in MR images: method and validation. IEEE Trans Med Imaging 13: 716–724
Zijdenbos A, Forghani R, Evans A (1998) Automatic quantification of MS lesions in 3D MRI brain data sets: Validation of INSECT. In: Wells WM, Colchester A, Delp S (eds) Proceedings of the 1st International conference on medical image computing and computer-assisted intervention – MICCAI '98. Lecture notes in computer science, Springer Verlag, vol 1496, pp 439–448

5 Clinical Magnetic Resonance Spectroscopy

Paul Van Hecke

CONTENTS

5.1 Introduction

Since the early days of the introduction of magnetic resonance as a clinical imaging modality, magnetic resonance spectroscopy (MRS) has been earmarked as a potentially useful clinical tool, able to provide biochemical information of tissues in a completely non-invasive way. The penetration of the technique into the daily clinical diagnosis has however been much slower than expected from the initial enthusiasm. Still, the progress is slow, is steady, and the quantity and reproducibility of data acquired in a number of pathologies are such that MRS is now being included as a diagnostic or of as a follow-up procedure in some examinations, as an essential adjunct to MRI and other imaging techniques (Danielsen and Ross 1998, Young and Cecil Charles 1996).

P. Van Hecke, MD, PhD
Department of Radiology, University Hospitals, Herestraat 49, 3000 Leuven, Belgium

5.2 Overview

The major asset of MRS is the ability to simultaneously observe and quantify, in a non-invasive way, a "spectrum" of molecules (metabolites) contained in a selected volume, rather than just those molecules, a priori selected for conventional chemical analysis, providing a "metabolic signature" of the tissue and offering the opportunity to detect new or unexpected metabolites. The drawback is the inherent lack of instrumental sensitivity of NMR, which prevents in vivo clinical observation of metabolites with tissue concentrations below about 1 mM. The number of observable brain metabolites is thus limited; in 1H spectroscopy it boils down to the well-known NAA, Cr+PCr, Cho, Lac, and lipids, and with adequate techniques also Ins, Glu, Gln, Glc, and a few others. In ^{31}P MRS it includes mainly Pi, PCr, ATP, PME and PDE. The diagnosis of cerebral diseases with MRS thus relies on the observation of variations of the concentration of this very limited number of molecules. These variations being moreover very similar for many diseases, the resulting lack of specificity is one of the major stumbling blocks preventing MRS becoming a fully fledged clinical diagnostic tool, the most striking example being the inability to achieve a reliable classification of cerebral tumours. To reach the latter goal, powerful statistical techniques based on pattern recognition and neural networks, requiring large and representative databases, are now explored in order to improve the classification performances of spectroscopic data.

Still, MRS has proved to be rather successful in intrapatient longitudinal studies, to assess the evolution of diseases, to provide a correlate with the severity of the disease, to follow the effect of medication and predict the clinical outcome. Also, regional deviations of brain metabolite patterns within a patient have allowed the detection of regional abnormalities not observed with MRI, such as in MS, in encephalopathies and in stroke, providing biochemical markers for the evolution of the disease or the response to a treatment, which are much more sensitive than MRI diagnosis. Intrapatient hemispheric asymmetries in brain metabolite distribution detected by MRS are the basis for the successful and highly specific, non-invasive lateralization of the epileptic focus in epilepsy.

A number of recent trends in MRS methodology are expected to contribute to an improved adaptation of the technique to the needs of the clinical user. The most obvious shift is that from phosphorus to proton spectroscopy. The major reason is that any clinical MR scanner can easily be adapted to perform proton spectroscopy. The advantages of proton spectroscopy are manyfold. Proton resonates at the highest frequency, resulting in the highest possible NMR signal amplitude in a given magnetic field, allowing for smaller selected volumes, and better spatial resolution than with phosphorus MR (for the same examination time); also, protons are present in all metabolites, while phosphorus is not. In general, proton spectroscopy turns out to be more sensitive to metabolic abnormalities than ^{31}P spectroscopy, due to more pronounced changes in metabolite concentrations in proton spectra.

The drawback of proton spectroscopy is the need to suppress the huge water signal which overshadows the weak metabolite signals (factor 10,000), and to achieve a good shim procedure to optimize the field homogeneity in order to be able to resolve the various metabolite spectral lines which in a proton spectrum are all very close together. These requirements are satisfactorily implemented on recent MR scanners.

Another trend is towards the simultaneous acquisition of a 2D array of voxels in a plane which, besides the complete spectral information within each of those voxels, also provides a 2D map of a particular metabolite within the selected plane, with a spatial resolution determined by the size of the voxel (spectroscopic imaging, SI). The technique is presently being extended to 3D. The superior sensitivity of protons allows for voxel sizes down to 1 ml, or even less in 2D. This resolution is insufficient for detailed metabolic studies of small tumours, but is sufficient to provide useful information in large tumours and in diffuse abnormalities, such as in epilepsy, stroke, degenerative diseases, and others. The drawback is a prolonged acquisition for very small voxel sizes and, more important, the need for a good homogeneity of the static and rf excitation magnetic fields over the whole plane; regions with large susceptibility gradients due to air- or bone-tissue interfaces will unavoidably lead to degraded spectra and distortions in the metabolic map. These difficulties limit for the moment the general use of the 2D technique for clinical applications. Also contamination of the spectrum by the large signal from the lipids of the subdural fat is being taken care of in all recent equipment by the use of saturation blocks.

Another trend is the use in proton MRS of short echo times in both single-voxel and SI techniques for the detection of more exotic molecules (Ins, Glu, Gln, Glc), which can add to the diagnostic power and/or the understanding of the biochemical process. The quality of these spectra is satisfactory for a qualitative appraisal of the spectral content but the accurate quantitative determination of metabolite concentrations is a formidable task due to strong and broad baseline components arising from signals from macromolecules, and to the complexity of the spectrum arising from the many and weak overlapping lines due to J-coupling. For a majority of clinical studies the long echo-time (135 or 270 ms) sequence still provides adequate information obtained after simple and straightforward quantification, a major consideration for the clinical user.

A growing number of studies have demonstrated the need to measure and report metabolite concentrations in absolute terms (mmol/kg) rather than as ratios relative to one of the peaks of the spectrum, taken as a reference. In proton spectroscopy, this reference is often PCr+Cr, in 31P sometimes ATP, both metabolites which are expected to show few regional and pathological variations. This is of course not always justified and erroneous conclusions can be drawn on the basis of this assumption. Several methods have been proposed for the absolute quantification of metabolite concentrations. They rely on the use of an external or an internal reference (such as the water signal in 1H spectroscopy), which both require an additional measurement. In proton MRS, the internal water reference approach is usually favoured in view of its ease and because the water signal originates from the same voxel; drawbacks are that the water signal may not necessarily originate from the same tissue compartment, and the water concentration may change in pathological tissue, all requiring additional corrections.

The issue of the mere calculation of the intensity of the MR signal (FID or echo) in the time domain, or the spectral peak after Fourier transform in the frequency domain, has received increased attention during recent years and various algorithms are being developed for automated and accurate quantification of the noisy and overlapping spectroscopy signals. Absolute quantification remains a time-consuming task, requiring expert operators. If absolute quantification is needed to obtain a good insight into the biochemical processes which underlie the pathogenesis of the disease, relative quantification based on simple ratios of metabolite amplitudes usually fulfill the needs of many clinical studies such as the longitudinal monitoring of a disease or a treatment, the detection of intrapatient regional variations, the discrimination of a group of patients from healthy controls or even the classification of lesions based on advanced pattern recognition techniques.

In summary, such technical and methodological developments in signal acquisition and processing should contribute to shape MRS into a more reliable and versatile tool for both clinical and the research applications.

Recent advances in major clinical applications of in vivo MRS are briefly reviewed in the following sections. Experimental studies on animals and high-resolution in vitro studies on cells and body fluids have been excluded from this survey.

5.3 Specific Applications

5.3.1 Tumours

Spectroscopy is capable of differentiating normal from pathologic brain and it generally provides tissue specificity greater than that of imaging (Doyle et al. 1999; Castilloand Kwock 1998; Kaibara et al. 1998). Still, detailed tissue characterization of brain tumours from MR spectra remains largely unsatisfactory, even controversial in some cases. Reasons have to be found in the large variation of metabolic characteristics within each type of tumour and within patient groups, and in their limited changes within a metabolite, leading to large overlaps and precluding diagnostic accuracy. Improvement could be expected from a better spatial resolution at the acquisition, which in the past has often been insufficient to match the spatial inhomogeneity of most tumours, combined with 2D SI. Absolute metabolite concentrations, rather than relative concentrations, could further contribute to a more accurate characterization of tumours (Mader et al. 1996). Recent spectroscopy studies of intracranial tumours have merely confirmed earlier observations. The general trends in 31P MRS of tumours include elevated PME, PDE and Pi relative to NTP, and alkaline pH (Maldonado et al. 1998). In 1H MRS the general trend includes, relative to Cr+PCr, a reduced or absent NAA, and an increased Cho signal, the latter being higher in HG than in LG gliomas (Shimizu et al. 1996; Tien et al. 1996; Negendank et al. 1996; Falini et al. 1996). The increase of Cho might be used as a marker of malignity (Speck et al. 1996) or of malignant degeneration in cerebral gliomas (Tedeschi et al. 1997). Similar trends are found in pediatric tumours (Byrd et al. 1996; Taylor et al. 1996; Byrd et al. 1996; Tzika et al. 1996; Girard et al. 1998; Lazareff et al. 1998; Taylor et al. 1998). In pediatric low-grade gliomas the persistent high Cho was reported to be predictive for tumor growth (Lazareff et al. 1998). These trends could even be observed at 0.5 T (Prost et al. 1997). Meningiomas usually show the highest Cho levels, as well as an alanine signal, which allow their differentiation from gliomas. Lac is elevated in the core of malignant gliomas and free lipids have been observed in most HG gliomas and malignant tumours (Furuya et al. 1997; Gotsis et al. 1996). Proton and phosphorus spectroscopy detect metabolic changes, prior to changes on MRI, in radiosensitive tumours following radiotherapy, and the absence of such changes in resistant tumours (Tomoi et al. 1997; Yoshino et al. 1996). They may distinguish radiation necrosis from recurrent tumours (Kizu et al. 1998; Grand et al. 1997). Radiation therapy and chemotherapy have been shown to induce metabolic changes in tissue remote from the tumour (Waldrop et al. 1998). In children, 1H MRS has been claimed to differentiate various types of suprasellar (Sutton et al. 1997) tumours. Intracranial tuberculomas (Gupta et al. 1996; Gupta and Roy 1999), abscesses (Remy et al. 1995), and cystic masses (Chang et al. 1998) can be differentiated from tumours using 1H MRS.

Major improvements in the categorization of tumours, according to stage and type, for daily clinical diagnosis, could be expected from automated classification methods (based on pattern recognition and neural networks), making use of a set of in vivo spectroscopic data, possibly in combination with data from imaging and from clinical observations (for a review see Hagberg 1998).

5.3.2 Ischaemia

The combination of newer MR techniques such as diffusion, perfusion, functional and spectroscopic

MR imaging provide the clinicians with much more precise information on localization, severity and potential reversibility of ischaemia. Spectroscopy contributes to the evaluation of the initial metabolic damage in the acute phase and the subsequent progress towards recovery or further degeneration, being in some cases prognostic for later neurological outcome (Berry et al. 1998; van der Grond and Mali 1998). Recent proton spectroscopy studies confirm the general observation of a decrease of NAA and an increase of Lac in the acute and subacute phase (Caplan 1997; Saunders et al. 1997). These metabolic changes correlate to a variable extent with the stroke score, the reduced blood flow, the lesion extent and the clinical outcome (Federico et al. 1996; Kamada et al. 1997; Lauriero et al. 1996; van der Grond et al. 1996; Wardlaw et al. 1998). The use of absolute metabolite concentrations rather than metabolite ratios has been emphasized in view of the observed simultaneous decrease of NAA and Cr in acute as well as in chronic ischaemic lesions (Harada et al. 1997), even in the hemisphere contralateral to the infarct; the increased water content after stroke has to be taken into account for such absolute quantification (Gideon et al. 1999). In the acute and subacute phase, lipids and macromolecules have been observed and persist much longer than lactate (Hwang et al. 1996; Saunders et al. 1997). An important finding is that, in acute stroke, Lac is elevated while NAA remains largely unchanged in regions around the hyperintense T2 area, pointing to ischaemic regions at risk (Morishita et al. 1997; Gillard et al. 1996). Likewise, in patients with stenosis of the internal carotid artery, with no visible infarcts on MRI, NAA/Cho was found to be lower than normal in the symptomatic hemisphere, and normal in the contralateral one, and to recover after carotid endarterectomy only when no Lac was detected before (van der Grond et al. 1996). Likewise, flow measurements in the ICA and MCA combined with NAA/Cho measurements in the MCA territory can be used to identify patients with insufficient perfusion to maintain cellular integrity (van der Grond et al. 1999).

In perinatal asphyxia, earlier 31P studies demonstrated delayed impairment of cerebral energy metabolism (decreased ATP and PCr content) and were shown to significantly improve the predictability of later neurological outcome (Martin et al. 1996). More recently, proton spectroscopy has shown Lac accumulation and decline in NAA (Huppi and Barnes 1997; Saliba et al. 1997) as well as a decline in Cho and an elevation of all metabolite T2s in central grey matter (Cady 1996). The elevated Lac/NAA ratio measured at birth seems to be indicative for a poor long-term prognosis (Groenendaal et al. 1996; Penrice et al. 1996), in agreement with the detection of Lac later than 1 month after birth in children with abnormal neurodevelopment outcome at 1 year of age (Hanrahan et al. 1998). Similar prognostic results may be achieved in hypoxia after near drowning (Dubowitz et al. 1998).

5.3.3 Epilepsy

MRI and MR based volumetry are techniques of choice for the non-invasive evaluation of patients with intractable epilepsy as the hippocampal atrophy detected on MR images has been shown to correlate with the EEG localization of ictal onset. The need for non-invasive techniques that can provide insight into the metabolic abnormalities associated with the epileptonic focus has triggered a large number of MR spectroscopy studies which have been the subject of reviews (Duncan 1997; Hajek et al. 1998; Jackson and Connelly 1996; King and Batuch 1998; Kuzniecky 1997; Laxer 1997; Sitoh and Tien 1998). Proton MRS has been shown to be extremely sensitive in the detection and lateralization of unilateral and bilateral metabolic abnormalities in patients with TLE. This was further confirmed by recent studies on large groups of patients for which the combination of MRS and MRI data was highly concordant with EEG and PET (Achten et al. 1998; Cendes et al. 1997; Constantinidis et al. 1996; Cross et al. 1997; Gadian et al. 1996; Holopainen et al. 1997; Knowlton et al. 1997; Kuzniecky et al. 1998; Lu et al. 1997). Temporal lobe abnormalities were found in both epileptic children with and without febrile convulsions (Holopainen et al. 1998). The decreased ratio NAA/Cho+Cr was in general the most sensitive parameter for lateralization, when combined with an asymmetry index (Achten et al. 1997; Cross et al. 1996; Thompson et al. 1998). There are indications that the reduction in NAA correlates with the seizure frequency (Garcia et al. 1997; Kuzniecky et al. 1997); correlation with hippocampal volume is contradictory. Recent work also demonstrates abnormal NAA concentrations contralateral to the EEG defined focus (Duc et al. 1998; Ende et al. 1997). Interestingly, MRS also provides evidence of decreased temporal NAA ratios in TLE patients with no abnormality on MRI (Connelly et al. 1998; Woermann et al. 1999). NAA can revert to normal values on the side of surgery in patients who become seizure free, and act as a marker of physiologic dysfunction associated with seizure (CENDES et al. 1997); contralateral recovery after surgery has also been reported (HUGG et al. 1996). In extratemporal epilepsy NAA ratios are also significantly decreased, providing evidence for widespread neuronal damage/dysfunction, greatest in the region of the seizure focus (STANLEY et al. 1998). On the other hand, NAA was not reduced in the hippocampus of patients with neocortical epilepsy (VERMATHEN et al. 1997). 1H MRS can be used to monitor the effects of the anti-epilepsy drugs vigabatrin (PETROFF et al. 1998; NOVOTNY et al. 1999; WEBER et al. 1999), gabapentin (PETROFF et al. 1996), topiramate (PETROFF et al. 1999) and valproate (PETROFF et al. 1999) on brain GABA and homocarnosine levels, which are associated with seizure control. The use of ^{31}P spectroscopy is limited by a lower signal-to-noise ratio and spatial resolution. The few recent studies have confirmed the increase in inorganic phosphate and decrease in PME in the epileptogenic temporal lobe, and to a lesser extent also in the contralateral lobe (VAN DER GROND et al. 1998). High-field studies achieved satisfactory lateralization in TLE using the PCr/Pi and ATP/Pi ratios (CHU et al. 1998).

5.3.4 Neurodegenerative Diseases

5.3.4.1 *Alzheimer's Disease*

The challenge for MRS is to differentiate Alzheimer's disease (AD) from normal aging. Recent studies confirm the significant decrease in Alzheimer of NAA levels in hippocampal, temporal, frontal, occipital and mesial grey matter and in white matter (HEUN et al. 1997; TEDESCHI et al. 1996; SCHUFF et al. 1998; SCHUFF et al. 1997). Short-echo time 1H MRS reveals increased myo-inositol levels in AD GM and the thus decreased NAA/Ins ratio contributes to a much better differentiation of AD from normal cerebral aging (PARNETTI et al. 1997; HEUN et al. 1997). The reduced NAA and increased mI seem to correlate with cognitive functions and the extent of atrophy (ROSE et al. 1999). Findings on Cho and Cr lack consistency. 1H MRS can also aid in distinguishing between AD and frontotemporal dementia (ERNST et al. 1997), subcortical ischaemic vascular dementia (KATTAPONG et al. 1996; MACKAY et al. 1996), and other dementias. 31P MRS studies have provided less consistent results, most tending to reveal alterations in membrane phospholipid metabolism (increased levels of phosphoesters) and some in high-energy phosphate metabolism (decreased phosphocreatine levels) (PETTEGREW et al. 1997; GONZALEZ et al. 1996).

5.3.4.2 *Parkinson's Disease*

Proton magnetic resonance is, as well as PET and SPECT, useful to help distinguish Parkinson's disease (PD) from atypical syndromes (BROOKS 1997; DAVIE 1998), such as multiple system atrophy (FEDERICO et al. 1997) and progressive supranuclear palsy (FEDERICO et al. 1997; AOTSUKA et al. 1997; TEDESCHI et al. 1997), where NAA/Cr is decreased in the lentiform nucleus compared to the normal value in idiopathic PD. In general, no significant differences in metabolite ratios have been found between PD patients and control healthy subjects in the globus pallidus, putamen (CRUZ et al. 1997), lentiform nucleus (CLARKE et al. 1997), or occipital lobe. Still, some studies report significant neuronal laterality in PD with unilateral symptoms, based on a reduction of NAA/Cr in the substantia nigra and putamen-GP in the symptomatic side (CHOE et al. 1998). Also NAA/Cho was found to be reduced in the putamen contralateral to the most affected side in drug-naive but not in a levodopa-treated IPD group, compared to healthy controls, which may provide a reversible marker of neuronal dysfunction in the striatum (ELLIS et al. 1997). Decreased temporoparietal NAA/Cr and Cho/Cr haven been reported in severely affected patients (TAYLOR et al. 1999).

5.3.4.3 *Amyotrophic Lateral Sclerosis*

1H NMR measurements of NAA reflect degeneration of lower motor neurons in the spinal cord and brainstem, and of upper motor neurons in the motor cortex of amyotrophic lateral sclerosis (ALS) patients. Indeed, NAA levels are found to be reduced in the sensorimotor cortex, the centrum semiovale and the anterior internal capsule, while unchanged in the frontal, parietal and mesial grey matter, in the cerebellum (BLOCK et al 1998; ROONEY et al. 1998; GIROUD et al. 1996) and in the motor subcortical white matter (ELLIS et al. 1998). Cho and Cr levels remain unaltered (GREDAL et al. 1997). More recently, reduced NAA, as well as elevated glutamate were demonstrated in the brainstem (pons and medulla) (CWIK et al. 1998; PIORO 1997). Finally, corticomotor NAA was shown to recover within a few weeks of riluzole therapy, a glutamate antagonist, suggesting a possible role for monitoring therapeutic response in ALS (KALRA et al. 1998).

5.3.5 Multiple Sclerosis

Although T2 weighted imaging is the standard diagnostic tool for the sensitive detection of multiple sclerosis (MS) lesions, it lacks pathological specificity and correlation with clinical disability. This has prompted the exploration of other techniques that would provide a better insight into lesion development. 1H MRS is now developing as a promising tool since many studies have shown evidence that the NAA level provides a specific index of axonal damage or dysfunction, which more strongly correlates with disability (Berry et al. 1998; Arnold et al. 1998; Miller et al. 1998b; Matthews et al. 1996; Miller et al. 1996a). Longitudinal studies have demonstrated that NAA is a useful marker for the evaluation of the progression of the disease (De et al. 1998; Narayana et al. 1998) and of the response to therapeutic treatment (Sarchielli et al. 1998). Although serial studies generally show irreversible decreases in NAA, mainly in progressive MS, decreases in acute lesions can be reversible. It has now been largely demonstrated that metabolic abnormalities extend beyond the lesion borders into the NAWM on MRI images. The decreased NAA/Cr ratio is interpreted as a reduction of NAA, which can be understood as axonal degeneration originating in axonal interruption in the lesions subsequent to inflammation and demyelination (Davie et al. 1997; Schiepers et al. 1997; Clanet and Berry 1998; Fu et al. 1998; Matthews et al. 1998; Tourbah et al. 1996). A few studies using absolute quantification have pointed out that the reduced NAA/Cr originated in an increase in Cr, consistent with the presence of gliosis in NAWM (Pan et al. 1996; Rooney et al. 1997), while still others find a constant Cr level (Sarchielli et al. 1999). As to the other metabolites detected with 1H MRS, choline is found to be increased early in the demyelination process, due to the release of choline containing membrane phospholipids during active myelin breakdown, after which it returns to nearly normal levels. Increases have been found in myo-inositol in most lesions and in visible lipids and in a composite peak (between 2.1 and 2.6 ppm) in acute lesions (Falini et al. 1998; Hirsch et al. 1996; Landtblom et al. 1996).

5.3.6 Human Immunodeficiency Virus Infection

In human immunodeficiency virus infection (HIV), MRS has a role in the early diagnosis of HIV encephalopathies, in the differential diagnosis of HIV encephalopathies versus psychiatric symptoms and versus other brain lesions and in the follow-up of response to therapy (Paley et al. 1996; Vion et al. 1998). Proton MR has been used for all MRS studies of the last few years. The metabolic abnormalities found with MRS in HIV patients (decreased NAA/Cr and NAA/Cho) reflect a diffuse rather than a regional process, not limited to the brain lesions visible with MRI (Alonso et al. 1996; Marcus et al. 1998), also in children (Lu et al. 1996; Salvan et al. 1998). Asymptomatic HIV infected patients present an abnormal metabolic profile (decreased NAA/Cr and NAA/Cho, and elevated conglomerate of amino acid peaks, between 2.1 and 2.6 ppm), which enable their differentiation to some extent from low and high risk HIV negative individuals (Jarvik et al. 1996; Salvan et al. 1997; Wilkinson et al. 1997). Progressive multifocal leukoencephalopathies have been studied in HIV patients (Chang et al. 1997; Iranzo et al. 1999) and claimed to be differentiated from HIV related encephalopathies (Simone et al. 1998). All studies agree that the onset of the HIV associated dementia complex is characterized by a raise in Cho, while the MRI findings are still normal, and later on by a decrease in NAA, which reflects brain damage (Cecil and Lenkinski 1998; Laubenberger et al. 1996; Lopez et al. 1997; Meyerhoff et al. 1999; Moller et al. 1999; Tracey et al. 1996). In general, metabolic abnormalities correlate with the severity of neurological and neuropsychological assessment (Goodkin et al. 1997; Harrison et al. 1998). As to the role of MRS in HIV therapy follow-up, NAA was observed to return to normal values subsequent to antiretroviral therapy, pointing to reversible neuronal dysfunction (Pavlakis et al. 1998; Salvan et al. 1997; Wilkinson et al. 1997).

5.3.7 Hepatic Encephalopathy

Chronic encephalopathy (HE) is usually diagnosed on clinical grounds, whereas subclinical HE (SCHE) requires neuropsychological tests. Various recent studies using short-time proton spectroscopy have confirmed the findings of earlier work and have identified both HE and SCHE patients by decreased cerebral concentrations of *myo*-inositol (mI) and choline (Cho) and increased concentrations of glutamine (Gln) (Bluml et al. 1998; Ross et al. 1996). The decreased mI has been interpreted as reflecting disturbances in cerebral osmoregulation. Patients with cirrhosis but without evidence for clinical HE present the same characteristic metabolic alterations; moreover the changes in mI, Cho and Gln seem in general to correlate with the clinical and neuropsychological status of HE (GEISSLER et al. 1997; LAUBENBERGER et al. 1997). Although HE is potentially reversible, spectroscopy studies after liver transplantation show that mI levels remain low and Gln levels high, albeit less pronounced (HUDA et al. 1998; THOMAS et al. 1998), while TIPS further worsens the difference with healthy subjects (KOSTLER 1998; NAGELE et al. 1999). Metabolite levels were found to be sensitive markers of lactulose therapy of HE (HASELER et al. 1998). NAA levels are normal in HE and SCHE. A recent 31P quantitative study reported reduced levels of cerebral nucleoside triphosphate, inorganic phosphate and phosphocreatine (BLUML et al. 1998), consistent with disturbed cerebral energy metabolism and at odds with previous studies reporting unchanged ATP levels relative to a supposedly constant level of PCr (MORGAN 1996).

5.3.8 Metabolic Diseases

MR spectroscopy is ideally suited to detecting inborn abnormalities of cerebral metabolism, and to monitor the effect of treatment and the progression of disease. High-resolution NMR spectroscopy of body fluids (plasma, urine, CSF) is a powerful technique providing a complete fingerprint of the metabolic pattern of the disease and is a promising diagnostic tool, albeit at present underestimated. In vivo NMR applications are limited to diseases involving changes in detectable metabolites (NAA, Cr, Cho, Ins in 1H MRS) or the visible accumulation of normally undetected brain metabolites (Lac, Gln, Ac). In the early days, abnormal metabolite concentrations were detected in the majority of metabolite diseases (peroxisomal, lysosomal, mitochondrial, amino acid, carbohydrate and primary grey and white matter diseases), such as increases of NAA in Canavan's disease, of glutamine in ornithine carbamoyl transferase deficiency, and of lactate in lactic acidoses of various origins (for reviews see GADIAN and LEONARD 1996; WANG AND ZIMMERMAN 1998) (see Fig. 22.9). Recent work has confirmed and extended these findings (LAM et al. 1998). Several studies of guanidinoacetate methyltransferase deficiency, an inborn error of creatine synthesis (SCHULZE et al. 1997), have reported the reduction or absence of brain creatine and the accumulation of guanidoacetic acid, the precursor of creatine, in proton NMR and the decrease of PCr and the accumulation of guanidinoacetate phosphate in 31P NMR; treatment by oral creatine intake resulted in increased brain creatine and a striking improvement of the neurological symptoms (STOCKLER and HANEFELD 1997; GANESAN et al. 1997). Elevated glutamine and lactate were reported in metabolic stroke in carbamyl phosphate synthetase deficiency (SPERL et al. 1997), while decreased NAA was reported in methylenetetrahydrofolate reductase deficiency (ENGELBRECHT et al. 1997). In neuronal ceroid lipofuscinosis, the severity of the metabolic abnormalities (decreased NAA and increased Lac and Ins) were found to correlate with the clinical symptoms and the decreasing age of onset (complete loss of NAA in the infantile form, normal in the juvenile form) (BROCKMANN et al. 1996; SEITZ et al. 1998). In propionic acidemia MRS revealed decreased NAA and Ins and elevated gln/glu in the basal ganglia, although MRI was normal in some of the patients (BERGMAN et al. 1996). In isovaleric acidemia, proton MRS revealed increased Lac/NAA, and phosphorus MRS, decreased PCr/Pi, which both returned to normal values after treatment, correlating with the neurological recovery (LOREK et al. 1996). In 3-hydroxy-3-methylglutaryl coenzyme A lyase (HMG CoA), the decreased NAA and increased Cho and Ins did correlate with the severity of the disease as evidenced from MRI (HUEMER et al. 1998; VAN DER Knaap et al. 1998). Intracerebral Lac and NAA were shown to recover to normal values upon biotin treatment in a patient with biotinidase deficiency (SCHURMANN et al. 1997). Finally various studies of mitochondrial myopathy, encephalopathy, lactic acidosis, strokes (MELAS), all show an increase in Lac, irrespective of a variety of MRI findings (CLARK et al. 1996) and a decrease in NAA, which recovers after the stroke, in agreement with the improved clinical status. After treatment with sodium dichloroacetate, the Lac/Cr ratio decreases in stroke regions, correlating with clinical improvement (PAVLAKIS et al. 1998). Similarly, children with cerebral energy deficiency due to enzyme deficiency show high Lac and normal NAA, in contrast to asphyxic children with high Lac, which correlates with clinical grade, and low NAA (KUGEL et al. 1998).

5.3.8.1 Adrenoleukodystrophy

Normal appearing white matter in adrenoleukodystrophy (ALD) was found to have decreased NAA/Cr and NAA/Cho and increased Cho/Cr and Ins/Cr compared to normals, which indicates onset of demyelination and neurological deterioration, before detection on MR images, while in the affected hyperintense WM the corresponding changes are much more pronounced, including increased Ins and appearance of Lac, reflecting the active demyelination process (Pouwels et al. 1998; Rajanayagam et al. 1997; Tourbah et al. 1997) (see Fig. 22.10). Metabolic changes seem to correlate with the severity of the demyelination process and the neurological involvement (Engelbrecht et al. 1997). After treatment (bone marrow transplantation), metabolite ratios recovered to values closer to normal (Rajanayagam et al. 1996). In children showing no further neurological deterioration, nor demyelination for long periods, the metabolic pattern revealed moderate NAA and Cho reduction, almost normal Ins and no Lac, in contrast to the above metabolic pattern observed in progressive ALD (Korenke et al. 1996).

5.3.8.2 Phenylketonuria

1H MRS can be used to measure the increased intracerebral phenylalanine concentration in patients. Increased sensitivity to measurement of Phe levels below 1 mmol/kg was obtained using short TE difference spectroscopy (phenylketonuria vs. normal) and larger volumes. Brain Phe levels were found to be 2–3 times smaller than blood plasma levels, without significant regional variations (Moller et al. 1997; Pietz et al. 1996). Individual level variations could be related to differences in the kinetics of Phe uptake (Moller et al. 1998). The non-invasive measurement of intracerebral Phe levels can thus be used to monitor compliance to and effects of various therapies and for correlation with neuropsychologic status. Continued supplementation of large neutral amino acids was shown to block brain Phe influx (Pietz et al. 1999). Other main metabolite concentrations are not significantly different from those in healthy persons.

5.3.9 Schizophrenia

Many 31P NMR studies in schizophrenics have confirmed the initial finding of reduced PME and increased PDE in dorsolateral prefrontal cortex (McClure et al. 1998, and references therein until 1997; Hinsberger et al. 1997; Kegeles et al. 1998; Shioiri et al. 1997), and also in parietal cortex (Bluml et al. 1999; Potwarka et al. 1999), albeit contradicted by others (Volz et al. 1998). These findings would support the hypothesis of an abnormal membrane phospholipid metabolism as evidenced by a reduced membrane synthesis (PME) and increased membrane breakdown (PDE), which is found in the first episode, as well as in medicated and chronic patients, suggesting that these alterations may reflect trait markers. In temporal lobes, only left side increased PDE has been reported (Fukuzako et al. 1996). Most in vivo 1H NMR studies have shown decreased NAA levels in bilateral frontal and temporal cortex and in the hippocampus (McClure et al. 1998, and references therein until 1997; Bertolino et al. 1998; Callicott et al. 1998; Cecil et al. 1999; Deicken et al. 1998; Thomas et al. 1998). Studies reported decreased NAA in the left thalamus (Heimberg et al. 1998), in the anterior cingulate (Deicken et al. 1997) and decreased NAA/Cho (and increased left Cho) in the basal ganglia (Fujimoto et al. 1996; Shioiri et al. 1996). Other regions have normal metabolite patterns (Bluml et al. 1999). The interpretation of the decreased NAA requires a careful treatment of the data since spectroscopic volumes may contain a mix of grey and white matter in which NAA behaves differently, requiring an accurate segmentation of brain tissue (Lim et al. 1998). The level of NAA decrease in general does not correlate with medication, clinical symptom scales, or duration of the disease. Finally, results on glutamate levels in prefrontal cortex are quite disparate, with a tendency towards decreased levels after medication (Bartha et al. 1997; Choe et al. 1996; Stanley et al. 1996).

References

Achten E, Boon P, Van-De Kerckhove T et al. (1997) Value of single-voxel proton MR spectroscopy in temporal lobe epilepsy. AJNR Am J Neuroradiol 18: 1131–1139

Achten E, Santens P, Boon P et al. (1998) Single-voxel proton MR spectroscopy and positron emission tomography for lateralization of refractory temporal lobe epilepsy [see comments]. AJNR Am J Neuroradiol 19: 1–8

Alonso J, Rovira A, Capellades J et al. (1996) Cerebral proton spectroscopy of people infected with the human immunodeficiency virus. Med Clin Barc 107: 361–365

Arnold DL, Wolinsky JS, Matthews PM et al. (1998) The use of magnetic resonance spectroscopy in the evaluation of the natural history of multiple sclerosis. J Neurol Neurosurg Psychiatry 64 Suppl 1: S94–101

Aotsuka A, Shinotoh H, Hattori T (1997) Magnetic resonance spectroscopy in Parkinson's disease and multiple system atrophy. Nippon Rinsho 55: 249–254

Bartha R, Williamson PC, Drost DJ et al. (1997) Measurement of glutamate and glutamine in the medial prefrontal cortex of never-treated schizophrenic patients and healthy controls by proton magnetic resonance spectroscopy. Arch Gen Psychiatry 54: 959–965

Bergman AJ, Van-der Knaap MS, Smeitink JA et al. (1996) Magnetic resonance imaging and spectroscopy of the brain in propionic acidemia: clinical and biochemical considerations. Pediatr Res 40: 404–409
Berry I, Ranjeva JP, Duthil P et al. (1998a) Diffusion and perfusion MRI, measurements of acute stroke events and outcome: present practice and future hope. Cerebrovasc Dis 8 Suppl 2: 8–16
Berry I, Ranjeva JP, Manelfe C et al. (1998b) Magnetic resonance imaging of multiple sclerosis lesions. Rev Neurol (Paris) 154: 607–617
Bertolino A, Callicott JH, Elman I et al. (1998a) Regionally specific neuronal pathology in untreated patients with schizophrenia: a proton magnetic resonance spectroscopic imaging study. Biol Psychiatry 43: 641–648
Bertolino A, Kumra S, Callicott JH et al. (1998b) Common pattern of cortical pathology in childhood-onset and adult-onset schizophrenia as identified by proton magnetic resonance spectroscopic imaging. Am J Psychiatry 155: 1376–1383
Block W, Karitzky J, Traber F et al. (1998) Proton magnetic resonance spectroscopy of the primary motor cortex in patients with motor neuron disease: subgroup analysis and follow-up measurements [see comments]. Arch Neurol 55: 931–936
Bluml S, Zuckerman E, Tan J et al. (1998) Proton-decoupled 31P magnetic resonance spectroscopy reveals osmotic and metabolic disturbances in human hepatic encephalopathy. J Neurochem 71: 1564–1576
Bluml S, Tan J, Harris K et al. (1999) Quantitative proton-decoupled P-31 MRS of the schizophrenic brain in vivo. J Comput Assist Tomogr 23: 272–275
Brockmann K, Pouwels PJ, Christen HJ et al. (1996) Localized proton magnetic resonance spectroscopy of cerebral metabolic disturbances in children with neuronal ceroid lipofuscinosis. Neuropediatrics 27: 242–248
Brooks DJ (1997) Advances in imaging Parkinson's disease [editorial]. Curr Opin Neurol 10: 327–331
Byrd SE, Tomita T, Palka PS et al. (1996) Magnetic resonance spectroscopy (MRS) in the evaluation of pediatric brain tumors. Part II: Clinical analysis. J Natl Med Assoc 88: 717–723
Cady EB (1996) Metabolite concentrations and relaxation in perinatal cerebral hypoxic-ischemic injury. Neurochem Res 21: 1043–1052
Callicott JH, Egan MF, Bertolino A et al. (1998) Hippocampal N-acetyl aspartate in unaffected siblings of patients with schizophrenia: A possible intermediate neurobiological phenotype. Biol Psychiatry 44: 941–950
Caplan LR (1997) New therapies for stroke. Arch Neurol 54: 1222–1224
Castillo M, Kwock L (1998) Proton MR spectroscopy of common brain tumors. Neuroimaging Clin North Am 8: 733–752
Cecil KM, Lenkinski RE (1998) Proton MR spectroscopy in inflammatory and infectious brain disorders. Neuroimaging Clin North Am 8: 863–880
Cecil KM, Lenkinski RE, Gur RE et al. (1999) Proton magnetic resonance spectroscopy in the frontal and temporal lobes of neuroleptic naive patients with schizophrenia. Neuropsychopharmacology 20: 131–140
Cendes F, Andermann F, Dubeau F et al. (1997a) Normalization of neuronal metabolic dysfunction after surgery for temporal lobe epilepsy. Evidence from proton MR spectroscopic imaging. Neurology 49: 1525–1533
Cendes F, Caramanos Z, Andermann F et al. (1997b) Proton magnetic resonance spectroscopic imaging and magnetic resonance imaging volumetry in the lateralization of temporal lobe epilepsy: a series of 100 patients. Ann Neurol 42: 737–746
Chang L, Ernst T, Tornatore C et al. (1997) Metabolite abnormalities in progressive multifocal leukoencephalopathy by proton magnetic resonance spectroscopy. Neurology 48: 836–845
Chang KH, Song IC, Kim SH et al. (1998) In vivo single-voxel proton MR spectroscopy in intracranial cystic masses [see comments]. AJNR Am J Neuroradiol 19: 401–405
Choe BY, Suh TS, Shinn KS et al. (1996) Observation of metabolic changes in chronic schizophrenia after neuroleptic treatment by in vivo hydrogen magnetic resonance spectroscopy. Invest Radiol 31: 345–352
Choe BY, Park JW, Lee KS et al. (1998) Neuronal laterality in Parkinson's disease with unilateral symptom by in vivo 1H magnetic resonance spectroscopy. Invest Radiol 33: 450–455
Chu WJ, Hetherington HP, Kuzniecky RI et al. (1998) Lateralization of human temporal lobe epilepsy by 31P NMR spectroscopic imaging at 4.1 T. Neurology 51: 472–479
Clanet M, Berry I (1998) Magnetic resonance imaging in multiple sclerosis. Curr Opin Neurol 11: 299–303
Clark JM, Marks MP, Adalsteinsson E et al. (1996) MELAS: Clinical and pathologic correlations with MRI, xenon/CT, and MR spectroscopy. Neurology 46: 223–227
Clarke CE, Lowry M, Horsman A (1997) Unchanged basal ganglia N-acetylaspartate and glutamate in idiopathic Parkinson's disease measured by proton magnetic resonance spectroscopy. Mov Disord 12: 297–301
Connelly A, Van Paesschen W, Porter DA et al. (1998) Proton magnetic resonance spectroscopy in MRI-negative temporal lobe epilepsy. Neurology 51: 61–66
Constantinidis I, Malko JA, Peterman SB et al. (1996) Evaluation of 1H magnetic resonance spectroscopic imaging as a diagnostic tool for the lateralization of epileptogenic seizure foci. Br J Radiol 69: 15–24
Cross JH, Connelly A, Jackson GD et al. (1996) Proton magnetic resonance spectroscopy in children with temporal lobe epilepsy. Ann Neurol 39: 107–113
Cross JH, Gordon I, Connelly A et al. (1997) Interictal 99Tc(m) HMPAO SPECT and 1H MRS in children with temporal lobe epilepsy. Epilepsia 38: 338–345
Cruz CJ, Aminoff MJ, Meyerhoff DJ et al. (1997) Proton MR spectroscopic imaging of the striatum in Parkinson's disease. Magn Reson Imaging 15: 619–624
Cwik VA, Hanstock CC, Allen PS et al. (1998) Estimation of brainstem neuronal loss in amyotrophic lateral sclerosis with in vivo proton magnetic resonance spectroscopy. Neurology 50: 72–77
Danielsen ER, Ross B (eds) (1998) Magnetic resonance spetroscopy diagnosis of neurological diseases. Marcel Dekker, New York Basel
Davie CA, Barker GJ, Thompson AJ et al. (1997) 1H magnetic resonance spectroscopy of chronic cerebral white matter lesions and normal appearing white matter in multiple sclerosis. J Neurol Neurosurg Psychiatry 63: 736–742
Davie C (1998) The role of spectroscopy in parkinsonism [editorial]. Mov Disord 13: 2–4
Deicken RF, Zhou L, Schuff N et al. (1997) Proton magnetic resonance spectroscopy of the anterior cingulate region in schizophrenia. Schizophr Res 27: 65–71

Deicken RF, Zhou L, Schuff N et al. (1998) Hippocampal neuronal dysfunction in schizophrenia as measured by proton magnetic resonance spectroscopy. Biol Psychiatry 43: 483–488

De Stefano N, Matthews PM, Fu L et al. (1998) Axonal damage correlates with disability in patients with relapsing-remitting multiple sclerosis. Results of a longitudinal magnetic resonance spectroscopy study. Brain 121: 1469–1477

Doyle VL, Barton SJ, Griffiths JR (1999) P-31 and H-1 MRS of human cancer. Curr Sci 76: 772–776

Dubowitz DJ, Bluml S, Arcinue E et al. (1998) MR of hypoxic encephalopathy in children after near drowning: correlation with quantitative proton MR spectroscopy and clinical outcome. AJNR Am J Neuroradiol 19: 1617–1627

Duc CO, Trabesinger AH, Weber OM et al. (1998) Quantitative H-1 MRS in the evaluation of mesial temporal lobe epilepsy in vivo. Magn Reson Imaging 16: 969–979

Duncan JS (1997) Imaging and epilepsy. Brain 120: 339–377

Ellis CM, Lemmens G, Williams SC et al. (1997) Changes in putamen N-acetylaspartate and choline ratios in untreated and levodopa-treated Parkinson's disease: a proton magnetic resonance spectroscopy study. Neurology 49: 438–444

Ellis CM, Simmons A, Andrews C et al. (1998) A proton magnetic resonance spectroscopic study in ALS: Correlation with clinical findings. Neurology 51: 1104–1109

Ende GR, Laxer KD, Knowlton RC et al. (1997) Temporal lobe epilepsy: bilateral hippocampal metabolite changes revealed at proton MR spectroscopic imaging. Radiology 202: 809–817

Engelbrecht V, Rassek M, Gartner J et al. (1997a) The value of new MRI techniques in adrenoleukodystrophy. Pediatr Radiol 27: 207–215

Engelbrecht V, Rassek M, Huismann J et al. (1997b) MR and proton MR spectroscopy of the brain in hyperhomocysteinemia caused by methylenetetrahydrofolate reductase deficiency. AJNR Am J Neuroradiol 18: 536–539

Ernst T, Chang L, Melchor R et al. (1997) Frontotemporal dementia and early Alzheimer disease: differentiation with frontal lobe H-1 MR spectroscopy. Radiology 203: 829–836

Falini A, Calabrese G, Origgi D et al. (1996) Proton magnetic resonance spectroscopy and intracranial tumours: clinical perspectives. J Neurol 243: 706–714

Falini A, Calabrese G, Filippi M et al. (1998) Benign versus secondary-progressive multiple sclerosis: the potential role of proton MR spectroscopy in defining the nature of disability. AJNR Am J Neuroradiol 19: 223–229

Federico F, Simone IL, Conte C et al. (1996) Prognostic significance of metabolic changes detected by proton magnetic resonance spectroscopy in ischaemic stroke. J Neurol 243: 241–247

Federico F, Simone IL, Lucivero V et al. (1997a) Proton magnetic resonance spectroscopy in Parkinson's disease and atypical parkinsonian disorders. Mov Disord 12: 903–909

Federico F, Simone IL, Lucivero V et al. (1997b) Proton magnetic resonance spectroscopy in Parkinson's disease and progressive supranuclear palsy. J Neurol Neurosurg Psychiatry 62: 239–242

Fu L, Matthews PM, De Stefano N et al. (1998) Imaging axonal damage of normal-appearing white matter in multiple sclerosis. Brain 121: 103–113

Fujimoto T, Nakano T, Takano T et al. (1996) Proton magnetic resonance spectroscopy of basal ganglia in chronic schizophrenia. Biol Psychiatry 40: 14–18

Fukuzako H, Fukuzako T, Takeuchi K et al. (1996) Phosphorus magnetic resonance spectroscopy in schizophrenia: correlation between membrane phospholipid metabolism in the temporal lobe and positive symptoms. Prog Neuropsychopharmacol Biol Psychiatry 20: 629–640

Furuya S, Naruse S, Ide M et al. (1997) Evaluation of metabolic heterogeneity in brain tumors using 1H-chemical shift imaging method. NMR Biomed 10: 25–30

Gadian DG, Leonard JV (1996) The role of magnetic resonance spectroscopy in the investigation of lactic acidosis and inborn errors of energy metabolism. J Inherit Metab Dis 19: 548–552

Gadian DG, Isaacs EB, Cross JH et al. (1996) Lateralization of brain function in childhood revealed by magnetic resonance spectroscopy. Neurology 46: 974–977

Ganesan V, Johnson A, Connelly A et al. (1997) Guanidinoacetate methyltransferase deficiency: new clinical features. Pediatr Neurol 17: 155–157

Garcia PA, Laxer KD, van-der Grond J et al. (1997) Correlation of seizure frequency with N-acetyl-aspartate levels determined by 1H magnetic resonance spectroscopic imaging. Magn Reson Imaging 15: 475–478

Geissler A, Lock G, Frund R et al. (1997) Cerebral abnormalities in patients with cirrhosis detected by proton magnetic resonance spectroscopy and magnetic resonance imaging. Hepatology 25: 48–54

Gideon P, Rosenbaum S, Sperling B et al. (1999) MR-visible brain water content in human acute stroke. Magn Reson Imaging 17: 301–304

Gillard JH, Barker PB, van Zijl PC et al. (1996) Proton MR spectroscopy in acute middle cerebral artery stroke. AJNR Am J Neuroradiol 17: 873–886

Girard N, Wang ZJ, Erbetta A et al. (1998) Prognostic value of proton MR spectroscopy of cerebral hemisphere tumors in children. Neuroradiology 40: 121–125

Giroud M, Walker P, Bernard D et al. (1996) Reduced brain N-acetyl-aspartate in frontal lobes suggests neuronal loss in patients with amyotrophic lateral sclerosis. Neurol Res 18: 241–243

Gonzalez RG, Guimaraes AR, Moore GJ et al. (1996) Quantitative in vivo 31P magnetic resonance spectroscopy of Alzheimer disease. Alzheimer Dis Assoc Disord 10: 46–52

Goodkin K, Wilkie FL, Concha M et al. (1997) Subtle neuropsychological impairment and minor cognitive-motor disorder in HIV-1 infection. Neuroradiological, neurophysiological, neuroimmunological, and virological correlates. Neuroimaging Clin North Am 7: 561–579

Gotsis ED, Fountas K, Kapsalaki E et al. (1996) In vivo proton MR spectroscopy: the diagnostic possibilities of lipid resonances in brain tumors. Anticancer Res 16: 1565–1567

Grand S, Esteve F, Remy C et al. (1997) Proton magnetic resonance spectroscopy: a metabolic approach of cerebral tumors and their follow-up after external radiation therapy. Rev Med Interne 18: 865–875

Gredal O, Rosenbaum S, Topp S et al. (1997) Quantification of brain metabolites in amyotrophic lateral sclerosis by localized proton magnetic resonance spectroscopy. Neurology 48: 878–881

Groenendaal F, van-der Grond J, van Haastert IC et al. (1996) Findings in cerebral proton spin resonance spectroscopy in newborn infants with asphyxia, and psychomotor development. Ned Tijdschr Geneeskd 140: 255–259

Gupta RK, Roy R, Dev R et al. (1996) Finger printing of Mycobacterium tuberculosis in patients with intracranial tuberculomas by using in vivo, ex vivo, and in vitro magnetic resonance spectroscopy. Magn Reson Med 36: 829–833

Gupta RK, Roy R (1999) Magnetic resonance imaging and spectroscopy of intracranial tuberculomas. Curr Sci 76: 783–788

Hagberg G (1998) From magnetic resonance spectroscopy to classification of tumors. A review of pattern recognition methods. NMR Biomed 11: 148–156

Hajek M, Dezortova M, Komarek V (1998) 1H MR spectroscopy in patients with mesial temporal epilepsy. MAGMA 7: 95–114

Hanrahan JD, Cox IJ, Edwards AD et al. (1998) Persistent increases in cerebral lactate concentration after birth asphyxia. Pediatr Res 44: 304–311

Harada M, Miyoshi H, Ootsuka H et al. (1997) Accuracy and clinical utility of quantitative proton magnetic resonance spectroscopy (MRS) on phantom and chronic cerebral ischemia. Nippon Igaku Hoshasen Gakkai Zasshi 57: 487–492

Harrison MJ, Newman SP, Hall CM et al. (1998) Evidence of CNS impairment in HIV infection: clinical, neuropsychological, EEG, and MRI/MRS study. J Neurol Neurosurg Psychiatry 65: 301–307

Haseler LJ, Sibbitt WL, Mojtahedzadeh HN et al. (1998) Proton MR spectroscopic measurement of neurometabolites in hepatic encephalopathy during oral lactulose therapy. AJNR Am J Neuroradiol 19: 1681–1686

Heimberg C, Komoroski RA, Lawson WB et al. (1998) Regional proton magnetic resonance spectroscopy in schizophrenia and exploration of drug effect. Psychiatry Res 83: 105–115

Heun R, Schlegel S, Graf MM et al. (1997) Proton magnetic resonance spectroscopy in dementia of Alzheimer type. Int J Geriatr Psychiatry 12: 349–358

Hinsberger AD, Williamson PC, Carr TJ et al. (1997) Magnetic resonance imaging volumetric and phosphorus 31 magnetic resonance spectroscopy measurements in schizophrenia. J Psychiatry Neurosci 22: 111–117

Hirsch JA, Lenkinski RE, Grossman RI (1996) MR spectroscopy in the evaluation of enhancing lesions in the brain in multiple sclerosis. AJNR Am J Neuroradiol 17: 1829–1836

Holopainen IE, Lundbom NM, Metsahonkala EL et al. (1997) Temporal lobe pathology in epilepsy: proton magnetic resonance spectroscopy and positron emission tomography study. Pediatr Neurol 16: 98–104

Holopainen IE, Valtonen ME, Komu ME et al. (1998) Proton spectroscopy in children with epilepsy and febrile convulsions. Pediatr Neurol 19: 93–99

Huda A, Guze BH, Thomas MA et al. (1998) Clinical correlation of neuropsychological tests with H-1 magnetic resonance spectroscopy in hepatic encephalopathy. Psychosom Med 60: 550–556

Huemer M, Muehl A, Wandl VK et al. (1998) Stroke-like encephalopathy in an infant with 3-hydroxy-3-methylglutaryl-coenzyme A lyase deficiency. Eur J Pediatr 157: 743–746

Hugg JW, Kuzniecky RI, Gilliam FG et al. (1996) Normalization of contralateral metabolic function following temporal lobectomy demonstrated by 1H magnetic resonance spectroscopic imaging. Ann Neurol 40: 236–239

Huppi PS, Barnes PD (1997) Magnetic resonance techniques in the evaluation of the newborn brain. Clin Perinatol 24: 693–723

Hwang JH, Graham GD, Behar KL et al. (1996) Short echo time proton magnetic resonance spectroscopic imaging of macromolecule and metabolite signal intensities in the human brain. Magn Reson Med 35: 633–639

Iranzo A, Moreno A, Pujol J et al. (1999) Proton magnetic resonance spectroscopy pattern of progressive multifocal leukoencephalopathy in AIDS. J Neurol Neurosurg Psychiatry 66: 520–523

Jackson GD, Connelly A (1996) Magnetic resonance imaging and spectroscopy. Curr Opin Neurol 9: 82–88

Jarvik JG, Lenkinski RE, Saykin AJ et al. (1996) Proton spectroscopy in asymptomatic HIV-infected adults: initial results in a prospective cohort study. J Acquir Immune Defic Syndr Hum Retrovirol 13: 247–253

Kaibara T, Tyson RL, Sutherland GR (1998) Human cerebral neoplasms studied using MR spectroscopy: a review. Biochem Cell Biol 76: 477–486

Kalra S, Cashman NR, Genge A et al. (1998) Recovery of N-acetylaspartate in corticomotor neurons of patients with ALS after riluzole therapy. Neuroreport 9: 1757–1761

Kamada K, Houkin K, Iwasaki Y et al. (1997) Metabolic and neurological patterns in chronic cerebral infarction: a single-voxel 1H-MR spectroscopy study. Neuroradiology 39: 560–565

Kattapong VJ, Brooks WM, Wesley MH et al. (1996) Proton magnetic resonance spectroscopy of vascular- and Alzheimer-type dementia. Arch Neurol 53: 678–680

Kegeles LS, Humaran TJ, Mann JJ (1998) In vivo neurochemistry of the brain in schizophrenia as revealed by magnetic resonance spectroscopy. Biol Psychiatry 44: 382–398

King D, Batuch GH (1998) Magnetic resonance imaging and temporal lobe epilepsy. Acta Neurol Scand 98: 217–223

Kizu O, Naruse S, Furuya S et al. (1998) Application of proton chemical shift imaging in monitoring of gamma knife radiosurgery on brain tumors. Magn Reson Imaging 16: 197–204

Knowlton RC, Laxer KD, Ende G et al. (1997) Presurgical multimodality neuroimaging in electroencephalographic lateralized temporal lobe epilepsy. Ann Neurol 42: 829–837

Korenke GC, Pouwels PJ, Frahm J et al. (1996) Arrested cerebral adrenoleukodystrophy: a clinical and proton magnetic resonance spectroscopy study in three patients. Pediatr Neurol 15: 103–107

Kostler H (1998) Proton magnetic resonance spectroscopy in portal-systemic encephalopathy. Metab Brain Dis 13: 291–301

Kugel H, Heindel W, Roth B et al. (1998) Proton MR spectroscopy in infants with cerebral energy deficiency due to hypoxia and metabolic disorders. Acta Radiol 39: 701–710

Kuzniecky R (1997) Magnetic resonance and functional magnetic resonance imaging: tools for the study of human epilepsy. Curr Opin Neurol 10: 88–91

Kuzniecky R, Hugg JW, Hetherington H et al. (1998) Relative utility of 1H spectroscopic imaging and hippocampal volumetry in the lateralization of mesial temporal lobe epilepsy. Neurology 51: 66–71

Lam WW, Wang ZJ, Zhao H et al. (1998) 1H MR spectroscopy of the basal ganglia in childhood: a semiquantitative analysis. Neuroradiology 40: 315–323

Landtblom AM, Sjoqvist L, Soderfeldt B et al. (1996) Proton MR spectroscopy and MR imaging in acute and chronic multiple sclerosis–ringlike appearances in acute plaques. Acta Radiol 37: 278–287

Laubenberger J, Haussinger D, Bayer S et al. (1996) HIV-related metabolic abnormalities in the brain: depiction with proton MR spectroscopy with short echo times. Radiology 199: 805–810

Laubenberger J, Haussinger D, Bayer S et al. (1997) Proton magnetic resonance spectroscopy of the brain in symptomatic and asymptomatic patients with liver cirrhosis [see comments]. Gastroenterology 112: 1610–1616

Lauriero F, Federico F, Rubini G et al. (1996) 99Tcm-HMPAO SPET and 1H-MRS (proton magnetic resonance spectroscopy) in patients with ischaemic cerebral infarction. Nucl Med Commun 17: 140–146

Laxer KD (1997) Clinical applications of magnetic resonance spectroscopy. Epilepsia 38 Suppl 4: S13-S17

Lazareff JA, Bockhorst KH, Curran J et al. (1998) Pediatric low-grade gliomas: prognosis with proton magnetic resonance spectroscopic imaging. Neurosurgery 43: 809–817

Lim KO, Adalsteinsson E, Spielman D et al. (1998) Proton magnetic resonance spectroscopic imaging of cortical gray and white matter in schizophrenia. Arch Gen Psychiatry 55: 346–352

Lopez VD, Lenkinski RE, Frank I (1997) Biochemical changes in the frontal lobe of HIV-infected individuals detected by magnetic resonance spectroscopy. Proc Natl Acad Sci USA 94: 9854–9859

Lorek AK, Penrice JM, Cady EB et al. (1996) Cerebral energy metabolism in isovaleric acidaemia. Arch Dis Child Fetal Neonatal Ed 74: F211-F213

Lu D, Pavlakis SG, Frank Y et al. (1996) Proton MR spectroscopy of the basal ganglia in healthy children and children with AIDS. Radiology 199: 423–428

Lu D, Margouleff C, Rubin E et al. (1997) Temporal lobe epilepsy: correlation of proton magnetic resonance spectroscopy and 18F-fluorodeoxyglucose positron emission tomography. Magn Reson Med 37: 18–23

McClure RJ, Keshavan MS, Pettegrew JW (1998) Chemical and physiologic brain imaging in schizophrenia. Psychiatr Clin North Am 21: 93–122

MacKay S, Ezekiel F, Di SV et al. (1996) Alzheimer disease and subcortical ischemic vascular dementia: evaluation by combining MR imaging segmentation and H-1 MR spectroscopic imaging. Radiology 198: 537–545

Mader I, Roser W, Hagberg G et al. (1996) Proton chemical shift imaging, metabolic maps, and single voxel spectroscopy of glial brain tumors. MAGMA 4: 139–150

Maldonado X, Alonso J, Giralt J et al. (1998) 31Phosphorus magnetic resonance spectroscopy in the assessment of head and neck tumors. Int J Radiat Oncol Biol Phys 40: 309–312

Marcus CD, Taylor RS, Sargentoni J et al. (1998) 1H MR spectroscopy of the brain in HIV-1-seropositive subjects: evidence for diffuse metabolic abnormalities. Metab Brain Dis 13: 123–136

Martin E, Buchli R, Ritter S et al. (1996) Diagnostic and prognostic value of cerebral 31P magnetic resonance spectroscopy in neonates with perinatal asphyxia. Pediatr Res 40: 749–758

Matthews PM, Pioro E, Narayanan S et al. (1996) Assessment of lesion pathology in multiple sclerosis using quantitative MRI morphometry and magnetic resonance spectroscopy. Brain 119: 715–722

Matthews PM, De Stefano N, Narayanan S et al. (1998) Putting magnetic resonance spectroscopy studies in context: axonal damage and disability in multiple sclerosis. Semin Neurol 18: 327–336

Mathews VP, Barker PB, Blackband SJ et al. (1995) Cerebral metabolites in patients with acute and subacute strokes: concentrations determined by quantitative proton MR spectroscopy. AJR Am J Roentgenol 165: 633–638

Meyerhoff DJ, Bloomer C, Cardenas V et al. (1999) Elevated subcortical choline metabolites in cognitively and clinically asymptomatic HIV+ patients. Neurology 52: 995–1003

Miller DH, Albert PS, Barkhof F et al. (1996) Guidelines for the use of magnetic resonance techniques in monitoring the treatment of multiple sclerosis. US National MS Society Task Force. Ann Neurol 39: 6–16

Miller DH, Grossman RI, Reingold SC et al. (1998) The role of magnetic resonance techniques in understanding and managing multiple sclerosis. Brain 121: 3–24

Moller HE, Weglage J, Wiedermann D et al. (1997) Kinetics of phenylalanine transport at the human blood-brain barrier investigated in vivo. Brain Res 778: 329–337

Moller HE, Weglage J, Wiedermann D et al. (1998) Blood-brain barrier phenylalanine transport and individual vulnerability in phenylketonuria. J Cereb Blood Flow Metab 18: 1184–1191

Moller HE, Vermathen P, Lentschig MG et al. (1999) Metabolic characterization of AIDS dementia complex by spectroscopic imaging. J Magn Reson Imaging 9: 10–18

Morgan MY (1996) Noninvasive neuroinvestigation in liver disease. Semin Liver Dis 16: 293–314

Morishita H, Naruse S, Furuya S et al. (1997) Evaluation of cerebral ischemia with metabolic image by using 3D-CSI–comparing with SPECT and PET. Nippon Rinsho 55: 1762–1767

Nagele T, Seeger U, Pereira P et al. (1999) Proton magnetic resonance spectroscopy to monitor the concentration changes of cerebral metabolites after TIPS implantation. Rofo Fortschr Geb Rontgenstr Neuen Bildgeb Verfahr 170: 298–303

Narayana PA, Doyle TJ, Lai D et al. (1998) Serial proton magnetic resonance spectroscopic imaging, contrast-enhanced magnetic resonance imaging, and quantitative lesion volumetry in multiple sclerosis. Ann Neurol 43: 56–71

Negendank WG, Sauter R, Brown TR et al. (1996) Proton magnetic resonance spectroscopy in patients with glial tumors: a multicenter study. J Neurosurg 84: 449–458

Novotny EJ, Hyder F, Shevell M et al. (1999) GABA changes with vigabatrin in the developing human brain. Epilepsia 40: 462–466

Paley M, Cozzone PJ, Alonso J et al. (1996) A multicenter proton magnetic resonance spectroscopy study of neurological complications of AIDS. AIDS Res Hum Retroviruses 12: 213–222

Pan JW, Hetherington HP, Vaughan JT et al. (1996) Evaluation of multiple sclerosis by 1H spectroscopic imaging at 4.1 T. Magn Reson Med 36: 72–77

Parnetti L, Tarducci R, Presciutti O et al. (1997) Proton magnetic resonance spectroscopy can differentiate Alzheimer's disease from normal aging. Mech Ageing Dev 97: 9–14

Pavlakis SG, Kingsley PB, Kaplan GP et al. (1998) Magnetic resonance spectroscopy: use in monitoring MELAS treatment. Arch Neurol 55: 849–852

Pavlakis SG, Lu D, Frank Y et al. (1998) Brain lactate and N-acetylaspartate in pediatric AIDS encephalopathy. AJNR Am J Neuroradiol 19: 383–385
Penrice J, Cady EB, Lorek A et al. (1996) Proton magnetic resonance spectroscopy of the brain in normal preterm and term infants, and early changes after perinatal hypoxia-ischemia. Pediatr Res 40: 6–14
Pettegrew JW, Klunk WE, Panchalingam K et al. (1997) Magnetic resonance spectroscopic changes in Alzheimer's disease. Ann N Y Acad Sci 826: 282–306
Petroff OA, Rothman DL, Behar KL et al. (1996) The effect of gabapentin on brain gamma-aminobutyric acid in patients with epilepsy. Ann Neurol 39: 95–99
Petroff OA, Mattson RH, Behar KL et al. (1998) Vigabatrin increases human brain homocarnosine and improves seizure control. Ann Neurol 44: 948–952
Petroff OA, Hyder F, Mattson RH et al. (1999a) Topiramate increases brain GABA, homocarnosine, and pyrrolidinone in patients with epilepsy [see comments]. Neurology 52: 473–478
Petroff OAC, Rothman DL, Behar KL et al. (1999b) Effects of valproate and other antiepileptic drugs on brain glutamate, glutamine, and GABA in patients with refractory complex partial seizures. Seizure 8: 120–127
Pietz J, Kreis R, Schmidt H et al. (1996) Phenylketonuria: findings at MR imaging and localized in vivo H-1 MR spectroscopy of the brain in patients with early treatment. Radiology 201: 413–420
Pietz J, Kreis R, Rupp A et al. (1999) Large neutral amino acids block phenylalanine transport into brain tissue in patients with phenylketonuria. J Clin Investig 103: 1169–1178
Pioro EP (1997) MR spectroscopy in amyotrophic lateral sclerosis/motor neuron disease. J Neurol Sci 152 Suppl 1: S49–S53
Potwarka JJ, Drost DJ, Williamson PC et al. (1999) A H-1-decoupled P-31 chemical shift imaging study of medicated schizophrenic patients and healthy controls. Biol Psychiatry 45: 687–693
Pouwels PJ, Kruse B, Korenke GC et al. (1998) Quantitative proton magnetic resonance spectroscopy of childhood adrenoleukodystrophy. Neuropediatrics 29: 254–264
Prost R, Haughton V, Li SJ (1997) Brain tumors: localized H-1 MR spectroscopy at 0.5 T. Radiology 204: 235–238
Rajanayagam V, Grad J, Krivit W et al. (1996) Proton MR spectroscopy of childhood adrenoleukodystrophy. AJNR Am J Neuroradiol 17: 1013–1024
Rajanayagam V, Balthazor M, Shapiro EG et al. (1997) Proton MR spectroscopy and neuropsychological testing in adrenoleukodystrophy. AJNR Am J Neuroradiol 18: 1909–1914
Remy C, Grand S, Lai ES et al. (1995) 1H MRS of human brain abscesses in vivo and in vitro. Magn Reson Med 34: 508–514
Rooney WD, Goodkin DE, Schuff N et al. (1997) 1H MRSI of normal appearing white matter in multiple sclerosis. Mult Scler 3: 231–237
Rooney WD, Miller RG, Gelinas D et al. (1998) Decreased N-acetylaspartate in motor cortex and corticospinal tract in ALS. Neurology 50: 1800–1805
Rose SE, de-Zubicaray GI, Wang D et al. (1999) A 1H MRS study of probable Alzheimer's disease and normal aging: implications for longitudinal monitoring of dementia progression. Magn Reson Imaging 17: 291–299
Ross BD, Danielsen ER, Bluml S (1996) Proton magnetic resonance spectroscopy: the new gold standard for diagnosis of clinical and subclinical hepatic encephalopathy? Dig Dis 14 Suppl 1: 30–39
Saliba E, Barantin L, Akoka S et al. (1997) (Circulation and cerebral metabolism in neonatal hypoxia-ischemia. J Gynecol Obstet Biol Reprod Paris 26: 465–469
Salvan AM, Vion DJ, Confort GS et al. (1997a) Brain proton magnetic resonance spectroscopy in HIV-related encephalopathy: identification of evolving metabolic patterns in relation to dementia and therapy. AIDS Res Hum Retroviruses 13: 1055–1066
Salvan AM, Vion DJ, Confort GS et al. (1997b) Cerebral metabolic alterations in human immunodeficiency virus-related encephalopathy detected by proton magnetic resonance spectroscopy. Comparison between sequences using short and long echo times. Invest Radiol 32: 485–495
Salvan AM, Lamoureux S, Michel G et al. (1998) Localized proton magnetic resonance spectroscopy of the brain in children infected with human immunodeficiency virus with and without encephalopathy. Pediatr Res 44: 755–762
Sarchielli P, Presciutti O, Pelliccioli GP et al. (1999) Absolute quantification of brain metabolites by proton magnetic resonance spectroscopy in normal-appearing white matter of multiple sclerosis patients. Brain 122 Part 3: 513–521
Sarchielli P, Presciutti O, Tarducci R et al. (1998) 1H-MRS in patients with multiple sclerosis undergoing treatment with interferon beta-1a: results of a preliminary study. J Neurol Neurosurg Psychiatry 64: 204–212
Saunders DE, Howe FA, van-den Boogaart A et al. (1997) Discrimination of metabolite from lipid and macromolecule resonances in cerebral infarction in humans using short echo proton spectroscopy. J Magn Reson Imaging 7: 1116–1121
Schiepers C, Van Hecke P, Vandenberghe R et al. (1997) Positron emission tomography, magnetic resonance imaging and proton NMR spectroscopy of white matter in multiple sclerosis. Mult Scler 3: 8–17
Seitz D, Grodd W, Schwab A et al. (1998) MR imaging and localized proton MR spectroscopy in late infantile neuronal ceroid lipofuscinosis. AJNR Am J Neuroradiol 19: 1373–1377
Shimizu H, Kumabe T, Tominaga T et al. (1996) Noninvasive evaluation of malignancy of brain tumors with proton MR spectroscopy. AJNR Am J Neuroradiol 17: 737–747
Shioiri T, Hamakawa H, Kato T et al. (1996) Proton magnetic resonance spectroscopy of the basal ganglia in patients with schizophrenia: a preliminary report. Schizophr Res 22: 19–26
Shioiri T, Someya T, Murashita J et al. (1997) Multiple regression analysis of relationship between frontal lobe phosphorus metabolism and clinical symptoms in patients with schizophrenia. Psychiatry Res 76: 113–122
Schuff N, Amend D, Ezekiel F et al. (1997) Changes of hippocampal N-acetyl aspartate and volume in Alzheimer's disease. A proton MR spectroscopic imaging and MRI study. Neurology 49: 1513–1521
Schuff N, Amend DL, Meyerhoff DJ et al. (1998) Alzheimer disease: quantitative H-1 MR spectroscopic imaging of frontoparietal brain. Radiology 207: 91–102
Schulze A, Hess T, Wevers R et al. (1997) Creatine deficiency syndrome caused by guanidinoacetate methyltransferase deficiency: diagnostic tools for a new inborn error of metabolism [see comments]. J Pediatr 131: 626–631

Schurmann M, Engelbrecht V, Lohmeier K et al. (1997) Cerebral metabolic changes in biotinidase deficiency. J Inherit Metab Dis 20: 755–760

Simone IL, Federico F, Tortorella C et al. (1998) Localised 1H-MR spectroscopy for metabolic characterisation of diffuse and focal brain lesions in patients infected with HIV. J Neurol Neurosurg Psychiatry 64: 516–523

Sitoh YY, Tien RD (1998) Neuroimaging in epilepsy. J Magn Reson Imaging 8: 277–288

Speck O, Thiel T, Hennig J (1996) Grading and therapy monitoring of astrocytomas with 1H-spectroscopy: preliminary study. Anticancer Res 16: 1581–1585

Sperl W, Felber S, Skladal D et al. (1997) Metabolic stroke in carbamyl phosphate synthetase deficiency. Neuropediatrics 28: 229–234

Stanley JA, Williamson PC, Drost DJ et al. (1996) An in vivo proton magnetic resonance spectroscopy study of schizophrenia patients. Schizophr Bull 22: 597–609

Stanley JA, Cendes F, Dubeau F et al. (1998) Proton magnetic resonance spectroscopic imaging in patients with extratemporal epilepsy. Epilepsia 39: 267–273

Stockler S, Hanefeld F (1997) Guanidinoacetate methyltransferase deficiency: a newly recognized inborn error of creatine biosynthesis. Wien Klin Wochenschr 109: 86–88

Sutton LN, Wang ZJ, Wehrli SL et al. (1997) Proton spectroscopy of suprasellar tumors in pediatric patients. Neurosurgery 41: 388–394

Taylor JS, Langston JW, Reddick WE et al. (1996) Clinical value of proton magnetic resonance spectroscopy for differentiating recurrent or residual brain tumor from delayed cerebral necrosis. Int J Radiat Oncol Biol Phys 36: 1251–1261

Taylor JS, Ogg RJ, Langston JW (1998) Proton MR spectroscopy of pediatric brain tumors. Neuroimaging Clin North Am 8: 753–779

Taylor RS, Turjanski N, Bhattacharya S et al. (1999) A proton magnetic resonance spectroscopy study of the striatum and cerebral cortex in Parkinson's disease. Metab Brain Dis 14: 45–55

Tedeschi G, Bertolino A, Lundbom N et al. (1996) Cortical and subcortical chemical pathology in Alzheimer's disease as assessed by multislice proton magnetic resonance spectroscopic imaging. Neurology 47: 696–704

Tedeschi G, Litvan I, Bonavita S et al. (1997a) Proton magnetic resonance spectroscopic imaging in progressive supranuclear palsy, Parkinson's disease and corticobasal degeneration. Brain 120: 1541–1552

Tedeschi G, Lundbom N, Raman R et al. (1997b) Increased choline signal coinciding with malignant degeneration of cerebral gliomas: a serial proton magnetic resonance spectroscopy imaging study. J Neurosurg 87: 516–524

Thomas MA, Huda A, Guze B et al. (1998a) Cerebral 1H MR spectroscopy and neuropsychologic status of patients with hepatic encephalopathy. AJR Am J Roentgenol 171: 1123–1130

Thomas MA, Ke Y, Levitt J et al. (1998b) Preliminary study of frontal lobe 1H MR spectroscopy in childhood-onset schizophrenia. J Magn Reson Imaging 8: 841–846

Thompson JE, Castillo M, Kwock L et al. (1998) Usefulness of proton MR spectroscopy in the evaluation of temporal lobe epilepsy. AJR Am J Roentgenol 170: 771–776

Tien RD, Lai PH, Smith JS et al. (1996) Single-voxel proton brain spectroscopy exam (PROBE/SV) in patients with primary brain tumors. AJR Am J Roentgenol 167: 201–209

Tomoi M, Kimura H, Yoshida M et al. (1997) Alterations of lactate (+lipid) concentration in brain tumors with in vivo hydrogen magnetic resonance spectroscopy during radiotherapy. Invest Radiol 32: 288–296

Tourbah A, Stievenart JL, Iba ZM et al. (1996) In vivo localized NMR proton spectroscopy of normal appearing white matter in patients with multiple sclerosis. J Neuroradiol 23: 49–55

Tourbah A, Stievenart JL, Iba ZM et al. (1997) Localized proton magnetic resonance spectroscopy in patients with adult adrenoleukodystrophy. Increase of choline compounds in normal appearing white matter. Arch Neurol 54: 586–592

Tracey I, Carr CA, Guimaraes AR et al. (1996) Brain choline-containing compounds are elevated in HIV-positive patients before the onset of AIDS dementia complex: A proton magnetic resonance spectroscopic study [published erratum appears in Neurology 1996 Jun;46(6):1787]. Neurology 46: 783–788

Tzika AA, Vigneron DB, Dunn RS et al. (1996) Intracranial tumors in children: small single-voxel proton MR spectroscopy using short- and long-echo sequences. Neuroradiology 38: 254–263

van der Grond J, Balm R, Klijn CJ et al. (1996) Cerebral metabolism of patients with stenosis of the internal carotid artery before and after endarterectomy. J Cereb Blood Flow Metab 16: 320–326

van der Grond J, Gerson JR, Laxer KD et al. (1998) Regional distribution of interictal 31P metabolic changes in patients with temporal lobe epilepsy. Epilepsia 39: 527–536

van der Grond J, Mali WP (1998) Multifunctional magnetic resonance imaging of cerebrovascular disease. Eur Radiol 8: 726–738

van der Grond J, van-Everdingen KJ, Eikelboom BC et al. (1999) Assessment of borderzone ischemia with a combined MR imaging-MR angiography-MR spectroscopy protocol. J Magn Reson Imaging 9: 1–9

van-der Knaap M, Bakker HD, Valk J (1998) MR imaging and proton spectroscopy in 3-hydroxy-3-methylglutaryl coenzyme A lyase deficiency. AJNR Am J Neuroradiol 19: 378–382

Vermathen P, Ende G, Laxer KD et al. (1997) Hippocampal N-acetylaspartate in neocortical epilepsy and mesial temporal lobe epilepsy. Ann Neurol 42: 194–199

Vion DJ, Salvan AM, Confort GS et al. (1998) Brain proton magnetic resonance spectroscopy. Indications for diagnosis and follow-up of HIV-related encephalopathy in the adult. Presse Med 27: 1398–1405

Volz HP, Rzanny R, Rossger G et al. (1998) 31Phosphorus magnetic resonance spectroscopy of the dorsolateral prefrontal region in schizophrenics–a study including 50 patients and 36 controls. Biol Psychiatry 44: 399–404

Waldrop SM, Davis PC, Padgett CA et al. (1998) Treatment of brain tumors in children is associated with abnormal MR spectroscopic ratios in brain tissue remote from the tumor site [see comments]. AJNR Am J Neuroradiol 19: 963–970

Wang ZJ, Zimmerman RA (1998) Proton MR spectroscopy of pediatric brain metabolic disorders. Neuroimaging Clin North Am 8: 781–807

Wardlaw JM, Marshall I, Wild J et al. (1998) Studies of acute ischemic stroke with proton magnetic resonance spectroscopy: relation between time from onset, neurological deficit, metabolite abnormalities in the infarct, blood flow, and clinical outcome. Stroke 29: 1618–1624

Weber OM, Verhagen A, Duc CO et al. (1999) Effects of vigabatrin intake on brain GABA activity as monitored by spectrally edited magnetic resonance spectroscopy and positron emission tomography. Magn Reson Imaging 17: 417–425

Wilkinson ID, Lunn S, Miszkiel KA et al. (1997a) Proton MRS and quantitative MRI assessment of the short term neurological response to antiretroviral therapy in AIDS. J Neurol Neurosurg Psychiatry 63: 477–482

Wilkinson ID, Miller RF, Miszkiel KA et al. (1997b) Cerebral proton magnetic resonance spectroscopy in asymptomatic HIV infection. AIDS 11: 289–295

Woermann FG, McLean MA, Bartlett PA et al. (1999) Short echo time single-voxel 1H magnetic resonance spectroscopy in magnetic resonance imaging-negative temporal lobe epilepsy: different biochemical profile compared with hippocampal sclerosis. Ann Neurol 45: 369–376

Yoshino E, Ohmori Y, Imahori Y et al. (1996) Irradiation effects on the metabolism of metastatic brain tumors: analysis by positron emission tomography and 1H-magnetic resonance spectroscopy. Stereotact Funct Neurosurg 66 Suppl 1: 240–259

Young IR, Cecil Charles H (eds) (1996) MR spectroscopy – clinical applications and techniques. Martin Dunitz, London

6 Recent Advances in MR Contrast Media

VINCENT DOUSSET

CONTENTS

6.1 Introduction

The need for contrast agents in MR imaging has been challenged over the past decade. The contrast obtained spontaneously between tissues does not appear sufficient for diagnosis or for the characterization of the nature and function of pathological processes. Today, small size molecules of gadolinium are widely used in a clinical setting and a large variety of contrasts can be obtained. New contrast agents are appearing with the goal of providing more specific information.

V. DOUSSET, MD, PhD
Service de Neuroradiologie, CHU Pellegrin, Place Amélie Raba-Léon, 33076 Bordeaux Cédex, France

6.2 Gadolinium Enhancement

6.2.1 Principle of Gadolinium Enhancement

A contrast mechanism is commonly exploited by the administration of contrast agents based on the paramagnetic atom, gadolinium (Gd). Such a paramagnetic substance, if in close proximity to water, will cause a shortening of both T1 and T2 relaxation times, with the shortening of T1 being the dominant effect. Due to the shortened T1 relaxation times in areas where Gd is in close proximity to water, these areas become hyperintense on T1 W images compared with identical images made without the administration of gadolinium. Gadolinium chelates do not cross the intact blood-brain barrier (BBB) because of the tight junctions between endothelial cells. Therefore, enhancement in T1 W images following the infusion of contrast agent demonstrates breakdown of the BBB or the presence of a neovascularisation lacking tight junctions.

6.2.2 Pulse Sequences using Gadolinium

6.2.2.1 Spin-Echo and Gradient-Echo Sequences

A large variety of T1 weighted sequences are available to demonstrate the T1 shortening induced by gadolinium in pathological processes. Refocused spin-echo (SE) sequences are the most commonly used of these sequences. They have several advantages over other sequences such as gradient-echo (GE) sequences. The 180° pulse compensates for local field inhomogeneities, thus inducing a reduction of magnetic susceptibility based artifacts at the air/tissue and tissue/bone interfaces. Furthermore, contrast between enhancing and non-enhancing tissues is better with SE than GE.

Gradient-echo imaging is mostly used in T1-weighted volume acquisition with a slice thickness of 1–2 mm, which can be displayed in the three-dimensional fashion. This is of major interest when investigating a patient for stereotaxy. It is also helpful to gain time in routine post-contrast imaging.

6.2.2.2
Fat Suppression Techniques

In the investigation of head and neck, including the orbit, it is sometimes useful to suppress the signal from fat. This is of particular importance on post-gadolinium imaging (Fig. 6.1). Two techniques are currently the most often used to suppress the signal of fat: the short tau inversion recovery (STIR) and the frequency-selective saturation pulse usually called fat-sat. In the former, the achievement of fat suppression lies on the time of the inversion time (TI), which is chosen such that the longitudinal magnetization of fat is zero when the 90° pulse of the spin echo sequence is applied. The value of TI for a given tissue changes with the field strength. At 1.5 Tesla, the TI for fat suppression is around 150 ms. However, the STIR-induced fat suppression technique is not suitable when using gadolinium. The shortened T1 of water molecules in the vicinity of gadolinium become closer to the T1 of fat. Thus, the TI of the STIR sequence may induce a suppression of the signal from both fat molecules and the water molecules in the vicinity of gadolinium. When using gadolinium, the most commonly used fat suppression technique is the fat-sat or chem-sat technique. Fat and water molecules resonate at frequencies that are separated by about 215 Hz (at 1.5 Tesla). Saturation of fat refers to the application of a narrow-bandwidth 90° saturation pulse at the frequency of fat molecules. If this pulse is followed by the SE sequence, the signal of fat is not detected whereas water protons are unaffected by the saturation pulse. This implies that the water molecule in the vicinity of the gadolinium molecule will not be affected by the saturation pulse. Thus, the fat-sat technique appears the technique of choice for improving contrast between fat and gadolinium enhancing tissues. Nevertheless, the fat-sat technique has some drawbacks, mostly because magnetic field inhomogeneities may cause shifts of the water and fat resonance frequencies, resulting in inefficient fat suppression.

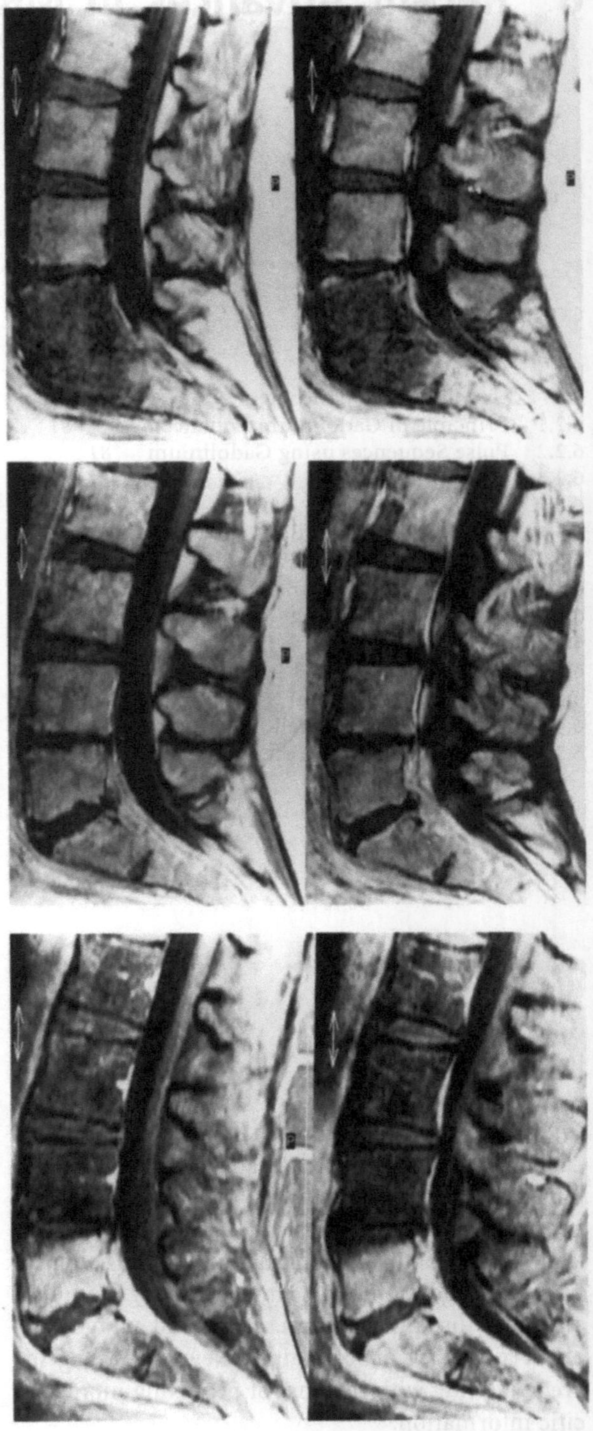

Fig. 6.1a–c. Gadolinium enhancement using fat suppression on T1-weighted images. **a–c** Spondylitis at L5–S1 level. **a** T1-weighted image; **b** T1-weighted image with gadolinium; **c** T1-weighted image with gadolinium and fat suppression. Note the pseudonormalization of the image when using gadolinium without fat suppression

6.2.2.3
Magnetization Transfer

The usefulness of magnetization transfer contrast (MTC) has been proven to increase the contrast between gadolinium-enhanced tissues and non-enhancing tissues. The principle of MTC lies in the difference of magnetic-field induced frequencies of free water protons and macromolecule bound water protons (Wolff and Balaban 1989). Between the two pools of protons, there is continuous through-space dipole-dipole cross-relaxation or chemical exchanges. In some tissues such as muscles, white matter (WM) and gray matter (GM), the rate of exchange is very high because the macromolecules have numerous surface sites where exchanges between the two pools are possible. However, in other tissues such as fat or cerebrospinal fluid the rate of exchange is very low or non-existent, either because the surface sites of exchanges are rare or because the macromolecules are absent. Based on the Forsen and Hoffman (1963) experiment, the saturation of macromolecular bound water protons induces a reduction in the magnetization of exchanging free water protons. This means that when using a saturating pulse at the frequency of non-visible macromolecule bound water protons, one may induce a decrease in signal of the MR-visible free water protons. The loss of signal is proportional to the amount and quality of exchanging sites. In tissues such as muscles, WM and GM, the signal may decrease by up to 50%–60% according to the technique used (Dousset et al. 1992). The most widely used technique to induce magnetization transfer is called the off-resonance technique. A saturation pulse at the frequency of the bound water proton (i.e., from 1000 to 5000 Hz at a distance from the free water proton frequency) is generated immediately before the imaging sequence. The saturation does not directly affect the "visible" free water protons. However, at the time of signal collection, the transfer of energy from the macromolecular bound water protons to the free water protons induced a loss of signal intensity in the resulting image. On the other hand, the pathway of proton-electron relaxation induced by gadolinium to the free water molecule is almost totally unaffected by the MTC pulse (Huot et al. 1997). Thus when using the MTC imaging technique in the presence of gadolinium, the contrast between gadolinium-enhanced lesions and non-enhancing WM and GM is strongly increased.

The most useful clinical application of MTC with gadolinium is in the detection of lesions at the level of the meninges. The decreased signal intensity of the normal brain parenchyma increases the contrast with pathological enhancing meninges. This might be the determinant for the diagnosis of carcinomatous or granulomatous meningitis (Runge et al. 1995). We routinely use MTC with gadolinium when meningitis is suspected (Fig. 6.2).

The most attractive clinical application is in the detection of gadolinium enhancing brain parenchyma lesions when the presence of enhancement or when the number of lesions is critical for the therapeutic strategy. This may be the case for many pathological conditions such as for the detection of brain metastases, for the therapeutic assessment in multiple sclerosis or in infectious lesions, etc. One drawback is the relative enhancement induced by the MTC to the parenchymal lesions prior to the injection of gadolinium. Because most lesions in the CNS are accompanied by an increase of free water molecules and scattered macromolecules, the rate of MT

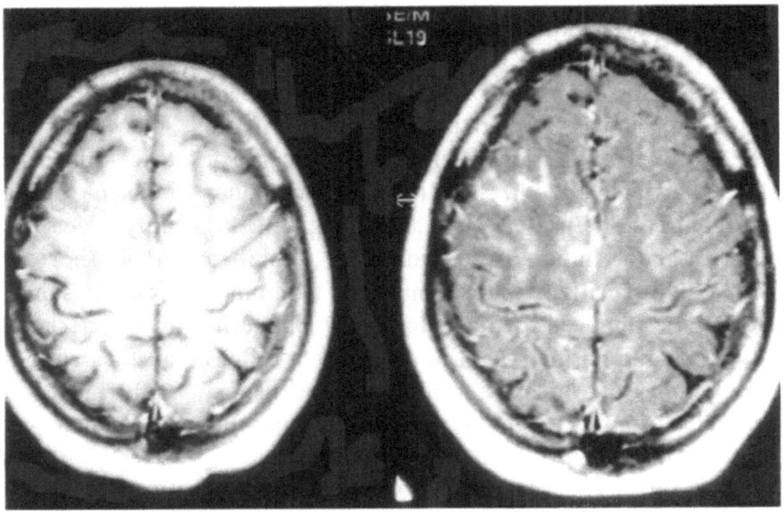

Fig. 6.2. Gadolinium enhancement using magnetization transfer on T1-weighted images. *Left* T1-weighted image with gadolinium, *right* T1-weighted image with gadolinium and magnetization transfer. Contrast between normal brain and meninges is enhanced using magnetization transfer in a case of metastatic meningitis

in those lesions is less than in the normal WM and GM. Thus, on MTC images prior to the administration of gadolinium those lesions may appear slightly hyperintense to GM and WM. To avoid a false diagnosis of gadolinium uptake, it is highly recommended to acquire images with MTC before and after the administration of gadolinium. It is not clear cut yet if MTC should be routinely used with gadolinium for parenchymal lesions. At our institute, we formally recommend the use of MTC with gadolinium when imaging the meninges and in some cases of parenchymal lesions when the confirmation of enhancement is required.

6.2.2.4 Ultra-Fast Imaging for Hemodynamic Evaluation

There are several MRI techniques proposed to evaluate the hemodynamic conditions of the CNS. The most robust in a clinical setting uses the magnetic susceptibility changes induced by the passage of concentrated gadolinium through the capillary beds. The so-called perfusion imaging (or hemodynamic-weighted MRI) requires the injection of a bolus of gadolinium using a single (0.1 mmol/kg) or a double dose. The dephasing of nearby protons results in a transient decrease in signal intensity on T2-weighted or T2*-weighted images (Rosen et al. 1991). This is possible only during the first passage of gadolinium through the capillary beds and on condition that the gadolinium stays in the vessel lumen. In the normal brain and in some pathological conditions such as acute stroke, the presence of the intact blood-brain barrier (BBB) allows the contrast agent to remain in the blood stream. The decrease of signal intensity is inversely proportional to the concentration of gadolinium in the vessel lumen. Thus, on T2-weighted or T2*-weighted images, regions of decreased perfusion will appear more intense relative to regions of normal perfusion. The temporal resolution of the sequence is of importance. The time for a concentrated bolus to pass through the capillary bed in the CNS is around 10–15 s. In order to draw the curve of the signal intensity, ultra-fast imaging techniques are required. The use of echoplanar imaging (EPI) allows a good temporal resolution to be combined with a high sensitivity to local magnetic field inhomogeneities induced by the gadolinium. This technique is based on the repetition of gradient echoes (the number of which determines the EPI factor) generated by powerful gradients. The EPI factor may be set such that during one repetition time the k-space is filled. This technique is called single-shot EPI. Combined with rapid reconstruction techniques, the EPI allows an image to be obtained every second or even less. However, the spatial resolution is much lower than for routine imaging. Other techniques such as the PRESTO technique may combine good temporal and spatial resolutions.

From the curve obtained by the decreased signal intensity induced by the first passage of concentrated gadolinium, one may calculate several parameters that may be pertinent to describe the hemodynamic conditions of the parenchyma. In affected regions with reduced perfusion, the time for gadolinium to reach the tissue and the time to the maximum decrease in signal intensity are delayed, the mean transit time (MTT) is longer, and the relative cerebral blood volume (rCBV) and cerebral blood flow (rCBF) are normal or reduced. Maps of these parameters are obtained based on a pixel by pixel calculation. However, one must be aware that the values of MTT, CBF and CBV are relative and not true (Sorensen et al. 1999). They allow the comparison of normal from hemodynamically modified areas (Fig. 6.3).

Beside the early assessment of hemodynamically compromised areas during the early phase of ischemia, the use of perfusion imaging remains under evaluation for other clinical conditions. If the BBB is ruptured, the leakage of gadolinium in the interstitial space changes the curve of the signal intensity produced by the concentrated gadolinium in the capillary beds. It usually leads to an underestimation of the perfusion parameters. However, from complex calculations that integrate the perfusion and the enhancement curves, the vascularity of some lesions such as tumors may be assessed. Thus, the characterization of vascularity may be useful to differentiate tumor versus treatment-related changes, to assess tumor grade or to test the efficacy of anti-angiogenesis drug therapy.

6.2.2.5 Gadolinium Bolus Tracking for MR Angiography

A new approach in MR angiography (MRA) involved three-dimensional (3D) imaging during the rapid bolus of contrast media. By administering gadolinium chelates intravenously, the T1 of blood is considerably shortened compared to that of background tissue. It is then possible to image the arteries directly. For neck vessels, the technique allows from the aortic arch to the circle of Willis to be covered (Fig. 6.4). This technique may have a tremendous impact on the management of patients with atherosclerotic vessels and may reduce the practice of conventional invasive angiography.

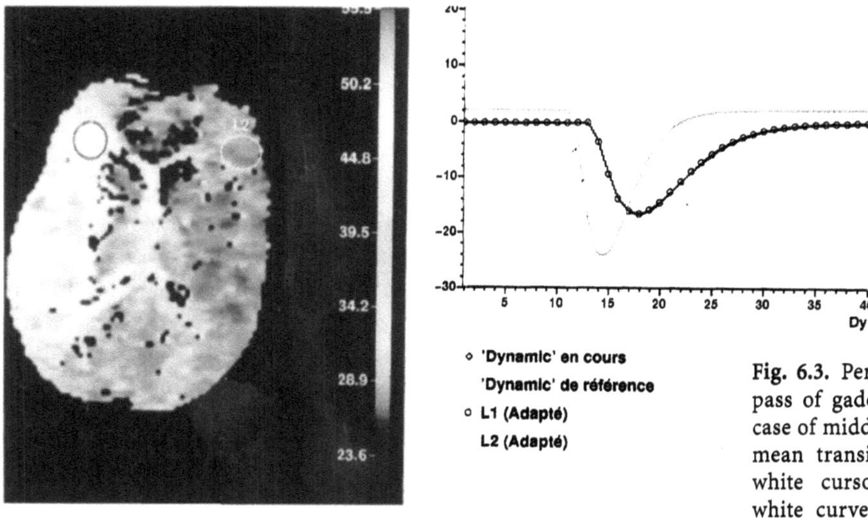

Fig. 6.3. Perfusion imaging using the first pass of gadolinium through the brain in a case of middle cerebral artery stroke. Map of mean transit time (MTT) with black and white cursors. Corresponding black and white curves (*right*) indicate the dynamic passage of gadolinium in the regions of interest. Note that the black curve shows a delay in the bolus arrival and a reduction of the height of the curve in the affected area

6.2.3 Gadolinium Dose

The dose of 0.1 mmol/kg chelates of gadolinium has been set up previously based on combined inocuity and diagnostic efficacy. However, many studies have demonstrated that at higher doses the conspicuity and the number of enhancing lesions dramatically improve. It is now proposed to use a triple dose of gadolinium in some conditions that are explained above in the magnetization transfer section of this chapter. The major drawback of increasing the dose of gadolinium is the cost of the procedure. Routinely, there is no need to increase the dose of gadolinium and the use of magnetization transfer should be preferred. For perfusion imaging or for gadolinium bolus tracking based MR angiography, increasing the dose of gadolinium might be useful to increase the signal to noise ratio.

6.3 Blood-Pool Agents

6.3.1 Principle and Potential Applications

The characterization of the vascular compartment of tissues including small and large vessels might be of importance for the evaluation of many diseases. Blood pool agents (BPA) are molecules of large size which remain for a longer time in the vascular bed in comparison to the small-molecular gadolinium che-

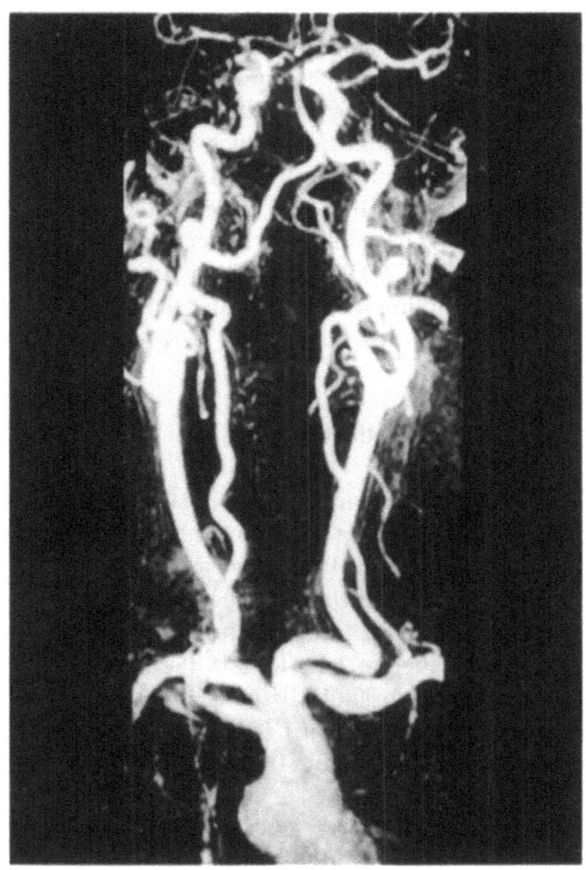

Fig. 6.4. MR angiography of the neck vessels using bolus tracking of gadolinium during the first pass on a heavily T1-weighted sequence. Note that the aortic arch and the circle of Willis are visualized

lates. Most of the BPA molecules which are currently tested in humans are gadolinium-based macromolecules. They might be interesting to investigate the arterial vasculature and perform angiography in steady state conditions. However, as with the injection of gadolinium chelates, the venous enhancement may produce some overlaps between arteries and veins. Imaging of coronary and pulmonary veins is promising. Another application is the evaluation of tumor vascular beds. Anti-angiogenesis therapies might be proposed and controlled based on such analysis. Finally, with BPA, the evaluation of the input function for perfusion imaging could help to quantify the perfusion parameters such as the blood flow which is hardly determined with dynamic susceptibility imaging using the first pass of gadolinium chelates.

6.3.2 Gadolinium-Based BPA

Several compounds are currently being tested in phase I–III studies. MS325 is a lipophilic DTPA gadolinium BPA which has the property of a transitory non-covalent coupling with the albumin of blood. This gives an equilibrium which allows the compound to remain a long time in the blood. Other gadolinium-based BPA are large molecules composed of several gadolinium molecules: Gadomere 17 composed of DTPA-gadolinium dendrimer and DOTA-gadolinium macromolecular monomer.

6.3.3 Superparamagnetic BPA

Ultra-small particle iron oxides (USPIO) are molecules of 20–40 nm size. They have a long blood half-life (several hours or days) because they are cleared from the blood by the cells of the mononuclear phagocytic system. In comparison to superparamagnetic iron oxide particles (SPIO), the liver Kupffer cells do not remove quickly the USPIO from blood.

BPA may be based on USPIO. The NC100150 is currently being tested for MR coronary angiography (Taylor et al. 1999). Such contrast agents produce a T1 and T2* effect whereas gadolinium-based BPA produce mostly a strong T1 effect.

6.4 Macrophage Imaging

6.4.1 USPIO

USPIO are dextran-coated iron oxide nanoparticles that are internalized into a variety of cells, among which are cells of the mononuclear phagocytic system (Weissleder et al. 1990, 1997; Bonnemain 1998). Due to the presence of iron, they produce a susceptibility effect that is observable on T2- and T2*-weighted images as low signal intensity. At lower concentrations they produce a T1 effect seen as a high signal intensity on T1-weighted images.

The ability of USPIO to accumulate in the cytoplasm of macrophagic cells makes it possible to investigate the presence of such cells in normal or pathological conditions. Potential applications include the visualisation of normal lymph nodes in MR lymphographia, the macrophagic uptake in pathological conditions of the CNS and the uptake from macrophagic cells in the atherosclerotic vessel wall. In addition, USPIO have been observed in C6 glioma cells implanted in the rat brain, several hours after IV injection of the contrast agent (Zimmer et al. 1995).

6.4.2 USPIO and Neck MR Lymphography

The most advanced application is for human MR lymphography (Anzai et al. 1994; Guimareas et al. 1994). USPIO are being tested in phase III studies. The contrast agent is given by intravenous infusion over 30 min. The MR imaging is performed 24 h later. Normal lymph nodes may exhibit a decreased signal intensity on T2*-weighted images whereas metastatic lymph nodes do not exhibit the presence of the contrast agent or only partially. This application could be very helpful in the evaluation of the lymph node spread of numerous neoplasms (Harisinghani et al. 1999). For head and neck imaging, it may help to solve the problem of staging the disease and may contribute to the therapeutic strategy.

6.4.3 USPIO in the Central Nervous System

Within the brain, macrophagic cells originate from two pools: hematogenous or bone-marrow-derived (monocytes) and activated microglia. In the early phases of many pathological conditions such as inflammation, demyelination, trauma or infection, the CNS exhibits intense macrophage activity (MARTIN and MCFARLAND 1995).

Since USPIO particles are taken up by macrophages in the mononuclear phagocyte system, macrophages with USPIO burden might be detectable by MRI in inflammatory sites within the CNS, several hours after IV injection of the contrast agent (DOUSSET et al. 1999).

Several experimental studies have been conducted on a model of multiple sclerosis (MS), experimental autoimmune encephalomyelitis (EAE) (DOUSSET et al. 1999a). Lesions of low signal intensity were seen on T2-weighted images 24 h after USPIO intravenous injection (Fig. 6.5). Pathological analysis demonstrated that the contrast agents were located in the cytoplasm of cells with macrophagic features. Interestingly, the comparison with gadolinium enhancement showed that EAE lesion with USPIO uptake might not be enhanced by gadolinium chelates (DOUSSET et al. 1999b). Thus, it might be possible that non-ruptured blood-brain barrier is permeable to USPIO loaded blood cells of macrophagic activity.

The contrast agent has been tested recently by our group on MS patients and the preliminary results are promising. Several clinical applications could be tested to characterize the macrophagic activity in many diseases of the CNS.

Although professional phagocytic cells such as blood monocytes and tissue macrophages are the most robust candidates for USPIO imaging, other cells seem to have the ability to capture the USPIO in vivo or in vitro. An experimental study by ZIMMER et al. (1995) on glial C6 implanted tumors has shown that the USPIO might be taken up by tumor cells. The recent report on human glial tumor also appears interesting (SCOTT ENOCHS et al. 1999). Moreover, by using USPIO, T cells have been tagged in vitro and visualized in vivo after their direct injection in rat testicle. The same strategy has been applied to oligodendrocytes in focal lesions of the rat spinal cord (BULTE et al. 1999). In such cases, MRI has the potential role to control the cell activity in a given tissue.

6.4.4 USPIO and Vessel Wall

In a recent report, it has been nicely demonstrated that USPIO loaded endothelial cells may colonize the vessel wall when driven by electromagnetic forces applied around the damaged portion (CONSIGNY et al. 1999).

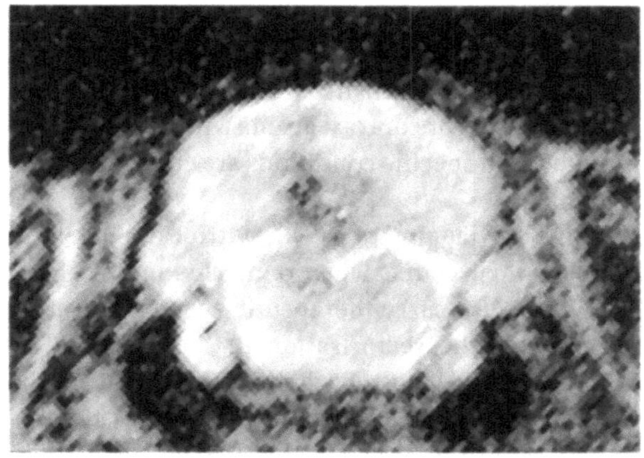

Fig. 6.5. Ultra small particle iron oxide (UPSIO) in acute experimental allergic encephalomyelitis. Coronal T2-weighted image at the level of the posterior fossa obtained 24 h after UPSIO injection. Due to the magnetic susceptibility effect, the lesions appear hypointense in the cerebellum. The contrast agent is located within the macrophages that are present in the lesion

Another experimental study on rabbit atherosclerotic lesions has shown that macrophages of the lipidic lesions may be detectable using USPIO (RUEHM et al. 1999). This could be of special interest to distinguish between active and non-active atherosclerotic lesions. It can be important in the management of atherosclerotic lesions of the carotid that are suspected to cause embolisms. It also could help to better understand in vivo the pathophysiology of such a lesion.

6.5 Strategies and Contrast Agents for the Future

Many other strategies using contrast agents may be proposed. First, the characterization of specific cells could be a step forward for in vivo imaging. The major problem is to reach the membrane receptors without modifying their biological properties and to obtain a detectable signal. Contrast agents coupled to cell membrane specific receptor antibodies have been used to characterize the surface cell. So far, this technique has not been successful for human use.

Second, the concept of a contrast agent that only reveals the pathological sites that are not positive elsewhere could dramatically help the imaging analysis. It could also help to investigate the whole body and determine the sites of disseminated diseases. It has been proposed to call these contrast agents "intelligent contrast agents" (Mikawa et al. 1999). Calcium sensitive, pH sensitive, temperature sensitive contrast agents or contrast agents with a blocker that is removed in specific conditions are currently in development.

Third, the tagging of cells in vitro can be helpful to follow their course when reinjected in vivo. Such cells could also carry therapeutic agents, thus making possible the vectorization to specific sites. By MRI one could control whether the target of the therapy has been reached, or by using focused ultrasound coupled to MRI, the therapeutic agent could be delivered on the specific sites of the disease.

References

Anzai Y, Blackwell KE, Hirschowitz SL et al. (1994) Initial clinical experience with dextran-coated superparamagnetic iron oxide for detection of lymph node metastases in patients with head and neck cancer. Radiology 192: 709–715

Bonnemain B (1998) Superparamagnetic agents in magnetic resonance imaging: physicochemical characteristics and clinical applications. A review. J Drug Target 6: 167–174

Dousset V, Grossman R, Ramer K et al. (1992) Experimental allergic encephalomyelitis and multiple sclerosis: lesion characterization with magnetization transfer imaging. Radiology 182: 483–491

Dousset V, Delalande C, Ballarino L et al. (1999a) In vivo macrophage activity imaging in the central nervous system detected by magnetic resonance. Magn Reson Med 41: 329–333

Dousset V, Ballarino L, Delalande C et al. (1999b) Comparison of ultrasmall particles of iron oxide (USPIO) T2-weighted, conventional T2-weighted and gadolinium-enhanced T1-weighted MR images in rats with experimental autoimmune encephalomyelitis. AJNR Am J Neuroradiol 20: 223–227

Forsén S, Hoffman RA (1963) Study of moderately rapid chemical exchange reactions by means of nuclear magnetic double resonance. J Chem Phys 39: 2892–2901

Guimareas R, Clément O, Bittoun J et al. (1994) MR lymphography with superparamagnetic iron nanoparticles in rats: pathologic basis for contrast enhancement. AJR Am J Roentgenol 162: 201–207

Huot P, Dousset V, Hatier E et al. (1997) Improvement of post-gadolinium contrast with magnetization transfer. Eur Radiol 7 (Suppl. 5): S174-S177

Harisinghani MG, Saini S, Weissleder R et al. (1999) MR lymphangiography using ultrasmall superparamagnetic iron oxide in patients with primary abdominal and pelvic malignancies: radiographic-pathologic correlation. AJR Am J Roentgenol 172: 1347–1351

Martin R, McFarland H (1995) Immunological aspects of experimental allergic encephalomyelitis and multiple sclerosis. Crit Rev Clin Lab Sci 32: 121–182

Mikawa M, Miwa T, Akaike T et al. (1999) An intelligent MRI contrast agent for tumor sensing. Proceedings of the International Society for Magnetic Resonance in Medicine, p 344

Rosen BR, Belliveau JW, Aronen HJ et al. (1991) Susceptibility contrast imaging of cerebral blood volume: human experience. Magn Reson Med 22: 293–299

Ruehm SG, Quick HH, Corot C et al. (1999) MR imaging of atherosclerotic plaque with ultrasmall super paramagnetic iron oxide (USPIO) in hyperlipidemic rabbits. Proceedings of the International Society for Magnetic Resonance in Medicine, p 81

Runge VM, Wells JW, Williams NM et al. (1995) Detectability of early brain meningitis with magnetic resonance imaging. Invest Radiol 30: 484–495

Scott Enochs W, Harsh G, Hochberg F et al. (1999) Improved delineation of human brain tumors on MR images using a long-circulating, superparamagnetic iron oxide agent. JMRI 9: 228–232

Sorensen AG, Copen WA, Ostergaard L et al. (1999) Hyperacute stroke: simultaneous measurement of relative cerebral blood volume, relative cerebral blood flow, and mean tissue transit time. Radiology 210: 519–527

Taylor AM, Panting JR, Keegan J et al. (1999) Safety and preliminary findings with the intravascular contrast agent NC100150 injection for MR coronary angiography. JMRI 9: 220–227

Weissleder R, Elizondo G, Wittenberg J et al. (1990) Ultrasmall superparamagnetic iron oxide: characterization of a new class contrast agents for MR imaging. Radiology 175: 494–498

Weissleder R, Cheng H-C, Bogdanova A et al. (1997) Magnetically labeled cells can be detected by MR imaging. JMRI 7: 258–263

Wolff SD, Balaban RS (1989) Magnetization transfer contrast (MTC) and tissue water proton relaxation in vivo. Magn Reson Med 10: 135–144

Zimmer C, Weissleder R, Poss K et al. (1995) MR imaging of phagocytosis in experimental gliomas. Radiology 197: 533–538

Brain

7 Guidelines for Brain MR Imaging

PHILIPPE DEMAEREL

CONTENTS

7.1 Introduction

MR imaging is the examination of choice in brain imaging but there is still limited evidence of effectiveness in regard to its impact on patient management. There is clearly a need for research on this topic.

Is there still a role for computed tomography (CT) in brain imaging? Can we define clinical protocols for brain MR imaging? Do we routinely need intravenous contrast agents? These and other questions will be addressed in this chapter, which serves as an introduction to the second part of this book. Several topics will be discussed more in detail in other chapters.

7.2 The Status of MR imaging

Radiology certainly plays a role in the rising health care costs. In an ideal world the introduction of a new (and better) imaging technique should result in a reduction of the health care costs and an improvement of the quality of care. Technology assessment will play a key role in reaching this goal.

Most of us are convinced that MR imaging is at least as effective as CT but few studies have compared both techniques in terms of cost, intermediate outcome and effects on quality of life. One study on the cost-effectiveness of neuroimaging, in the United States, for patients with equivocal neurological symptoms showed that only CT was cost-effective for most patients (MUSHLIN et al. 1997). The cost-effectiveness of MR imaging improved as the likelihood of an underlying disease increased. Australian data have shown savings in the diagnosis of several conditions for which MR imaging was known to be promising through eliminating more invasive examinations and the sometimes associated need for hospitalization (CROWE and HAILEY 1989). Technology assessment must be rapid were it only because the field of radiology changes rapidly and slow assessments would produce results that are no longer up-to-date. But, it is not easy to evaluate the impact of an imaging technique on the clinical decision. Imaging will never be obtained in isolation but will be part of several investigations considered by the clinician in reaching a decision on management of the patient (see Chap. 1). The decision-making process is complex.

Most published comparisons between CT and MR imaging consider pathological conditions while it is clear that the determination of clinical guidelines for an imaging technique and the proof of effectiveness must be based on clinical indications.

There is a growing interest for this kind of research in radiology. It is important to realize that technology assessment is not simple and requires a rigorous methodology (HAILEY and McDONALD 1996, SUNSHINE and MCNEIL 1997).

An interesting paper on the effect of brain MR imaging on diagnosis, diagnostic work-up, therapy and prognosis in 103 inpatients revealed important conclusions (HIRSCH et al. 1996). MR imaging ruled out a diagnosis or suggested a new one in 63% of cases. The presumptive clinical diagnoses included

PH. DEMAEREL, MD, PhD
Consultant Neuroradiologist, Department of Radiology, University Hospitals, Herestraat 49, 3000 Leuven, Belgium

stroke (27%), tumor (26%), infection (10%), hemorrhage (6%), vasculitis (4%) and other diseases (27%). The MR examination confirmed the existence of or determined the extent of known disease in 38%. Changes in diagnostic work-up and therapy planning occurred 24% and 34% of the time. According to the referring physician, MR imaging had an effect on prognosis 47% of the time. These findings reflect the impact of MR imaging on the clinical assessment and provide indirect evidence for societal efficacy of brain MR imaging.

7.3 When to Order CT or MR imaging?

Neuroimaging plays a crucial role in the diagnosis of central nervous system disorders. Although MR imaging is being increasingly used in the diagnostic and therapeutic work-up, computed tomography still offers some advantages. CT has been shown to be excellent for the evaluation of bony structures, calcification, ossification and acute hemorrhage. The use of contrast agents will be discussed in Sect. 7.6. The role of imaging techniques in assessing the spine and spinal cord is discussed in Chap. 25.

It is evident that the indications for CT will depend on the availability of MR imaging. One important factor to consider with respect to which imaging examination to choose for the evaluation of the patient is the efficacy of a particular imaging modality with regard to diagnosing a specific disease process. Advantages of MR imaging include high spatial and contrast resolution, multiplanar imaging capability and lack of ionizing radiation and iodinated contrast agents. On the other hand MR imaging may be contraindicated in some patients because of the presence of ferromagnetic implants/foreign bodies or claustrophobia. MR imaging requires more cooperation from patients and patient motion always results in image artifacts. Ideally if the access to MR imaging were unrestricted, one would expect the number of CT examinations to decrease dramatically. But, it is much more difficult to provide straightforward guidelines when the availability of MR imaging is limited. Often this situation will lead to the duplication of information from another procedure while it should be the purpose to replace or complement a procedure. CT will be requested to avoid the waiting list for MR imaging and to exclude major abnormalities, but in a varying percentage of patients MR imaging will subsequently be requested. In our experience this happens in up to 30% of patients. It is therefore clear that practice guidelines are mandatory.

At this moment, CT remains the examination of choice in acute trauma and intensive care patients because of the monitoring equipment, life support and traction devices that these patients often need. The location of CT close to the emergency department is another advantage because the risk associated with the transportation of these patients is often underestimated. It often concerns the exclusion of intracranial bleeding or edema. It is, however, important to realize that a normal CT in these situations does not exclude abnormalities. MR imaging is indicated in these patients as soon as it is feasible in order to exclude smaller axonal shearing injuries and/or brain contusion.

The role of CT in the assessment of stroke is changing. Until the mid-nineties the wait and see policy meant that these patients underwent only CT in order to exclude an intracranial bleeding. The increasing interest in intraarterial thrombolysis is changing the approach of stroke. The possible role of diffusion/perfusion MR imaging in selecting the patients who may benefit from thrombolysis is being investigated (see Chaps. 8, 10). It has been suggested that these techniques could demonstrate the "penumbra," corresponding to that part of the brain that is compromised but still may recover if reperfusion is obtained rapidly.

CT is also indicated in patients who cannot have MR imaging for one of the above mentioned reasons.

Overall MR imaging is superior in the evaluation of most diseases and this is particularly true in neuropediatrics. State of the art imaging of the pituitary gland and orbit is discussed in Chaps. 19 and 20.

7.4 The Battlefield of Pulse Sequences

Multiple sequences are available and similar techniques may have different names according to the different vendors. Does the ideal standard procedure exist? Do we routinely need T1-weighted images? Can we replace conventional spin-echo techniques by fast spin-echo techniques? What is the role of fluid attenuated inversion recovery sequences? These questions play an important role in daily practice.

The two major groups of sequences are the spin-echo (SE) and the gradient-echo (GE) sequences. A more detailed discussion can be found in Chap. 3.

The conventional spin-echo (CSE) technique belongs to the first group. The inversion recovery (IR), short tau inversion recovery (STIR) and fluid attenuated inversion recovery sequence belong to the same group but are obtained with magnetization preparation. Rapid acquisition with relaxation enhancement (RARE) belongs to the SE group with multi-echo technique. This technique formed the basis for the fast SE (FSE) and turbo SE (TSE) techniques. Using TSE or FSE techniques, the fat appears hyperintense as compared with the CSE techniques and the sequence is characterized by a better contrast and spatial resolution. Due to a limited sensitivity to susceptibility differences, blood degradation products are less well observed.

The turbo IR, fast fluid attenuated inversion recovery (FLAIR) and turboFLAIR belong to the group of SE sequences using multi-echo techniques with magnetization preparation. A FLAIR sequence produces heavily T2-weighted images, while simultaneously suppressing the signal from cerebrospinal fluid, by applying an inversion pulse with a long recovery time between this pulse and the start of the measurement. The successful implementation of RARE acquisition schemes meant a significant reduction of the time of measurement. The technique has been used in most pathological conditions and proved particularly useful to document periventricular and subcortical abnormalities (Fig. 7.1). But one should be careful when interpreting FLAIR images. Artifacts are often present in the posterior fossa. Occasionally the FLAIR image may be less clear than the T2 weighted and proton density images (Fig. 7.2).

Spin-echo single-shot techniques without (HASTE and RARE) and with (IR-HASTE and IR-RARE) magnetization preparation have been used in the differentiation of epidermoid tumors and arachnoid cysts and in the detection intratumoral cysts or necrosis in solid lesions (IKUSHIMA et al. 1997).

The GE sequences belong to the second group.

Compared with CSE, the 180° refocusing pulse is omitted in a GE sequence of the fast low-angle shot (FLASH). The result is a T2*-weighted sequence resulting in a higher sensitivity to susceptibility artifacts but being at the same time more appropriate to studying blood degradation products such as deoxyhemoglobin and hemosiderin. The difference between FLASH and FISP (fast imaging with steady precession) lies in the build-up of a steady state for the transverse magnetization, which is only present

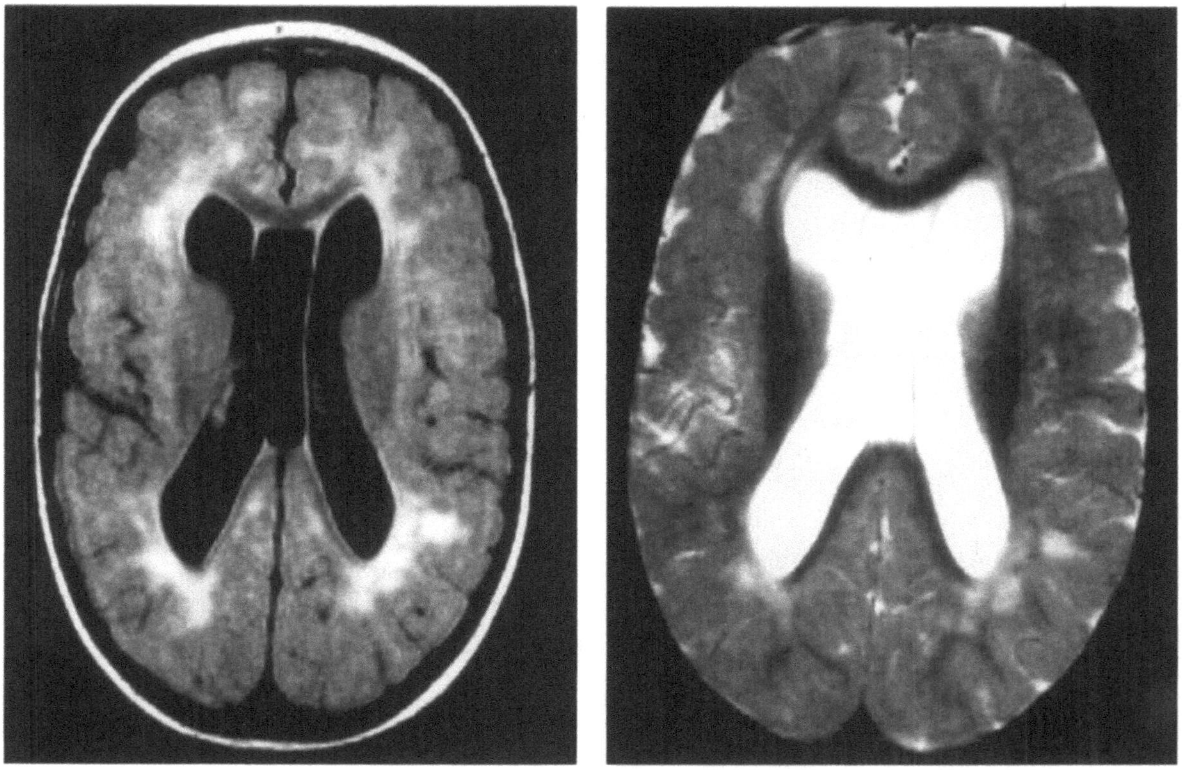

a b

Fig. 7.1a,b. Axial fast FLAIR (**a**) and DESTIR T2 weighted (**b**) MR images in a child with polymicrogyria. The white matter involvement is more clearly seen on the fast FLAIR image

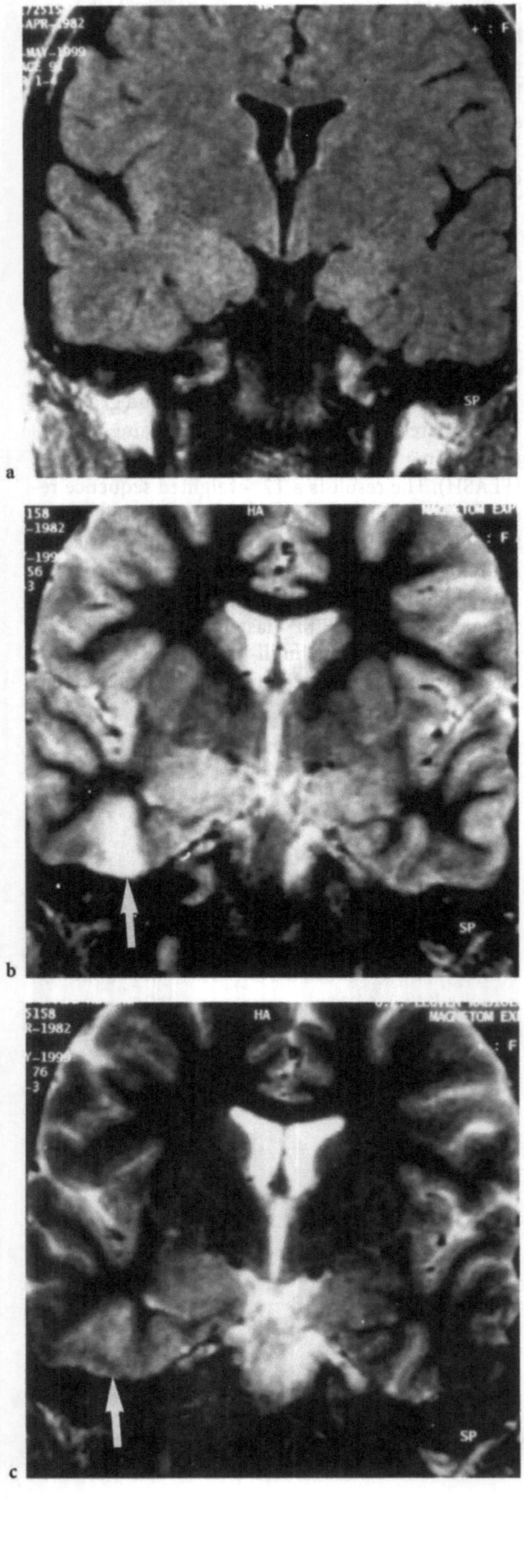

Fig. 7.2a–c. Coronal fast FLAIR (a), proton density (b) and T2 weighted (c) DESTIR images in a patient with focal cortical dysplasia. Note the poor visualization on the fast FLAIR image

in the latter. A sequence derived from the FISP technique is the constructive interference in steady state (CISS) (Casselman et al. 1993). This sequence consists of the addition of two sequences with an alternation of the RF phase with disappearance of the interference patterns (see Chap. 3). The heavy T2-weighting of steady-state gradient-echo techniques with spin-echo sampling has been used to obtain MR-cisternographic images for detection of cerebrospinal fluid leaks (Eberhardt et al. 1997). Fast spin-echo images with fat suppression, using coronal and sagittal 3-mm interleaved contiguous slices, of the sinuses and petrous bones showed a significant correlation with the surgical findings (El Gammal et al. 1998). Thin-section coronal CT is useful as it may help in focusing the MR cisternographic examination.

Another group of GE techniques is those with a preparation of magnetization. The combination of the shortest possible repetition time (TR), a low flip angle and an inversion pulse prior to the rapid acquisition was called snapshotFLASH. The three-dimensional version of this technique was called magnetization prepared rapid acquired gradient echoes (MPRAGE).

Echo planar imaging is the best known single-shot GE sequence. The classical concept uses a single excitation pulse followed by multiple phase-encoded gradient-echoes. This ultrafast technique can acquire an image in 30–100 ms. Their most promising clinical applications include diffusion and perfusion imaging and functional imaging. The major disadvantages are the magnetic susceptibility and chemical shift artifacts. Diffusion-weighted imaging is being increasingly used in clinical practice. The best known application is probably acute stroke (see Chap. 10 and Lutsep et al. 1997). It allows the early detection of even the smallest ischemic lesions and the differentiation of new from older lesions. New software releases give instantaneously an ADC map together with the diffusion-weighted images (Fig. 7.3). But its application in brain abscess, multiple sclerosis, tumors and Creutzfeldt-Jakob has been reported too. It may allow the differentiation between cytotoxic and vasogenic edema (Fig. 7.4). Diffusion-weighted images may also be sensitive to the detec-

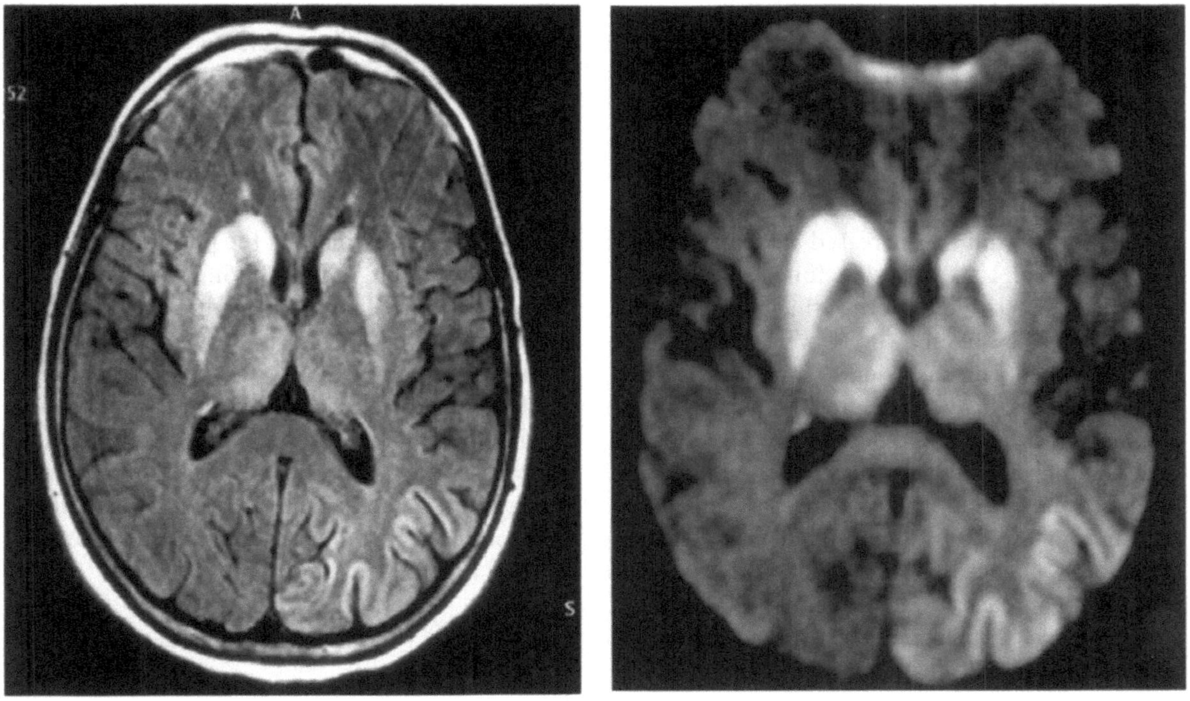

a b

Fig. 7.3a,b. Axial diffusion weighted (**a**) MR image and apparent diffusion coefficient (ADC) map (**b**) showing an infarct in the posterior cerebral artery territory 2 h after the insult. Note the low ADC

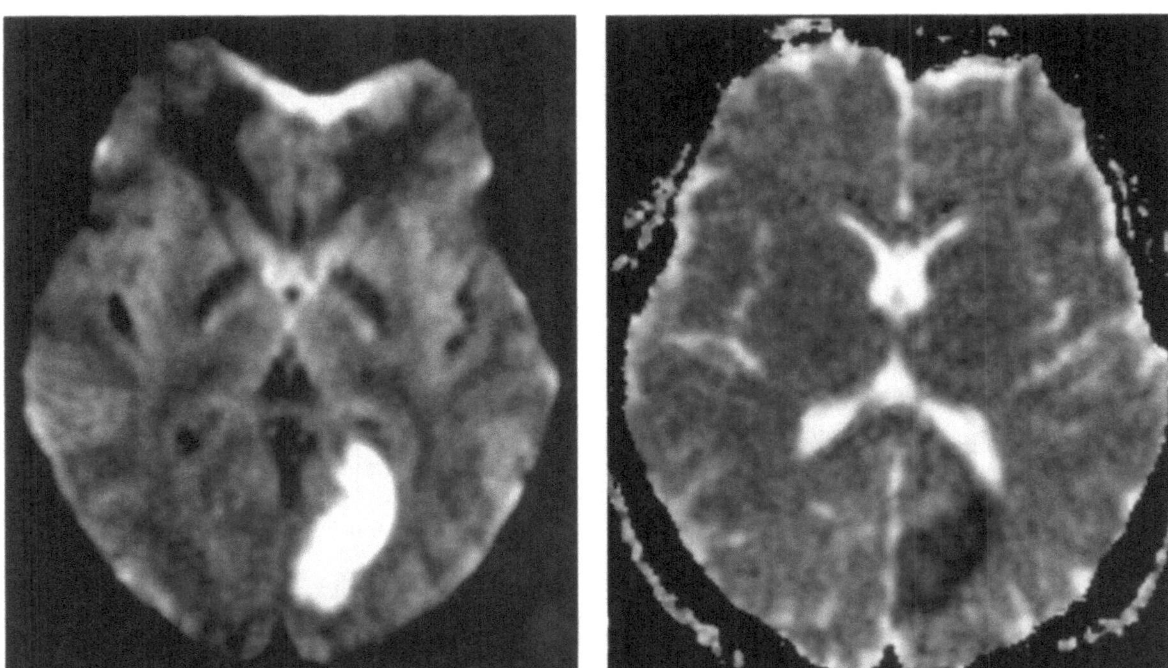

a b

Fig. 7.4a,b. Axial FLAIR (**a**) and diffusion-weighted (**b**) MR images showing the involvement of the caudate heads and lentiform nuclei in a patient with Creutzfeldt-Jakob disease. The involvement of the left temporal and occipital cortex is much better seen on the diffusion-weighted image tion of myelin-edema, which is associated with vacuolating myelinopathy (see Chap. 22).

It is very difficult to define the ideal routine protocol. The easiest and for a long time the most widely used protocol consists of a T1- and a proton-density and T2-weighted SE sequence. Turbo spin echo or FSE has not replaced CSE despite the reduced measurement time and the increased spatial resolution (Norbash et al. 1992) (Fig. 7.5). If it has been decided to use FSE techniques for routine brain imaging, one should also obtain a GE T2-weighted sequence whenever there is a suspicion of a hemorrhagic lesion. Examples include imaging following cranial trauma, hypertension and hematoma (Fig. 7.6). The combination of a high resolution T2-weighted FSE sequence and a fast FLAIR sequence is a valuable alternative to the classical proton density and T2-weighted sequence. The gradient- and spin-echo (GRASE) approach produce heavily T2-weighted images while further reducing the measurement time relative to FSE imaging (Fellner et al. 1997). The image quality and the contrast spectrum of GRASE imaging remain slightly inferior to that of FSE.

One could easily develop a fast imaging protocol consisting of, e.g., 5 min imaging time in two different planes. The efficacy of such a rapid imaging protocol was shown in the screening of children and adolescents with suspected intracranial tumors (Medina et al. 1998). The final diagnosis included a wide variety of diseases. The sensitivity of the fast screening protocol was 100%, the specificity 92.6% and the false positive rate 7.2%.

CSE, FSE and fastFLAIR have been compared in evaluation of the lesion load in multiple sclerosis (Yousry et al. 1997). FSE (TR=2500 ms) was better than CSE (TR=3000 ms) particularly in cortical and subcortical areas, fastFLAIR was far better than CSE except for the assessment of the posterior fossa and fastFLAIR was better than FSE. Single-shot EPI techniques have been assessed in multiple sclerosis and an echo time of 45 ms has been recommended (Wolansky et al. 1998).

T1-weighted sequences often do not contribute to the diagnosis. Because fat, methemoglobin, venous thrombosis, calcification and cortical laminar necrosis may return a high signal on pre-contrast images, their routine acquisition is recommended (Boyko et al. 1992) (Fig. 7.7).

7.5 Clinical Protocols for Brain Imaging

In the near future it will become increasingly important to define fixed protocols for MR imaging in order to optimize efficacy and efficiency in daily practice (see Chap. 1). First it will be necessary to define the routine brain MR protocol to image the patient presenting with non-specific neurological signs or symptoms. In a second step standard proto-

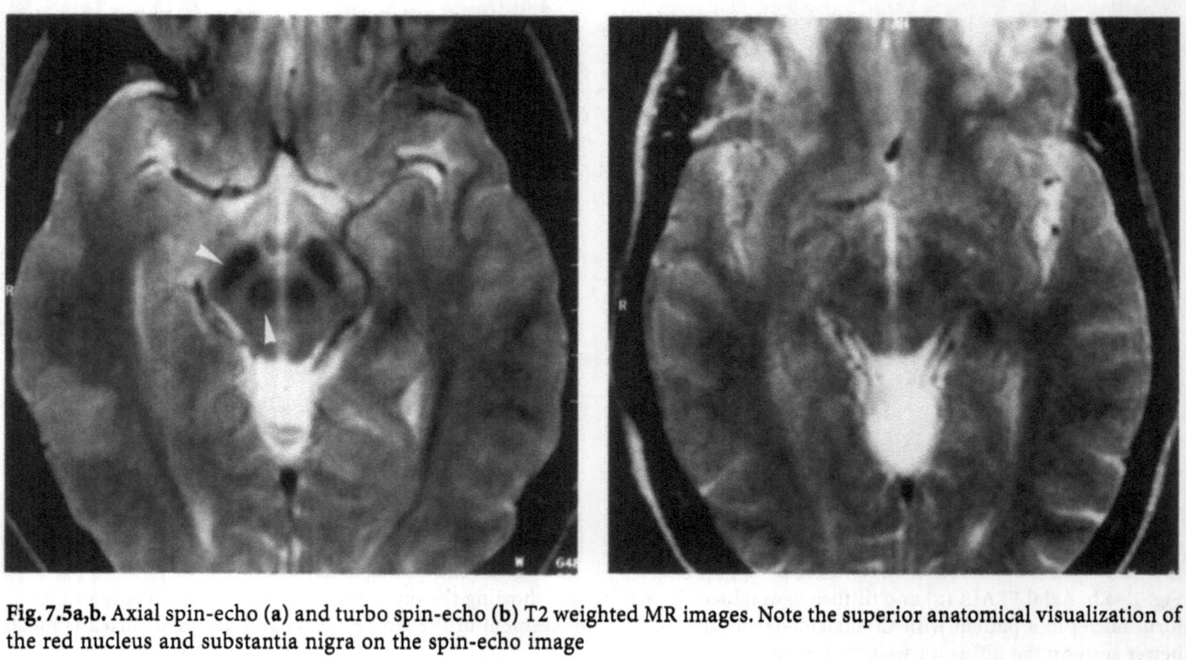

a b

Fig. 7.5a,b. Axial spin-echo (**a**) and turbo spin-echo (**b**) T2 weighted MR images. Note the superior anatomical visualization of the red nucleus and substantia nigra on the spin-echo image

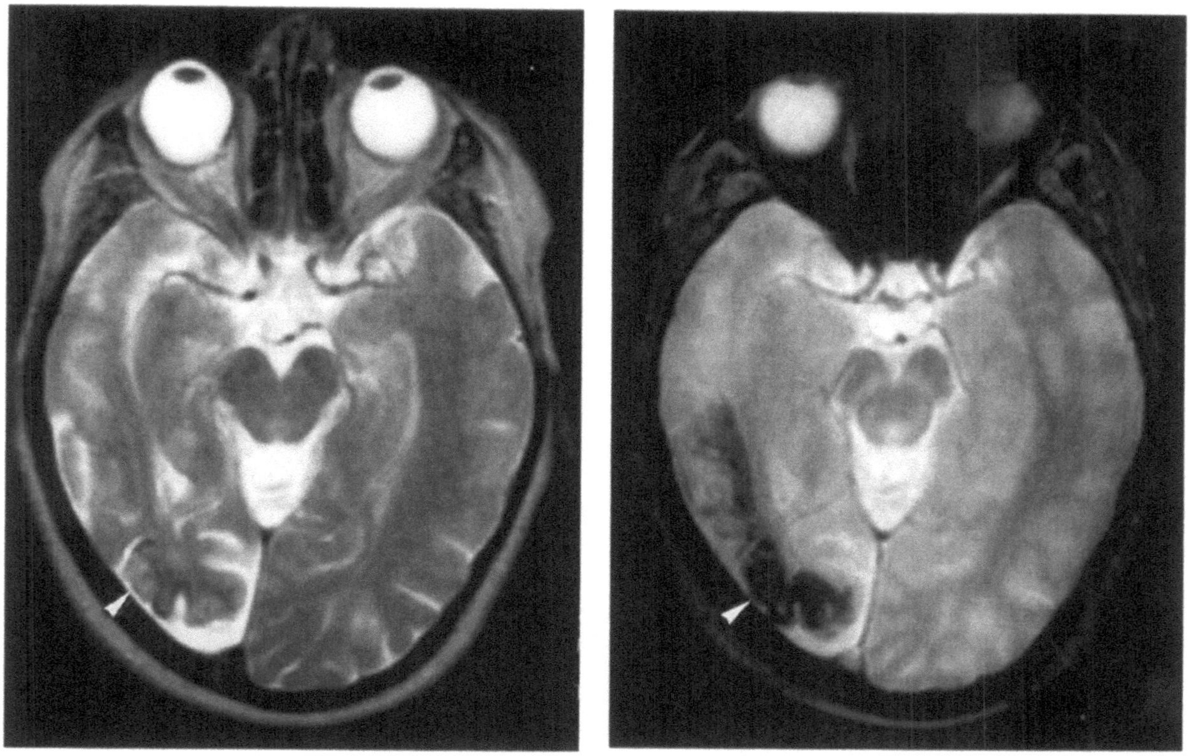

a b

Fig. 7.6a,b. Axial turbo spin-echo (**a**) and gradient-echo (**b**) T2 weighted MR images in a patient with an hemorrhagic infarct in the right middle cerebral artery territory

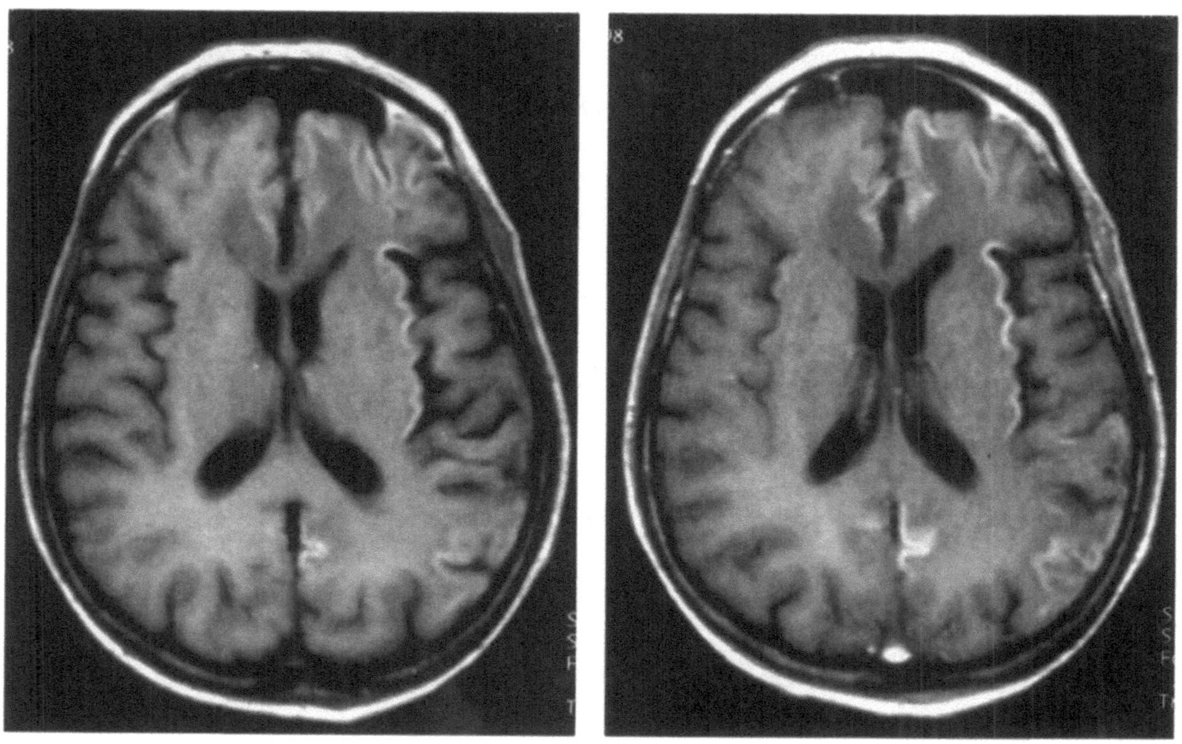

a b

Fig. 7.7a,b. Axial pre- (**a**) and postcontrast (**b**) MR images in a patient with cortical laminar necrosis. Note the limited enhancement cols for imaging patients with various conditions should be developed.

The applications of MR angiography will be discussed in Chaps. 12 and 13.

7.5.1 Multiple Sclerosis

In the past axial and sagittal proton density and T2-weighted spin-echo images have been recommended. Contrast enhanced examinations are more sensitive than either clinical examination or T2-weighted MR imaging in detecting disease activity and can potentially separate clinical groups. The FLAIR sequence is a useful sequence in assessing patients with the clinical suspicion of MS.

Guidelines for the use of MR technique in monitoring the treatment of MS are available from the literature (Miller et al. 1996). Serial MR imaging at 6- to 12-month intervals is a useful secondary end point in providing an index of pathological progression. Contrast enhanced examinations are more sensitive than either clinical examination or T2-weighted MR imaging in detecting disease activity and can potentially separate clinical groups. But enhancement in MS cannot be viewed as an all or none phenomenon. The enhancement of lesions depends on the type of MS and the blood brain barrier breakdown plays a less important role over time when there is evolution to the secondary progressive stage. The enhancement may precede the abnormalities on T2-weighted images and the clinical findings. The availability of diffusion-weighted images may add to our understanding of the pathogenesis of recent MS plaques (Fig. 7.8). It should be mentioned that the normal window of enhancement varies from 2 to 8 weeks and that MS plaques may enhance up to 4 months. The dosage of contrast agent, magnetization transfer and delayed imaging all play a role in imaging patients with MS.

A more extensive discussion follows in Chap. 16, which is dedicated to imaging in multiple sclerosis.

7.5.2 Epilepsy

Chapter 14 will review the latest novelties in imaging epilepsy. Multiplanar imaging plays an important role in assessing the temporal lobe. Three dimensional T1 weighted volumetric imaging is necessary in the search for small cortical abnormalities (see Chap. 14) and to perform volume measurements of structures such as the hippocampus.

7.5.3 Pituitary Gland

Several imaging protocols have been suggested in assessing the pituitary gland and surrounding structures and these are reviewed in Chap. 19. When a mass is suspected, thin coronal and sagittal T1-weighted pre- and postcontrast images will demonstrate the lesion and an additional MR angiogram of the intracranial arteries may be useful preoperatively.

When there is a clinical suspicion of microadenoma, the same protocol may be sufficient. The use of a coronal T2-weighted sequence, dynamic imaging and delayed imaging are helpful in depicting microadenomas which may have remained undetected (Fig. 7.9).

7.5.4 Venous Thrombosis

Most cases of dural sinus thrombosis will be easily depicted on T1-weighted images in the three different planes. An additional proton density and a T2-weighted sequence are recommended. Venous MR angiography may be useful in confirming this diagnosis.

7.5.5 Trauma

If there is a history of cranial trauma, a cranial CT will usually be requested. If cranial CT remains normal in the presence of neurological symptoms, brain MR imaging is recommended. The examination should include axial proton density and T2-weighted images, T1-weighted images (to detect a small subdural hematoma) in one or several planes, gradient echo T2-weighted images (to detect hemosiderin deposits) and, if available, diffusion weighted images (see Chap. 8).

7.5.6 Tumor

Advances in imaging tumors are discussed in Chapter 9.

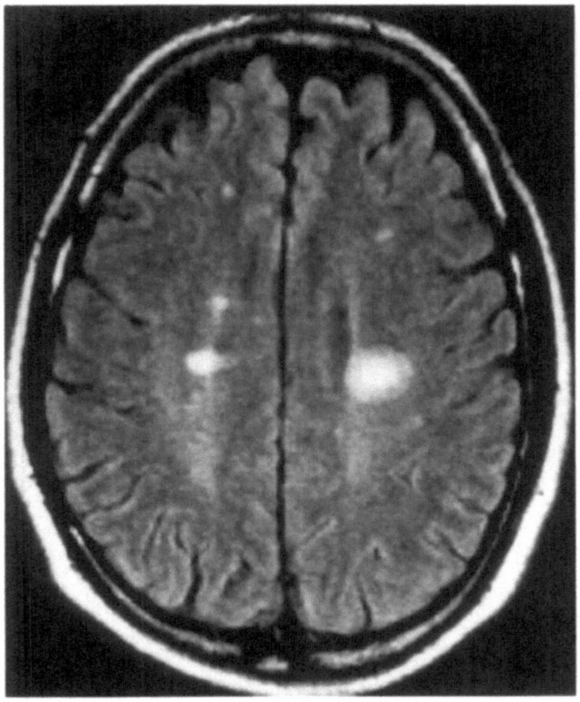
a

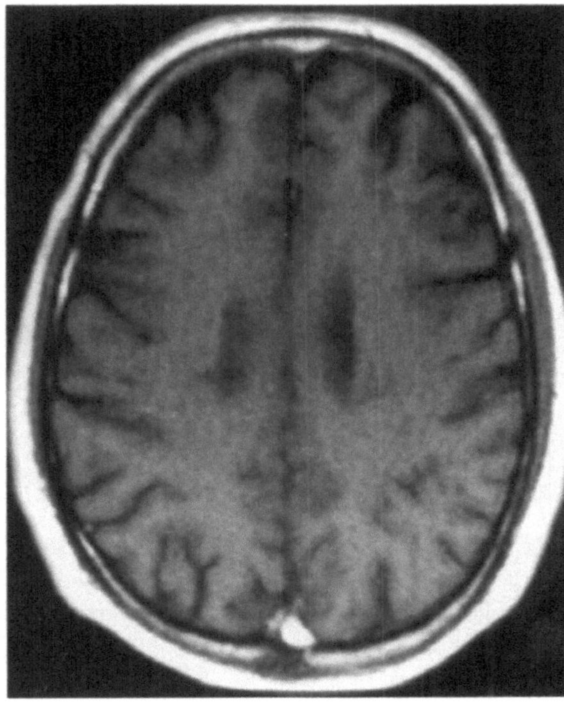
b

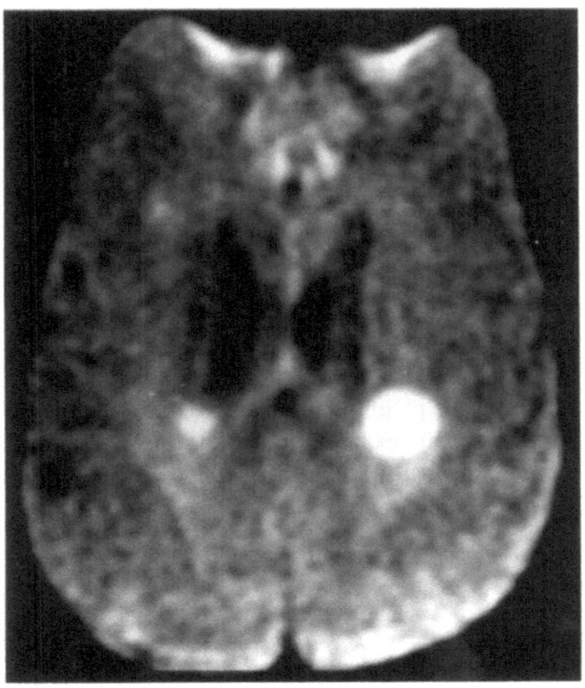
c

Fig. 7.8a–c. Axial fast FLAIR (**a**), gadolinium-enhanced T1 weighted spin-echo (**b**) and diffusion-weighted (**c**) MR images. The non-enhancing lesion, visible on diffusion-weighted images, corresponded to the presenting clinical signs

7.5.7 Stroke

The approach to imaging a patient presenting with a stroke is rapidly changing. Chapter 10 is devoted to imaging brain ischemia. The approach mainly depends on the available therapy and the available time window.

7.5.8 Sensorineural Hearing Loss

It has been demonstrated that unenhanced FSE MR imaging of the internal auditory canal and cerebellopontine angle provides high resolution images at low cost (ALLEN et al. 1996). The authors showed that there was no statistically significant difference be-

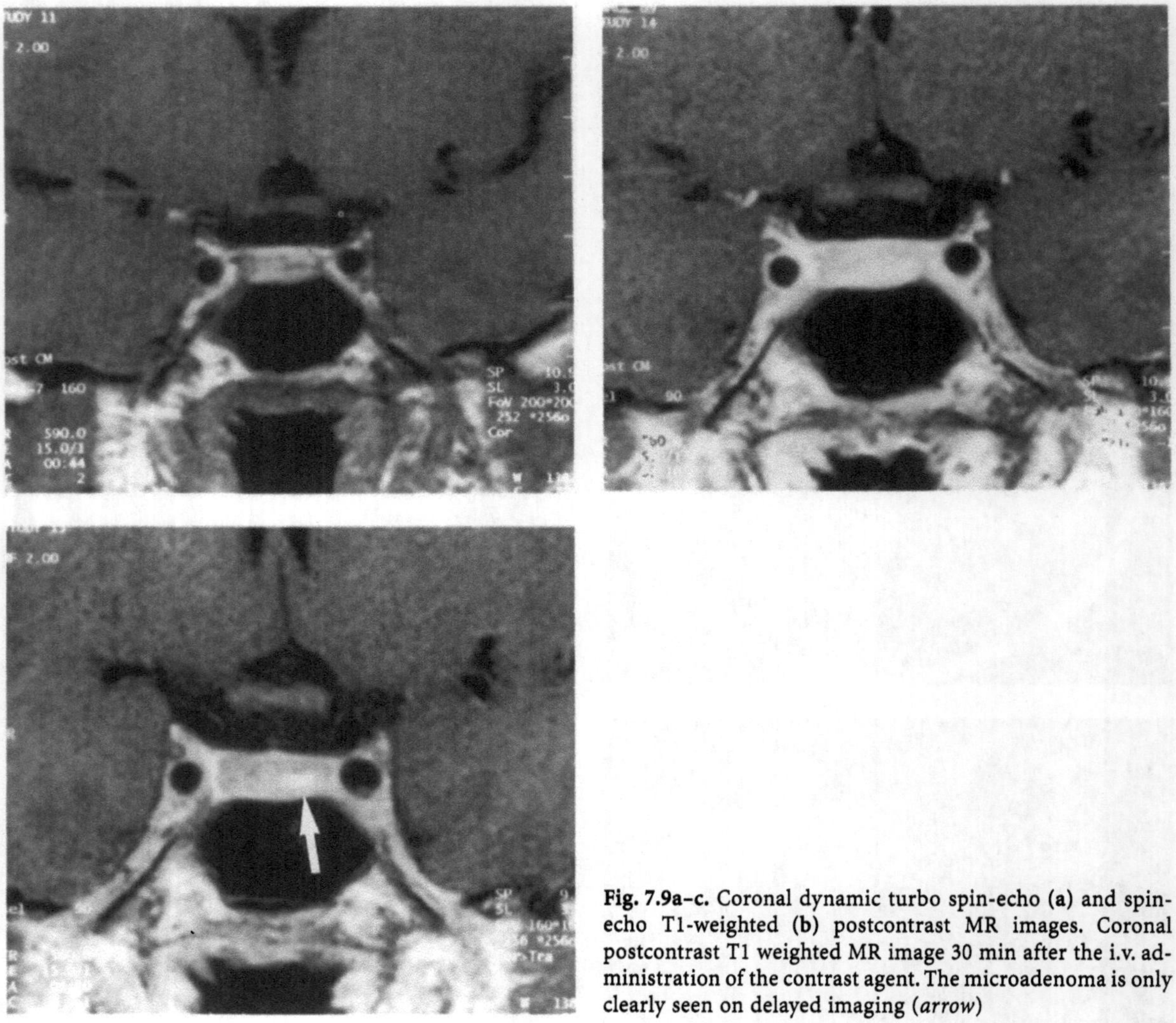

a b c

Fig. 7.9a–c. Coronal dynamic turbo spin-echo (**a**) and spin-echo T1-weighted (**b**) postcontrast MR images. Coronal postcontrast T1 weighted MR image 30 min after the i.v. administration of the contrast agent. The microadenoma is only clearly seen on delayed imaging (*arrow*)

tween enhanced T1-weighted CSE images and unenhanced high resolution FSE MR techniques in the detection of acoustic schwannoma.

The CISS sequence provides high resolution 1-mm slices of the internal auditory canal. If this cost-effective approach is used, ideally the radiologist should be available during the examination for a timely determination of whether contrast is needed.

In another study FSE MR imaging proved the most cost-effective method to screen patients presenting with sudden sensorineural hearing loss (Daniels et al. 1998). Compared with the traditional brain stem response testing including contrast-enhanced MR imaging, there was a 54% reduction in screening costs.

A possible consensus could be to use the non-contrast protocol in patients at low risk of having an acoustic schwannoma, i.e., when there is only slight asymmetrical hearing loss or unilateral tinnitus. When the suspicion is high, such as after extensive neurotological examinations, contrast enhanced scans are probably recommended.

7.6 Guidelines for the Use of Intravenous Contrast Agents

In an ideal world with no medical costs and infinite availability of resources, one would probably recommend the use of Gd-chelates in all patients. In our world, with increasing cost containment pressures and with limited imager availability, this approach is not feasible. Apart from the cost of the contrast agent, one should also consider the additional examination time.

In this paragraph several topics will be dealt with. Do we routinely need intravenous contrast agents? Do we need pre-contrast T1 weighted images? What dose of contrast do we need and at what time is post-contrast imaging recommended? Is the contrast enhancement dependent on the type of sequence and the field strength?

The issue of new contrast agents such as specific agents targeted to specific tissue or disease and ultrasmall superparamagnetic iron oxide particles is addressed in Chap. 6.

The safety and utility of gadolinium (Gd) chelates in brain imaging has been thoroughly documented in the adult and in the pediatric population (ELSTER et al. 1990). The clinical efficacy or the probability that the patient's outcome may improve remains largely unknown.

The general indications for IV Gd chelates are to (1) reveal the presence or absence of enhancing lesions, (2) to evaluate the extent of enhancement and (3) to characterize the pattern of enhancement. It is important to realize that the absence of enhancement can be an important new finding.

The clinical utility of Gd chelates has been studied in large patient series with routine administration of contrast agents. In approximately 20% of the patients enhancing lesions were observed but new or additional lesions were seen in only 3–4% of the patients (ELSTER et al. 1989). The enhancement of a lesion was judged useful in approximately 15–20%. It is important too to emphasize that the absence of enhancement was judged useful in another 15–20% of the patients.

Knowing these figures, it is clear that evidence-based guidelines for the application of contrast are needed. Recently it was demonstrated that no rigorous studies exist on the sensitivity and specificity of contrast agents (BRESLAU et al. 1999). The authors identified 108 articles that evaluated contrast agent efficacy for a minimum of 20 patients per study. The authors concluded that the clinical efficacy of contrast agents remains unproved and that neuroradiologists will have to apply robust methodologies to measure the diagnostic accuracy of contrast agents. The recommendations given here summarize the state-of-the-art on this topic together with our personal experience.

Recently we defined guidelines on the use of contrast agents in brain CT. Using four guidelines, we were able to reduce our average number of contrast enhanced scans from approximately 60% to 20%, without affecting the quality of service to the patient (DEMAEREL et al. 1998). These guidelines include (1) screening for brain metastasis in the presence of a primary tumor, (2) documented systemic diseases with central nervous system involvement such as neurofibromatosis, phakomatosis, lymphoproliferative diseases, infectious disease, (3) prior cranial neurosurgery or chemotherapy/radiotherapy and (4) presence of a suspicious abnormality on the unenhanced scan. It may be interesting to subtract the pre- and postcontrast scans (MELHEM et al. 1999).

These guidelines can be used for brain MR imaging too (Figs. 7.10, 7.11). We suggest a fifth guideline when considering MR imaging, i.e., cranial nerve palsy.

The currently recommended clinical dose of contrast is 0.1 mmol/kg body weight and the volume injected is 0.2 ml/kg. The dose can be reduced 50% in the diagnostic work-up of microadenoma because of the intrinsic contrast of the parasellar tissues and the kinetics of the contrast agent. Increasing the dose to 0.2 and 0.3 mmol/kg body weight results in an increased lesion enhancement, tissue contrast, border definition and lesion detection of respectively 15% and 43% compared with single dose (VAN DIJK et al. 1997). This technique has mainly been used in the detection of metastases. Routine administration of triple dose in all cases of suspected brain metastases is certainly not helpful (SZE et al.1998). Apart from the increased cost, the disadvantage is the increased number of false positive results (such as the detection of small vascular structures and/or flow artifacts around the brainstem and in the posterior fossa). Therefore triple dose of Gd chelates should be reserved for patients with equivocal findings or solitary metastases. The alternative and cheaper approach, with almost comparable findings in terms of lesion conspicuity and detection, is the use of magnetization transfer imaging.

In intracranial hematoma, which can return a high signal, the comparison between pre- and post-contrast scans can be difficult. The demonstration of nodular enhancement is suggestive of an underlying lesion while rim enhancement is more commonly seen in pure hematoma.

Magnetization transfer has been used successfully in multiple sclerosis, viral (meningo)encephalitis, low grade tumor and metastases (MATHEWS et al. 1997). Magnetization transfer influences the intrinsic property of normal tissue, which results in a decreased tissue signal. An observable reduction in magnetization of water can be obtained by saturating the macromolecular component of tissues, i.e., the bound hydrogen pool with an MT pulse of an appropriate radiofrequency. This is achieved by an exchange of longitudinal magnetization between the

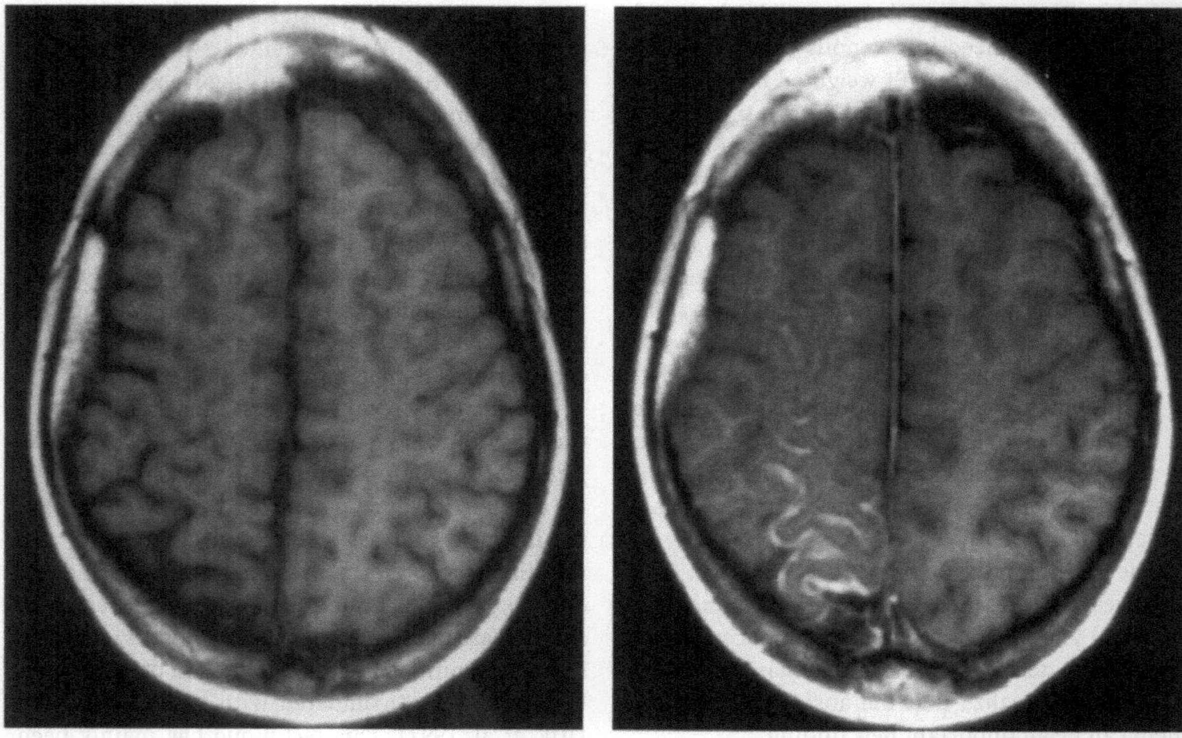

Fig. 7.10a,b. Axial pre- (a) and postcontrast scan in a child with Sturge-Weber syndrome demonstrating leptomeningeal angiomatosis

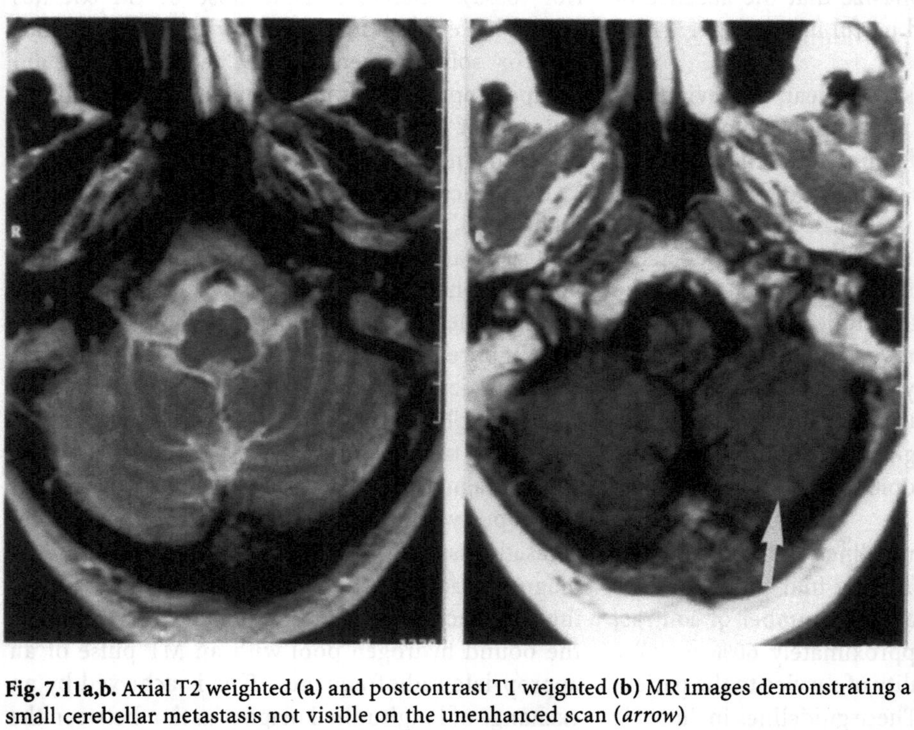

Fig. 7.11a,b. Axial T2 weighted (a) and postcontrast T1 weighted (b) MR images demonstrating a small cerebellar metastasis not visible on the unenhanced scan (*arrow*)

bound and the free hydrogen pool. The signal of normal brain, containing more bound protons, will be suppressed while pathology, containing more free protons, will be more easily depicted (Fig. 7.12). MT is highly sensitive to differential MT ratios which account for the typical gray/white matter reversal and high signal intensity of the basal ganglia observed on non-contrast T1-weighted images with MT. For this reason it is mandatory to obtain pre-contrast images with MT in order to avoid a false positive diagnosis on the post-contrast scan with MT (MEYER et al. 1997). Attempts to replace standard dose conventional T1 weighted sequences by half-dose enhanced MT have failed as comparable results between the two techniques were observed in only 50% of cases (HAN et al. 1998).

Gadolinium-enhanced fast FLAIR images were inferior to conventional T1 weighted images and are therefore not recommended (MELHEM et al. 1998).

Several publications have dealt with the relationship between magnetic field strength and contrast enhancement. There is a trend toward increasing enhancement with field strength and dose (RINCK and MULLER 1999). Gradient-echo sequences show a lower contrast-to-noise ratio than spin-echo sequences (Fig. 7.13). MT 3D gradient-echo MR imag-

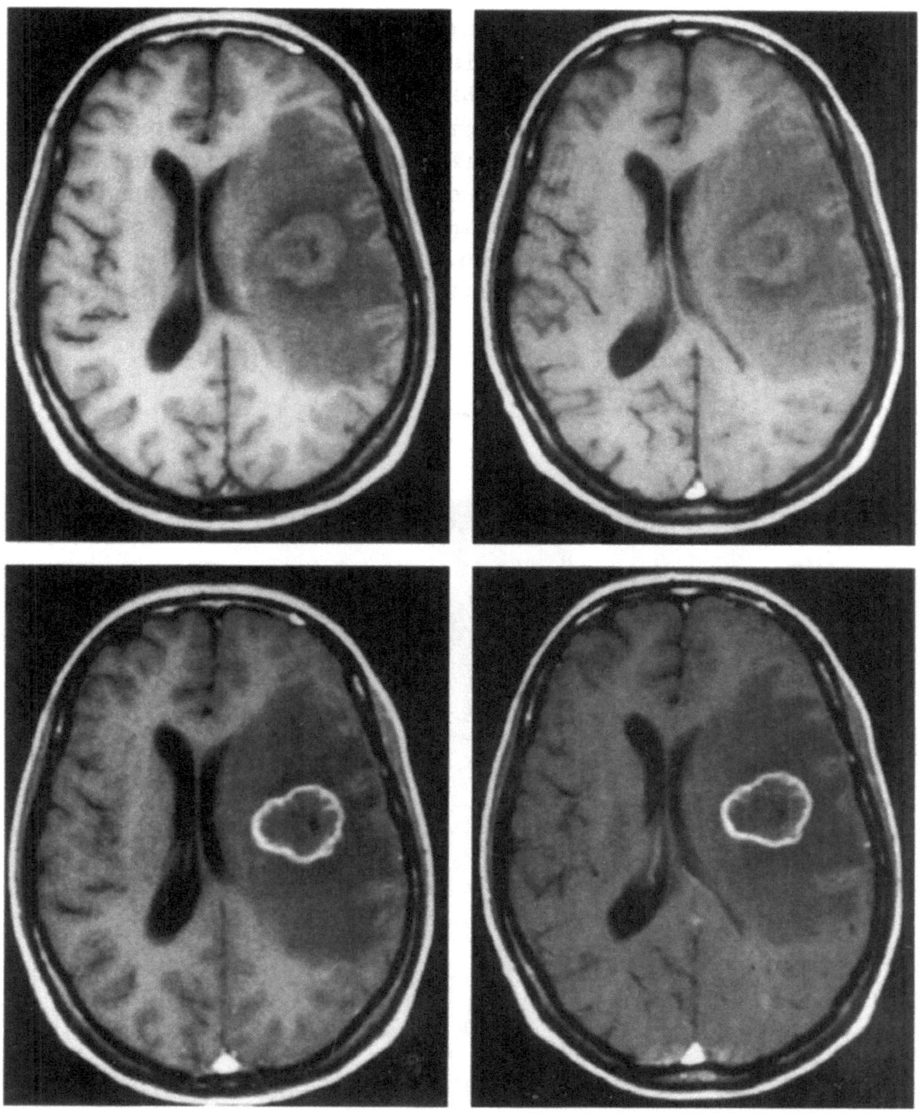

Fig. 7.12. Axial pre- and postcontrast T1 weighted MR images without (*left*) and with (*right*) magnetization transfer showing the sharper delineation of the metastasis on the magnetization transfer images

ing improves the contrast between enhancing lesion and background white matter compared with T1-weighted 3D gradient-echo and spin-echo imaging without MT. The advantage over MT T1-weighted spin-echo sequences consists of the spatial resolution and image coverage (Finelli et al. 1998).

Delayed imaging has been recommended in multiple sclerosis and in the diagnostic work-up of microadenoma. The optimal imaging time is 23 min but it can vary from 15 to 60 min after the injection of the contrast agent.

Intrathecal gadopentetate dimeglumine injection has not yet received worldwide legal approval but appears to be promising in selected indications (see Chap. 31).

7.7 Conclusion

The greatest advantage of modern neuroimaging is that the patient endures a less unpleasant experience and runs less risk. There is little evidence that the outcome for patients has significantly improved. In deciding which technique to use, one should take into account the cost, availability, inconvenience and risk associated with a given imaging technique.

Compared to a decade ago, there is at least a tenfold increase in the number of available pulse sequences. It is clear that one of the challenges of the coming years will be the definition of evidence based guidelines for radiological practice. At this moment these guidelines are almost non-existent. Time-efficient protocols with high diagnostic performance are mandatory in order to cope with the increasing financial constraints. The guidelines should be managed by a radiologist.

An example of the choices of imaging procedures the clinician has to make when confronted with a given clinical problem has been summarized by the Royal College of Radiologists in a booklet that is regularly updated (The Royal College of Radiologists 1998).

The Royal College of Radiologists' recommendation is that if you are in doubt as to whether an investigation is required or which investigation is best, it makes sense to ask the radiologist, who, like other consultants, will know much more about their specialty than those whose primary interests are in other fields.

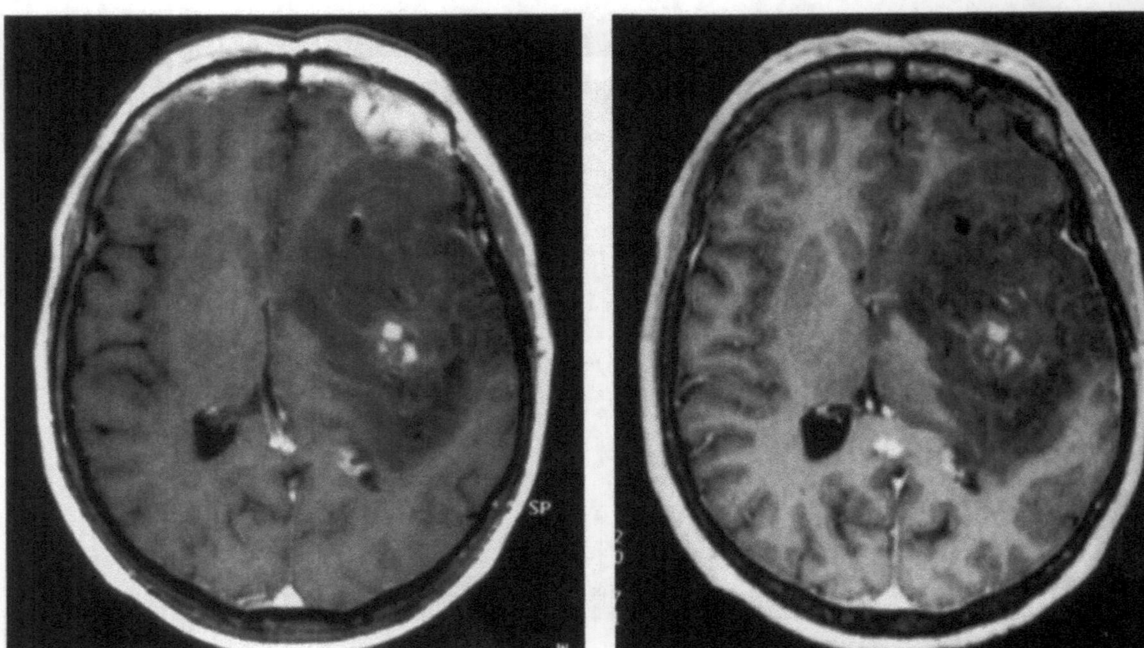

a b

Fig. 7.13a,b. Axial T1 weighted spin-echo (**a**) and reformated MPRAGE contrast-enhanced (**b**) MR images showing the superior contrast-to-noise on the spin-echo image

References

Allen RW, Harnsberger HR, Shelton C, King B, Bell DA, Miller R, Parkin JL, Appelbaum RI, Parker D (1996) Low cost high-resloution fast spin-echo MR imaging of acoustic schwannoma: an alternative to conventional spin-echo MR? Am J Neuroradiol 17: 1205–1210

Boyko OB, Burger PC, Shelburne JD, Ingram P (1992) Nonheme mechanisms for T1 shortening: pathologic, CT, and MR elucidation. Am J Neuroradiol 13: 1439–1445

Breslau J, Jarvik JG, Haynor DR, Longstreth WT, Kent DL, Maravilla KR (1999) MR contrast media in neuroimaging: a critical review of the literature. Am J Neuroradiol 20: 670–675

Casselman JW, Kuhweide R, Ampe W, Meeus L, Steyaert L (1993) Pathology of the mebranous labyrinth: comparison of T1- and T2-weighted and gadolinium-enhanced spin-echo and 3DFT-CISS imaging. Am J Neuroradiol 14: 59–69

Crowe BL, Hailey DM (1989) Collection of cost data from public hospitals' MRI units. In: Selby Smith C (ed) Economics and Health 1988. Monash University, Melbourne, pp 274–289

Daniels RL, Shelton C, Harnsberger HR (1998) Ultra high resolution non enhanced fast spin echo magnetic resonance imaging: cost-effective screening for acoustic neuroma in patients with sudden sensorineural hearing loss. Otolaryngol Head Neck Surg 119: 36–49

Demaerel Ph, Buelens C, Wilms G, Baert AL (1998) Cranial CT revisited: do we really need contrast enhancement? Eur Radiol 8: 1447–1451

Eberhardt KE, Hollenbach HP, Deimling M, Tomandl BF, Huk WJ (1997) MR cisternography: a new method for the diagnosis of CSF fistulae. Eur Radiol 7: 1485–1491

El Gammal TE, Sobol W, Wadlington VR, Sillers MJ, Crews C, Fisher III WS, Lee JY (1998) Cerebrospinal fluid fistula: detection with MR cisternography. Am J Neuroradiol 19: 627–631

Elster AD, Moody DM, Ball MR, Laster DW (1989) Is Gd-DTPA required for routine cranial MR imaging? 173: 231–238

Elster AD (1990) Cranial MR imaging with Gd-DTPA in neonates and young infants: preliminary experience. Radiology 176: 225–230

Fellner F, Fellner C, Held P, Schmitt R (1997) Comparison of spin-echo MR pulse sequences for imaging of the brain. Am J Neuroradiol 18: 1618–1625

Finelli DA, Hurst GC, Gullapalli RP (1998) T1 weighted three dimensional magnetization transfer MR of the brain: improved lesion contrast enhancement. Am J Neuroradiol 19: 59–64

Han D, Chang K-H, Han MH, Cho JY, Han SW, Kim HD, Scong SO (1998) Half dose gadolinium-enhanced MR imaging with magnetization-trasnfer technique in brain tumors. Am J Roentgenol 170: 189–193

Hailey D, McDonald I (1996) The assessment of diagnostic imaging technologies: a policy perspective. Health Policy 36: 185–197

Hirsch JA, Langlotz CP, Lee J, Tanio CP, Grossman RI, Schulman KA (1996) Clinical assessment of MR of the brain in non surgical patients. Am J Neuroradiol 17: 1245–1253

Ikushima I, Korogi Y, Yamashita Y, Yi T, Hamatake S, Sugahara T, Shigematsu Y, Takahashi M (1997) Evaluation of intracranial lesions with inversion recovery half-Fourier single-shot turbo spin-echo MR: initial observations. Am J Neuroradiol 18: 421–426

Lutsep HL, Albers GW, DeCrespigny A, Kamat GN, Marks MP, Moseley ME (1997) Clinical utility of diffusion-weighted magnetic resonance imaging in the assessment of ischemic stroke. Ann Neurol 41: 574–580

Matthews VP, Caldemeyer KS, Ulmer JL, Nguyen H, Yuh WTC (1997) Effects of contrast dose, delayed imaging and magnetization transfer saturation on gadolinium enhanced imaging of brain lesions. J Magn Reson Imaging 7: 14–22

Medina LS, Zurakowski D, Strife KR, Robertson RL, Young Poussaint T, Barnes PD (1998) Efficacy of fast screening MR in children and adolescents with suspected intracranial tumors. Am J Neuroradiol 19: 529–534

Melhem ER, Bert RJ, Walker RE (1998) Usefulness of optimized gadolinium-enhanced fluid attenuation inversion recovery MR imaging in revealing lesions of the brain. Am J Roentgenol 171: 803–807

Melhem ER, Mehta NR (1999) Dynamic T1 weighted MR imaging: the role of digital subtraction in the demonstration of enhancing brain lesions. J Magn Reson Imaging 9: 503–508

Meyer JR, Androux RW, Salamon N, Rabin B, Callahan C, Parrish TB, Prager J, Russell EJ (1997) Contrast-enhanced magnetization transfer MR of the brain: importance of pre contrast images. Am J Neuroradiol 18: 1515–1521

Miller DH, Albert PS, Barkhof F, Francis G, Frank JA, Hodgkinson S, Lublin FD, Paty DW, Reingold SC, Simon J (1996) Guidelines for the use of magnetic resonance techniques in monitoring the treatment of multiple sclerosis. Ann Neurol 39: 6–16

Mushlin AI, Mooney C, Holloway RG, Detsky AS, Mattson DH, Phelps CE (1997) The cost-effectiveness of magnetic resonance imaging for patients with equivocal neurological symptoms. Int J Technol Assess 13: 21–34

Norbash AM, Glover GH, Enzmann DR (1992) Intracerebral lesion contrast with spin-echo and fast spin-echo pulse sequences. Radiology 185: 661–665

Rinck PA, Muller RN (1999) Field strength and dose dependence of contrast enhancement by gadolinium-based MR contrast agents. Eur Radiol 9: 998–1004

Royal College of Radiologists (1998) Making the best use of a department of clinical radiology. Guidelines for doctors. 4th ed. London: Royal College of Radiologists

Sze G, Johnson C, Kawamura Y, Goldberg SN, Lange R, Friedland RJ, Wolf RJ (1998) Comparison of single and triple dose contrast material in the MR screening of brain metastases. Am J Neuroradiol 19: 821–828

Sunshine JH, McNeil BJ (1997) Rapid method for rigorous assessment of radiologic imaging technologies. Radiology 202: 549–557

Van Dijk P, Sijens PE, Schmitz PIM, Oudkerk M (1997) Gd-enhanced MR imaging of brain metastases: contrast as a function of dose and lesion size. Magn Reson Imaging 15: 535–541

Wolansky LJ, Chong S, Liu WC, Kang E, Simpson SW, Karimi S, Akbari H (1999) Single-shot echo-planar imaging of multiple sclerosis: effects of varying echo-time. Neuroradiology 41: 163–166

Yousry TA, Filippi M, Becker C, Horsfield MA, Voltz R (1997) Comparison of MR pulse sequences in the detection of multiple sclerosis lesions. Am J Neuroradiol 18: 959–963

8 Emergencies in Brain Imaging

MARGARET D. HOURIHAN

CONTENTS

8.1 Introduction

Neurological disease is very common. It accounts for about a fifth of admissions to hospitals in the United Kingdom. Most of these admissions are emergencies. At the time of admission the clinical history available may be poor or unobtainable and the diagnosis not apparent. Physical examination may be more informative in suggesting a diagnosis or differential but generally imaging has a central role in substantiating any clinical diagnosis and guiding the clinical management of these patients. In most situations, whether the patients are admitted as a result of trauma or medical emergency, computed tomography (CT) is the initial and definitive investigation. A 24-h service should be provided.

Guidelines are available to identify which patients are in need of an urgent scan, those who are at risk and others who can wait until the normal working day (THE SOCIETY OF BRITISH NEUROLOGICAL SURGEONS 1998).

An unenhanced CT scan can:

- Detect the immediate effects of trauma
- Differentiate between haemorrhage and ischaemia as the cause of acute stroke
- Delineate a mass lesion causing a decrease in the level of consciousness
- Demonstrate evidence of raised intracranial pressure (ICP) which would contraindicate a lumbar puncture.

Contrast enhanced CT of the brain is not often indicated in the emergency situation, but in some cases can establish a definitive diagnosis.

Magnetic resonance imaging (MRI) is usually performed either to provide diagnostic confirmation in specific clinical situations, such as suspected herpes encephalitis or cerebral venous thrombosis, or to confirm whether a patient with a recent onset of stroke is a candidate for thrombolysis, although it has been suggested that MRI should be considered as the initial investigation in other emergency situations (CAMPBELL and ZIMMERMAN 1998).

8.2 Imaging Strategies

Traditionally, computed tomography (CT) is the initial imaging performed on patients with an acute neurological presentation. This approach has reflected the availability of CT, and the speed at which examinations can be performed on these patients who are often unstable clinically and may be ventilated. Current helical CT scanners allow faster acquisition with more slices performed in a given time without running into the problems of tube overheating. As MRI becomes more readily available and with the developments in sequence technology, e.g. fast spin echo (FSE) and echo planar imaging (EPI) which allow fast scan times, it can be argued that MRI should be used as the first line investigation for patients presenting with acute neurological emergencies.

MRI is a more sensitive technique and therefore improves diagnostic accuracy, resulting in more rapid institution of appropriate treatment and improved

M.D. HOURIHAN, MD
Consultant Neuroradiologist, Radiology Directorate, University Hospital of Wales, Heath Park, Cardiff, CF4 4XW, UK

outcome for the patient. One frequently stated reason why CT has been favoured over MRI in the acute situation is that MRI had been shown previously to be insensitive in detecting hyperacute intracranial haemorrhage and acute subarachnoid haemorrhage (SAH), important diagnoses to make in the emergency situation as many scans are performed on patients admitted with stroke, where the primary aim is to differentiate between ischaemic stroke and stroke secondary to haemorrhage, or with sudden onset of headache and meningism when SAH is suspected. These clinical diagnoses can be investigated if the more recently developed sequences are performed; gradient-echo sequences, in addition to the routine sequences in the former and a fluid attenuated inversion recovery sequence (FLAIR) in the latter.

The goal of emergency scanning is to obtain the information necessary to make the diagnosis without delay.

Routine CT protocols should include contiguous 3- to 5-mm-thick slices, through the posterior fossa from the skull base (below the level of the cerebellar tonsils) and 8- to 10-mm-thick slices to the vertex. These are displayed at routine brain settings: window width (W) 100–150/level (L) 30–50. Additional bone and intermediate settings are indicated in trauma cases to identify skull fractures and small extra axial collections respectively. Intravenous contrast is rarely indicated except to increase the specificity of the diagnosis when a mass lesion has been demonstrated or venous thrombosis is suspected. CT angiography (CTA) necessitates the timed bolus injection of intravenous contrast and can be useful in the assessment of cerebral perfusion in patients admitted with stroke, and in the demonstration of the intracranial vessels when an aneurysm is suspected. This may obviate the need to perform conventional cerebral angiography in an emergency situation. The protocols for CTA are discussed in Chap. 12.

Routine MRI protocols vary depending on the magnetic field strength, machine capabilities and suspected clinical diagnosis. Generally sagittal T1-weighted and axial proton density (PD) and T2-weighted sequences are performed initially. If cerebral venous thrombosis is suspected, additional T2-weighted coronal and 2D phase contrast (PC) MR venography in both the sagittal and axial planes are performed. Gradient-echo (GE) sequences are more sensitive for intracerebral haemorrhage and FLAIR sequences for SAH. Diffusion-weighted (DWI) and perfusion-weighted (PWI) imaging is one focus of current research in early imaging for stroke; DWI scans become abnormal within minutes of the acute event. MR angiography (MRA) has a role to play in the detection of intracranial aneurysms. To image these, 3D time-of-flight (TOF) MRA is performed unless the standard T2-weighted scan demonstrates a giant aneurysm or a large haematoma when PC MRA is performed.

When a patient presents with a large intraparenchymal haematoma which may need evacuation and the possibility of an underlying vascular lesion, such as an aneurysm or arteriovenous malformation (AVM) is raised, catheter cerebral angiography is indicated prior to surgery. However, with the availability of CTA or MRA, the need for an invasive angiogram may be obviated when neurosurgeons will undertake surgery on an aneurysm demonstrated on CTA or MRA. MRI with MRA is the investigation of choice for patients presenting with a painful third nerve palsy when the possibility of a posterior communicating artery aneurysm is raised.

8.3 Medical Emergencies

Imaging staff must be familiar with the common causes of symptom complexes when planning the investigation on a patient admitted with an acute non-traumatic neurological problem. The patient admitted with the sudden onset of a new focal neurological deficit usually has a stroke; the sudden onset of the worst headache ever experienced, the feeling that they have been hit at the back of the neck is typical for SAH; headache with a focal deficit proceeding to impaired consciousness in a postpartum female is often due to cerebral venous thrombosis. In some of these clinical circumstances, if the patient can cooperate, MRI would be the imaging modality of choice if available. Recent advances in imaging technology influencing neurological emergencies will be reviewed.

8.3.1 Stroke

Amongst the most recent and exciting advances in emergency neuroimaging are those related to the imaging and management of patients admitted with acute stroke. The role of imaging is twofold. Firstly, to confirm the clinical diagnosis of ischaemic stroke and to exclude haemorrhage and other structural abnormalities such as tumour which can also present as stroke. CT imaging has attained, and is likely to maintain, a central role in stroke triage because it is widely accessible to most stroke patients and it is highly sensitive in demonstrating haemorrhagic stroke. The appearance, within 3 h of stroke onset, of a significant brain volume involvement with CT density alteration (hypodensity), combined with subtle mass effect, are considered to be sensitive indicators of irreversible injury and of increased haemorrhagic risk if reperfused (VON KUMMER et al. 1995).

Many conditions mimic stroke and there are published series where the condition is misdiagnosed. LIBMAN et al. (1995) reviewed patients who were misdiagnosed (19%) to see if there were clinical variables to alert the clinician to a stroke mimic. Although univariate analysis showed that decreased level of consciousness and normal eye movements increased the odds of stroke mimic and abnormal visual fields, diastolic blood pressure greater than 90 mmHg, atrial fibrillation on ECG and history of angina decreased the odds of stroke mimic; the sensitivity for predicting the mimics was only 21%, the specificity 96%. There were 18 different conditions that mimicked stroke. The most common of these were seizure (16.7%), systemic infection (16.7%), brain tumour (15.4%), toxic/metabolic disturbance (12.8%) and positional vertigo (6.4%).

When a decision has to be made as to whether to enter a patient into a course of treatment that has potential side effects, it is important to have accurate information available from appropriate imaging and some of the conditions that present with a focal neurological deficit may not be excluded by CT. Prospective studies comparing conventional CT and MRI in hyperacute stroke, within the 6 h, were essentially equivalent in detecting infarct (MOHR et al. 1995). If MRI is performed acutely the features of a hyperacute haematoma are iso- to mildly hyperintensity on T1-weighted and hyperintensity on T2-weighted images. The hallmark on finding MRI is peripheral hypointensity on GE images.

Diffusion-weighted magnetic resonance imaging (DWI) is the most accurate tool available for the diagnosis or exclusion of acute infarction (BAREST et al. 1998). Its availability has changed the management of their patients presenting as emergencies with stroke. DWI is abnormal within 30–90 min of acute stroke with the area of acute ischaemic infarction, in which there is reduced diffusion of water molecules, appearing hyperintense (bright) (Fig. 8.1). If DWI is normal, acute stroke is excluded and the patient is not necessarily admitted. Despite a specificity of 100% and a sensitivity of 94%, LÖVBLAD et al. (1998) concluded that a negative scan did not rule out an ischaemic pathogenesis, when scanning patients within 6 h of symptom onset. Others suggest a note of caution if the DWI MR is abnormal as other factors may also cause hyperintensity, and failure to consider these factors will result in errors of diagnosis (WARACH et al. 1997). Standard T2-weighted MRI should always be performed as other causes of stroke can be identified, e.g. arterial dissection, which is the cause of stroke in 5–20% of young patients.

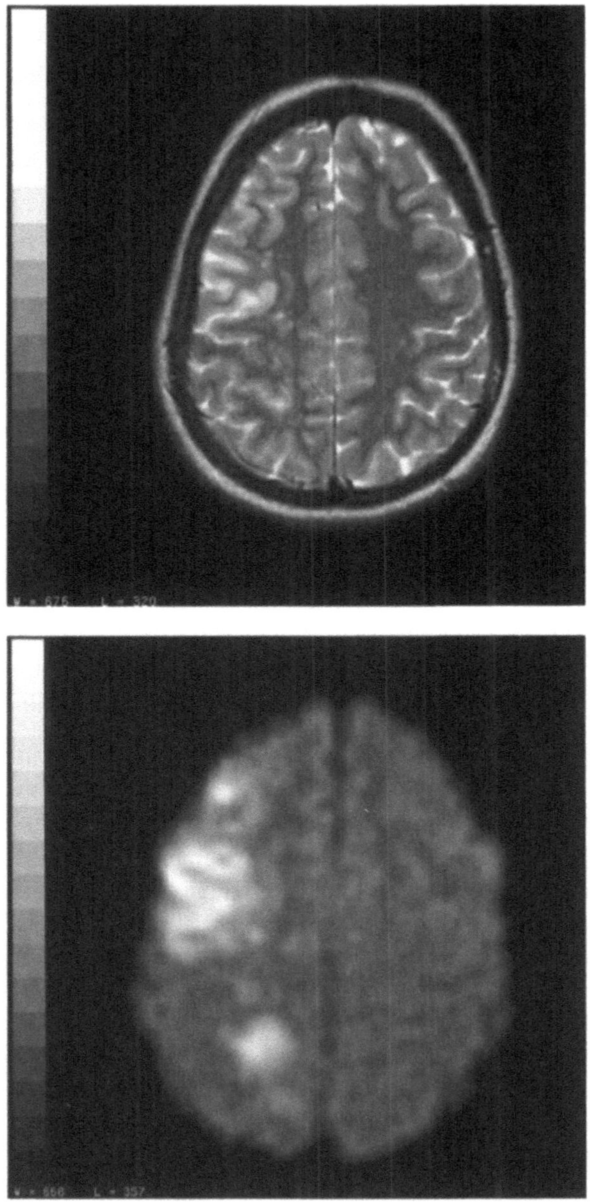

a

b

Fig. 8.1a,b. A 16-year-old schoolgirl presented with a sudden onset of left sided hemiparesis. **a** T2-weighted MRI demonstrates cortical swelling and hyperintensity in the right frontal and parietal lobes. **b** DWI MR confirms the presence of middle cerebral artery distribution infarcts

Secondly, with effective therapeutic options now available for the ischaemic stroke patient, it is important to provide an imaging technique that can rapidly differentiate between the ischaemic penumbra of tissue at risk, and tissue already infarcted tissue. Knowing whether an ischaemic insult is still reversible or already irreversible provides the essential understanding of how aggressively the efforts towards reperfusion should be pursued. The current challenge in imaging is to identify which of the imaging techniques are capable of confirming accurately and quickly the presence and volume of the ischaemic penumbra at the time of presentation following the acute infarction.

Research is proceeding along three imaging pathways:

- Diffusion/perfusion weighted MRI
- CT perfusion techniques
- Xenon-enhanced CT

Availability of the above techniques for emergency neuroimaging is a major factor, which has influenced the research in this field. As helical CT scanners become more commonplace the emergency use of CT angiography becomes a real possibility. The imaging algorithm would comprise an unenhanced CT examination to provide information regarding acute haemorrhage, followed by a helical CT scan during bolus infusion of intravenous contrast to provide high resolution anatomical definition of intracranial vessels. The information is immediately available. The 2D images can delineate perfusion defects. When the data set is postprocessed, CT angiograms of the circle of Willis can be assessed to identify any site of arterial occlusion so that the appropriate treatment can be instigated. Quantitative maps of perfused cerebral blood volume can be attained from these data sets (Hunter et al. 1998). These represent maps of contrast delivery to those vessels still receiving blood despite ischaemia or infarction. They show the perfused brain. The threshold levels that distinguish salvageable tissue from dead tissue or tissue destined to die have yet to be defined. The technique improves the sensitivity of CT to early ischaemia in some cases.

Perfusion-weighted magnetic resonance imaging (PWI) is a dynamic contrast enhanced technique that requires rapid imaging. It measures the signal change that accompanies the passage of a bolus of paramagnetic contrast medium through the brain. DWI demonstrates the ischaemic core. The combination of PWI with DWI is more informative than DWI alone (Sorensen et al. 1996). Tissue with abnormal perfusion outside the core represents the ischaemic penumbra tissue at risk, in which there is still the potential to prevent infarction if treated. If the DWI scan is abnormal but PWI normal the tissue has been reperfused already, possibly through collaterals. If the DWI and the PWI defects match then reperfusion has not taken place by the time of imaging and there may be a therapeutic window. When the PWI is larger than the DWI, unless there is therapeutic intervention, the DWI enlarges to the size to match the PWI (Barest et al. 1998). These techniques are becoming increasingly important in the diagnosis and management of acute stroke.

Currently the best and most quantifiable technique for determining tissue at risk is xenon-enhanced CT (XeCT). This technique measures cerebral blood flow (CBF) in regions of interest throughout the brain. Performing XeCT on patients with middle cerebral artery occlusion between 1 and 6 h after the onset of ischaemic stroke, Kaufmann et al. (1999) observed that the ischaemic penumbra had blood flow values of between 7 and 20 $cm^3/100g/min$ and the severely ischaemic core CBF ≤ 6 $cm^3/100g/min$. The preliminary results of this technique suggest it will be useful because therapeutic efforts to provide reperfusion up to and beyond 6 h after the onset of stroke may be rewarding if there is a known threshold value of cerebral perfusion below which it is unlikely that the involved brain is viable. In the absence of perfusion, efforts at reperfusion are unlikely to provide any benefit. The main limitation of XeCT is availability. It is a relatively cheap option, which can be added on to most helical CT scanners but currently there are not many systems installed worldwide. Also patients need to cooperate and keep still for the scans, and stroke patients are often confused and move. If this technique is to be used to provide essential information in acute stroke management, more systems must be installed, comparative prospective studies performed and more effective strategies to minimise motion artefact will be needed.

8.3.2 Subarachnoid Haemorrhage (SAH)

Although headache is commonly experienced and is rarely significant, the sudden onset of a severe headache in a previously well patient, especially when associated with meningism, may be associated with significant pathology and requires further investigation. When there are other neurological signs, such as a decreased level of consciousness, this should be performed immediately. The diagnosis of SAH is considered in the above clinical setting and the role of imaging is to confirm the presence of an SAH and, where possible, direct the next imaging investigation, cerebral angiography, toward the probable location of the ruptured intracranial aneurysm. CT is the initial investigation of choice, being positive in about 90% of cases of SAH within the first 24 h. If the CT is negative, the diagnosis cannot be excluded and a lumbar puncture (LP) has to be performed. The CT scan can also confirm there is no contraindication to LP such as an intracranial mass lesion or signs of raised intracranial pressure. While CT is rapid, accurate and a simple test for the detection of subarachnoid haemorrhage, Campbell and Zimmerman (1998) have found that MR is more sensitive than CT in the detection of non-traumatic acute SAH when a FLAIR sequence is performed. On FLAIR images, normal cerebrospinal fluid (CSF) is dark because of an inversion pulse timed to null CSF signal; bloody CSF is not nulled because its T1 relaxation time is shortened by the components of haemoglobin and it is hyperintense to normal CSF (Fig. 8.2). SAH is also hyperintense to brain parenchyma on FLAIR because it has a longer T2 relaxation time. Acute SAH is therefore more conspicuous on MR FLAIR images than on CT. In subacute or chronic SAH when the CT may be falsely negative, FLAIR or gradient echo imaging remains positive (Noguchi et al. 1997). The use of MR could replace an LP to confirm the presence of subacute or chronic SAH when CT scan is negative. The detection of SAH on MRI is sensitive but not specific. Other processes such as meningitis or slow arterial flow can produce sulcal hyperintensity that can mimic SAH on FLAIR sequences. Other authors have reported that FLAIR MRI also identifies acute and subacute intraventricular haemorrhage in the lateral ventricles with high sensitivity and specificity (Bakshi et al. 1998). Although it is useful for detecting third and fourth ventricular haemorrhage, the images may be compromised by artefacts.

MRI will not quickly replace CT in the routine investigation of patients suspected of having SAH or intraparenchymal or ventricular haemorrhage. It does, however, have a role to play in subacute or chronic cases where the CT may have returned to normal.

Although catheter cerebral angiography is usually the next imaging investigation once the clinical diagnosis of SAH has been confirmed, this investigation is not without risk and the non-invasive techniques of CTA and MRA are currently being assessed. In a recent study, MRI combined with MRA detected 75% of all aneurysms and 95% of aneurysms greater than 3 mm (Atlas et al. 1997). Our own experience comparing MRA and digital subtraction cerebral angiography in a prospective study of 50 patients with proven SAH showed a sensitivity of 91% and a specificity of 89% (unpublished data). With the availability of helical CT and the potential for performing

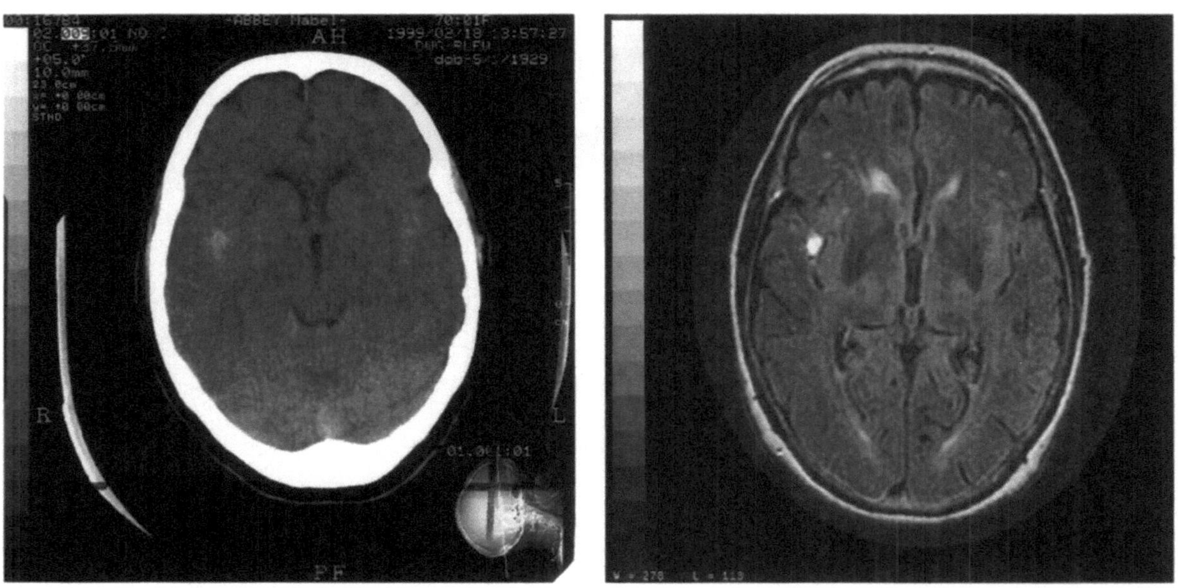

a b

Fig. 8.2a,b. A 70-year-old male patient presented with SAH. **a** CT demonstrated diffuse SAH but predominantly on the right side in the sylvian fissure. **b** FLAIR MRI 8 days later demonstrates hyperintensity in the right sylvian fissure, secondary to this localised collection of blood

CTA of the intracranial circulation the role of this investigation in the preoperative investigation of patients with acute SAH will evolve. It can be completed quickly, safely and inexpensively. The examination can be performed after the diagnostic CT scan and the 3D models generated to display the cause of the SAH. Studies comparing CTA and digital subtraction angiography in the detection of circle of Willis aneurysms in patients with acute SAH have been encouraging (Vieco et al. 1995). This technique is particularly helpful when patients present with a decreased level of consciousness or coma, secondary to a large intraparenchymal haematoma and subarachnoid haemorrhage from an underlying aneurysm, and need to go to theatre urgently to have the haematoma evacuated (Fig. 8.3). The exact role of CTA in patients with SAH or suspected aneurysms is still under evaluation but it is a reasonable alternative to MRA for aneurysm detection. Whether CTA or other non-invasive imaging can replace catheter angiography in the future remains undecided.

8.3.3 Venous Thrombosis

The clinical presentation of patients with thrombosis of a dural venous sinus or cortical veins is variable. The thrombus can occur secondary to many medical conditions such as infection, trauma, tu-

a

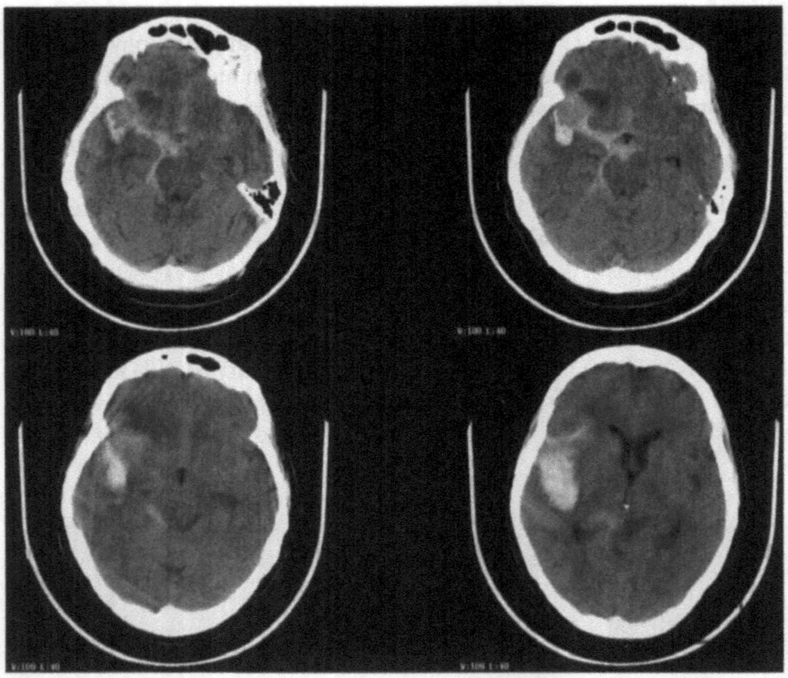

b

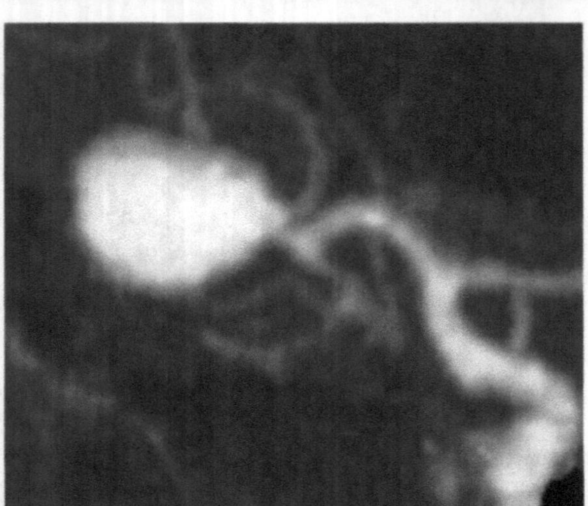

Fig. 8.3a,b. An 80-year-old female presented with sudden onset of headache and decreasing level of consciousness. **a** CT demonstrates a right sylvian haematoma. **b** CTA demonstrates the underlying right middle cerebral artery aneurysm

mour, dehydration or systemic hypercoagulability (including pregnancy and oral contraceptive pill use). Patients can present with headache, secondary to raised intracranial pressure, seizures, focal deficits due to infarction or decreased level of consciousness. This condition is underdiagnosed and the neuroradiologist is often the first person to suggest it as a diagnosis (Provenzale et al. 1998). Although the early clinical course is frequently mild with thrombosis involving one or more dural sinuses, the condition may progress and the late clinical course, when cortical venous thrombosis and infarction occurs, can carry significant morbidity and mortality unless appropriate therapy is commenced. On an unenhanced CT the diagnosis is suspected when hyperdensity is seen in the superior sagittal sinus or in a thrombosed cortical vein. Venous infarction can occur secondary to this and it is frequently near the mid line and often haemorrhagic. If there is diffuse cerebral swelling the ventricles may be small. The diagnosis can be confirmed by contrast enhanced CT where an empty delta sign is observed in the thrombus filled dual sinus; however, if the diagnosis is suspected clinically or on the unenhanced CT, MRI is indicated as it is a more sensitive technique. The normal flow void in the dural sinuses is replaced by abnormal signal which is usually hyperintense on both T1-weighted and T2-weighted images. Care must be taken, however, as depending on the age of the clot the MRI signal characteristics vary and in the acute stage it is hypointense on T2-weighted images, and may look like a normal flow void. In addition to the standard MR sequences, coronal T2-weighted sequence and 2D PC MR venography in the sagittal and axial planes are acquired. The latter will demonstrate absence of the normal bright signal from the involved sinuses. This most commonly affects the superior sagittal sinus followed by, in decreasing order of involvement, the lateral sinus, cerebral veins, straight sinus and cerebellar veins. The complications of venous thrombosis such as venous infarction and diffuse brain swelling can also be diagnosed with MRI. Prior to the advent of MRI, cerebral venous thrombosis was difficult to diagnose.

8.3.4 Intracranial Infection

When intracranial infection is suspected the instigation of prompt and appropriate treatment is mandatory to ensure a successful clinical outcome. Although an LP can be performed in a suspected case of meningitis, with no adverse neurological signs, if CT is readily available it should be performed prior to the LP to exclude evidence of raised intracranial pressure, obstructive hydrocephalus or a mass lesion. Different infective agents have different, and sometimes characteristic, findings on CT and MRI. MRI is particularly useful in confirming the clinical diagnosis of acute viral herpes simplex encephalitis. This usually affects the temporal and frontal lobes and early on in the course of the disease hyperintensity is identified on T2-weighted, proton density or FLAIR MR images, when the CT is either negative or the relevant images are degraded by artefact from the adjacent bone (Fig. 8.4). Small subdural empyemas are often difficult to identify on CT as they are parallel to the inner table of the skull (Fig. 8.5). These must be drained urgently since antibiotics alone are ineffective in their treatment. That MRI better demonstrates these collections can be useful to convince a neurosurgeon that the empyema is present and should be drained.

8.3.5 Posterior Reversible Encephalopathy Syndrome

In the posterior reversible encephalopathy syndrome (PRES) patients present with nausea and vomiting, headache, visual disturbances, seizures and a depressed mental state. This condition has also been called hypertensive encephalopathy as these patients have an acute elevation of blood pressure, reversible vasoreactive oedema (RVT) and alternatively posterior leukoencephalopathy syndrome because of the clinical and imaging features seen in this condition. The elevated systemic blood pressure overrides the normal autoregulation of intracranial blood pressure leading to exudation of serum (vasogenic oedema). This has a predeliction for the posterior brain so oedema of the subcortical white matter of the parietal and occipital lobes is a common involvement and of the anterior portions of the brain less common (Fig. 8.6). There may be involvement of the thalami, brainstem and cerebellum. Imaging helps to make the correct diagnosis and, as MRI is more sensitive than CT in detecting vasogenic oedema, is the investigation of choice. Similar clinical and imaging findings are found in eclampsia, with cyclosporin, and with the drug toxicities. The findings resolve rapidly with treatment of the elevated blood pressure or removing the causative agent, but deterioration progressing to infarction, haemorrhage and permanent neurological deficit may occur if it is not treated promptly.

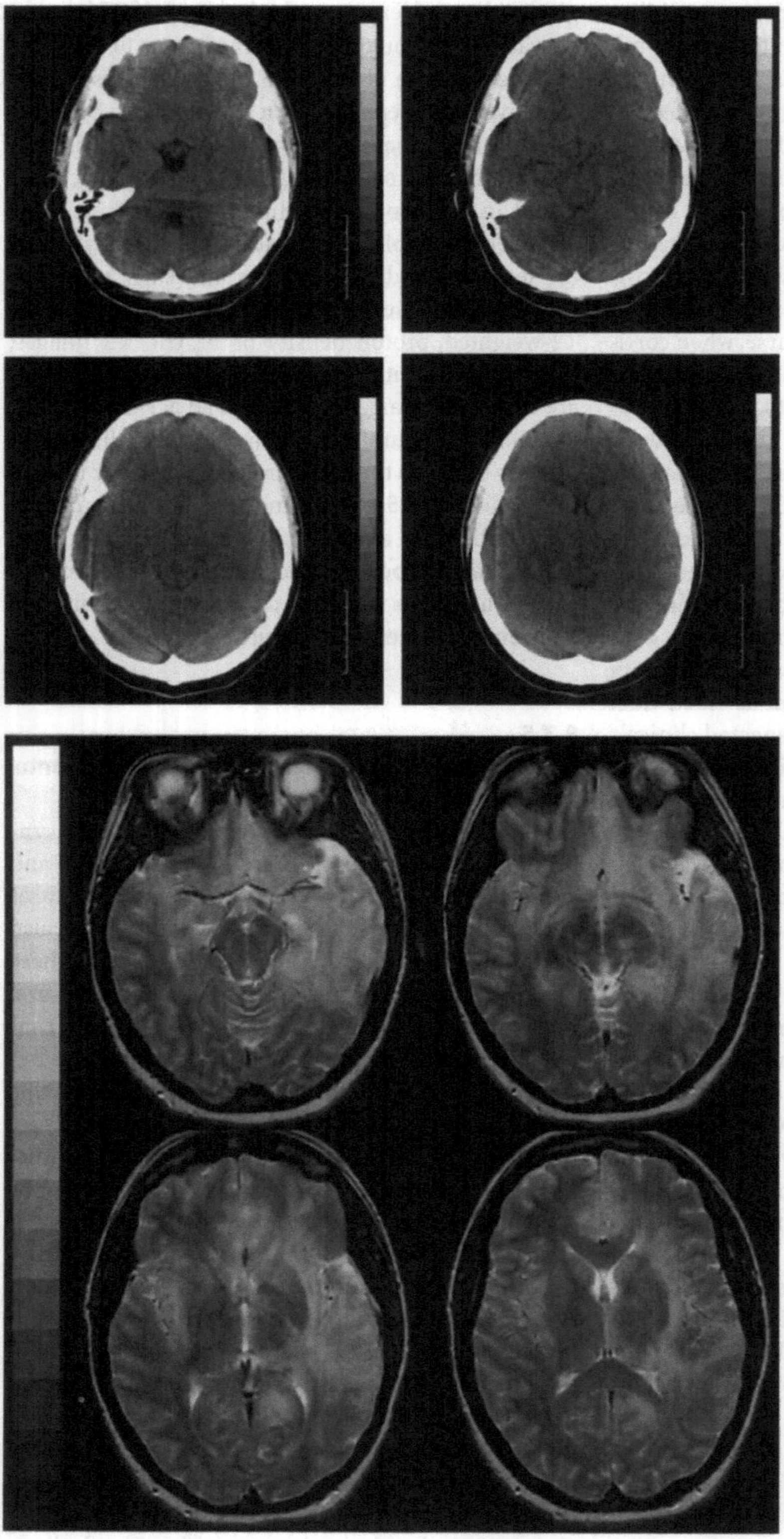

Fig. 8.4a,b. A 28-year-old female with a prodromal viral illness presented with a decreasing level of consciousness and fits. **a** CT was unremarkable. **b** T2-weighted MEI 2 days later demonstrates extensive high signal in the left temporal lobe extending into the inferior frontal lobe and involving the insular cortex bilaterally and the cingulate gyri bilaterally

8.4 Imaging in Trauma

The advent of computed tomography (CT) in the early 1970s revolutionised the diagnosis and management of head trauma patients, and this is still the case. With helical CT there are additional benefits for efficient evaluation of multiple areas without encountering problems of tube heating. CT must be available in all hospitals admitting trauma and acutely ill patients, and a 24-h service is required. Unenhanced cranial CT is fast and accurate at detecting and locating significant neurosurgical haematomas. Images must be obtained at three window width (*W*)/level (*L*) settings to evaluate: the soft tissues of the brain (*W*=100–150, *L*=30–50), bone (*W*=3000, *L*=500) and an intermediate window (*W*=150–200, *L*=50–100) to identify skull fractures and small subdural or extradural haematomas respectively. The scout view must be examined to look for fractures, although these can be missed if they are in line with the scan plane and/or foreign bodies. Assess the scalp for the coup site where a skull fracture and extradural may be seen, and the contracoup site for the parenchymal injury. Acute cranial trauma affects all ages and is the leading cause of death in those under 40 years of age. It is also the cause of significant morbidity so that prompt and effective management is essential, including imaging.

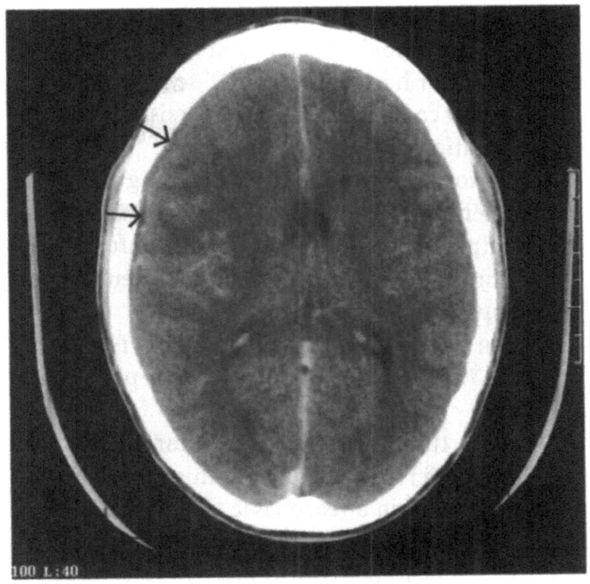

Fig. 8.5. A 21-year-old male with a past history of sinusitis treated with antibiotics presented with headaches. Enhanced CT demonstrates a subtle subdural empyema (*arrow*)

It is important that there are guidelines for CT in head injured patients. Current guidelines have been reviewed and revised by The Society of British Neurological Surgeons (1998).

a 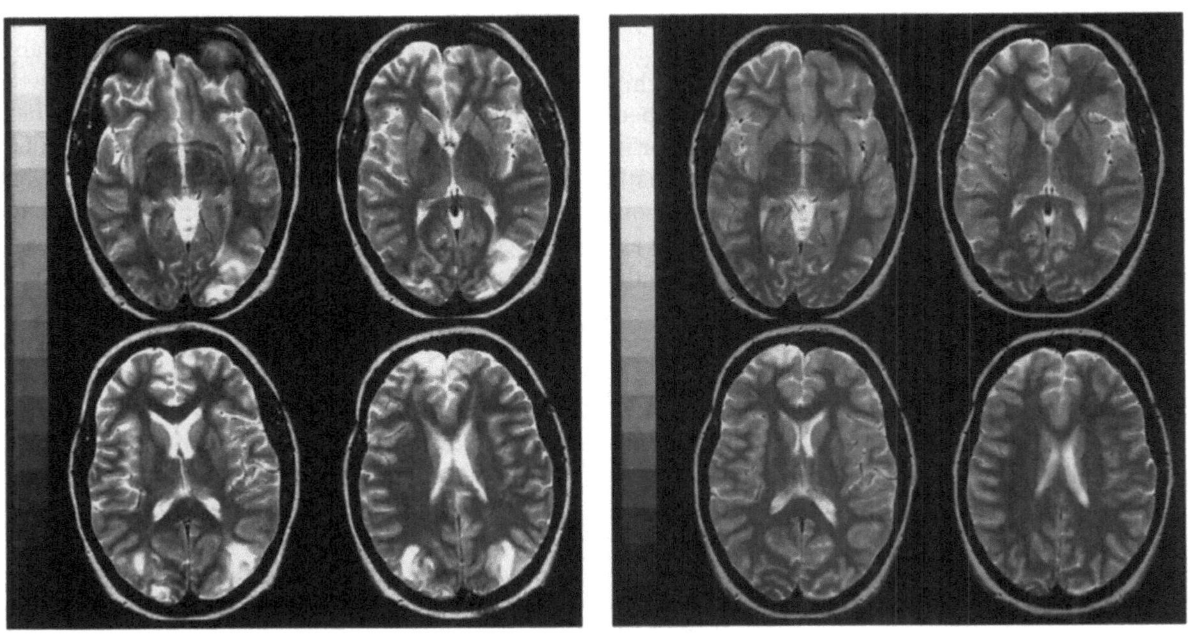 b

Fig. 8.6a,b. A 28-year-old female presented at 30 weeks gestation with eclampsia and fits. **a** MRI demonstrates vasogenic oedema mainly involving the posterior parieto-occipital lobes. **b** Two months following delivery, the scan is normal

Two categories of patients are defined:

1. Those that should be referred to the neurosurgeon and/or have an urgent CT scan
   - Glasgow coma score < than 9 persisting after resuscitation
   - Deteriorating consciousness or progressive focal neurological deficits
   - Fracture of the skull with any of: confusion, deteriorating consciousness, fits or neurological symptoms and signs
   - Open injury – depressed compound fracture of skull vault, base of skull fracture or penetrating injury
   - Patient fulfils criteria for CT scan of the head within referring hospital but this cannot be performed within a reasonable time (e.g. 2–4 h).

2. CT of the head performed prior to referral to the neurosurgeons. In this group the CT scan should be performed urgently (within 2–4 h) on patients of all ages with any of the following criteria:
   - Full consciousness but with a skull fracture
   - Fits without a skull fracture
   - Confusion or neurological symptoms/signs persisting after initial assessment and resuscitation
   - Unstable systemic state precluding transfer to neurosurgery
   - Diagnosis uncertain
   - Tense fontanelle or suture diastasis in a child
   - Significant head injury requiring general anaesthesia.

These guidelines can be used for adults and children and are evidence based from results of prospectively studied cohorts. This evidence concerns principally the estimation of the risk of a traumatic intracranial haematoma. A depressed level of consciousness and the presence of a skull fracture are the main factors, which can be determined when the patient is assessed in the emergency department that identify the risk that a patient has of having or developing a surgically significant intracranial haematoma.

CT is less sensitive when performed on patients with severe anaemia or who suffer from disseminated intravascular coagulopathy when acute haematomas may be isodense or low density. MRI is more sensitive in these situations.

MRI is indicated when there is a discrepancy between the patient's clinical condition and CT findings. CT may be unremarkable and the likely diagnosis is that the patient has a diffuse axonal injury (DAI) secondary to a rotational injury. DAI usually affects the lobar white matter, corpus callosum and brainstem. Gradient-echo imaging is more sensitive at detecting the haemorrhagic component of this injury. Cortical contusions and brainstem injuries are also better seen on MRI.

8.5 Conclusion

CT will remain the imaging modality of choice for the investigation of most patients presenting to the emergency department because of its availability and because it is quick to perform. It can detect haemorrhage, mass lesions, signs of raised intracranial pressure, cerebral oedema and brain herniation accurately. The information obtained can direct the management pathway for most patients presenting as emergencies. Guidelines are available as to which patients who have had traumatic brain injury should be scanned. Patients with acute medical neurological problems, such as the sudden onset of severe headache where an SAH is suspected, decreasing level of consciousness which may be secondary to a focal intracranial mass lesion (infarct, haemorrhage, tumour, abscess) or a diffuse process (cerebral oedema), should be scanned as a matter of urgency. The exact timing of the imaging on patients presenting with the sudden onset of focal neurological signs depends on the suspected clinical diagnosis and whether the result of imaging will change the management of that patient and also the time course of the clinical picture, which if progressive identifies the patient that needs to be imaged urgently. If an LP is indicated to confirm the clinical diagnosis, e.g. meningitis and there is a clinical contraindication to LP, urgent imaging is necessary. CTA has an increasing role to play in the evaluation of emergency patients with intraparenchymal and subarachnoid haemorrhage, to assess the possibility of an underlying vascular cause, such as an aneurysm, prior to evacuation of the haematoma, and also if there is a contraindication to catheter cerebral angiography. MRI is becoming increasingly available. When the suspected clinical diagnosis is posterior reversible encephalopathy syndrome (hypertensive encephalopathy), herpes simplex encephalitis, subdural empyema or venous thrombosis, MRI is a more sensitive investigation and should be performed in the first instance, provided there is no contraindication to MRI and the patient can cooperate for the scan. MRI is likely to lead to an earlier accurate diagnosis, and allow prompt institution of appropriate treatment with resultant improvement in patient outcome. CT will continue to play a central role in acute stroke management. XeCT provides quantifiable information about the threshold levels of cerebral blood flow necessary to ensure cerebral tissue viability, but it is not widely available. CT perfusion techniques and DWI/PWI MRI will play important roles in the assessment of patients who have had a confirmed diagnosis of ischaemic stroke when thrombolysis treatment is being considered.

References

Atlas SW, Sheppard L, Goldberg HI, Hurst RW, Listerud J, Flamm E (1997) Intracranial aneurysms: detection and characterization with MR angiography with use of an advanced post processing technique in a blinded-reader study. Radiology 20: 807–814

Bakshi R, Kamran S, Kinkel PR et al. (1999) Fluid-attenuated inversion-recovery MR imaging in acute and subacute cerebral intraventricular haemorrhage. Am J Neuroradiol 20: 629–636

Barest GD, Sorensen AG, Gonzalez RG (1998) Magnetic resonance imaging of cerebral infarction. Top Magn Reson Imaging 9: 199–207

Campbell BG, Zimmerman RD (1998) Emergency magnetic resonance of the brain. Top Magn Reson Imaging 9: 208–227

Hunter GJ, Hamberg LM, Ponzo JA et al. (1998) Assessment of cerebral perfusion and arterial anatomy in hyperacute stroke with three-dimensional functional CT: early clinical results. Am J Neuroradiol 19: 29–37

Kaufmann AM, Firlik AD, Fukui MB, Wechsler LR, Jungries CA, Yonas H (1999) Ischaemic core and penumbra in human stroke. Stroke 30: 93–99

Libman RB, Wirkowski E, Alvir J, Rao TH (1995) Conditions that mimic stroke in the emergency department. Arch Neurol 52: 1119–1122

Lövblad KO, Laubach HJ, Baird AE et al. (1998) Clinical experience with diffusion-weighted MR in patients with acute stroke. Am J Neuroradiol 19: 1061–1066

Mohr JP, Biller J, Hilal SK et al. (1995) Magnetic resonance versus computed tomographic imaging in acute stroke. Stroke 26: 807–812

Noguchi K, Ogawa T, Seto H et al. (1997) Subacute and chronic subarachnoid haemorrhage: diagnosis with fluid-attenuated inversion-recovery MR imaging Radiology 203: 257–262

Provenzale JM, Joseph GJ, Barboriak DP (1998) Dural sinus thrombosis: findings on CT and MR images and diagnostic pitfalls Am J Roentgenol 170: 777–783

Sorensen AG, Buonanno FS, Gonzalez RG et al. (1996) Hyperacute stroke: evaluation with combined multisection diffusion-weighted and hemodynamically weighted echo-planar MR imaging. Radiology 199: 391–401

The Society of British Neurological Surgeons (1998) Guidelines for the initial management of head injuries: recommendations for the Society of British Neurological Surgeons. Br J Neurosurg 14: 349–352

Vieco PT, Shuman WP (1995) A comparison of CT angiography and digital subtraction angiography in the detection of Circle of Willis aneurysms in patients with acute subarachnoid haemorrhage. Am J Roentgenol 165: 425–430

Von Kummer R, Bozzao L, Manelfe C (eds) (1995) Early CT diagnosis of hemispheric brain infarction. Berlin, Springer

Warach S, Boska M, Welch KMA (1997) Pitfalls and potential of clinical diffusion-weighted MR imaging in acute stroke. Stroke 28: 481–482

9 Recent Developments in Brain Tumour Diagnosis

GUY WILMS, STEFAN SUNAERT, PATRICK FLAMEN

CONTENTS

9.1 Introduction

The introduction of magnetic resonance imaging (MRI) in the mid-eighties was a major step forward in the diagnosis and pretherapeutic set-up of brain tumors. As compared to computed tomography (CT), which was considered as the gold standard up to then, MRI offered several advantages.

First, MRI has a definite higher sensitivity for pathological changes in the brain parenchyma. Lesions with comparable absorption coefficients for X-rays can be invisible on CT. The classical example here is of course the "plaque" of multiple sclerosis, but tumors too can be missed on CT for the same reason. With MRI, the high water content of most glial and other tumors leads to an obvious hyperintensity on T2-weighted images.

G. WILMS, MD, PhD
Professor, Department of Radiology, University Hospitals, Herestraat 49, 3000 Leuven, Belgium
S. SUNAERT, MD
Department of Radiology, University Hospitals, Herestraat 49, 3000 Leuven, Belgium
P. FLAMEN, MD
Department of Nuklear Medicine, University Hospitals, Herestraat 49, 3000 Leuven, Belgium

A second advantage is the higher contrast resolution obtained with MRI. This allows better detection of smaller lesions and better study of the morphology of the mass. The higher anatomic detail, with excellent differentiation between gray and white matter, leads to a better understanding of the lesions' topography. After intravenous injection of paramagnetic contrast media, smaller foci of contrast enhancement can be detected. The degree and pattern of enhancement can better be appreciated.

On CT, lesions in the posterior fossa, and more specifically in the brainstem, are easily missed due to beam-hardening artifacts from bone. Streak artifacts can mask lesions adjacent to bone. In a similar way contrast enhancement can be hard to appreciate in the vicinity of bone, such as the convexity and the internal auditory canal due to the intrinsic hyperdensity of bone. On MRI cortical bone returns no signal, so that artifacts from bone are non-existent. Therefore the structures of the posterior fossa, cerebellum and brainstem, as well as the infratentorial and supratentorial superficial cortical structures, are very well displayed on the different imaging sequences. After intravenous injection of paramagnetic contrast agents, enhancing and thus T1-hyperintense lesions stand out excellently against the absent signal and thus black image of the bone. This allows easy detection of intracanalicular acoustic schwannomas and superficial carcinomatous meningitis.

Another major advantage of MRI over CT is the ease of obtaining multiplanar imaging and reconstructable 3D datasets, without the necessity of repositioning the patient. This enables more appropriate imaging planes for specific anatomic areas such as the hypophysis (coronal and sagittal views), the brainstem (sagittal incidence), the cerebellopontine angle (axial and coronal views), etc. Furthermore it allows the exact spatial topographical localization of tumors and better estimation of the lesions' volume and extent. Correlation with other imaging modalities such as tomography, reconstructed CT or angiography is possible in the same imaging planes.

Despite these obvious advantages of MRI, some shortcomings became rapidly evident. Some smaller lesions such as micrometastases were missed, leading to false negative screening examinations. In the same way, doses of paramagnetic contrast media were judged too low or too high. Differentiation between tumor and peritumoral edema was not always easy, especially at the edges of contrast enhancing lesions with heavy repercussion on the determination of the radiation field. Differentiation between benign and malignant tumors appeared less accurate than initially thought. In the case of a ring-enhancing lesion, differentiation between tumor, abscess and other lesions was difficult. Mass effect or edema with distortion and effacing of local sulcal anatomy could hamper exact topographical localization of tumoral lesions, especially with regard to eloquent areas such as the motor or speech cortex. An exact stereotactic approach of tumoral lesions was difficult due to image distortion. In the follow-up of patients treated with surgery, radiotherapy, chemotherapy or a combination of these therapies, one of the major drawbacks remained the exact determination of the tumor volume. Finally in the follow-up of patients treated with radiotherapy, differentiation between recurrent tumor and radiation necrosis was difficult. Clinical and fundamental research in the last 5 years has therefore aimed at answering these shortcomings.

9.2 MR and New Tumoral Entities

In 1993 the World Health Organization (WHO) profoundly revised the histologic typing of tumors of the central nervous system (Kleihues et al. 1993). Besides changes in the classification of the known tumors, new entities were added. Since these lesions were described in the era of MRI, their imaging characteristics were very rapidly reported. On the other hand their discovery was greatly facilitated by the higher sensitivity of soft-tissue changes by MRI. The lesions are mostly benign and occur in children or young adults. They concern new types of neuronal and mixed neuronal-glial tumors such as: dysembryoplastic neuroepithelial tumor, desmoplastic infantile ganglioglioma and central neurocytoma and a new subtype of focal astrocytoma, the so-called pleiomorphic xanthoastrocytoma.

The dysembryoplastic neuroepithelial tumor (DNT) has a mixed glial-neuronal origin. The tumor is composed of oligodendrocyte-like cells located in a myxoid matrix. It is typically a supratentorial intracortical tumor mostly situated in the temporal lobe and manifests as intractable epilepsy in children. On MR besides the cortical and temporal location, a typical feature is the multicystic nature referring to the myxoid matrix with strongly hyperintense cysts, due to the high protein content. Approximately half of the solid DNT elements show enhancement (Koeller et al. 1992).

The desmoplastic infantile ganglioglioma (Fig. 9.1) is also a mixed glial-neuronal tumor. The typical appearance is a frontal or parietal predominantly cystic tumor, with a solid part abutting the meningeal surface. On MR the cystic component is isointense with CSF. The peripheral nodule is broad based on the surface. Enhancement of the solid nodule and possible intracystic septa is intense (Rypens et al. 1996).

Central neurocytoma (Fig. 9.2) is composed of cells with ultrastructural features of neurons. It appears as a well-circumscribed mass in the lateral ventricles near the foramen of Monro with a charac-

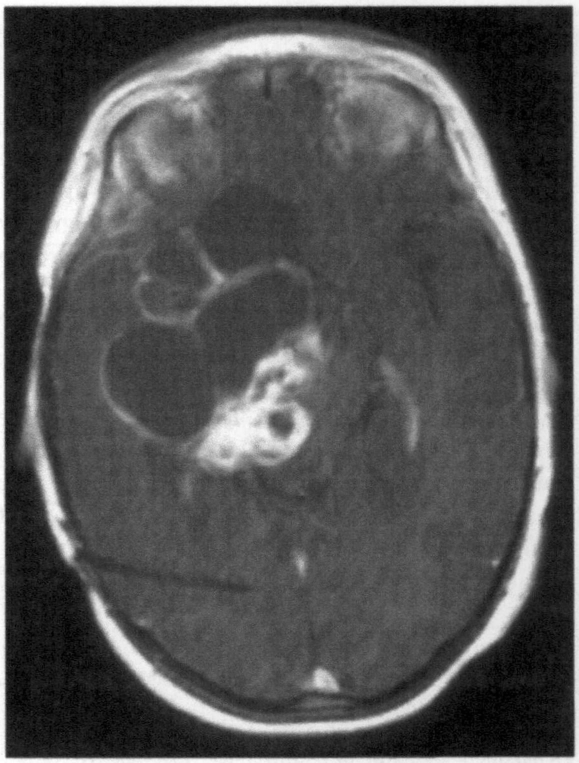

Fig. 9.1. Desmoplastic infantile ganglioglioma. Transverse T1-weighted spin-echo gadolinium-enhanced image. Huge multicystic ring-enhancing lesion in the right frontotemporal region. Solid portions invading the brainstem

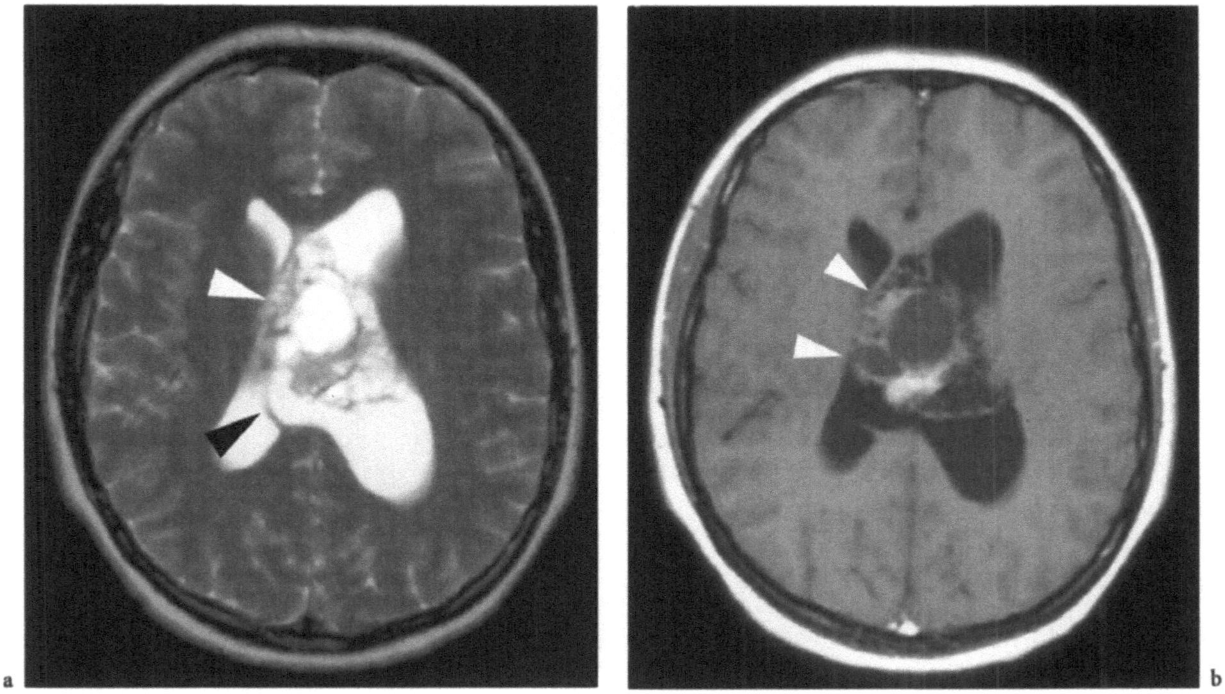

Fig. 9.2a,b. Central neurocytoma. **a** Transverse T2-weighted spin-echo image (TR=5000, TE=125 ms). **b** Transverse Gd-enhanced T1-weighted spin-echo image (TR=600, TE=15 ms). Solid tumor with multiple small and larger intratumoral cysts in the left lateral ventricle. Note broad implantation on the septum pellucidum (*arrowheads*)

teristic attachment to the septum pellucidum. Cysts, calcification and necrosis are common. On MR the attachment to the septum pellucidum or the broad-based attachment to the superolateral ventricular wall is well visualized on multiplanar images. The tumor is isointense to gray matter on T1- and T2-weighted images, with inlaying small cysts and calcification. Contrast enhancement is mild (GOERGEN et al. 1992).

The pleiomorphic xanthoastrocytoma is superficially located with a solid nodule that is intimately related to the meninges, frequently with an underlying cyst. The epitheton "xantho" refers to the content of xanthomatous lipid vacuoles present in pleiomorphic astrocytes. On MR the lesion is hypointense on T1-weighted images and hyperintense on T2-weighted images. The nodule and the overlying meninges enhance markedly so that the lesion is frequently mistaken for a meningioma or, if cystic, for a pilocytic astrocytoma (RIPPE et al. 1992). Angiographic external carotid artery supply can further add to the confusion with meningioma.

9.3 Paramagnetic Contrast Dosage and Background Signal Suppression

Much attention was paid in the recent literature to the influence of the dose of paramagnetic contrast media on the detection of smaller lesions and the determination of the extent of larger brain tumors.

Most brain metastases larger than 10 mm are easily visible on T2-weighted images due to accompanying edema. Lesions smaller than 10 mm can be invisible on conventional T2-weighted sequences. Moreover they can be missed even after the injection of paramagnetic contrast media. Detection of small lesions is important, since resection of a solitary metastasis or treatment of multiple lesions with chemo- or radiotherapy can markedly improve the survival and quality of life of patients. Here it was demonstrated that a cumulative triple dose study is more effective than the standard dose of 0.1 mmol/kg in the detection of metastases smaller than 10 mm. Delayed imaging after the injection of a standard dose improves the detection rate too, but to a lesser extent (YUH et al. 1995, 1997) (Fig. 9.3).

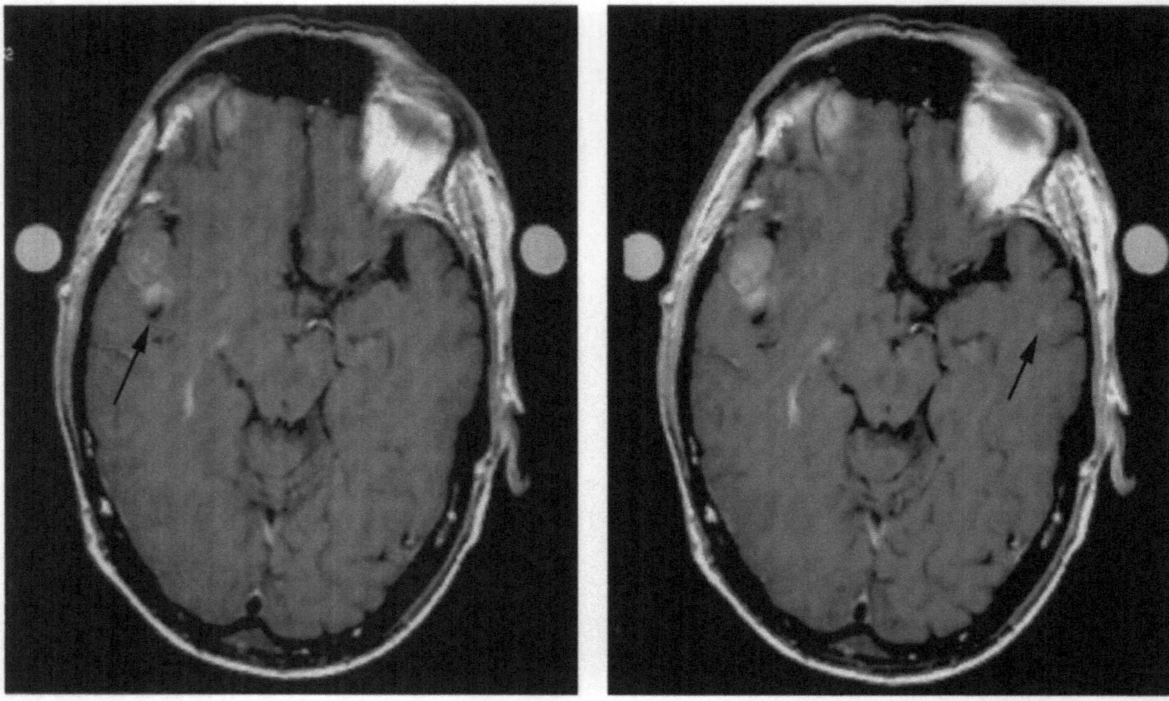

Fig. 9.3a,b. Use of triple dose in the search for cerebral metastases. a Transverse T1-weighted spin-echo image (TR=700, TE=14 ms) after a single contrast dose. Metastatic lesion in the right temporal lobe (*arrow*). No lesion is seen in the left temporal lobe. b After double contrast dose. Small additional metastasis (*arrow*) is seen in the left temporal lobe. Case courtesy of L. van den Hauwe and P. Parizel, University Hospitals, Antwerp, Belgium

Further studies analyzed the effect of the combination of contrast injection and suppression of the background signal by the application of a magnetization transfer (MT) pulse (Finelli et al. 1998; Knauth et al. 1996; Ramadan et al. 1997). It was shown that MT improved the contrast between enhancing lesions and background white matter. Furthermore standard dose MT T1-weighted spin-echo MR studies were equivalent to triple dose T1-weighted sequences. Triple dose MT T1-weighted studies further increase lesion-to-white matter contrast but without showing additional lesions. On the other hand, the combination of MT with half-dose gadolinium-enhanced MR proved inferior to standard dose-enhanced conventional MR imaging (Han et al. 1998).

Another point of interest was the effect of higher contrast doses on the delineation of gliomas. It is known that in most tumors the extent of signal abnormalities on T2-weighted images is larger than the area of contrast enhancement. Pathological studies on biopsies of malignant gliomas though have demonstrated that tumoral cells are found beyond the area of enhancement. With triple doses of paramagnetic contrast agents the area of enhancement seems greater than with the conventional dose and extends clearly in the peritumoral edema as seen on T2-weighted images and sometimes even beyond this area. This is explained by the authors by an increased contrast pooling of the higher doses of contrast in the intravascular space of gliomas with partially intact blood-brain barrier (Maley et al. 1998; Yuh et al. 1994a,b).

In other tumors, on the contrary, the standard contrast dose seems to be too high. For the study of acoustic schwannoma, for instance, a fractional dose of one-half (0.05 mmol/kg) seems to lead to an intense enhancement with sufficient lesion to background ratio (Nguyen et al. 1995). Microadenomas of the pituitary gland show a very rapid take-up of the contrast agent and therefore a smaller dose is sufficient.-

9.4 Role of Diffusion-Weighted MR (DWI) in the Diagnosis of Brain Tumors

Diffusion-weighted MR (DWI) is a new MR technique based on the natural sensitivity of MRI to motion, in this case random or "brownian" motion (KRABBE et al. 1997). Using diffusion-sensitizing gradient pulses, the diffusion effect can be enhanced, leading to dephasing and hence attenuation of the MR signal. The most common clinical application is the early detection of cerebral infarcts, before the appearance of T2 hyperintensity and the differentiation of old from recent infarcts.

Diffusion-weighted MR imaging has been used to distinguish the tumor core from edema, cysts or necrosis (KRABBE et al. 1997). The areas of enhancing tumor on conventional gadolinium-enhanced MRI were found to be markedly hyperintense on diffusion-weighted images, whereas peritumoral edema is not. In the same way, cysts with a high protein content that resemble solid tumors on conventional spin-echo sequences are easily recognized on diffusion-weighted MR imaging.

Several authors have stressed the value of diffusion-weighted MR imaging in the differential diagnosis of ring-enhancing lesions (KIM et al. 1998; NOGUCHI et al. 1999). Brain abscesses show restricted diffusion (Fig. 9.4), due to the presence of pus, cellular debris and bacteria and therefore return markedly hyperintense signal. Necrotic or cystic brain tumors, such as malignant gliomas and metastases, have a more fluid content and therefore are hypointense on diffusion-weighted MR imaging (Fig. 9.5). Although this finding is useful, exceptions to this rule have been reported.

Other authors found higher diffusion in the enhancing portions of malignant gliomas and in the surrounding edema than in the enhancing portions and surrounding edema of cerebral metastases. This might avoid unnecessary searches for a primary tumor in patients with doubtful findings on conventional spin-echo images (KUCHARCZYK et al. 1997; SUGAHARA et al. 1999).

According to recent reports, diffusion-weighted MR imaging seems of great value in the differentiation between pediatric fossa posterior tumors (KLISCH et al. 1999; ZIMMERMAN et al. 1999). It is known that on conventional spin-echo images "everything can resemble everything." Pediatric primitive neuroectodermal tumors or PNETs have a tendency to strong hyperintensity on diffusion-weighted MR images, whereas other tumors such as low-grade astrocytomas are hypointense. The high signal in diffusion-weighted MR imaging is probably due to dense cell packing. In addition the appearance on images

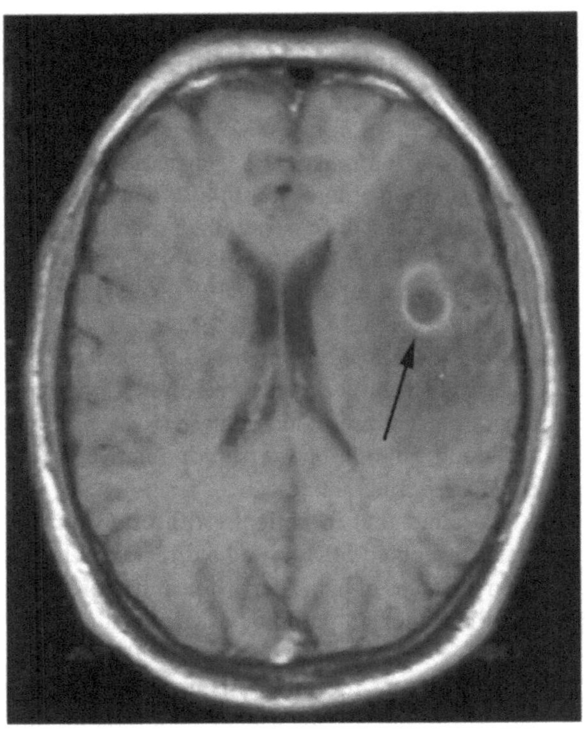
a

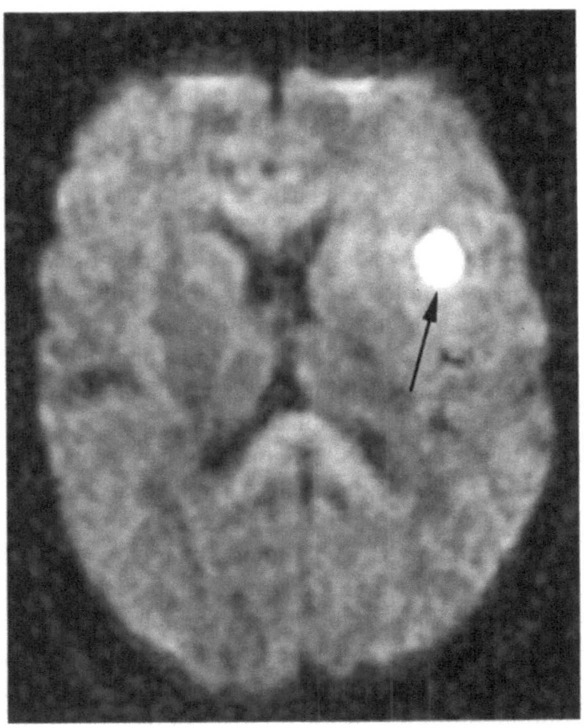
b

Fig. 9.4a,b. Brain abscess. **a** Transverse gadolinium-enhanced T1-weighted spin-echo image. Rounded lesion (*arrow*) in the left frontal lobe surrounded by edema. Ring-enhancement of the lesion. **b** Transverse diffusion-weighted EPI image. The center of the lesion is hyperintense (*arrow*)

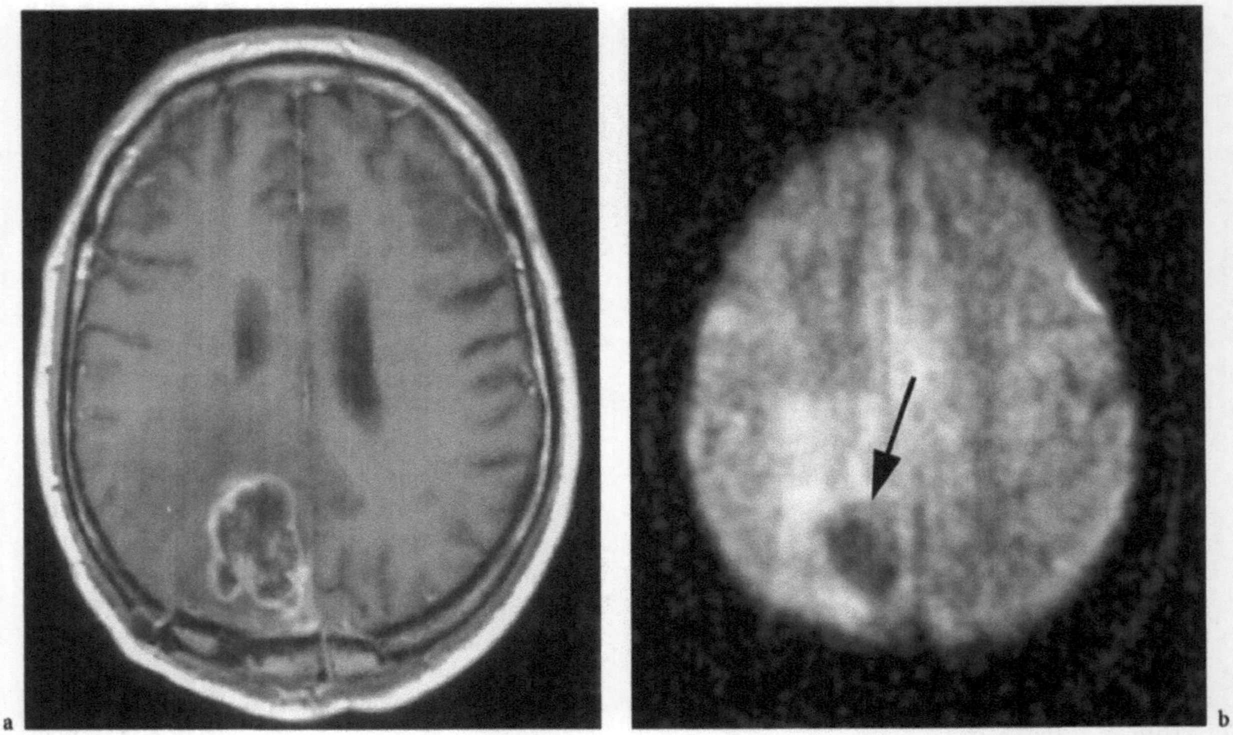

Fig. 9.5a,b. Metastasis. **a** Transverse T1-weighted gadolinium-enhanced spin-echo image. Ring-enhancing lesion in the right parieto-occipital region. **b** Transverse diffusion-weighted EPI image. The center of the lesion is hypointense (*arrow*)

obtained with fluid attenuation recovery (FLAIR) is different too, PNETs being isointense while gliomatous tumors tend to be hyperintense. Supratentorial PNETs show the same behavior as their infratentorial counterparts.

The same hypercellularity as in PNET is found in cerebral lymphoma (Fig. 9.6). Therefore it is not surprising that these lesions show hyperintensity on diffusion-weighted MR imaging. This finding of the correlation of high signal on diffusion-weighted MR imaging and high cellularity might be of utmost importance in the selection of the targets of biopsy or the determination of radiation fields.

Diffusion-weighted MR imaging can be used in the differential diagnosis of arachnoid cysts and epidermoid cysts (Ikushima et al. 1997; Tsuruda et al. 1990). Both are extraaxial tumors that have a predilection for the cerebellopontine or parasellar cisterns, show long T1 and T2 and are non-enhancing. On diffusion-weighted MR imaging epidermoid cysts (Fig. 9.7) are hyperintense due to restricted motion of protons by the presence of membranes of densely layered epithelium. In arachnoid cysts (Fig. 9.8) water motion is free and hence the lesions are hypointense (Tsuruda et al. 1990).

9.5 Perfusion Imaging and Brain Tumors

The combination of ultrafast MR sequences and bolus injection of paramagnetic contrast agents provides information about cerebral perfusion (Knopp et al. 1999). The administration of paramagnetic contrast agents leads to susceptibility effects with a decrease in signal intensity on T2* images that can easily be measured. In patients with brain tumors, this allows the evaluation of tissue blood flow and microvascular volume, mostly measured as the ratio of maximum cerebral blood volume (rCBV), a ratio of the blood volume of the tumor relative to the contralateral white matter.

It was found that in patients with brain tumors perfusion-weighted MR showed a direct correlation between the areas of hyperperfusion and aggressiveness of the tumor on pathology (Knopp et al. 1999; Lam et al. 1999; Sugahara et al. 1998) (Figs. 9.9, 9.10). Considering the different prognosis and response to therapy between anaplastic glioma and glioblastoma that may show similar imaging characteristics on MR, determination of the perfusion of these tumors might have practical implications for

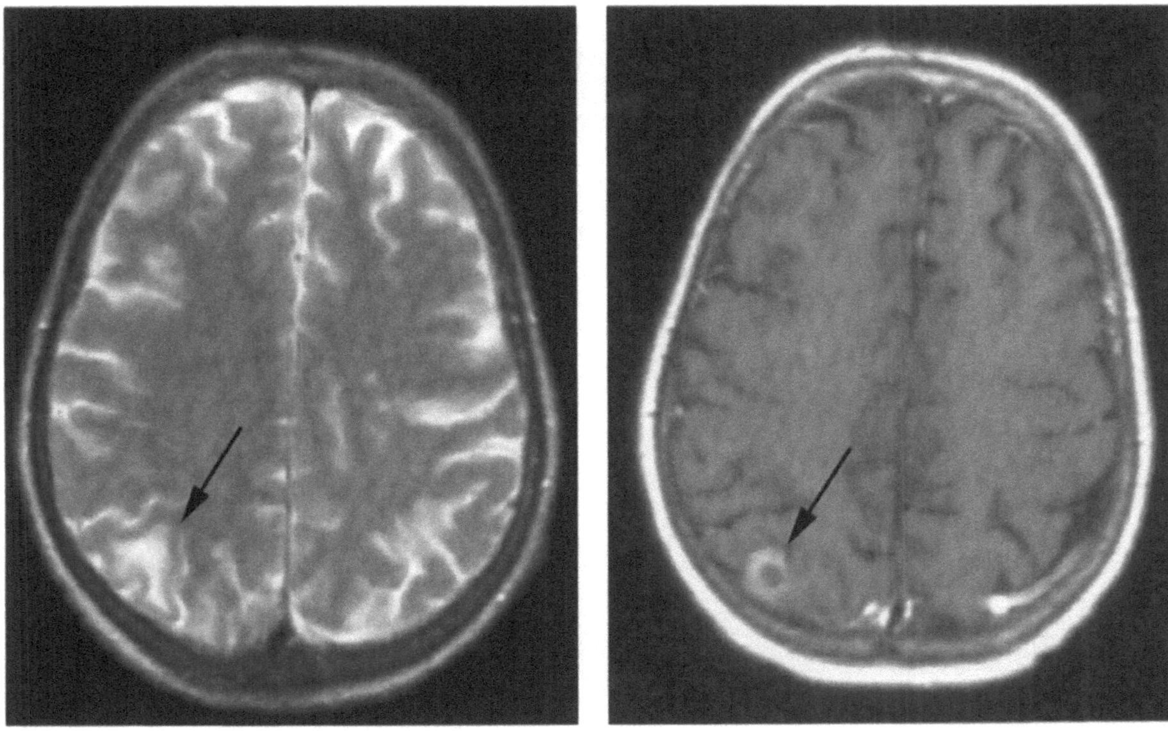

a b

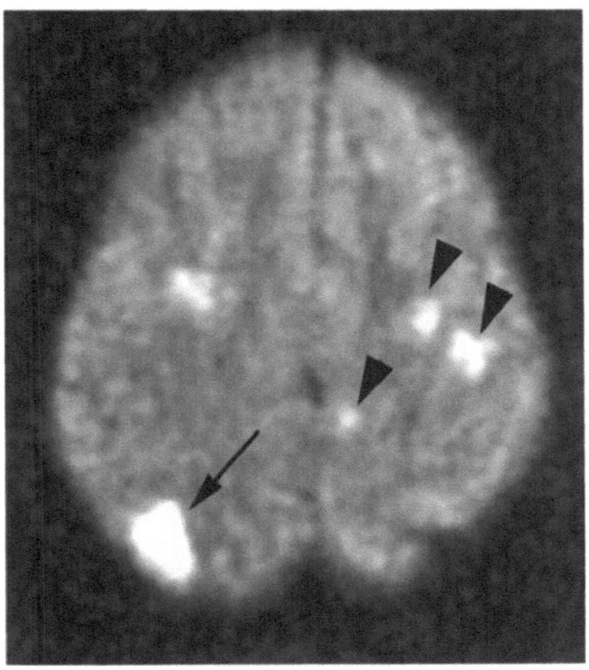

c

Fig. 9.6a–c. Lymphoma. **a** Transverse T2-weighted (TR=3380, TE=90 ms) spin-echo image. Hyperintense lesion (*arrow*) in the right parietal region. **b** Transverse gadolinium-enhanced spin-echo image. Enhancement of the lesion (*arrow*). **c** Transverse diffusion-weighted EPI image. The lesion (*arrow*) is hypertense. Note appearance of additional lesions (*arrowheads*)

therapy. Moreover there was a correlation between the tumoral perfusion and its enhancement and its histologic vascularity. This might reflect the amount of tumor angiogenesis. Since with perfusion imaging the total vascular bed is imaged there is also a correlation between the maximum rCBV ratios and angiographic hypervascularity. An rCBV ratio of 4.30 correlates with angiographic hypervascularity. The determination of the areas of maximal perfusion allows targeting biopsies in order to obtain the most representative specimens. The technique may also guide radiotherapy planning by demonstrating the border between active tumor and normal brain or surrounding edema. Finally it is obvious that perfusion MR will be able to differentiate between relapsing neoplasm and radiation necrosis.

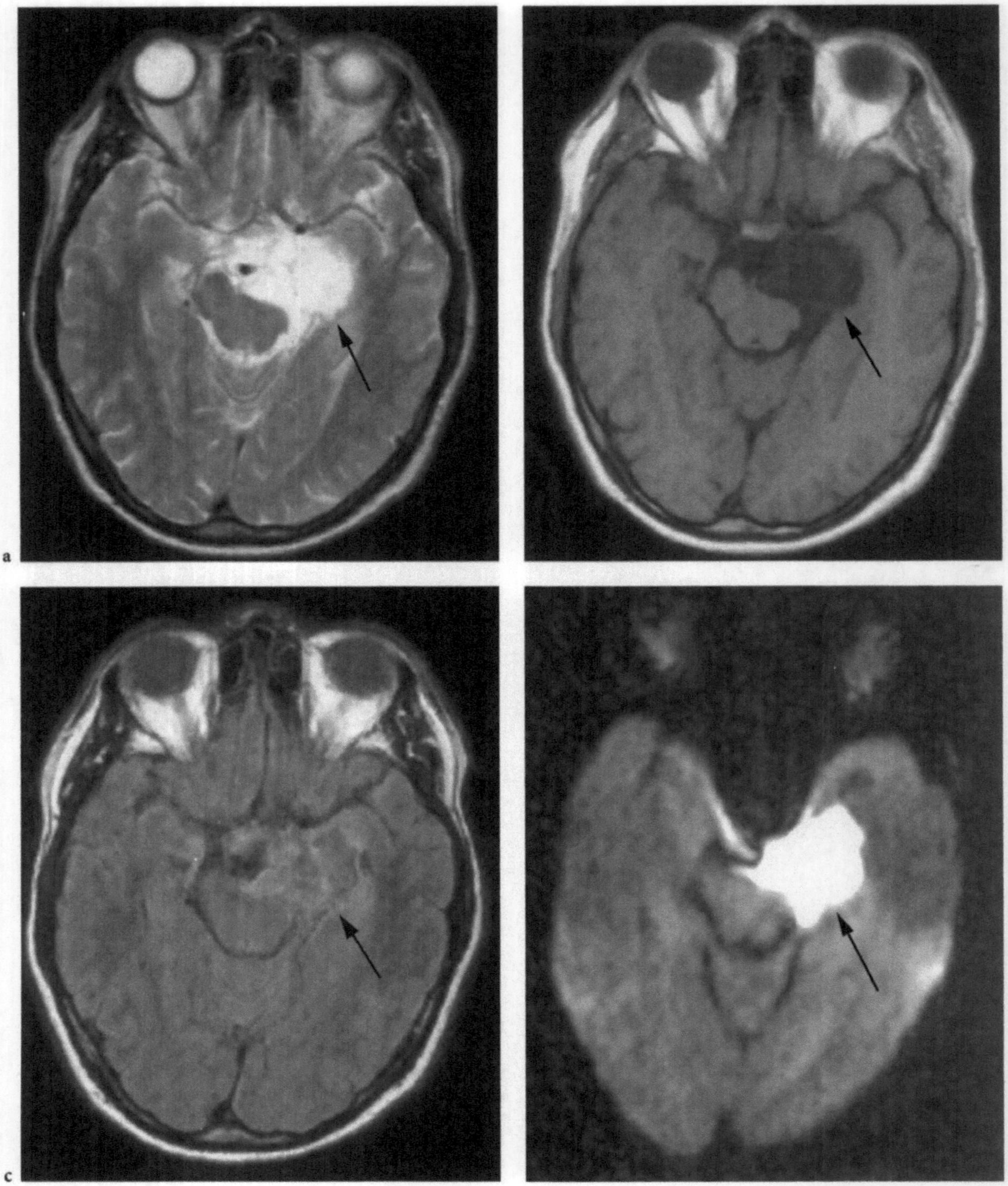

Fig. 9.7a–d. Epidermoid cyst. **a** Transverse T2-weighted (TR=3380, TE=90 ms) spin-echo image. Inhomogeneously hyperintense lesion (*arrow*) in the right prepontine cistern with extension to the temporal fossa. Some intralesional strands are visible. Note brainstem compression. **b** Transverse T1-weighted (TR=560, TE=15 ms) spin-echo image at the same level. The lesion is hypointense (*arrow*). **c** Transverse T2-weighted image with fluid suppression (TR=6500, TE=105 ms, TI=180 ms) at the same level. The fluid in the eyeball and the subarachnoid spaces is suppressed. The lesion (*arrow*) remains hyperintense. **d** Transverse diffusion-weighted EPI image. Lesion remains hyperintense (*arrow*)

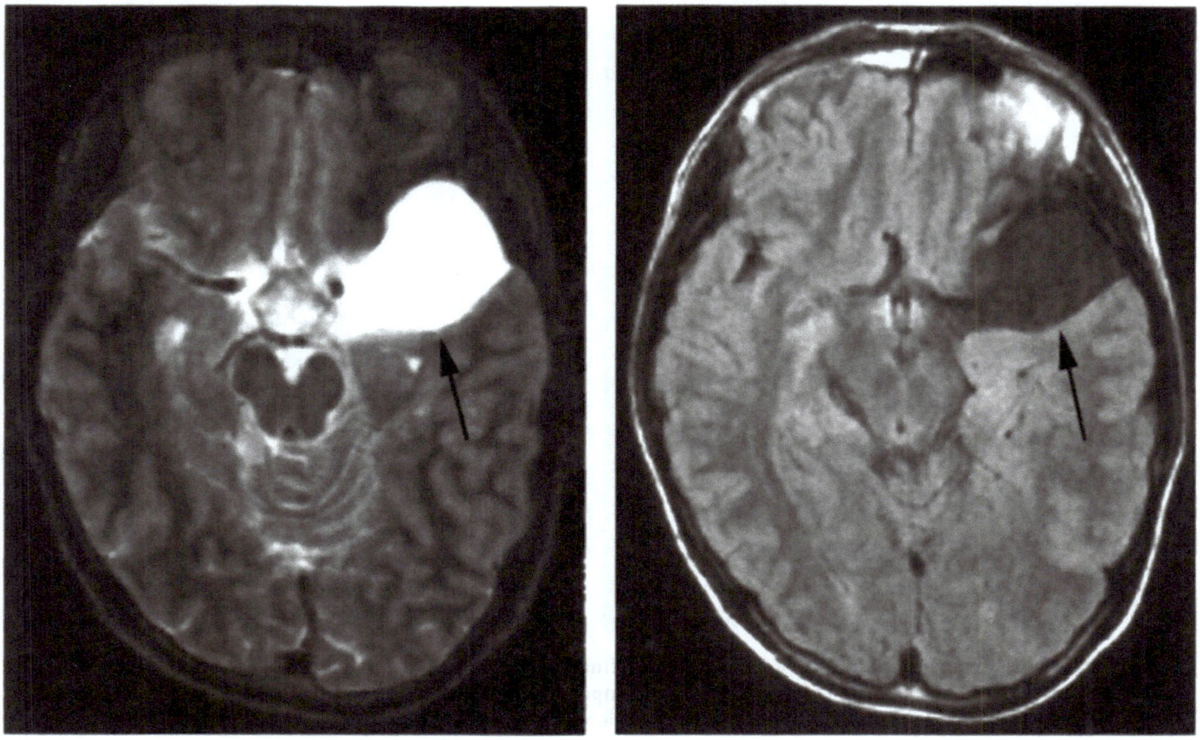

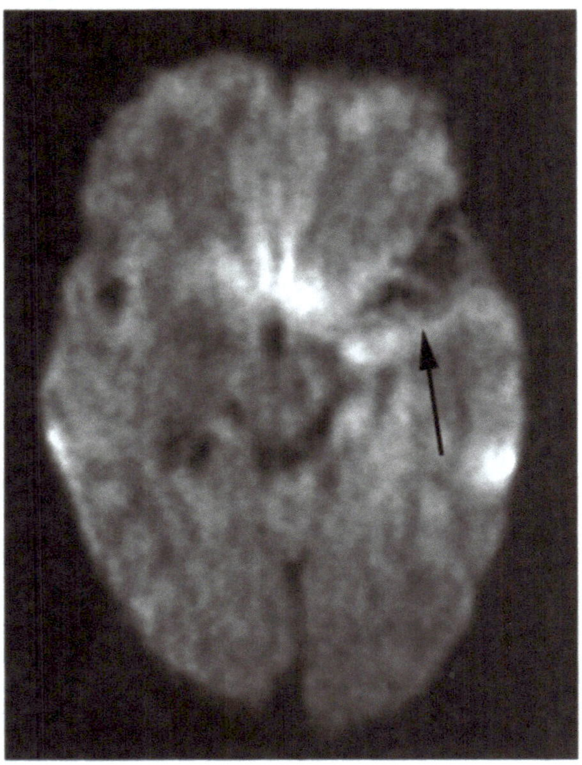

Fig. 9.8a–c. Arachnoid cyst of the left temporal fossa. **a** Transverse T2-weighted (TR=5000, TE=85 ms) spin-echo image. Strongly hyperintense lesion (*arrow*) in the left temporal fossa, suggesting a fluid containing cyst. **b** Transverse T2-weighted image with fluid suppression (TR=6500, TE=105 ms, TI=2340 ms). The signal in the lesion is suppressed, confirming the aqueous nature of the lesion. **c** Transverse diffusion-weighted EPI sequence. No signal in the lesion (*arrow*), pointing to normal diffusion

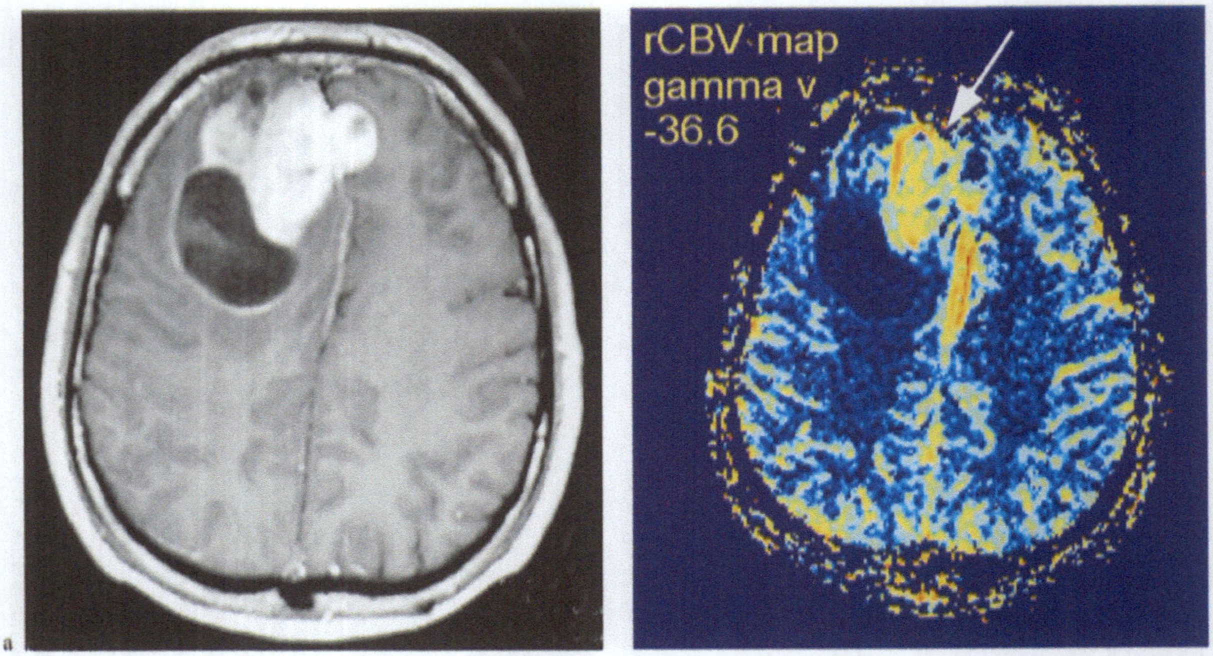

Fig. 9.9a,b. Glioblastoma: perfusion MRI. **a** Transverse gadolinium enhanced T1-weighted spin-echo image (TR=600, TE=14 ms). Right frontal strongly enhancing tumor. Note cystic component. **b** Perfusion MR: relative cerebral blood volume (rCBV) map after gamma variate correction. There is good correlation between the hyperperfused areas on rCBC map (*arrow*) and the contrast enhancement on spin-echo sequences. Case courtesy of T. Stadnik and M. Osteaux, AZ-VUB, Brussels, Belgium

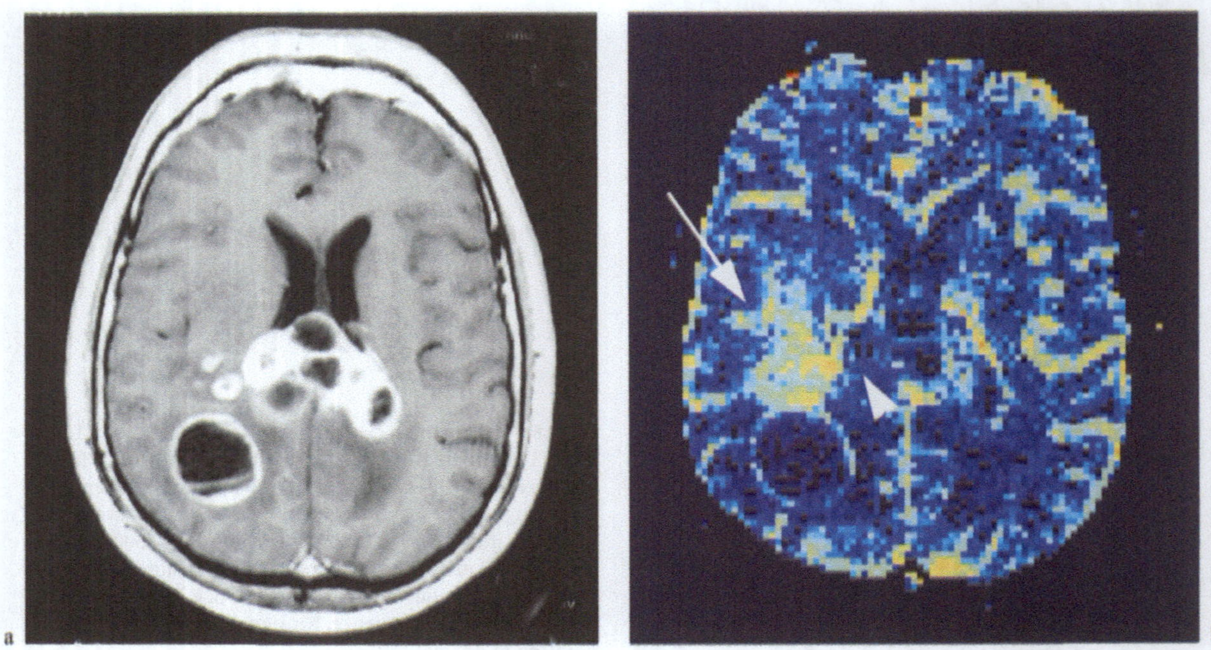

Fig. 9.10a,b. Glioblastoma of the corpus callosum: perfusion MR. **a** Transverse gadolinium enhanced T1-weighted spin-echo image (TR=600, TE=14 ms). Multifocal, multicystic enhancing lesion in the splenium of the corpus callosum, extending to the right parieto-occipital lobe and to a lesser extent to the left. Note solid enhancing portions. **b** Perfusion MR: rCBV map after gamma variate correction. The highest perfusion is seen in an area with less enhancement on enhanced spin-echo images (*arrow*). Other enhancing portions are less perfused (*arrowhead*). Biopsy in the hyperperfused non-enhancing zone indicated glioblastoma. In the enhancing zone no signs of malignancy were present. Case courtesy of T. Stadnik and M. Osteaux, AZ-VUB, Brussels, Belgium

In patients with acquired immunodeficiency syndrome (AIDS), perfusion MR might allow differentiation between toxoplasmosis and lymphoma (Ernst et al. 1998). Toxoplasmosis lesions are poorly vascular and the surrounding edema shows vasoconstriction with reduced rCBV. In lymphoma necrotic areas and the surrounding edema show the same hypoperfusion, but these tumors always show areas of increased blood volume, correlating with hypervascularity of the active neoplastic process. In this way for the differentiation between toxoplasmosis and lymphoma, perfusion MR might guide the biopsy. Ultimately, combined with clinical and laboratory findings, perfusion MR might replace biopsy, avoiding complications in patients at risk.

Finally, preliminary results suggest that perfusion MR might be of importance in evaluating the pathophysiological changes of therapeutic drugs on tumoral tissue. Dramatic acute changes in rCBV were seen in brain tumors after glucocorticoid administration, reflecting acute changes in blood-tumor barrier (Østergaard et al. 1999).

9.6 Functional MR and Brain Tumor Diagnosis and Topography

The exact topographical location of brain tumors with regard to functional anatomic areas is of the utmost importance for several reasons. First it helps to understand patients' symptomatology and to correlate the MR images with the observed neurologic deficit. Further it can determine the operability of a tumoral lesion so that the lesion can be removed without functional deficit. In the same way it can predict the functional deficit if aggressive surgical debulking is considered or postulate possible clinical worsening in case of tumor growth. Finally it can guide stereotactic biopsy or surgery (Roux et al. 1999; Holodny et al. 1999; Dymarkowski et al. 1998).

Functional MRI (fMRI) has proved to be a very useful tool in the visualization of neuronal activity in humans ("the brain at function") both in normal volunteers as in patients with brain tumors and other lesions, providing patients' clinical status does not interfere with active cooperation in the MR study. The technique visualizes the physiological changes in oxy- and deoxyhemoglobin concentration in small cortical blood vessels during neuronal activation. The increase in the metabolism of neurons during activation leads to an initial increase in oxygen extraction, rapidly followed by an increase in regional cerebral blood flow resulting in an increased oxy-/deoxyhemoglobin ratio (Sunaert et al. 1998). The drop in the concentration of the paramagnetic deoxyhemoglobin leads to a focal increase in 'T2*' signal that can be visualized by MRI. Therefore the technique is called "blood oxygenation level dependent" or "BOLD."

Considering the various tumor locations different activation paradigms have to be used to activate the cortex in the neighborhood of the tumor. For the perirolandic area, according to the location of the tumor, sensorimotor tasks of the hands (mid-rolandic), feet (paramedian) or tongue (low situated) are used (Dymarkowski et al. 1998). For left insular and lower parietal lesions auditory and phonological paradigms are used to localize the speech and hearing areas (Roux et al. 1999). Visual stimuli attempt to activate the visual cortex in relation to occipital tumors.

Tasks, engaging short- and long-term memory, are employed to visualize (medial) temporal lobe function in relation to temporal tumors. In this way it can be determined whether a functional area is located adjacent to the lesion, is at a distance from it or projects within the tumor. In a clinical setting this proved to be of special importance in tumors with severe mass effect with fainting of sulcal anatomy due to accompanying edema (Achten et al. 1999; Dymarkowski et al. 1998). In these lesions the anatomical landmarks are distorted so that accurate localization on a purely morphological basis is hampered. Here, fMRI allows the exact localization of the tumor with respect to the visualized activity in eloquent functional regions so that the local anatomic relations can be recognized (Fig. 9.11). In larger series fMRI was successfully used to predict the operability or functional inoperability of brain tumors in different locations (Fig. 9.12). Therefore fMRI can contribute to more efficient surgical removal of both benign and malignant brain tumors with an increase in patient survival and a decrease in surgical morbidity.

9.7 Image Guided Neurosurgery of Cerebral Tumors

Advances in medical imaging, more specifically the advent of MR, have had a huge impact on daily neurosurgical practice. The guiding of neurosurgical

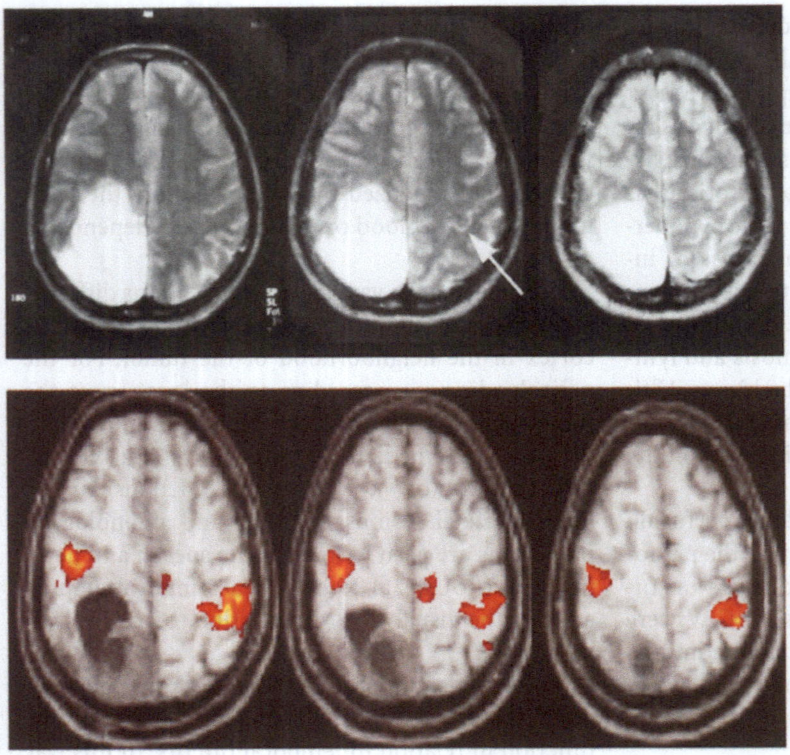

a

b

Fig. 9.11a,b. Functional MRI in a patient with glioblastoma multiforme and distortion of anatomic landmarks. **a** T2-weighted axial sections: hyperintense right parietal lesion. Along the left central sulcus an "inverted omega" shape (*arrow*) can be identified, which has been shown to correspond to the motor cortex of the hand (Yousri et al. Brain 1997; 120:141–57). This landmark is no longer visible in the right hemisphere due to the mass effect of the parietal lesion. Based on these images the right motor cortex was thought to be adjacent to or even included in the lesion. **b** Statistical parametric map of bilateral finger tapping alternated with rest. The sensorimotor cortex activation is *displayed in red*. It is clearly displaced anteriorly by the lesion and, in contrast to the presumed findings from image **a**, revealed not to be adjacent to the lesion, but operable

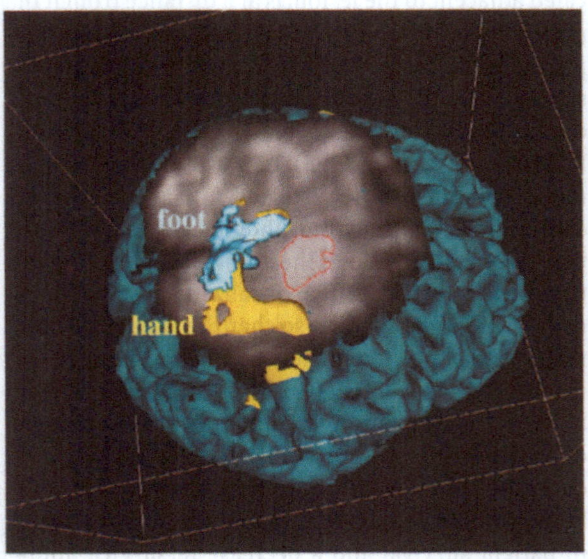

a

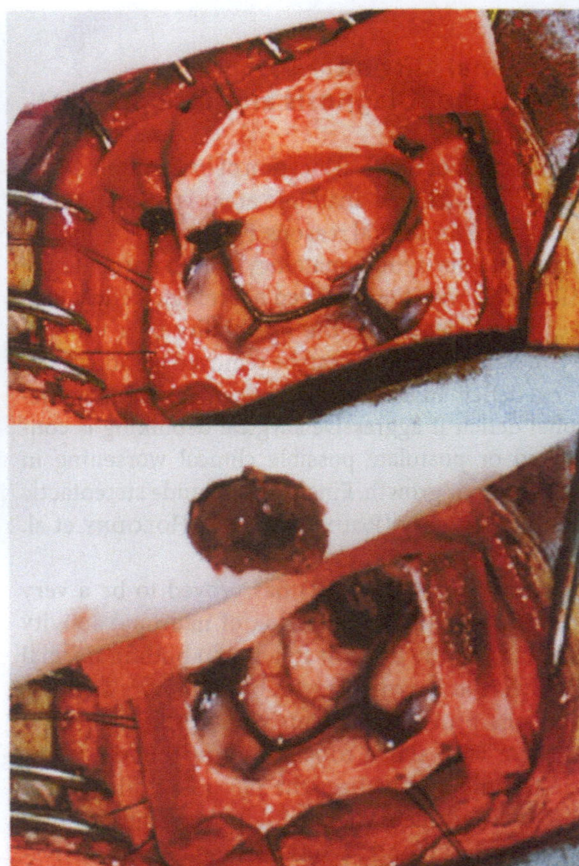

b

Fig. 9.12a,b. Functional MRI in a patient with a left frontal metastasis. **a** Three-dimensional surface reconstruction of the brain of a patient presenting with a metastatic lesion (*red outline*). The primary sensorimotor regions of the hand (*yellow*) and the foot (*blue*) were obtained with an alternation of movement of the hand/foot versus rest. The lesion was situated in the superior frontal gyrus and was separated from the sensorimotor activations by the precentral sulcus. **b** Intraoperative view. The precentral sulcus can be seen. The lesion was surgically removed, without harming the activated regions. The patient had a normal sensorimotor function immediately postoperatively interventions with images has gained widespread acceptance with the aim of improving surgical results in terms of smaller craniotomies, better preservation of eloquent cortex, less brain retraction and thus finally better patient outcome. These image guided neurosurgical techniques include frame-based stereotaxy or stereotactic biopsy and intraoperative MR (ALEXANDER et al. 1997; DIPIERRO et al. 1999; KUCHARCZYK et al. 1997).

Frame-based stereotaxy is the most widely practiced image-guided neurosurgical technique. This technique registers the coordinates of intracranial structures by means of a rigid frame attached to the skull. Several stereotactic frames became commercially available, each with their own advantages and disadvantages (DIPIERRO et al. 1999). The most frequent indication of frame-based stereotaxy is the biopsy of intracranial lesions with high surgical risk due to deep location or location in eloquent cortex (MCDONALD et al. 1999). The final aim of the technique is to obtain a pathological diagnosis with reduced morbidity of the patient and with reduced cost. In some centers frame based stereotactic biopsies are even performed on an outpatient basis. The positive diagnosis rate as reported in the literature exceeds 90%. Failure of the biopsy diagnosis is mainly due to the aspecificity of inflammatory lesions and sampling error in neoplastic lesions with undergrading of the tumor. Complication rate is as low as 5% and mostly consists of hemorrhage.

Other applications of frame-based stereotaxy include location of a tumor before craniotomy, aspiration of cystic tumors to relieve mass effect and symptomatic compression and interstitial brachytherapy (LEWIN et al. 1998).

Stereotactic guidance can also be obtained in a frameless way with devices tracking the position of the surgical instruments relative to the patient's head. Without the encumbrance of the solid and immobile skull-frame combination the indications of image-guided surgery can be extended to open craniotomy (VILLALOBOS et al. 1999). The most common application is the resection of deep cerebral and skull base tumors. The major indications are the roadmapping to the lesion, the definition of the completeness of resection and the avoidance of critical structures (MATSUMOTO et al. 1995).

The main technical challenge of using MR for the planning of stereotactic neurosurgical interventions is the correction of geometric distortion (HARDY et al. 1998; MICHIELS et al. 1994). The causes of geometric distortion can be grouped into three categories: (a) the MR imager, (b) the stereotactic localizer frame and (c) the patient. Main magnetic field inhomogeneities, imperfect slice or volume selection pulses, non-linearity of the magnetic field gradients and eddy currents mainly cause the imager-dependent distortion. The stereotactic localizer frame must, of course, be mechanically accurate and MR compatible, but, in addition, the choice of the liquid in the localizer rods is very important, in particular with respect to visibility for all imaging sequences and distortion caused by chemical shift. The patient-dependent distortion is due to magnetic susceptibility variations, chemical shift and blood flow; the first two are proportional to the main magnetic field. For MR angiography, it was shown that a 3D sequence is mandatory, because it allows the compensation of the flow-induced distortion in both the phase-encoding and the slice-encoding direction.

The major disadvantage of stereotactic neurosurgery of brain tumors lies in spatial errors due to shifts occurring during progressive removal of the tumor bulk, since the stereotactic information relies solely on preoperative images. This disadvantage can be overcome by intraoperative MR, offering the possibility of repeated imaging of altered surgical situations at different stages of the intervention (SCHWARTZ et al. 1999).

Intraoperative MR can be used to guide and confirm intralesional needle placement or to follow aspiration of cystic tumors (SCHWARTZ et al. 1998; TRONNIER et al. 1997). It is useful in determining the completeness of surgical resection, since in up to one-third of cases residual enhancing tumor might be seen when the surgeon thought complete removal had been achieved (KNAUTH et al. 1998).

9.8 Note: Positron Emission Tomography (PET) in Brain Tumors

P. FLAMEN

PET offers the unique opportunity to measure brain tissue metabolism in vivo. Several positron-emitting radioisotopes, including ^{15}O, ^{11}C, ^{13}N, and ^{18}F, can be incorporated into biologically significant natural compounds.

Dedicated positron tomographs can then measure, in a fully quantitative way, the degree of accumulation of these tracers in normal and/or neoplastic tissue, thereby assessing specific elements of tissue metabolism, such as glucose utilization, perfusion and blood volume, amino acid uptake, protein synthesis, DNA synthesis, oxygenation and hypoxia. Therefore, PET will certainly continue to offer unique opportunities for fundamental research on several elements of tumor metabolism. On the other hand, PET has some established clinical indications providing metabolic information complementary to the purely structural data obtained through conventional brain tumor imaging. These indications include the preoperative assessment of tumor volume, grading and prognosis, and the postoperative diagnosis of tumor recurrence. Anatomic (CT/MRI) and metabolic images (PET) provide essentially complementary information. Therefore, spatial registration of both sets of images is elementary for correct interpretation and optimal clinical integration. This can be done visually or, preferably, using various computerized methods that are becoming more readily available. At the present time, two positron-labeled tracers play the key roles in brain PET: ^{18}F-fluorodeoxyglucose (FGD) for the assessment of cerebral glucose metabolism and ^{11}C-methionine (MET) for the study of protein metabolism (Delbeke et al. 1995; DiChiro et al. 1982; Kaschten et al. 1998; Ogawa et al. 1993, 1996). The rationale of the use of these tracers for cancer imaging is that malignantly transformed cells express intensified levels of glucose and/or amino acid metabolism, resulting in an increased intracellular accumulation of these tracers. This allows a differentiation between benign and malignant lesions on a purely metabolic basis. Moreover PET provides essential information on prognosis as the intensity of the tracer uptake is correlated with the degree of malignancy of the lesions.

PET can be used for the delineation of brain tumor volume. Although CT and MRI are unsurpassed diagnostic modalities for the detection of brain tumors, they are limited in the differentiation of tumor tissue from edematous and necrotic tissue. This could result in imperfect delineation of the tumor volume, especially in low-grade malignancies or in post-therapeutic conditions. Using PET, both FDG and MET accumulate intensely in primary malignant brain tumors, independent of the integrity of the blood-brain barrier. However, MET is certainly the preferred tracer in this indication because it provides much higher tumor-to-normal brain contrast compared to FDG, based on the much lower physiologic brain uptake of MET. It has been reported that in most cases of cerebral glioma the area of increased MET is larger than that of the enhanced area on CT scans (Kaschten et al. 1998). Therefore, PET, essentially with CT/MRI registration, certainly has a clinical role in surgical and radiotherapy planning, or biopsy guidance.

PET can also be used for tumor grading and prognosis (Figs. 9.13, 9.14). A significant correlation of

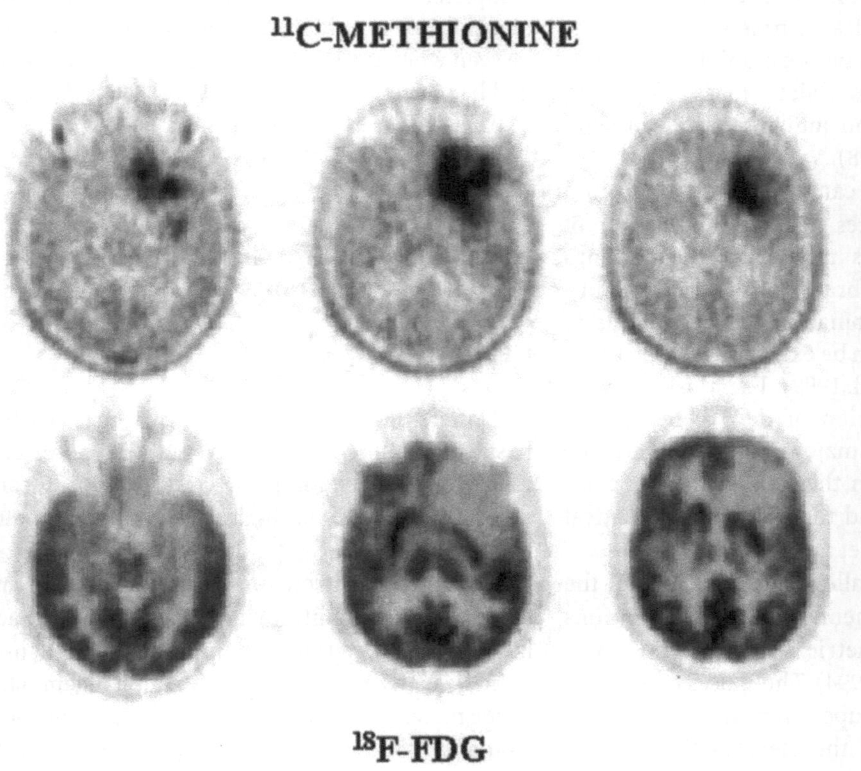

Fig. 9.13. PET scan in high-grade glioma. A 39-year-old male patient with a history of a trepanation of a glioma grade II located in the frontal left cortex. A follow-up CT scan indicated tumor growth. The PET images show intensely increased accumulation of both ^{11}C-methionine and ^{18}F-FDG in the left fronto-temporal and parietal region, which is highly suspicious of a high grade (III or IV) tumor recurrence. A stereotactic biopsy was performed and pathology found glioblastoma multiforme

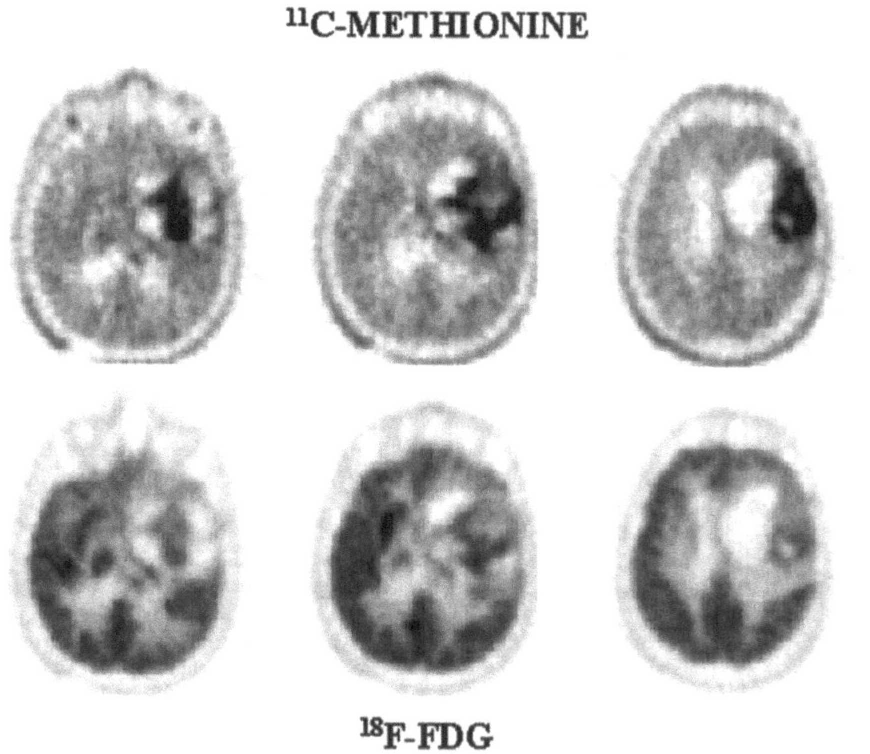

Fig. 9.14. PET scan in low-grade glioma. A 48-year-old male patient with a low-grade (II) oligoastrocytoma located in the left frontotemporal area. A follow-up MRI reported abnormal contrast capture in the tumor, suspected of malignant degeneration. The PET images show intensely increased accumulation of ^{11}C-methionine in the left frontal lobe. However, no increased ^{18}F-FDG uptake was found in that area, indicating the absence of a high-grade tumor component. The PET findings were confirmed by clinical follow-up

tumor uptake and histologic grade and prognosis in patients with glioma has been reported with FDG and, to a lesser degree, with MET (Alavi et al. 1998; Delbeke et al. 1995; Francavilla et al. 1989). PET can thus be used for the differentiation of high-grade gliomas from low-grade or benign lesions. The clinical applications related to this fundamental observation are the diagnosis of malignant degeneration of low-grade gliomas, and the differentiation of high-grade tumor recurrence from radiochemonecrosis (Patronas et al. 1982). Moreover, as uptake is related to the grade of malignancy, PET can help to indicate the most appropriate site for stereotactic biopsy.

Finally, PET can be used for therapy monitoring. PET offers the possibility of studying the metabolic effects of chemotherapeutic or radiotherapeutic treatments before any structural response can be measured using the conventional imaging modalities. This metabolic response assessment can be important in patient management as it provides a basis for early therapeutic adjustments. Newer, more specific agents for the assessment of brain tumor growth characteristics, such as ^{11}C-thymidine and ^{11}C-choline, are becoming available, and will probably become the preferred tracers in this indication.

References

Achten E, Jackson GD, Cameron JA, Abbott DF, Stella DL, Fabinyi GCA (1999) Presurgical evaluation of the motor hand area with functional MR imaging in patients with tumors and dysplastic lesions. Radiology 210: 529–538

Alavi JB, Alavi A, Chawluk J et al. (1988) Positron emission tomography in patients with gliomas: a predictor of prognosis. Cancer 62: 1074–1078

Alexander E, Moriarty TM, Kikinis R, Black PM, Jolesz FM (1997) The present and future role of intraoperative MRI in neurosurgical procedures. Stereotact Funct Neurosurg 68(1–4 Pt 1): 10–17

Delbeke D, Meyerowitz C, Lapidus R et al. (1995) Optimal cutoff levels of F-18 Fluorodeoxyglucose uptake in the differentiation of low-grade from high-grade brain tumors with PET. Radiology 195: 47–52

DiChiro G, DeLaPaz RL, Brooks RA et al. (1982) Glucose utilization of cerebral gliomas measured by (18F) fluorodeoxyglucose and positron emission tomography. Neurology 32: 1323–1329

DiPierro CG, Francel PC, Jackson TR, Kamiryo T, Laws ER Jr (1999) Optimizing accuracy in magnetic resonance imaging-guided stereotaxis: a technique with validation based on the anterior commissure-posterior commissure line. J Neurosurg 90: 94–100

Dymarkowski S, Sunaert S, Van Oostende S et al. (1998) Functional MRI of the brain: localization of eloquent cortex in focal brain lesion therapy. Eur Radiol 8: 1573–1580

Ernst TM, Chang L, Witt MD et al. (1998) Cerebral toxoplasmosis and lymphoma in AIDS: perfusion MR imaging experience in 13 patients. Radiology 208: 663–669

Finelli DA, Hurst GC, Gullapalli RP (1998) T1-weighted three-dimensional magnetization transfer MR of the brain: improved lesion contrast enhancement. Am J Neuroradiol 19: 59–64

Francavilla TL, Miletich RS, DiChiro G et al. (1989) Positron emission tomography in the detection of malignant degeneration of low-grade gliomas. Neurosurgery 24: 1–5

Goergen SK, Gonzales MF, McLean CA (1992) Intraventricular neurocytoma: radiologic features and review of the literature. Radiology 182: 787–792

Han D, Chang KH, Han MH et al. (1998) Half-dose gadolinium-enhanced MR imaging with magnetization transfer technique in brain tumors: comparison with conventional contrast-enhanced MR imaging. Am J Roentgenol AJR 170: 189–193

Hardy P, Barnett G (1998) Spatial distortion in magnetic resonance imaging: impact on stereotactic localization. In: Textbook of Stereotactic and Functional Neurosurgery. McGraw-Hill, New York, pp 271–280

Holodny AI, Schulder M, Liu WC, Maldjian JA, Kalnin AJ (1999) Decrease BOLD functional MR activation of the motor and sensory cortices adjacent to a glioblastoma multiforme: implications for image-guided neurosurgery. Am J Neuroradiol 20: 609–612

Ikushima I, Korogi Y, Hirai T et al. (1997) MR of epidermoids with a variety of pulse sequences. Am J Neuroradiol 18: 1359–1363

Kaschten B, Stevenaert A, Sadzot B et al. (1998) Preoperative evaluation of 54 gliomas by PET with fluorine-18-fluorodeoxyglucose and/or carbon-11-methionine. J Nucl Med 39: 778–785

Kim YJ, Chang KH, Song IC et al. (1998) Brain abscess and necrotic or cystic brain tumor: discrimination with signal intensity on diffusion-weighted MR imaging. Am J Roentgenol AJR 171: 1487–1490

Kleihues P, Burger PC, Scheithauer BW (1993) Histologic typing of tumours of the central nervous system. Springer, Berlin Heidelberg New York, p 21

Klisch J, Husstedt H, Hennings S et al. (1999) Supratentorial primitive neuroectodermal tumors (PNETs) and diffusion-weighted MRI. Presented at the 25th Congress of the ESNR, September 7–11, 1999, Vienna, Austria. Neuroradiology 41: 38–39

Knauth M, Forsting M, Hartmann M, Heiland S, Balzer T, Sartor K (1996) MR enhancement of brain lesions: increased contrast dose compared with magnetization transfer. Am J Neuroradiol 17: 1853–1859

Knauth M, Wirtz CR, Tronnier VM, Staubert A, Kunze S, Sartor K (1998) Intraoperative magnetic resonance tomography for control of extent of neurosurgical operations. Radiologe 38: 218–224

Knopp EA, Cha S, Johnson G et al. (1999) Echo planar perfusion imaging in the evaluation and management of patients with intracranial neoplasms: the NYU experience. Presented at the 25th Congress of the ESNR, September 7–11, 1999, Vienna, Austria. Neuroradiology 41: 39

Koeller KK, Dillon WP (1992) Dysembryoplastic neuroepithelial tumors: MR appearance. Am J Neuroradiol 13: 1319–1325

Krabbe K, Gideon P, Wagn P, Hansen U, Thomsen C, Madsen F (1997) MR diffusion imaging of human intracranial tumours. Neuroradiology 39: 483–489

Kucharczyk W, Bernstein M (1997) Do the benefits of image guidance in neurosurgery justify the costs? From stereotaxy to intraoperative MR. Am J Neuroradiol 18: 1855–1859

Lam LL, Cha S, Kopp EA et al. (1999) Cerebral gangliogliomas: dynamic contrast-enhanced perfusion MR imaging and histopathologic correlation. Presented at the 25th Congress of the ESNR, September 7–11, 1999, Vienna, Austria. Neuroradiology 41: 38

Lewin JS, Petersilge CA, Hatem SF et al. (1998) Interactive MR imaging-guided biopsy and aspiration with a modified clinical C-arm system. Am J Roentgenol AJR 170: 1593–1601

Maley JE, Yuh WT (1998) Contrast dosage in the neuroimaging of brain tumors. Principles and indications. Magn Reson Imaging Clin N Am 6: 113–124

Matsumoto K, Higashi H, Tomita S, Furuta T, Ohmoto T (1995) Resection of deep-seated gliomas using neuroimaging for stereotactic placement of guidance catheters. Neurol Med Chir Tokyo 35: 148–155

McDonald JD, Chong BW, Lewine JD et al. (1999) Integration of preoperative and intraoperative functional brain mapping in a frameless stereotactic environment for lesions near eloquent cortex. J Neurosurg 90: 591–598

Michiels J, Bosmans H, Pelgrims P et al. (1994) On the problem of geometric distortion in magnetic resonance images for stereotactic neurosurgery. J Magn Reson Imaging 12: 749–764

Nguyen HD, Simonson TM, Fisher DJ et al. (1995) MR evaluation of acoustic schwannoma with fractional contrast dose. J Comput Assist Tomogr 19: 23–27

Noguchi K, Watanabe N, Nagayoshi T et al. (1999) Role of diffusion-weighted echo-planar MRI in distinguishing between brain abscess and tumour: a preliminary report. Neuroradiology 41: 171–174

Ogawa T, Inugami A, Hatazawa J et al. (1996) Clinical positron emission tomography for brain tumors: comparison of fluorodeoxyglucose F-18 and L-methyl-11c-methionine. Am J Neuroradiology 17: 345–353

Ogawa T, Shishido F, Kanno I et al. (1993) Cerebral glioma: evaluation with methionine PET. Radiology 186: 45–53

Østergaard L, Hochberg FH, Rabinov JD et al. (1999) Early changes measured by magnetic resonance imaging in cerebral blood flow, blood volume, and blood-brain barrier permeability following dexamethasone treatment in patients with brain tumors. J Neurosurg 90: 300–305

Patronas NJ, Di Chiro G, Broioks RA et al. (1982) Work in progress: (18F)-fluorodeoxyglucose and positron emission tomography in the evaluation of radiation necrosis of the brain. Radiology 144: 885–889

Ramadan UA, Aronen HJ, Tanttu JI et al. (1997) Improvement of brain lesion detection at 0.1 T by simultaneous use of Gd-DTPA and magnetization transfer imaging. MRM 37: 268–274

Rippe DJ, Boyko OB, Radi M, Worth R, Fuller GN (1992) MRI of temporal lobe pleomorphic xanthoastrocytoma. J Comput Assist Tomogr 16: 856–859

Roux FE, Boulanouar K, Ibarrola D et al. (1999) Importance and limitations of the validation of functional MRI of motor function and language using preoperative cortical stimulation. J Neuroradiol 26: 82–88

Rypens F, Esteban MJ, Lellouch-Fagnou C, Renier D, Baraton J, Brunelle F (1996) Desmoplastic supratentorial neuroepithelial tumours of childhood: imaging in 5 patients. Neuroradiology 38: 165–168

Schuierer G, Reimer P, Tigges A, Peters PE (1996) Perfusion studies with paramagnetic contrast media and rapid pulse sequences in cerebrovascular diseases and brain tumors. Radiologe 36: 107–114

Schwartz RB, Hsu L, Black PM et al. (1998) Evaluation of intracranial cysts by intraoperative MR. J Magn Reson Imaging 8: 807–813

Schwartz RB, Hsu L, Wong TZ et al. (1999) Intraoperative MR imaging guidance for intracranial neurosurgery: experience with the first 200 cases. Radiology 211: 477–488

Sugahara T, Korogi Y, Kochi M et al. (1998) Correlation of MR imaging-determined cerebral blood volume maps with histologic and angiographic determination of vascularity of gliomas. Am J Roentgenol AJR 171: 1479–1486

Sugahara T, Korogi Y, Kochi M et al. (1999) Usefulness of diffusion-weighted MRI with echo-planar technique in the evaluation of cellularity in gliomas. J Magn Reson Imaging 9: 53–60

Sunaert S, Dymarkowski S, Van Oostende S, Van Hecke P, Wilms G, Marchal G (1998) Functional magnetic resonance imaging (fMRI) visualises the brain at work. Acta Neurol Belg 98: 8–16

Tronnier VM, Wirtz CR, Knauth M et al. (1997) Intraoperative diagnostic and interventional magnetic resonance imaging in neurosurgery. Neurosurgery 40: 891–900

Tsuruda JS, Chew WM, Moseley ME, Norman D (1990) Diffusion-weighted MR imaging of the brain: value of differentiating between extraaxial cysts and epidermoid tumors. Am J Neuroradiol 11: 925–931

Villalobos H, Germano IM (1999) Clinical evaluation of multimodality registration in frameless stereotaxy. Comput Aided Surg 4: 45–49

Yuh WT, Halloran JI, Mayr NA, Fisher DJ, Nguyen HD, Simonson TM (1994a) Dose of contrast material in the MR imaging evaluation of central nervous system tumors. J Magn Reson Imaging 4: 243–249

Yuh WT, Nguyen HD, Tali ET et al. (1994b) Delineation of gliomas with various doses of MR contrast material. Am J Neuroradiol 15: 983–989

Yuh WT, Parker JR, Carvlin MJ (1997) Indication-related dosing for magnetic resonance contrast media. Eur Radiol 7: 269–275

Yuh WTC, Tali ET, Nguyen HD, Simonson TM, Mayr NA, Fisher DJ (1995) The effect of contrast dose, imaging time, and lesion size in the MR detection of intracerebral metastasis. Am J Neuroradiol 16: 373–380

Zimmerman RA, Erdem E, Bilaniuk LT, Hunter JV, Sutton LN, Rorke LB (1999) Diffusion weighted imaging (DWI) and fluid attenuated inversion recovery (FLAIR) imaging in the evaluation of primitive neuroectodermal tumors. Presented at the 25th Congress of the ESNR, September 7–11, 1999, Vienna, Austria. Neuroradiology 41: 39

10 Brain Ischemia

Olav Jansen, Peter D. Schellinger

CONTENTS

10.1 Introduction

For a long time acute stroke has been a disease without specific therapeutic options and most therapies were concentrated on a general medical stabilization in the acute setting. This more fatalistic approach has changed dramatically since several studies have shown the efficacy of recanalization therapies in acute ischemic stroke patients. Under these circumstances, neuroradiology with its new modalities has become a major player in the diagnostic work-up but also in the therapeutic approach of acute stroke patients. However, for those who are working with stroke patients, it has become essential not only to understand the technology of their diagnostic tools but also to have enough knowledge about the pathophysiology of stroke itself. With this growing knowledge on the neuroradiologist's part, and new techniques available, the neuroradiologist is able to look inside the ischemic disease and becomes a competent partner in the diagnostic and therapeutic discussion.

Stroke is the third leading cause of death in the industrial nations, with an incidence of 150–200/100,000/year and a threefold larger number of patients left with severe disabilities (WHO Task Force). Depending on the location of the lesion patients suffer from acute hemiparesis, aphasia or other focal neurological deficits. The stroke related lesion is more likely to be ischemic than hemorrhagic (85% vs 15%). Cerebral ischemia itself is more often focal than global and is most frequently caused by an acute occlusion of intracranial arteries due to an embolism from an extracranial vessel or from the heart. Less commonly, the cause for an ischemic lesion is an extracranial arterial occlusion resulting, sometimes combined with a drop in systemic arterial pressure, in a significant reduction of the cerebral blood flow (CBF). The normal gray matter blood flow is 0.8 ml/g/min in man. Brain function is preserved with a decrease of the CBF down to 0.25 ml/g/min, but is reversibly disturbed with flow rates between 0.25 and 0.15 ml/g/min. A decrease of the CBF to less than 0.15 ml/g/min results in damage of the morphological cell structure, which is irreversible depending on the time of ischemia (Astrup et al. 1981). The hemodynamic consequences of an acute cerebral artery occlusion and the resulting decrease of the CBF in the affected brain tissue vary because alterations in cerebral blood flow change with time, location, and potentially available collateral circulation. The latter seems to be the most important factor. Large artery-to-artery anastomoses through the circle of Willis, the external to internal carotid distributions (via the ophthalmic artery) and primarily the leptomeningeal collaterals offer relative protection and blood supply of the affected tissue. While in selected cases huge areas of the brain may be permanently supplied only by these collaterals, in other cases the absence or secondary failure of these collaterals leads to irreversible tissue damage. This vari-

O. Jansen, MD; P.D. Schellinger, MD
Department of Neuroradiology, University of Heidelberg Medical School, Im Neuenheimer Feld 400, 69120 Heidelberg, Germany

ability of the collateral status in each individual causes different morphological and clinical outcomes even in patients with the same occlusion localization.

The target for most therapeutic interventions for focal ischemia should be ischemic tissue that can respond to treatment and is not irreversibly injured. Such tissue will be defined as potentially salvageable ischemic tissue and must be distinguished from non-salvageable ischemic tissue, which has evolved to a status in which recovery is no longer possible. The characterization of potentially reversible versus irreversible ischemic tissue is based on the ischemic penumbra hypothesis (Astrup et al. 1981). In extension of this hypothesis three areas in an ischemic tissue can be differentiated: the central infarct core, which contains already irreversible damaged tissue; the penumbra, a tissue with disturbed function but still salvageable; and a peripheral area with reduced CBF but preserved function (Fig. 10.1).

Reduction of the CBF causes energy depletion in the affected neurons. Breakdown of the Na^+/K^+ pump and secondary loss of the ion homeostasis result in an increase of the intracellular water content (cytotoxic edema). This cytotoxic edema leads to an increase of the cellular size and a shift of the cellular/extracellular relation. In this initial stage the overall water content does not increase significantly, so that there is no great mass effect within the first 24 h. Because of the greater resistance of endothelial cells, the disruption of the blood-brain barrier occurs later than the neuronal damage. The maximal increase

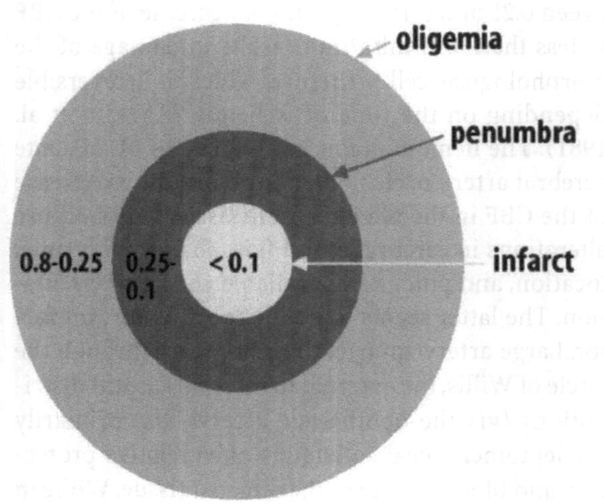

Fig. 10.1. Recent concept of the three-compartment model of ischemic brain tissue: the infarct core is irreversibly damaged, the penumbra zone shows disturbed function but is still salvageable, and the oligemic zone has preserved function and morphology (numbers indicate the CBF in ml/g/min)

of the water content occurs 3–4 days after the ischemic event resulting in a maximal mass effect at that point of time. Nevertheless, even during the first hours after the arterial occlusion a very slight increase of the total water content can be measured experimentally (Schlaug et al. 1997).

In specific, four important questions concerning this concept should be answered by an optimal diagnostic procedure before any aggressive therapeutic approach (i.e., thrombolysis) is undertaken:

1. Does the patient have an acute cerebral ischemia or is another underlying pathology responsible for the stroke symptoms (e.g., intracerebral hemorrhage, tumor)?
2. Is there already an area of irreversibly damaged ischemic tissue and what is the size of this infarct core?
3. Is there a tissue of risk ("penumbra"), which can be preserved from damage by therapeutic intervention and what is the size of this area?
4. Is the vessel which is responsible for the ischemia still occluded or is there already a spontaneous recanalization?

The ideal imaging modality will be able to answer all of these questions within an acceptable amount of time before a specific treatment is started.

10.2 Recent Developments in Therapeutic Strategies in Acute Ischemic Stroke

In the following chapter recent studies on new therapeutic concepts, which are implemented in hyperacute ischemic stroke such as thrombolysis and neuroprotection, will be discussed. Severe middle cerebral artery (MCA) infarctions or so called "malignant" MCA infarctions have a poor prognosis with medical treatment alone and generally are associated with a mortality of 80% (Hacke et al. 1994, 1995, 1996). Escalating forms of therapy such as hemicraniectomy and hypothermia for those patients with severe ischemic strokes, who are not suitable for thrombolytic therapy, have been studied in smaller series.

10.2.1 Intravenous Thrombolysis

To date there have been several large, randomized, placebo-controlled multicenter trials of intravenous thrombolytic therapy in acute ischemic stroke. The use of intravenous streptokinase within 6 h after stroke onset was evaluated in three trials, all of which had to be terminated prematurely because of an excessive rate of symptomatic intracerebral hemorrhage (ICH) and mortality in the treatment arm (Donnan et al. 1995). Three other randomized, placebo-controlled multicenter trials investigated the effect of recombinant tissue plasminogen activator (alteplase, rt-PA) in acute ischemic stroke. The National Institute of Neurological Disorders and Stroke (NINDS) trial showed that treatment with rt-PA within 3 h after symptom onset (dosage 0.9 mg/kg, 10% bolus, 1 h infusion time) led to an increase of 12% in the patient group with a good functional outcome [Modified Rankin Scale (mRS) $\leqslant$1] although there was a tenfold increase in symptomatic hemorrhage. These results led to FDA approval of rt-PA for acute ischemic stroke for the 3 h time window in the USA. At the same time a European trial multicenter trial (ECASS I) evaluated rt-PA in acute stroke patients in a 6-h time window with a higher dosage of 1.1 mg/kg body weight (Hacke et al. 1995). The intention-to-treat analysis (all patients who were randomized and included in the protocol) could not show an advantage for rt-PA over placebo in this study. A target group analysis (all patients who met the inclusion criteria according to the predefined protocol) yielded the same positive results as the NINDS study, thus suggesting a statistically significant benefit for patients treated with rt-PA. There was no statistical difference between the 0–3 h and 3–6 h cohort in ECASS I regarding mortality, hemorrhage or outcome (Steiner et al. 1998).

The results of NINDS and ECASS I led to the design of ECASS II with the primary endpoint being a difference in the functional outcome (mRS 0 and 1) at day 90 (Hacke et al. 1998). In ECASS II a lower dose of 0.9 mg/kg was chosen to match NINDS criteria, the time window again being 6 h after symptom onset. To reduce the rate of ICH, more rigorous CT criteria and guidelines for blood pressure control were implemented. A total number of 800 patients were randomized, roughly 400 to each arm (treatment vs placebo). At 90 days there was no difference in mortality between treatment and placebo arm (10.5% vs 10.7%) with an excess in mortality due to secondary hemorrhage in the treated patients and an excess in mortality due to edema in the placebo arm. ECASS II yielded negative results regarding the primary endpoint with a 3.7% absolute difference (P=0.277) between rt-PA and placebo arm. However, a post hoc analysis with an alternative dichotomization for an independent outcome (mRS 0–2) showed an absolute difference of 8.3% (P=0.024) between rt-PA and placebo. A preliminary metaanalysis of the NINDS, ECASS I and II data utilizing more than 1000 patients per study arm shows an odds ratio of 0.63 for a functionally dependent or dead outcome (mRS 3–6) and 0.68 for an unfavorable outcome (mRS 2–6) for all time windows and dosages, and 0.55 for a dependent or dead outcome (mRS 3–6) in the 3-h time window with a 0.9 mg/kg dose (more than 400 patients per study arm). This translates into 90 events (reduction in death or disability; mRS 3–6) per 1000 patients treated (number needed to treat = 11) for all time windows and doses, and 140 events (reduction in death or disability; mRS 3–6) per 1000 patients treated (number needed to treat = 7) for the 3-h time window and 0.9-mg/kg dose. It must be mentioned, however, that another multicenter trial investigating the effect of rt-PA in the 3- to 5-h time window could not show any benefit in the treated patients. Therefore, only the 0.9-mg/kg dose rt-PA in the treatment of acute stroke within 3 h after symptom onset is proven to be safe and clinically effective.

10.2.2 Intraarterial Thrombolysis

The rationale for an intraarterial approach to recanalize an occluded cerebral vessel is the presumably higher recanalization rate than with the intravenous application of rt-PA or urokinase. Unfortunately, there exists no exact data on the spontaneous, intravenous and intraarterial recanalization rates. In older studies with small patient cohorts, the spontaneous and intravenous recanalization rates are estimated at 10%–20% and 50%–60% respectively (Mori et al. 1992). Studies with a small patient series, in whom intraarterial thrombolysis was performed, reported recanalization rates from 50% (Mori et al. 1988) to 90% (Zeumer et al. 1985, 1993). Recently, an intraarterial thrombolysis study, which used prourokinase, randomized 180 patients, and showed a recanalization rate of 67%, was presented. These authors showed that intraarterial thrombolysis with prourokinase was of benefit for patients with acute ischemic stroke in the 6-h time window. Presently, however, the intraarterial approach, which is more invasive and therefore has more potential complications, should be reserved for patients in whom recanalization cannot be achieved otherwise, i.e., patients with occlusion of the carotid-T. Another possibility is the add-on approach in patients with a large tissue at risk as assessed by stroke MRI and a time window exceeding 3 h, where a reduced dose intravenous thrombolysis may be initiated and an interventional procedure subsequently is performed to achieve vessel recanalization.

Vessel occlusions in the posterior circulation on the other hand justify the primary angiographic approach, as permanent occlusion of the basilar artery is nearly always associated with a fatal outcome (Brandt et al. 1995). Also, there is no definite time window for thrombolytic therapy in the posterior circulation as long as there are no extensive infarctions seen on CT or stroke MRI studies (Brandt et al. 1996).

10.2.3 Neuroprotection

In theory, neuroprotectants may enlarge the narrow time window for successful recanalization therapy or save brain tissue in the ischemic penumbra until a sufficient collateral flow is established (Hacke et al. 1996). More than 70 different substances with encouraging results in animal experiments (Davis et al. 1995) have been investigated in clinical trials; none, however, was shown to be of any benefit regarding survival rate or outcome. To date the only neuroprotectant with a potential benefit but still inconsistent data in multicenter trials is lubeluzole, which may reduce mortality and improve outcome when given to acute stroke patients with un- to moderate severe deficits within 6 h (Diener et al. 1998). Despite the discouraging results to date, an effective neuroprotectant would be a worthwhile addition to the present armament against the devastating consequences of acute ischemic stroke.

10.2.4 Decompressive Surgery

In space occupying MCA infarction intractable brain edema, midline shift and subsequent herniation with brainstem compromise lead to a mortality of approximately 80% in these stroke patients (Hacke et al. 1996). Steiner et al. showed that the survival rate of patients with MCA infarction undergoing intubation can exceed 30% (Steiner et al. 1997). Nevertheless, all medical treatment including the use of hyperventilation, osmodiuretics, barbiturates and TRIS buffer has not been shown to improve outcome in patients with raised ICP due to severe MCA stroke (Schellinger et al. 1998; Schwab et al. 1997).

There is strong animal experimental evidence that decompressive surgery not only reduces mortality but also improves outcome in survivors (Forsting et al. 1995; Doerfler et al. 1996). Two patient series with decompressive surgery for malignant MCA infarction have been reported (Rieke et al. 1995; Schwab et al. 1998). The surgical technique required the removal of a large bone flap (minimum diameter 12 cm), fixation of the dura at the bone edges to prevent epidural bleeding, insertion of a dural patch (duroplasty) to gain more space for the swelling brain, no resection of infarcted brain tissue, and invasive measurement of ICP by intraparenchymal probes (Hacke et al. 1996a,b). In the earlier series by Rieke et al. in 1995, 32 patients were operated upon with clinical deterioration within a mean time interval from symptom onset of 39 h. Mortality was reduced to 34.4% with the majority of survivors only mildly to moderately disabled [median Barthel index (BI) 62/100]. In the second series by Schwab et al., the mean time interval to surgery was 21 h, mortality only 16% and the median outcome BI was 68.8. The time of NCCU stay was significantly reduced to 7.4 days. Compared to a patient group (*N*=56) with malignant MCA infarctions and a natural course without surgical intervention (mortality 78%, median outcome BI 60, mean length of NCCU stay 12.6 days), these results favor early decompressive surgery in patients with space occupying MCA infarctions. A multicenter study for hemicraniectomy in acute ischemic stroke, where patients are randomized on admission and operated on or medically treated upon deterioration, is underway in the USA (Frank et al. 1999).

10.2.5 Hypothermia

It is well known that profound but also mild to moderate (28–34°C) hypothermia has a neuroprotective effect. Severe management problems such as cardiac arrhythmia, shivering, pulmonal infections, coagulation disorders, and electrolyte disturbances, however, have restricted the use of therapeutic hypothermia (Schwab et al. 1998). Animal experiments showed that infarct volumes can be reduced by up to 90% after focal cerebral ischemia (Busto et al. 1987). Schwab et al. induced hypothermia of 33°C in 25 patients with large MCA infarctions for 48–72 h. Passive rewarming was allowed over 24 h (Schwab et al. 1998). The mortality in this investigation was 44% (11/25) as compared to a control group of medically treated patients with a mortality of 78%. Complications included severe pneumonias in 40% of the patients and asymptomatic thrombopenia and pancreatitis. The most severe complication, however, was an intractable increase in ICP in some patients (all of whom died), which shows that the maximum amount of brain edema may only be delayed but not decreased. Further multicenter studies are necessary to evaluate this very promising treatment for malignant MCA infarctions.

10.3 CT Diagnosis in Early Ischemic Stroke

Either in newer textbooks or in recent papers in highly rated non-neuroradiological journals it is considered that CT is negative with regard to ischemic tissue changes during the first 12 h after symptom onset (GILMAN 1998a,b). However, during the last 5 years it has been generally accepted in the neuroradiological community that CT can demonstrate early infarct signs within the first 6 h after stroke. With the availability of high-quality CT scanners more and more investigators reported their positive CT findings in early ischemic stroke. The sensitivity of these findings vary in a huge range from 12% to 92%, depending on the infarct signs, the exact time window of the investigated population, and the authors.

The most common sign of an early infarct is the gray matter hypodensity, which develops in the early stages of an infarction and can be subtle and difficult to depict. The development of an extracellular edema can be recognized even in the first hours after stroke onset and is due to a masking of cortical or deep nuclear structures. This phenomenon can be demonstrated best in cases of an acute occlusion of the main stem of the middle cerebral artery (M1 occlusion), where the parenchymal hypodensity shows up first in terminal artery supply areas like the basal ganglia (BOZZAO et al. 1989; VON KUMMER et al. 1995; VON KUMMER et al. 1996). Depending on the origin of the recurrent artery of Heubner, this hypodensity also involves the caput of the caudate nucleus. In cases with insufficient leptomeningeal collaterals the primary hypodensity involves cortical structures, i.e., the insula, which is known as the "loss of the insular ribbon sign" (TRUWIT et al. 1990), or other territories of the middle cerebral artery (Fig. 10.2).

The incidence of hypodensities in patients with acute stroke is reported in a wide range and certainly depends on the part of patients with a major vessel occlusion (i.e., M1 segment). More recent studies have reported incidences of early CT signs of infarction between 53% and 92% within the first 6 h for all acute stroke patients (VON KUMMER et al. 1995; HOROWITZ et al. 1991; TOMURA et al. 1988; VON KUMMER et al. 1994). In patients with a M1 segment occlusion the incidence of a parenchymal hypodensity is reported with 68% within the first 2 h but increases to 89% in the 3rd h after symptom onset and up to 100% thereafter (VON KUMMER et al. 1994). A reversibility of these early hypodensities has not been reported; however, there is an association between the size of early hypodensities and the risk of a secondary hemorrhage (BOZZAO et al. 1991) and clinical outcome. VON KUMMER (1994) showed that early parenchymal hypodensity covering more than an estimated 50% of the MCA territory is a specific finding associated with a mortality of 85%. The same findings could be confirmed by the ECASS trial: mortali-

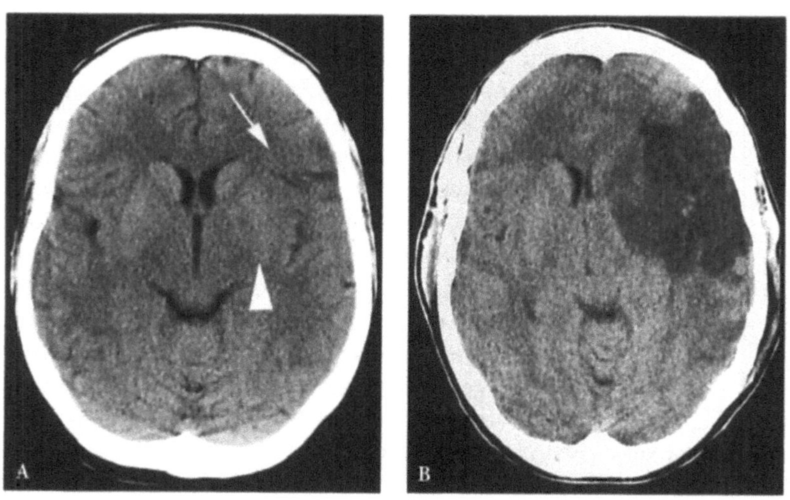

Fig. 10.2A,B. Forty-five-year-old patient with acute right-sided hemiparesis and aphasia for 4 h. CT shows slight hypodensity of the left lentiform nucleus and the insular cortex ("loss of the insular ribbon") (**A**). Second CT scan 48 h after the onset of symptoms demonstrates marked hypodensity of part of the MCA territory with local mass effect (**B**)

ty was 13% in patients without hypodensity, 23% in patients with parenchymal hypodensity less than 33% of the MCA territory, and 49% in patients with an early hypodensity exceeding 33% of the MCA territory (HACKE et al. 1995). Confirmed by both ECASS trials I and II, it has been clearly demonstrated that the clinical response to intravenous rt-PA in patients with ischemic stroke can be predicted on the basis of initial CT findings. These studies showed that in patients with a small area of hypoattenuation (<33% of the MCA territory) treatment increased the chance of a good clinical outcome. In patients with a normal baseline CT scan or in patients with a large area of hypoattenuation (>33% of the MCA territory) rt-PA had no benefit but increased the risk for a fatal brain hemorrhage (VON KUMMER et al. 1997).

Focal brain swelling of the ischemic territory leads to a sulcal effacement, which can be recognized best by direct comparison of the two hemispheres. Although severe brain swelling occurs more in the acute (12–24 h) or subacute (>24 h) stage of an ischemia, it can also be demonstrated within the first 6 h after stroke in 12%–41% of stroke patients (HOROWITZ et al. 1991; VON KUMMER et al. 1995).

The hyperdense middle cerebral artery sign (HMCAS) is defined as a part of the MCA denser than other parts of the vessel or its counterpart, not attributable to calcification, as shown on unenhanced CT (TOMSICK et al. 1990, 1996). This sign describes the visualization of the thrombus itself within the vessel and can of course also be described in other vessels of the circle of Willis (Fig. 10.3). The HMCAS is present

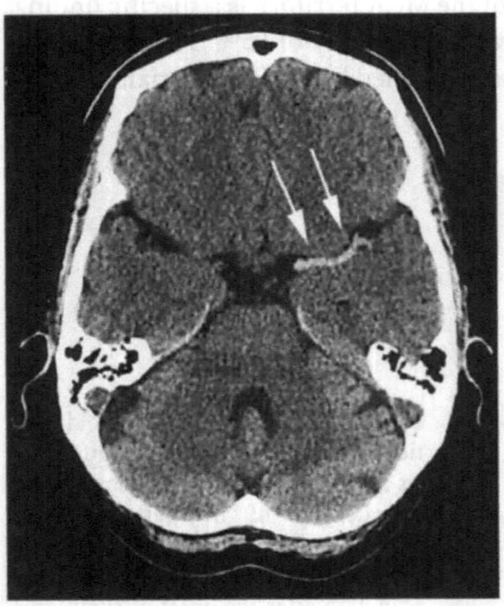

Fig. 10.3. CT scan 2 h after onset of symptoms shows hyperdensity of the entire left MCA in relation to the right MCA (HMCAS, hyperdense middle cerebral artery sign)

in 40–60% of patients with angiographically proven MCA occlusion of any type (VON KUMMER et al. 1994; TOMSICK et al. 1990; LEYS et al. 1992). In a primarily unselected population of stroke patients the HMCAS was found in about 17%, but was associated with severe brain ischemia and poor clinical outcome (MANELFE et al. 1999). Nevertheless, the same study showed that patients with an HMCAS may benefit from thrombolysis when they do not show a large hypodensity in the initial CT scan.

While several studies have shown the usefulness of early CT findings to select patients before intravenous thrombolytic therapy, other studies demonstrated that physicians including general radiologists and neurologists do not uniformly achieve a sufficient level of sensitivity for identification of CT contraindications for thrombolytic therapy (i.e., intracerebral hemorrhage or early signs of ischemia) (SCHRIGER et al. 1998). However, the recognition of early infarct signs by CT can be trained and the positive effect of training in reading CT scans of hyperacute stroke patients has recently been demonstrated in a large trial (VON KUMMER et al. 1998).

CT angiography (CTA) by using spiral CT nowadays is a widely available tool to evaluate the circle of Willis. In acute ischemic stroke patients this technique can provide accurate information on stenoses or occlusions in the basal arteries of the brain (KNAUTH et al. 1997; SHRIER et al. 1997). The method is non-invasive, safe and independent from the grade of experience of the investigator (in contrast to Doppler sonography). In a large series of stroke patients none had any immediate adverse reactions after administration of the intravenous nonionic iodinated contrast material (SHRIER et al. 1997). While older studies reported an increase of the infarct size after administration of iodinated contrast material, a recently published experimental study clearly demonstrated that bolus injection of nonionic contrast material does not affect infarction volume or worsen the symptoms of cerebral ischemia (DOERFLER et al. 1998). CTA is superior to Doppler sonography in the assessment of basilar artery patency in patients with the syndrome of an acute basilar artery ischemia, particularly in patients with distal basilar artery occlusion (BRANDT et al. 1999). In addition to the assessment of a major vessel occlusion, CTA has the potential to deliver information about the quality of the collateral circulation. In patients with good leptomeningeal collaterals contrast enhancement in arterial branches beyond the occlusion occurs. This degree of enhancement can be taken as an estimate of the collateral blood flow (Fig. 10.4) (KNAUTH et al.

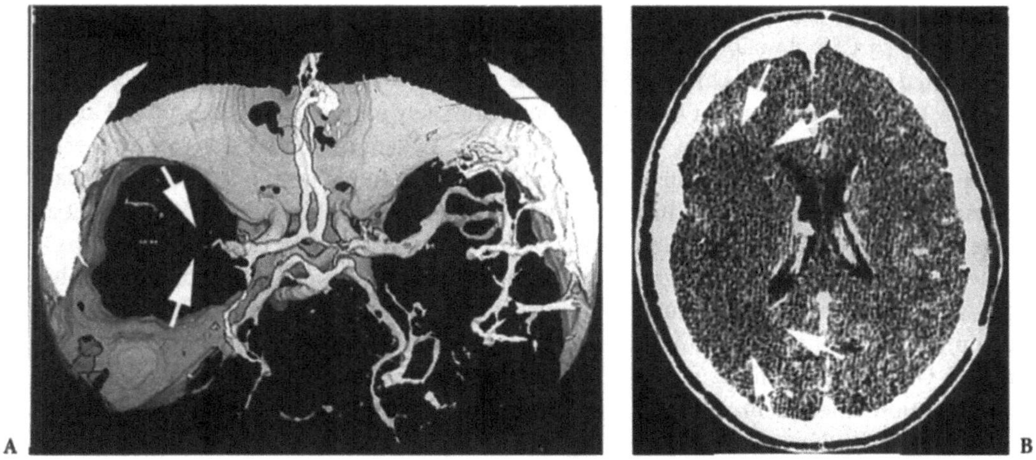

Fig. 10.4A,B. CT angiography in a case of hyperacute (<6 h) occlusion of the right MCA. 3D reconstruction demonstrates the occlusion site (**A**) while the source images show an large area of reduced vascular enhancement (**B**), which can be taken as an area with insufficient supply by collaterals

1996; WILDERMUTH et al. 1998). However, CTA has its limitations and is less reliable in demonstrating branch occlusions of the middle cerebral artery or other smaller vessels distally to the circle of Willis (KNAUTH et al. 1996; SHRIER et al. 1997).

Dynamic CT during first pass of an iodine contrast bolus by unidirectional X-ray tube rotation results in images which can be used to construct functional maps of cerebral blood volume (CBV), cerebral blood flow (CBF) or time to peak enhancement (TTP). These functional maps of perfusion CT provide a high-resolution tool, which enables the physician to visualize cerebrovascular parameters and their changes in acute stroke patients (HAMBERG et al. 1996a,b). Areas with reduced CBF can be shown immediately after vessel occlusion with high contrast to areas with normal perfusion. In a recently published study, perfusion CT was performed within 6 h of symptom onset in 32 patients with acute stroke symptoms. Comparison with SPECT, performed immediately after perfusion CT, and follow-up CT showed a good correspondence in 81% of the patients. However, in three patients the ischemia was located outside the scanning level of perfusion CT and was therefore missed (KOENIG et al. 1998). This demonstrates the actual disadvantages of the method, because with each bolus injection only one brain section can be evaluated. It is possible to obtain a second or third bolus injection to perform another perfusion CT; however, it is impossible to evaluate the total brain. Future developments in CT technology, including dynamic scanning with multisection data acquisition (multislice CT), may further increase the value of this technique and provide information about the three-dimensional extent of cerebral ischemia. Electron beam computed tomography is also able to perform multislice dynamic CT with calculation of absolute CBV and CBF. In a small series of 11 patients with acute stroke symptoms this technique demonstrated reduced CBV and CBF in the 4 patients with proven infarcts on follow-up CT. Disadvantages were caused by high image noise, limiting the demarcation of ischemic tissue (BRUNING et al. 1998).

10.4 MRI in Early Ischemic Stroke

10.4.1 Diffusion-Weighted Imaging (DWI)

Since the description of early findings in acute experimental ischemic stroke with diffusion weighted imaging (DWI), it has been predicted that this technique might become an important tool for the identification of very early ischemic injury in patients (MOSELEY et al. 1990). In the last 5 years several clinical works have been published showing the feasibility of this motion sensitive technique even in patients with an acute stroke. Since the availability of echo-planar imaging (EPI) on clinical scanner systems, DWI can be performed more and more in the clinical routine. With EPI technique and its higher gradients and shorter imaging time (images obtained on the order of 100 ms) whole brain DWI scans can be acquired in a matter of seconds. Bulk motion artifacts caused by head movement or by physiological motion, such as CSF flow and brain pulsation, can be eliminated with the EPI technique, making DWI applicable to any stroke patient who has no contraindication for MR (WARACH et al. 1995). DWI is sensitive to the microscopic motion of water protons (molecular movement of Brown). In a DWI weighted image structures with fast diffusion are dark, structures with slower diffusion are bright. By acquiring images with different diffusion values, the apparent diffusion coefficient (ADC) and ADC maps can be calculated. On these ADC maps structures with a high diffusion coefficient (normal brain) are bright, structures with lower coefficients (ischemic tissue) are dark (Fig. 10.5).

Failure of sodium potassium ATPase function leads to a rapid shift of water from extracellular to intracellular compartments (cytotoxic edema) in the area of acute infarct (MOSELEY et al. 1990). The increase of the intracellular space causes a net drop in the ADC value. A hyperacute infarction becomes hyperintense in early DWI and dark in ADC maps (WARACH et al. 1995), and can be detected with this technique within minutes after vessel occlusion, whereas standard (i.e., T2-weighted) MR images have not the capability to detect an acute infarction within the first 6 h (MOHR et al. 1995). SCHWAMM and colleagues reported their findings in 14 acute stroke patients, in which they obtained serial DWI starting within 13 h of symptom onset and repeated imaging after 8, 24, 36 and 48 h and 7 days and >42 days after first imaging. The mean relative ADC (ADCr = relative to the normal brain) of the initial lesion was 0.73; the mean time to minimum ADCr was 33 h. ADCr exceeded 1 after 42 days (SCHWAMM et al. 1998).

While an early ischemic injury becomes bright in DWI, unfortunately not all bright areas in DWI are ischemic lesions. Other factors may also cause hyperintensity in the DWI and failure to consider these factors will result in errors in diagnosis (WARACH et al. 1997). Signal intensity in DWI can be affected by (1) diffusion anisotropy, (2) the amount of regional hyperintensity on the images without diffusion weighting (T2-shine-through-mechanism) and (3) susceptibility artifacts. The first two problems can be solved by using either diffusion isotropy and/or by calculating and interpreting the ADC value/maps consequently. The third problem is easily recognizable and should not pose a problem for anyone sufficiently experienced in MRI interpretation (ULUG et al. 1997).

The hypothesis that hyperintensities in DWI demonstrate areas of increased intracellular space is now generally accepted. The reversibility of these hyperintensities in the clinical setting is still a matter of discussion. In animal experiments it was shown that transient decreases of the ADC in the ischemic border zone exist with a variation in recovery time. It is thought that these areas of transient ADC decreases represent the ischemic penumbra (ROTHER et al. 1996), which therefore could completely recover. Reversible changes in the ADC have also been shown in other than ischemic diseases, for instance in severe transient hypoglycemia (HASEGAWA et al. 1994). In clinical studies with acute stroke patients full recovery of DWI abnormalities was only reported in single cases (KIDWELL et al. 1999; TONG et al. 1998),

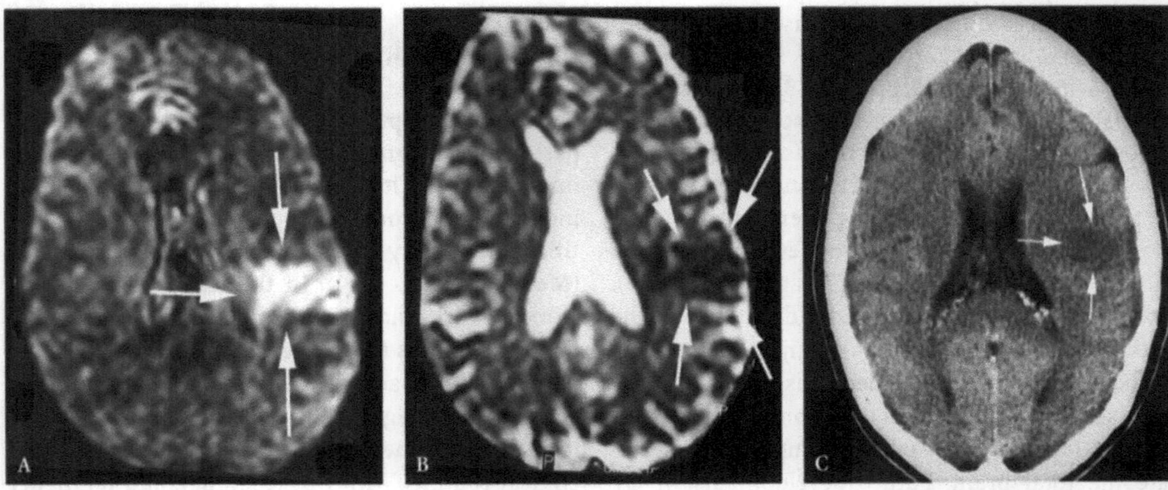

Fig. 10.5A–C. Patient with an M2 branch occlusion 2.5 h after symptom onset. Diffusion weighted image (DWI) shows the area with cytotoxic edema and reduced diffusion brightness (**A**); on the ADC map this area appears dark (**B**). CT scan 27 h later shows an infarct with identical dimensions (**C**)

leading to the opinion that in the acute clinical setting DWI abnormalities can be interpreted as irreversibly damaged areas (Jansen et al. 1999). However, in a recently published small series with patients undergoing successful thrombolysis, the partial reversibility of DWI changes could be demonstrated. At the moment, the question if and how much DWI changes in acute ischemic stroke patients are reversible cannot be answered with certainty.

10.4.2 Perfusion-Weighted Imaging (PWI)

Perfusion-weighted imaging (PWI) makes use of the signal loss that occurs during the dynamic tracking of the first pass of an intravenous paramagnetic contrast agent. A concentration-time-course is consequently derived voxel-by-voxel. Different hemodynamic parameters such as relative mean transit time (rMTT) and relative cerebral blood volume (rCBV) and flow (rCBF) can then be calculated and displayed as perfusion maps from the entire brain (Belliveau et al. 1990). Although PWI is not able to measure absolute CBV or CBF values, relative maps, however, demonstrate areas of minor perfusion in comparison to the unaffected brain. With a two section technique a simultaneous creation of concentration time curves in the brain-feeding arteries (i.e., internal carotid artery) and in the brain tissue can be acquired. In this way the arterial input function can be measured and absolute regional CBF and CBV values calculated. The perfusion data with this technique are in good agreement with data from PET studies, but have the disadvantage that only one section of the brain can be measured. In the clinical routine this method has not yet been established.

Perfusion images are usually obtained with an EPI spin-echo sequence. The contrast bolus is administered with an injector via a large-bore cannula in the antecubital fossa (i.e., 0.1 mmol/kg). The total imaging time is approximately between 1 and 2 min with an additional time needed for postprocessing the hemodynamic maps. The rMTT maps usually show perfusion deficits of a greater volume and with a clearer distinction to the unaffected tissue than other hemodynamic measurements (Barber et al. 1998). In the daily routine many centers only use the rMTT maps as a basis to describe the hemodynamic situation in an acute stroke patient. Hemodynamic imaging cannot only be used to describe the area of reduced perfusion in an acute stroke patient, but also to obtain relative hemodynamic information in patients with stenosis at the brain-feeding vessels (i.e., ICA stenosis) or during the angiographic tolerance test of an ICA occlusion.

10.4.3 Multimodal MRI Approach in Acute Ischemic Stroke Patients

In the beginning of rapid and functional MR imaging, several groups tried to answer the most relevant questions in the acute stroke patient with one of the described techniques alone. Especially DWI seemed to have enough potential to differentiate between the irreversibly damaged infarct core and the still salvageable penumbra or another kind of tissue at risk. However, these attempts were not successful and the concept of a multimodal MRI approach was created (Moseley et al. 1991).

The protocol contains a regular fast T2 weighted image, magnetic resonance angiography (MRA), DWI and PWI. This combination of PWI, DWI and MRA with regular T2-weighted imaging is the most practicable and promising stroke imaging protocol (Fig. 10.6).

The regular T2 image is obtained to rule out severe non-ischemic lesions and to show older vascular lesions either of micro- or macroangiopathic etiology.

MRA has been well accepted as a reliable method to demonstrate vessel occlusion in the arteries of the circle of Willis. To save time, a very short sequence with reduced resolution is used. However, the quality of the MRA should be good enough to completely evaluate the major brain vessels and also the proximal parts of the M2 segments of the MCA. Instead of a TOF-MRA with reduced resolution, PC angiography with only a few sections in the coronal plane can be obtained. The slab thickness must be large enough to demonstrate the patency or occlusion of the major brain vessels.

The common approach with PWI and DWI in acute stroke patients presumes a simplification in the interpretation of the data from these techniques. In this concept it is speculated that DWI lesions present irreversible damaged tissue – the infarct core. PWI and especially the rMTT maps demonstrate the area of minor perfusion in patients with acute vessel occlusion. The correlation of DWI lesions with PWI lesions results either in a match (PWI = DWI) or in a mismatch (PWI>DWI; PWI<DWI) (Fig. 10.7). It is speculated that the mismatch area (with PWI>DWI) represents a tissue at

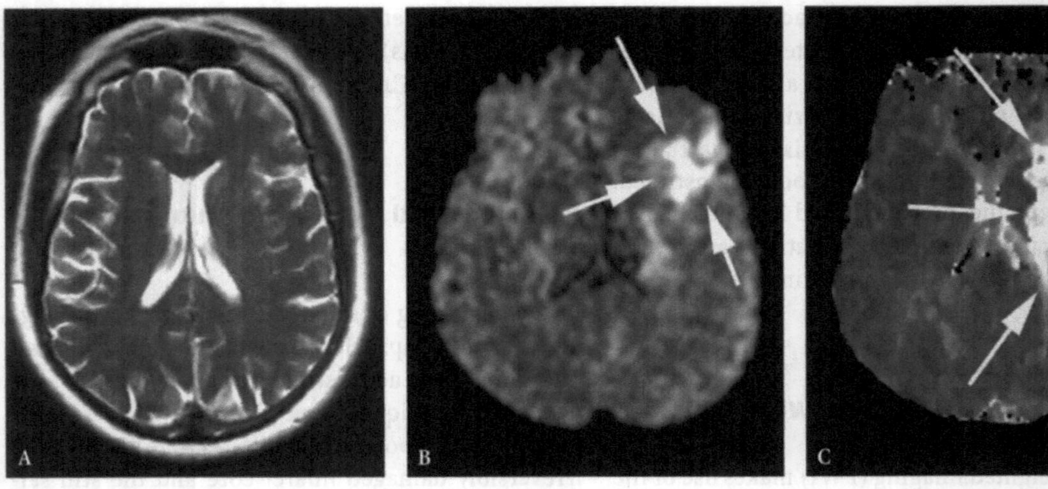

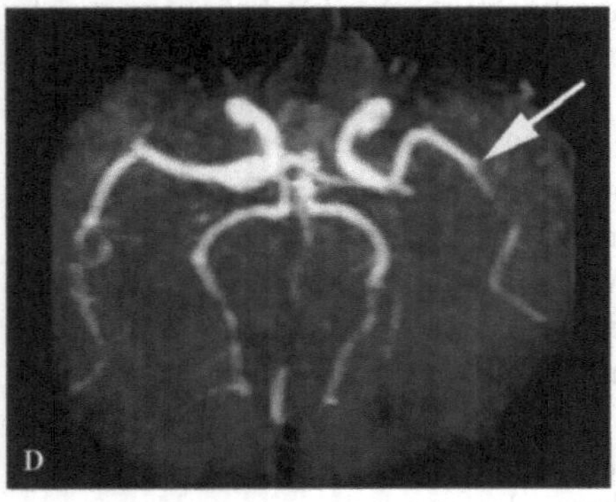

Fig. 10.6A–D. Multimodal stroke MRI in a patient 3 h after onset of left hemispheric symptoms: T2-weighted image is normal (**A**). DWI shows an ischemic lesion in the left frontal insular (**B**). PWI shows an abnormal perfusion of nearly the entire MCA territory. This mismatch between DWI and PWI demonstrates a large tissue at risk. MRA demonstrates a partial occlusion of the distal left MCA (**D**)

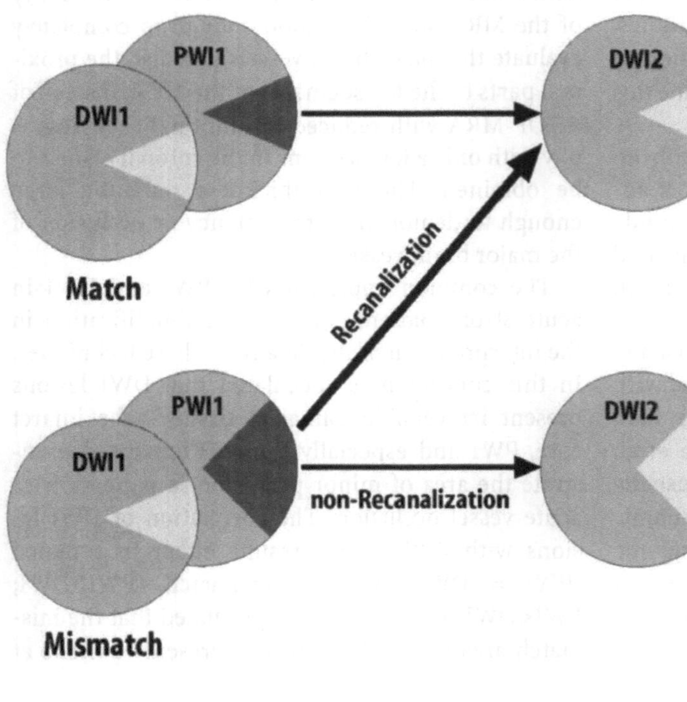

Fig. 10.7. Concept of match and mismatch based on the correlation between PWI and DWI in acute stroke patients. Match patients do not have a tissue at risk and no increase in infarct size: the DWI lesion on day 2 after stroke has nearly the same size as on day 1. Mismatch patients do have a tissue at risk, which can be preserved from infarction by early recanalization. In case of non-recanalization the tissue at risk can be damaged and the infarct size increases from day 1 to day 2

risk, which is at risk of infarction. In these patients the area of abnormal and reduced perfusion is larger than the already damaged area. With increase of the edema or slight decrease of systemic blood pressure, patients with a mismatch have a high risk of larger infarctions at follow-up due to secondary failure of leptomeningeal collaterals. However, in mismatch patients with a successful recanalization or maintaining patency of sufficient collaterals, the tissue at risk can be saved from infarction. Patients with a match between PWI and DWI do not show a tissue at risk. In these patients the whole infarct has already developed and in those cases with no additional vascular event the infarct size should not grow significantly during the follow-up in comparison to the initial DWI lesion. The third group of patients show a mismatch with PWI smaller than DWI. This kind of *inverse* mismatch is not very often observed in hyperacute and acute patients (Tong et al. 1998; Jansen et al. 1999) and occurs in cases with a spontaneous recanalization. The perfusion in the already damaged tissue (DWI lesions) has improved or normalized and there is no risk of an increase of the infarct size.

Combined PWI and DWI has the potential to be more powerful than either study alone in predicting infarct outcome (Sorensen et al. 1996). Both PWI and DWI are highly correlated with severity of neurological deficit by 24-h NIHSS score and T2 weighted stroke size at day 7 (Tong et al. 1998). In another study acute PWI lesions correlated with acute neurological state, clinical outcome and final infarct volume, while DWI lesions correlated less robustly with the acute neurological state, but correlated well with clinical outcome and final infarct volume (Barber et al. 1998) These findings advocated the concept that combined PWI and DWI can define potentially salvageable tissue at risk. In a recently published series of 35 patients it could be clearly shown that patients with a mismatch of more than 20% between PWI and DWI showed a highly statistical benefit in clinical outcome and final infarct size, when the occluded vessel was recanalized in comparison to patients with a mismatch but without early recanalization (Jansen et al. 1999) (Fig. 10.8).

The quotient of PWI/DWI measures the size of the tissue at risk in acute stroke patients. The concept of "time is brain", i.e., a reduction of salvageable brain tissue with progressing time, is shown by comparing this quotient with the time window between stroke onset and MR investigation in an acute stroke population. This comparison shows a continuous decrease of the quotient over time and demonstrates that a multimodal stroke MRI is able to show that "time is brain" (Fig. 10.9). However, the same figure shows that there are patients far beyond the 6-h window, who have a significant tissue at risk. These data challenge the concept of a rigid and universal time window for the treatment of acute ischemic stroke (Baron et al. 1995).

Primary intracerebral hemorrhage is the main differential diagnosis in hyperacute stroke patients (15%) and must be ruled out before any treatment of ischemic stroke can be initiated. A number of previous studies claimed that MRI is insensitive to the detection of acute intracranial hemorrhage. However, these studies were performed at a low field strength (<0.6 T) and the results seemed to be not valid at higher field strengths (>1 T). While animal experimental data already demonstrated the potential of MRI to demonstrate even hyperacute hemorrhages, this suggestion was proven clinically in two published series recently (Patel et al. 1996; Schellinger et al. 1999). These results show that MRI with susceptibility weighted sequences (T2*-weighted gradient echo sequences) is sensitive to hyperacute hemorrhage within the first hours after stroke onset, and that MR can be used as an adequate screening tool for primary intraparenchymal hemorrhage (Fig. 10.10). It is postulated that radiologists who are experienced with MR imaging of acute stroke patients and therefore trained to interpret the different appearances of hyperacute stroke imaging do not need an additional CT scan to exclude intracerebral hemorrhage, when stroke MRI has been performed. Multimodal stroke MRI will be more cost-effective and less time-consuming as opposed to CT and Doppler ultrasound to rule out hemorrhage and vessel occlusion followed by stroke MRI to demonstrate infarct core and tissue at risk (Patel et al. 1996; Schellinger et al. 1999). However, this experience should be proven with a larger patient group before it is generally recommendable.

Acute subarachnoid hemorrhage (SAH) is another disease which rarely can present with stroke-like symptoms and it is requested from some authors that an optimal stroke imaging modality should be able to rule out SAH, although most patients with acute SAH have typical symptoms, which can easily be differentiated from ischemic or hemorrhagic stroke. To demonstrate acute SAH by MRI, FLAIR sequences have been found to be highly sensitive at low field strengths. At higher field strengths flow artifacts on FLAIR images may be mistaken for SAH. This misinterpretation can be avoided by acquisition of additional proton density weighted (PDW) images (Wiesmann et al. 1999). However, in unclear cases

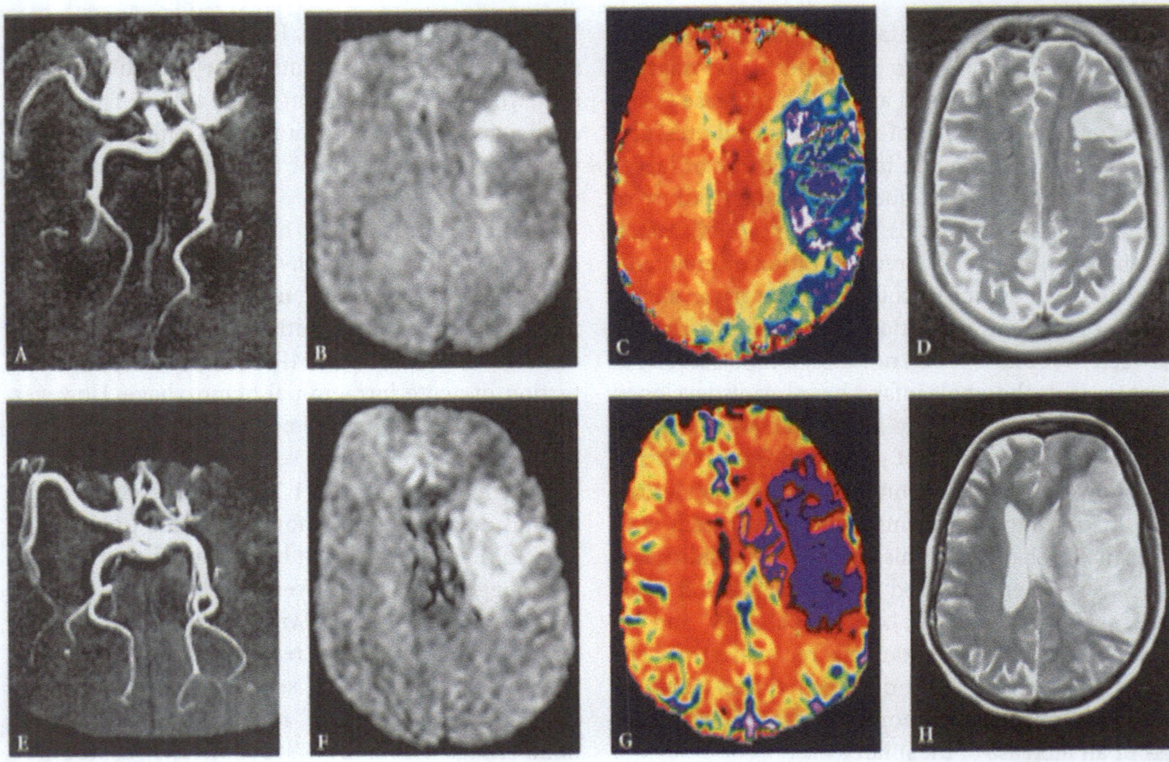

Fig. 10.8A–H. Forty-six-year-old patient 2 h 30 min after onset of left hemispheric symptoms. MRA (**A**) shows left middle cerebral artery (*MCA*) occlusion (+). DWI (**B**) shows a small area of ischemically injured tissue in the left frontal lobe, while PWI (**C**) shows a disturbed perfusion in most of the MCA territory. After early recanalization T2-weighted image on day 5 (**D**) reveals only a small left frontal infarct. Patient had a NIHSS of 1 at day 90. E–I 49-year-old patient 2 h after onset of left hemispheric symptoms. MRA (**E**) shows left MCA occlusion (+). DWI (**F**) shows medium sized area of injury in left basal ganglia, while PWI (**G**) again shows a disturbed perfusion of most of the MCA territory. Early thrombolysis failed in MCA recanalization. T2WI (**H**) on day5 shows an infarct that involves nearly the entire left MCA territory. Patient had a NIHSS of 7 at day 90

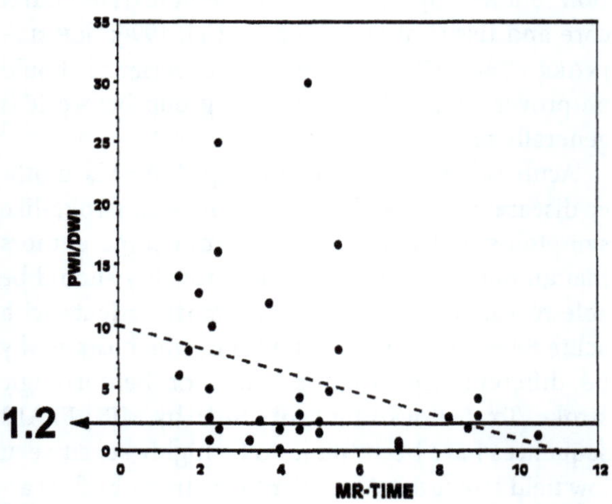

Fig. 10.9. Correlation between PWI/DWI and time of the MRI scan (hours) after onset of symptoms in an acute stroke population. 1.2 defines the cut-off value of a 20% mismatch between PWI and DWI

or in patients highly suspicious of having acute SAH a CT scan and facultatively lumbar puncture should be performed.

Proton magnetic resonance spectroscopy has been used in the assessment of stroke patients. Typically an elevated lactate and a decreased *N*-acetylaspartate, believed to be a neuronal marker, were observed in stroke patients, using single-voxel spectroscopy techniques. Single-voxel techniques, however, do not provide information regarding the spatial distribution and extent of metabolic abnormalities, and require that the location of the ischemic or infarcted region be already known or visible on MR images. In small recently published series it has been shown that spectroscopy imaging is feasible for imaging patients with acute stroke and more studies are on the way to prove if this technique can identify tissue at risk or even the penumbra (Gillard et al. 1996). More details about the use of spectroscopy is stroke patients can be found in Chap. 5.

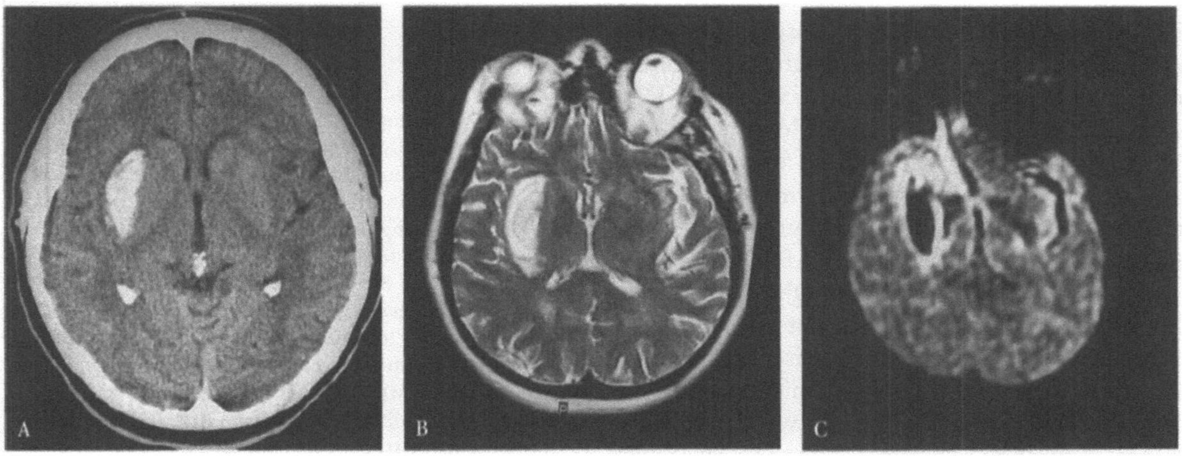

Fig. 10.10A–C. Patient with primary intracerebral hemorrhage 4 h after symptom onset. The initial CT demonstrates the hemorrhage in the right lateral lentiform nucleus (**A**). MRI was performed 20 min after CT scan and shows an unspecific hyperintensity in the T2-weighted spin-echo image (**B**), but a dark lesion with an hyperintense halo in the susceptibility EPI-FLAIR image (**C**), which has been shown to be a typical appearance of hyperacute intracerebral hemorrhage

10.5 PET and SPECT in Acute Ischemic Stroke

The uptake of the tracer HMPAO in the brain tissue is proportional to the actual cerebral blood flow. For this reason HMPAO is regarded as a perfusion-reflecting tracer and HMPAO-SPECT can be used in acute cerebral ischemia to detect areas of abnormal perfusion. The focal absence of HMPAO is a hallmark of arterial occlusion. This information can be acquired within an imaging time of 20 min, but an additional time of 30–60 min is necessary for preparation of the tracer. Images can be interpreted on a visual or semiquantitative basis using a region-to-cerebellar ratio or asymmetry index, but no quantitative data on CBV or CBF can be obtained with SPECT. However, one investigator showed that patients with an extensive deep ischemia on HMPAO-SPECT have a high risk of secondary hemorrhage if local intraarterial thrombolysis is performed (Ueda et al. 1994).

SPECT with HMPAO can be interesting in prospective clinical treatment studies, because the tracer remains trapped in the tissue, allowing reproducible imaging during the first 4 h because of minimal washout from the brain. Therefore study designs with application of the tracer prior to treatment and secondary SPECT-imaging are possible without a large time delay (Alexandrov et al. 1997).

PET is the only validated method to measure the absolute CBV or CBF. Using quantitative multitracer PET studies it is possible to visualize the irreversibly damaged tissue, the penumbra and also the area of oligemia in an acute ischemic stroke patient. However, absolute quantitation of the CBF requires knowledge of the arterial input function, which can only be obtained by continuous arterial blood sampling during the PET study. This requires placement of arterial lines, which is contraindicated in patients who may be potential candidates for thrombolytic therapy. Moreover, quantitative PET studies require very complex logistics, which is usually not possible for an around-the-clock service. Additionally, in the case of an acute interventional treatment quantitative PET will consume unacceptable time. All these arguments stand for the problems associated with integration of PET into an aggressive treatment concept of acute ischemic stroke. Since quantitative measures of CBF could not be obtained in acute stroke patients, Heiss and colleagues (1997) used the relative regional tracer uptake of (^{15}O)-H_2O to estimate the level of residual blood flow in the affected hemisphere. In 12 patients they demonstrated that this technique can semiquantitatively demonstrate critically hypoperfused tissue, which can be preserved from infarction by early reperfusion. However, as with stroke MRI, this technique can not *directly* delineate the penumbra but can demonstrate a tissue at risk only.

10.6 Conclusion

With the advent of sufficient therapies for acute ischemic stroke the availability of accurate brain imaging information assumes an increasingly important role in patient management. Currently, CT is still the most widely used brain imaging technique in acute stroke patients. Whereas new knowledge about early infarct signs and contraindications for thrombolysis are important, CT remains primarily a tool to rule out intracerebral hemorrhage. Standard MRI techniques are also of limited value but DWI and PWI in combination with MRA and T2-weighted MRI (stroke MRI) have several important attributes: (1) they demonstrate location and extent of the ischemic area; (2) they show the region of disturbed microvascular perfusion; (3) they demonstrate major vessel occlusions; and (4) they can rule out hemorrhage or tumor, which may be responsible for stroke-like symptoms.

Several studies on these new MRI techniques in acute ischemic stroke patients suggest that a so-called "diffusion-perfusion-mismatch" may identify a tissue at risk, which can be preserved from damage by adjuvant therapy. This region of mismatch is not identical with the ischemic penumbra but may be used as an indicator for the still salvageable tissue in case of sufficient therapy. Smaller series documented the feasibility of DWI-PWI studies in patients treated with rt-PA and the potential of this technique to identify patients who benefit from early successful recanalization (Jansen et al. 1999; Marks et al. 1999). This remains to be established by appropriately designed multicenter studies. Besides the clinical use of these techniques – identifying patients who should undergo aggressive therapeutic strategies – multimodal stroke MRI will have a significant impact on stroke trial design and implementation. The possibility of determining very early stroke subtypes and of focusing a trial on certain stroke patients will certainly decrease the needed patient population and simultaneously increase the study power (Fisher et al. 1999). CT angiography and CT-based perfusion, the latter now possible with a new CT generation, are also promising techniques and it is suggested that CT will be of continued utility and value for the diagnosis of acute ischemic stroke. However, the advantages of stroke MRI for depicting early parenchymal injury during the initial period after stroke are evident. For those who have the capacity to perform early stroke MRI, this method may be the imaging modality of choice in acute stroke patients, especially since susceptibility-weighted MRI sequences can reliably detect intracerebral hemorrhage. PET and SPECT are of use to answer certain questions under research aspects but will probably not have the potential to become an initial standard diagnostic tool in acute stroke patients.

References

Alexandrov AV, Masdeu JC, Devous Sr MD, Black SE, Grotta JC (1997) Brain single-photon emission CT with HMPAO and safety of thrombolytic therapy in acute ischemic stroke. Proceedings of the meeting of the SPECT Safe Thrombolysis Study Collaborators and the members of the Brain Imaging Council of the Society of Nuclear Medicine. Stroke 28: 1830–1834

Astrup J, Siesj+ B, Symon L (1981) Thresholds in cerebral ischemia – the ischemic penumbra. Stroke 12: 723–725

Barber PA, Darby DG, Desmond PM et al. (1998) Prediction of stroke outcome with echoplanar perfusion- and diffusion-weighted MRI. Neurology 51: 418–426

Baron JC, vonKummer R, delZoppo GJ (1995) Treatment of acute ischemic stroke. Challenging the concept of a rigid and universal time window. Stroke 26: 2219–2221

Belliveau JW, Rosen BR, Kantor HL et al. (1990) Functional cerebral imaging by susceptibility-contrast NMR. Magn Reson Med 14: 538–546

Bozzao L, Bastianello S, Fantozzi LM, Angeloni U, Argentino C, Fieschi C (1989) Correlation of angiographic and sequential CT findings in patients with evolving cerebral infarction. AJNR 10: 1215–1222

Bozzao L, Angeloni U, Bastianello S, Fantozzi LM, Pierallini A, Fieschi C (1991) Early angiographic and CT findings in patients with hemorrhagic infarction in the distribution of the middle cerebral artery. AJNR 12: 1115–1121

Brandt T, Thie A, Caplan LR, Hacke W (1995) Infarcts in the brain areas supplied by the posterior cerebral artery. Clinical aspects, pathogenesis and prognosis. Nervenarzt 66: 267–274

Brandt T, von Kummer R, Muller Kuppers M, Hacke W (1996) Thrombolytic therapy of acute basilar artery occlusion. Variables affecting recanalization and outcome. Stroke 27: 875–881

Brandt T, Knauth M, Wildermuth S et al. (1999) CT angiography and Doppler sonography for emergency assessment in acute basilar artery ischemia. Stroke 30: 606–612

Bruning R, Penzkofer H, Schopf U et al. (1998) Calculation of absolute cerebral blood volume and cerebral blood flow by means of electron-beam computed tomography (EBT) in acute ischemia. Radiologe 38: 1054–1059

Busto R, Dietrich WD, Globus MY-T et al. (1987) Small differences in intraischemic brain temperature critically determine the extent of ischemic injury. J Cereb Blood Flow Metab 7: 729–738

Davis M, Mendelow AD, Perry RH, Chambers IR, James OF (1995) Experimental stroke and neuroprotection in the aging rat brain. Stroke 26: 1072–1078

Diener HC (1998) Multinational randomised controlled trial of lubelozole in acute ischaemic stroke. Cerebrovasc Dis 8: 172–181

Doerfler A, Forsting M, Reith W et al. (1996) Decompressive surgery in a rat model of "malignant" cerebral hemispherical stroke: experimental support for an aggressive therapeutic approach. J Neurosurg 85: 853–859

Doerfler A, Engelhorn T, von Kummer R et al. (1998) Are iodinated contrast agents detrimental in acute cerebral ischemia? An experimental study in rats. Radiology 206: 211–217

Donnan GA, Davis SM, Chambers BR et al. (1995) Trials of streptokinase in severe acute ischaemic stroke. Lancet 345: 578–579

Fisher M, Albers GW (1999) Applications of diffusion-perfusion magnetic resonance imaging in acute ischemic stroke. Neurology 52: 1750–1756

Forsting M, Reith W, Schabitz WR et al. (1995) Decompressive craniectomy for cerebral infarction. An experimental study in rats. Stroke 26: 259–264

Frank JI, Krieger D, Chyatte D, Cancian S (1999) HEADD-FIRST: Hemicraniectomy and durotomy upon deterioration from massive hemispheric infarctions. A proposed multicenter, prospective, randomized study. 24th American Heart Association International Conference on Stroke and Cerebral Circulation. Nashville, Tennessee, USA

Gillard JH, Barker PB, van Zijl PC, Bryan RN, Oppenheimer SM (1996) Proton MR spectroscopy in acute middle cerebral artery stroke. AJNR 17: 873–886

Gilman S (1998) Imaging the brain. First of two parts. N Engl J Med 338: 812–820

Gilman S (1998) Imaging the brain. Second of two parts. N Engl J Med 338: 889–896

Hacke W, Schwab S, DeGeorgia M (1994) Intensive care of acute ischemic stroke. Cerebrovasc Dis 4: 384–392

Hacke W, Kaste M, Fieschi C et al. (1995) Intravenous thrombolysis with recombinant tissue plasminogen activator for acute hemispheric stroke. The European Cooperative Acute Stroke Study. JAMA 274: 1017–1025

Hacke W, Stingele R, Steiner T, Schuchardt V, Schwab S (1995) Critical care of acute ischemic stroke. Intensive Care Med 21: 856–862

Hacke W, Schwab S, Horn M, Spranger M, De Georgia M, von Kummer R (1996) 'Malignant' middle cerebral artery territory infarction: clinical course and prognostic signs. Arch Neurol 53: 309–315

Hacke W, Steiner T, Schwab S (1996) Critical management of the acute stroke: Medical and surgical therapy. In: Batjer HH, Caplan LR, Freiberg L, Greenlee RG, Jr., Kopitnik TH, Jr. and Young WL (eds) Cerebrovascular Disease. Lippincott-Raven, Hagerstown, pp 523–533

Hacke W, Kaste M, Fieschi C et al. (1998) Randomised double-blind placebo-controlled trial of thrombolytic therapy with intravenous alteplase in acute ischaemic stroke (ECASS II). Lancet 352: 1245–1251

Hamberg LM, Hunter GJ, Halpern EF, Hoop B, Gazelle GS, Wolf GL (1996) Quantitative high-resolution measurement of cerebrovascular physiology with slip-ring CT. AJNR 17: 639–650

Hamberg LM, Hunter GJ, Kierstead D, Lo EH, Gilberto-Gonzalez R, Wolf GL (1996) Measurement of cerebral blood volume with subtraction three-dimensional functional CT. AJNR 17: 1861–1869

Hasegawa Y, Fisher M, Latour LL, Dardzinski BJ, Sotak CH (1994) MRI diffusion mapping of reversible and irreversible ischemic injury in focal brain ischemia. Neurology 44: 1484–1490

Heiss WD, Grond M, Thiel A et al. (1998) Tissue at risk of infarction rescued by early reperfusion: a positron emission tomography study in systemic recombinant tissue plasminogen activator thrombolysis of acute stroke. J Cerebr Blood Flow Met 18: 1298–1307

Horowitz SH, Zito JL, Donnarumma R, Patel M, Alvir J (1991) Computed tomographic-angiographic findings within the first five hours of cerebral infarction. Stroke 22: 1245–1253

Jansen O, Schellinger PD, Fiebach JB, Hacke W, Sartor K (1999) Early recanalization in acute ischemic stroke saves tissue at risk defined by MRI. Lancet 353: 2036–2037

Kidwell CS, Alger JR, Di Salle F et al. (1999) Diffusion MRI in patients with transient ischemic attacks. Stroke 30: 1174–1180

Knauth M, Forsting M, Hartmann M, Heiland S, Balzer T, Sartor K (1996) MR enhancement of brain lesions: Increased contrast dose compared with magnetization transfer. AJNR 17: 1853–1859

Knauth M, Kummer Rv, Jansen O, Haehnel S, Doerfler A, Sartor K (1997) Potential of CT angiography in acute ischemic stroke. AJNR 18: 1001–1010

Koenig M, Klotz E, Luka B, Venderink DJ, Spittler JF, Heuser L (1998) Perfusion CT of the brain: diagnostic approach for early detection of ischemic stroke. Radiology 209: 85–93

Leys D, Pruvo JP, Godefroy O, Rondepierre P, Leclerc X (1992) Prevalence and significance of hyperdense middle cerebral artery in acute stroke. Stroke 23: 317–324

Manelfe C, Larrue V, von Kummer R et al. (1999) Association of hyperdense middle cerebral artery sign with clinical outcome in patients treated with tissue plasminogen activator. Stroke 30: 769–772

Marks MP, Tong D, Beaulieu C, Albers G, de Crespigny A, Moseley ME (1999) Evaluation of early reperfusion and IV rt-PA therapy using diffusion- and perfusion-weighted MRI. Neurology 52: 1792–1798

Mohr JP, Biller J, Hilal SK et al. (1995) Magnetic resonance versus computed tomographic imaging in acute stroke. Stroke 26: 807–812

Mori E, Tabuchi M, Yoshida T, Yamadori A (1988) Intracarotid urokinase with thromboembolic occlusion of the middle cerebral artery. Stroke 19: 802–812

Mori E, Yoneda Y, Tabuchi M et al. (1992) Intravenous recombinant tissue plasminogen activator in acute carotid artery territory stroke. Neurology 42: 976–982

Moseley ME, Kucharczyk J, Mintorovitch J et al. (1990) Diffusion-weighted MR imaging of acute stroke: correlation with T2-weighted and magnetic susceptibility-enhanced MR imaging in cats. AJNR 11: 423–429

Moseley ME, Wendland MF, Kucharczyk J (1991) Magnetic resonance imaging of diffusion and perfusion. Top Magn Reson Imaging 3: 50–67

Multicenter Acute Stroke Trial - Europe Study Group (1996) Thrombolytic therapy with streptokinase in acute ischaemic stroke. N Engl J Med 335: 145–150

Multicentre Acute Stroke Trial - Italy (MAST-I) Group (1995) Randomized controlled trial of streptokinase, aspirin, and combination of both in treatment of acute ischaemic stroke. Lancet 356: 1509–1514

Patel MR, Edelman RR, Warach S (1996) Detection of hyperacute primary intraparenchymal hemorrhage by magnetic resonance imaging. Stroke 27: 2321–2324

PROACT II Investigators (1999) PROACT II: Recombinant prourokinase (r-ProUK) in acute cerebral thromboembolism. Initial trial results. 24th American Heart Association International Conference on Stroke and Cerebral Circulation. Nashville, Tennessee, USA

Rieke K, Schwab S, Krieger D, von Kummer R, Aschoff A, Schuchardt V, Hacke W (1995) Decompressive surgery in space-occupying hemispheric infarction: results of an open, prospective trial. Crit Care Med 23: 1576–1587

Rother J, de Crespigny AJ, H DA, Iwai K, Moseley ME (1996) Recovery of apparent diffusion coefficient after ischemia-induced spreading depression relates to cerebral perfusion gradient. Stroke 27: 980–986

Schellinger P, Steiner T (1998) Emergency and intensive-care treatment after a stroke. Recommendations of the European Consensus Group. Nervenarzt 69: 530–539

Schellinger PD, Jansen O, Fiebach JB, Hacke W, Sartor K (1999) A standardized MRI stroke protocol: comparison with CT in hyperacute intracerebral hemorrhage. Stroke 30: 765–768

Schlaug G, Siewert B, Benfield A, Edelman RR, Warach S (1997) Time course of the apparent diffusion coefficient (ADC) abnormality in human stroke. Neurology 49: 113–119

Schriger DL, Kalafut M, Starkman S, Krueger M, Saver JL (1998) Cranial computed tomography interpretation in acute stroke: physician accuracy in determining eligibility for thrombolytic therapy. JAMA 279: 1293–1297

Schwab S, Spranger M, Schwarz S, Hacke W (1997) Barbiturate coma in severe hemispheric stroke: useful or obsolete? Neurology 48: 1608–1613

Schwab S, Steiner T, Aschoff A et al. ( ) Early hemicraniectomy in patients with complete middle cerebral artery infarction. Stroke 29: 1888–1893

Schwab S, Schwarz S, Spranger M, Keller E, Bertram M, Hacke W (1998) Moderate hypothermia in the treatment of patients with severe middle cerebral artery infarction. Stroke 29: 2461–2466

Schwamm LH, Koroshetz WJ, Sorensen AG et al. (1998) Time course of lesion development in patients with acute stroke. Serial diffusion- and hemodynamic-weighted magnetic resonance imaging. Stroke 29: 2268–2276

Shrier DA, Tanaka H, Numaguchi Y, Konno S, Patel U, Shibata D (1997) CT angiography in the evaluation of acute stroke. AJNR 18: 1011–1020

Sorensen AG, Buonanno FS, Gonzalez RG et al. (1996) Hyperacute stroke: evaluation with combined multisection diffusion-weighted and hemodynamically weighted echo-planar MR imaging. Radiology 199: 391–401

Steiner T, Mendoza G, De Georgia M et al. (1997) Prognosis of stroke patients requiring mechanical ventilation in a neurological critical care unit. Stroke 28: 711–715

Steiner T, Bluhmki E, Kaste M et al. (1998) The ECASS 3-hour cohort. Secondary analysis of ECASS data by time stratification. Cerebrovasc Dis 8: 198–203

The ATLANTIS Stroke Study Investigators (1999) The ATLANTIS rt-PA (Alteplase) acute stroke trial: final results. 24th American Heart Association International Conference on Stroke and Cerebral Circulation. Nashville, Tennessee, USA

The National Institute of Neurological Disorders and Stroke rt-PA Stroke Study Group. Tissue plasminogen activator for acute ischemic stroke. N Engl J Med 333: 1581–1587

Tomsick TA, Brott TG, Chambers AA et al. (1990) Hyperdense middle cerebral artery sign on CT: efficacy in detecting middle cerebral artery thrombosis. AJNR 11: 473–477

Tomsick T, Brott T, Barsan W et al. (1996) Prognostic value of the hyperdense middle cerebral artery sign and stroke scale score before ultraearly thrombolytic therapy. AJNR 17: 1–7

Tomura N, Uemura K, Inugami A, Fujita H, Higano S, Shishido F (1988) Early CT finding in cerebral infarction: obscuration of the lentiform nucleus. Radiology 168: 463–467

Tong DC, Yenari MA, Albers GW, M OB, Marks MP, Moseley ME (1998) Correlation of perfusion- and diffusion-weighted MRI with NIHSS score in acute (<6.5 hour) ischemic stroke. Neurology 50: 864–870

Truwit CL, Barkovich AJ, Gean-Marton A, Hibri N, Norman D (1990) Loss of the insular ribbon: another early CT sign of acute middle cerebral artery infarction. Radiology 176: 801–806

Ueda T, Hatakeyama T, Kumon Y, Sakaki S, Uraoka T (1994) Evaluation of risk of hemorrhagic transformation in local intra-arterial thrombolysis in acute ischemic stroke by initial SPECT. Stroke 25: 298–303

Ulug AM, Beauchamp Jr N, Bryan RN, van Zijl PCM (1997) Absolute quantitation of diffusion constants in human. stroke 28: 483–490

von Kummer R, Meyding-Lamade U, Forsting M et al. (1994) Sensitivity and prognostic value of early CT in occlusion of the middle cerebral artery trunk. AJNR 15: 9–15

von Kummer R, Bozzao L, Manelfe C (eds) (1995) Early CT diagnosis of hemispheric brain infarction (1st ed). Springer Verlag, Berlin, pp 1–95

von Kummer R, Nolte PN, Schnittger H, Thron A, Ringelstein EB (1996) Detectability of cerebral hemisphere ischaemic infarcts by CT within 6 h of stroke. Neuroradiology 38: 31–33

von Kummer R, Allen KL, Holle R et al. (1997) Acute stroke: usefulness of early CT findings before thrombolytic therapy. Radiology 205: 327–333

von Kummer R (1998) Effect of training in reading CT scans on patient selection for ECASS II. Neurology 51(Suppl 3): S50-S52

Warach S, Gaa J, Siewert B, Wielopolski P, Edelman RR (1995) Acute human stroke studied by whole brain echo planar diffusion-weighted magnetic resonance imaging. Ann Neurol 37: 231–241

Warach S, Boska M, Welch KM (1997) Pitfalls and potential of clinical diffusion-weighted MR imaging in acute stroke. Stroke 28: 481–482

WHO Task Force (1989) Recommendations on stroke prevention, diagnosis, and therapy. Report of the WHO Task Force on stroke and other cerebrovascular disorders. Stroke 20: 1407–1431

Wiesmann M, Mayer T, Yousry I et al. (1999) Comparison of FLAIR and Fast Spin-Echo MR Imaging at 1.5 T for detection of acute subarachnoid hemorrhage. Joint Annual Meeting of the American Society of Neuroradiology. San Diego, CA, USA

Wildermuth S, Knauth M, Brandt T, Winter R, Sartor K, Hacke W (1998) Role of CT angiography in patient selection for thrombolytic therapy in acute hemispheric stroke. Stroke 29: 935–938

Zeumer H (1985) Vascular recanalizing technique in interventional neuroradiology. J Neurol 231: 287–294

Zeumer H, Freitag HJ, Zanella F, Thie A, Arning C (1993) Local intra-arterial fibrinolytic therapy in patients with stroke: urokinase versus recombinant tissue plasminogen activator (r-TPA). Neuroradiology 35: 159–162

11 Vascular Malformations of the Brain

WENDY J. TAYLOR

CONTENTS

11.1 Introduction

Vascular malformations of the central nervous system present an interesting group of disorders to the neuroradiologist. The term covers a spectrum of abnormalities, some of which represent an extreme variant of normal anatomical disposition, and others which require treatment. Methods of investigation are therefore tailored to the expected outcome for the patient. Some of the vascular malformations are associated with vascular pathology elsewhere in the body and are a reflection of a generalised disorder of vascular modelling and repair. This should be borne in mind when developing a strategy for investigation.

11.2 Classification

11.2.1 Developmental Venous Anomalies (Venous Angioma) and False Vascular Malformations

Developmental venous anomalies are not malformations of the venous system, but represent a variability in the venous drainage pattern of the cerebral white matter (BORDEN et al. 1995; HUBER et al. 1991; KUKER et al. 1997; LASJAUNIAS et al. 1989; LEE et al. 1996; PEEBLES and VIECO 1997; ZOUAOUI et al. 1995). There are two principal patterns: the superficial developmental anomalies (DVAs) which drain the deeper medullary veins into the cortical venous system, and the deep DVAs which drain the subcortical venous system via a deep DVA to the deep venous system (Fig. 11.1).

They are not to be confused with collateral venous drainage pathways that open up in response to occlusion of normal venous pathways, nor do they require any treatment.

Coincidental association of DVAs with cavernomas is described (CHAIX et al. 1996) (Fig. 11.3) and MRI and MRA have shown their coincidence as being as relatively frequent (ZOUAOUI et al. 1995). DVAs have also been found in conjunction with other vascular anomalies (HUBER 1991) including dermal haemangioma, Klippel-Trenauny syndrome, spinal dural fistulae and cerebral arterial aneurysms.

Sinus pericranii is a variant of cerebral venous drainage to the extracranial venous system through

W. J. TAYLOR, MD
Consultant Neuroradiologist, Lysholm Radiological Department, The National Hospital for Neurology and Neurosurgery, Queen Square, London, WC1N 3BG, UK; and Great Ormond Street Hospital for Children, Great Ormond Street, London, WC1N 3JH, UK

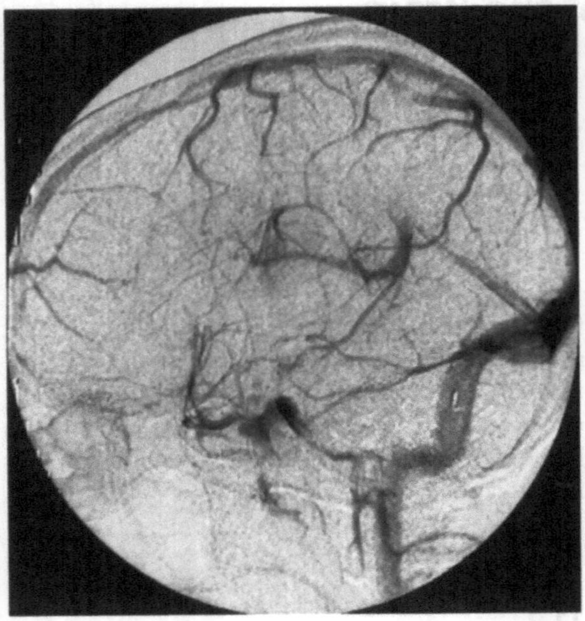

Fig. 11.1. Developmental venous anomaly of the subcortical venous system draining to the deep venous system

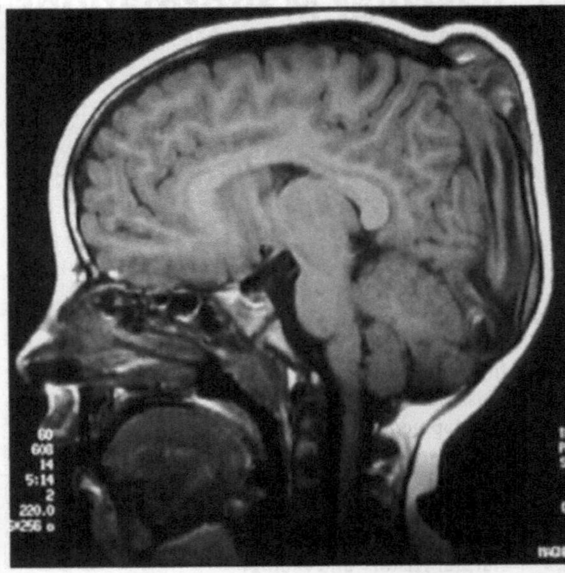

Fig. 11.2. Sagittal T1 SE sequence demonstrating transosseous cranial drainage in sinus pericranii

an osseous defect in the skull in the midline (Fig. 11.2). It is associated with partial agenesis of the superior sagittal sinus. It may be associated with other venous anomalies, and any form of treatment should only be undertaken after careful consideration of the brain venous drainage, as its exclusion from the circulation may cause venous infarction.

11.2.2
Cerebral Cavernoma

Cavernomata are an enigmatic disorder. Pathologically they consist of cavernous spaces filled with blood and present as a result of peripheral haemorrhage. Cavernous angiomata are vascular malformations mostly located in the central nervous system and characterised by enlarged capillary cavities without intervening brain parenchyma (Houtteville 1997).

Prevalence of cerebral cavernoma is approximately 0.5% in the general population. They can be sporadic or familial. Genes associated with the disorder have been mapped to the long arm of chromosome 7 (Dubovsky et al. 1995; Gil-Nagel et al. 1996; Gunel et al. 1996; Johnson et al. 1995; Polymeropoulos et al. 1997), two others on the short arm of chromosome 7 and also the long arm of chromosome 3 (Craig et al. 1998). They may be inherited in an autosomal dominant form in as much as 50% of cases. Most cavernomata have a relatively benign course, but some seem to repeatedly rebleed. A previous haemorrhage (Kondziolka et al. 1995) and infratentorial location (Curling et al. 1991) are the main prognostic factors for occurrence of haemorrhage. They can be familial and multiple, associated with DVAs and also with the development of arteriovenous malformations (Lasjaunias 1989). Clinical symptoms include seizures, haemorrhage and focal neurological deficits (see later). Cavernomata are found in all age groups and all locations and multiple in approximately 2–3% of cases (Voigt and Yasargil 1976). A specific clinical syndrome is not associated with their occurrence, but their course is acute or subacute. Microscopic calcification is found in 11% of cases and on MR they show as a focal area of haemorrhage (acute, chronic or mixed) (Voigt and Yasargil 1976) (Fig. 11.4). There is no pathological circulation on formal angiography, but they can be demonstrated by their displacement of local vessels and mass effect in some cases.

11.2.3
Capillary Venous Malformations

Capillary venous malformations, port wine stains and telangiectasias are sometimes associated with intracranial vascular abnormalities.

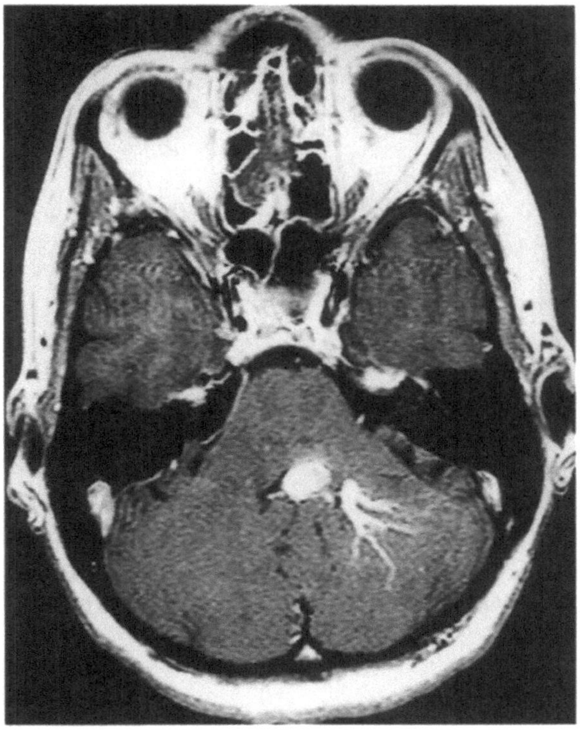

Fig. 11.3. Contrast enhanced axial T1 SE sequence demonstrating coincidental DVA with cavernoma

Sturge Weber syndrome affects approximately 1–2% of patients with facial port wine stains. The embryonic linkage lies in the cell origins of the facial and intracranial mesoderm. From the work of Couly on chick/quail chimeras the origins and destinations of mesodermal tissue in the head show the linkages of cell lines and the endothelial cells in this region derived from neural crest mesenchyme. Sturge Weber syndrome is characterised by cortical venous thrombosis and capillary venous proliferation. This is associated with prominent transmedullary venous drainage and often an enlarged choroid plexus. Impaired venous drainage results in cortical calcification and leukoencephalomalacia (Fig. 11.5).

When the lesions overlie the spine they may be associated with spinal dysraphism or a myelomeric arteriovenous shunt.

Skin telangiectasias are also venous abnormalities and are known to be associated with intracranial vascular lesions. Hereditary haemorrhagic telangiectasia is implicated in some patients with subpial arteriovenous shunts occurring in either the brain or the spinal cord.

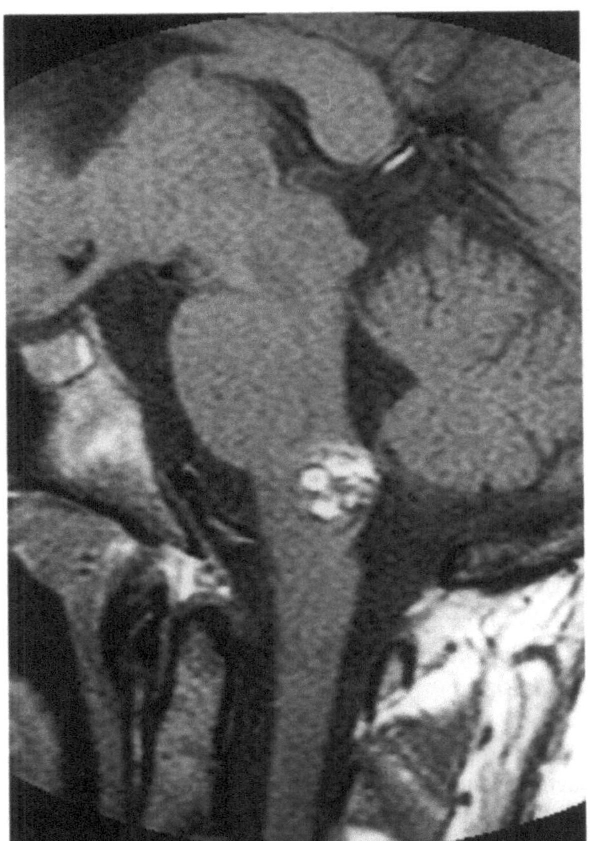

a

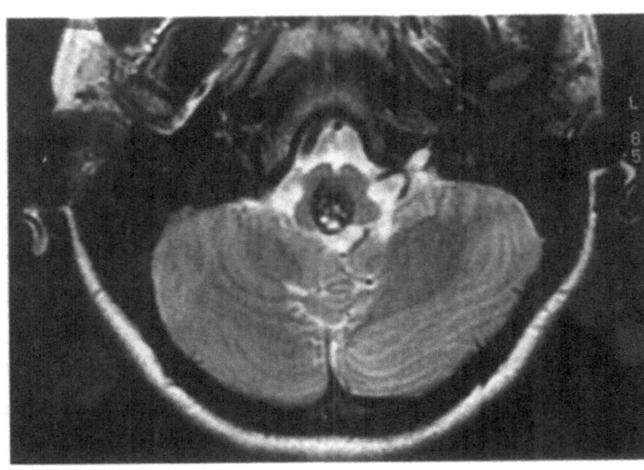

b

Fig. 11.4. a Sagittal T1 SE sequence of a brain stem cavernoma showing heterogeneous increase in signal, suggestive of recent haemorrhage. **b** Axial T2 weighted image with low signal components of haemosiderin deposition confirming previous haemorrhage

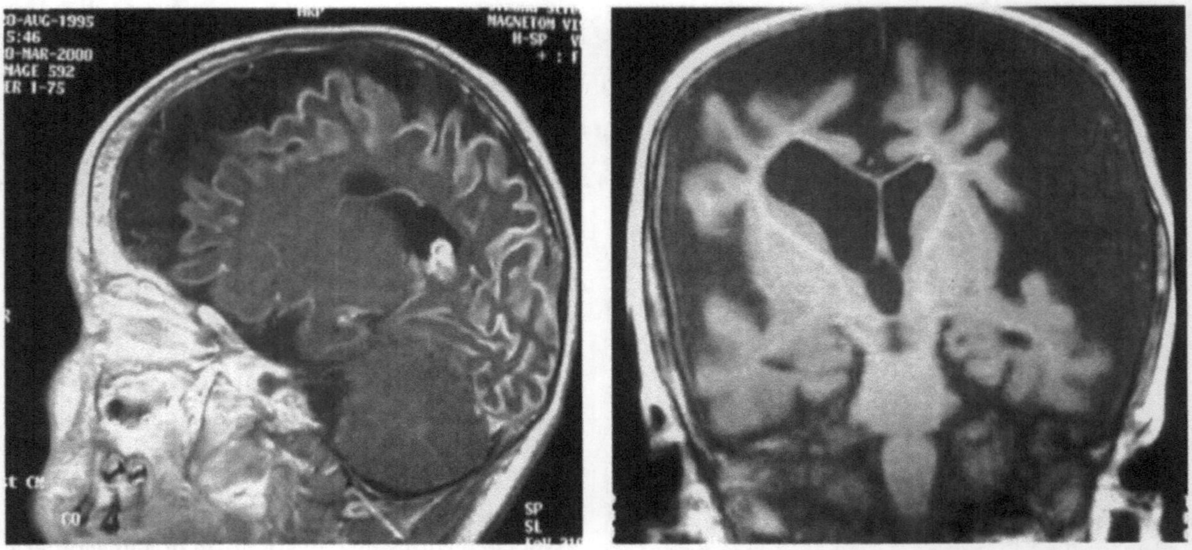

a b

Fig. 11.5. a Sagittal T1 SE sequence after administration of intravenous gadolinium demonstrating leptomeningeal enhancement, prominent choroid plexus, and generalised cerebral atrophic change. b Coronal T1 SE sequence confirming profound cerebral atrophy

11.2.4 Arteriovenous Shunts

General Comments

Arteriovenous malformations (AVM) have been variously classified according to pathology, demography, topography, and haemodynamic or anatomoclinical features. Depending on the type of therapy that is being considered (conservative, endovascular, radiosurgical or neurosurgical), the different classifications have their different uses. However, to contribute to the understanding of the behaviour and natural history of these abnormalities, they are best considered as abnormal arteriovenous shunts, which may be single or multiple, and located in any of the spaces of the brain (that is the subarachnoid, subpial or subdural spaces). The effects of these shunts on the surrounding normal vasculature also should be recognised. This can be recognised as a kind of perinidal hypervascularity which represents a normal brain vasculature (which would not normally be visible at the level of resolution that can be observed under normal circumstances, but which is carrying increased blood flow which is sumped into the abnormal shunt). As this is *normal* vasculature, which is carrying abnormal flow, it should not be a target for any treatment and can be seen to regress after correct disconnection of the arteriovenous shunt.

On the arterial side, abnormal high flow may induce flow-related aneurysms, typically on the feeding vessels (Fig. 11.6), although aneurysms on unrelated vessels may also be associated. These flow related aneurysms can show spontaneous regression when the flow in the vessel is reduced. On the venous side, the vessels respond by dilatation, then kinking, stenosis and eventually occlusion (Fig. 11.7). These vessels may then rupture.

There may also be intranidal aneurysms (Fig. 11.8), which may be either venous or arterial and these may also rupture. Following rupture of these vessels there may be residual 'false' aneurysm which is really a haematoma cavity connected to the vascular system (Fig. 11.9).

The time course of the lesion is also important to understand to try and ensure that adverse features that can be handled are in fact done so in a way which may have a positive effect on the natural history. In analysing AVM in this way they can be subclassified in a sensible fashion.

Although this chapter deals with brain vascular malformations, all the general comments relating to arteriovenous shunts can apply equally to the spinal cord.

11.2.4.1 Arteriovenous Shunts Apparent Antenatally or at Birth

There appear very few developmentally apparent arteriovenous shunts present at birth. These includes multiple arteriovenous shunts at the choroidal level (arising in the subarachnoid space) giving rise to the

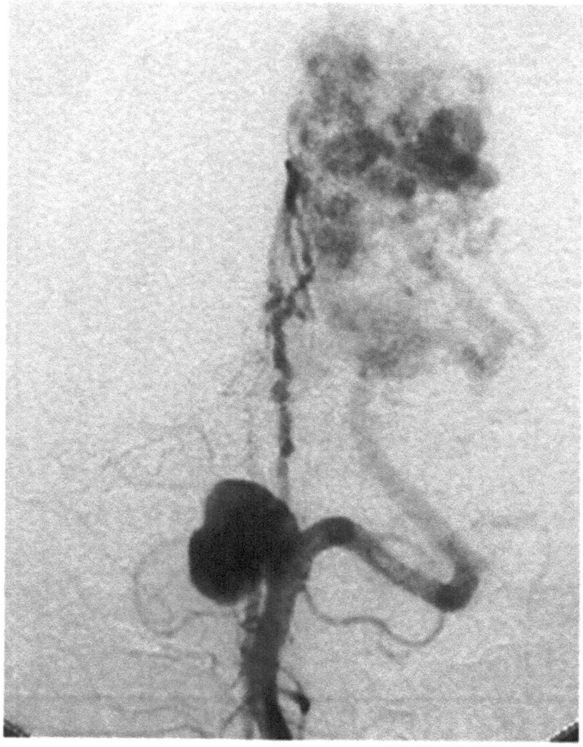

Fig. 11.6. Angiographic AP view of a left vertebral injection demonstrating hypertrophy of the left posterior cerebral artery with an associated aneurysm at the basilar tip

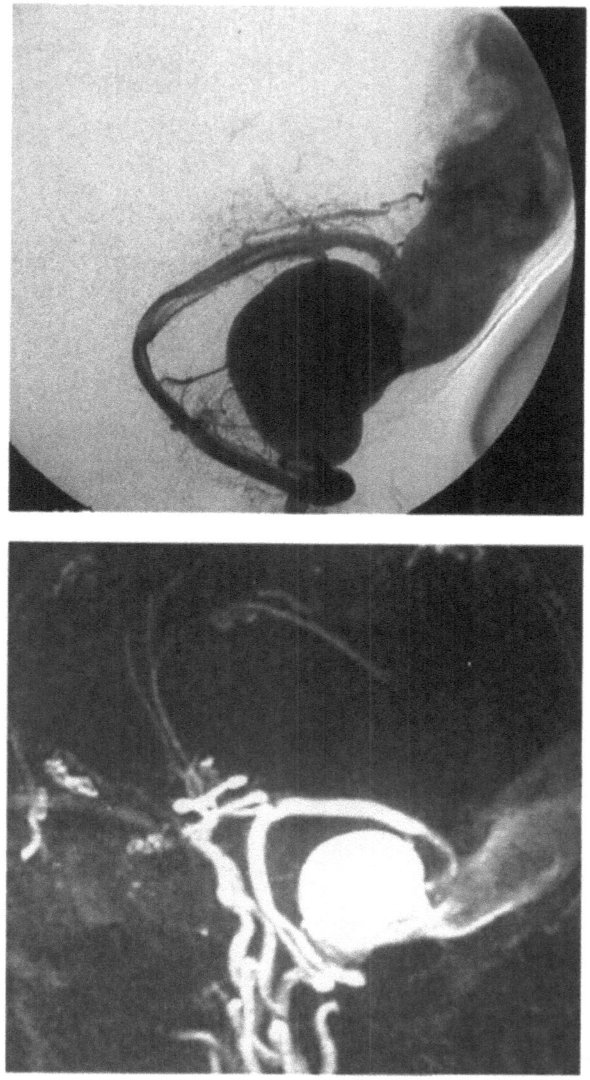

Fig. 11.7. a Lateral view of a left vertebral artery injection demonstrating gross venous ectasia and stenosis with reflux into the superior sagittal sinus with turbulent flow. b Phase contrast MRA demonstrating the same abnormality

better known 'vein of Galen' malformations. Others include intradural shunts associated with a malformed dural sinus. Rarely a subpial arteriovenous shunt presents in the neonatal period. All these shunts have two effects. One is systemic and related to the size of the shunt. These children present with varying degrees of cardiac failure. The other effect is on the maturation of the normal venous system (which is not mature until 2 years of age). In the presence of a shunt there tends to be a progressive occlusion of major outflow tracts at the skull base and in some cases jugular bulb occlusion (Fig. 11.9).

11.2.4.2 Subpial Shunts

The prevalence of cerebral arteriovenous malformations is quoted as 0.14% to 0.8% in a population per year (Jellinger 1986; Wilkins and Rengachary 1985).

Commonly subpial shunts first become manifest in early adult life (often with sporadic and sometimes unconnected neurological clinical events commencing in puberty). These lesions are usually isolated but may be multifocal in up to 10% (Willinsky et al. 1990). Even less common is the association of cerebral and spinal arteriovenous malformations (Hoffman et al. 1976; Mazza et al. 1989; Parkinson and West 1977). They are usually multiple shunts in one location either fed by several separate arteries or multiple vessels arising from the side of a single artery. They induce a surrounding angioectasia which can be difficult to isolate from the true lesion, but which regresses once correct treatment has been instituted. These lesions also provoke changes in the venous system draining the area and may affect the surrounding normal venous vessels.

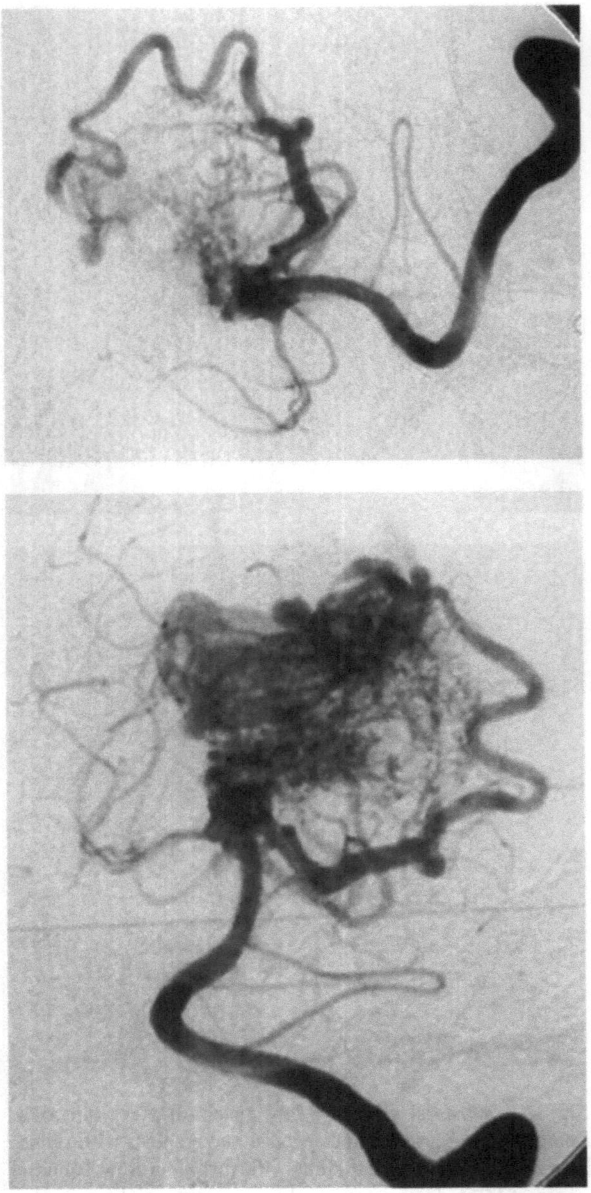

a

b

Fig. 11.8a,b. A 45-year-old male with history of previous subarachnoid haemorrhage and mild right hemiparesis. **a** Left vertebral artery injection early arterial phase showing thalamic AVM demonstrating intranidal aneurysms supplied by posterior cerebral artery and perforating branches. **b** Later arterial phase

These lesions may be related to a known genetic disorder, such as hereditary haemorrhagic telangiectasia (HHT), but usually there is no, as yet, identified abnormality. Subpial shunts represent the most common type of disorder that is encountered in clinical practice (Fig. 11.10).

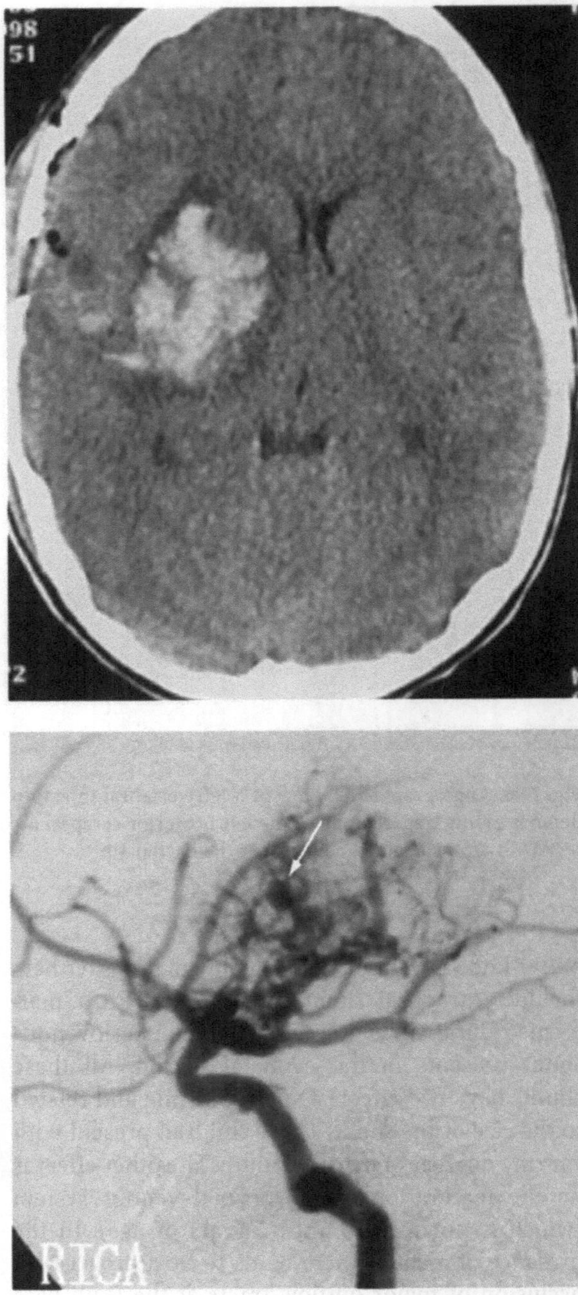

a

b

Fig. 11.9a,b. Previously well 15-year-old girl, presenting with spontaneous intracerebral haemorrhage. **a** Non-enhanced axial CT demonstrating residual haematoma following surgical decompression. **b** Right carotid artery injection, lateral view, at time of intracerebral haemorrhage demonstrating false aneurysm

11.2.4.3
Dural Arteriovenous Shunts

Shunts at this level occur throughout life from an antenatal presentation through to an adult. Understanding is incomplete and there have been topo-

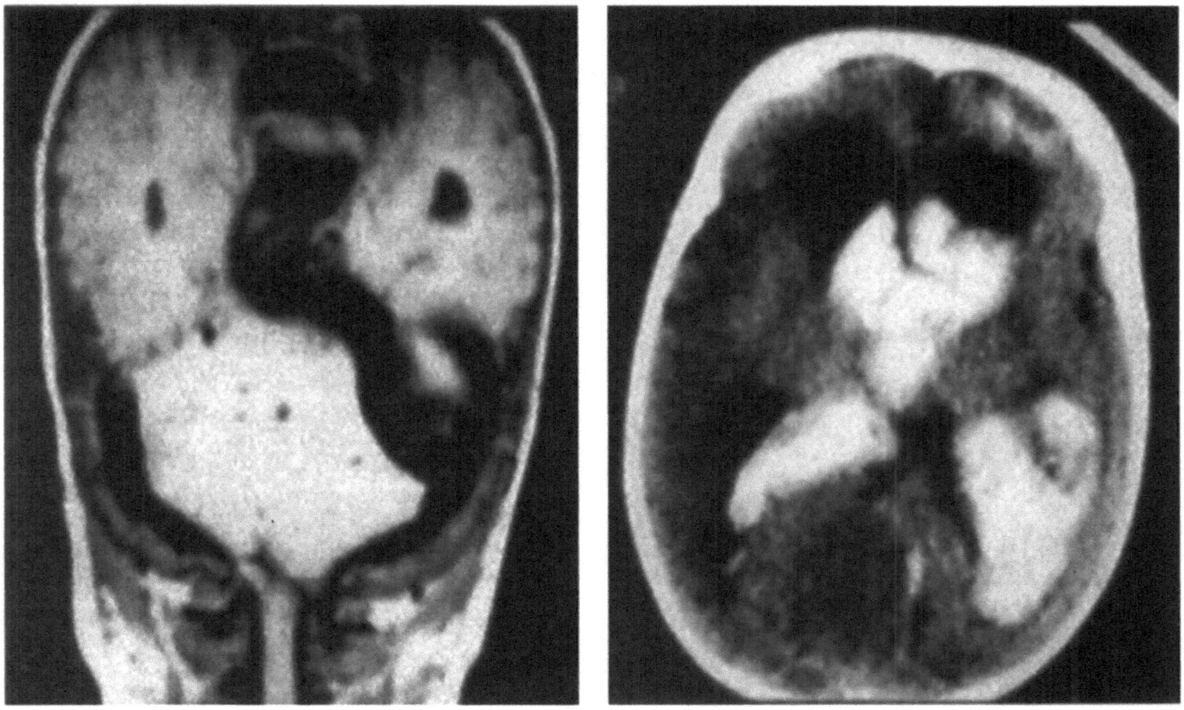

Fig. 11.10a,b. A 1-month-old girl presenting with a generalised seizure and macrocrania. **a** Coronal T1 SE sequence demonstrating a hugely ballooned dural sinus with decrease in flow and partial thrombosis. **b** Axial CT scan 1 month later. Bilateral venous infarction with intraventricular haemorrhage. (Note: this appears in Prof. Pierre Lasjaunias' book: *Vascular Diseases in Neonates, Infants and Children*; 1997, but it is originally my photo)

graphic and anatomoclinical classifications of these disease groups in an attempt to identify the risk factors for each patient. Essentially, there appear to be some important factors that need to be established to establish a prognosis. Features which represent a poor outcome for the patient include pial venous reflux, inadequate collateral venous drainage in the presence of venous outlet occlusion, and location of a shunt at the midline. Impaired venous exit can precipitate a rapid onset of encepahlomalacia and venous ischaemia in the immature brain and cerebral oedema and haemorrhage in the mature brain.

Shunts at the level of the cavernous sinus, which is developmentally related to the notochord/spinal column, and shunts which occur at the level of the dural sinuses, which have tissue origins in cranial mesenchyme, may have a different biology and pathology.

11.2.4.3.1 Dural Sinus Arteriovenous Shunts

Dural Sinus Malformation. These shunts may involve the midline at the level of the torcular or may be lateralised. Presentation in a neonatal age group demonstrate an often high flow direct arteriovenous (AV) shunt between dural arteries and a 'malformed' sinus which appears to have no proper communication with the jugular bulb. The sinuses are thus ballooned and contain very sluggish blood flow. There is typically very little normal cerebral venous drainage and these children die rapidly (Fig. 11.10). There are few therapeutic options unless the shunt is very lateralised in which case disconnection may be possible (Fig. 11.11).

Infantile Dural Arteriovenous Malformations. These are multifocal high flow low-pressure shunts, which occur in the presence of normally formed sinuses, although these may become secondarily occluded at the skull base. They tend to present in childhood when there is a multifocal AV shunt with a myriad of feeding dural arteries to normal sinuses that are progressively occluding at the skull base due to the vasculopathic effects of high flow. These children will present with the clinical effects of venous hypertension, and may have ocular symptoms, macrocrania, and venous ischaemia of the cerebral hemispheres. Their prognosis is extremely poor (Fig. 11.12).

These shunts may well have been induced by 'something' at some stage during development or re-

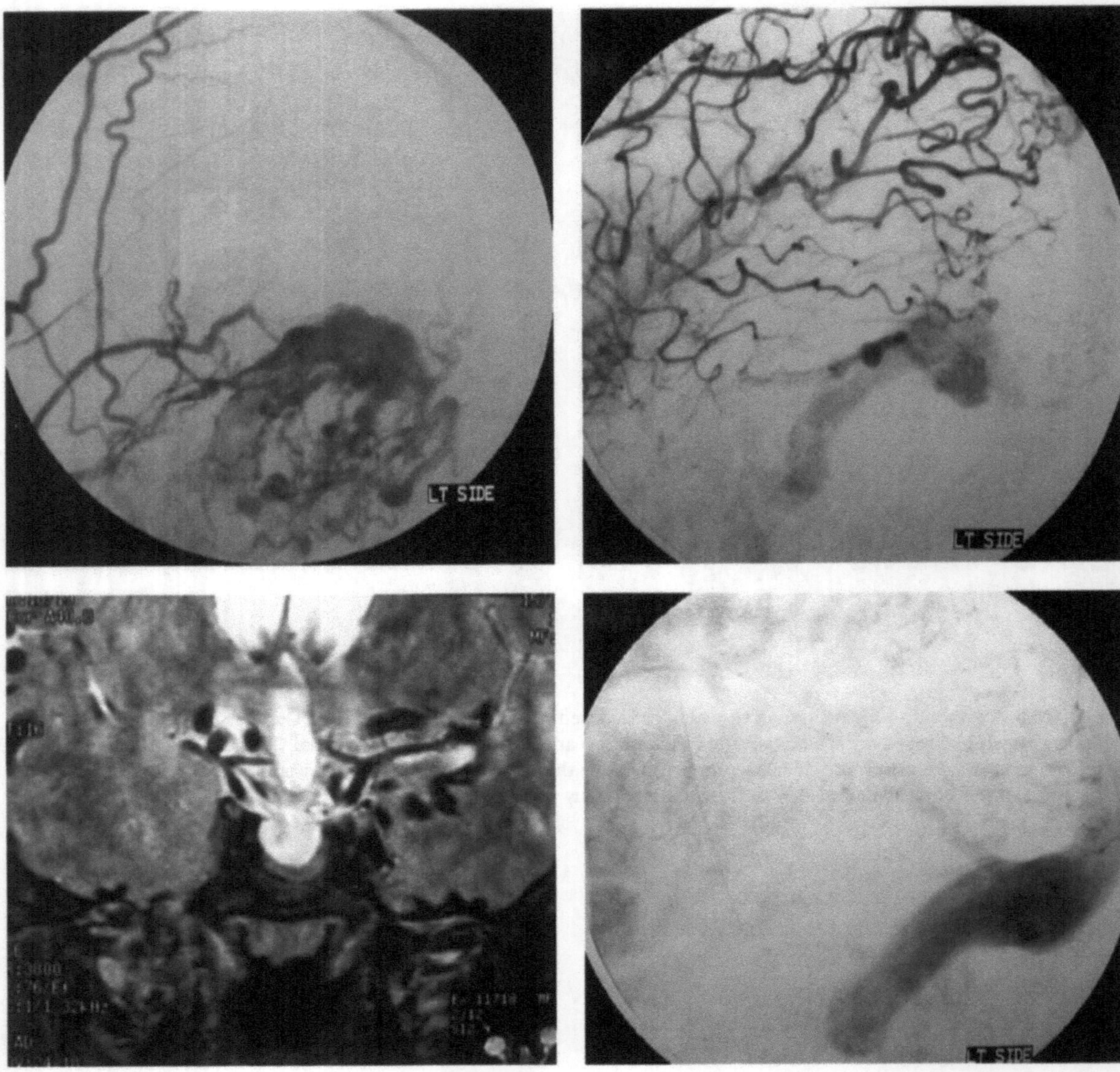

a b c d

Fig. 11.11a–d. A 15-year-old boy, presenting with visual failure. **a** Left external carotid injection demonstrating dural fistula to the left transverse and sigmoid sinus. **b** Left internal carotid injection demonstrating secondarily induced pial shunts. **c** Coronal MR demonstrating venous congestion and ventricular megaly with distortion of the optic chiasm by the ballooned third ventricle. **d** Late venous phase of left internal carotid injection showing occlusion of the jugular bulb

modelling in infancy, but whether this is at a level of genetic expression, or triggered by external factors is not known.

Adult Type Dural Arteriovenous Shunts. These shunts occur in all ages, but are the typically recognised and described shunts. The sinuses are anatomically normally developed and there is often associated thrombosis. Symptoms again depend on location and the degree of venous impairment of the brain as a consequence.

Table 11.1 summarises a classification of these types of shunts.

11.2.4.3.2
Induced Dural Arteriovenous Shunts

Other dural shunts are recognised as being induced by external factors. These include induced shunts by high sinus blood flow velocities from AV shunts in the subpial space or subarachnoid space (Fig. 11.13).

There are in addition shunts that may be induced by thrombosis and seem to be related either to a previous history of infection or trauma (Fig. 11.13). Often there is no such history and their true aetiology remains unknown. These are slow flow intradural shunts that find venous exits in all available venous pathways and are classified by this. They have a be-

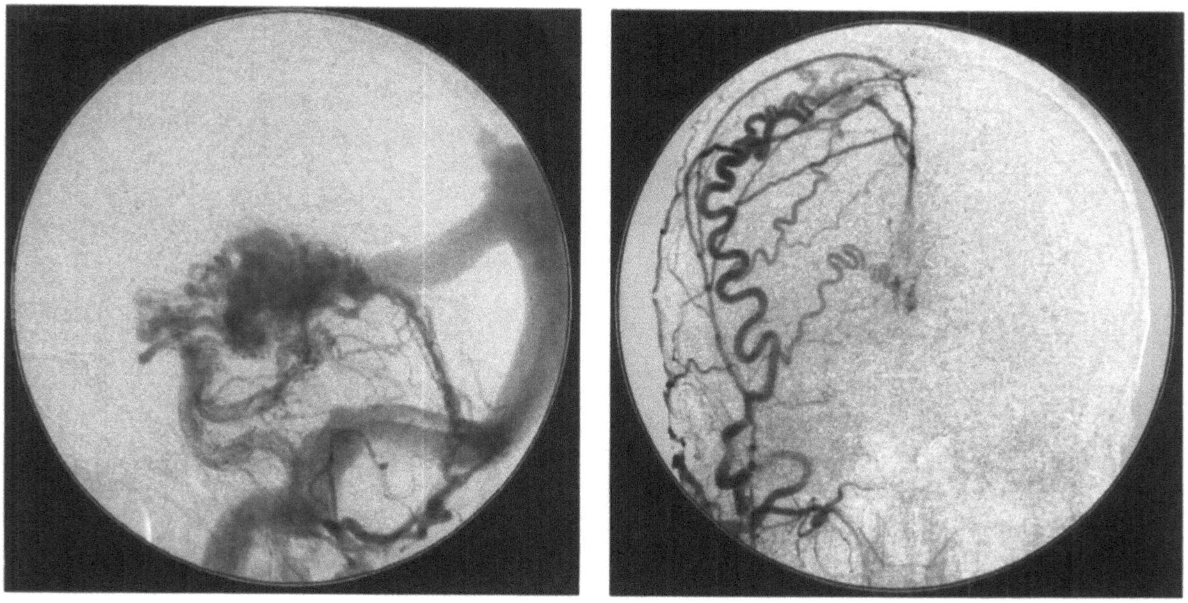

Fig. 11.12a,b. Choroidal type vein of Galen malformation. a Left vertebral injection with induced dural shunt. b Right external carotid artery injection of the same patient

Table 11.1. Classification of adult dural type arterial venous shunts: Djinjian and Merlands classification

Group I	DAVM drains immediately into a sinus or meningeal vein, with preservation of normal flow direction
Group II	Drainage of DAVM to a sinus but accompanied by reflux into cortical veins or another sinus
Group III	Direct drainage into cortical veins with retro grade flow
Group IV	Drainage into a venous lake

nign course relatively speaking, although if the shunts utilise pial venous routes there is an increased risk of intracranial haemorrhage.

Topographic Classification of Cerebral Arteriovenous Malformations (CAVM). The topographic classification of CAVM evolved initially from the basis of brain evolution and its vascular system formulated by Ask-Upmark in 1938 and was modified by a neurosurgeon, Yasargil. Whilst this classification takes into account the intrinsic blood supply of the AVM and its venous drainage, the evolution of understanding has been primarily from a neurosurgical perspective with a view to surgical extirpation. Thus the classification takes into account whether the lesion is supra or infratentorial and where within these regions the abnormality lies, clearly of great importance when planning a surgical approach. A different approach to analysis, however, is required for the endovascular therapy (Muller-Forell and Valavanis 1995). Triplanar MR is invaluable at precisely locating the AVM in relation to the normal brain structures and further subclassification has been described by Valavanis and Yasargil (1998). Three main subtypes of cortical AVM are described, sulcal, gyral and mixed. Their arterial supply is from the subpial vessels coursing over the brain surface and if their AVM lies only within the sulcus may also take additional supply from the meningeal vessels. Gyral AVM are located within a gyrus and have a surface covering of cortex (Fig. 11.14) (they therefore do not have a meningeal supply). The arterial supply is from cortical, corticomedullary and medullary arteries that also supply normal brain distal to the AVM and extension towards the ventricular margin may take additional supply from basal perforating arteries.

Some extensive 'AVM' described as a diffuse AVM by Valavanis are really a diffuse proliferative angiopathy that involves all vessels supplying, often large, regions of the brain. They are not amenable to any form of treatment without causing injury to brain tissue (Fig. 11.15).

Locations of AVM in the deep structures of the brain may be essentially located in the basal cisterns and fissures and are subarachnoid in location. They are supplied from the choroidal arteries and perforating arteries and are often amenable to endovascular disconnection. Other deep AVM are to be found

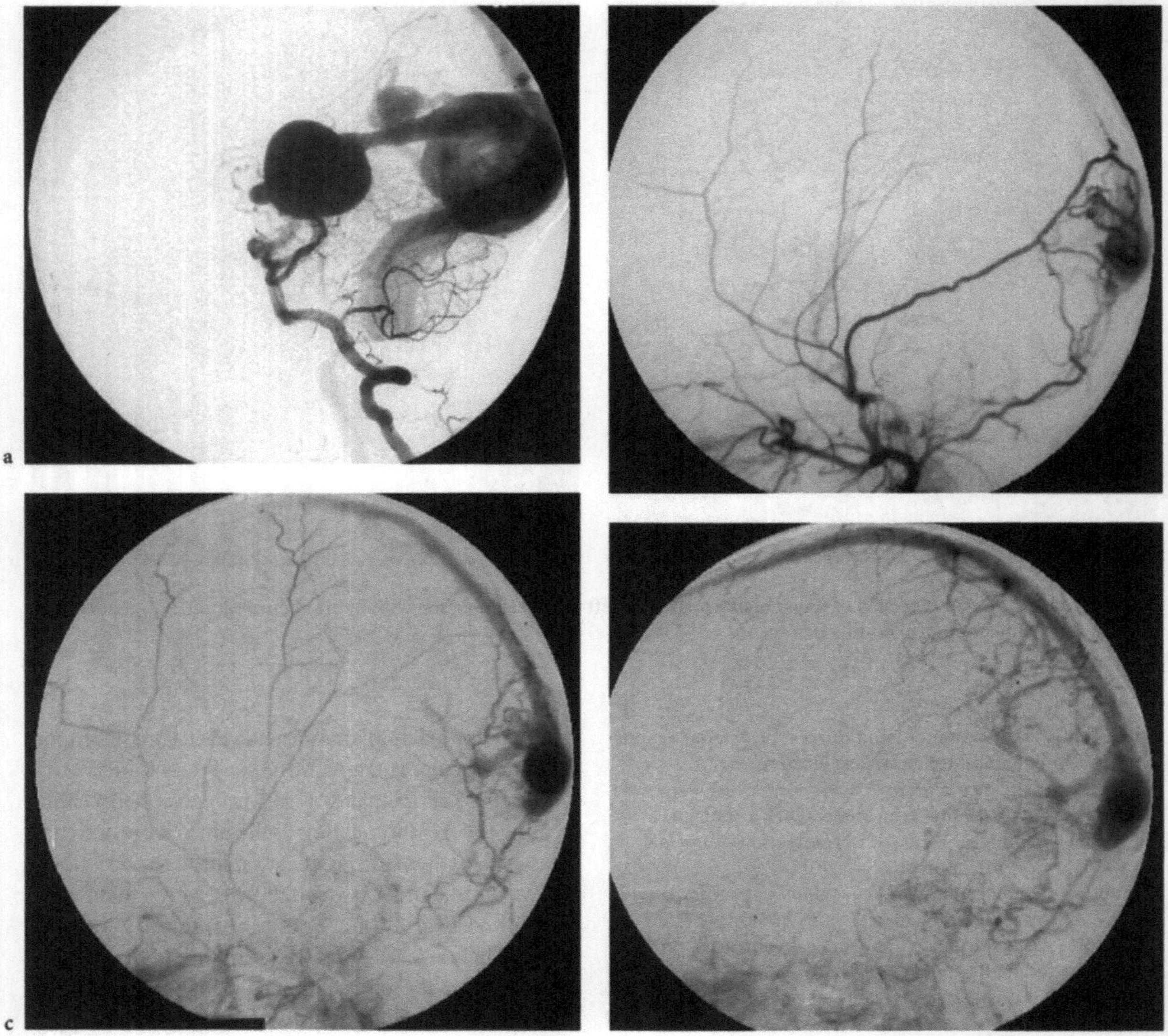

Fig. 11.13a–d. A 5-month-old baby with vein of Galen malformation. a Initial angiography, already demonstrating jugular bulb stenosis and reflux into the superior sagittal sinus. b Left external carotid injection demonstrating induced dural shunt secondary to dural sinus occlusion. c Gross reflux into the superior sagittal sinus. d Pial venous reflux into the cortical veins

in the deep brain structures, basal ganglia, thalamus, hypothalamus internal capsule, limbic system and septum pellucidum (Fig. 11.16).

Table 11.2 summarises the topographic classification of brain AVM.

11.2.4.4 False Subpial Arteriovenous Shunts

Proliferative Angiopathy. Whilst the term diffuse proliferative angiopathy has been included in the overall topographic classification of subpial AVM, it seems very likely that this subgroup represents a completely separate group of disorder. There is at present no published work on this subgroup firmly establishing its distinctness although several authors have alluded to it (Lasjaunias, personal communication). Certainly, it is hypothetically feasible to consider a field change in the sensibility of a vascular territory to vascular endothelial growth factors that modulate the response of the vasculature to growth and repair, resulting in an abnormal morphology. Typically, there is a diffuse cortical network and there is an associated transdural supply. Most patients present in childhood and may have headaches, which can be controlled by embolising the dural supply, and may have seizures or neurological deficit. No aetiology has so far been identified (see Fig. 11.15).

Induced Pial Shunts Secondary to Dural Sinus High Flow Lesions. These abnormalities develop in re-

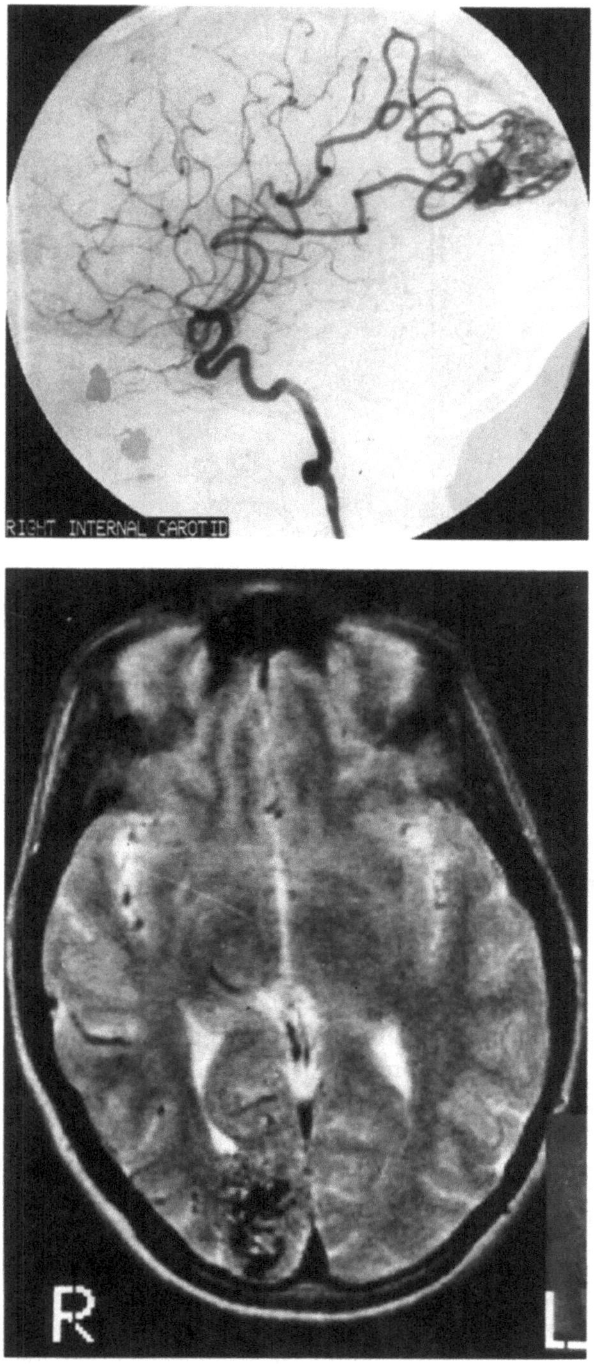

Fig. 11.14a,b. A 35-year-old woman presenting with seizures. **a** Right internal carotid injection, demonstrating gyral type AVM. **b** Axial MR image of the same patient

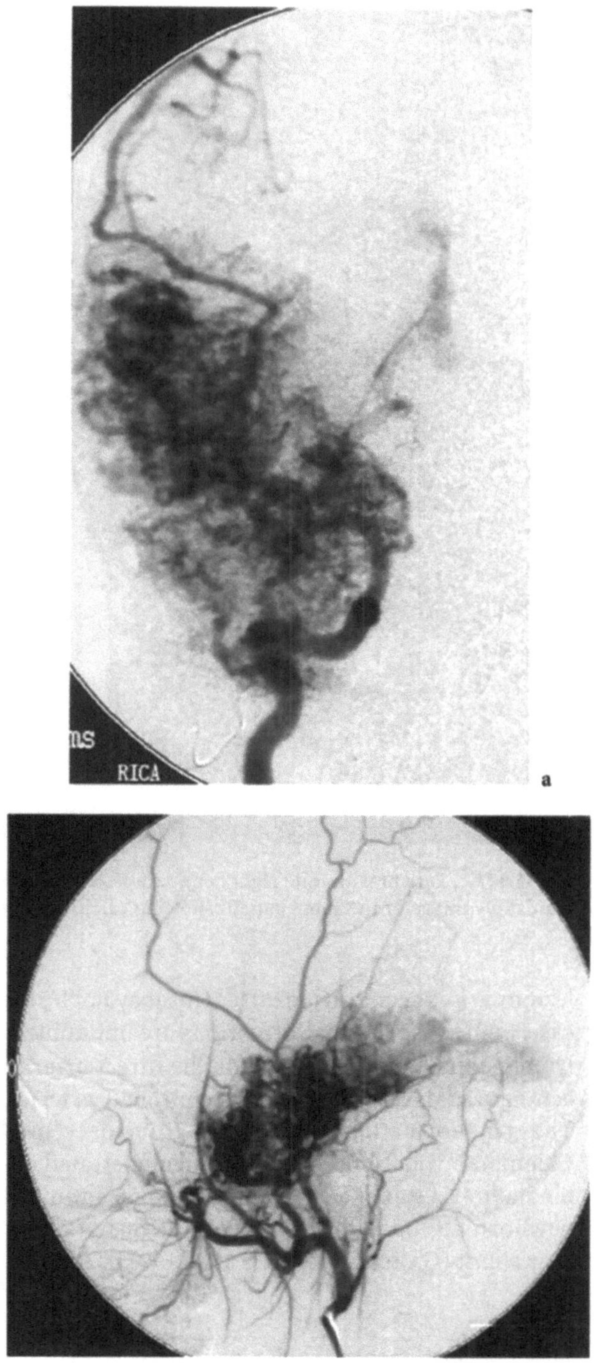

Fig. 11.15. a Right internal carotid injection showing diffuse proliferative angiopathy. **b** Right external carotid injection in the same patient

sponse to high flow dural shunts (see Fig. 11.11b), and have all the characteristics of subpial arteriovenous shunts. They can show regression after treatment of the dural lesion. They do not need treatment themselves.

11.3 Natural History and Biology of Arteriovenous Shunts

In considering the natural history of vascular malformations, it has long been believed that all these

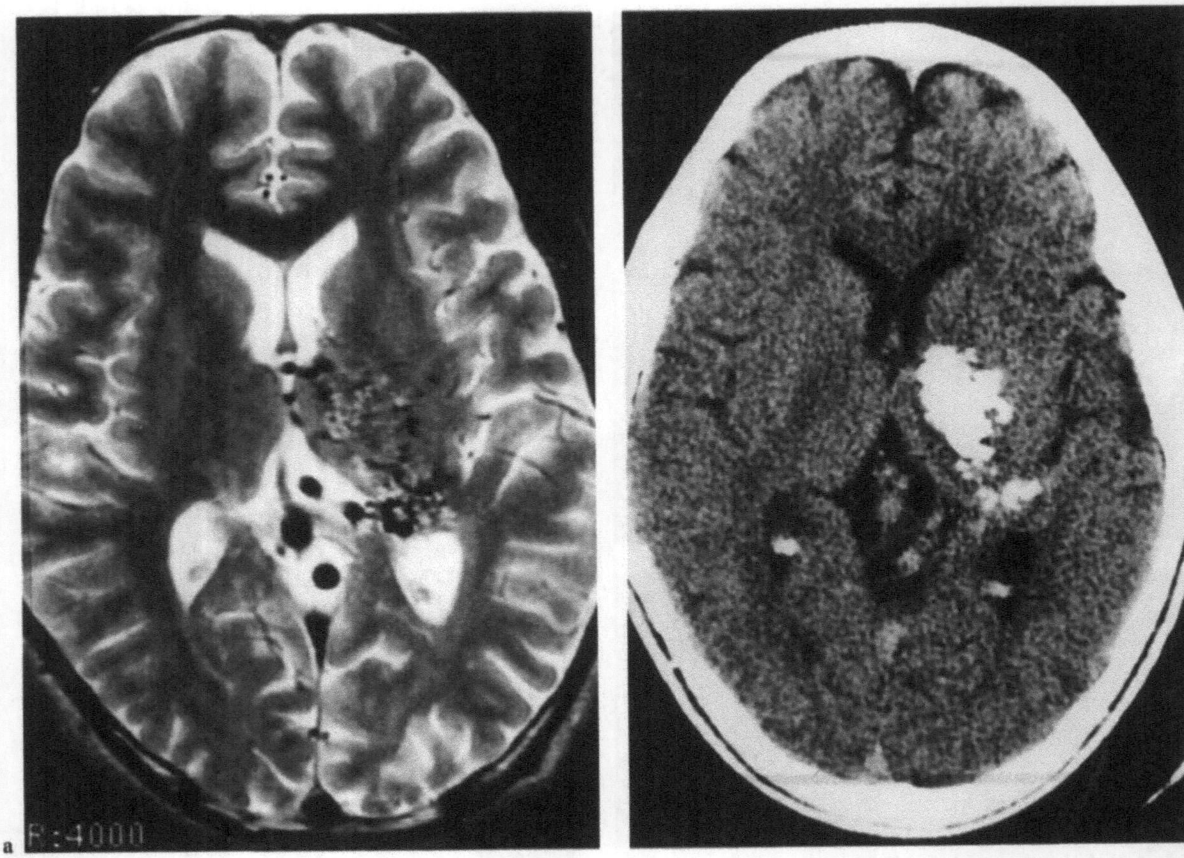

a b

Fig. 11.16a,b. Patient with mild right hemiparesis. **a** Axial MR image demonstrating left thalamic AVM. **b** Axial non-enhanced cranial CT image of the same patient showing calcification of the same lesion

lesions are congenital in nature. This may not be the case. Some vascular malformations are undoubtedly congenital, and these include the direct arteriovenous fistulae that affect the choroidal arteries. These malformations, known as a group as 'vein of Galen malformations', have been demonstrated antenatally (Campi et al. 1996) and can present in the newborn period with the systemic effects of a high flow shunt (Garcia-Monaco et al. 1991). Other direct fistulae in the pial arteries may present in a similar fashion, but they are extremely rare and for the most part are not manifest until childhood or early adult life. There have never been reported abnormalities in antenatal studies that have become manifest in later years.

Table 11.2. Topographic classification of cerebral arteriovenous malformation

A. Convexity or superficial AVM (72%)[a]	
1. Sulcal AVM	28%
2. Gyral AVM	12%
3. Mixed sulco/gyral	29%
4. Diffuse proliferative angiopathy	3%
B. Deep or central AVM (26%)	
1. Subarachnoid (fissural/cisternal)	12%
2. Parenchymal	7%
3. Choroid plexus	1%
4. Mixed	6%

Other diseases are known to be hereditary. Hereditary haemorrhagic telangiectasia (HHT) has been shown to be associated with various mutations in the gene for endoglin on chromosome 9q3 (Shovlin et al. 1994). HHT is recognised as being associated with multifocal arteriovenous malformations and direct arteriovenous fistulae. Neurofibromatosis type 1, which has been shown to be associated with stenosis, occlusions, aneurysms and direct fistulae, has a gene mutation on chromosome 17q11 (Riccardi 1989) and familial cavernomas have been associated with a mutation on chromosome 7q (Dubovsky 1995).

Given a growing understanding of the contribution that genetic mutation has in producing vascular abnormalities and the lack of evidence that the more common lesions are present antenatally, it would seem plausible to postulate that vascular abnormalities can emerge over time. Additionally, it can be demonstrated that vessels that are 'normal' will produce pathological changes when subjected to abnormal stresses. Thus an artery that is carrying an abnormal flow will normally enlarge but is capable of producing flow related aneurysms that can regress when the flow is reduced (Redekop et al. 1998). The aneurysms only rarely seem to rupture. Similarly veins carrying abnormal flow at unusually high pressure will dilate, but may also kink and produce stenoses and eventually occlusions. These pathophysiological responses tend to develop over time (Fig. 11.17).

For the most part the brain lives in symbiosis with abnormal vasculature and symptoms only occur when there is a loss of cerebral compliance with the abnormal vascular structure. The symptoms that are produced relate to a temporary dysfunction of neural tissue (i.e. seizures) or a more permanent loss of function related to loss or death of cerebral tissue. These events can be triggered by abnormal perfusion of the brain or destruction by haemorrhage. Much has been written about 'arterial steal' (Homan et al. 1986; Marks et al. 1991) as a cause of symptoms in patients with cerebral AVM but doubt about this as a real phenomenon has also been raised by various authors (Bederson et al. 1991). Another hypothesis relating to disruption of normal perfusion is the effect of venous hypertension on brain substance. In an immature brain, the presence of venous hypertension in combination with high output cardiac failure can precipitate a rapid onset of severe widespread encephalomalacia (Fig. 11.18). In a mature brain, venous hypertension can be associated with loss of normal function, seizure activity and deficit if there is a venous haemorrhagic infarct.

Haemorrhage can be the result of different factors. Abnormal blood vessels may rupture. Normal vessels that are under abnormal stresses may rupture (Mansmann et al. 2000; Meisel et al. 2000). The effects of a bleed depend on the location and quantity of blood. The sequelae of such an event may result in gliosis and haemosiderin deposition locally, which may act as a seizure focus and produce irreversible neurological damage.

The nature and relationship of clinical events to the pathological changes are different for abnormal vessels in different spaces in the brain. They are also related to the timing and evolution of the pathology.

11.4 Clinical Presentation

Introduction. For the most part in this chapter, discussion of the various abnormalities is categorised by pathology and anatomical location. However, this is not a useful way of approaching the subject when it comes to the management of patients. In this section, assessment by age group best deals with the clinical presentation of abnormalities.

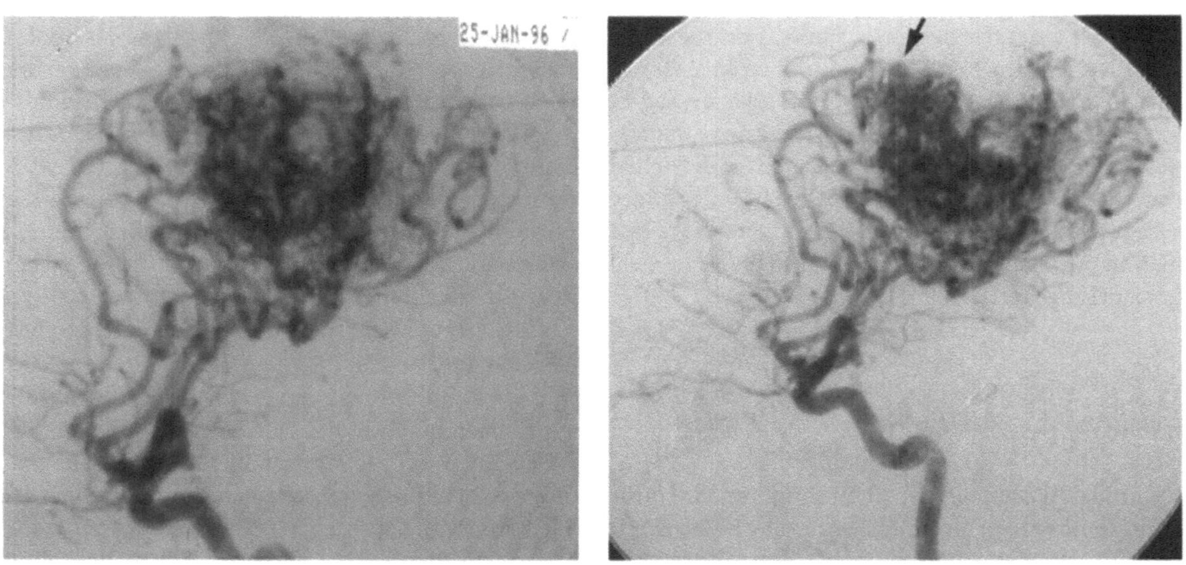

a b

Fig. 11.17. a A young adult patient in 1996: right internal carotid injection. **b** In 1999, showing the development of an intranidal aneurysm over time

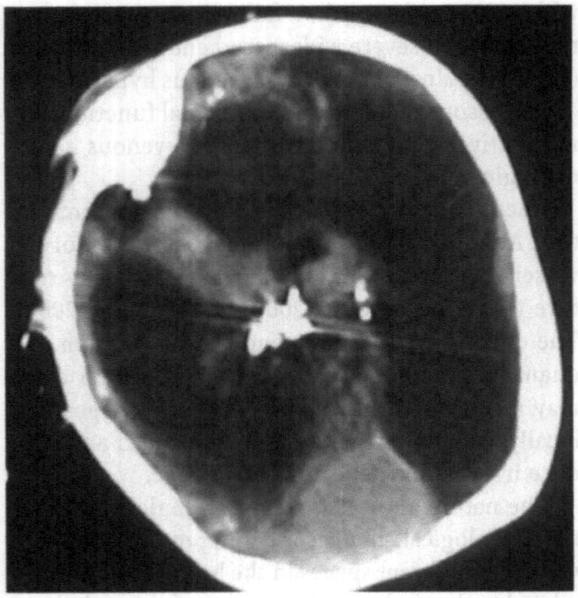

Fig. 11.18. Axial non-enhanced cranial CT demonstrating severe encephelomalacia despite successful disconnection of the high flow shunt

11.4.1
Neonatal

For the most part only the embryonic malformations present in the neonate and these include the vein of Galen malformation, the dural sinus malformation and in extremely rare instances the subpial arteriovenous shunts. The lesions that present in the neonate are the high flow shunts and produce a high output cardiac failure and, rapidly, multisystem failure. Apart from the deleterious effects on the body, these lesions are associated with a rapid onset of encephalomalacia, the 'melting brain' as described by LASJAUNIAS (see Fig. 11.18). The dural sinus malformations, because they are associated with virtual occlusion of the venous outlets of the brain, produce a large head with ventriculomegaly and seizures that may be the herald of local ischaemic damage or focal haemorrhages.

11.4.2
Infant

Choroidal AV shunts, subpial AV shunts and infantile dural shunts are principally manifest by high venous pressure. As the venous system is not mature until about 2 years of age, these children cannot adequately absorb brain water and show a progressive increase in head circumference. Partly because the head is heavy, they have poor head control, but they often begin to show mild developmental delay. If alternative routes of cerebral venous drainage are patent, by cavernous capture, then prominent facial collateral veins begin to be visible. If treatment is instituted promptly, these children will develop normally, but if treatment is delayed until later, then some permanent developmental deficit occurs, and the brain shows subependymal atrophy.

11.4.3
Child

Most children these days are diagnosed before childhood if they have subarachnoid (Galenic) or dural high flow shunts. Those that escape the attentions of a paediatrician present as an end stage of chronic venous hypertension, pial venous congestion and progressive venous occlusion leading to focal ischaemic infarction that may be haemorrhagic. In addition to the accumulated abnormalities of the infant, these children begin to have focal neurological signs and often begin to have seizures. This is the result of white matter ischaemia, calcification and haemorrhage (Fig. 11.19). There is often a prominent facial collateral drainage and epistaxis. Because there is high venous pressure in the posterior fossa, there may be perimedullary venous drainage and cerebellar tonsillar prolapse.

In most series, haemorrhage is the commonest presenting symptom of a subpial AVM in the child population. HLADKY et al. (1994) in his series quotes an incidence of 80%. LASJAUNIAS and TERBRUGGE (1997) quote over 50% in his series. These haemorrhagic events may cause focal deficit or seizures depending on location of the bleed. The expected natural history of such an event would depend on the cause of the bleed (venous stenosis or thrombosis, arterial aneurysmal rupture, etc.) and the long term vascular modelling of the lesion.

Other sorts of vascular lesions become manifest in the infant and childhood period.

Cavernous haemangiomas may reveal themselves with a haemorrhage, and then the deficit that occurs is dependent on the location of the lesion. There is often considerable improvement with time as the haematoma reabsorbs; however, if the lesion is in the brain stem, there can be lasting significant neurological damage.

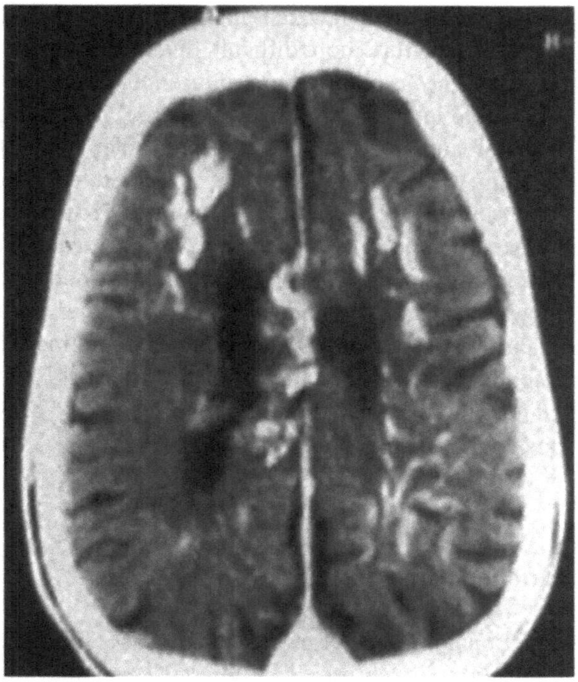

Fig. 11.19. Axial non-enhanced cranial CT demonstrating deep white matter calcification secondary to venous ischaemia

11.4.4 Adult

Symptoms of subpial shunts in the young adult age group fall into three broad categories based on disturbed haemodynamics and, sometimes, focal haemorrhages. About one-half of cerebral AVM present with a haemorrhage and one-third as a seizure disorder. Depending on the location of the shunt there is also often a subtle focal neurology, a mild paresis or sensory neglect for example.

Disorders that are primarily veno-occlusive (dural AV shunts) may have no focal symptoms, but may reveal themselves by a slow decline in intellectual function.

Prognosis for first haemorrhages is surprisingly good, with over 75% of patients making a complete recovery (Karlsson et al. 1997).

The onset of clinical symptoms is a sign of loss of cerebral compliance and symbiosis. As these lesions are evolving, there is a tendency for the symptomatology to worsen over time, but the time course for each patient is highly individual.

11.5 Methods of Investigation

11.5.1 Computerised Axial Tomography and Magnetic Resonance Imaging (CT and MR)

CT examination remains the commonest method of discovery of a vascular abnormality in the brain as it is the most widely available tool and in use as a general screening method for patients presenting with a variety of symptoms, both specific and non-specific. Acute haemorrhage, subarachnoid blood and calcification are all readily identifiable on a non-enhanced CT scan. A contrast enhanced CT scan may render visible abnormal configurations of blood vessels.

Magnetic resonance (MR) scanning is also an extensively used tool for assessment of the cerebral parenchyme, and planar imaging permits the relationship and morphology of abnormal vessels to be visualised more clearly. This is only of relevance if there is any consideration for treatment.

11.5.2 Computerised Tomographic Angiography (CTA) and Magnetic Resonance Angiography (MRA)

CTA and MRA can also demonstrate vessels, but have relatively poor spatial resolution and no temporal resolution when compared to conventional intra-arterial angiography.

3D time of flight (TOF) MRA is well suited to demonstrating high velocity flow in the major feeding vessels and nidus of a cerebral AVM. The advantages of 3D TOF are excellent spatial resolution, efficient scan time yielding a favourable signal-to-noise ratio, reduced complex flow signal loss and clearly visible T1-weighted anatomy. However, its primary limitation is loss of signal from saturation effects in vessels or structures with slow flow (Pernicone et al. 1992). Slower flow within compartments of the nidus and in draining veins may therefore remain undetected. Contrast enhanced MRA using a 3D fast spin echo (FSE) or 3D TOF MRA sequences have been shown to improve the visibility of the slow flow components of AVMs (Fig. 11.20). Gadolinium shortens the T1 relaxation time of blood, which increases intravascular signal, making it less dependent on laminar flow. The resulting short T1 of blood permits sequences with very short TRs and subsequently short acquisition times, avoiding problems with

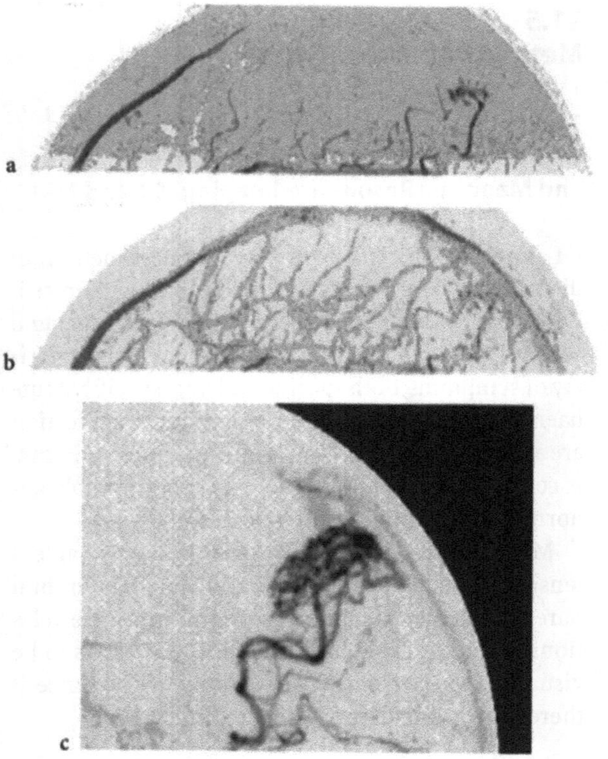

Fig. 11.20. **a** 3D fast SE (FSE). **b** Contrast enhanced 3D FSE demonstrating a succal AVM. **c** Intra-arterial digital subtraction angiography of the same lesion

saturation effects. This can also be achieved with phase contrast (PC) MRA, which is, however, more time-consuming. It may be necessary to repeat the PC MRA sequence a number of times with different velocity windows to show arterial and venous components equally well. Additional information can be obtained about the direction and velocity of flow within different compartments of the AVM (Brant-Zawadzki and Heiserman 1997).

CT angiography (CTA) represents a variation of spiral CT scanning. Thin section axial images are acquired during the injection of contrast medium bolus, typically at a rate of 3–4 ml s^{-1}. During this period, simultaneous rotation of the CT tube and movement of the scanning table take place. Images can be post-processed to create both surface-shaded displays and maximum intensity projections. CTA has, so far, not been widely used for the investigation of cerebral AVMs although there have been anecdotal reports. CTA demonstrates well the site, anatomical classification and size of the AVM as well as numbers of arterial feeders and draining veins (Jäger et al. 1999). One particular difficulty associated with CTA is the lack of temporal resolution. This means that both arterial and venous phases are seen on the same image, often obscuring each other, which makes interpretation of the AVM structure more difficult. In addition, operator experience is required to produce reliable and reproducible images. CTA involves the use of ionising radiation and an iodine-based intravascular contrast medium, which is a disadvantage compared to MRA. Its advantages are that it is quick, requires less patient cooperation and is less sensitive to slow or turbulent flow. Acquisition is based on true volumetric data and allows calculation of nidus volumes together with quantification of embolisation volumes, assuming the embolic material is of a high enough Hounsfield unit value to be thresholded out separately from the contrasted intranidal blood.

11.5.3 Functional Imaging

Functional imaging of patients with AVMs has been reported relatively rarely. Studies fall roughly into two categories: measurement of regional cerebral blood flow (rCBF) and similar quantities, and localisation of neurological function. In the latter case, PET and functional MRI have been used to demonstrate the motor strip (Grafton et al. 1994; Latchaw et al. 1995; Maldjian et al. 1996; Okazawa et al. 1995) or language areas (Leblanc et al. 1992) adjacent to an AVM. fMRI has also shown in a small number of cases that there is activity within the nidus (Maldjian 1996).

Regional CBF can be measured in several ways, including xenon-CT, gadolinium first-pass MR, SPECT and PET. Xenon-CT consistently shows a reduced CBF on the ipsilateral side (Marks 1988; Okabe 1983; Roost 1996; Tarr 1990, 1991), while PET has shown no significant difference in CBF but a reduction in oxygen metabolism on the affected side (Tyler et al. 1989). Recently SPECT has been used before and after embolisation (Sugita et al. 1993) or removal (Takeshita et al. 1994) of the AVM, and has shown reduced perfusion within the nidus and in tissues adjacent to the AVM in some patients. Postoperative perfusion changes were heterogeneous within the group (Takeshita 1994), but suggested that SPECT is useful to measure cerebral perfusion. Gd-MR may be difficult to use in AVMs, because the high concentration of gadolinium causes an extensive susceptibility artefact over the adjacent areas of brain (Moore et al. 1999). However, new developments in MR contrast agents will almost certainly lead to useful studies with this technique, which of course has the advantage of not involving a radiation dose to the patient.

11.5.4 Cerebral Angiography

Cerebral angiography is indicated when important information about the angioarchitecture of the lesion and a temporal resolution of the passage of contrast through the lesion is required. It is useful in the demonstration of flow related arterial aneurysms, intranidal aneurysms, false arterial and venous aneurysms, venous stenoses and occlusions and pial venous reflux into normal cerebral veins. Temporal resolution may demonstrate severely delayed transit of contrast medium through normal cerebral parenchyme, and accumulation and slow washout of contrast in false aneurysms.

If the lesion is to be treated by stereotactic methods then it is possible to perform cerebral angiography with a stereotactic frame in situ to permit an accurate assessment of the size of the lesion.

Angiography remains the definitive investigation in the assessment and follow-up of cerebral AVM.

11.6 Treatment Strategies

The aim of offering treatments for abnormal vascular lesions of the brain of course must depend on the type of abnormality and the age of the patient. In the youngest of patients, the aim of treatment is to reduce the high flow shunt and to normalise cardiac failure, in the growing child the aim is to protect normal brain development. The situation is less clear in the older patients, because we have to be clear that the risks and benefits of treatment are in the right order of magnitude as opposed to the natural history of the disease. This means that an absolute understanding of the natural history of the lesion and of the actual risk of interference is strictly understood. As with many areas in medicine, this is, at best, an inexact science, and in truth often as not we do really know whether or not treatments are really going to significantly change the outcome for the patient. This is all compounded by a non-unified language and idiosyncratic approach to treatments. There is also a strong tendency within all therapists to view the lesion rather than the patient and whereas a 'total cure' by surgical, endovascular or radiation means may in fact spell permanent neurological morbidity for the patient. The majority of lesions that present in adult life cannot be cured. This is either because of their size or their location and the risks of removing them outweigh the risks of leaving them there. However, it does appear that a careful approach and partial targeted treatment may be beneficial to the patient. This, for example, could be the exclusion of a false aneurysm within a lesion that is known to have previously bled. Small lesions can be cured by either a radiosurgery or surgical extirpation.

11.6.1 Forms of Treatment

11.6.1.1 Surgery

The role of the neurosurgeon in the management of vascular abnormalities of the brain depends on local practice and expertise. There are some centres that offer a strong surgical practice, whilst other centres rely more on endovascular techniques or on radiosurgery. With new image guidance techniques it is possible to obtain more accurate localisation of the lesion, permitting a more successful and safe extirpation. At the National Hospital for Neurology and Neurosurgery it is possible to perform superselective angiography with microcatheters on the operating table during surgery and this has been useful to locate small leashes of vessels precisely that would be difficult to find without risking causing extensive damage. Small peripheral CAVM, some cavernomas, and sometimes dural shunts can be successfully treated by neurosurgeons. The advantage of surgery is that if complete and affected without complication the patient is cured from the risk of future haemorrhage.

11.6.1.2 Radiosurgery

Radiosurgery employs one of two methods, that is either a gamma knife or a linear accelerator to deliver a radiation dose to the nidus of the lesion. Most use a stereotaxic frame firmly attached to the patient's skull to accurately localise the AVM within a framework, but more recent developments include frameless stereotaxy methods of localisation (Picard et al. 1997; Soderman et al. 1998). The lesion should ideally be under 2 cm^3 and the dose delivered approximately 25 Gy. As the volume of the lesion increases, the amount of radiation delivered to surrounding normal brain increases and if the dose is not dropped, then radiation damage is more likely to occur. Therefore, the efficacy of radiosurgery falls with increasing size of the lesion. Radiation causes an obliterative arteriopathy of the vasa vasorum of the abnormal vessels (Lunsford et al. 1998) and over a time (typically 2–3 years) the abnormal vessels occlude. This, of course, means that a patient will not be protected from haemorrhage in the interim (Pollock et al. 1996). Postradiation imaging changes are common in treated patients occurring in 20 out of 72 patients in Flikinger's series and are symptomatic in just under half of the patients. Most imaging changes resolve over time and consist of perilesional low density on CT or high T2 signal on MR imaging. There is often perilesional enhancement termed 'supernova' by Lunsford (Lunsford 1998; Flickinger et al. 1992). One of the more gratifying aspects of management of vascular malformations by this method is the objectivity in which the volume treated and dose applied are accurately known, making it possible to accurately predict probabilities of cure and complication rates (Karlsson et al. 1997).

11.6.2 Endovascular Treatments

In Europe most endovascular treatments are offered by neuroradiologists. This is not so in all countries, where endovascular treatments are performed by neurosurgeons as in Japan. Abnormal vessels are selectively obliterated with a variety of agents including cyanoacrylate polymers, polyvinyl alcohol particles, small coils, large coils and even ethanol. Whatever the agent, they can cause damage if they are not deposited correctly. They can be difficult to use and require an understanding of the therapeutic target and goal of treatment.

Complete cure is rare by an endovascular route. An emerging concept is the sensitive and judicious disconnection of perceived potential angioarchitectural risk for the patient. This may of course only involve a tiny portion of the lesion, for example an intranidal fistula or false aneurysm, but it appears that this sort of approach may actually ultimately improve the patients' outcomes over natural history.

11.7 Conclusion

These lesions are a clinical subject, and their understanding through imagery over time tells a story of their effects on the brain and the symbiotic nature the brain has with many of the abnormalities. It is only by taking an overview in this way that the story of vascular malformations can be told. There is nothing esoteric about the images, nothing difficult, except perhaps to understand that they have an evolving life and to have the patience and powers of observation to witness these things. They present a fascinating mystery and our ability to really effectively treat them lies in the Dark Ages, as in the case of drainage of pleural abscesses before the era of antibiotic treatment. With greater understanding at a molecular and genetic level, we will be able to deliver more precise and elegant management strategies for our enduring patients.

References

Bederson JB, Wiestler OD, Brustle O, Roth P, Frick R, Yasargil MG (1991) Intracranial venous hypertension and the effects of venous outflow obstruction in a rat model of arteriovenous fistula. Neurosurgery 29: 341–350

Borden NM, Khayata MH, Dean BL, Flom RA (1995) Unusual pattern of a deep developmental venous anomaly on CT and MR studies. J Comput Assist Tomogr 19: 885–889

Brant-Zawadzki M, Heiserman J (1997) The roles of MR angiography, CT angiography, and sonography in vascular imaging of the head and neck. AJNR 18: 1820–1825

Campi A, Scotti G, Filippi M, Gerevini S, Strigimi F, Lasjaunias P (1996) Antenatal diagnosis of vein of Galen aneurysmal malformation: MR study of fetal brain and postnatal follow-up. Neuroradiology 38: 87–90

Chaix Y, Grouteau E, Sevely A, Boetto S, Carriere JP (1996) [Association of venous angioma and cavernoma of the posterior fossa]. Arch Pediatr 3: 685–688

Craig HD, Gunel M, Cepeda O et al. (1998) Multilocus linkage identifies two new loci for a mendelian form of stroke, cerebral cavernous malformation, at 7p15–13 and 3q25.2–27. Hum Mol Genet 7: 1851–1858

Curling OD, Kelly D, Elster A (1991) An analysis of natural history of cavernous haemangiomas. J Neurosurg 75: 702–708

Dubovsky J, Zabramski JM, Kurth J et al. (1995) A gene responsible for cavernous malformations of the brain maps to chromosome 7q. Hum Mol Genet 4: 453–458

Flickinger JC, Lunsford LD, Kondziolka D et al. (1992) Radiosurgery and brain tolerance: an analysis of neurodiagnostic imaging changes after gamma knife radiosurgery for arteriovenous malformations. Int J Radiat Oncol Biol Phys 23: 19–26

Garcia-Monaco R, De Victor D, Mann C, Hannedouche A, TerBrugge K, Lasjaunias P (1991) Congestive cardiac manifestations from cerebrocranial arteriovenous shunts. Endovascular management in 30 children. Childs Nerv Syst 7: 48–52

Gil-Nagel A, Dubovsky J, Wilcox K et al. (1996) Familial cerebral cavernous angioma: a gene localised to a 15 cM interval on chromosome 7q. Ann Neurol 39: 807–810

Grafton S, Martin N, Mazziotta JC (1994) Localization of motor areas adjacent to arteriovenous malformations. A positron emission tomographic study. J Neuroimaging 4: 97–103

Gunel M, Awad IA, Finberg K et al. (1996) A founder mutation as a cause of cerebral cavernous malformation in Hispanic Americans. N Engl J Med 334: 946–951

Gunel M, Awad IA, Finberg K et al. (1996) Genetic heterogeneity of inherited cerebral cavernous malformation. Neurosurgery 38: 1265–1271
Hladky J, Lejeune J, Blond S, Pruvo J, Dhellemmes P (1994) Cerebral arteriovenous malformations in children: report in 62 cases. Childs Nerv Syst 10: 328–333
Hoffman J, Mohr G, Kusunoki T (1976) Multiple arteriovenous malformations of the spinal cord and brain in a child: case report. Childs Brain 2: 317–324
Homan RW, Devous MD Sr, Stokely EM, Bonte FJ (1986) Quantification of intracerebral steal in patients with arteriovenous malformation. Arch Neurol 43: 779–785
Houtteville JP (1997) Brain cavernoma: a dynamic lesion. Surg Neurol 48: 610–614
Huber G, Piepgras U, Henkes H, Faubert C (1991) [Venous anomalies of the brain. The clinical significance of the so-called venous angioma]. Radiologe 31: 274–282
Jäger H, Grieve J, Moore E, Kitchen N, Taylor W (1999) Comparison of CTA and intra-arterial DSA in patients with cerebral AVMs. Neuroradiology 41: 227–228
Jellinger K (1986) Vascular malformations of the ventral nervous system: a morphological overview. Neurosurg Rev 9: 177–216
Johnson E, Lyer L, Rich S et al. (1995) Refined localisation of the cerebral cavenous malformation gene (CCM1) to a 4-cM interval of chromosome 7q contained in a well defined YAC Contig. Genome Res 5: 368–380
Karlsson B, Lax I, Soderman M (1997) Factors influencing the risk for complications following Gamma Knife radiosurgery of cerebral arteriovenous malformations. Radiother Oncol 43: 275–280
Karlsson B, Lundquist C, Johansson A, Steiner L (1997) Annual risk for the first haemorrhage from untreated arteriovenous malformations. Minim Invasive Neurosurg 40: 40–46
Kondziolka D, Lunsford L, Kestle J (1995) The natural history of cerebral cavernous malformations. J Neurosurg 83: 820–824
Kuker W, Mull M, Thron A (1997) Developmental venous anomalies of the posterior fossa with transpontine drainage: report of 3 cases. Eur Radiol 7: 913–917
Lasjaunias P, TerBrugge K (1997) Vascular Diseases in Neonates, Infants and Children. Springer Verlag, Berlin Heidelberg New York
Lasjaunias P, TerBrugge K, Rodesch G et al. (1989) [True and false cerebral venous malformations. Venous pseudo-angiomas and cavernous hemangiomas]. Neurochirurgie 35: 132–139
Latchaw R, Hu X, Ugurbil K (1995) Functional magnetic resonance imaging as a management tool for cerebral arteriovenous malformations. Neurosurgery 37: 619–625
Leblanc R, Meyer E, Bub D (1992) Language localization with activation positron emission tomography scanning. Neurosurgery 31: 369–373
Lee C, Pennington MA, Kenney CM 3rd (1996) MR evaluation of developmental venous anomalies: medullary venous anatomy of venous angiomas. AJNR 17: 61–70
Lunsford LD, Kondziolka D, Maitz A, Flickinger JC (1998) Black holes, white dwarfs and supernovas: imaging after radiosurgery. Stereotact Funct Neurosurg 70 Suppl 1: 2–10
Maldjian J, Atlas S, Howard R 2nd et al. (1996) Functional magnetic resonance imaging of regional brain activity in patients with intracerebral arteriovenous malformations before surgical or endovascular therapy. J Neurosurg 84: 477–483
Mansmann U, Meisel J, Brock M, Rodesch G, Alvarez H, Lasjaunias P (2000) Factors associated with intracranial hemorrhage in cases of cerebral arteriovenous malformation. Neurosurgery 46: 272–281
Marks M, O'Donahue J, Fabricant JI et al. (1988) Cerebral blood flow evaluation of arteriovenous malformations with stable xenon CT. AJNR 9: 1169–1175
Marks MP, Lane B, Steinberg G, Chang P (1991) Vascular characteristics of intracerebral arteriovenous malformations in patients with clinical steal. AJNR 12: 489–496
Mazza C, Scienza R, Bernardin BD, Beltramello A, Bontempini L, Dapian R (1989) Malformations caverneuse de l'enfant. Neuorchirurgie 35: 106–108
Meisel HJ, Mansmann U, Alvarez H, Rodesch G, Brock M, Lasjaunias P (2000) Cerebral arteriovenous malformations and associated aneurysms: analysis of 305 cases from a series of 662 patients [In Process Citation]. Neurosurgery 46: 793–802
Moore E, Jager R, Grieve J (1999) Private communication.
Muller-Forell W, Valavanis A (1995) How angioarchitecture of cerebral arteriovenous malformations should influence the therapeutic considerations. Minim Invasive Neurosurg 38: 32–40
Okabe T, Meyer J, Okayasu H et al. (1983) Xenon-enhanced CT CBF measurements in cerebral AVM's before and after excision. Contribution to pathogenesis and treatment. J Neurosurg 59: 21–31
Okazawa H, Yonekura Y, Sadato N (1995) Delayed data acquisition for optimal PET activation studies with oxygen-15-water in cerebral arteriovenous malformation. J Nucl Med 36: 2149–2153
Parkinson D, West M (1977) Spontaneous subarachnoid haemorrhage first from an intracranial and then from a spinal arteriovenous malformation: case report. J Neurosurg 47: 965–968
Peebles TR, Vieco PT (1997) Intracranial developmental venous anomalies: diagnosis using CT angiography. J Comput Assist Tomogr 21: 582–586
Pernicone J, Siebert J, Cooper T, Potchen M (1992) Magnetic Resonance Angiography. In: Grainger R, Allison D (eds) Diagnostic Imaging in Radiology. 2nd ed. Churchill Livingstone, New York, pp 2410–2423
Picard L, Maurincomme E, Soderman M et al. (1997) X-ray angiography in stereotactic conditions: techniques and interest for interventional neuroradiology. Stereotact Funct Neurosurg 68: 117–120
Pollock BE, Flickinger JC, Lunsford LD, Bissonette DJ, Kondziolka D (1996) Hemorrhage risk after stereotactic radiosurgery of cerebral arteriovenous malformations. Neurosurgery 38: 652–661
Polymeropoulos M, Hurko O, Hsu F et al. (1997) Linkage of the locus for cerebral cavernous haemangiomas to human chromosome 7q in four families of Mexican-American descent. Neurology 48: 752–757
Redekop G, TerBrugge K, Montanera W, Willinsky R (1998) Arterial aneurysms associated with cerebral arteriovenous malformations: classification, incidence, and risk of hemorrhage. J Neurosurg 89: 539–546
Riccardi VM (1989) Genetic alterations and growth factors in the pathogenesis of von Recklinghausen neurofibromatosis. Neurofibromatosis 2: 292–298
Roost DV, Schramm J, Solymosi L, Hartmann A (1996) Presence and removal of arteriovenous malformation: Impact

of regional cerebral blood flow, as assessed with xenon/CT. Acta Neurol Scand Suppl 166: 136–138

Shovlin CL, Hughes JM, Tuddenham EG et al. (1994) A gene for hereditary haemorrhagic telangiectasia maps to chromosome 9q3. Nat Genet 6: 205–209

Soderman M, Picard C, Ericson K (1998) An algorithm for correction of distortion in stereotaxic digital subtraction angiography. Neuroradiology 40: 277–282

Sugita M, Takahashi A, Ogawa A, Yoshimoto T (1993) Improvement of cerebral blood flow and clinical symptoms associated with embolization of a large arteriovenous malformation: case report. Neurosurgery 33: 748–751

Takeshita G, Toyama H, Nakane K et al. (1994) Evaluation of regional cerebral blood flow changes on perifocal brain tissue SPECT before and after removal of arteriovenous malformations. Nucl Med Commun 15: 461–468

Tarr R, Johnson D, Horton J (1991) Impaired cerebral vasoreactivity after embolization of arteriovenous malformations: assessment with serial acetazolamide challenge xenon CT. AJNR 12: 417–423

Tarr R, Johnson D, Rutigliano M (1990) Use of acetazolamide-challenge xenon CT in the assessment of cerebral blood flow dynamics in patients with arteriovenous malformations. AJNR 11: 441–448

Tyler J, Leblanc R, Meyer E et al. (1989) Hemodynamic and metabolic effects of cerebral arteriovenous malformations studied by positron emission tomography. Stroke 20: 890–898

Valavanis A, Yasargil MG (1998) The endovascular treatment of brain arteriovenous malformations. Adv Tech Stand Neurosurg 24: 131–214

Voigt K, Yasargil MG (1976) Cerebral cavernous haemangiomas or cavernomas. Incidence, pathology, localization, diagnosis, clinical features and treatment. Review of the literature and report of an unusual case. Neurochirurgia (Stuttg) 19: 59–68

Wilkins R, Rengachary S (eds) (1985) Intracranial Arteriovenous Malformations. McGraw Hill, New York

Willinsky R, Lasjaunias P, TerBrugge K, Burrows P (1990) Multiple cerebral arteriovenous malformations. Review of our experience from 203 patients with cerebral vascular lesions. Neuroradiology 32: 207–210

Zouaoui A, Maillard JC, Ganthier V, Chedid G, Dangeard S (1995) [Modern imaging in cerebral vein angioma]. J Neuroradiol 22: 86–102

Zouaoui A, Maillard JC, Ganthier V, Chedid G, Dangeard S (1995) [Modern imaging in cerebral vein angioma]. J Neuroradiol 22: 86–102

12 Role of Intracranial CT and MR Angiography

Shawn Halpin, Max Ryan

CONTENTS

12.1 Introduction

The holy grail for CTA and MRA of the intracranial vasculature is to replace catheter angiography as the primary imaging modality for the investigation of the cerebral vascular diseases, in particular in the search for berry aneurysms. In order to achieve this, the computed techniques must have sensitivity and specificity at least equal to digital subtraction angiography (DSA) (i.e. they must replace invasive techniques as the gold standard by which other techniques are measured), and must also allow adequate surgical or neuro-interventional planning. For example, the neck of the aneurysm must be definitively displayed, and the presence of neighbouring small vessels depicted. Since both neurosurgeons and interventional neuroradiologists will approach an anterior communicating artery aneurysm from the side of its maximum inflow, the imaging technique must be able to demonstrate flow dynamics around a lesion with the same temporal resolution as DSA.

Cross-sectional techniques have some inherent advantages and disadvantages when compared to DSA. On the positive side, and most importantly, they do not carry the morbidity and mortality inherent to DSA. They do, however, provide the opportunity to display the intracranial vasculature in any imaging plane and demonstrate normal brain anatomy around aneurysms. For example, they may enable a surgeon to plan his or her approach to an aneurysm which compresses the optic chiasm.

On the other hand, it is difficult to achieve quantification of flow within an aneurysm or AVM without complex algorithms and lengthy scans, and many radiologists appreciate the chance to assess the practical difficulties of vascular access by performing diagnostic angiography prior to intervention.

The bulk of this chapter will deal with the role of CTA and MRA in the search for, and in the demonstration of, berry aneurysms. In order to discuss this topic, it is first necessary to appreciate the clinical context, and then to understand the techniques themselves, their strengths and weaknesses, as well as their merits when compared to each other and to DSA. Of course cerebral CTA and MRA are used to demonstrate many other lesions, and these will be discussed in the final sections of the chapter, but due to the constraints of space, and their lesser clinical importance, the greater part of this chapter will deal with aneurysms.

12.2 Clinical Context

In the Western world, subarachnoid haemorrhage affects approximately 10–20 per 100,000 population per annum (Wiebers et al. 1992; Sekhar et al. 1982).

S. Halpin, MRCP, FRCR; M. Ryan, FFR RCSI, FRCR
Department of Radiology, University Hospital of Wales, Heath Park, Cardiff, CF4 4XW, UK

When caused by rupture of an aneurysm, at least half of the affected individuals will die, and 25% will live with serious neurological sequelae. Only 25% will recover completely or with minimal disability (Hashi 1997; Fogelholm 1981; Sarti 1991). Kassel et al. (1984) reported deaths in 27.3% of patients presenting to hospital, vegetative states in 2.2%, and moderate to severe sequelae in 14.1%; his figures did not include those patients who died instantly or before reaching hospital.

Cerebral aneurysms are present in a surprisingly large number of people, and have been reported to be found in 1–5% of the general population (Hashi 1997; Juvela et al. 1993). If an individual has an aneurysm, then the chance of it rupturing varies according to its size and location. Although it has recently been reported that the annual risk of rupture is between 1 and 2% (Juvela et al. 1993), more recent data (Wiebers et al. 1998) has suggested an annual rupture rate of less than 0.05% for aneurysms less than 1 cm in diameter, and a rate of approximately 0.5% per annum for aneurysms larger than this. Although contested by some neurosurgeons, these figures are almost certainly correct: from the above data, approximately 100 in a population of 1 million people will suffer SAH each year. If 2% of that population have an aneurysm, then the yearly risk of rupture for each individual is 0.05%. Moreover, at least 25% of patients with SAH will have a second aneurysm or multiple aneurysms. If a second aneurysm is within reach of the ruptured aneurysm, it is usual for a neurosurgeon to clip both at the same operation.

Once a patient with SAH has reached hospital, the commonest cause of death is a second haemorrhage. This is most likely in the first 24–48 h following the initial SAH, but remains a frequent phenomenon for the first 2 weeks. Mortality increases by 50% with each rebleed (Khanna et al. 1996). Deterioration in the 2nd week is more likely to be due to delayed ischaemic deficit (DID), a clinical phenomenon of cerebral ischaemia associated with vasospasm of the major cerebral vessels. Neurosurgical intervention between day 4 and day 10 may be complicated by, or may precipitate, DID, and so neurosurgeons prefer to operate either on day 1 or 2 following SAH, or alternatively to delay surgery until after day 10. The international co-operative study randomised patients with aneurysmal SAH between early and late intervention, and found no difference in outcome between the two groups (except in a retrospective subset of US patients where young patients with good clinical condition were found to benefit from early surgery) (Kassell et al. 1984). Current clinical management in most centres is to operate early on young and good grade patients, and to delay operating on elderly or poor grade patients.

DSA has been, and remains, the mainstay of investigation of patients with SAH. It represents the gold standard for the detection of cerebral aneurysms, but current experience demonstrates that it is not 100% accurate. Even in the best of hands, errors of commission, omission, or perception will occasionally occur, and there is no doubt that even faultless angiography will occasionally fail to demonstrate an aneurysm due to temporary thrombosis or spasm at its neck (Kaim et al. 1996).

DSA carries a small but definite risk with around 0.5% of patients suffering persisting neurological deficit (Heiserman et al. 1994), and is associated with an increased risk of rebleeding when performed within 6 h of SAH (Inagawa 1994, Saitoh et al. 1995). The risks of DSA are probably greater in the elderly or ill population (O'Leary et al. 1989).

Catheter angiography provides information not only of the location of an aneurysm, but also its neck size, its relationship to other vessels, and the pattern of inflow of blood. This is particularly important in dealing with anterior communicating artery aneurysms, as a surgeon or neuro-interventionalist will approach these from the side of maximal inflow. The challenge for CTA and MRA is to demonstrate all aneurysms, incidental and ruptured, at least as well as DSA, and to accurately depict their flow characteristics.

12.3 MRA Acquisition Parameters

12.3.1 Time of Flight MRA

Three dimensional time of flight (TOF) is the current primary MRA tool in the search for a berry aneurysm with sensitivities of approximately 95%. Although an explanation of the physics of TOF MRA is outside the scope of this chapter, it should be understood that the technique relies on a saturation pulse, usually a fast gradient echo sequence with flow compensation, which is applied to a slab of tissue. Repetition time (TR) is much less than the T1 of tissue, resulting in suppression of longitudinal magnetisation and hence signal from the slab, while inflowing blood, which has not been subject to the saturation pulse, generates high signal. To achieve maximum angiographic contrast, the inflow must be laminar, rapid, and perpendicular to the acquisition plane.

To avoid saturation of inflowing blood and subsequent loss of signal, the TR and TE must be as low as achievable, and the slab should be small, or alternatively multiple overlapping small slabs (MOTSA) can be used (ANDERSON and LEE 1993; DAVIS et al. 1994). Since T1 recovery is more rapid at low field strengths, and signal to noise ratios are lower, MRA is generally more successful in a high field system. Good results have been reported, however, for mid-field systems, despite their inherent restrictions in acquisition volume and spatial resolution (GRANDIN et al. 1998). On our 1.5 T GE Signa Echospeed system, we use a TOF fast spoiled GRASS MOTSA technique: TR/TE = 38/3.1, matrix 256×192; flip angle 25, receive bandwidth 16 MHz, field of view 20×16 cm; with two overlapping slabs of 32 1.4-mm slices. The slabs overlap by 6 mm, and by angling the slabs we can acquire data through the whole circle of Willis, including the origins of the posterior inferior cerebellar arteries and the middle cerebral artery bifurcations in approximately 5 min. Several additional steps are taken to maximise signal from these vessels. Firstly, flow compensation is essential to TOF angiography. Flow compensation techniques work by applying triplets or quadruplets of gradients which tend to correct first and second order motion artefact: moving protons tend to fall out of phase with each other, causing a reduction in signal, and these groups of gradients attempt to restore the phase of protons moving with constant velocity or acceleration (LAUB and KAISER 1988). Secondly, background signal should be minimised. This is done by optimising the flip angle. Larger flip angles produce better background suppression, but also tend to rapidly saturate blood traversing the volume. Some manufacturers use a variable or tailored flip angle which varies across the thickness of the volume, and has the effect of compensating for the reduction of signal often seen at the far end of the volume due to saturation of inflowing blood. This technique is termed TONE (tilted optimised non-saturating excitation), and is especially useful in reducing the seam between adjacent slabs (PURDY et al. 1992). Further background suppression is obtained by a magnetisation transfer pulse which reduces signal from all but free fluid protons (WOLFF et al. 1992), and this has the effect of making small and more distal vessels visible. Thirdly, since venous blood flow is in the opposite direction to arterial blood, a presaturation band applied above the imaged volume will suppress venous signal, and this is particularly useful when examining the cavernous carotid artery which is surrounded by venous channels.

Unfortunately, the conditions of rapid laminar flow perpendicular to the imaged volume are often not met in clinical practice, and where conditions are less than ideal, signal is lost. The major factors in signal loss in TOF MRA are saturation of slow flow, and dephasing of spins due to turbulent flow or flow in the plane of the volume. The ideal situation to develop these conditions is in a large or giant aneurysm, where blood swirls around before leaving the aneurysm to pass along the vascular tree (Fig. 12.1). 3D TOF MRA usually fails to adequately demonstrate the neck of a giant aneurysm, and lack of signal homogeneity within the sac can give a false impression regarding the true size of the aneurysm. Furthermore complex flow can be misinterpreted as intraluminal thrombus and vice versa (BRUGIERES et al. 1998; DE JESUS 1997). For this reason, alternative techniques such as 2D and 3D phase contrast MRA (HUSTON III et al. 1991, 1994), 2D GRE MRA, (BRUGIERES et al. 1993) have been suggested in the assessment of giant aneurysms.

Acute SAH presents another pitfall in the TOF MRA detection of aneurysms. Once extravasated, haemoglobin degrades to methaemoglobin, which can persist for days or weeks within the subarachnoid space. Methaemoglobin has a much shorter T1 than brain tissue, and so it is not adequately suppressed by the TOF sequence. High signal from methaemoglobin can be mistaken for flow within an aneurysm, or can obscure such flow (HUSTON 1994).

Recently, interpolation algorithms have been introduced to increase the apparent resolution of MRA data, or to reconstruct data in a smaller effective slice thickness (CHUNG et al. 1999). These techniques allow shorter scan times for the same apparent resolu-

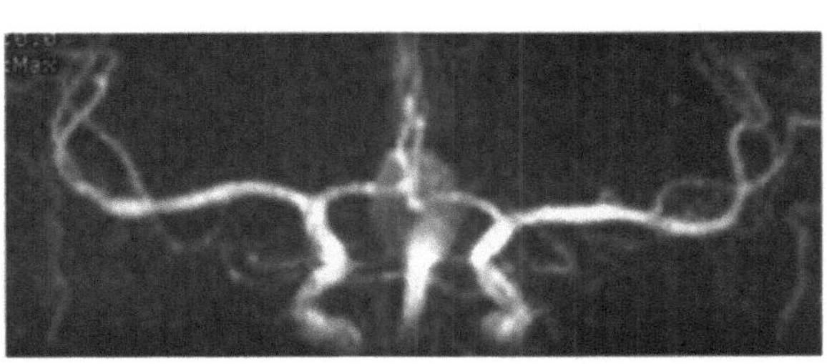

Fig. 12.1. AP projection from a MIP projection of a 3D TOF MRA. There is a large basilar aneurysm. The in-flow jet maintains bright signal but turbulent and in-plain flow within the rest of the aneurysm have caused signal drop out, obscuring the neck region. This does not allow adequate pre-operative assessment of the neck

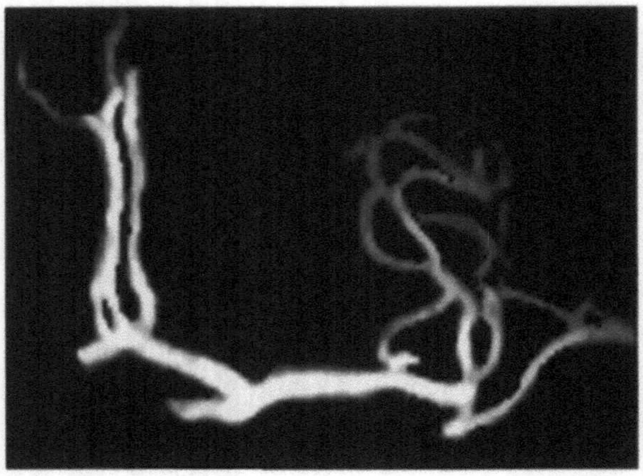

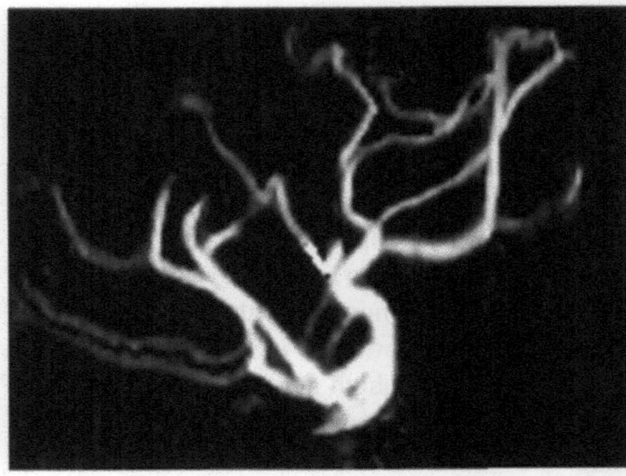

Fig. 12.2a,b. AP oblique (**a**) and lateral oblique (**b**) views from a MIP projection from a MRA dataset. By using progressive volumes of interest, views are obtained to mimic DSA projections. These minimise vessel overlap, and are acceptable and familiar to our neurosurgeons

tion. We use a zero interpolation (ZIP) algorithm routinely, both in plane and between slices, to increase apparent resolution and to allow thinner slice reconstruction respectively (Fig. 12.3).

12.3.2 Phase Contrast MRA

Phase Contrast (PC) MRA still has a limited role in the assessment of cerebral aneurysms. It is essentially a subtraction technique, which relies on the differences in phase between a stationary proton and an inflowing proton to create an image. In comparison to TOF MRA, it gives better background suppression and this optimises the differences between flowing and stationary tissue. Data is acquired in three planes on two separate occasions, with opposite phase encoding. When one is subtracted from the other, the resulting differences in phase are displayed. These phase differences are proportional to flow velocity, and to accurately reconstruct an angiogram, the computer must be told the approximate flow velocity within the target vessel. A velocity encoding of 50 cm/s, for example, will optimally demonstrate middle cerebral artery flow, while a velocity encoding of 15 cm/s will better demonstrate the slower flow found in veins or some giant aneurysms (Turski et al. 1993).

Parameters for 3D PC MRA on our Signa are: TR/TE 23/14; flip angle 15; field of view 23 cm; matrix 256×192; slice thickness 2 mm; 64 partitions, acquisition time 8 min.

The great problem with PC MRA is that the sequences have traditionally taken too long to acquire, and therefore have been limited by movement artefact. Several studies have shown this technique to be less sensitive than TOF in demonstrating small cerebral aneurysms (Ikawa et al. 1994; Huston III et al. 1994). PC MRA is, however, useful in detecting sluggish flow in slow flow or in giant aneurysms that may not be shown by the TOF technique, and may demonstrate aneurysms in the presence of surrounding methaemoglobin because of the subtraction inherent to the technique (Fig. 12.2).

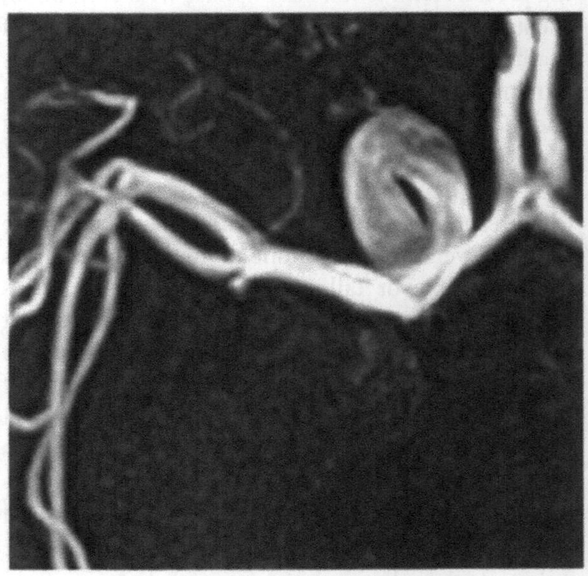

Fig. 12.3. MIP projection from an MRA data search using an image enhancement system filter and zip interpolation. A volume of interest has been drawn around the right internal carotid artery territory. A small right middle cerebral artery trifurcation aneurysm is clearly demonstrated projecting posteriorly

PC MRA is commonly used to demonstrate flow in the dural sinuses as it is less sensitive to saturation effects than TOF MRA and therefore provides improved demonstration of venous blood flow in cortical veins and dural sinuses. By setting a low velocity encoding, and using a 2D technique, the major cerebral veins can be demonstrated in less than 2 min.

CELLERINI et al. (1999) reported 3D and 2D PC MRA findings in 13 patients with dural arteriovenous fistula and found the PC technique to be better than MRI alone in the demonstration of fistula sites and their feeding arteries, as well as in demonstrating stenosis or occlusion of the dural sinuses. The same authors also describe how 2D PC MRA can demonstrate flow reversal, for example, in dural sinuses or the superior ophthalmic vein.

Slow velocity encoding PC MRA is also of benefit for evaluating venous malformations such as venous angioma. IKEDA et al. (1998) and AOKI et al. (1998) demonstrated how velocity coded colour MRA using a colour code from the data obtained from velocity phase images of PC MRA could be used to add flow direction information to MR angiograms. The technique was said to be particularly useful in distinguishing veins from arteries, and to demonstrate flow changes such as those seen in the subclavian steal syndrome.

12.3.3 Gadolinium Enhancement in Cerebral MRA

The use of gadolinium chelates has some theoretical advantages in the search for a berry aneurysm. Contrast enhancement reduces artefact due to slow flow and allows the detection of smaller, more distal middle cerebral arteries than unenhanced TOF or PC MRA alone, but its effect is greater for veins than for arteries, and a major side effect is a large increase in venous and background signal, partially nullifying the improved depiction of small vessels, but more importantly obscuring the cavernous carotid arteries because of the increased signal from the cavernous sinuses (ANDERSON and LEE 1993). As yet, there are no published studies to indicate improved sensitivity or specificity of contrast enhanced MRA over TOF or PC MRA alone in the cerebral circulation.

Contrast enhancement does not lessen artefact due to turbulent flow, and so probably will not improve neck depiction of giant aneurysms or distinguish thrombus from complex flow. However, the blood brain barrier and the long period of significant T1 reduction of blood induced by gadolinium may lead to development of very high resolution MRA techniques in the future (PARKER et al. 1998).

Other MRA techniques such as black blood MRA, which uses the phenomenon of flow voids seen in major arteries on a volumetric T2 weighted image to create an angiographic image via a minimum intensity projection (EL GAMMAL and BROOKES 1991), and adiabatic fast passage, which uses a 180° pulse to tag blood which then flows into the imaged volume (SARDASHTI et al. 1990), are seldom used in clinical practice and will not be further discussed.

12.4 CTA Acquisition Parameters

CTA techniques have evolved dramatically since the evolution of helical CT. The main advantages of the helical technique are its speed, and the volumetric nature of the data it acquires. This allows data acquisition through the circle of Willis during the period of maximal arterial contrast enhancement, thus minimizing both patient motion and venous enhancement. At our institution, using a GE HiSpeed CTI scanner, we use 40 1-s rotations, with 1 mm collimation and 1:1 pitch starting 25 s after a 150 ml bolus of iohexol 300 injected at 3 ml/s. Other parameters include a 512×512 matrix, 16-cm field of view, 140 kV, and 125 mA. Some scanners permit angling the gantry for the acquisition, which allows coverage of the entire circle of Willis from the origin of the posterior inferior cerebellar arteries to the middle cerebral artery bifurcations. If this option is not available without image degradation, then asking the patient to flex their neck as far as is comfortable has the same effect.

In order to obtain optimal images of the cavernous and supraclinoid internal carotid arteries, venous opacification must be minimised, and arterial opacification maximised. Arterial contrast medium concentrations can be optimised and contrast dose kept to a minimum by techniques which predict the time from injection to peak arterial contrast medium concentration. This is most easily done by carrying out a dynamic scan at one location, such as the cavernous carotid artery, injecting a relatively small amount of contrast medium, and creating a time-density curve to calculate the time to peak contrast enhancement. Such software is standard on all major CT installations. This calculated time delay is then applied to the diagnostic scan (PUSKAS 1996; NAKIJIMA et al. 1998).

CTA and subsequent maximum intensity projection (MIP) image data are hampered by beam hardening artefact from the dense bone of the skull base and vault, and some authors have recommended a subtraction technique to deal with this. Such a method requires no movement between the mask scan and the CTA scan, and this must be accomplished by fixing the patient's head firmly to the scanner table (Imakita et al. 1998). In our experience, such a technique is unnecessary, and we prefer to remove the skull vault from the image dataset by thresholding and electronically cutting out any remaining bone.

12.5 Display and Post Processing

With both CTA and MRA it is vital to view the source images, since this will clarify or exclude many artefacts and prevent common errors in interpretation. This is particularly important in MRA datasets, where in the presence of subarachnoid haemorrhage, high signal from methaemoglobin can easily be confused with vascular anatomy.

The commonest post processing protocol for both modalities is the maximum intensity projection (MIP). MIP takes bright pixels from each image, and summates this data to make an angiographic projection, which can then be rotated, cropped, or further modified to exclude unwanted data or to improve the subjective image quality. The MIP data are a type of projection image, where a set of slices from a 2D or 3D acquisition are reduced or collapsed into a single image. In its simplest form, a projection image is like transferring each of the images onto a sheet of glass, and then stacking up the sheets to see the angiogram (Anderson 1993). The problem with this is that the background noise from each slice summates, and tends to obscure smaller vessels.

The MIP algorithm goes a step further: by transferring only the brightest, or maximum intensity, pixels to each virtual sheet, so that the resultant projection is almost free of background, and small vessels stand out clearly. It is standard radiological practice to produce views from more than one direction; hence several MIP projections are calculated. In its most simple form, this would involve a number of projections at 10–15° intervals around a vertical axis. We have found this simplistic approach to be both misleading and inaccurate. In a conventional angiogram, overlapping vessels, or an aneurysm close to a vessel, will result in a double density, and this sign is widely used in the interpretation of DSA. In a MIP projection, however, since intensities are by definition at maximum, there is no double density, and a small aneurysm can be hidden by an overlapping vessel. It is therefore necessary that simple MIP projections are avoided. In the assessment of a MIP projection, we prescribe a number of volumes of interest, and individually and interactively examine these using multiple projections and angles. We routinely start with a volume of interest drawn around the right internal carotid artery, the ipsilateral middle cerebral artery, and the anterior communicating complex. Once this has been assessed, we create six to eight projections which mimic standard angiographic views, and which best show the neck of an aneurysm. These are then electronically smoothed and/or edge enhanced and imaged onto hard copy film (Fig. 12.2). We then go on to do the same process for the left cerebral circulation and the posterior circulation. The resulting films are acceptable to our neurosurgical colleagues because they are familiar with the appearance of the projections. We believe it is vital that the images are interactively examined and created by an experienced neuroradiologist, and not by a technician alone, as we have seen several mistakes made by the latter approach.

Even when assessed by an expert, MIP projections can be subject to signal loss or artefact. If the background is noisy, and contains high density or high intensity pixels, these can summate to make the background in the projection appear greater than that in the individual slices (Anderson et al. 1990). Examining the individual slices that make up the angiographic dataset will often demonstrate small vessels not apparent on the MIP itself.

Since blood velocity is slightly higher at the centre of a vessel than it is along the vessel wall, pixels at the edge of a vessel will tend to be of lower intensity on an MRA MIP, and this effect can be exaggerated by partial volume averaging at the margin of a vessel. MRA MIPs can therefore underestimate the true lumen size of a vascular structure, and this can be further complicated by signal loss from saturation or dephasing. CTA MIPs suffer less from this phenomenon: there may be some partial volume effects, but the contrast medium concentration and resultant CT density are identical across the width of the vessel.

Cortical bone gives no signal on MRI, but high density on CT images. Several techniques are available to remove bone from CTA datasets and to allow projections which are not obscured by bone. The simplest of these is to set a density threshold whereby pixels above or below predefined values are omitted from the dataset and the subsequent MIP. This can be done with an automated program (Hope et al. 1995), or by manually specifying the threshold values to be used. An upper limit of 350–450 Hounsfield units will extract nearly all bone densities from the dataset (Zouaoui et al. 1997). Some authors in addition have advocated using a lower threshold as well, to reduce background noise (Nakajima et al. 1998), but in our experience this will often exclude small vessels from the MIP projection, particularly when these have been partial volume averaged to an artificially low density.

An alternative to the conventional MIP projection is surface shading or surface rendering. This is a projection technique where only the outer surface of the vessel lumen is displayed. These images can have a very natural appearance, particularly when colours are applied, and can convey some 3D information (Cline et al. 1991). However, most authors prefer MIP to surface shading because the latter technique may be more user dependent (Zouaoui et al. 1997). Hope et al. have reported that the surface shaded technique is more prone to the possibility of confusing high attenuation clot with intravascular contrast medium. Other authors emphasise that surface shaded displays are best reserved for aneurysms larger than 1 cm in diameter, and that surface rendering can hide small aneurysms which can be mixed in with neighbouring bone (Zouaoui et al. 1997; Ogawa et al. 1996; Schwartz et al. 1994).

More recently, a volume rendering technique has been devised and assessed in the cerebral circulation (Johnson et al. 1996; Korogi et al. 1999). This technique uses information from all voxels within a volume, avoiding the loss of information that is inherent to MIP and surface shaded displays, and provides greater control over the display of structures with varying attenuation. Relative voxel attenuation is conveyed by means of a grey scale in the final image, and the images maintain the original spatial relationships of their CT datasets, as well as a 3D appearance. Korogi et al. (1999) have claimed that this method is substantially better at demonstrating very small aneurysms – i.e. those less than 3 mm in diameter, but their method included 0.8 mm CT collimation, automated triggering of the data acquisition by detection of the arrival of the contrast bolus, stereoscopic display of the volume rendered images, and colour overlays, and so the exact contribution of volume rendering per se to their results is questionable.

There are some theoretical advantages in abandoning projection methods in favour of multiplanar reconstruction (MPR). Such a technique avoids the difficulties of the MIP projection, and the possibility of an exaggerated background, by reformatting the data to show thin sections in any desired plane. Thin section reformats also avoid problems with overlapping vessels. This is particularly successful in the assessment of very small branches and aneurysms (Chung et al. 1999).

Finally, an endovascular or endoscopic perspective can be gained by software available from some manufacturers. The Navigator technique enables the radiologist to look at the neck of an aneurysm as if from the inside (Fig. 12.5). This can be surprisingly useful in assessing the neck region in depicting small branches arising from the dome of an aneurysm, or very close to its neck, but the quality of the images obtained are, in our experience, highly user dependent.

There has been recent interest in the use of raw data or MIP data filtering to improve subjective image quality. We have found that the use of Image Enhancement Systems (IES, California, USA) filters can dramatically improve image quality, in particular 3D image quality not apparent on the MRA raw data. This improvement in image quality is achieved without affecting the final radiological diagnosis (Halpin et al. 1997) either positively or negatively (Fig. 12.6). Most MR system manufacturers have image filtering algorithms either built in and hidden within their system, or available as an optional and user controllable feature.

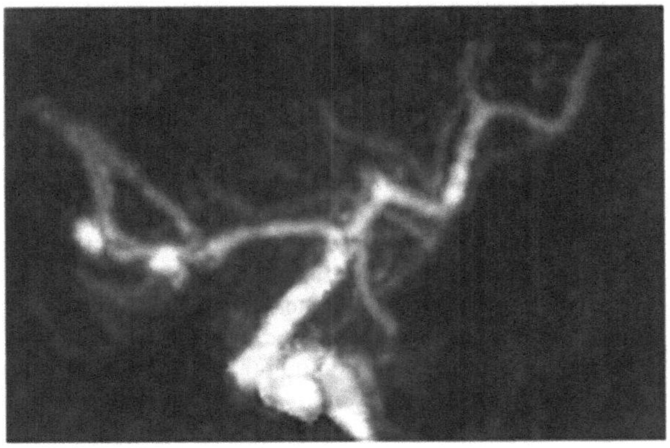

Fig. 12.4. MIP projection from a CT angiogram produced at the original diagnostic scan for a patient with acute subarachnoid haemorrhage. The source images have been interactively examined and by using volumes of interest this AP oblique projection of the left internal carotid territory has been produced. There are two aneurysms, one at the anterior communicating artery and a second on a more distal anterior cerebral artery branch. Assessment and display of such volumes of interest in this manner has been highly successful and acceptable to both radiologists and neurosurgeons

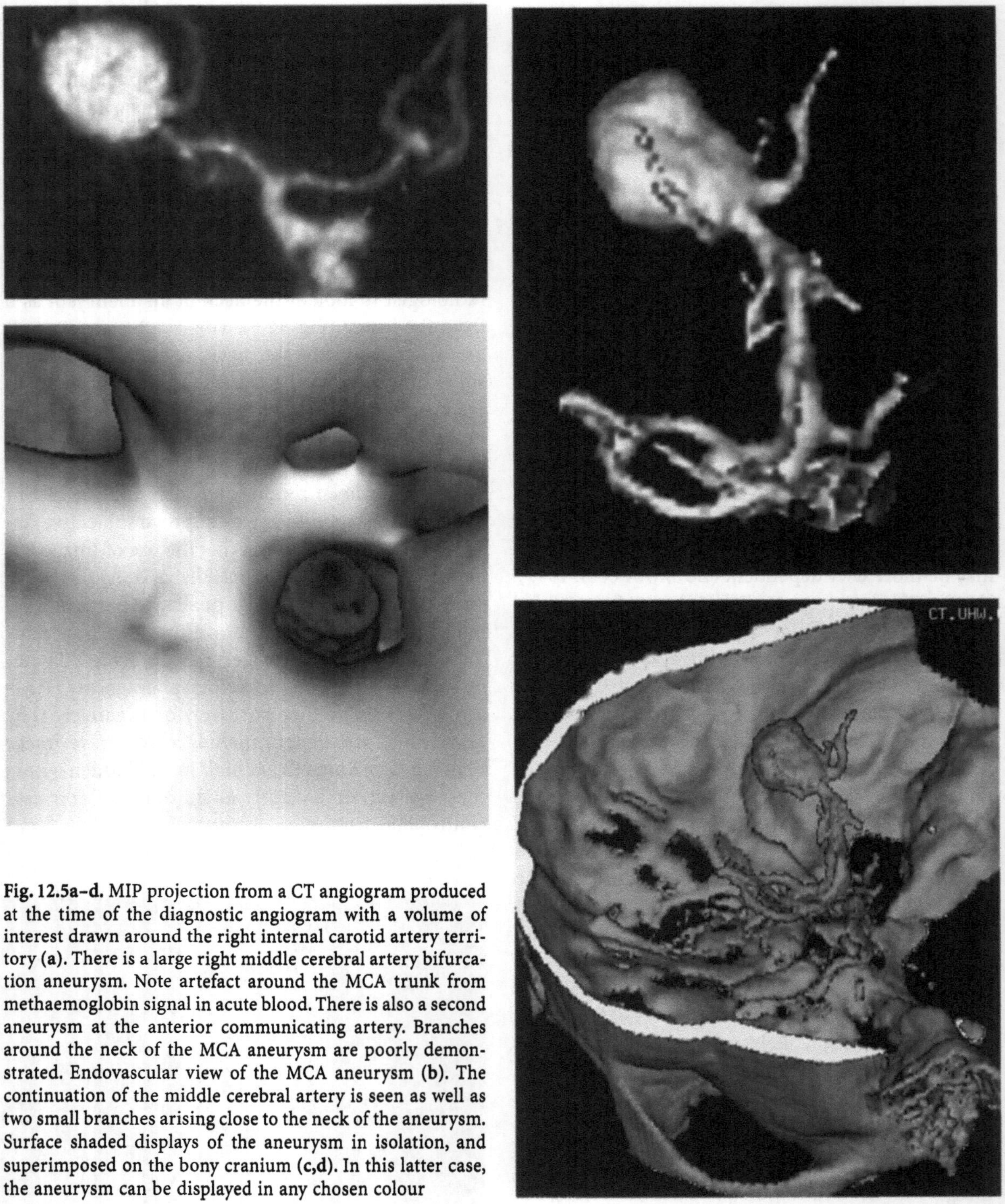

Fig. 12.5a–d. MIP projection from a CT angiogram produced at the time of the diagnostic angiogram with a volume of interest drawn around the right internal carotid artery territory (**a**). There is a large right middle cerebral artery bifurcation aneurysm. Note artefact around the MCA trunk from methaemoglobin signal in acute blood. There is also a second aneurysm at the anterior communicating artery. Branches around the neck of the MCA aneurysm are poorly demonstrated. Endovascular view of the MCA aneurysm (**b**). The continuation of the middle cerebral artery is seen as well as two small branches arising close to the neck of the aneurysm. Surface shaded displays of the aneurysm in isolation, and superimposed on the bony cranium (**c**,**d**). In this latter case, the aneurysm can be displayed in any chosen colour

12.6 Comparisons with DSA

A large number of studies have compared the sensitivity and specificity of CTA and MRA with DSA and/or with each other. DSA is the commonly accepted gold standard, but it must be remembered that even DSA is not 100% sensitive when compared to surgical findings or post mortem examination. Several studies have used a forced decision method, compelling radiologists to answer yes or no to the question, is there an aneurysm? Although scientifically valid this does not reflect real life practice where a radiologist will readily state when he or she is unable to come to a definite conclusion, perhaps due to patient motion or other artefact. In this situation, many of us a 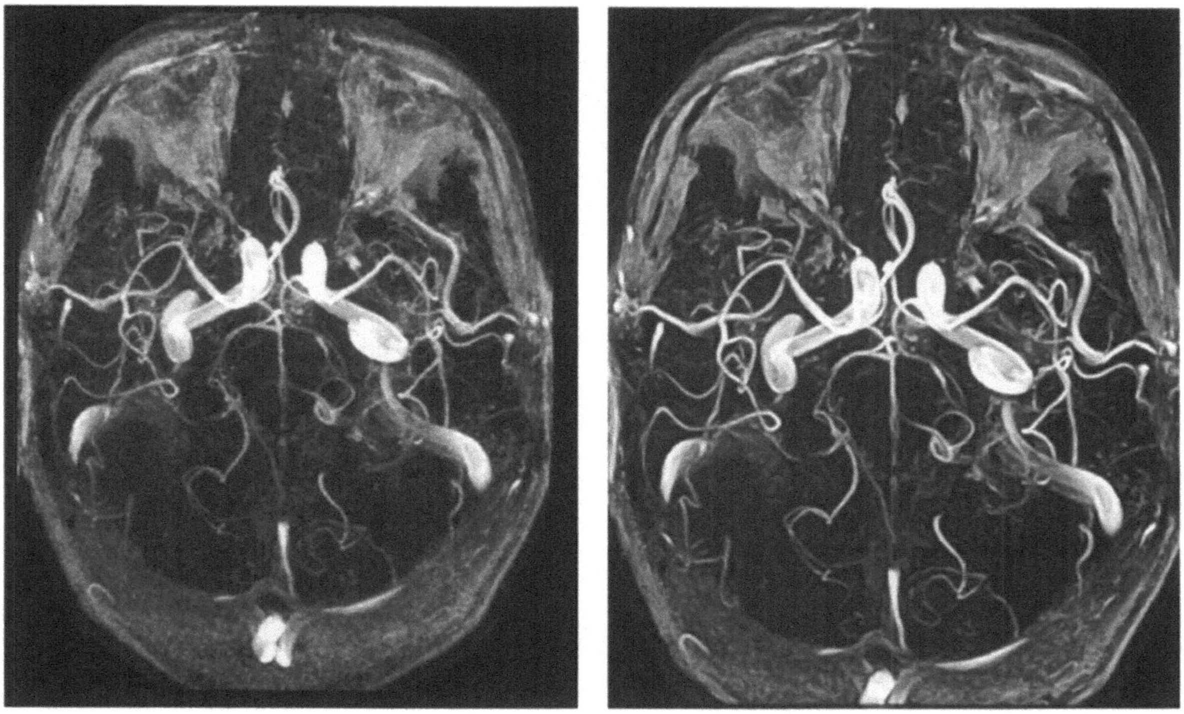 b

Fig. 12.6a,b. MIP projection from 3D TOF MRA before (**a**) and after (**b**) image filtering using the Image Enhancement System algorithm. **b** shows increased clarity of large and small vessels and a better apparent 3D effect

will seek a second opinion from a colleague. These factors hold especially true when comparing the specificity of the techniques. It is a cardinal error in neuroradiology to send a surgeon to perform a craniotomy for an aneurysm which is not really present, and all of us work very hard to ensure this never happens. Often if there is doubt, we will either repeat the angiogram on another day, or resort to an additional study like CTA or MRA to confirm or refute equivocal angiographic findings. And so one of the most worrying aspects of the following comparative studies is the relatively large number of false positive studies. We hope that day to day reality would not permit these in clinical practice.

12.6.1 MRA versus DSA

Studies from the early 1990s compared TOF or PC MRA with DSA and found sensitivities of 85–95% for the detection of ruptured aneurysms, and of aneurysms greater than 5 mm in diameter (Schuierer et al. 1992; Anzalone et al. 1995; Huston 1994; Stock et al. 1995), with specificity at or close to 100%. Aneurysms smaller than 5 mm in diameter have been more difficult to detect and Huston (1994) found an overall sensitivity for detecting all aneurysms, including those shown by DSA to be less than 3 mm in size, of only 55%. Our own experience at this time was similar. In a prospective blinded study of patients with subarachnoid haemorrhage, we found a sensitivity of 94% for ruptured aneurysms, but only 74% for unruptured or incidental aneurysms within the same cohort, and a specificity of 96% (Roberts, Halpin and Hourihan, unpublished data). This finding is crucial, since a neurosurgeon will often clip a second, unruptured, aneurysm at the same craniotomy as the ruptured aneurysm. More recent studies, with slightly improved technologies, have shown improvement. Grandin et al. reported an overall sensitivity of MRA on a 0.5 T unit as 91% and specificity of 100%. This cohort included 89 aneurysms, of which 25 were less than 5 mm in size.

Chung et al. (1999) reported 100% sensitivity for MRA when compared to DSA, using a section interpolation technique, and MPR as well as MIP. This was not a prospective comparison, however: the authors compared the data of 30 patients in whom MRA had detected at least one aneurysm with subsequent DSA, and so a sensitivity of 100% was almost to be predicted. Nevertheless among the 39 aneurysms seen at MRA, 21 were ruptured and 18 were incidental (not all the patients had SAH), and 12 were less than 2 mm in size, and so these results must be seen as encouraging.

There are a few reports of MRA failing to detect either a large ruptured aneurysm (TURTZ et al. 1995), or a very small one which went on to cause SAH at a later date (VANNINEN et al. 1996). Many such errors can be seen in retrospect to have been due to a failure of adequate interrogation of the MRA datasets, or their interpretation, but we feel that a small number of such errors are inevitable.

12.6.2 CTA versus DSA

Data from earlier studies is similar to the experience with MRA. SCHWARTZ et al. (1994) reported sensitivity of CTA to be identical to MRA at 87%. HOPE et al. (1996) found a sensitivity of CTA when prospectively compared to DSA of 90%, but a specificity of only 50%. Sensitivity for the detection of aneurysms less than 5 mm in diameter fell to 79%. OGAWA et al. (1996) reported a sensitivity of only 70%, failing to detect a significant number of small aneurysms. ANDERSON et al. (1997) reported a sensitivity and a specificity of 86% and 90% respectively. More recently, however, the published results have been improving. ROHNERT et al. (1998) reported a 93% sensitivity and a 100% specificity, and ZOUAOUI et al. (1997) reported sensitivity and specificity of 100% and stated that CTA detected all aneurysms shown on DSA, as well as two additional aneurysms which were found on CTA, and surgically confirmed, but were not seen on DSA.

12.7 Associated Lesions

CTA and MRA techniques are approaching sensitivities acceptable for detecting aneurysms in the acute situation; in addition there is growing evidence that these modalities may be able to fulfil the other essential roles in the management of aneurysmal subarachnoid haemorrhage.

The depiction of the aneurysm neck anatomy is crucial to the neurosurgeon and neuro-interventionalist. We have found MRA to be extremely unreliable in this regard, and have stopped using the technique prior to embolisation of brain aneurysms because the information gained was often inaccurate. CTA, however, does not suffer from the same signal loss at the neck of moderate or large aneurysms, and we agree with the reports that suggest CTA is a reliable method of measuring the true diameter of an aneurysm's lumen, and assessing its neck. LENHART et al. (1997) reported that CTA was superior to DSA in the demonstration of the neck, shape, and direction of an aneurysm, and others have found similar results (NG et al. 1997; HARRISON et al. 1997; PREDA et al. 1998; VELTHUIS 1998).

Flow around an anterior communicating artery can be assessed with CTA and MRA. VELTHUIS et al. found that the dominant side of filling of these aneurysms could be predicted with 100% accuracy based on asymmetric size of the proximal (A1) portion of the anterior cerebral arteries, asymmetric aneurysm location, or both. MRA algorithms exist for determining the inflow to these aneurysms, which can be derived by placing a presaturation pulse over each internal carotid artery in turn, to see which results in non-visualisation of the aneurysm.

Both pre- and postsurgical vasospasm can be reliably detected with CTA and MRA (TAKAGI et al. 1998; ZOUAOUI et al. 1997; TAMATANI et al. 1997). MRA can be used to follow up patients who have had an aneurysm clipped, but extreme caution must be exercised in doing this, and our current policy is only to perform MRI on patients who have undergone aneurysm surgery if we have written evidence that the clip used was MR compatible, and even then only if no other modality is likely to provide sufficient information. Despite the fact that the clips are not ferromagnetic, they cause sufficient susceptibility artefact to create a large signal void, which obscures the neighbouring vessels. CTA, however, successfully images these cerebral vessels after such surgery, and the expected artefact from aneurysm clips does not present a problem, as it can be taken out of the dataset by thresholding (ZOUAUOI et al. 1997; VIECO et al. 1995). MRA is the better technique to follow up patients after coil embolisation, because artefact from the platinum coils is less than that from clips. Inspection of the individual partitions allows determination of neck remnants with reasonable accuracy (GONNER et al. 1998).

12.8 CTA and MRA in Vascular Malformations

The goals of angiography in the assessment of cerebral arteriovenous malformations (AVM) are to define the arterial supply and venous drainage; demonstrate the size and location of the nidus; identify the presence and the dynamics of any arteriovenous shunts; locate any aneurysms proximal to, or within, the nidus; and assess the haemodynamic impact of the lesion on the surrounding brain. MRI alone can accomplish much of this. MRI is an excellent tool for demonstrating the location of even small AVMs, and can demonstrate angiographically occult lesions such as cavernous haemangiomas.

MRA techniques have been described using a combination of TOF MRA, to outline the abnormal vessels, and PC MRA to quantify flow within the relevant arteries and veins (Turski et al. 1993). This method can produce elegant surface shaded displays of AVMs within the cerebral substance, and go some way towards measuring the arteriovenous shunt by calculating flow velocity within the draining veins, and is almost certainly adequate for those small lesions which will be treated by stereotactic radiosurgery (Nussel et al. 1991; Anzalone et al. 1998). Tanaka et al. (1997) found that CTA detected more veins, but fewer arteries, than MRA.

Larger AVMs, however, or those to be treated by embolisation, require a much more detailed vascular assessment. The approach taken by an interventional neuroradiologist is to perform an endovascular exploration of the AVM using a microcatheter, and then to target the initial embolisation against those pedicles which have the most dangerous angioarchitecture – intranidal aneurysms, pseudoaneurysms, high flow fistulae, and venous ectasias. As yet MRA cannot match DSA in this respect. In addition some types of AVM are very difficult to locate with MRA and CTA. These include micro AVMs, where there may only be a single fistulous connection from one normal sized artery into a relatively small vein, these are hard enough to identify on DSA, and the presence of early venous filling is a major clue to their presence. CTA and MRA do not as yet provide a simple, easily attainable method for detecting these small shunts.

The other group of brain AVM which is notoriously difficult to detect on MRA or CTA is the dural arteriovenous fistula. These may have both a dural and pial supply, but if present the pial vessels are usually small. Phase contrast studies seem to be the most reliable in their detection, but in the event of a normal CT or MR study, we always proceed to selective internal and external carotid arteriography if a dural AVF is suspected.

MRA or CTA can be used successfully and interchangeably to follow up AVMs which have been treated with radiosurgery, but one cannot guarantee complete abolition of an arteriovenous shunt without the temporal data provided by arteriography.

12.9 CTA and MRA in Vascular Stenosis and Occlusion

There has been recent renewed interest in the emergency treatment of cerebrovascular thrombosis, with the emergence of the "brain attack" examination. This is beyond the scope of this chapter, but in essence the MR protocol uses diffusion and perfusion imaging to detect areas of ischaemic but not infarcted brain. When MRA is added to this exam, a complete vascular and physiological work up is provided in the one visit, and the complete brain attack protocol, including MRA, can be concluded in around 15 min of scanning time. Identification of intracranial vascular stenosis or occlusion allows early consideration of systemic or local fibrinolysis. MRA has been shown to be 100% sensitive and 95% specific in the detection of cerebrovascular occlusion, and 86% sensitive and specific for stenosis (Stock et al. 1995). We feel these results are good enough to allow us not to perform cerebral angiography in acute stroke unless we intend to proceed with local fibrinolysis. The CTA technique has a lesser role in brain attack, but xenon CT and CTA can provide similar information.

12.10 MRA and CTA in Brain Tumours

Several authors have proposed the use of CTA or MRA to provide better surgical planning of superficial or deep cerebral tumours (Pant et al. 1997; Tetsumura et al. 1999; Kadota et al. 1998). Such techniques show most, but not all, of the relevant feeding arteries and veins, and when combined with further display techniques such as surface shaded display with colour, or stereoscopic display, can provide superb images. Whether neurosurgical outcome is influenced by such techniques has not been assessed. Most UK neurosurgical centres have abandoned cerebral angiography in the work up of patients with glioma, but these display methods may generate further interest.

12.11
Assessment of the Circle of Willis

Both CTA and MRA show high accuracy in determining the competence of the circle of Willis (Stock et al. 1996). A sensitivity of 89% with a specificity of 88% has been reported for MRA, using MIP and source images. When compared to DSA, PC MRA has the advantage of giving information regarding the direction of flow in the anterior and posterior communicating arteries, and can also be used to calculate flow volume rates, which in turn have some value in predicting cerebral ischaemia (Anderson et al. 1993). Flow coding images are part of the source data for PC MRA, and this technique can readily be applied to the assessment of flow around an anterior communicating artery.

12.12
Population Screening

In Japan, there has been considerable interest in using MRA to screen the whole population for the presence of cerebral aneurysms. This involves a short hospital admission for a full clinical assessment and a scan, and has been termed "Brain Dock" (Hashi 1997). Given that some data suggests that both CTA and MRA have a relatively low sensitivity for the detection of unruptured aneurysms, the small chance of an aneurysm rupturing in an individual; and the surprisingly high morbidity associated with clipping of unruptured aneurysms (Wiebers et al. 1998), it is not surprising that it has been estimated that in Japan it costs $690,000 to save a life at 5 years under such a screening programme (Linuma et al. 1998). It has been suggested that CTA or MRA can be reliably used in the screening of siblings where there is a family history of subarachnoid haemorrhage (Raaymakers et al. 1998). However, with current technology, one cannot absolutely exclude an incidental aneurysm, nor prevent the later development of a new aneurysm. The screening process can only represent a snapshot in a lifetime of risk of subarachnoid haemorrhage. The recent report of a serum marker lipoprotein (a) defining a group at particularly high risk of developing an aneurysm in affected families is encouraging, and may help define a future high risk population to be screened (Phillips et al. 1997).

The choice between CTA and MRA is difficult, and different centres will make different decisions based on local availability and quality of equipment, as well as personal expertise. Given first rate CT and MR hardware and software, the radiologist will have to consider which modality is likely to produce the most accurate answer in his or her hands. Although MRA is attractive due to the lack of ionising radiation or intravenous contrast media, CTA has made considerable inroads into territory once the domain of MRA. Our personal experience is that CTA images are quicker, and a little easier to acquire. We have adopted a protocol of obtaining CTA in every patient who presents to our department with SAH. This is particularly convenient, since all these patients will have a diagnostic CT scan. We have been very impressed with the accuracy of CTA in the detection of cerebral lesions; to date no significant lesions have been missed. Nor have there been any false positive examinations. We have not, however, abandoned DSA, which is still performed on all patients prior to neurosurgical clipping, and more reports need to be published showing 100% sensitivity in the detection of small aneurysms.

In the event of a patient presenting from elsewhere with CT proven SAH, we use DSA as our investigation of first choice. If this is negative, we use CTA as the confirmatory examination. MRA, at our institution, is used for the screening of high-risk groups, such as professional boxers, or families with an inherited tendency to aneurysm formation. We also use MRA to follow up patients with small or questionable lesions.

We have only recently had the capacity to gain 1024×1024 matrix MRA images, and it cannot be long before CTA and/or MRA succeed DSA as the gold standard for imaging the cerebral vasculature.

References

Anderson CM, Saloner D, Tsuruda JS, Shapeero LG, Lee RE (1990) Artifacts in Maximum Intensity Projection display of MR angiographs. Am J Roentgenol 154: 623–629
Anderson C, Lee RE (1993) Time of Flight angiography in clinical magnetic resonance angiography. In: Anderson CM, Edelman RR, Turski PA (eds). Raven Press, New York
Anderson CM, Turski PA, Edelman RR (1993) Flow quantification. In: Anderson CM, Edelman RR, Turski PA (eds) Clinical magnetic resonance angiography. Raven Press, New York
Anderson CM, Lee RE (1993) Time of Flight angiography in clinical magnetic resonance angiography. In: Anderson CM, Edelman RR, Turski PA (eds). Raven Press, New York
Anzalone N, Tirulzi F, Scotti G (1995) Acute subarachnoid haemorrhage 3D MR angiography verses DSA. Neuroradiology 37: 257–261

Anzalone N, Scomazzoni F, Starda L, Patay Z, Scotti G (1998) Intracranial vascular malformations. Eur Radiol 8: 685–690

Aoki S, Osawa S, Yoshioka N, Yamashita H, Kumagai H, Araki T (1998) Velocity coded colour MR angiography. Am J Neuroradiol 19: 691–693

Cellerini M, Mascalchi M, Mangiafico S et al. (1999) Phase contrast MR angiography of intracranial dural arteriovenous fistulae. Neuroradiology 41: 487–492

Chung TS, Joo JY, Lee SK, Chien D, Laub G (1999) Evaluation of cerebral aneurysms with high resolution MR angiography using a section interpolation technique: correlation with digital subtraction angiography. Am J Neuroradiol 20: 229–235

Cline H, Lorensen W, Souza S (1991) 3D surface rendered MR images of the brain and its vasculature. J Comput Assist Tomogr 15: 103–107

Davis WL, Blatter DD, Harnsberger HR, Parker DL (1994) Intracranial MR angiography: comparison of single volume 3D time of flight and multiple overlapping thin slab acquisition techniques. Am J Roentgenol 163: 915–920

De Jesus O, Rifkinson N (1997) Magnetic resonance angiography of giant aneurysms. Pitfalls and surgical implications. PR Health Science Journal 16: 131–135

El Gammal T, Brooks B (1991) Conventional MR neuro-angiography. Am J Roentgnol 156: 1075–1080

Fogelholm R (1981) Subarachnoid haemorrhage in middle Finland; incidents, early prognosis and indications for neurosurgical treatment. Stroke 12: 296–301

Gonner F, Heid O, Nicholi G, Baumgartner W, Schroth T (1998) MR angiography with ultra short echo time in cerebral aneurysms treated with Guglielmi detachable coils. Am J Neuroradiol 19: 1324–1328

Grandin CB, Mathurin P, Duprez T et al. (1998) Diagnosis of intracranial aneurysms: accuracy of MR angiography and 0.5 T. Am J Neuroradiol 19: 245–252

Halpin SFS, Hourihan MD, Chawda S, Bourne MW (1998) The affect of scan data filtering on image quality. Presented at the American Society of Neuroradiology, Seattle

Harrison M, Johnson B, Gardner G, Welling B (1997) Preliminary results on the management of unruptured intracranial aneurysms with MRA and CTA. Neurosurgery 40: 947–955

Hashi K (1997) Present status of brain. Doc Neurol Med 47: 549–554

Juveal S, Porras M, Heiskanen O (1993) Natural history of unruptured intracranial aneurysm: a longterm follow up study. J Neurosurg 79: 174–182

Heiserman JE, Dean BL, Hodak JA (1994) Neurologic complications of cerebral angiography. Am J Neuroradiol 15: 1401–1407

Hope JKA, Wilson JL, Thomson FJ (1996) 3D CT angiography in the detection and characterisation of intracranial berry aneurysms. Am J Neuroradiol 17: 439–445

Huston J III, Rufenacht DA, Ehman RL, Wiebers DO (1991) Intracranial aneurysms and vascular malformations: comparison of time of flight and phase contrast MR angiography. Radiology 181: 721–730

Huston J III, Nichols DA, Luetmer PH et al. (1994) Blinded prospective evaluation of sensitivity of MR angiography to known intracranial aneurysms: importance of aneurysm size. Am J Neuroradiol 15: 1607–1614

Huston J III, Nichols DA, Luetmer PH et al. (1994) Blinded prospective evaluation of sensitivity of MR angiography to known intracranial aneurysms: importance of aneurysm size. Am J Neuroradiol 15: 1607–1614

Imakita S, Onishi Y, Hashimoto T, Motosugi S (1998) Subtraction CT angiography with controlled orbit helical scanning for detection of intracranial aneurysms. Am J Neuroradiol 19: 291–295

Ikawa F, Sumida M, Uozumi T et al. (1994) Comparison of 3D phase contrast magnetic resonance angiography with 3D time of flight magnetic resonance angiography in cerebral aneurysms. Surg Neurol 42: 287–292

Ikeda K, Hatanaka N, Kinoshita M, Kuwajima A (1998) Cerebral venous angioma detected by slow velocity coding phase contrast MRA. No To Shinkei 50: 459–462

Inagawa T (1994) Ultra early rebleeding within 6 hours after aneurysmal rupture. Surg Neurol 42: 130–134

Kassell NF, Torner JC (1984) The international co-operative study of timing of aneurysm surgery – an update. Stroke 15: 566–570

Kim A, Proske M, Tirsch E, Von Waymann A, Radu EW, Steinbrich W (1996) Value of repeat angiography in cases of unexplained subarachnoid haemorrhage. Acta Neurol Scand 93: 366–373

Khanna RK, Malik G M, Qureshi N (1996) Predicting outcome following surgical treatment of unruptured intracranial aneurysms; a proposed grading system. J Neurosurg 84: 49–54

Laub GA, Kiser WA (1998) MR angiography with gradient motion refocussing. J Comput Assist Tomogr 12: 377–382

Lenhart M, Bretchneider T, Gmeinwieser J, Ellrich O, Feuerbach S (1997) Cerebral CT angiography in the diagnosis of acute subarachnoid haemorrhage. Acta Radiol 38: 791–796

Linuma T, Tatelo Y, Furuse M (1998) Re-estimation of cost performance for mass screening for unruptured intracranial aneurysms using MR angiography. Japan J Magnresonmed 18: 243–246

Nakajima Y, Yoshimine T, Yoshida H, Sakasishita K, Okamoto M (1998) Computerised tomography angiography of ruptured cerebral aneurysms: factors affecting time to maximum contrast concentration. J Neurosurg 88: 663–669

Nussel F, Wegmuller H, Huber P (1991) Comparison of magnetic resonance angiography and conventional angiography cerebral arteriovenous malformations. Neuroradiology 33: 56–61

Ng SH, Wong H, Ko S et al. (1997) CT angiography of intracranial aneurysms: advantages and pitfalls. Eur J Radiol 25: 141–149

Ogawa T, Okudera T, Nogukhi K, Sasaki N, Yasui N (1996) Cerebral aneurysms evaluation with three dimensional CT angiography. Am J Neuroradiol 17: 447–454

O'Leary DH, Mattle H, Potter JE (1989) Atheromatous pseudo-occlusion of the internal carotid artery. Stroke 20: 1168–1173

Pant B, Sumida M, Kurisu K, Arita K, Kutsuma M, Uozumi T (1997) Usefulness of 2D time of flight MRA combined with surface anatomy scanning for convexities lesions. Neurosurg Rev 20: 108–113

Parker DL, Tsuruda JS, Goodridge KC, Alexander AL, Boswell HR (1998) Contrast enhanced magnetic resonance angiography of cerebral arteries. A review. Invest Radiol 33: 560–572

Perdy D, Cadena G, Laub F (1992) The design of variable tip angle slab selection (TONE) pulses for improved 3D MR angiography. In: Proceedings 11th Annual Meeting of the

Society of Magnetic Resonance in Medicine. Berlin: The Society of Magnetic Resonance in Medicine, p 882
Phillips J, Roberts G, Bolger C et al. (1997) A potential biological marker for unruptured intracranial aneurysms. Neurosurgery 40: 112–115
Preta L, Gaetani P, Dore R, Fulle I, Infuso L, Campani R (1998) Spiral CTA and surgical correlations in the evaluation of intracranial aneurysms. Eur Radiol 8: 739–745
Puskas Z, Schuierer G (1996) Determination of blood circulation time for optimising contrast medium opacification in CT angiography. Radiologe 36: 750–757
Raaymakers TW, Rankel GK, Ramos LM (1998) Initial and follow up screening for aneurysms in families with aneurysmal subarachnoid haemorrhage. Neurology 51: 1125–1130
Rohnert W, Hanig V, Hietschold V, Abolmaali N (1998) Detection of aneurysms in subarachnoid haemorrhage CTA verses DSA. Aktuel Radiol 8: 63–70
Saitoh H, Hayakawa K, Nishimura K (1995) Re-rupture of cerebral aneurysms during angiography. Am J Neuroradiol 16: 539–542
Sarti C, Tuomilehto J, Salomaa V (1991) Epidemiology of subarachnoid haemorrhage in Finland from 1983–1985. Stroke 22: 848–853
Sardashti M, Schwartzberg DG, Stomp GP, Dickson WT (1990) Spin labelling angiography of the carotid by presaturation and simplified adiabatic inversion. Magn Reson Med 15: 192–200
Turski PA, Korosec FA (1993) Phase contrast angiography in clinical magnetic resonance angiography. In: Anderson CM, Edelman RR, Turski PA (eds). Raven Press
Schwartz RB, Tice HM, Hootem SM, Hsu RTL, Stieg PE (1994) Evaluation of cerebral aneurysms with helical CT correlation with conventional angiography and MR angiography. Radiology 192: 717–722
Schuierer G, Huck WJ, Laub G (1992) Magnetic resonance angiography of intracranial aneurysms comparison with intra-arterial DSA. Neuroradiology 35: 50–54
Sekhar LN, Heros RC (1981) Origin growth and rupture of sacular aneurysms: a review. Neurosurgery 8: 248–260
Stock KW, Radue AW, Jacob AL, Bao XS, Steinbrich W (1995) Intracranial arteries: prospective blinded comparative study of MRA and DSA. Radiology 195: 451–456
Takagi R, Hayashi H, Isayama K, Ikeda Y, Teramoto A (1998) 3D CTA of intracranial vasospasm following SAH. Neuroradiology 40: 631–635
Tanaka H, Numaguchi Y, Konno S, Shrir D, Patel U (1997) Initial experience with helical CT and 3D reconstruction in therapeutic planning of cerebral AVMS: comparison with 3D TOF MRA and DSA. J Comput Assist Tomogr 21: 811–817
Tanatani S, Sasaki O, Takeuchi S, Fujii Y, Tanaka R (1997) Detection of delayed cerebral vasospasm after rupture of intracranial aneurysms by MRA. Neurosurgery 40: 748–753
Tetsumlmura A, Yoshino M, Yamada I, Sasaki T (1999) Head and neck haemangiomas: contrast enhanced 3D MRA. Neuroradiology 41: 140–143
Turski P (1993) Magnetic resonance angiography of vascular malformations in clinical magnetic resonance angiography. In: Anderson CM, Edelman RR, Turski PA (eds). Raven Press, New York
Turtz A, Allen D, Koenigsberg R, Goldman H (1995) Non visualisation of a large cerebral aneurysm despite high resolution MRA. J Neurosurg 82: 294–295
Vanninen RL, Hernesniemi JA, Puranen M, Ronkinen A (1996) Magnetic resonance angiographic screening for asymptomatic intracranial aneurysms: the problem of false negatives: technical case report. Neurosurgery 38: 836–841
Velthuis BK, Rankel G, Ramos L, Vandertop W, Van Leeuwen M (1998) Subarachnoid haemorrhage: aneurysm detection and pre-operative evaluation with CTA. Radiology 208: 423–430
Vieco P, Lauren E, Gross C (1996) CT angiography in the examination of patients with aneurysm clips. Am J Neuroradiol 17: 455–457
Wiebers DO (1998) Unruptured intracranial aneurysms – risk of rupture and risks of surgical intervention. New Engl J Med 339: 1725–1733
Wiebers DO, Torner JC, Meissner I (1992) Impact of unruptured intracranial aneurysms on public health in the United States. Stroke 23: 1416–1419
Zouaoui A, Sahel M, Marro B, Clemenceau S, Dargent N, Marsault C (1997) 3D computed telegraphic angiography in detection of cerebral aneurysms in acute subarachnoid haemorrhage. Neurosurgery 41: 125–130

13 Role of Extracranial CT and MR Angiography

ANDREW G. CLIFTON

CONTENTS

13.1 Introduction

Angiography, either conventional catheter angiography or non-invasive techniques such as CT and MR angiography and ultrasound, is used for the investigation of arterial and venous pathology in the neck. Its primary use is for the evaluation of the presence and severity of carotid stenosis. Other conditions such as vertebral artery stenosis and occlusion, carotid and vertebral artery dissection and fibromuscular dysplasia are less common but easily detectable with conventional angiography and, as will be discussed below, are becoming increasingly reliably evaluated by non-invasive imaging.

13.2 Carotid Artery Disease

13.2.1 Conventional Angiography

The ideal investigation is non-invasive, has no morbidity, is of low cost and has a high sensitivity and specificity. All non-invasive tests strive to achieve this ideal. Conventional angiography, the gold standard, is invasive and has morbidity. Complications/morbidity include the following:

1. Local at the puncture site: complications are related to catheter size and repeated punctures, with a low incidence of complications in angiograms performed by neuroradiologists due to the use of increasingly small catheters (4 and 5 French) and good haemostasis. Less careful workers using larger catheters have a higher rate of haematoma and pseudoaneurysm formation (PRYOR et al. 1996).
2. Systemic complications: contrast reactions are much less common with isotonic non-ionic contrast and with the use of steroids in allergic subjects.
3. Neurological transient global amnesia, cortical blindness, confusional states and dementia: these occur rarely and are possibly due to contrast toxicity or secondary to microscopic air emboli. This has been studied in humans and sheep with transcranial Doppler. The number of emboli is reduced if the contrast is allowed to stand (MARKUS et al. 1993).
4. Stroke: there are variable rates reported in the literature. Conventional angiography is relatively safe in patients without atherosclerotic disease. BERENSTEIN reports that in the 4 years from 1992 to 1995, in 1802 angiograms, complications occurred in four procedures, three with temporary neurological deficit (0.17%) and one permanent neurological deficit (0.05%) (PRYOR et al. 1996). Our own audit of 100 consecutive patients showed no neurological deficit (CLIFTON 1999).

There are two studies looking at patients with cerebrovascular disease:

1. THE ASYMPTOMATIC CAROTID ATHEROSCLEROSIS STUDY (ACAS) (EXECUTIVE COMMITTEE FOR ASYMPTOMATIC CAROTID ATHEROSCLEROSIS STUDY 1995) reports the combined complication rate for carotid endarterectomy and angiography

A.G. CLIFTON, MD
Consultant Neuroradiologist, Atkinson Morley's Hospital, Copse Hill, Wimbledon, London, SW20 0NE, UK

was 2.3% at 30 days, with 1.2% angiographic strokes. This is in asymptomatic patients.

2. Heiserman et al. report a 1.6% stroke rate in patients undergoing angiography following stroke or TIA (Heiserman et al. 1994). This is significant morbidity. The risk is higher in older patients, hypertensives, diabetics, smokers and patients with tortuous vessels. It is also higher with longer examination times. This is precisely the group of patients who are likely to be undergoing investigation for carotid artery stenosis.

13.2.2 Why the Need for Non-invasive Imaging?

The majority of patients being investigated are those with carotid stenosis. Severe atherosclerotic stenosis of the carotid artery causes 10% of all ischaemic strokes (Foulkes et al. 1988). Some of these strokes go unheralded but many are preceded by transient ischaemic attack (TIA) or minor stroke. Detection of significant carotid artery stenosis after a TIA or stroke provides the opportunity for specific targeted treatment to prevent further stroke. The risk of stroke following recent symptoms of a TIA is about 8% in the 1st year and then 5% per annum (Dennis et al. 1990), but in medically treated patients with severe carotid stenosis the risk increases by up to 28% over 2 years (Brown and Humphrey 1992). Two large multicentre clinical trials, the European Carotid Surgery Trial (ECST) and the North American Symptomatic Carotid Endarterectomy Trial (NASCET), have convincingly demonstrated that the risks of stroke are significantly reduced by carotid endarterectomy in medically fit patients with recent symptoms from severe carotid stenosis (European Carotid Surgery Trialists Collaborative Group 1998; North American Symptomatic Carotid Endarterectomy Trial Collaborators 1991).

Carotid angioplasty and stenting is an alternative to carotid endarterectomy (Clifton 1998). Recent studies show angioplasty/stenting may have a similar morbidity to conventional endarterectomy. Further trials are under way in the USA. The Carotid Revascularisation Endarterectomy versus Stent Trial (CREST) is about to start in the USA. This is a multi-centre randomised controlled trial to contrast efficacy of carotid artery stenting versus carotid endarterectomy in preventing stroke, myocardial infarction or death during a 30-day peri-procedural period and ipsilateral stroke during a 4-year follow-up in patients with symptomatic extracranial stenosis greater than 70%. A bid for funding by the CAVATAS group for a similar European-based trial is currently (July 1999) being made. If successful, this trial will start in early 2000.

As there is now proven surgical treatment for severe carotid stenosis, an increasing number of patients with TIA or stroke are being investigated. As discussed above, angiography has significant morbidity which is expensive and may require an inpatient stay. A proven non-invasive imaging technique would be the ideal alternative. It is thus imperative that non-invasive techniques are accurate, i.e. have appropriate sensitivity and specificity in detecting surgically significant stenoses. Are we now at a stage where non-invasive studies can replace angiography, either alone or as a combination of two techniques? Our practice at Atkinson Morley's Hospital is to combine screening with ultrasound, followed by magnetic resonance angiography (MRA) if the ultrasound detects a significant stenosis (Fig. 13.1).

Doppler sonography is popular because it is readily available and cheap. One of the main criticisms of the technique, however, is of operator variability and it is important that each operator is validated. Our operators were validated with conventional angiography but in these days of non-invasive imaging, new operators may need to be validated against MRA. Other limitations of Doppler sonography include the inability to view the high cervical carotid, problems with tortuous and heavily calcified vessels and the inability to visualise the distal cervical ICA and the intracranial vasculature, as well as the aortic arch and great vessel origins. Doppler will, however, exclude the 80% of patients with TIAs who do not have carotid stenosis (Sidhu and Allan 1997). A positive study can then be confirmed with an MRA study. The combination of both results has been shown to give sensitivities of 100% and specificities between 90% and 98%, and this is based on data from 1995 and before (De Marco et al. 1996). Further technological improvements in ultrasound and MRI, as discussed below, should improve these figures. If there is discordance between the two tests, conventional angiography is performed. We perform angiography in less than 5% of patients, although other authors report angiography rates of 16%–21% (Patel et al. 1995; Nicholas et al. 1995; Kent et al. 1995). This is too high in our experience and presumably is because advances in technology since 1995 have made MRA more accurate.

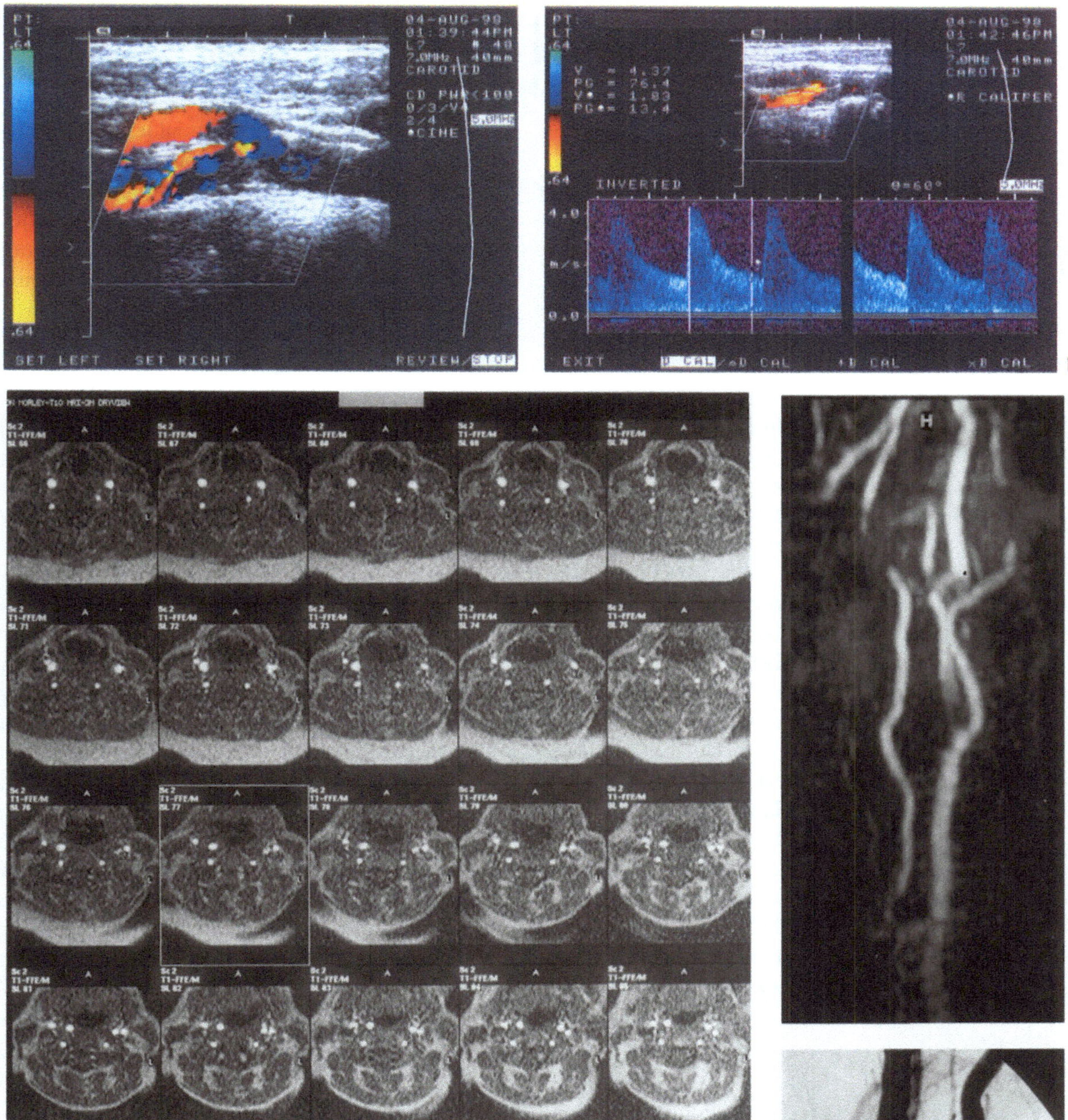

a b c d

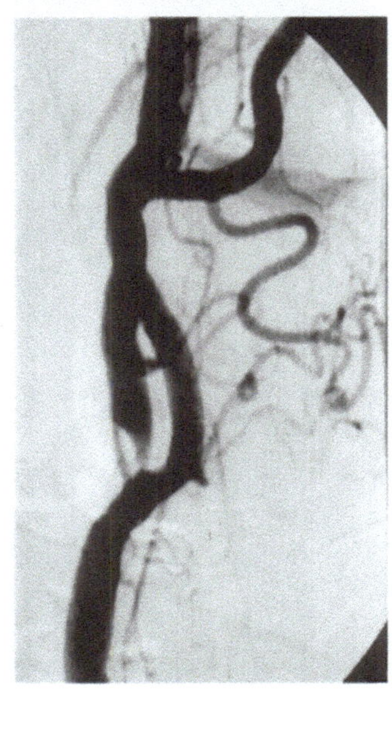

e

Fig. 13.1a–e. Colour duplex ultrasound showing soft plaque and narrowing of the right carotid bifurcation by at least 90% (**a**). Doppler analysis showing peak systolic velocity of over 4 m/s, indicating a stenosis greater than 90% (**b**). MRA 2D time of flight source images showing decrease in signal from the left internal carotid artery just after the bifurcation, consistent with the stenosis (**c**). MIP projection showing tight stenosis to the internal carotid artery origin (**d**). Selective internal carotid artery digital subtraction angiogram, confirming the tight stenosis to the origin of the internal carotid artery. (Angiogram was performed precarotid angioplasty)(**e**)

13.2.3 Magnetic Resonance Angiography: the Advantages and its Pitfalls

1. Plaque morphology: None of the non-invasive forms of imaging are accurate in identifying ulcers or other supposed forms of unstable plaque and indeed there is controversy as to the relationship of plaque morphology to symptoms (Sidhu and Allan 1997; Holdsworth et al. 1995).
2. Overestimation of stenosis and artefacts: Turbulent flow can cause pseudo-stenosis in the normal bulbous bifurcation, and a tight focal stenosis can cause distal turbulence and a large flow gap mimicking a long 2- to 3-cm stenosis (Fig. 13.2). Swallowing or motion can cause severe artefact. Any metal such as clips or a stent can markedly degrade image. As always, review of the source images with the postprocessing images (maximum intensity projection – MIP) is essential.
3. Differentiation of complete occlusion of the ICA from a very severe stenosis or string sign: This is important as a complete occlusion is treated medically but a very severe, greater than 95% stenosis with a string sign is treated surgically (Fig. 13.3). MR angiography is 100% sensitive and specific in differentiating carotid occlusion from a string sign. It is vital, as always, to analyse the source images particularly looking for flow at the skull base and following the signal caudally down to the CCA. It can be easy to confuse the string flow from a very severely stenosed ICA with an ECA branch on the MIP image if it is looked at in isolation (Currie et al. 1994).
4. Tandem lesions and intracranial lesions: There is controversy in the vascular surgical community as to whether it is worth looking for tandem lesions. Many surgeons are happy to operate just using ultrasound or by following a similar protocol to that advocated by our unit, i.e. ultrasound followed by MRA if the ultrasound detects a stenosis. Other surgeons require full conventional angiography, including views of the origins of the great vessels and intracranial circulation. When conventional angiography is used, especially with selective common carotid artery injections, intracranial stenoses are easily and accurately detected. Distal stenoses of the distal cervical ICA are poorly detected using ultrasound, sometimes being suggested by the presence of damped flow at the bifurcation. Intracranial stenoses are not detected by conventional bifurcation ultrasound. There is limited efficacy of detection of some intracranial stenoses, particularly middle cerebral artery stenoses, using transcranial Doppler. Transcranial Doppler is not routinely performed on most patients undergoing screening for carotid stenosis. Some centres do, however, perform cerebral reactivity with carbon dioxide on known stenoses prior to endarterectomy. MRA is relatively sensitive, particularly with severe stenoses. MIP projection should be interpreted with care. Stenoses are often greatly overestimated and tortuous vessels coursing in and out of the scan plane can also suggest stenosis when it is not really there.

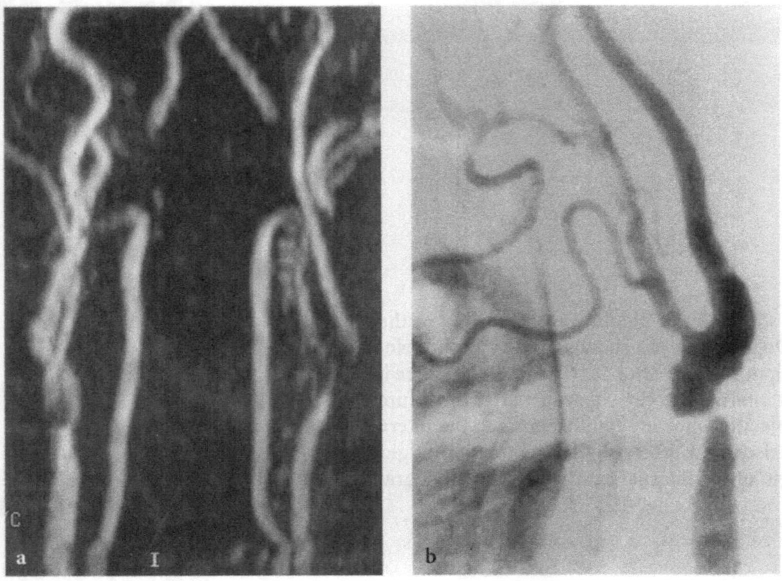

Fig. 13.2a,b. MIP image showing tight stenosis of both internal carotid origins (**a**). *On the left*, the stenosis appears to extend from the distal common carotid into both internal and external carotid arteries. However, this is artefact due to distal turbulence causing a large flow gap. The angiogram, performed pre-angioplasty, showing a very tight focal stenosis of the distal CCA (**b**)

In our experience of several hundred conventional angiograms for carotid bifurcation disease, significant tandem stenosis is rare. We do not routinely image the intracranial circulation with MRA. Similar arguments apply to the origin of the great vessels from the aortic arch, where the incidence of stenoses in this region has been quoted as high as 5% (Brant-Zawadzki 1997). Success in imaging the aortic arch has been poor to date but the newer techniques involving gadolinium-enhanced MR (discussed below) show great promise.

13.2.3.1
Techniques

Until recently, the mainstay of MR angiography has been time of flight or phase contrast angiography. The objective in both techniques is to maximise the signal from rapidly flowing blood and to minimise signal from background stationary tissues. An excellent review of the physics of the two techniques is given by Keller (1996) and by Rosovsky et al. (1996) and this will not be discussed further in detail here.

a b c

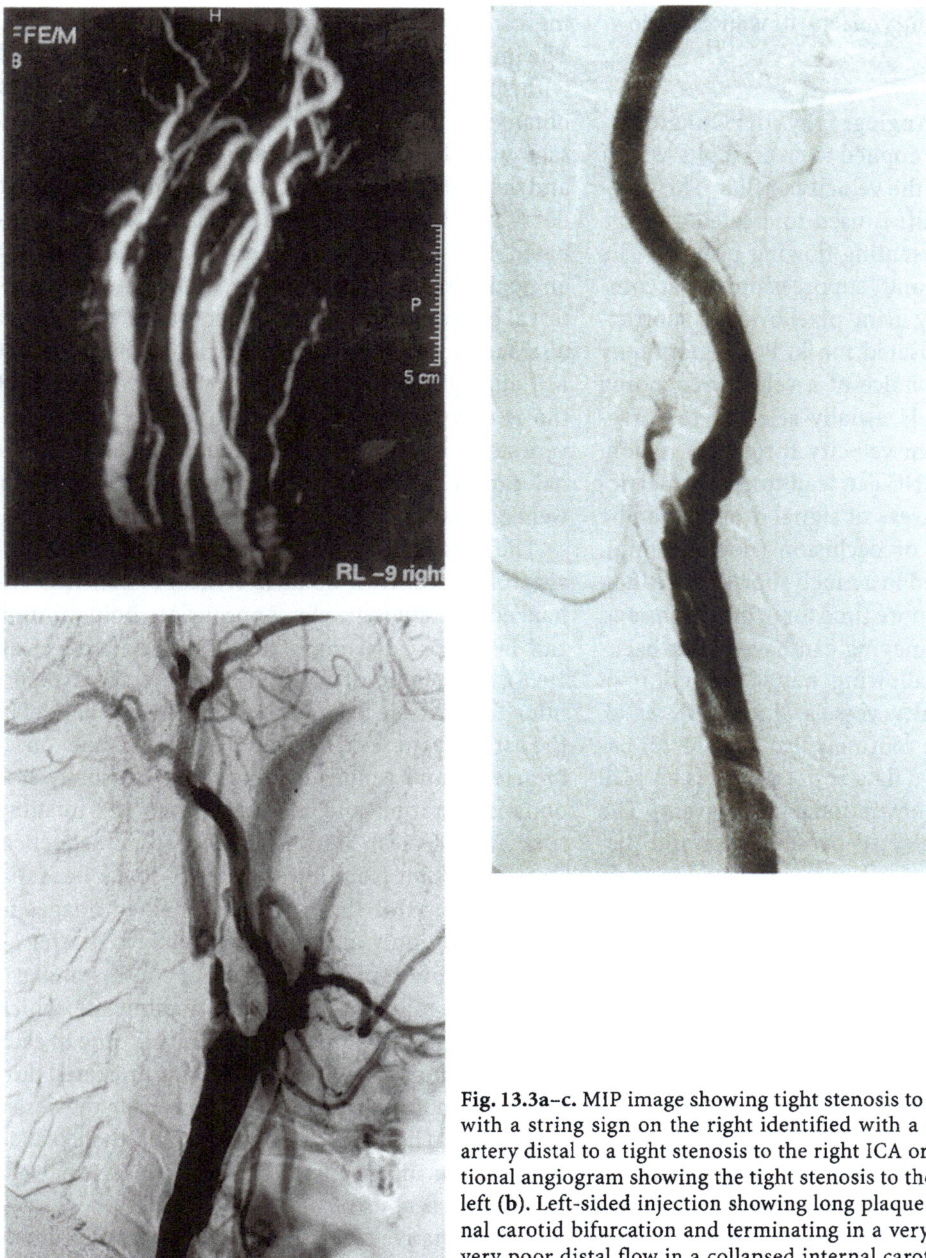

Fig. 13.3a–c. MIP image showing tight stenosis to the origin of the left ECA, with a string sign on the right identified with a collapsed internal carotid artery distal to a tight stenosis to the right ICA origin (**a**). Selective conventional angiogram showing the tight stenosis to the origin of the ECA on the left (**b**). Left-sided injection showing long plaque commencing at the internal carotid bifurcation and terminating in a very tight focal stenosis, with very poor distal flow in a collapsed internal carotid artery distally (**c**)

Time of flight. There are two forms: two dimensional (2D ToF) and three dimensional (3D TOF). In TOF or inflow imaging, the background protons are suppressed and the inflowing protons with full longitudinal magnetisation enter the excitation volume and generate a strong signal. The difference in longitudinal magnetisation between the stationary saturated background tissue and unsaturated incoming blood generates high intensity within vessels, a phenomenon known as flow-related enhancement (Bradley and Waluch 1985; Bradley et al. 1984). In 2D TOF, protons are excited slice by slice, and with 3D TOF, a larger volume is imaged. 2D TOF is most commonly used for carotid imaging due to its superior flow-related enhancement.

Phased Contrast (PC) Angiography. In PC angiography, a magnetic field is applied to create a phase shift that is proportional to the velocity of flow. The magnitude of the phase shift is used to create an image with high signal representing flowing protons. The second step, background suppression, is accomplished mathematically using pixel by pixel subtraction of a flow compensated mask. PC angiography requires the use and choice of a velocity encoding factor (VENC) which is usually selected to correspond to the maximum velocity through a region. Incorrect choice of VENC can lead to errors, particularly aliasing where areas of signal dropout can be mistaken for stenosis or occlusion (flow aliasing). ToF imaging is acquired in a much shorter time than PC imaging, allowing more time for acquisitions and better resolution. PC imaging can have better background suppression, allowing better depiction of slower flow and smaller vessels (Enzmann et al. 1994; Atlas 1994). We routinely use 2D TOF for carotid imaging. The final data is presented as an MIP which looks like a conventional angiogram. The brightest pixels are selected by computer and displayed. The data can be further manipulated to show both carotids and vertebrals or each individual vessel. It is, of course, essential to review the MIP images with the source images, otherwise errors can be made, particularly, as discussed above, in distinguishing occlusion from near occlusion.

Contrast-Enhanced MR Angiography. It is obvious from my discussion above that traditional TOF MR angiography cannot yet replace catheter angiography with two non-invasive tests (either MR then ultrasound or ultrasound then MR) needed and with conventional angiography being required in up to 25% of cases. The next leap forward is gadolinium-enhanced MR angiography. This technique is now available on the latest generation of MR scanners, but will not be widely available in the UK for many years. Contrast-enhanced MR angiography may be the leap forward in eliminating the use of conventional angiography (Rofsky and Adelman 1998; Bowen 1999; Ackerman et al. 1999; Foo et al. 1999) (Fig. 13.4).

Software and hardware development has now reached a stage where gadolinium-enhanced MR is a practical and straightforward technique to use, even in busy units. Remonda et al. elegantly describe the technique and compare first-pass MR angiography with conventional DSA in patients suspected of having carotid artery stenosis (Remonda et al. 1998). The images were acquired without a breath hold and with manual injection of contrast. The 3D images obtained during the arterial phase of the bolus passage were identified by means of visual inspection and that data set was subtracted from the pre-contrast data set, after the background signal of fat was eliminated. MIP images were generated. The time for 3D angiography was only 5–10 min. In their study, the interval between conventional angiography and 3D MR angiography was less than 24 h. Grading of stenoses at MR angiography agreed with that at DSA in 92% of the 44 carotid arteries. In 18 carotid arteries with severe stenosis (70–99%), agreement was 94%. All internal carotid occlusions (n=7) or pseudo-occlusions were accurately detected with MR angiography.

The timing from the start of acquisition to the arrival of the contrast bolus is critical in contrast-enhanced MR angiography. Appropriate bolus timing can be achieved using a timing bolus (Kim et al. 1998). A test bolus of gadolinium is injected to determine transit time from venous injection to arrival in the carotid arteries. The time window between onset of arterial and venous enhancement is usually seconds in duration and is shorter than the imaging time in a typical 3D MR angiographic sequence. Data collection from lower order K space needs to occur during this time window for fined images to demonstrate only arterial enhancement. Kim et al. timed the course of a small bolus of contrast material from the injection site to the imaging site, which provides a good estimate of true transit time in each patient. A small 1- to 2-ml bolus is administered during a fast multiphase 2D acquisition near the vessel of interest. The MR scan operator has then just to identify the image number where the arterial enhancement is at its peak.

An alternative is to use an automated bolus detection and scan-triggering scheme such as SMARTPREP (GE Medical Systems, Milwaukee, Wisconsin,

USA) (Foo et al. 1997; Ho and Foo 1998). Similar systems are available from other manufacturers and are included in the basic package or as an add-on to all current generation MR scanners. The MR SMARTPREP system uses a tracking pulse sequence to continuously monitor the MR signal from the user-prescribed volume of interest. This can be the aortic arch or the common carotid artery. As the signal from this region increases because of the arrival of contrast material in the arteries, the pulse sequence controller checks to see if the signal intensity amplitude threshold values are exceeded. Once the measured signal intensity exceeds the threshold values, the pulse sequence controller automatically begins data acquisition. The advantage of this technique is that it is already readily available and easy to use.

Alternatives to the above 3D techniques in which the acquisition of the centre of the K space is timed to coincide with the arrival of the contrast bolus in the imaging region of interest have been described (Melhem et al. 1999). Melhem et al. describe a technique which allows 3D time-resolved MR angiography with a reduced need for precise timing or the need to account for intravascular transit times of the contrast bolus. Their technique involves obtaining a first-pass contrast bolus tracking 3D MR angiogram, implemented using a single-shot T1 weighted turbo field echo readout technique. The acquisition is modified by a keyhole scheme that improves the temporal resolution in dynamic MR imaging by a factor of 2.2. A full sampling of K space prior to intravenous administration of contrast is followed by truncated sampling limited to the segment of K space sensitive to changes in image contrast (central 46 phase-encoded lines of K space). Optimal visualisation of the contrast bolus is achieved by image subtraction using the first image (full K space sampling) as a reference. They concluded this technique

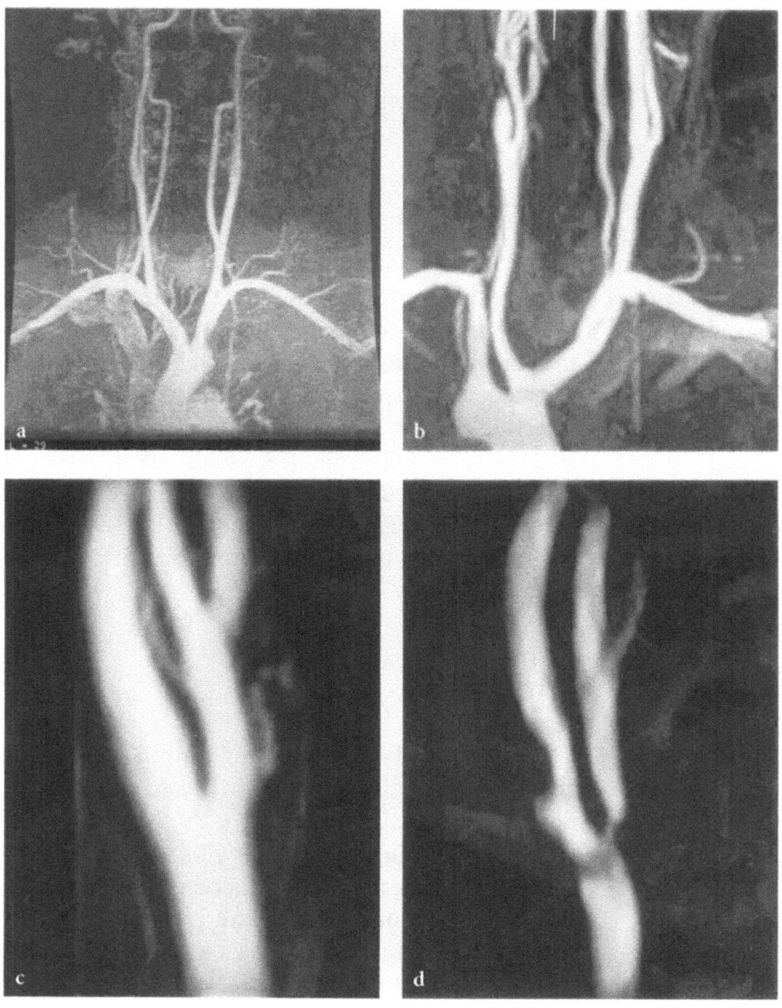

Fig. 13.4a–d. Contrast enhanced (gadolinium) fast gradient echo 3D time of flight imaging, using a neurovascular array coil (anterior element), showing the aortic arch, the origins of both vertebral arteries, and both common internal and external carotid arteries up to the skull base **(a)** (A normal study.) (Courtesy of Dr. S. Halpin, University of Wales). Contrast enhanced (gadolinium) 3D time of flight study showing complete occlusion at the right carotid bifurcation **(b)**. (Courtesy of Professor P. Griffiths, University of Sheffield). Standard gadolinium-enhanced 3D ToF cervical vessels in which the individual carotids have been dissected out and reprojected, showing (this figure) normal left bifurcation **(c)**. (Courtesy of Professor P. Griffiths, University of Sheffield). Same case, right side: there is a moderate stenosis of the right internal carotid artery and a tight stenosis of the external carotid artery. An ulcer cavity is shown on the internal carotid artery and there is some loss of signal at the bifurcation due to turbulent flow **(d)**. (Courtesy of Professor P. Griffiths, University of Sheffield)

could reliably time resolve carotid arteries from jugular veins, and has the potential to more accurately represent vascular luminal narrowing as compared to TOF MR angiography.

Another method that does not rely on the timing of the arrival of the contrast bolus is to use the method proposed by Korosec et al. (1996), the 3D time-resolved imaging of contrast kinetics (3D-TRICKS). This technique produces images of higher spatial resolution. It uses a fast 3D acquisition sequence sampling the central K space more than the outer K space.

13.2.3.2 Postprocessing

Postprocessing packages such as the GE Advantage Navigator for Advantage Workstation bring a new dimension to MR angiography. Endoluminal 3D surface shadow images show endoscopic perspectives based on ray casting algorithms. With the help of a fisheye lens and point-focal light cones, visible images are approached by the user. Through threshold value technology, vessel walls (opaque image elements) become visible. Passing through the lumen is done stage by stage or finally in an automatic cine mode (Fig. 13.5).

13.2.4 CT Angiography

In the UK, CT angiography is not widely used for evaluation of the extracranial carotid vessels. This is in part due to the widespread use and availability of ultrasound and, as discussed above, the widespread

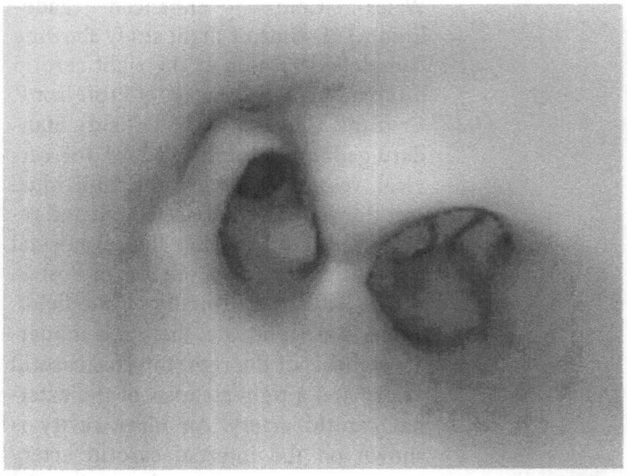

Fig. 13.5. Endoluminal 3D surface shadow imaging showing an endoscopic view of the carotid bifurcation. (Courtesy of Dr. S. Halpin, University of Wales)

acceptance of ultrasound. However, as most departments when installing a new scanner or replacing an existing one almost invariably install a helical scanner, the technique is being used more widely. This is certainly the case where MR angiography is not available on site or has limited availability or is of poor quality.

The advantages of CT as opposed to MR are that it is less claustrophobic and can be used in patients with aneurysm clips (intracranial) or other ferrous metal implants, as well as in patients with cardiac pacemakers. The main disadvantage over MR is the need to inject up to 120 ml of IV contrast through a power injector.

My own view is that CT angiography should not be used as a primary investigation for carotid stenosis but should be used, like MR angiography, to confirm the degree of stenosis detected by ultrasound. The literature comparing CT angiography of the extracranial carotid artery with ultrasound, MR angiography and conventional angiography shows that CT angiography has good sensitivity and specificity in detecting significant stenosis as well as in distinguishing stenosis from occlusion. Sensitivity and specificity has been stated to be at or near 100% (Vieco 1998; Link et al. 1997).

13.2.4.1 Technique

An excellent review of the technical aspects of CT angiography is given by Kuszyk and Fishman (1998). Images are usually obtained from well below the carotid bifurcation to the skull base. Contrast is injected into an antecubital vein using a pressure injection (usually 100 ml non-ionic contrast – we use iohexol 300) at 3–4 ml/s). A small test injection is given whilst scanning at the approximate carotid bifurcation, e.g. at C3/4. The peak of the curve generated indicates the optimal time for acquisition in the diagnostic study.

13.2.4.2 Postprocessing

The most popular methods for carotid studies are shaded surface display (SSD), MIP and volume rendering.

In SSD imaging (Vieco 1998; Kuszyk and Fishman 1998) a threshold is set whereby densities below an arbitrary Hounsfield unit are excluded from the model. The remaining data are viewed as if the surfaces of the model are illuminated from a point source.

MIP imaging is also widely available and evaluates each voxel along a line from the viewer's eye through the image and selects the maximum voxel value as the value of the corresponding display pixel. A disadvantage of the MIP technique is that high density calcification in plaques may obscure the vessel lumen, making stenosis assessment difficult.

A more advanced technique is volume rendering (MARCUS et al. 1999; KUSZYK and FISHMAN 1998). The drawback of this technique has been that it is slow but recent advances in computer hardware have overcome this problem. Volume rendering renders the entire volume of data rather than just surfaces of maximum intensity voxels. The recent paper by MARCUS et al. found that the volume rendering technique (VRT) was valuable for grading carotid arterial stenosis. It also provided excellent visualisation of the lumen in calcified vessels, allowing for accurate assessment of high attenuation circumferential atheromatous plaques. They suggest VRT is used rather than SSD when calcification is seen on the source images, avoiding time consuming segmentation or subtraction.

13.3 Vertebral Artery Disease

One-quarter of all ischaemic strokes occur in the posterior circulation (BAMFORD et al. 1991). Twenty per cent of posterior circulation infarcts are thought to be cardio-embolic in origin and a further 20% due to intra-arterial embolism, usually from the vertebral artery (CAPLAN 1993). In a postmortem study examining the mechanism underlying the occlusion of branches of the posterior circulation, 70% of vertebral and basilar occlusions were related to tight arterial stenoses. Embolism had occurred from a more proximal stenosis in a further 10% (CASTAIGNE et al. 1973). In a more recent series of 35 consecutive patients with occipital infarction, six had vertebral atheroma with presumed distal atheroma (PESSIN et al. 1987). Imaging of the arteries of the posterior circulation is often not considered because of the perception that it will not alter patient management. CRAWLEY et al. looked at 53 patients with conventional vertebral angiography (CRAWLEY et al. 1998b). This was significantly abnormal in 32 patients (60%). Five (9%) had vertebral artery dissections, nine (17%) had unilateral vertebral artery occlusion, two had a basilar artery disease, 16 (30%) had vertebral artery stenosis, 12 stenoses were considered suitable for percutaneous transluminal angioplasty (23%), and 11 patients were anti-coagulated (21%). There was no significant correlation between clinical features, site of infarct or the presence of carotid stenosis that would have allowed the prediction of the findings in the posterior circulation. The results indicated that using vertebral angiography to investigate posterior circulation ischaemia will identify a significant number of potentially treatable lesions.

If an occlusive lesion is found, it may be treatable by angioplasty or stenting (CRAWLEY et al. 1998a) and, in many cases, anti-coagulation is considered.

As discussed above, like carotid angiography, vertebral angiography is not without risk, is invasive and is expensive. A good non-invasive technique is needed. MRA has been reported to be highly sensitive and specific (97% and 98.9% respectively) compared with catheter angiography in identifying stenoses and occlusions in the posterior circulation. The sensitivity of Doppler ultrasound is less (76.4%) but the specificity identical. My own view is that gadolinium enhanced MRA will be the imaging technique of choice but that this will initially have to be validated by comparison with conventional angiography. In our experience, neither MRA nor duplex ultrasound is sufficiently sensitive to stenosis at the origin of the vertebral artery (the commonest site to find lesions suitable for PTA) to be used as a screening procedure at present (Fig. 13.7).

13.4 Other Non-Atheromatous Vascular Diseases in the Neck

These include dissection of the carotid and vertebral arteries, fibromuscular dysplasia, trauma and radiation arteritis (RUSSO et al. 1996).

Dissection. With the advent of MR imaging, this is an increasingly recognised condition. It causes around 2% of all strokes but up to 20% of strokes in younger patients (PROVENZALE 1995). Dissection may be post-traumatic, spontaneous or secondary to conditions such as fibromuscular dysplasia. A dissection is a haemorrhage within the media which narrows or occludes the lumen and may be a source for emboli. MR findings of carotid dissection (usually T1 and T2 axial images, with fat-suppressed images often being useful for confirmation) are usually characteristic, making conventional angiography unnecessary (Fig. 13.8).

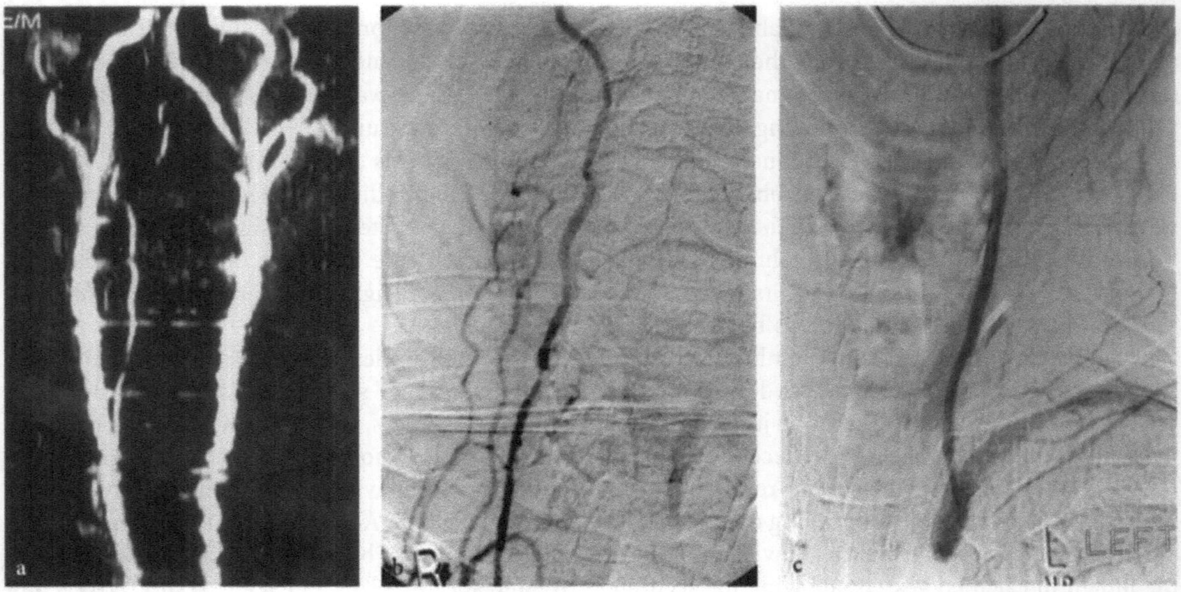

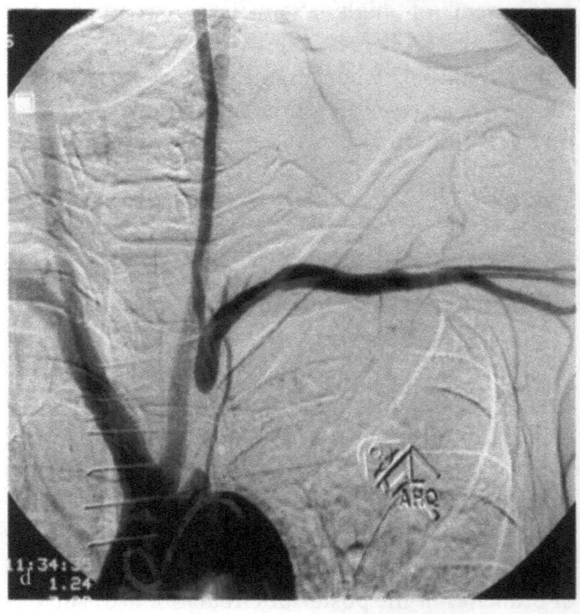

Fig. 13.6a–d. 2D time of flight MIP image of the neck vessels showing cranial flow in the right vertebral with a focal stenosis in the mid-cervical segment (**a**). No flow is seen in the cervical segment of the dominant vertebral on this study. The vertebral origins are not seen clearly on this standard 2D time of flight acquisition. Selective angiography to the right subclavian with views of the right vertebral confirming a tight stenosis to the right cervical segment of the vertebral artery (**b**). Delayed image of an angiogram, obtained from injection of the left common carotid artery, showing retrograde filling of the left vertebral artery which fills in its upper cervical segment via muscular collaterals from the external carotid artery (**c**). Angiogram showing the true anatomy in this case (**d**). Simultaneous injections into the aortic arch and the left subclavian via a brachial approach show total occlusion of the proximal subclavian artery. Due to the poor calibre of the right vertebral artery on angiography, both cranial flow into the distal cervical and intracranial segments of the left vertebral and retrograde flow down the right cervical vertebral artery were from collaterals from the external carotid artery on the left

On MR, the flow void from the narrowed lumen of the ICA is surrounded by a crescent of high signal, i.e. the haematoma. MRA elegantly shows the length of stenosis. Ultrasound can show the intimal flap and evidence of occlusion and differential flows in true and false lumens but has limitations in its ability to view the more distal ICA. There is very limited experience with CT angiography. Our own policy is to perform conventional MR of the brain and neck with MRA, and also to perform duplex ultrasonography. If the diagnosis of dissection is not clear cut, conventional angiography is performed.

Non-invasive imaging is much less sensitive for vertebral dissection, particularly where one vertebral is dominant. As there can be difficulty in distinguishing an atretic vessel from a dissected or occluded vessel on MR and ultrasound, we usually perform angiography.

Fibromuscular dysplasia. Catheter angiography is the imaging method of choice. MR can identify severe lesions but is as yet much less sensitive. MR artefacts may also mimic lesions (Heiserman et al. 1992).

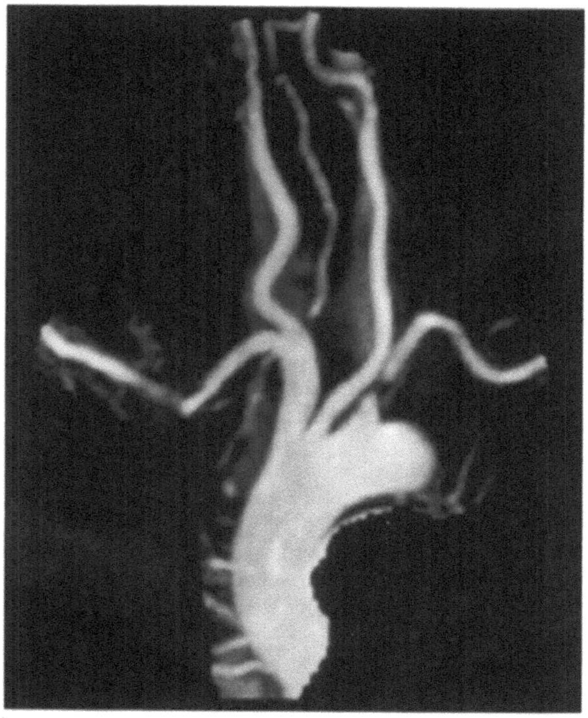

Fig. 13.7. Fast gadolinium image, 3D time of flight, using a neurovascular array coil showing tight stenosis to the proximal left subclavian artery. (This is a different patient from Fig. 13.5.) (Courtesy of Dr. S. Halpin, University of Wales)

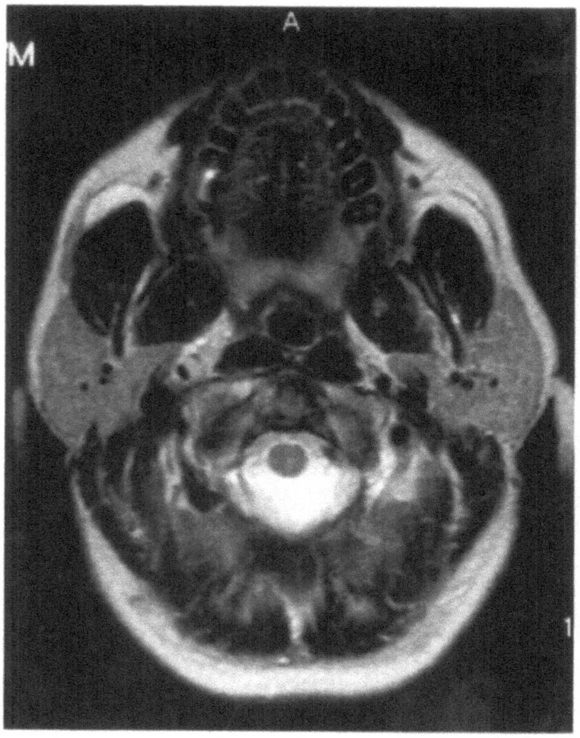

a

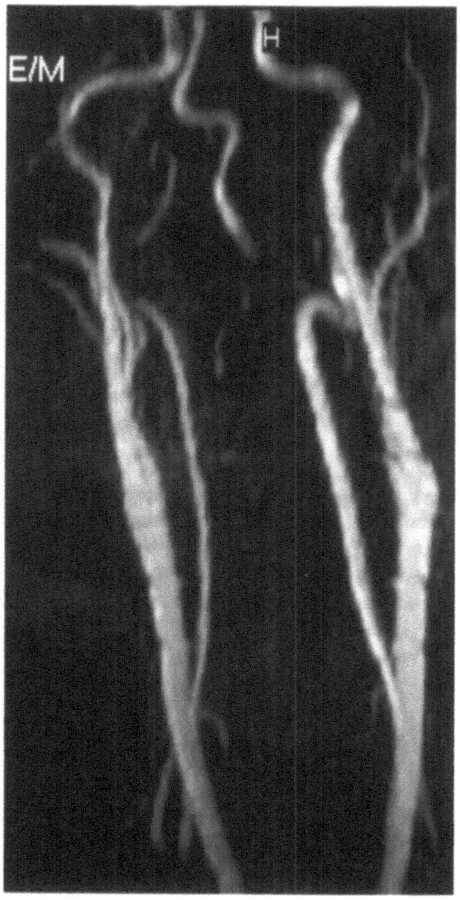

b

Fig. 13.8a,b. Axial T2 weighted image through the skull base showing narrowing of the lumen of the right internal carotid artery with a surrounding crescent of high signal, consistent with the intramural haematoma (**a**). The MRA sequence shows narrowing of the distal cervical carotid at this level as compared to the left (**b**)

References

Ackerman RH, Candia MR, May Z (1999) Editorial: Technical advances and clinical progress in carotid diagnosis. AJNR 20: 187–189

Atlas SW (1994) MR angiography in neurologic disease. Radiology 193: 1–16

Bamford J, Sandercock P, Dennis M et al. (1991) Classification and natural history of clinically identifiable subtypes of cerebral infarction. Lancet 337: 1521–1526

Bowen B (1999) Editorial: The carotid artery through a keyhole. AJNR 20: 186–187

Bradley WG, Waluch V (1985) Blood flow: magnetic resonance imaging. Radiology 154: 443–450

Bradley WG, Waluch V, Lai K et al. (1984) Appearance of rapidly flowing blood on MRI. AJR 143: 1167–1174

Brant-Zawadzki M (1997) The roles of MR angiography, CT angiography and sonography in vascular imaging of the head and neck. AJNR 18: 1820–1825

Brown MM, Humphrey PRD (1992) Carotid endarterectomy, recommendations for management of transient ischaemic attack and ischaemic stroke. BMJ 305: 1071–1074

Caplan LR (1993) Brain embolism revisited. Neurology 43: 1281–1287

Castaigne P, Lhermitte F, Gautier JC et al. (1973) Arterial occlusions in the vertebrobasilar system: a study of 44 patients with post mortem data. Brain 96: 133–154

Clifton AG (1998) Results of CAVATAS study. Presented at WIN, Val d'Isere (January 1998) and BSNR, Cork (October 1998)

Clifton AG (1999) Imaging of the carotid bifurcation. Personal communication/presentation given to the Diagnostic Neuroradiology Forum, Atkinson Morley's Hospital (February 1999)

Crawley F, Brown MM, Clifton AG (1998a) Angioplasty and stenting in the carotid and vertebral arteries. Postgrad Med J 74: 7–10

Crawley F, Clifton A, Brown MM (1998b) Treatable lesions demonstrated on vertebral angiography for posterior circulation ischaemic events. Br J Radiol 71: 1266–1270

Currie IC, Murphy KP, Jones AJ et al. (1994) Magnetic resonance angiography of IADSA for diagnosis of carotid pseudo-occlusion. Eur J Vasc Surg 8: 562–566

De Marco JK, Schonfield S, Wesbey G (1996) Can non-invasive studies replace conventional angiography in the preoperative evaluation of carotid stenosis. Neuroimaging Clin North Am 6: 911–929

Dennis M, Bamford J, Sandercock P et al. (1990) Prognosis of transient ischaemic attacks in the Oxfordshire stroke project. Stroke 21: 848–853

Enzmann DR, Ross MR, Marks M et al. (1994) Blood flow in major cerebral arteries measured by phase contrast angiography. AJNR 15: 123–129

European Carotid Surgery Trialists Collaborative Group (1998) Randomised trial of endarterectomy for recently symptomatic carotid stenosis: final results of the MRC European Carotid Surgery Trial (ECST). Lancet 351: 1379–1387

Executive Committee for the Asymptomatic Carotid Atherosclerosis Study (1995) Endarterectomy for asymptomatic carotid artery stenosis. J Am Med Assoc 273: 1421–1428

Foo TKF, Saranathan M, Prince MK et al. (1997) Automated detection of bolus arrival and initiation of data acquisition in fast, three dimensional, Gadolinium-enhanced angiography. Radiology 203: 275–280

Foo TKF, Ho VB, Choyke PL (1999) Contrast-enhanced carotid MR angiography (imaging principles and physics). Neuroimaging Clin North Am: Fast scan and echo planar MR imaging, 9: 263–284

Foulkes MA, Wolf PA, Price TR et al. (1988) The stroke data bank, design, methods and baseline characteristics. Stroke 19: 547–554

Heiserman JE, Drayer BP, Frake EK et al. (1992) MR angiography of cervical fibromuscular dysplasia. AJNR 13: 1454–1451

Heiserman JE, Dean BL, Hodak JA et al. (1994) Neurological complications of cerebral angiography. Am J Neuroradiol 15: 1401–1407

Holdsworth RJ, McCallum PT, Bryce JS et al. (1995) Symptoms, stenosis and carotid plaque morphology: is plaque morphology relevant? Eur J Vasc Surg 9: 80–85

Ho VB, Foo TKF (1998) Optimisation of Gadolinium-enhanced magnetic resonance angiography using an automated bolus detection algorithm (MR SMARTPREP). Invest Radiol 33: 515–523

Keller PJ (1996) Magnetic resonance angiography of the neck: technical issues. Neuroimaging Clin North Am (Imaging of carotid artery disease) 6: 853–861

Kent KC, Kuntz KM, Patel MR et al. (1995) Peri-operative imaging strategies for carotid endarterectomy: an analysis of morbidity and cost effectiveness in symptomatic patients. JAMA 274: 888–893

Kim JK, Farb R, Wright GA (1998) Test bolus examination in the carotid artery at dynamic Gadolinium-enhanced MR angiography. Radiology 206: 283–289

Korosec FR, Frague R, Grist TM et al. (1996) Time-resolved contrast enhanced 3D MR angiography. Magn Reson Med 36: 345–351

Kuszyk BS, Fishman EK (1998) Technical aspects of CT angiography. Semin Ultrasound CT MRI 19: 383–393

Link J, Brossman J, Penselin V et al. (1997) Common carotid artery bifurcation: preliminary results of CT angiography and color-coded duplex sonography compared with digital subtraction angiography. Am J Roentgenol 168: 361–365

Marcus C, Ladam-Marcus VJ, Bigot J-L et al. (1999) Carotid arterial stenosis, evaluation at CT angiography with the volume-rendering technique. Radiology 211: 775–780

Markus H, Loh A, Israel D et al. (1993) Microscopic air embolization during cerebral angiography and strategies for its removal. Lancet 341: 784–787

Melhem ER, Caruthers SD, Faddoul SG et al. (1999) Use of 3D MR angiography for tracking a contrast bolus in the carotid artery. AJNR 20: 263–266

Nicholas GG, Osborne AM, Jaffe JW et al. (1995) Carotid artery stenosis: pre-operative non-invasive evaluation in a community hospital. J Vasc Surg 22: 9–16

North American Symptomatic Carotid Endarterectomy Trial Collaborators (1991) Beneficial effects of carotid endarterectomy in symptomatic patients with high grade stenoses. N Eng J Med 325: 445–453

Patel MR, Kuntz KM, Klufas RA et al. (1995) Pre-operative assessment of the carotid bifurcation. Can magnetic resonance angiography and duplex ultrasonography replace contrast arteriography. Stroke 26: 1753–1758

Pessin MS, Lathi ES, Cohen MB et al. (1987) Clinical features and mechanisms of occipital infarction. Ann Neurol 21: 290–299
Provenzale JM (1995) Dissection of the internal carotid and vertebral arteries: imaging features. Am J Roentgenol 165: 1099–1104
Pryor JC, Setton A, Nelson PK et al. (1996) Complications of diagnostic cerebral angiography and tips on its avoidance. Neuroimaging Clin North Am (Cerebral angiography) 6: 751–758
Remonda L, Heed O, Silroth G (1998) Carotid artery stenosis, occlusion and pseudo-occlusion: first-pass Gadolinium-enhanced, three dimensional MR angiography – preliminary study. Radiology 209: 95–102
Rofsky NM, Adelman MA (1998) Gadolinium-enhanced MR angiography of the carotid arteries: a small step, a giant leap. Radiology 209: 31–34
Rosovsky MA, Litt AW, Krinsky MD (1996) Magnetic resonance carotid angiography of the neck (clinical implications). Neuroimaging Clin North Am (Imaging of carotid artery disease) 6: 863–874
Russo CP, Smoker WRK (1996) Non-atheromatous carotid artery disease. Neuroimaging Clin North Am 6: 811–830
Sidhu PS, Allan PL (1997) Review II: Ultrasound assessment of internal carotid artery stenosis. Clin Radiol 52: 654–658
Vieco PT (1998) CT angiography of the carotid artery. Neuroimaging Clin North Am 8: 593–605

14 MR Imaging Strategies in Epilepsy

ERIC ACHTEN

CONTENTS

14.1 Introduction

14.1.1 Definition

Epilepsy is one of the most common neurological diseases. Epileptic seizures (ENGEL 1989) may occur as a result of intercurrent events such as fever, hypoglycemia, acute central nervous system infections and the like, and are then termed occasional seizures. When they recur spontaneously without known cause, they constitute epilepsy. "Epilepsy" is a chronic condition in which occasional seizures tend to occur repeatedly as a result of either structural brain damage or of an intrinsic functional propensity to have seizures.

A classification of epileptic seizures has been adopted by the International League Against Epilepsy (ILAE) based on the distinction between partial seizures, in which the first electrophysiological and clinical symptoms indicate activation of a small part of a single hemisphere, and generalized seizures, in which the first electroclinical changes indicate involvement of both hemispheres (COMMISSION ON CLASSIFICATION AND TERMINOLOGY OF THE INTERNATIONAL LEAGUE AGAINST EPILEPSY 1981). When partial seizures occur without altered consciousness they are termed simple partial seizures (SPS); otherwise they are termed complex partial seizures (CPE).

E. ACHTEN, MD, PhD
MR Department, University Hospital Gent, De Pintelaan 185, 9000 Gent, Belgium

14.1.2 Pathology

The pathology of epilepsy is extremely diverse and seizures may occur in patients with almost any pathological process: brain malformations, tumors (Fig. 14.1), acquired traumatic lesions (Fig. 14.2) and vascular lesions. Table 14.1 lists the most important brain disorders that may be amenable with surgical intervention. Mesial temporal sclerosis with damage to the hippocampus, glial scarring and atrophy is a well recognized entity that may result from prolonged febrile seizures or convulsive status epilepticus and accompanying systemic disturbances (hypotension, fever, hypoglycemia, etc.) (BABB et al. 1993). This entity is often the substrate of temporal lobe epilepsy (TLE). TLE is the dominant form of com-

Table 14.1. Disorders that may be treatable by surgery

Genetic and developmental disorders
Sturge-Weber-Dimitri syndrome
Neurofibromatosis
Tuberous sclerosis
Congenital porencephalic cyst
Congenital tumor
Neuronal migration disorders: cortical dysplasias, hemimegalencephaly, etc.
Acquired disorders
Rasmussen's encephalitis
Tumor: primary and metastasis
Infectious lesions: meningitis, abscess, encephalitis
Subarachnoid hemorrhage
Stroke
Trauma
Mesial temporal sclerosis

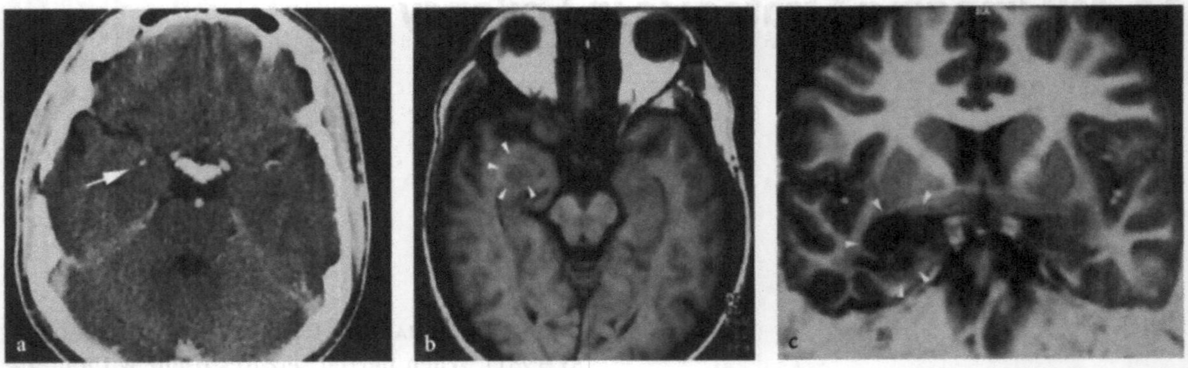

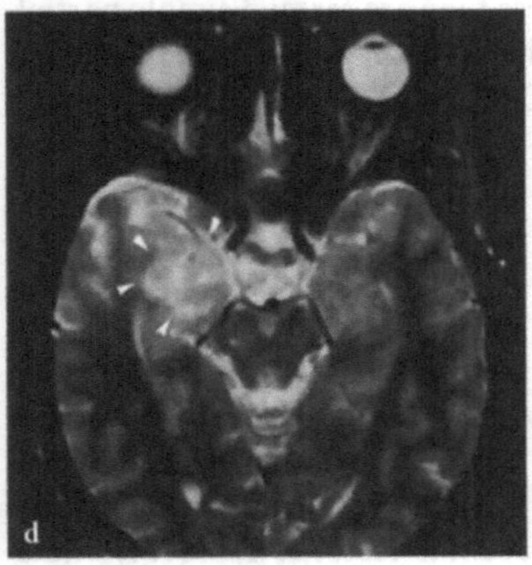

Fig. 14.1a–d. CT and MR exam of a patient with recent onset complex partial epilepsy (CPE). The images were taken after a second seizure. The only abnormality visible on the CT study (**a**) is the small punctate calcification (*arrow*) in the right amygdala region. T1 W (**b**) and T2 W (**c**) spin-echo images make finding the small low grade glioma in the right amygdala much easier (*arrowheads*). The coronal T1 W inversion recovery image (**d**) yielded the highest contrast and facilitated dose calculations for brachytherapy

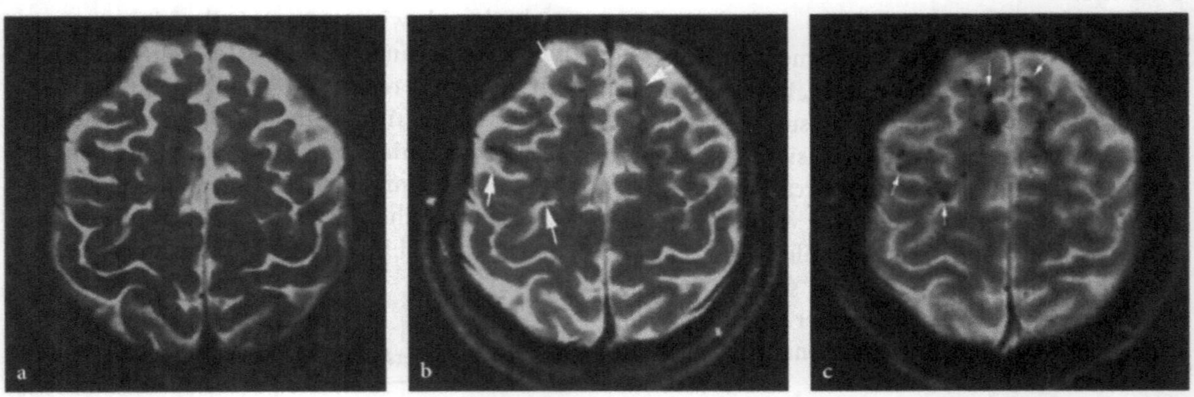

Fig. 14.2a–c. Subject with CPE of the frontal type. The hemosiderin deposits (*arrows*) are not at all visible on the turbo-T2 W image (**a**). SE T2 W images (**b**) are more sensitive and, in this case, because a closed head trauma was in the personal history of this patient, gradient-echo T2*W images (**c**) were also acquired because they are most sensitive for hemosiderin

plex partial epilepsy and accounts for 70% or more (see below).

Cortical dysplasias (Fig. 14.3) are not specific for epilepsy but are more often seen in epileptic brains. The more marked abnormalities include migration disorders which can be diffuse (from lissencephaly to laminar subcortical heterotopias) or focal (hemimegencephaly, bilateral opercular polymicrogyria, focal dysplasias).

14.2 Neuroimaging

14.2.1 Occasional Seizures

Occasional seizures are rather frequent. About 5–10% of the population will have an epileptic seizure during their life time (Berg et al. 1996). Although in

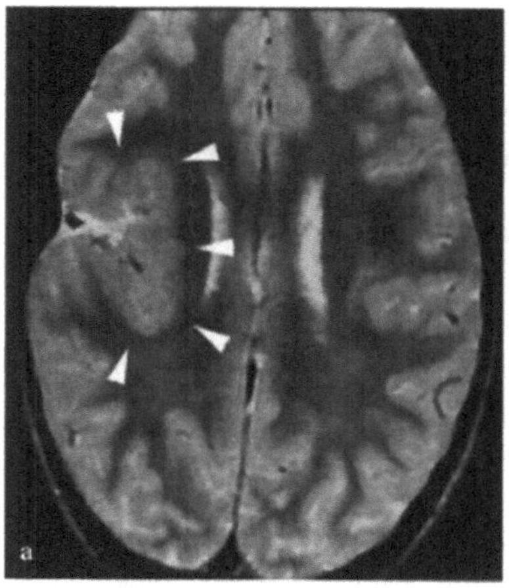
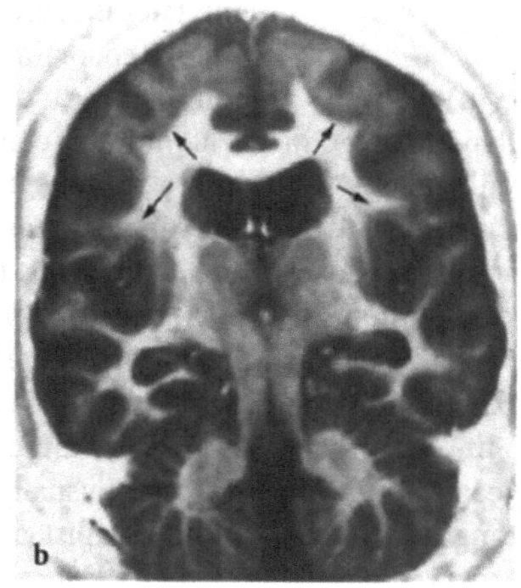

Fig. 14.3a,b. Patients with cortical dysplasias often suffer from seizures. MR is currently the best imaging technique to find such abnormalities in the brain. The T2 W image on the left (**a**) shows a focal area of polymicrogyria in the right suprarolandic area (*arrowheads*). *On the right* (**b**) is a coronal T1 W inversion recovery image through the brain of a young female patient with mental retardation and epilepsy. A distinct subcortical band of abnormally migrated neural tissue is clearly seen (*arrows*) in this case of band heterotopia

many instances this is a single event, many of these patients will be referred for neuroimaging. Imaging guidelines here depend on the age of the patient and the clinical and paraclinical findings.

Children and young adults with one occasional seizure, a negative history, and no paraclinical abnormalities can be screened using standard MR imaging, but the yield is rather poor. Standard brain screening with MR in our department consists of standard spin-echo (SE) proton-density (PD), T2-weighted (T2 W) and T1-weighted (T1 W) images followed by a set of coronal fast- or turbo-T2 W and sagittal SE T1 W images. Occasionally a lesion will be found and appropriate action can be taken (Fig. 14.4). Patients with a medical history of trauma also have to be screened for hemosiderin deposits using a gradient-echo T2*-weighted sequence.

When seizures recur, imaging is definitely indicated. MR imaging with the "as required" use of intravenous gadolinium will rule out pathology that may be treatable by surgery. The use of gadolinium for epilepsy referrals is controversial (Sanders et al. 1995) and is best guided by the findings on axial and coronal T2 W images. I would recommend the use of intravenous contrast in patients with a strong suspicion of infectious or metastatic disease even when the axial T2 W and T1 W screening is negative. Patients over age 55 years are also screened with the use of intravenous gadolinium to rule out possible metastasis. In such cases, a screening exam is performed and after gadolinium administration the axial T1 W images are repeated. If any lesion enhances, additional T1 W images are acquired with different orientation.

Patients with persistent neurological deficits or altered mental status after acute seizure activity will often also be referred for imaging. Here focal gyral swelling and contrast enhancement are frequent findings. The differential diagnosis should include postictal change, reversible ischemia, complicated migraine and resolved inflammation of infection (Silverstein and Alexander 1998).

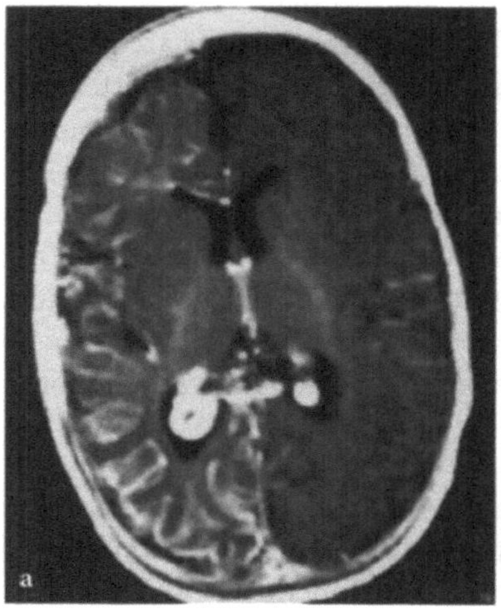
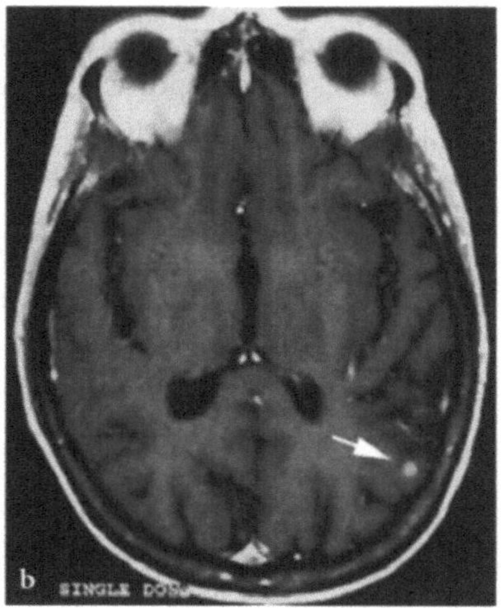

Fig. 14.4a,b. Although gadolinium is seldom used to screen patients with epilepsy, it is mandatory in specific situations. Some examples: *on the left* (**a**) an axial T1 W image in a patient with Sturge Weber syndrome. *On the right* (**b**), a patient with a breast malignancy and recent onset epilepsy. The solitary small subcortical metastasis in the left supramarginal region was only visible after gadolinium administration (*arrow*)

14.2.2 Chronic Generalized Epilepsy

Patients with chronic generalized epilepsy or certain epileptic syndromes with generalized seizures can seldom be helped with a surgical intervention (PHILLIPS and SAKAS 1996). A partial or complete callosotomy is about the only thing that can be done to diminish the spread of epileptic discharges. This usually reduces the severity of the seizures, improves the quality of life and diminishes the secondary damage to the brain. Neuroimaging can help in the preoperative planning of the callosotomy and can be useful in checking the result after surgery.

Nevertheless, every individual developing what might be considered seizures should have an MR screening exam to rule out pathology amenable for treatment.

Some lesions on imaging studies found in chronic epilepsy patients are probably due to antiepileptic drug toxicity. This was described by KIM et al. (1999). These authors found discrete, focal, ovoid, nonhemorrhagic lesions in the splenium of the corpus callosum of six patients with chronic epilepsy and inferred that these lesions represented reversible demyelination related to antiepileptic drug toxicity.

14.2.3 Complex Partial Epilepsy

According to the literature, about 25% of epilepsy patients will become refractory to medical treatment (WARD 1983) and for those with partial seizures, surgery is an effective alternative treatment (ENGEL 1989). The role of neuroimaging becomes very important here for the determination of the actual site of epileptic origin. This includes the identification of lesions that may be amenable for tailored resection, the objectivation of lateralization in TLE by detecting lateralized damage to the hippocampus or temporal neocortical regions, and the detection of often microscopic cortical abnormalities in case of extratemporal complex partial epilepsy (ETLE). We also would like to establish the relationship between the seizure focus and eloquent cortex when resection in such regions is mandatory.

Macroscopic lesions amenable for tailored resection in any part of the brain are easily detected with MR imaging (with or without the administration of intravenous gadolinium) and a reasonable differential diagnosis can usually be proposed. The surgeon or radiotherapist also needs accurate information concerning the localization of the lesion. MR imaging can also be used to guide a stereotactic approach for biopsy and microscopic resection (PANNEK and OPPEL 1999).

When no macroscopic lesions are found in a chronic partial epilepsy patient refractory to medical treatment, he or she becomes a candidate for "epilepsy surgery." This is the surgical removal of the seizure focus. The patient is then entered in an extensive presurgical evaluation program including: neurological exam, interictal scalp EEG, video-EEG monitoring (BOON et al. 1994) neuropsychological testing (JONES-GOTMAN et al. 1993), neuroimaging (ACHTEN et al. 1995), metabolic mapping (HENRY et al. 1993) and MR spectroscopy (ACHTEN et al. 1997) in order to localize and lateralize the initial seizure activity. In a joint setting, the results of all of these tests are discussed to reach a consensus as to where the seizure activity originates. When a consensus is reached as a result of congruent findings of the non-invasive test battery, the patient can go to surgery when the results of the WADA test (IAP or intracarotid amythal procedure) are acceptable (RAUSCH et al. 1993). In the case of TLE as a result of mesiotemporal sclerosis, a modified anterior temporal lobectomy and partial hippocampectomy is performed (FRIED et al. 1993). In more difficult cases where conflicting results of the non-invasive tests are present, depth electrode studies will have to be performed (SPENCER 1991). The aims of improving non-invasive localization of the seizure focus are:

1. To diminish the use of DE studies
2. To diminish the number of cases where doubt remains as a result of non-conclusive presurgical evaluation
3. To diminish possible postoperative functional deficits

Magnetic resonance imaging (BRONEN et al. 1991; JACK et al.1992; JACKSON et al. 1993, 1994; MEINERS et al. 1999) (anatomical and functional) and possibly

Table 14.2. Generalized epilepsy: disorders and syndromes (not exhaustive) (Lechtenberg 1998)

Juvenile myoclonic epilepsy
Childhood absence epilepsy
Juvenile absence epilepsy
West's syndrome
Lennox-Gastaut syndrome
Benign familial neonatal convulsions
Benign (rolandic) epilepsy of childhood
Early myoclonic encephalopathy
Severe myoclonic epilepsy of childhood
Myoclonic epilepsy of Unverricht-Lunborg type

magnetic resonance spectroscopy (Matthews et al. 1990; Connelly et al. 1994; Gadian et al. 1994; Giroud et al. 1994; Woermann et al. 1999) play a key role in the preoperative management of such patients.

14.2.3.1
Temporal lobe epilepsy (TLE)

As many as 70% of the patients with CPE refractory to medical treatment have temporal lobe epilepsy. The main purpose of MR examinations here is to detect hippocampal damage with high sensitivity and specificity. Three important features are characteristic of hippocampal damage: decreased volume, signal changes and structural changes (Achten et al. 1995). Structural changes are often associated with extensive gliosis and this will also cause signal changes on T2 W and T1 W images. From pathological studies, we know that volume loss and gliotic changes often extend beyond the hippocampus into the adjacent temporal lobe (Henry et al. 1993).

We tested all of the available techniques that were currently used for this purpose in 1991. Tilted coronal T1WIR images were more sensitive for detecting hippocampal pathology than T2 W coronal imaging, volume measurements and T2 mapping (Achten et al. 1995). T1WIR images have a very high gray-white matter contrast and excellent signal to noise. Therefore, the internal hippocampal microarchitecture (Fig. 14.5) can be seen. The visibility of this microstructure is canceled when gliosis is present (Fig. 14.6). When this is the only abnormality present, we have termed this minimal structural loss (MSL). In patients with TLE, these gliotic changes are often present. This study resulted in a decision tree for the localization and lateralization of hippocampal damage in patients with TLE (Fig. 14.7).

The detection of the internal structure of the hippocampus is probably also possible with the use of very high resolution fast-spin-echo sequences (using 512 matrices and high S/N). The use of a true inversion recovery sequence was inspired by the fact that these real-part phase corrected images better depict the very small anatomical details of the hippocampus than the modulus images of normal sequences.

In one of our studies, we found MSL as seen on T1WIR images a very sensitive marker for hippocampal gliosis, but that minimal gliosis does not always lead to seizures (Achten et al. 1995). Indeed, disruption of the internal morphology of the hippocampus on paracoronal T1WIR images was the only qualitative abnormality found in four of our patients but one subject with MSL associated with a parahippocampal hamartoma on the ipsilateral side remains seizure free after tumor removal; the HC was left untouched (Fig. 14.8). Two other patients were consistently lateralized with MSL as the only abnormality; one had surgery and remains seizure free. MSL was also present in the contralateral non-epileptic hippocampus of two patients with lateralized TLE, one with a mass lesion. In these, all imaging sequences demonstrated more severe pathology in the hippocampus on the side of epileptic activity. The HC ipsilateral to the EEG focus has been removed, and they remain seizure free. The association of hippocampal damage when foreign tis-

a 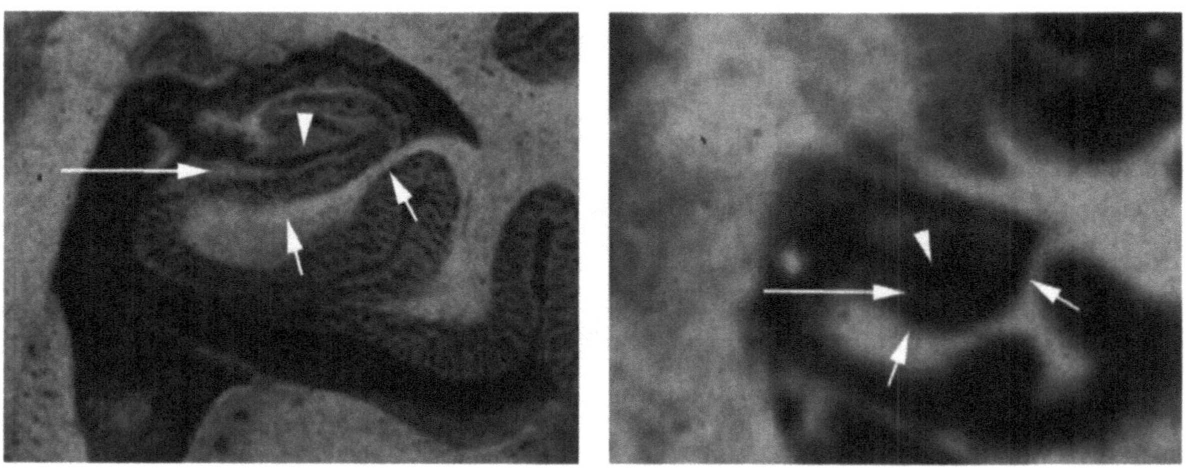 b

Fig. 14.5a,b. The power of inversion recovery T1 W images. *On the left* (**a**) an anatomical slice through the body of the left hippocampus and mesiotemporal region, *on the right* a corresponding T1 W inversion recovery image (**b**). The microarchitecture of the hippocampus can easily be recognized: cornu Ammonis (*arrows*) and dentate gyrus (*arrowhead*) mainly contain neurons and have gray matter signal. In between is a layer of white matter tracts (*long arrow*)

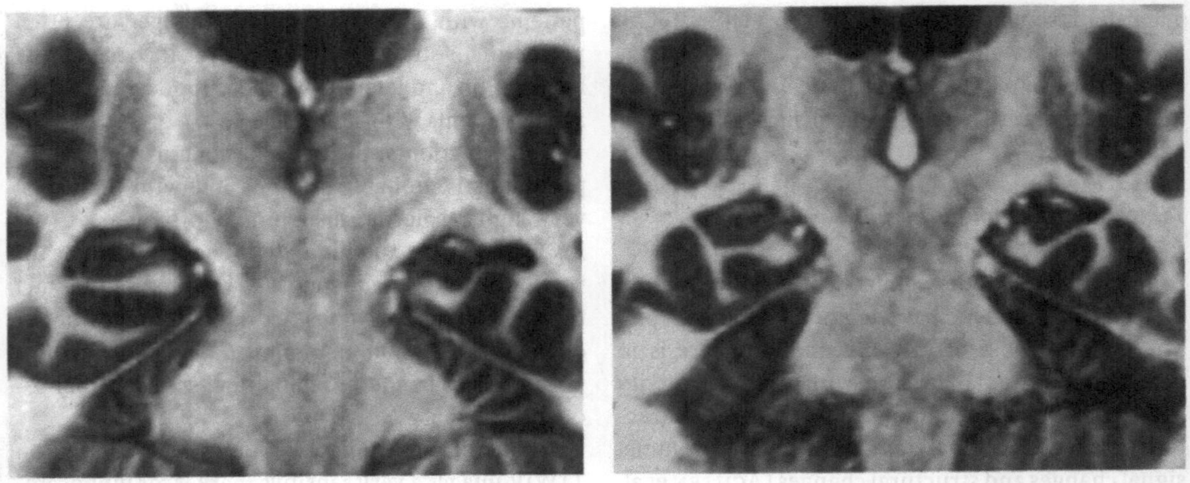

a b

Fig. 14.6a,b. Two examples of a damaged left hippocampus. *On the left* (**a**) a patient with classical imaging findings in hippocampal sclerosis: volume loss, decreased signal and effacement of the internal structure. *On the right* (**b**) a patient with only minimal structural loss (MSL), a more subtle form of hippocampal damage (see text). Note the well preserved internal architecture in the right hippocampus

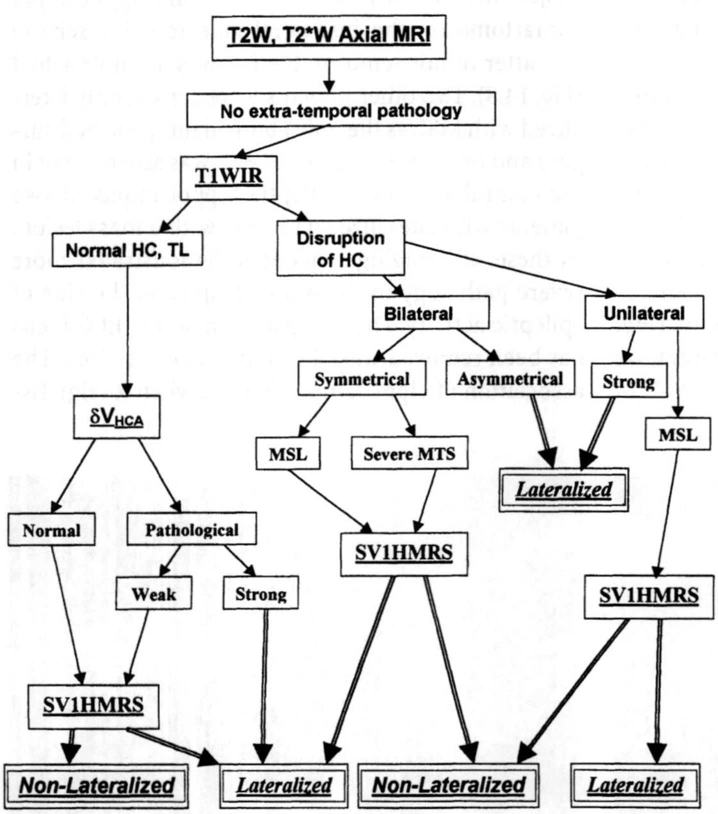

Fig. 14.7. Flow chart for MR in temporal lobe epilepsy (TLE) [*T1WIR* T1 W inversion recovery sequences, *HC* hippocampus, *TL* temporal lobe, *MSL* minimal structural loss, *MTS* mesial temporal sclerosis, *δ* VHCA left-to-right volume difference for hippocampus and amygdala together, *weak* beyond normal range (5–10%), *strong* beyond weak, *SV1HMRS* single voxel proton magnetic resonance spectroscopy]

sue lesions are present probably means that hippocampal scarring (ipsi- and/or contralateral) results from long-standing epilepsy. It remains to be proven if this is related to the frequency of secondary generalized seizures.

T2-mapping was not very sensitive in our study in depicting HC pathology. This technique continues to be used with success though (Jackson et al. 1993). Its use has been advocated to detect bilateral hippocampal abnormalities. We did not find elevated T2

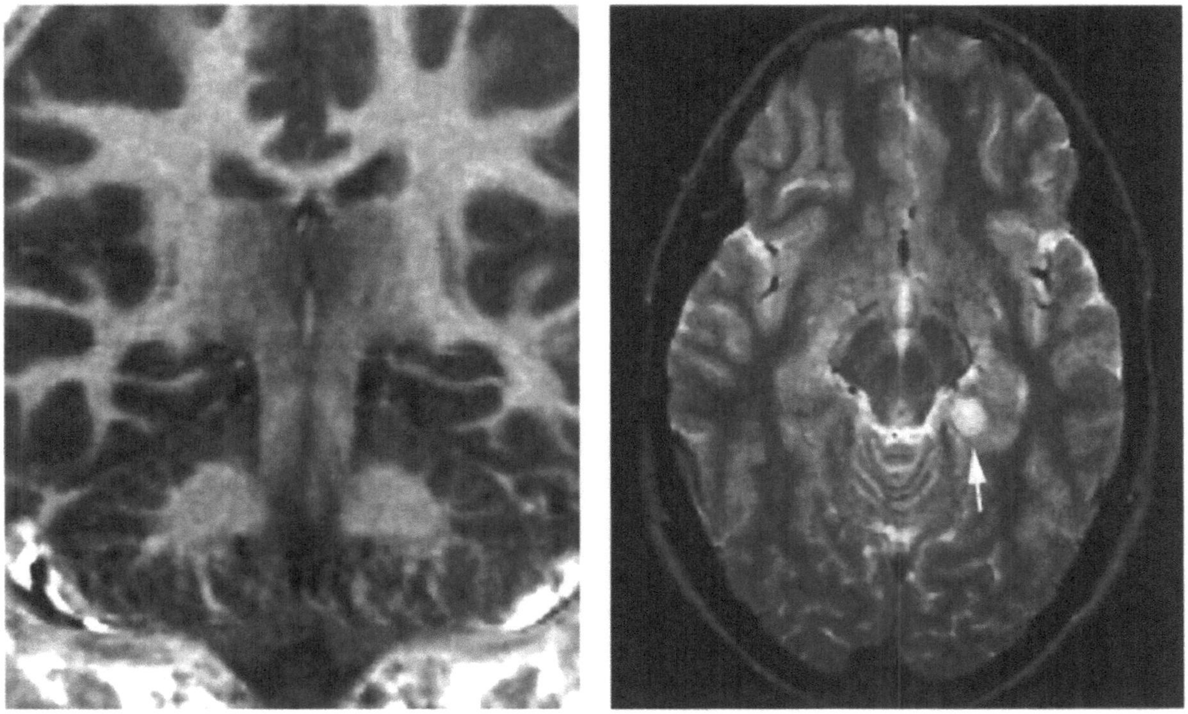

Fig. 14.8a,b. MSL in this patient's left hippocampus (shown on T1 W inversion recovery in **a** probably resulted from epilepsy that was caused by a parahippocampal hamartoma (*arrow in* **b**). The patient became seizure free after surgical removal of this hamartoma. The hippocampus was left untouched. The significance is that when unilateral MSL is the sole finding in a TLE patient, this has to be corroborated by other tests like spectroscopy or PET (see flowchart, Fig. 14.7)

values when T2 W images did not reveal a high signal, and T2 W image inspection was less sensitive than T1WIR imaging. An explanation could be that multislice techniques give less reproducible results than single slice techniques (GRÜNEWALD et al. 1994). The use of a multislice technique was inspired by the fact that we did not want to miss focal hippocampal pathology. Nevertheless, we feel that in our hands this technique does not give information that cannot be acquired with other sequences. On the other hand, we use MR spectroscopy to find bilateral temporal lobe abnormalities (see below).

Volume measurements remain important for quantitative control. When an intact hippocampal structure is shown by the T1WIR images, a clear pathological volume measurement could be the signature of diffuse neuronal loss without gliotic changes. But when the structure is lost on T1WIR images, volume differences can be misleading (ACHTEN et al. 1995). For volume measurements to be useful, a small intra- and interobserver variability is essential (CENDES et al. 1993; JACK 1994; ACHTEN et al. 1998a). We have conducted a study to test the variability of our method of manual ray-tracing (ACHTEN et al. 1998a) and measured a value of 3.6% for interobserver variability and 3.4% for intraobserver variability when measuring left-to-right volume difference of the combined HC and amygdala (δ VHCA). This compares favorably with what other authors found (CENDES et al. 1993; JACK 1994).

14.2.3.2
Proton Magnetic Resonance Spectrosopy (^{1}HMRS)

Whereas imaging can detect most structural abnormalities in the temporal lobes of patients with TLE, ^{1}HMRS and other metabolic sampling techniques can provide additional information concerning the pathological processes involved and their distribution. From PET studies, it became clear that metabolic abnormalities extend beyond the traditional hippocampal sclerosis area (ENGEL et al. 1982; RADTKE et al. 1990; SACKELLARES et al. 1990; HENRY et al. 1993) and from pathological studies more widespread abnormalities, many of them bilateral, have also been reported (ENGEL et al. 1982; BRUTON 1988; FALCONER 1974). Because it is still unclear to what extent these changes contribute to outcome after surgery, the role of single voxel or other ^{1}HMRS techniques is to find these abnormalities, for lateralization purposes, but also to reveal possible bilateral abnormalities.

Single voxel proton MR spectroscopy (SV1HMRS) techniques typically sample brain regions in the order of 10 ml. More recently, multivoxel techniques like chemical shift imaging (CSI) can acquire spectra from voxels as small as 1 ml. Usually, longer echo-time proton spectra (135 or 270 ms) are acquired and three metabolites can readily be discerned (Figs. 14.9, 14.10): *N*-Acetyl aspartate (NAA) at 2 ppm, choline compounds (Cho) at 3.2 ppm, creatine/phosphocreatine (Cr) at 3 ppm. Occasionally, a lactate (Lac) doublet is present at 1.3 ppm (not shown), but this is only the case in a short time span after a seizure (BREITER et al. 1994). Although more metabolites can be seen at shorter echo-times, the technical problems of acquiring and quantifying such spectra in vivo makes them less attractive for clinical use.

Because it was evident from several cell-culture studies that NAA was mainly present in neuronal cells and their precursors (URENJAK et al. 1993), the decrease of NAA that accompanies several disease states has been interpreted as neuronal loss or dysfunction. This was confirmed by a high-resolution proton spectroscopy study of extracts of human cerebral neoplasms (PEELING and SUTHERLAND 1992) where lower levels of NAA and gamma-aminobutyric acid (GABA) and a shift in the glutamate/glutamine ratio toward glutamine reflected neuronal loss. Creatine (Cr) and choline compounds (Cho) are also found in neurons and their progenitors, but evidence from the same studies suggests a much higher concentration in the glia.

Recent studies have shown that NAA as a marker for neuronal loss or dysfunction (URENJAK et al. 1993; CONNELLY et al. 1994; INCISA-DELLA-ROCCHETTA et al. 1995; ACHTEN et al. 1997) is often more decreased in afflicted TL. Many bilateral abnormalities were also found precluding the sensitivity of the technique in lateralization issues (CONNELLY et al. 1994; ACHTEN et al. 1997; CENDES et al. 1997). An increase in both Cho and Cr has also been reported (CONNELLY et al. 1994) although this was not supported by other authors (DUC et al. 1995; ACHTEN et al. 1997).

Because of the lack of an internal standard, it is rather difficult to calculate absolute concentrations of the metabolites present in the spectra, and therefore several metabolite ratios like NAA/(Cho+Cr) or the NAA/Cr ratios are calculated. We recently proved that the most consistent SV1HMRS parameter for concordant lateralization was the NAA/(Cho+Cr) ratio followed by the normalized concentration of NAA (ACHTEN et al. 1997). Although many bilateral abnormal ratios were found, the introduction of an adequate asymmetry index (AI) improved the lateralization capabilities of the technique.

An important question to be answered now is whether patients with discordant findings between different non-invasive tests can benefit from 1HMRS. It is well known that the outcome of sub-

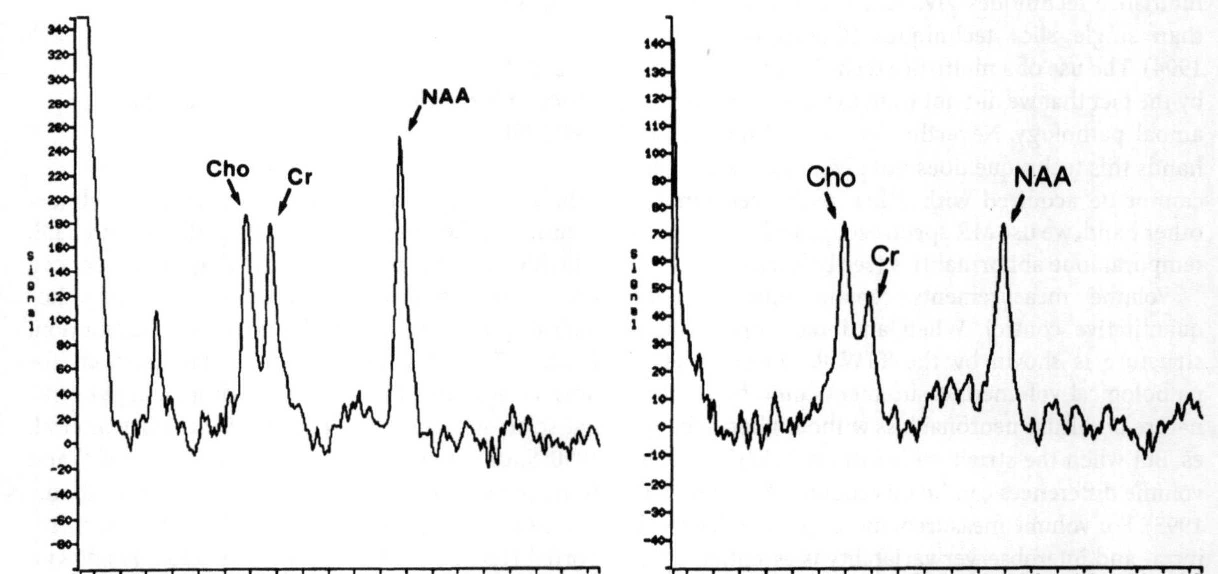

Fig. 14.9a,b. Single voxel proton spectra acquired from the mesial temporal areas of a left temporal lobe epilepsy patient with an echo-time of 135 ms. The spectrum from the right side (a) shows normal peak areas: *N*-acetyl-aspartate (*NAA*) at 2.01 ppm, creatine (*Cr*) at 3 ppm and choline compounds (*Cho*) at 3.2 ppm. A clear decrease of NAA is visible in the pathological temporal lobe (b) and a slight increase of Cho in respect to Cr as compared to the spectrum from the other side (a)

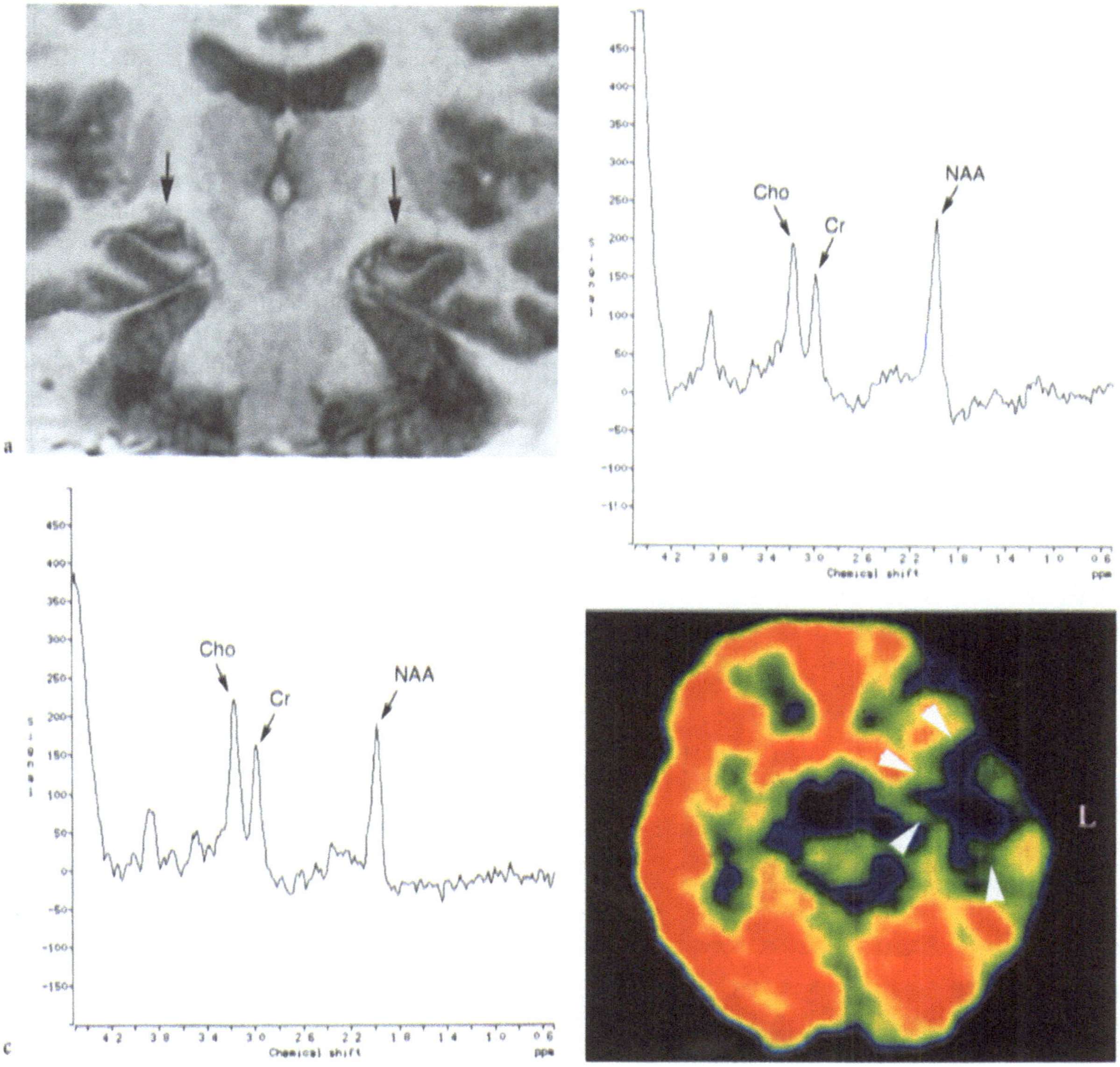

Fig. 14.10a–d. Bilateral TLE: lateralization with ictal and interictal EEG was not possible in this TLE patient because of short aura and a lot of muscle artifacts. T1 W inversion recovery images (**a**) showed bilateral hippocampal damage (*arrows*). SV1HMRS showed a normal spectral pattern *on the right side* (**b**) and a pathological pattern *on the left* with a decreased NAA/(Cho+Cr) ratio (**c**). An interictal 18FDG-PET study (**d**) showed a typical diffuse left temporal diminished tracer uptake (*arrowheads*): lateralization to the left side

jects with discordance between the EEG and the other non-invasive tests have a worse outcome after surgery than patients in whom all tests pointed to the same side (Boon et al. 1994b; Semah et al. 1995). It is tempting to rely on spectroscopy results for lateralization and possibly localization in patients with bilateral, minimal or no imaging abnormalities. We should be cautious when the EEG is not concordant though. Not enough cases with such problematic discordant findings have been studied for a definite answer about the value of 1HMRS.

Although several enigmas remain, SV1HMRS is part of the presurgical evaluation of TLE patients in our institution; it is performed in all. With the aid of a decision tree (Achten et al. 1995, 1997) (Fig. 14.7), lateralization issues are cleared. Lateralization with SV1HMRS, congruent with the EEG, reinforces the decision to go ahead with the surgical planning. In cases with only minimal unilateral, symmetrical bilateral or no imaging abnormalities, depth electrode (DE) studies are still always performed. But good results in some patients with clear lateralization with spectroscopy makes us optimistic in our belief that eventually such patients will benefit from the information and DE studies will no longer have to be performed in some (ACHTEN et al. 1997, 1998b).

14.2.3.4 Extratemporal Complex Partial Epilepsy (ETLE)

As said previously, 70% of the patients with complex partial epilepsy refractory to medical treatment have the temporal lobe variety. The remaining 30% have ETLE (Fig. 14.11). Here, lesions related to the foci are in most instances small and cannot be detected with current standard imaging techniques. High resolution surface coil MR imaging (GRANT et al. 1997), MR spectroscopy (STANLEY et al. 1998), functional MR imaging (SEECK et al. 1998), PET (DA SILVA et al. 1997) and magnetoencephalography (MEG) (ISHIBASHI et al. 1998) have been useful in demonstrating focal lesions that were below the threshold of conventional MR.

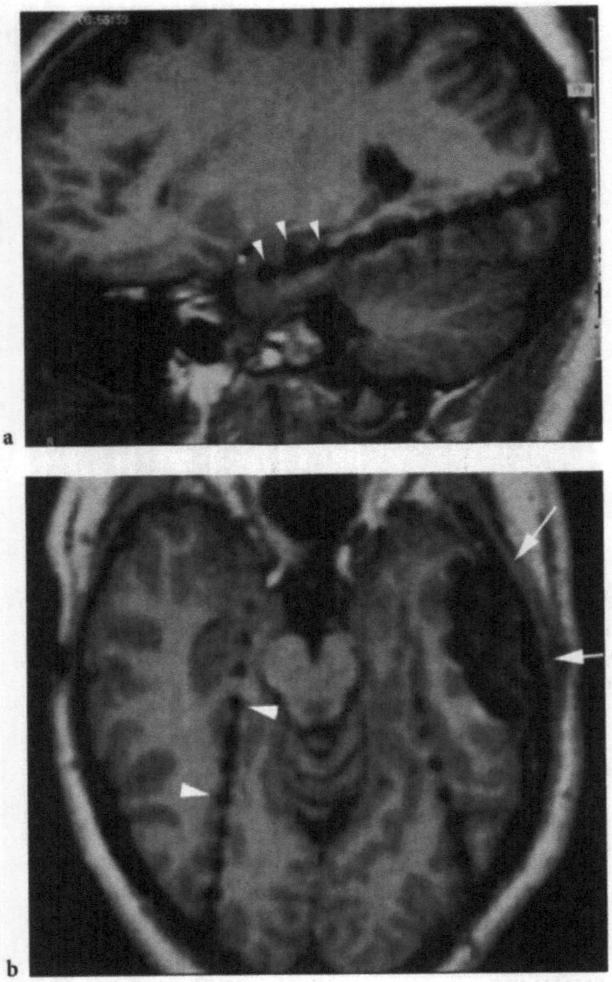

Fig. 14.11a,b. MR imaging is used to ascertain the correct positioning of depth electrodes and to know the exact position of the electrode contact points seen as small susceptibility artifacts (**a**, *arrowheads*). Subdural strips can also be seen (**b**) and in this case a small associated hematoma is present (*arrows*)

GRANT et al. (1997) compared standard head-coil studies and high resolution surface-coil imaging of the cerebral cortex and found improved detection and differentiation of focal cortical lesions in 64% of patients. When combined with EEG results, localization of the suspected epileptogenic zone or the detection of relevant prognostic information was improved in 85% of their cases.

STANLEY et al. (1998) used chemical shift imaging in patients with non-lesional ETLE and found evidence of widespread neuronal damage or dysfunction that was greatest in the region of seizure focus.

A new approach for non-invasive localization of focal epileptogenic discharges in patients considered for surgical treatment was recently proposed by SEECK et al. (1998). They used EEG-triggered functional MR imaging (fMRI) combined with EEG source localization to map the primary electrical epileptic source with high spatial resolution. EEG obtained in the MRI system allowed triggering of the fMRI acquisition by habitual epileptogenic discharges. This technique, although not possible in all patients because of the lack of sufficient interictal epileptic EEG signals, is very promising for certain patients with ETLE.

14.2.3.5 Imaging after Surgical Procedures

With MR imaging, the position of depth electrodes and cortical grids can easily and safely be defined (Fig. 14.12) (SILVERBUSCH et al. 1998). Although a certain theoretical risk for stimulation exists during MR imaging, none of the patients has ever complained or felt anything. This is due to the fact that low SAR (specific absorption rate) sequences are used (MPRAGE). By using MR imaging after the implantation of the electrodes, an accurate view is offered about their position and the presence of complications can be detected (hematomas).

In the future, the stereotactic guidance of the actual implantation should become possible with the use of real-time imaging in a dedicated MR scanner (e.g. special built open systems).

Recent reports also mention the possibility of using selective mesiotemporal radiosurgery as a therapy alternative to plain surgery in patients with TLE (REGIS et al. 1999). Although brachytherapy has

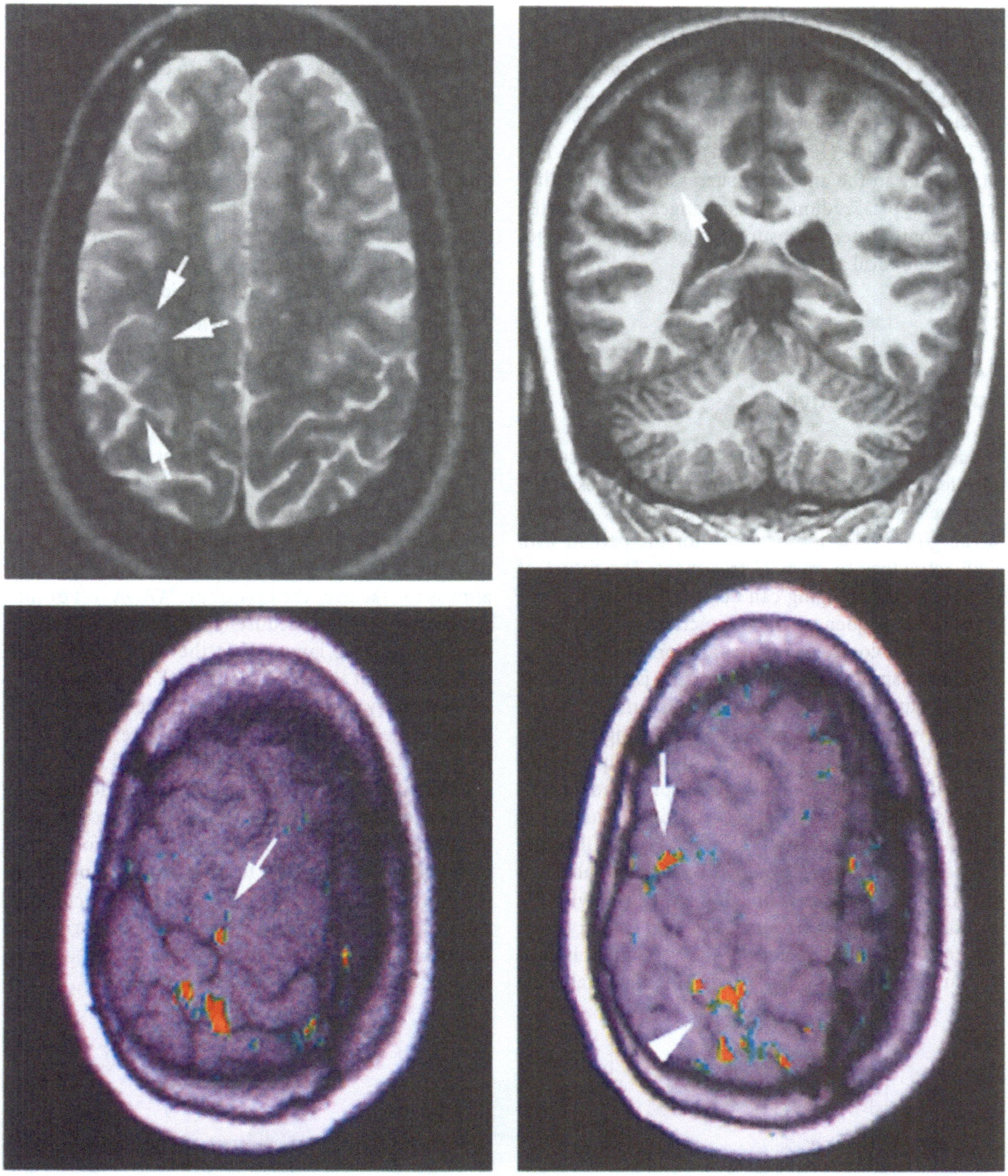

Fig. 14.12a–d. Alteration of the motor hand representation area in a dysplastic lesion in the right frontal lobe: axial T2 W (**a**) and T1 W (**b**) images show the lesion (*arrows*). The central sulcus is deformed and difficult to identify. Statistical parametrical maps (SPM) of the left hand motor function superimposed on oblique T1 W images (**c**,**d**) show motor activation at two locations in the border of the lesion (*solid arrow*). Activation of the sensory cortex for the hand (*open arrow*, **d**) and the posterior parietal cortex (Brodmann's areas 5 and 7) are also prominent. These activations were confirmed by Penfield stimulation

been tried in the past (Talairach et al. 1974), the technical difficulties related to the use of the radioelement led to the cessation of this approach. With the advent of the gamma knife, focal foreign tissue lesions causing epilepsy could be treated (Lindquist et al. 1991). Regis et al. (1999) treated one patient with TLE originating in the amygdala successfully with radiosurgery. Typical radionecrosis changes were reported at 10 months after radiosurgery. Later, these changes reverted to focal atrophy.

14.3 Future Perspectives

It has been said before, what is optimal today can be obsolete tomorrow. With this in mind, it is essential that we test and integrate new techniques into our presurgical evaluation program for the patient with CPE refractory to medical treatment. The future of structural MR imaging can be found in the application of fast sequences in conjunction with different kinds of MR contrast and preparation and the development of special coils. An interesting issue would be to find out if high resolution (0.3–0.5 mm in plane resolution) turbo-spin-echo (TSE) imaging in the titled coronal plane can depict the hippocampal anatomy better than the currently used spin-echo T1WIR images (0.8–1.0 mm in plan resolution). The use of fluid-attenuated inversion recovery (FLAIR) imaging may also contribute. No studies have been published that compare these new imaging modalities with the standard inversion recovery T1 W that we are using. On the other hand, a recent study found standard resolution TSE T2 W images in the titled coronal plane more sensitive than the T1WIR images in the detection of hippocampal sclerosis (Meiners et al. 1997).

A lot of effort has to be put into the refinement of imaging protocols to detect small structural abnormalities in patients with ETLE. Until now, structural MR imaging was not as sensitive in detecting lesions outside the temporal lobe. Image fusion between functional studies (multitracer SPECT and PET studies, and functional MRI) and high resolution (surface coil) MR imaging will definitely increase the yield in the detection of small cortical abnormalities because the structural MR imaging studies can then be focussed on the functional abnormality detected by nuclear medicine techniques (Engel et al. 1982; Sackellares et al. 1990; Henry et al. 1993; Berckovic et al. 1993; Da Silva et al. 1997; Stanley et al. 1998; Seeck et al. 1998; Ishibashi et al. 1998).

Another new technique with a great potential is functional MR imaging (fMRI). fMRI can teach us something about the functioning of the living human brain, but in epileptology one of the important aims is to take over the task of the WADA test or intracarotid amytal procedure (IAP) in a non-invasive way. Lateralizing language is the easier part (Van der Kallen et al. 1998; Yetkin et al. 1998), but mapping memory associated with the hippocampus and anterior mesial temporal lobe structures with fMRI is not yet possible. fMRI can also be used in the presurgical investigation of the relation of epileptogenic lesions to possible nearby eloquent cortex (Jack et al. 1994; Achten et al. 1999) (Fig. 14.13). Most interestingly, with a solution to problems arising when combining EEG and fMRI, this combined technique might be valuable in the detection of the origin of interictal spike-and-wave complexes or delta waves (Seeck et al. 1998).

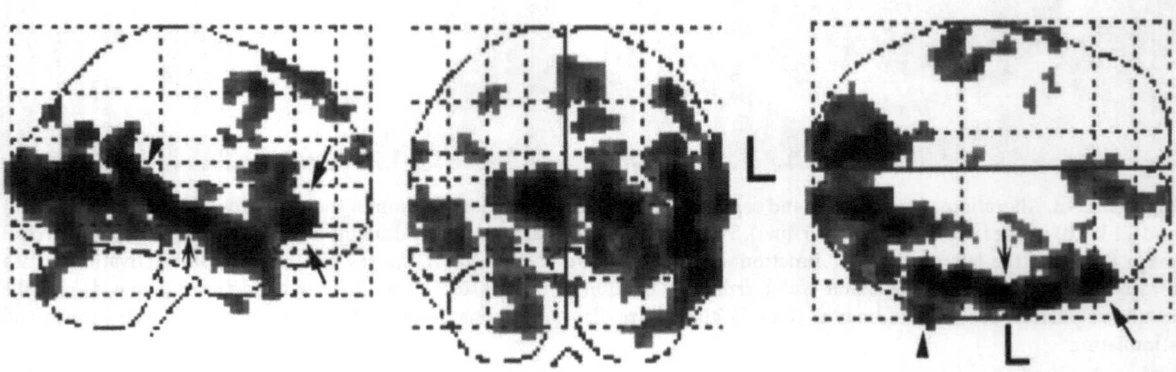

Fig. 14.13. MIPs of language related fMRI activation in a normal right handed subject. The statistical parametric maps (SPMs) are the result of the contrast between reading normal versus nonsense text and emphasize language related areas: left-sided Broca's area (*arrow*), mainly left sided Wernicke's area (*arrowhead*) and mainly left sided temporal areas related to language (*pointed arrow*). In the future, fMRI will probably be used for the non-invasive assessment of language and memory lateralization

With the use of the long echo-time of 135 ms used in many MRS studies, only three metabolites can be seen in the brains of chronic CPE patients. With the use of shorter echo-times, several more metabolites can be quantified (JACKSON et al. 1995; WOERMANN et al. 1999). Also, a better insight might be gained into the physiopathology of epilepsy with the use of absolute quantification (DANIELSEN and HENRIKSEN 1994). Whereas single voxel MRS techniques give little localizing information, chemical shift imaging, the multivoxel MRS technique, can give information about the spatial distribution of the spectroscopic abnormality and this technique will be more useful in ETLE where no clear structural abnormalities are found.

References

Achten E, Boon P, De Poorter J et al. (1995) An MR protocol for the pre-surgical work-up of patients with complex partial seizures of temporal lobe origin. Am J Neuroradiol 16: 1201–1213

Achten E, Boon P, Van De Kerckhove T, Caemaert J, De Reuck J, Kunnen M (1997) Value of single voxel proton MR spectroscopy in temporal lobe epilepsy. Am J Neuroradiol 18: 1131–1139

Achten E, Santens P, Boon P et al. (1998a) Single voxel proton MRS and 18FDG-PET in patients with refractory temporal lobe epilepsy. Am J Neuroradiol 19: 1–8

Achten E, Deblaere K, De Wagter C et al. (1998b) Intra- and interobserver variability of MR based volume measurements of the hippocampus and the amygdala using the manual ray-tracing method. Neuroradiology 40: 558–566

Achten E, Jackson GD, Cameron JA, Abbott DF, Stella DL, Fabinyi GCA (1999) Presurgical evaluation of the motor hand area with fMRI in patients with tumors and dysplastic lesions. Radiology 210: 529–538

Babb TL, Brown WJ (1993) Pathological findings in epilepsy. In: Engel JJ (ed) Surgical treatment of the epilepsies, 2nd ed. Raven Press, New York, pp 511–540

Berg AT, Test FM, Levy SR, Shinnar S (1996) The epidemiology of epilepsy: past, present and future. Neurol Clin 14: 383–398

Berkovic SF, Newton MR, Chiron C, Dulac O (1993) Single photon emission tomography. In: Engel JJ (ed) Surgical treatment of the epilepsies, 2nd ed. Raven Press, New York, pp 233–243

Boon P, De Reuck J, Drieghe C, De Bruycker K, Aers I, Pengel J (1994a) Long-term video-EEG monitoring revisisted; the value of the interictal and ictal video-EEG recording, a follow-up study. Eur Neurol 34: 33–39

Boon P, Calliauw L, De Reuck J et al. (1994) Clinical and neurophysiological correlations in patients with refractory partial epilepsy and intracranial structural lesions. Acta Neurochir 128: 68–83

Breiter SN, Arroyo S, Mathews VP, Lesser RP, Bryan RN, Barker PB (1994) Proton MR spectroscopy in patients with seizure disorders. Am J Neuroradiol 15: 373–384

Bronen RA, Cheung G, Charles JT (1991) Imaging findings in hippocampal sclerosis: correlation with pathology. Am J Neuroradiol 12: 933–940

Bruton CJ (1988) The neuropathology of temporal lobe epilepsy. Oxford University Press

Cendes F, Caramanos Z, Andermann F, Dubeau F, Arnold DL (1997) Proton magnetic resonance spectroscopic imaging and magnetic resonance imaging volumetry in the lateralization of temporal lobe epilepsy: a series of 100 patients. Ann Neurol 42: 737–746

Cendes F, Leproux F, Melanson D et al. (1993) MRI of amygdala and hippocampus in temporal lobe epilepsy. J Comput Assist Tomogr 17: 206–210

Commission on Classification and Terminology of the International League against Epilepsy: Proposal for revised clinical and electroencephalographic classification of epileptic seizures (1981) Epilepsia 22: 489–501

Connelly A, Jackson GD, Duncan JS, King MD, Gadian DG (1994) Magnetic resonance spectroscopy in temporal lobe epilepsy. Neurology 44: 1411–1417

Danielsen ER, Henriksen O (1994) Absolute quantitative proton NMR spectroscopy based on the amplitude of the local water suppression pulse. Quantification of brain water and metabolites. NMR Biomed 7: 311–318

Da Silva EA, Chugani DC, Muzik O, Chugani HT (1997) Identification of frontal lobe epileptic foci in children using positron emission tomography. Epilepsia 38: 1198–1208

Duc CO, Meier D, Golay XG, Weber OM, Wieser HG, Boesiger P (1995) Investigation of the temporal lobe epilepsy by quantitative 1H MRS of the hippocampus in vivo. Proceedings of the SMRM, Nice (France). Book of abstracts p 1829

Engel J Jr, Brown WJ, Kuhl DE, Phelps ME, Mazziota JC, Crandall PH (1982) Pathological findings underlying focal temporal lobe hypometabolism in partial epilepsy. Ann Neurol 12: 518–528

Engel J Jr (1989) Seizures and epilepsy. FA Davis, Philadelphia

Falconer MA (1974) Mesial temporal (Ammon's Horn) sclerosis as a common cause of epilepsy: aetiology, treatment and prevention. Lancet 2: 767–770

Fried I, Cascino GD (1993) Lesional surgery. In: Engel JJ (ed) Surgical treatment of the epilepsies, 2nd ed. Raven Press, New York, pp 501–509

Gadian DG, Connelly A, Duncan JS et al. (1994) 1H magnetic resonance spectroscopy in the investigation of intractable epilepsy. Acta Neurol Scand Suppl 152: 116–121

Giroud M, Walker P, Bernard D et al. (1994) Preliminary observations of metabolic characterization of bilateral temporal epileptic focus, using proton magnetic resonance spectroscopy. Three cases. Neurol Res 16: 481–483

Grant PE, Barkovich AJ, Wald LL, Dillon WP, Laxer KD, Vigneron DBSO (1997) High-resolution surface-coil MR of cortical lesions in medically refractory epilepsy: a prospective study. Am J Neuroradiol 18: 291–301

Grünewald RA, Jackson GD, Connelly A, Duncan JS (1994) MR detection of hippocampal disease in epilepsy: factors influencing T2 relaxion times. Am J Neuroradiol 15: 1149–1156

Henry TR, Chugani HT, Abou-Khalil BW, THeodore WH, Swartz BE (1993) Positron emission tomography. In: Engel JJ (ed) Surgical treatment of the epilepsies, 2nd ed. Raven Press, New York, pp 211–232

Incisa della Rocchetta A, Gadian DG et al. (1995) Verbal memory impairment after right temporal lobe surgery: role of contralateral damage as revealed by 1H magnetic resonance spectroscopy and T2 relaxometry. Neurology 45: 797–802

Ishibashi H, Morioka T, Shigeto H, Nishio S, Yamamoto T, Fukui MSO (1998) Three-dimensional localization of sub-

clinical ictal activity by magnetoencephalography: correlation with invasive monitoring. Surg Neurol 50: 157–163
Jack CR Jr, Sharbrough FW, Cascino GD, Hirschorn KA, O'Brien PC, Marsh WR (1992) Magnetic resonance image-based hippocampal volumetry: correlation with outcome after temporal lobectomy. Ann Neurol 31: 138–146
Jack CR Jr, Thompson RM, Butts RK et al. (1994) Sensory motor cortex: correlation of presurgical mapping with functional MR imaging and invasive cortical mapping. Radiology 190: 85–92
Jack-CR Jr (1994) MRI-based hippocampal volume measurements in epilepsy. Epilepsia 35: S21-S29
Jackson GD, Connelly A, Duncan JS, Grunewald R, Gadian GD (1993) Detection of hippocampal pathology in intractable partial epilepsy: increased sensitivity with quantitative T2 relaxometry. Neurology 43: 1793–1799
Jackson GD, Berkovic SF, Tress BM, Kalnins RM, Fabinyi GC, Bladin PF (1994) Hippocampal sclerosis can be reliably detected by magnetic resonance imaging. Neurology 40: 1869–1875
Jackson GD, Kuzniecky RI (1995) Magnetic resonance spectroscopy in epilepsy. In: Jackson GD, Kuzniecky RI (eds) Magnetic resonance in epilepsy. Raven Press, New York, pp 289–314
Jones-Gotman M, Smith ML, Zatorre RJ (1993) Neuropsychological testing for the localizing and lateralizing the epileptogenic region. In: Engel JJ (ed.) Surgical treatment of the epilepsies, 2nd ed. Raven Press, New York, pp 245–261
Kim SS, Chang KH, Kim ST et al. (1999) Focal lesion in the splenium of the corpus callosum in epileptic patients: antiepileptic drug toxicity? Am J Neuroradiol 20: 125–129
Lechtenberg R (1998) Generalized, partial and febrile seizures. In: Lechtenberg R, Schutta HS (eds) Neurology practice guidelines. Marcel Dekker Inc., New York, Basel, Hong Kong, pp 303–328
Lindquist C, Kilström L, Hellstrand E (1991) Functional neurosurgery: a future for the gamma knife? Stereotact Funct Neurosurg 57: 72–81
Matthews PM, Andermann F, Arnold DL (1990) A proton magnetic resonance spectroscopy study of focal epilepsy in humans. Neurology 40: 985–989
Meiners LC, Valk J, van Gils PG et al. (1997) Assessment of the preferred plane and sequence in the depiction of mesial temporal sclerosis using magnetic resonance imaging. Invest Radiol 32: 268–276
Meiners LC, Valk J, Jansen GH, Van Veelen CW (1999) MR contribution in surgery of epilepsy. Eur Radiol 9: 493–507
Pannek HW, Oppel F (1999) Minimally invasive lesionectomies through a stereotactically guided working sleeve. Neurol Res 21: 51–59
Peeling J, Sutherland G (1992) High-resolution 1H NMR spectroscopy studies of extracts of human cerebral neoplasms. Magn Reson Med 24: 23–36
Phillips J, Sakas DE (1996) Anterior callosotomy for intractable epilepsy: outcome in a series of twenty patients. Br J Neurosurg 10: 351–356
Radtke RA, Hoffman JM, Hanson MW, Walczak TS, Lewis DV, Coleman RE (1990) Temporal PET hypometabolism: predictor of positive outcome after temporal lobectomy. Epilepsia 31: 626
Rausch R, Silfvenius H, Wieser HG, Dodrill CB, Meador KJ, Jones-Gotman M (1993) Intra-arterial amytal procedures. In: Engel JJ (ed) Surgical treatment of the epilepsies, 2nd ed. Raven Press, New York, pp 341–357
Regis J, Semah F, Bryan RN et al. (1999) Early and delayed MR and PET changes after selective temporomesial radiosurgery in mesial temporal sclerosis. Am J Neuroradiol 20: 213–216
Sackellares JC, Siegel GL, Abou-Khalil BW et al. (1990) Differences between lateral and mesial temporal metabolism interictally in epilepsy of temporal origin. Neurology 40: 1420–1426
Sanders WP, Silbergleit R, Spickler EM, Barkley GL, Mehta BAAD (1995) Efficacy of gadolinium administration in magnetic resonance imaging screening of patients with complex partial seizures and results of a normal neurologic examination. Invest Radiol 30: 634–637
Seeck M, Lazeyras F, Michel CM et al. (1998) Non-invasive epileptic focus localization using EEG-triggered functional MRI and electromagnetic tomography. Electroencephalogr Clin Neurophysiol 106: 508–512
Semah F, Baulac M, Hasboun D et al. (1995) Is interictal temporal hypometabolism related to mesial temporal sclerosis? A positron emission tomography/magnetic resonance confrontation. Epilepsia 36: 447–456
Silberbusch MA, Rothman MI, Bergey GK, Zoarski GH, Zagardo MT (1998) Subdural grid implantation for intracranial EEG recording: CT and MR appearance. Am J Neuroradiol 19: 1089–1093
Silverstein AM, Alexander J (1998) Acute postictal cerebral imaging. Am J Neuroradiol 19: 1485–1488
Spencer SS (1991) Intracranial recording. In: Spencer DD, Spencer SS (eds) Epilepsy Surgery. Blackwell, Cambridge, pp 54–64
Stanley JA, Cendes F, Dubeau F, Andermann F, Arnold DLSO (1998) Proton magnetic resonance spectroscopic imaging in patients with extratemporal epilepsy. Epilepsia 39: 267–273
Talairach J, Bancaud J, Szikla G, Bonis A, Geler S, Vedrenne C (1974) Approche nouvelle de la neurochirurgie de l'épilepsie. Méthodologie stéréotaxique et résultats thérapeutiques. Presented at the Congrès Annuel de la Société de la Langue Française, Marseille, June 1974
Urenjak J, Williams SR, Gadian DG, Noble M (1993) Proton nuclear magnetic resonance spectroscopy unambiguously identifies different neural cell types. J Neurosci 13: 981–989
Van der Kallen BF, Morris GL, Yetkin FZ, van Erning LJ, Thijssen HO, Haughton VMSO (1998) Hemispheric language dominance studied with functional MR: preliminary study in healthy volunteers and patients with epilepsy. Am J Neuroradiol 19: 73–77
Ward AA Jr (1983) Perspectives of surgical therapy of epilepsy. In: Ward AA, Penry JK, Purura D (eds) Epilepsy ARNMD. Raven Press, New York, pp 371–390
Woermann FG, McLean MA, Bartlett PA, Parker GJ, Barker GJ, Duncan JS (1999) Short echo time single-voxel 1H magnetic resonance spectroscopy in magnetic resonance imaging-negative temporal lobe epilepsy: different biochemical profile compared with hippocampal sclerosis. Ann Neurol 45: 369–376
Yetkin FZ, Swanson S, Fischer M et al. (1998) Functional MR of frontal lobe activation: comparison with Wada language results. Am J Neuroradiol 19: 1095–1098

15 Degenerative Diseases

Mario Savoiardo, Marina Grisoli

CONTENTS

15.1 Introduction

The degenerative diseases of the central nervous system (CNS) are a heterogeneous group of disorders, genetically determined or with sporadic occurrence and unknown etiology, which may affect the brain and spinal cord with different mechanisms; they may involve the whole nervous system, but often exhibit a remarkable selectivity in affecting one system or another.

In several degenerative processes, the main pathological feature is loss of neurons with atrophy; atrophy may diffusely involve the brain, but, in many diseases, selectively affects cortical areas or deep nuclei and the fibers that originate from the involved cortical areas or nuclei degenerate. In other diseases, the white matter is probably primarily involved.

The pathological changes that characterize the different degenerative diseases of the CNS usually cause very subtle modifications of signal intensity in magnetic resonance imaging (MRI) studies. Nevertheless, in degenerative diseases the accurate observation of MRI studies in the search for these subtle signal abnormalities and of characteristic distribution of atrophic changes is the best possible way to reach a neuroradiological diagnosis.

Another problem with degenerative disorders of the CNS is that, in some groups of diseases, considerable overlapping in the distribution of tissue changes and signal abnormalities exists. In making a diagnosis, therefore, it is always necessary to correlate the MRI findings with the clinical presentation and with other neurophysiological, genetic, or laboratory studies. In addition to MRI, neuroradiology can also offer MR spectroscopy (MRS) and functional studies with positron emission tomography (PET) and single photon emission tomography (SPET). We shall try, however, to point out the characteristic MRI findings of the most common degenerative diseases of the CNS. We shall review dementing diseases, parkinsonian and other extrapyramidal disorders, cerebellar degenerative diseases, motor neuron disease, and degenerative disorders mainly affecting the pediatric population, such as neuroaxonal dystrophies and neuronal ceroid lipofuscinosis.

15.2 Dementia

Impairment of higher intellectual functions may be seen in several conditions and the search for a treat-

M. Savoiardo, MD; M. Grisoli, MD
Department of Neuroradiology, Istituto Nazionale Neurologico "C. Besta", Via Celoria 11, 20133 Milan, Italy

able cause makes medical evaluation and laboratory and neuroradiological studies necessary. We shall not discuss normal pressure hydrocephalus or multi-infarct dementia, but shall limit our description to Alzheimer's disease and frontotemporal dementia.

15.2.1 Alzheimer's Disease

Alzheimer's disease (AD) is the commonest cause of dementia and, with the prolongation of life, has become the commonest neurodegenerative disorder. It includes the cases that in the past had been classified as senile dementia, which have the same pathological substratum.

Diffuse cerebral atrophy with enlargement of the ventricles and sulci is seen in computed tomography (CT) and MRI studies; these changes are similar to those seen in normal aging. However, in AD there is also a selective vulnerability of the hippocampal formation that correlates with the marked involvement of memory, a characteristic of the disease. Therefore, atrophy of the mesial temporal structures leads to a more marked enlargement of the temporal horns and of the suprasellar, perimesencephalic, and sylvian cisterns (de Leon et al. 1993). The atrophic mesial temporal structures and the cortex of the insula may appear hyperintense in proton density and T2-weighted images (Braffman et al. 1991) (Fig. 15.1).

Selective atrophy of the hippocampal region is the principal feature of an MRI diagnosis of AD (Jack et al. 1992) and has become the object of quantitative evaluation in several volumetric MRI studies that have demonstrated a significant overlapping with other types of dementia (Laakso et al. 1996; Frisoni et al. 1999).

Other MRI features found in AD patients are signal changes in the subcortical and periventricular white matter, which are, however, seen less frequently than in multi-infarct dementia (Braffman et al. 1991; Osborn 1994).

1H-MRS studies have suggested that myoinositol is increased and *N*-acetylaspartate, a neuronal marker, is decreased in AD patients compared to controls (Miller et al. 1993). 1H-MRS has been used in the differential diagnosis between AD and other dementias (see Chap. 5). PET studies have shown a decreased glucose metabolism in AD patients. Ibanez et al. (1998) demonstrated that the decreased metabolism, which is mostly evident in inferior parietal, frontal, and lateral temporal cortex, is not simply related to atrophy, but that the glucose metabolic values remain lower in AD patients than in controls even after correction for atrophy.

Volumetric MRI studies, MRS and functional studies are of great value in a research setting, but in the single patient the simplest support to the diagnosis of AD remains the observation at MRI of diffuse atrophy with selective prevalence in the mesial temporal structures. The search for a simple discriminating linear measurement that may be used in routine studies remains elusive (Osborn 1994).

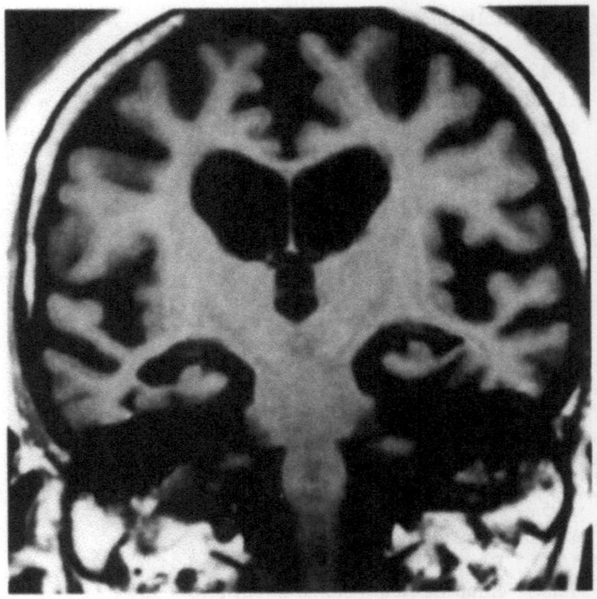
a

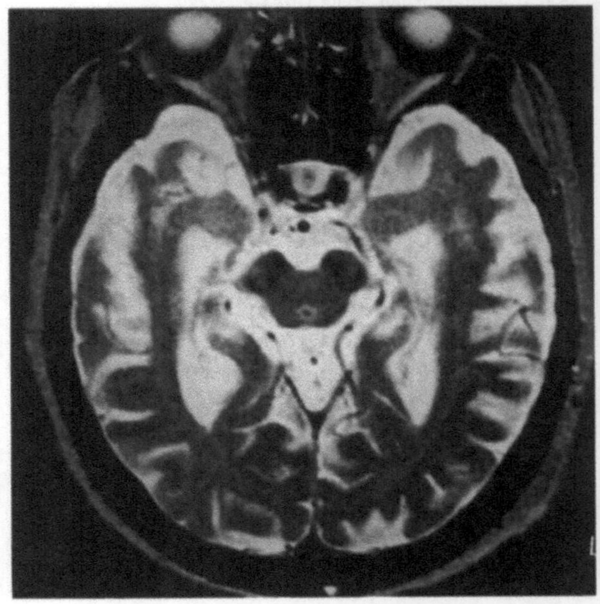
b

Fig. 15.1a,b. Alzheimer's disease. **a** T1-weighted coronal section demonstrates diffuse atrophy, more severe in the mesial temporal areas. **b** T2-weighted axial section shows enlargement of all the cisterns surrounding the temporal lobes; mild hyperintensity is present in the amygdala

15.2.2
Frontotemporal Dementia

Pick's disease and other forms of dementia lacking the histological features of Pick's disease but sharing the anatomical distribution and the clinical presentation (with prominent behavioral disturbances) are included under the denomination of frontotemporal dementia (FTD).

Prominent involvement of the frontal and temporal lobes, often asymmetrical, severe enough to cause the so-called "knife-edge" convolutions, is commonly known from pathological studies. In the neuroradiological literature, only a few articles have dealt with FTD or Pick's disease, investigating mostly the aspect of atrophy distribution with MRI volumetric studies or surface rendering techniques (Kitagaki et al. 1998; Frisoni et al. 1999). Only rarely have signal changes been described (Kitagaki et al. 1997).

We recently reviewed the MRI studies of 13 cases carrying the clinical diagnosis of FTD (2 confirmed by autopsy) and found a few aspects that may strongly support the clinical diagnosis (unpublished data, presented at the ENS Meeting, Milan, June 1999).

In the atrophic frontal and temporal lobes there is a progressive thinning of the cortex and loss of bulk of the underlying white matter that may lead to the "knife-blade" gyri. Atrophy may sometimes involve, to a lesser extent, the parietal lobes; particularly in these cases, the precentral and postcentral gyri stand out because they are not involved in atrophy. Similarly, it is known from pathology that the posterior part of the superior temporal convolution, T1, is spared. On MRI, the preservation of this gyrus is clearly seen; in addition, sparing of the Heschl gyrus and of the planum temporale in the depth of the sylvian fissure are clearly recognizable (Fig. 15.2).

The basal ganglia are atrophic; the head of the caudate nucleus is particularly thin, even more than that usually seen in Huntington's chorea, resulting in a remarkable enlargement of the frontal horns of the lateral ventricles, which are, in any case, widened in all their segments (Savoiardo et al., in press) (Fig. 15.2).

As a consequence of the frontal atrophy, there is degeneration of the frontopontine fibers that run in the medial part of the cerebral peduncles; atrophy of this part of the peduncles results in an enlargement of the interpeduncular cistern. Apart from this finding, there are no significant changes in posterior fossa.

In the cerebral atrophic areas, the signal intensity of the cortex and, even more, of the underlying white matter is increased in proton density and T2-weighted images (Fig. 15.2).

The hyperintensity gradually fades away in the posterior temporal and parietal regions; the optic radiations that do not degenerate maintain their normal signal intensity and, therefore, stand out against the abnormal background particularly in proton density images (Savoiardo et al., in press). Normal signal intensity is also maintained in the superior posterior temporal regions and in the precentral and postcentral gyri and subjacent white matter.

The severity of these findings has varied from case to case; it was most severe in the patient with the longest disease duration, examined shortly before death. This examination showed a marked progression of atrophy and signal changes in comparison with an MRI obtained early in the course of the disease.

In our series, atrophy of the frontal lobes was equal to or more marked than atrophy of the temporal lobes, but the opposite may occur in other forms of FTD; clear asymmetry was often not detectable.

It is interesting to note that three of our patients had some unusual features: two had, in addition to the typical findings described, a small midbrain with a concave superior profile, as is usually seen in progressive supranuclear palsy (PSP); one had a more marked parietal atrophy, and the atrophic changes were definitely more marked on one side. These findings were, therefore, similar to those observed in corticobasal degeneration (CBD); the patient, in fact, had a clinical picture with some mixed features pointing both to CBD and FTD, with prevalence of FTD. It should be remembered that FTD, PSP and CBD are all tauopathies and that cases with overlapping features do exist; MRI may be important not only in demonstrating the involved anatomical regions, thus supporting the clinical diagnosis, but also in showing the overlapping features in atypical cases, thus allowing better clinicoradiological correlations.

15.3
Parkinsonisms and Other Extrapyramidal Disorders

A remarkable amount of literature has been produced on Parkinson's disease, with some contrasting results on signal alterations in the substantia nigra, which becomes progressively atrophic. The main MRI finding is a loss of signal intensity in T2-weighted images in high-field MRI due to iron deposition, resulting in a reduction of the band with normal signal interposed between the substantia nigra and the red nuclei. A recent paper examines in detail the

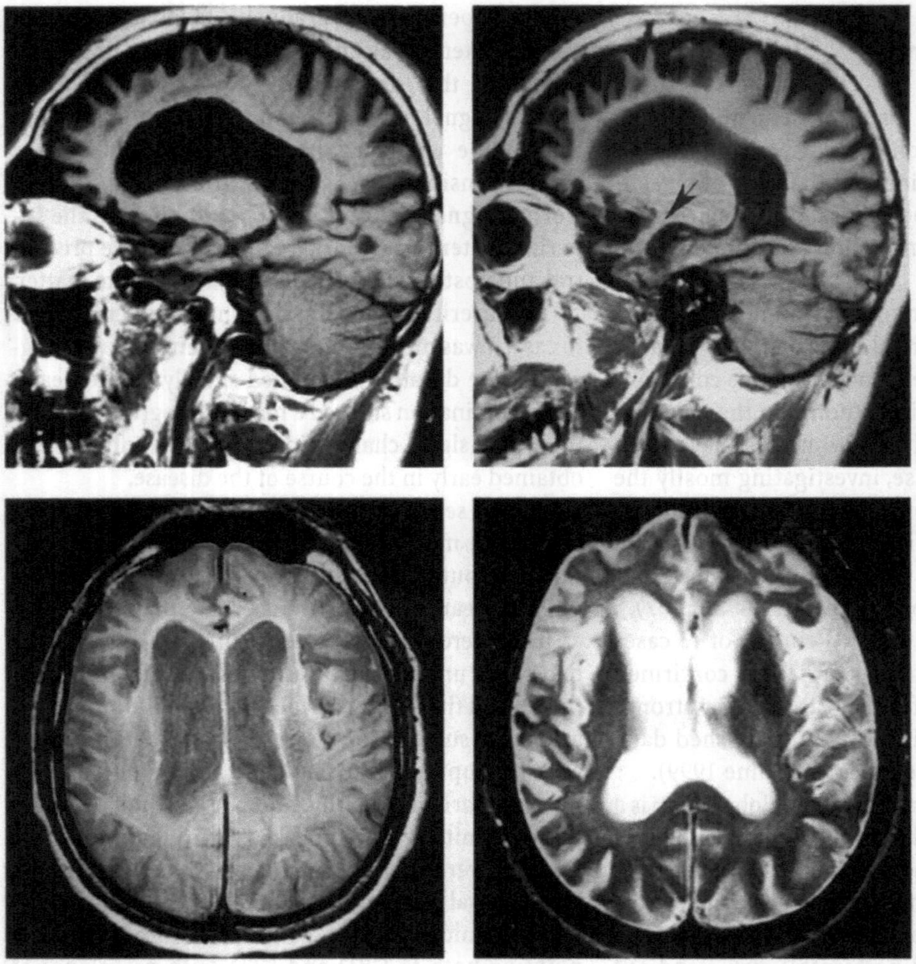

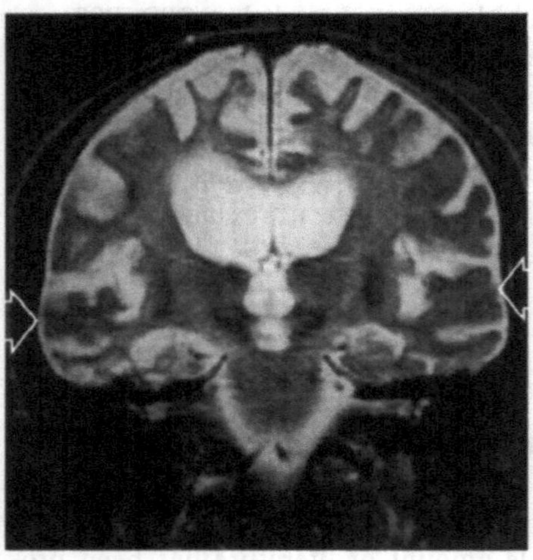

Fig. 15.2a–e. Frontotemporal dementia in a 55-year-old-man. **a,b** Sagittal T1-weighted sections show marked thinning of the frontal and temporal gyri with ventricular dilatation; ballooning of the temporal horn indicates atrophy of the amygdala (*arrow in* **b**). **c,d** Axial proton density and T2-weighted sections at adjacent levels demonstrate hyperintensity in the frontal regions fading backward; ballooning of the frontal horns is associated with severe atrophy of the heads of the caudate nuclei. **e** Coronal T2-weighted section on the posterior temporal lobes demonstrates severe temporal atrophy with preservation of T1 gyrus, planum temporale, and Heschl gyrus (*open arrows*)

effects of deposition of different forms of iron and speculates on the possible influences from iron and other paramagnetic substances such as neuromelanin in different nuclei in Parkinson's disease and multiple system atrophy (Vymazal et al. 1999).

Since the diagnosis of Parkinson's disease does not require an MRI examination, here we prefer to address another practical problem: in patients poorly responding to L-dopa, who might, therefore, have striatonigral degeneration (SND), which is a component of the multisystem atrophy (MSA), is it possible to recognize on MRI some features that may suggest the diagnosis of SND? Are there characteristic abnormalities that may allow the diagnosis of other

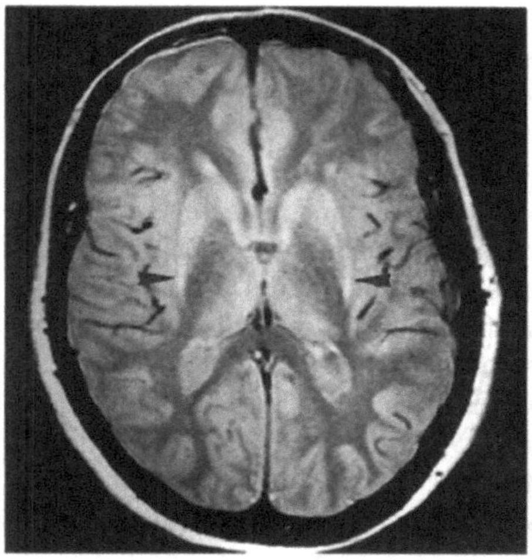

a

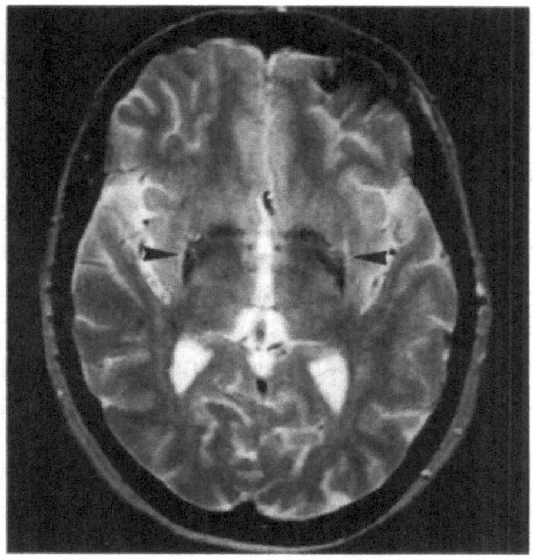

b

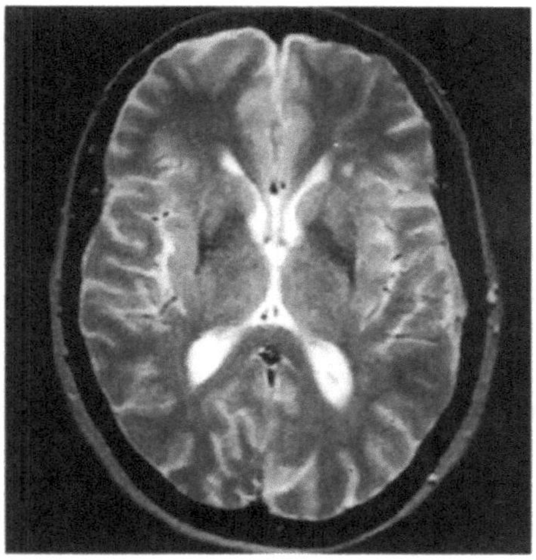

c

Fig. 15.3a–c. Multiple system atrophy, striatonigral degeneration type, in a 58-year-old woman; 1.5 T. **a** Axial proton density image shows slight hyperintensity in the posterior part of the putamina (*arrowheads*). **b,c** T2-weighted images at adjacent levels demonstrate putaminal hypointensity, more marked than in the pallida, with thin lateral rim of hyperintensity (*arrowheads*, **b**)

parkinsonisms not responding to L-dopa therapy, such as PSP or CBD?

We shall first examine MSA, with its components, namely SND and olivopontocerebellar atrophy (OPCA), and then PSP and CBD.

1H-MRS has been used in Parkinson's disease in order to help distinguish this entity from atypical syndromes such as progressive supranuclear palsy and multisystem atrophy (see Chap. 5).

15.3.1 Multisystem Atrophy – Striatonigral Degeneration

In MSA, multiple systems are involved: extrapyramidal, autonomic, and cerebellar, resulting in a complex symptomatology with parkinsonian features not responding to treatment, autonomic disturbances, and cerebellar and brainstem symptoms and signs. The term Shy-Drager disease is considered equivalent to MSA, but most of the time it refers to the combination of SND and autonomic failure. Since the pathological changes causing the autonomic failure are in the intermediolateral cell columns of the spinal cord, they cannot be detected by MRI; only PET studies have shown brain abnormalities associated with autonomic failure, namely hypometabolism in the frontal and temporal regions and thalami (PERANI et al. 1995). The abnormalities that may be detected by MRI in MSA are, therefore, essentially confined to the putamen in SND, to the pons, inferior olives and cerebellum in sporadic OPCA; lesions at both sites can be seen in MSA, but in a certain number of cases, clinical and pathological findings are restricted, at least in the initial stages of the disease, to the extrapyramidal or the cerebellar system.

In SND, the pathological findings involve substantia nigra, putamen and globus pallidus, but the most prominent changes, consisting in neuronal loss, loss of myelinated fibers, gliosis, and deposition of iron and pigments such as neuromelanin, are confined to the putamen and are more prominent in its posterior dorsolateral part (Borit et al. 1975; Fearnley and Lees 1990; Goto et al. 1996).

On low-field-intensity MRI (0.5 T or less), the signal changes seen in the putamen are increased signal intensity in proton density and T2-weighted images in the posterior part of the putamen, more marked laterally. On higher field intensity (1.5 T), the magnetic susceptibility effects of iron, neuromelanin and perhaps other elements cause a loss of signal intensity in T2-weighted images which masks the increased signal due to increased water content. The putamen, therefore, becomes largely hypointense in T2-weighted images, with a signal that is equal to or lower than that normally seen in the pallidum, where iron is normally present. A thin lateral rim on the margin of the putamen remains hyperintense, evidently free from iron deposits (Drayer et al. 1986; Pastakia et al. 1986; Savoiardo et al. 1989) (Fig. 15.3).

Minor changes are also present in the substantia nigra with smudging of hypointensity and decreased distance from the red nucleus (Savoiardo et al. 1989).

Several authors have investigated the sensitivity and specificity of the putaminal findings; when we reviewed a series of 42 cases with clinically diagnosed MSA (Testa et al. 1993), putaminal abnormalities were found in 9/9 cases with SND and in 17/20 cases with probable MSA and presence of both extrapyramidal and cerebellar signs. Other authors have found these abnormalities less frequently and, therefore, the sensitivity is variable in different series; the specificity of putaminal hyperintense rim combined with hypointensity is generally considered high, while specificity of hypointensity alone is lower (Schrag et al. 1998; Kraft et al. 1999). It should also be remembered that deposition of iron increases with age, and observation of some putaminal hypointensity in T2-weighted images in a normal subject over 70 years of age is common.

In summary, in a patient with parkinsonian features and doubtful response to L-dopa treatment, observation of hypointensity with a lateral hyperintense rim in T2-weighted images at high-field MRI strongly support the diagnosis of MSA-SND type.

15.3.2 Multisystem Atrophy – Olivopontocerebellar Atrophy

In sporadic OPCA, there is neuronal loss in the pontine nuclei; their fibers (transverse pontine fibers), which run mostly on the anterior and posterior margins of the basis pontis reaching the cerebellum through the middle cerebellar peduncles, degenerate. In the cerebellum, there is a marked loss of Purkinje cells and their fibers which project to the dentate nuclei, resulting in diffuse gliosis. The neurons of the dentate nuclei do not degenerate and their fibers which run in the superior cerebellar peduncles are therefore preserved. The corticospinal tracts and the pontine tegmentum are normal. In the medulla, retrograde cell loss of the inferior olives secondary to cortical cerebellar lesions is observed (Oppenheimer 1984).

Atrophy of the cerebellum, pons, and middle cerebellar peduncles with signal abnormalities in the degenerated structures is therefore expected on MRI in OPCA cases. In fact, not only can we demonstrate the signal abnormalities in the transverse pontine fibers, middle cerebellar peduncles and cerebellum, but we can recognize preservation of normal signal intensity in the corticospinal tracts and in the superior cerebellar peduncles, thus making the whole MRI picture very specific (Savoiardo et al. 1990) (Fig. 15.4).

In order to recognize the distribution of atrophy and the mild hyperintensity in proton density and T2-weighted images of the affected structures, observation in the appropriate sagittal, axial or coronal planes may be necessary.

In our review of 42 cases with MSA, we found characteristic posterior fossa abnormalities in all 13 patients with OPCA and in 13 of the 20 patients with combined parkinsonian and cerebellar features (3 alone and 10 combined with putaminal abnormalities) (Testa et al. 1993).

In their recent review of MSA patients, Schrag et al. (1998) found that all 16 cases with clinical diagnosis of OPCA type of MSA had the characteristic abnormalities in the brainstem and cerebellum (100% of sensitivity); the positive predictive value of these findings was higher than 90% both versus controls and versus idiopathic Parkinson's disease patients (Schrag et al. 1998).

In our opinion, in patients with suspected MSA, the observation on MRI of the posterior fossa changes described here and of the putaminal abnormalities described in SND makes the diagnosis of MSA certain, because it clearly demonstrates involvement of two different systems.

The pathological changes in some autosomal dominant cerebellar ataxias, namely spinocerebellar ataxia types 1, 2 and 3 (SCA-1, SCA-2, SCA-3), have many similarities with those described in sporadic OPCA; it is understandable, therefore, that similarities and overlapping may be observed on MRI. Clinical presentation and family history should obviously be taken into account before making a diagnosis.

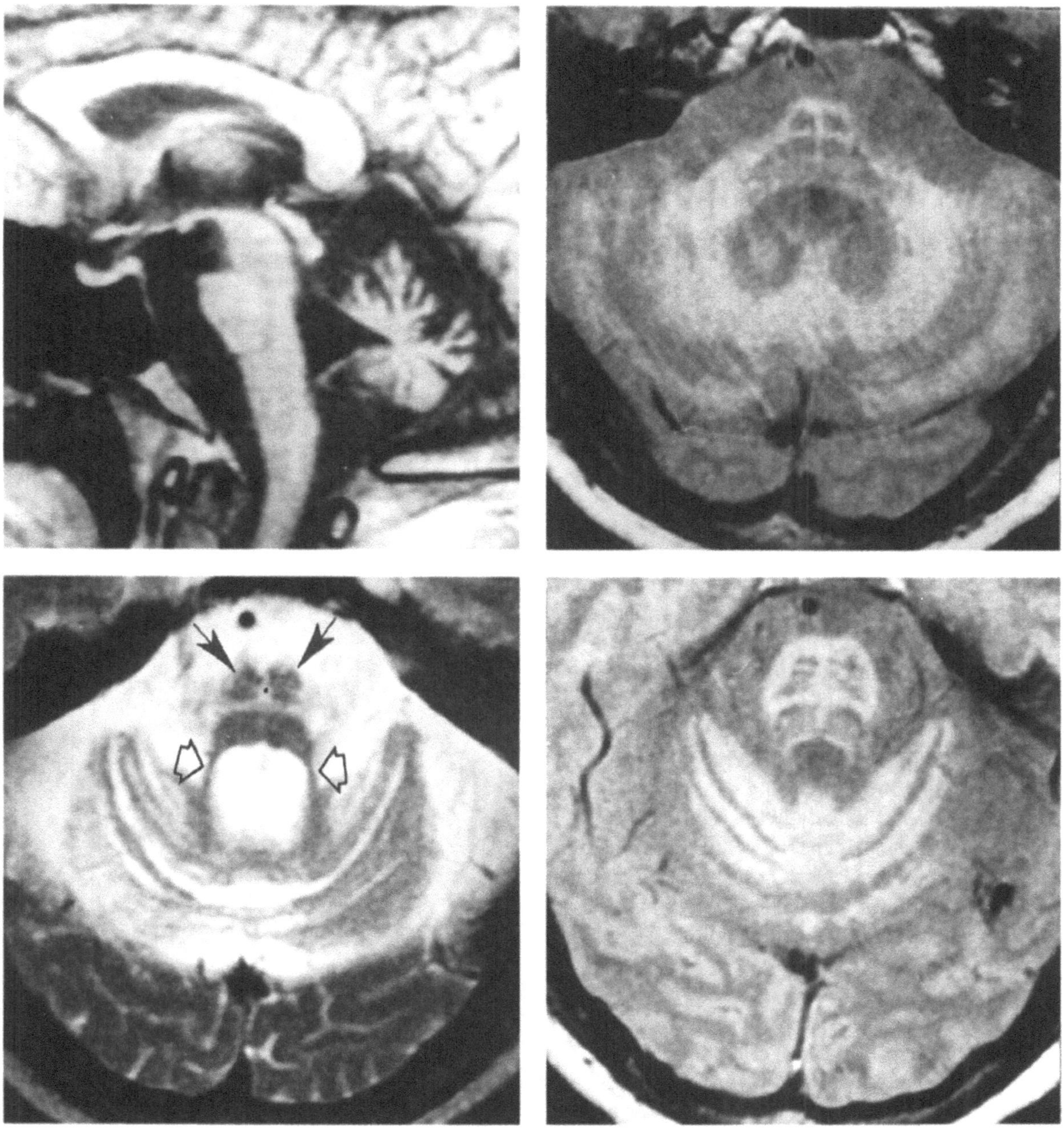

a b c d

Fig. 15.4a–d. Multiple system atrophy, olivopontocerebellar atrophy type. **a** Sagittal T1-weighted image shows atrophy of the pons, with flattening of its inferior profile (compare with Fig. 13.5a), cerebellar atrophy, and enlargement of the fourth ventricle. **b,c** Axial proton density and **d** T2-weighted images at different levels of the pons demonstrate increased signal intensity in the transverse pontine fibers, middle cerebellar peduncles and cerebellum; the pyramidal tracts (*arrows in* **d**), the tegmentum, and the superior cerebellar peduncles (*open arrows in* **d**) maintain normal signal intensity. Compare signal changes in posterior fossa with normal occipital lobes

15.3.3 Progressive Supranuclear Palsy

Progressive supranuclear palsy or Steele-Richardson-Olszewski syndrome is characterized by parkinsonism with age at onset over 40 years, supranuclear vertical gaze palsy, postural instability, late mild dementia, and poor response to L-dopa (LITVAN et al. 1996).

The pathological changes, neuronal loss, gliosis, loss of myelin, neurofibrillary tangles and granulovacuolar degeneration are mainly found in the periaqueductal area of the midbrain, which becomes progressively atrophic, but are also present in the globi pallidi, subthalamic nuclei, and pars compacta of the substantia nigra and may extend to the pontine tegmentum (YAGISHITA and ODA 1996; AIBA et al. 1997).

The MRI abnormalities are, therefore, found in these same areas. Atrophy of the midbrain is well demonstrated particularly in the midline sagittal section, with decrease of both sagittal and vertical diameters, enlargement of the aqueduct, and thinning of the quadrigeminal plate, mainly of the superior colliculi. The superior profile of the midbrain becomes flattened and then concave, with progressive enlargement of the third ventricle (Fig. 15.5).

In a recent review we made of 24 patients with clinical diagnosis of PSP, atrophy was present in 22 (91.7%), severe in 13, and slight in 9 (SAVOIARDO et al. in press).

Signal abnormalities are mild and consist of hyperintensity in proton density and T2-weighted images in the periaqueductal region of the midbrain; they are more visible in proton density and FLAIR images. In our series, midbrain signal abnormalities were present in 16 patients (66.7%) (Fig. 15.5).

In their detailed analysis of MRI and pathological findings, YAGISHITA and ODA (1996) were also able to demonstrate shrinkage and hyperintensity of the pallida and hyperintensity of the pontine tegmentum, occasional thinning of the pars compacta and, in one case, hyperintensity of the inferior olive.

A decreased signal in the substantia nigra with thinning of the pars compacta is a non-specific finding that may be seen both in Parkinson's disease and in parkinsonian disorders (PSP and SND) (YAGISHITA and ODA 1996).

Abnormalities in the putamen as seen in SND are not a feature of PSP. In one PSP brain we examined with postmortem MRI and Perls' stain, no iron was present in the putamen (SAVOIARDO et al. 1989); this finding, i.e., absence of iron, has been confirmed by other investigators (YAGISHITA and ODA 1996). Occasionally, decreased signal intensity in T2-weighted images consistent with iron deposition is seen in patients with PSP, but several patients are in their late sixties or over 70, and age may justify this finding. To our knowledge, no hyperintense lateral rim was ever reported in the putamen in PSP patients.

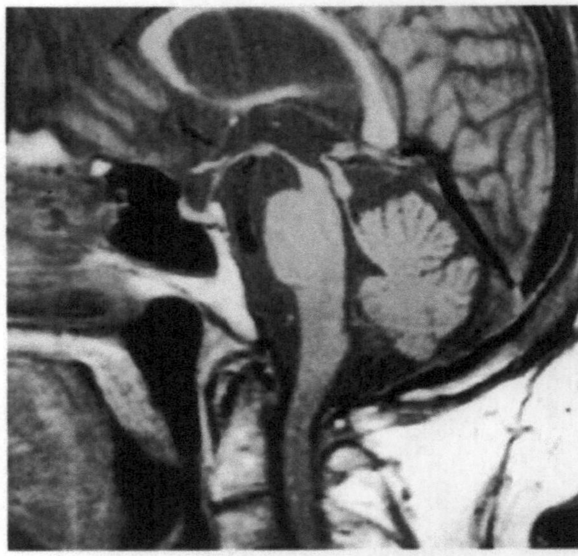

a

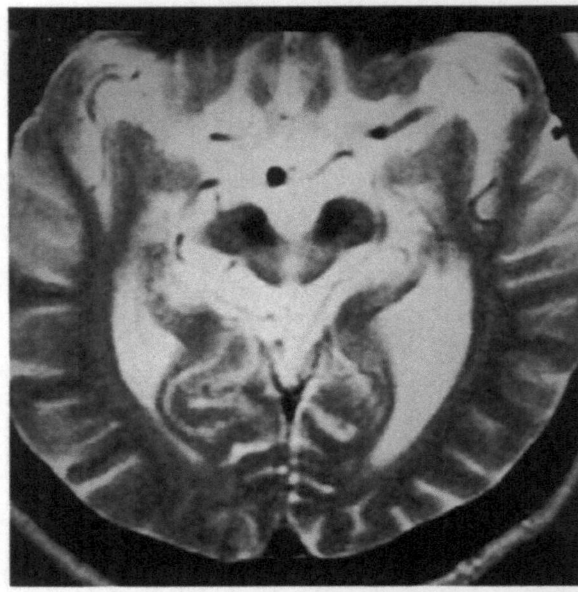

b

Fig. 15.5a,b. Progressive supranuclear palsy. **a** Midline sagittal T1-weighted section shows marked midbrain atrophy; compare with midbrain of Fig. 13.4a. **b** Atrophy is confirmed by T2-weighted axial section; diffuse hyperintensity is present in the tegmentum and tectum (compare with Fig. 13.1b)

15.3.4 Corticobasal Degeneration

Only in recent years has CBD been increasingly recognized. Clinically it is characterized by slowly progressive, asymmetric, akinetic-rigid syndrome with one or more of the following signs: ideomotor apraxia, myoclonus, cortical sensory deficit, and alien limb syndrome. There is no response to L-dopa treatment (LITVAN et al. 1997).

As asymmetry is a characteristic clinical feature, asymmetrical atrophy is the main MRI aspect.

In our series of 25 patients meeting the standard clinical criteria of CBD studied by MRI, asymmetrical atrophy, mostly involving the posterior frontal and parietal areas on the side contralateral to the

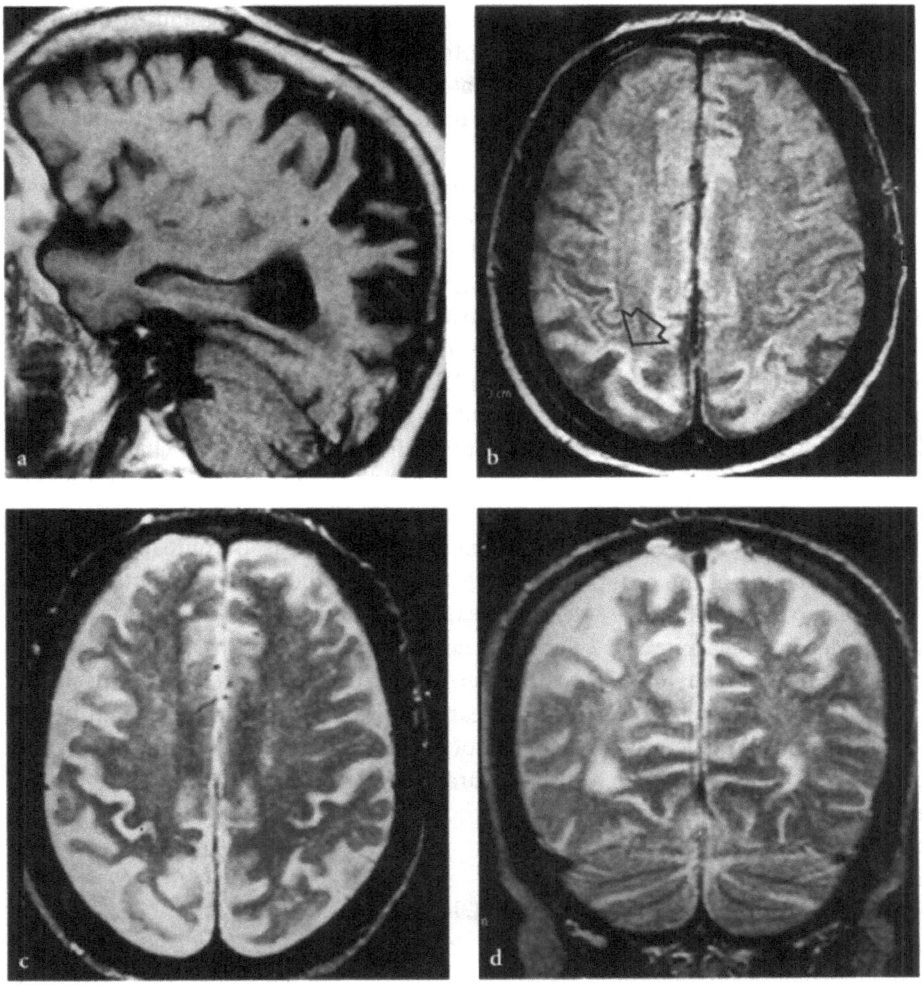

Fig. 15.6a–d. Corticobasal degeneration in a 65-year-old patient. **a** Sagittal T1-weighted image on the right cerebral hemisphere shows distribution of atrophy in the posterior frontal and mostly parietal region. **b,c** Proton density and T2-weighted axial images demonstrate asymmetrical atrophy, more marked on the right side, in a patient with left-sided symptoms; the right parietal cortex is slightly hyperintense in **b** (*open arrow*). **d** The coronal T2-weighted section confirms the prevalence of right parietal atrophy. Minimal hyperintensity is present in the subcortical white matter in the atrophic right parietal lobe. Rare hyperintense areas in the white matter of both cerebral hemispheres **(b–d)** are probably related to ischemic changes, consistent with the age of the patient

clinically most affected side, was seen in 24 (96%). On the most atrophic side, the ventricle was slightly larger and the sulci were dilated. Often the postcentral gyrus was particularly thin. The bulk of white matter was decreased. Occasionally, a slight increase in signal intensity in the thin cortex in the atrophic parietal area was seen in proton density or FLAIR images. No abnormalities were recognizable in T2-weighted images, probably because of overshadowing by the hyperintensity of the surrounding cerebrospinal fluid (CSF) (Savoiardo et al., in press). A minimal pallor sometimes extended to the subjacent white matter (Fig. 15.6).

It is interesting to note that when we reexamined the first few MRI studies of patients with CBD blind to the most affected side (alerted by the neurologist that asymmetrical atrophy was the main feature of CBD), we could easily identify the pathological hemisphere while the original report never mentioned asymmetry (Grisoli et al. 1995).

Even in CBD, at high-field MRI, putaminal hypointensity may occasionally be seen, but the hyperintense lateral rim was never found in our series.

Occasional hyperintensities in T2-weighted images in the periventricular or subcortical white matter were present, but not in excess of what is usually seen in a population of the same age.

The midbrain in CBD is normal; however, two of our patients had mild atrophy of the midbrain with minimal periaqueductal hyperintensity as seen in PSP: these cases might have the pathological findings of both diseases, although there were no clinical features pointing to PSP. Follow-up and possibly postmortem examination may clarify this point.

15.3.5 Huntington's Disease

Huntington's disease (HD) is an autosomal dominant, neurodegenerative disorder, clinically characterized by choreiform hyperkinesia, affective-emotional disturbances and intellectual deterioration, usually beginning between 35 and 45 years of age. A "rigid" variant may be seen, more commonly in young patients. The classic hyperkinetic form may evolve toward an akinetic state.

In HD, the brain is diffusely atrophic, with more marked atrophy in the basal ganglia, severely involving the head of the caudate nucleus and, even more, the putamen.

In neuroradiological studies, atrophy of the head of caudate nucleus has been recognized even with pneumoencephalograms because of flattening of the profile of the frontal horns of the lateral ventricles. The greater involvement of the putamen has been appreciated only by MRI volumetric studies (Harris et al. 1992).

Signal abnormalities consisting of slight hyperintensity in proton density and T2-weighted images in the atrophic neostriatum (head of caudate nucleus and putamen) were constantly found in the rigid variant (Savoiardo et al. 1991), possibly related to greater neuronal loss and gliosis.

Some patient with the classic hyperkinetic form also had neostriatal signal abnormalities. When the hyperkinetic patients were split into two groups, with or without signal abnormalities, it turned out that the patients with signal abnormalities were younger, with earlier disease onset, had more severe motor disability, fewer hyperkinesias, worse Mini-Mental State examination scores, and greater reduction of verbal fluency than the patients of the other group. In other words, neostriatal signal abnormalities correlated with greater motor and cognitive impairment, probably reflecting more severe anatomic damage (Oliva et al. 1993) (Fig. 15.7).

A more recent MRI volumetric study confirmed that measurement of putamen is the best discriminator of HD patients from healthy controls (Harris et al. 1996), while measures of caudate atrophy and SPET measures performed less well. A longitudinal MRI study demonstrated progressive basal ganglia atrophy in HD and indicated that age at onset of the disease and length of trinucleotide repeat correlated significantly with amount of volume change in caudate and total basal ganglia (Aylward et al. 1997).

A few PET and SPET studies have been performed in HD demonstrating decreased frontostriatal perfusion; a SPET-MRI investigation in patients with different disease duration demonstrated that prefrontal perfusion correlated with cognitive measures, motor cortical perfusion correlated with physical disability, and decrease in cortical perfusion occurred before evidence of atrophy on MRI in patients with short disease duration (Sax et al. 1996).

15.3.6 Wilson's Disease

Wilson's disease or hepatolenticular degeneration is an autosomal recessive disease of copper metabolism, which leads to accumulation of copper in several organs, mainly liver and brain. If untreated, Wilson's disease leads to death with cirrhosis of the liver. Presentation may be neurological, with various movement disorders, intellectual deterioration or

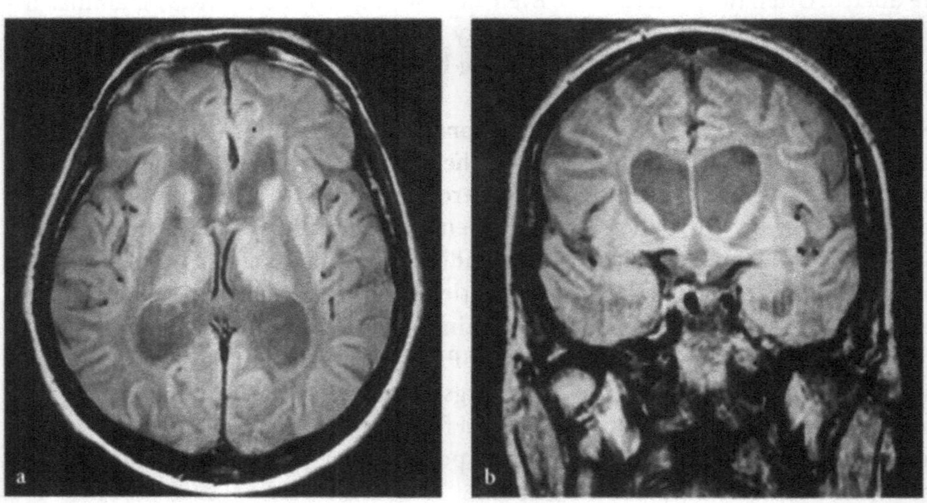

Fig. 15.7a,b. Huntington's disease, classic hyperkinetic form. **a** Axial, and **b** coronal proton density, images show atrophy of the putamina and caudate nuclei. Their signal intensity is barely increased; hyper-intensity is more marked in the rigid variant

behavioral disturbances. When the disease presents with only psychiatric problems, the diagnosis may be delayed and the neuroradiologist may be the first to suggest the correct diagnosis if he recognizes, on MRI, the characteristic findings of the disease. The MRI features of Wilson's disease, although variable, should be familiar, therefore, to the neuroradiologist.

Pathological changes mainly consist of shrinkage and light brown discoloration of the lenticular nuclei, where neuronal loss, degeneration of myelinated fibers, and vacuolization occur. These changes may be found in other nuclei, namely head of caudate nucleus, substantia nigra, and dentate nuclei. Marked astrocytic hyperplasia may be found in the basal ganglia, thalami, brainstem and cerebellum. More rarely the cerebral cortex and the white matter may be affected.

Copper deposition is limited to the basal ganglia, where microhemorrhages may also occur when severe destructive changes are present (Cumings 1948; Duchen and Jacobs 1984).

From these pathological changes, one may understand the MRI features: in T2-weighted images, two aspects may be seen, i.e., increased signal intensity related to increased water content from neuronal loss, gliosis, vacuolization, and decreased signal intensity from copper deposition and possibly hemosiderin, if microhemorrhages occurred.

Hyperintensities are more frequently observed and have greater extension (Fig. 15.8); they usually involve the neostriatum (head of caudate nucleus and putamen), the lateral part of the thalami, midbrain, pons, and dentate nuclei; rarely the globus pallidus (Fig. 15.8).

They may also involve white matter tracts, particularly the dentatorubrothalamic pathways, running from the dentate nucleus through the superior cerebellar peduncle to the contralateral red nucleus (which may also be abnormal) and then to the ventrolateral nucleus of the thalamus (and lateral thalamus is very often abnormal). Segments of the corticospinal tract and of the pontocerebellar tract,

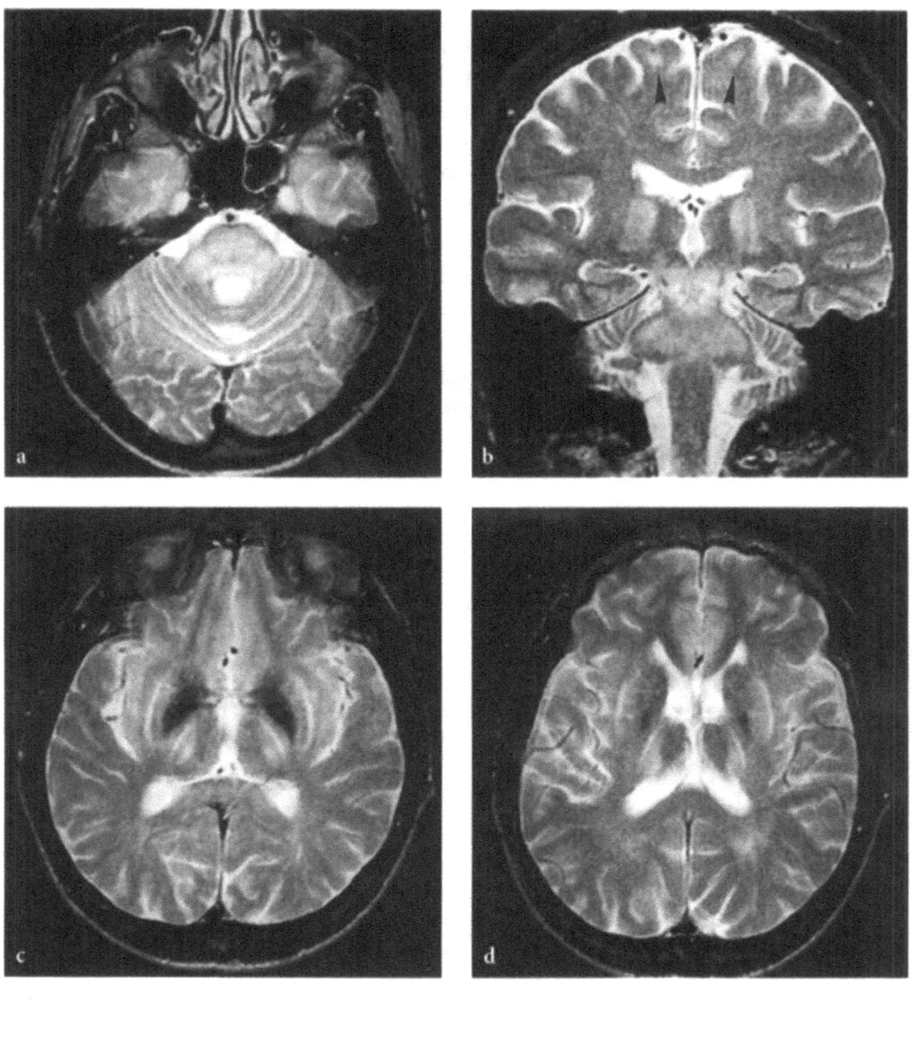

Fig. 15.8a–d. Wilson's disease in a 34-year-old man; 1.5 T, T2-weighted images. **a,b** Axial and coronal sections on the pons demonstrate moderate hyperintensity also involving the middle cerebellar peduncles; in **b** hyperintensity is also seen in the midbrain, lateral part of the thalami, and peripheral subcortical white matter (*arrowheads*). **c,d** Axial sections on the basal ganglia show pallidal hypointensity and hyperintensities in the lateral thalami and putamina with a markedly hyperintense lateral rim. In the thalami, this rim presumably corresponds to the reticular thalamic nucleus

which runs through the middle cerebellar peduncle, may also be involved (VAN WASSENAER-VAN HALL et al. 1995).

Hypointensities in T2-weighted images are more rare; when present, they are limited to the lentiform nucleus and head of caudate nucleus, sometimes only to the putamen. They may be surrounded by a hyperintense halo, with a somewhat swollen aspect of the nucleus, or may have a shrunken aspect in an atrophic nucleus (MAGALHAES et al. 1994; SAVOIARDO and GRISOLI 1998) (Fig. 15.8).

Modifications of signal abnormalities during D-penicillamine treatment were observed by ENGELBRECHT et al. (1995), who suggested iron deposition in exchange for copper.

T1-weighted images may show hypointensity in the most severely affected nuclei, particularly putamina, probably when destructive changes occur. However, they may also show hyperintensity in the pallida, as may be seen in patients with severe liver failure and portosystemic shunt (INOUE et al. 1991). The exact cause of T1-weighted pallidal hyperintensities in Wilson's disease is not completely clear; VAN WASSENAER-VAN HALL et al. (1996) call special attention to liver failure when these abnormalities and hyperintensity in T2-weighted images in the claustrum are present.

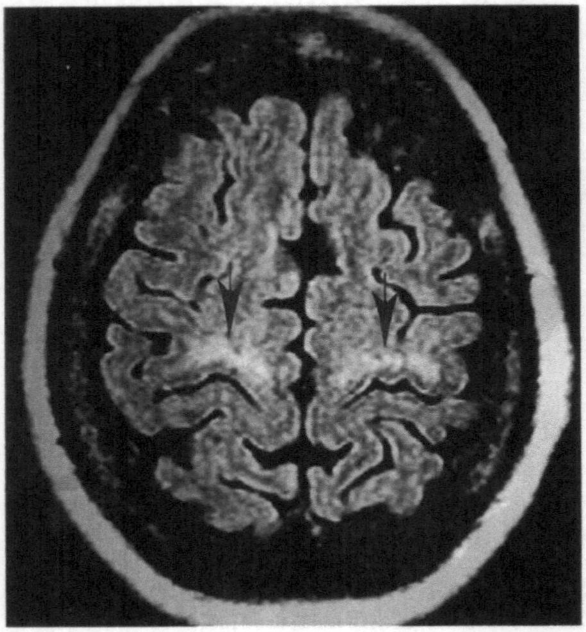

Fig. 15.9. Amyotrophic lateral sclerosis. Axial FLAIR section demonstrates slight hyperintensity of the white matter of the corticospinal tract in the center of the precentral gyrus (*arrows*)

15.4 Motor System

15.4.1 Amyotrophic Lateral Sclerosis

Amyotrophic lateral sclerosis (ALS) or motor neuron disease does not usually need neuroradiologic support for the diagnosis; occasionally, in the first stages of the disease, differential diagnosis can be entertained with spinal cord compression by cervical spondylosis, and MRI examination of the cervical spinal cord is commonly requested. Atrophy of the spinal cord may be demonstrated, but usually at an advanced stage of the disease.

Several MRI studies have investigated the brain for possible changes in the motor cortex and along the corticospinal tract.

A nearly constant decrease in signal intensity in T2-weighted images in the motor cortex related to iron deposits has been reported (OBA et al. 1993), but this abnormality has been considered non-specific by other authors; it is common in old age and in patients with cerebrovascular disease (HIRAI et al. 1996).

Increased signal intensity in T2-weighted images of the corticospinal tract from the precentral gyrus to the corona radiata, the posterior limb of the internal capsule and the central third of the cerebral peduncle has been observed in proton density and T2-weighted images in up to 70–75% of the cases (CARELLA et al. 1995; WARAGAI 1997); demonstration of signal abnormalities may vary during the evolution of the disease (Fig. 15.9).

A more specific finding has been observed by WARAGAI (1997) in a few patients with prominent upper motor neuron signs: hyperintensity in T1-weighted images along the corticospinal tract, possibly due to lipid-laden macrophages and accumulation of neurofilaments; this author also demonstrated some signal abnormalities in the spinal cord.

On brain MRI, slight hyperintensities along the corticospinal tract in T2-weighted images may occasionally be seen, however, in other diseases and in normal subjects; therefore, these signal abnormalities do not play a significant role in supporting the diagnosis of ALS. In an attempt to provide objective and quantitative information on the degeneration of the pyramidal tract in ALS, KATO et al. (1997) measured the magnetization-transfer ratios (MTRs) in the posterior limb of the internal capsule in nine ALS patients and in nine healthy volunteers, and found statistically significant differences. This study suggests that MTRs may be more useful and more sensitive than MR images in detecting subtle signs of early degeneration of the corticospinal tract in ALS patients.

In recent years, 1H-MRS has received greater attention than MRI in ALS investigation: although the *N*-acetylaspartate(NAA)/choline ratio or other metabolic peak area ratios may not be sensitive enough to detect early changes in ALS along the corticospinal tract (ELLIS et al. 1998), a significant decrease of NAA, exclusively expressed in neurons, has been found in ALS, proving that NAA measurement is a reliable, quantitative measurement of upper motor neuron dysfunction in ALS (ROONEY et al. 1998; BLOCK et al. 1998), also able to monitor reversal of metabolic changes after treatment with riluzole, a glutamate antagonist (KALRA et al. 1998).

15.5 Cerebellar System – Inherited Ataxias

Sporadic OPCA has already been discussed in the section on parkinsonisms because of its link with SND in MSA. We shall briefly review here the inherited ataxias.

The very broad field of inherited ataxias has attracted great interest in the last decade because of the enormous progression in molecular genetics that has allowed better understanding and reclassification of this group of diseases (HAMMANS 1996; HURKO 1997; DI DONATO 1998).

There are several reasons why the neuroradiologist is confused: ignorance of this new, complex classification, rarity of some genetic subtypes (absolute or relative to geographical areas), rarity of neuroradiological studies; in fact, most of the reports which also deal with MRI have appeared in the neurological literature. MRI may allow better "pathological"-clinical correlations, but the usefulness of these correlations in the general understanding of these disorders is questionable in view of the "substantial variability of brain and spinal cord pathological changes among families and within families with the same disease" (DI DONATO 1998).

A thorough review of this field would go beyond the limits of this chapter. We would only like to mention a few findings reported in some autosomal dominant cerebellar ataxias and briefly describe two autosomal recessive diseases, Friedreich's ataxia and ataxia-telangiectasia.

15.5.1 Autosomal Dominant Cerebellar Ataxia Type 1

Autosomal dominant cerebellar ataxia type 1 (ADCA I) is subdivided into different spinocerebellar ataxia types: SCA-1 to SCA-4 and SCA-6. SCA-1, SCA-2 and SCA-3 have been the object of a clinical and morphometric MRI analysis by BÜRK et al. (1996). These authors found that MRI, in combination with clinical and neurophysiologic studies, may help in distinguishing these diseases. Atrophy of SCA-2 patients was the most severe, and involved the pons, middle cerebellar peduncles and cerebellum as in OPCA. Brainstem and cerebellar changes in SCA-1 were similar, but more variable and less severe. SCA-3 patients had only mild brainstem and cerebellar atrophy. Putaminal and caudate volume was reduced in SCA-3 but with considerable overlap of the individual SCA-3 and control data (KLOCKGETHER et al. 1998).

It should be noted that Machado-Joseph disease, a disease first recognized in people of Azorean and Portuguese descent, has been found to be genetically an SCA-3. In a Japanese series of patients with this disease, which is the most common type of autosomal dominant spinocerebellar degeneration, MRI showed variable signal abnormalities, with the transverse pontine fibers hyperintense in proton density and T2-weighted images in 14 of 31 patients (45%), while these fibers were hyperintense in all 20 patients with sporadic OPCA, and not in any controls (MURATA et al. 1998b).

MRI studies in patients with SCA-6 have been reported: they had pure cerebellar atrophy, usually very severe, without significant abnormalities in the brainstem despite swallowing problems and ophthalmoplegia in many patients of one of the series (MURATA et al. 1998a; SCHÖLS et al. 1998). Since clinical manifestations of SCA-6 may appear late and the parents of the patients may have died before the appearance of clinical manifestations, the disease may be misdiagnosed as a sporadic disorder unless genetic testing is performed (SCHÖLS et al. 1998).

Considering the large phenotypic variation of Machado-Joseph disease (BÜRK et al. 1996) and of other dominant ataxias, and the variability of the pathological changes mentioned above (DI DONATO 1998), the MRI changes of these diseases should be verified in other large series.

15.5.2
Friedreich's Ataxia

In Friedreich's ataxia, slight neuronal loss in the dentate nuclei with consequent thinning of the superior cerebellar peduncles, and some loss of Purkinje cells, may be seen on pathological specimens, but most of the changes are in the spinal cord. In Friedreich's ataxia, the spinal cord is atrophic, with posterior columns, corticospinal and spinocerebellar tracts depleted of myelinated fibers and marked by gliosis (Adams and Victor 1993).

Since the MRI changes in the cerebellum are slight or minimal, and the main pathological changes are in the spinal cord, in a suspected case of Friedreich's ataxia it is mandatory to study the spinal cord, at least at cervical level (Gallucci et al. 1990). Because the patients usually have scoliosis, axial sections are often necessary to convincingly demonstrate the atrophy. In addition to atrophy, signal changes may be demonstrated, namely hyperintensity in proton density and T2-weighted images in the posterior columns (Mascalchi et al. 1994).

15.5.3
Ataxia-Telangiectasia

Ataxia-telangiectasia is a relatively frequent childhood ataxia which may present with, or be complicated by, recurrent pulmonary infections or sinusitis caused by an immunodeficient state characterized by decreased or absent immunoglobulin IgA. The typical oculocutaneous telangiectasias usually appear between 3 and 6 years of age and spread in a symmetrical fashion (Subramony 1998).

Brain MRI studies demonstrate severe cerebellar atrophy, often with inferior vermian hypoplasia, without signal abnormalities (Farina et al. 1994). Spinal cord examinations have not been described, but spinal cord atrophy should be seen, since involvement of the posterior columns and spinocerebellar tracts is recognized by the pathologist.

The main reason for mentioning ataxia-telangiectasia here is to recall that children or adolescents with this disease are also prone to develop lymphomas and leukemias, more rarely medulloblastomas and gliomas, and have an extreme radiation sensitivity (Hurko 1997).

15.6
Degenerative Diseases in Pediatric Age

Degenerative diseases are usually associated with adult or senile age. A few of the disorders discussed above may present during adolescence or childhood, particularly Wilson's disease and ataxia-telangiectasia. By separating the following diseases under this heading, we want to stress here that degenerative diseases do occur, unfortunately, also in children, and some are characteristic of the pediatric age.

We shall review the infantile neuroaxonal dystrophy and Hallervorden-Spatz disease, and the neuronal ceroid-lipofuscinosis.

15.6.1
Infantile Neuroaxonal Dystrophy

Infantile neuroaxonal dystrophy (INAD) is an inherited neurodegenerative disease with onset in the 1st or 2nd year of life, clinically characterized by psychomotor regression and hypotonia, which progress to tetraplegia, blindness, and dementia. Death usually occurs before the age of 10 years (Nardocci et al. 1999; Farina et al. 1999).

No biochemical marker is known. The pathological hallmark of the disease is the presence in the central and peripheral nervous systems of diffuse axonal swelling and "spheroid bodies" (i.e., the larger axonal swellings), containing different types of structured materials. Involvement of the peripheral nerves allows diagnosis by biopsy of the skin, nerve, conjunctiva, rectum, or muscle.

The MRI findings of INAD have been described in a few cases; recently a series of 11 cases from our institute has been reviewed (Farina et al. 1999): the most common finding was cerebellar atrophy, which progressed in follow-up examinations, with slightly increased signal intensity of the cerebellar cortex in proton density and T2-weighted images; rarely was hyperintensity of the dentate nuclei also seen. Mild hyperintensity of the supratentorial white matter, mostly in the posterior periventricular regions, probably indicated widespread neuroaxonal degeneration. The chiasm was usually thin, clearly atrophic in four.

An interesting finding observed in two of our patients and in a few other reported cases consisted of signal abnormalities in the globus pallidus similar to those observed in Hallervorden-Spatz disease (HSD), i.e., the "eye-of-the-tiger sign," with hypointensity in T2-weighted images, related to iron deposition; a similar hypointensity was also present in the substantia nigra. HSD is a neuroaxonal dystrophy and similarities are, therefore, not surprising; whether INAD and HSD represent phenotypes of the same disease is at present unknown (Farina et al. 1999).

15.6.2 Hallervorden-Spatz Disease

HSD is a rare neurologic disorder characterized by progressive dystonia, with prominent oromandibular involvement, mental deterioration, pyramidal signs, and retinal degeneration (Angelini et al. 1992). HSD is part of the neuroaxonal dystrophies, but the diagnosis cannot be obtained by skin or conjunctival biopsy because the pathological changes only involve the CNS and spare the peripheral nervous system. The gene locus associated with HSD has recently been identified on chromosome 20 (Taylor et al. 1996).

Characteristic findings observed on MRI may facilitate the diagnosis. In fact, the pathological changes in the pallida, known for many years, include deposition of iron, which gives a rusty brown discoloration to these nuclei.

Sethi et al. (1988) first called attention to what they called the "eye-of-the-tiger" sign, i.e., marked hypointensity of the pallida in T2-weighted images due to magnetic susceptibility effects from iron surrounding a central-medial area of high signal intensity. The nature of the pathological changes in this high signal area was unclear; previous pathological reports of HSD did not describe a definite "geographic" distribution of iron and other changes within the pallida.

We had observed an identical distribution of signal changes both at 0.5 T and 1.5 T in eight cases with clinical diagnosis of HSD; of course, hypointensity

a 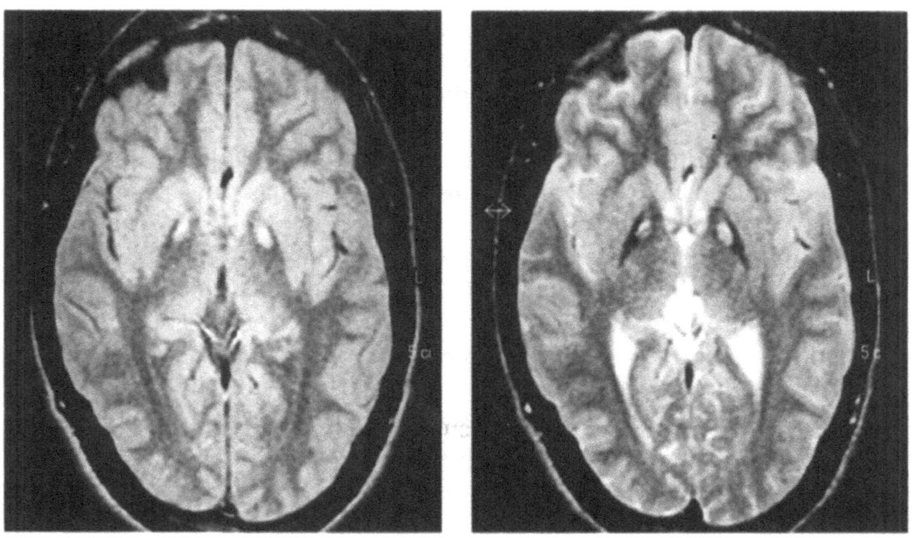 b

c 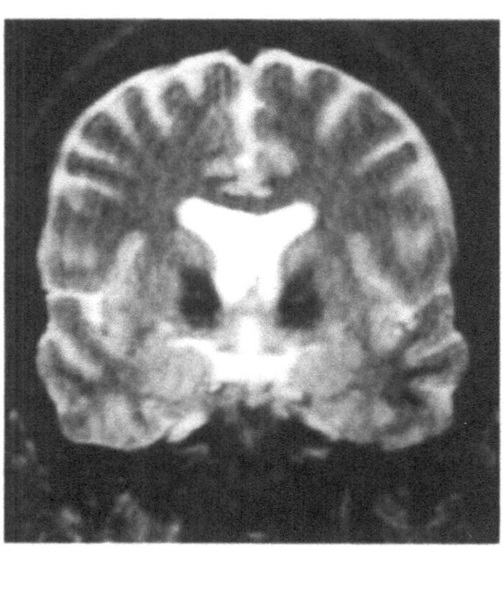

Fig. 15.10a–c. Hallervorden-Spatz disease. **a,b** Proton density and T2-weighted images at 0.5 T show a hyperintense area within the pallidum; despite the low field intensity, iron is enough to cause hypointensity in T2-weighted image. **c** At 1.5 T, coronal T2-weighted section, although disturbed by movement artifacts, shows marked hypointensity masking almost completely the hyperintense area due to iron was better demonstrated in 1.5 T studies, but central anteromedial hyperintensity was also well delineated in 0.5 T studies (Fig. 15.10).

We were able to eventually correlate these findings with the pathological examination of two brains of HSD patients studied by W.C. Halliday from Winnipeg, Canada: the low signal intensity corresponds to iron deposits in a dense tissue, while the high signal intensity of the eye-of-the-tiger sign corresponds to an area of loose tissue with vacuolization, with much less abundant iron deposits (Savoiardo et al. 1993).

A central spot of hypointensity within the high-signal area seen in some of our cases could correspond to an isolated area of mineralization, but this finding awaits pathological confirmation.

The pathological confirmation of a geographic distribution within the pallidum of the different histological changes of HSD makes the MRI findings very reliable for the diagnosis of HSD. However, the spectrum of signal abnormalities that can be encountered in neuroaxonal dystrophies is not yet known.

15.6.3 Neuronal Ceroid-Lipofuscinosis

Neuronal ceroid-lipofuscinoses are among the most common progressive encephalopathies of childhood and adolescence and are present throughout the world. The are divided into different forms according to age of onset (infantile, late infantile, juvenile, and adult types), with different eponyms. This separation is justified by different clinical phenotypes, which reflect their genetic heterogeneity; they are all inherited as autosomal recessive traits but the genes for the infantile and juvenile forms have been mapped on different chromosomes, 1 and 16, respectively (Autti et al. 1996).

Pathologically, they are characterized by cell loss and atrophy, especially in the cerebral cortex, and accumulation of ceroid and lipofuscin within numerous cell types. This accumulation allows diagnosis by electron microscopy examination of skin biopsy or circulating lymphocytes. In a series of juvenile and late infantile-type cases studied with postmortem MRI and histopathologically, loss of myelin and gliosis of various degrees were found mostly in the periventricular white matter; severe thalamic degeneration was found in the cases with the Jansky-Bielschowsky variant (Autti et al. 1997).

Without going into the details of the different clinical presentations, it is sufficient to mention here that severe psychomotor delay or regression, epilepsy, myoclonus, visual impairment from retinal degeneration or blindness characterize the disease. In the infantile form, microcephaly is present; in the adult form, myoclonus epilepsy, various degrees of dementia and motor disturbances are present, but visual function may be normal (Nardocci et al. 1995).

MRI findings are fairly characteristic. In the infantile form, cerebral atrophy with dilatation of ventricles and sulci is seen and is more marked than cerebellar atrophy. The corpus callosum is thin. Microcephaly is present. The most striking signal abnormality is hypointensity of the thalami in T2-weighted images, attributed, although without pathological proof, to deposition of iron, perhaps a non-specific response to degeneration, and to accumulation of lipofuscin (Vanhanen et al. 1994). Moderate periventricular and slight subcortical hyperintensity persists beyond the normal age for a change in signal intensity: the

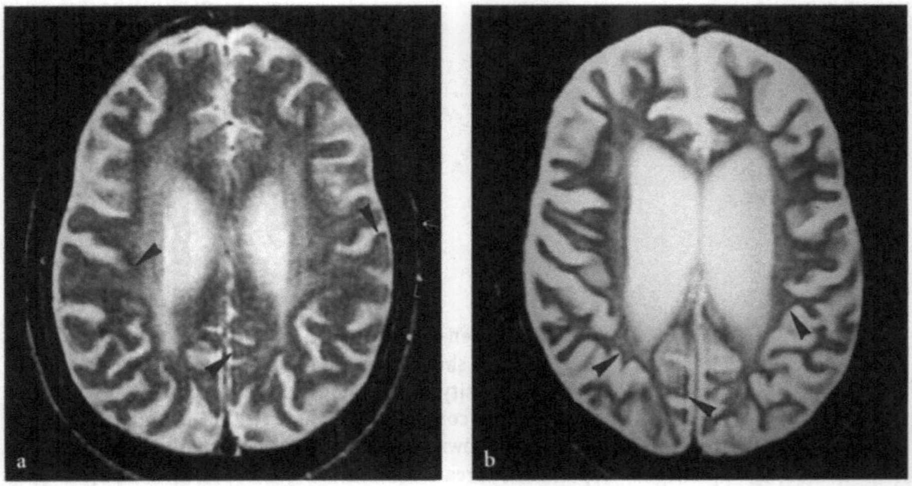

Fig. 15.11a,b. Neuronal ceroid-lipofuscinosis, juvenile type, in two different patients. **a** In a moderately advanced, and **b** in a severely advanced, case, T2-weighted axial sections show diffuse atrophy and white matter hyperintensity, more marked in the periventricular regions. Note the remarkable thinning of the cortex (*arrowheads*)

subcortical white matter remains hyperintense with respect to the cortex (VANHANEN et al. 1994).

In juvenile and adult forms, the most evident finding is progressive atrophy, more severe in the supratentorial than in the infratentorial compartment. The convolutions become thin and the bulk of the white matter decreases. The cortex becomes very thin; in a few cases we observed, this was particularly evident in the occipital areas and in the frontal gyri near the vertex, probably because the axial sections in this area cut the cortex perpendicularly. In advanced cases, the cortex was always hypointense in T2-weighted images with respect to the subcortical white matter (Fig. 15.11).

In less advanced cases, only slight hyperintensity was present in the periventricular white matter; this finding corresponds to myelin loss and gliosis demonstrated by AUTTI et al. (1997). Mild to moderate cerebral atrophy and a periventricular band of slight hyperintensity were the most common findings in a large Finnish series of juvenile neuronal ceroid-lipofuscinosis (AUTTI et al. 1996).

In our experience, observation of thinning of the cortex was the most important feature for suggesting the diagnosis, which was often correct.

Hypointensity in the thalami, characteristic of the infantile form, rapidly disappears with increasing age in the later onset forms.

15.7 Conclusion

The neuroradiologist is a clinician, a clinician working in a team. If this is true in all the fields of neuroradiology, it is even more important when he has to deal with degenerative disorders, sometimes rare and poorly known, in which the MRI changes may be subtle and, therefore, easily overlooked. Only a constant dialogue with the neurologist or the pediatric neurologist specifically interested in these disorders, and possibly the neuropathologist and geneticist, may lead to a more careful and sharper observation of the cases. Only if there is a constant feedback may the neuroradiologist enhance his diagnostic capability.

In degenerative and metabolic disorders, a good number of cases remain undefined. Nevertheless, the neuroradiologist can offer at least the indication of the areas involved, narrow the differential diagnosis and eliminate wrong hypotheses.

1H-MRS has just entered the field of degenerative diseases; functional studies will probably find their place, and correlations with neuropsychological testing will improve our understanding particularly of different types of dementia. A multidisciplinary approach is increasingly desirable; as in many other fields of medicine, it may more rapidly improve our knowledge regarding degenerative disorders and, in the end, make better care of the patients possible.

References

Adams RD, Victor M (1993) Principles of Neurology, 5th edn. McGraw-Hill, New York, pp 987–989

Aiba I, Hashizume Y, Yoshida M et al. (1997) Relationship between brainstem MRI and pathological findings in progressive supranuclear palsy- study in autopsy cases. J Neurol Sci 152: 210–217

Angelini L, Nardocci N, Rumi V et al. (1992) Hallervorden-Spatz disease: clinical and MRI study in eleven cases diagnosed in life. J Neurol 239: 417–425

Autti T, Raininko R, Vanhanen SL et al. (1996) MRI of neuronal ceroid lipofuscinosis. I Cranial MRI of 30 patients with juvenile neuronal ceroid lipofuscinosis. Neuroradiology 38: 476–482

Autti T, Raininko R, Santavuori P et al. (1997) MRI of neuronal ceroid lipofuscinosis. II Postmortem MRI and histopathological study of the brain in 16 cases of neuronal ceroid lipofuscinosis of juvenile or late infantile type. Neuroradiology 39: 371–377

Aylward EH, Li Q, Stine OC et al. (1997) Longitudinal change in basal ganglia volume in patients with Huntington's disease. Neurology 48: 394–399

Block W, Karitzky J, Traber F et al. (1998) Proton magnetic resonance spectroscopy of the primary motor cortex in patients with motor neuron disease: subgroup analysis and follow-up measurements. Arch Neurol 55: 931–936

Borit A, Rubinstein LJ, Urich H (1975) The striatonigral degenerations: putaminal pigments and nosology. Brain 98: 101–112

Braffman BH, Trojanowski JQ, Atlas SW (1991) The aging brain and neurodegenerative disorders. In: Atlas SW (ed) Magnetic resonance imaging of the brain and spine. Raven Press, New York, pp 567–624

Bürk K, Abele M, Fetter M et al. (1996) Autosomal dominant cerebellar ataxia type I. Clinical features and MRI in families with SCA 1, SCA 2 and SCA 3. Brain 119: 1497–1505

Carella F, Grisoli M, Savoiardo M et al. (1995) Magnetic resonance signal abnormalities along the pyramidal tracts in amyotrophic lateral sclerosis. Ital J Neurol Sci 16: 511–515

Cumings JN (1948) The copper and iron content of brain and liver in the normal and in hepato-lenticular degeneration. Brain 71: 410–415

de Leon MJ, Golomb J, Convit A et al. (1993) The radiologic prediction of Alzheimer disease: the atrophic hippocampal formation. Am J Neuroradiol 14: 897–906

Di Donato S (1998) The complex clinical and genetic classification of inherited ataxias. Ital J Neurol Sci 19: 335–343

Drayer BP, Olanow W, Burger P et al. (1986) Parkinson plus syndrome: diagnosis using high field MR imaging of brain iron. Radiology 159: 493–498

Duchen LW, Jakobs JM (1984) Nutritional deficiencies and metabolic disorders. In: Hume Adams J, Corsellis JAN, Duchen LW (eds) Greenfield's neuropathology, 4th edn. Wiley, New York, pp 573–626

Ellis CM, Simmons A, Andrews C et al. (1998) A proton magnetic resonance spectroscopic study in ALS: correlation with clinical findings. Neurology 51: 1104–1109

Engelbrecht V, Schlang G, Hefter H et al. (1995) MRI of the brain in Wilson disease: T2 signal loss under therapy. J Comput Assist Tomogr 19: 635–638

Farina L, Uggetti C, Ottolini A et al. (1994) Ataxia-telangiectasia: MR and CT findings. J Comput Assist Tomogr 18: 724–727

Farina L, Nardocci N, Bruzzone MG et al. (1999) Infantile neuroaxonal dystrophy: neuroradiological studies in 11 patients. Neuroradiology 41: 376–380

Fearnley JM, Lees AJ (1990) Striatonigral degeneration. A clinicopathological study. Brain 113: 1823–1842

Frisoni GB, Laakso MP, Beltramello A et al. (1999) Hippocampal and entorhinal cortex atrophy in frontotemporal dementia and Alzheimer's disease. Neurology 52: 91–100

Gallucci M, Splendiani A, Bozzao A et al. (1990) MR imaging of degenerative disorders of brain stem and cerebellum. Magn Reson Imaging 8: 117–122

Goto S, Matsumoto S, Ushio Y et al. (1996) Subregional loss of putaminal efferents to the basal ganglia output nuclei may cause parkinsonism in striatonigral degeneration. Neurology 47: 1032–1036

Grisoli M, Fetoni V, Savoiardo M et al. (1995) MRI in corticobasal degeneration. Eur J Neurol 2: 547–552

Hammans SR (1996) The inherited ataxias and the new genetics. J Neurol Neurosurg Psychiatry 61: 327–332

Harris GJ, Pearlson GD, Peyser CE et al. (1992) Putamen volume reduction on magnetic resonance imaging exceeds caudate changes in mild Huntington's disease. Ann Neurol 31: 69–75

Harris GJ, Aylward EH, Peyser CE et al. (1996) Single photon emission computed tomographic blood flow and magnetic resonance volume imaging of basal ganglia in Huntington's disease. Arch Neurol 53: 316–324

Hirai T, Korogi Y, Sakamoto Y et al. (1996) T2 shortening in the motor cortex: effect of aging and cerebrovascular diseases. Radiology 199: 799–803

Hurko O (1997) Recent advances in heritable ataxias. Ann Neurol 41: 4–6

Ibanez V, Pietrini P, Alexander GE et al. (1998) Regional glucose metabolic abnormalities are not the result of atrophy in Alzheimer's disease. Neurology 50: 1585–1593

Inoue E, Hori S, Narumi Y et al. (1991) Portal-systemic encephalopathy: presence of basal ganglia lesions with high signal intensity on MR images. Radiology 179: 551–555

Jack CR, Petersen RC, O'Brien PC et al. (1992) MR-based hippocampal volumetry in the diagnosis of Alzheimer's disease. Neurology 42: 183–188

Kalra S, Cashman NR, Genge A et al. (1998) Recovery of N-acetylaspartate in corticomotor neurons of patients with ALS after riluzole therapy. Neuroreport 9: 1757–1761

Kato Y, Matsumura K, Kinosade Y et al. (1997) Detection of pyramidal tract lesions in amyotrophic lateral sclerosis with magnetization-transfer measurements. Am J Neuroradiol 18: 1541–1547

Kitagaki H, Mori E, Hirono N et al. (1997) Alteration of white matter MR signal intensity in frontotemporal dementia. Am J Neuroradiol 18: 367–378

Kitagaki H, Mori E, Yamaji S et al. (1998) Frontotemporal dementia and Alzheimer disease: evaluation of cortical atrophy with automated hemispheric surface display generated with MR images. Radiology 208: 431–439

Klockgether T, Skalej M, Wedekind D et al. (1998) Autosomal dominant cerebellar ataxia type I. MRI-based volumetry of posterior fossa structures and basal ganglia in spinocerebellar ataxia types 1, 2 and 3. Brain 121: 1687–1693

Kraft E, Schwarz J, Trenkwalder C et al. (1999) The combination of hypointense and hyperintense signal changes on T2-weighted magnetic resonance imaging sequences. A specific marker of multiple system atrophy? Arch Neurol 56: 225–228

Laakso MP, Partanen K, Riekkinen P et al. (1996) Hippocampal volumes in Alzheimer's disease, Parkinson's disease with and without dementia, and in vascular dementia: an MRI study. Neurology 46: 678–681

Litvan I, Agid Y, Jankovic J et al. (1996) Accuracy of clinical criteria for the diagnosis of progressive supranuclear palsy (Steele-Richardson-Olszewski syndrome). Neurology 46: 922–930

Litvan I, Agid Y, Goetz C et al. (1997) Accuracy of the clinical diagnosis of corticobasal degeneration: a clinicopathologic study. Neurology 48: 119–125

Magalhaes ACA, Caramelli P, Menezes JR et al. (1994) Wilson's disease: MRI with clinical correlation. Neuroradiology 36: 97–100

Mascalchi M, Salvi F, Piacentini S et al. (1994) Friedreich's ataxia: MR findings involving the cervical portion of the spinal cord. AJR 163: 187–191

Miller BL, Moats RA, Shonk T et al. (1993) Alzheimer disease: depiction of increased cerebral myo-inositol with proton MR spectroscopy. Radiology 187: 433–437

Murata Y, Kawakami H, Yamaguchi S et al. (1998a) Characteristic magnetic resonance imaging findings in spinocerebellar ataxia 6. Arch Neurol 55: 1348–1352

Murata Y, Yamaguchi S, Kawakami H et al. (1998b) Characteristic magnetic resonance imaging findings in Machado-Joseph disease. Arch Neurol 55: 33–37

Nardocci N, Verga ML, Binelli S et al. (1995) Neuronal ceroid-lipofuscinosis: a clinical and morphological study of 19 patients. Am J Med Genetics 57: 137–141

Nardocci N, Zorzi G, Farina L et al. (1999) Infantile neuroaxonal dystrophy. Clinical spectrum and diagnostic criteria. Neurology 52: 1472–1478

Oba H, Araki T, Ohtomo K et al. (1993) Amyotrophic lateral sclerosis: T2 shortening in motor cortex at MR imaging. Radiology 189: 843–846

Oliva D, Carella M, Savoiardo M et al. (1993) Clinical and magnetic resonance features of the classic and akinetic-rigid variants of Huntington's disease. Arch Neurol 50: 17–19

Oppenheimer DR (1984) Diseases of the basal ganglia, cerebellum and motor neurons. In: Hume Adams J, Corsellis JAN, Duchen LW (eds) Greenfield's neuropathology, 4th edn. Wiley, New York, pp 699–747

Osborn AG (1994) Diagnostic neuroradiology (Chapter 18: Acquired metabolic, white matter, and degenerative diseases of the brain). Mosby, St Louis, pp 748–781

Pastakia B, Polinsky R, Di Chiro G et al. (1986) Multiple system atrophy (Shy-Drager syndrome): MR imaging . Radiology 159: 499–502

Perani D, Bressi S, Testa D et al. (1995) Clinical/metabolic correlations in multiple system atrophy. A fludeoxyglu-

cose F18 positron emission tomographic study. Arch Neurol 52: 179–185
Rooney WD, Miller RG, Gelinas D et al. (1998) Decreased N-acetylaspartate in motor cortex and corticospinal tract in ALS. Neurology 50: 1800–1805
Savoiardo M, Strada L, Girotti F et al.(1989) MR imaging in progressive supranuclear palsy and Shy-Drager syndrome. J Comput Assist Tomogr 13: 555–560
Savoiardo M, Strada L, Girotti F et al.(1990) Olivopontocerebellar atrophy: MR diagnosis and relationship to multisystem atrophy. Radiology 174: 693–696
Savoiardo M, Strada L, Oliva D et al.(1991) Abnormal MRI signal in the rigid form of Huntington's disease. J Neurol Neurosurg Psychiatry 54: 888–891
Savoiardo M, Halliday WC, Nardocci N et al. (1993) Hallervorden-Spatz disease: MR and pathologic findings. Am J Neuroradiol 14: 155–162
Savoiardo M, Grisoli M (1998) Magnetic resonance imaging of movement disorders. In: Jankovic J, Tolosa E (eds) Parkinson's disease and movement disorders. Williams & Wilkins, Baltimore, pp 967–990
Savoiardo M, Grisoli M, Girotti F (1999) Magnetic resonance imaging in CBD and related atypical parkinsonian disorders and dementias. In: Litvan I, Goetz C, Lang A (eds) Corticobasal degeneration: clinical and research aspects. "Advances in Neurology" series. Lippincott-Raven Publishers, Philadelphia, in press
Sax DS, Powsner R, Kim A et al. (1996) Evidence of cortical metabolic dysfunction in early Huntington's disease by single-photon-emission computed tomography. Mov Disord 11: 671–677
Schöls L, Krüger R, Amoiridis G et al. (1998) Spinocerebellar ataxia type 6: genotype and phenotype in German kindreds. J Neurol Neurosurg Psychiatry 64: 67–73
Schrag A, Kingsley D, Phatouros C et al. (1998) Clinical usefulness of magnetic resonance imaging in multiple system atrophy. J Neurol Neurosurg Psychiatry 65: 65–71
Sethi KD, Adams RJ, Loring DW et al. (1988) Hallervorden-Spatz syndrome: clinical and magnetic resonance imaging correlations. Ann Neurol 24: 692–694
Subramony SH (1998) The inherited ataxias. In: Jankovic J, Tolosa E (eds) Parkinson's disease and movement disorders. Williams & Wilkins, Baltimore, pp 887–907
Taylor TD, Litt M, Kramer P (1996) Homozygosity mapping of Hallervorden-Spatz syndrome to chromosome 20 p 12.3-p 13. Nat Genet 14: 479–481
Testa D, Savoiardo M, Fetoni V et al. (1993) Multiple system atrophy. Clinical and MR observations on 42 cases. Ital J Neurol Sci 14: 211–216
Vanhanen SL, Rainiko R, Santavuori P (1994) Early differential diagnosis of infantile neuronal ceroid lipofuscinosis, Rett syndrome and Krabbe disease by CT and MR. Am J Neuroradiol 15: 1443–1453
van Wassenaer-van Hall HN, van den Heuvel AG, Jansen GH et al. (1995) Cranial MR in Wilson disease. Abnormal white matter in extrapyramidal and pyramidal tracts. Am J Neuroradiol 16: 2021–2027
van Wassenaer-van Hall HN, van den Heuvel AG, Algra A et al. (1996) Wilson disease: findings at MR imaging and CT of the brain with clinical correlation. Radiology 198: 531–536
Vymazal J, Righini A, Brooks RA et al. (1999) T1 and T2 in the brain of healthy subjects, patients with Parkinson disease, and patients with multiple system atrophy: relation to iron content. Radiology 211: 489–495
Waragai M (1997) MRI and clinical features in amyotrophic lateral sclerosis. Neuroradiology 39: 847–851
Yagishita A, Oda M (1996) Progressive supranuclear palsy: MRI and pathological findings. Neuroradiology 38: 560–566

16 Multiple Sclerosis

Elisabeth Bergers, Frederik Barkhof

CONTENTS

16.1 Introduction

Multiple sclerosis (MS) is the most common neurological disease among young adults in temperate climates, with the onset usually between the ages of 20 and 40 years, affecting twice as many women as men. MS is a chronic inflammatory disease of the central nervous system (CNS), pathologically characterized by infiltration of immune cells into the CNS, localized myelin destruction, most likely due to autoimmune reactions against myelin proteins, and loss of oligodendrocytes and axons (Bruck et al. 1997; McDonald et al. 1992). Neurologically, MS is characterized by progressive disability of neurological functions, for example coordination, sensibility, pyramidal or urological functions. In MS, several specific patterns of the clinical disease course can be distinguished (Lublin and Reingold 1996) (Fig. 16.1).

In most patients the disease starts with a relapsing-remitting (RR) course, with full or incomplete recovery after attacks. The periods between relapses are characterized by a lack of disease progression. In a substantial proportion of RR-MS patients, a secondary progressive (SP) course develops. Progression is defined as continuous worsening of baseline disability without or between relapses. RR-MS is the most common course of the disease, initially occurring in up to 85% of the patients. Within 10 years, 50% (and within 25 years, 90%) of these patients enter the SP-MS phase. A small percentage of MS patients (10%) show a primary progressive (PP) disease course including paraparesis, hemiparesis, brainstem syndromes and visual loss, without relapses or remissions. Poser et al. (1983) defined clinical diagnostic criteria based on the number of neurological attacks, clinical, paraclinical and laboratory evidence. Four

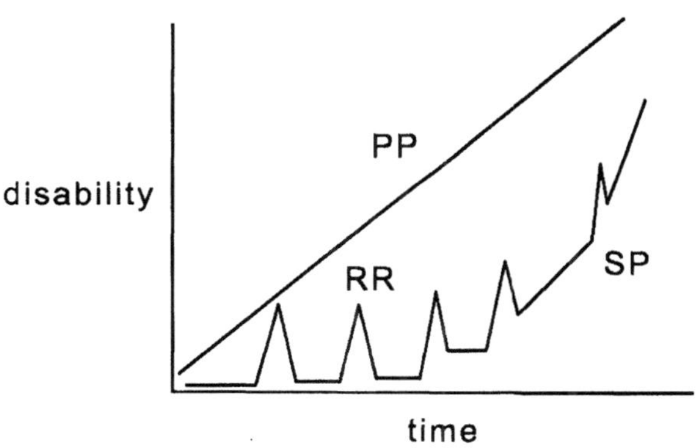

Fig. 16.1. Illustration of the three different MS courses. The relapsing remitting (RR) type. MS patients intermittently develop periods of neurological attacks and recover completely or incompletely. Between the attacks no progression of disability takes place. A substantial proportion of these patients will enter the secondary progressive (SP) phase in which the patients develop progression of disability between the neurological attacks. The primary progressive (PP) patients develop progression of disability from the start of the disease without relapses

E. Bergers, MD, PhD; F. Barkhof, MD, PhD
Department of Radiology, MR Centre for MS Research, Academic Hospital "Vrije Universiteit", PO Box 7057, 1007-MB Amsterdam, The Netherlands

groups are distinguished: clinically definite MS, laboratory supported definite MS, clinically probable MS and laboratory supported probable MS.

Magnetic resonance imaging (MRI) is the major confirmatory test for MS showing multiple white matter lesions in the brain. In comparison with computed tomography, MRI shows ten times as many lesions. At present, MRI is used in a diagnostic manner and for evaluation of new developments in treatment of MS (FILIPPI et al. 1998a). In this chapter we will discuss new MR developments with respect to MRI techniques, diagnostic work-up and non-conventional research techniques.

16.2 T2-Weighted MRI

16.2.1 Brain

On T2-weighted MRI, alterations in the composition of brain tissue will increase T2 relaxation times leading to a hyperintense signal in comparison with the surrounding grey and white matter. The most commonly used MRI sequence is a conventional dual-echo spin-echo (CSE), but also other sequences like turbo spin echo (TSE), fluid attenuated inversion recovery (FLAIR) or gradient echo (GE) have been employed. Figure 16.2 shows examples of brain imaging in MS patients using different sequences and Table 16.1 examples of different sequence parameters.

Dual-echo CSE is very sensitive for the detection of white matter lesions. However, with CSE some brain areas are more difficult to interpret and the acquisition time is relatively long. Unfortunately, the majority of alternative sequences do not increase the sensitivity to detect MS lesions. With TSE, similar numbers of lesions are detected in comparison to CSE (THORPE et al. 1994a), but the image formation of TSE is more complex, with increased incidental magnetic transfer effects.

On TSE, the signal of fat is higher and there are less susceptibility artefacts. The advantages of TSE are limited timewise with regard to proton density weighting, since the short echo time (TE) precludes the use of long echo-trains. In order to improve the contrast between normal appearing white matter and lesions, a magnetization transfer (MT) pulse can

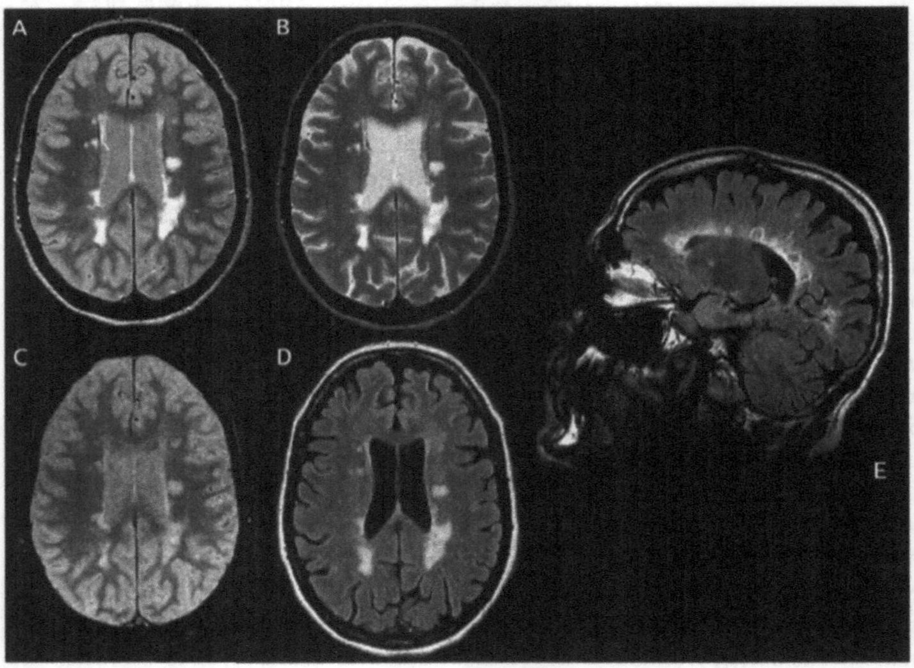

Fig. 16.2A–E. Illustrations of T2-weighted MR images of the brain of an MS patient obtained with different sequences. **A** Axial proton density weighted CSE image, **B** axial heavily T2-weighted CSE image, **C** axial GE image, and **D** an axial FLAIR image of the same patient at the same position in the brain. The white matter lesions, located typically periventricularly, are detectable with all techniques; however, the image quality of the GE is lower, which makes it more difficult to detect small lesions. On the axial FLAIR image the contrast between the ventricle and lesions is very clear in comparison to the proton density weighted image. The sagittal FLAIR image (E) is of another MS patient. It showed that the contrast between the corpus callosum and the lesions is very clear, which makes it easier to detect callosal lesions. Also juxtacortical lesions are easier to detect with FLAIR

be applied to suppress the background signal. However, the sensitivity of CSE and TSE for the detection of MS lesions does not benefit much from the added MT pulse (VAN WAESBERGHE et al. 1998a).

The sensitivity of echo-planar imaging and turbo gradient spin echo sequences is lower compared to CSE, with the advantage, however, of a marked reduction in image acquisition time.

However, the image quality obtained with such techniques is still relatively poor, and small lesions may be difficult to detect. Therefore, these techniques have to be reserved for uncooperative patients.

An exception is FLAIR, which has been found to be more sensitive for detection of supratentorial white matter lesions in MS patients than CSE (BARATTI et al. 1995; GAWNE et al. 1997a,b; HAJNAL et al. 1992; HASHEMI et al. 1995; RYDBERG et al. 1994; STEVENSON et al. 1997). The biggest advantage is the increased lesion to CSF contrast, since the CSF signal is nulled out, facilitating detection of periventricular lesions. Lesion to grey matter contrast can be higher on FLAIR than on TSE, which may also be favourable for detection of lesions in the cortex or basal ganglia. Lesion to white matter contrast is similar for FLAIR and TSE. A serious disadvantage of FLAIR is the poor sensitivity for detection of MS lesions in the infratentorial regions (BASTIANELLO et al. 1997), which is of concern since such lesions are typical for MS. Furthermore, part of the hyperintense lesions on T2-weighted images which are hypointense on T1-weighted images may become isointense on FLAIR (VAN WAESBERGHE et al. 1996b). However, for diagnostic purposes, FLAIR can be useful in addition to the SE sequences, for example in a sagittal plane showing small callosal lesions (Fig. 16.2E).

Lesions in the optic nerve can be visualized using a short tau inversion recovery (STIR) sequence or fat-suppressed T2-weighted SE sequence to reduce the orbital fat signal (GASS et al. 1996) (Fig. 16.3).

High signal lesions are seen in 80–90% of patients with optic neuritis (MILLER et al. 1993b; TIEN et al. 1991), but also in clinically unaffected nerves.

16.2.2 Spinal Cord

As for the brain, the most sensitive MRI sequence to image the spinal cord is a dual-echo CSE, but other sequences have also been applied. Several studies compared CSE with TSE (LYCKLAMA et al. 1996), STIR and FLAIR, but overall the CSE or TSE sequences seem to produce the most reliable images at present. In order to reduce motion artefacts of the spinal cord imaging, cardiac triggering and saturation of the thorax and abdomen can be applied to the CSE and TSE. Figure 16.4 shows examples of the different sequences and Table 16.1 shows examples of sequence parameters.

STIR (HITTMAIR et al. 1996; MASCALCHI et al 1993; THORPE et al. 1994b) results in a high lesion to cord contrast, but at the same time provides a poorer anatomical definition, more artefacts and a lower signal to noise ratio. It appears that when STIR is used in addition to TSE, approximately 25% more lesions are detected than with TSE alone. However, fast STIR shows more artefacts and cannot be used as a single technique. As for FLAIR, early studies reported that FLAIR might detect more lesions in the spinal cord (WHITE et al. 1992; THOMAS et al. 1993), but this was not confirmed by others (HITTMAIR et al. 1996; KEIPER et al. 1997; STEVENSON et al. 1997).

Although successful in obtaining CSF suppression, the sensitivity of lesion detection was in the latter studies much lower than for the CSE.

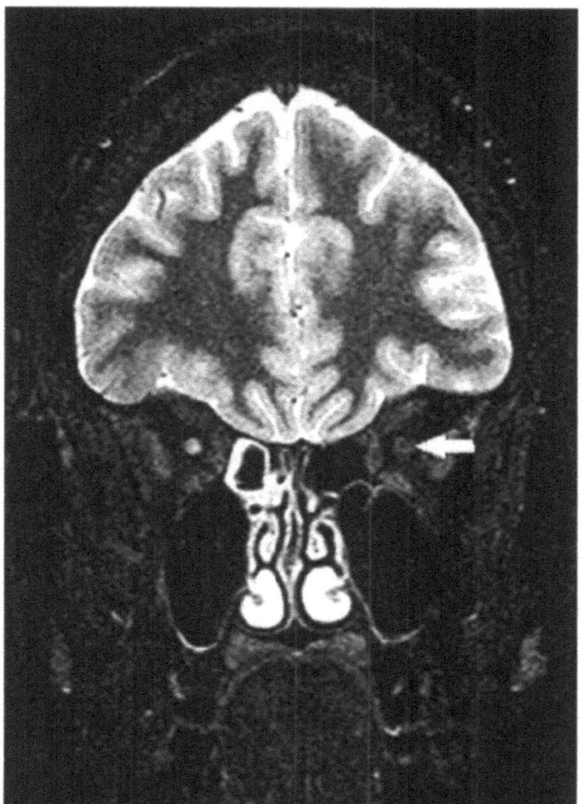

Fig. 16.3. Illustration of a STIR image in a patient with right sided optic neuritis. Note that the right optic nerve is hyperintense in contrast to the left one (*arrow*), which has the normal (low) signal intensity of white matter

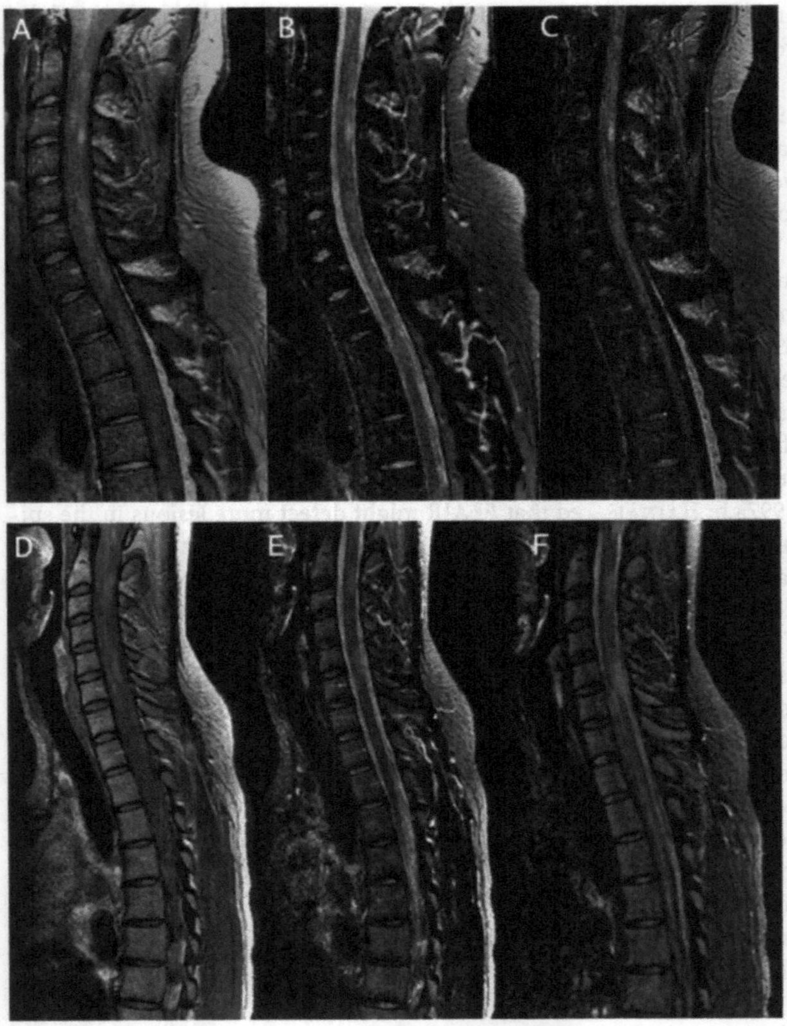

Fig. 16.4A–F. Illustrations of sagittal T2-weighted spinal cord MR images obtained with different sequences. **A** Proton density weighted CSE, **B** heavily T2-weighted CSE, and **C** FLAIR images of an MS patient. Focal lesions are detected on all sequences, but the proton density and heavily T2-weighted images show more focal lesions. Note the poor quality of the FLAIR image. **D** Proton density weighted CSE, **E** heavily T2-weighted CSE and **F** STIR image of another MS patient. The focal lesions are observed on all sequences, but the lesion to cord contrast is highest for STIR. However, STIR is more influenced by motion artefacts than CSE. Therefore, STIR can only be used in addition to CSE

Axial imaging of the spinal cord is more difficult than sagittal imaging mostly due to CSF pulsations. Sequences used are TSE and GE. The quality of gradient echo images can be much improved by the application of an MT presaturation pulse (Finelli et al. 1994; Lycklama et al. 1996).

16.3 T1-Weighted MRI

16.3.1 Brain

T1-weighted conventional SE is used for brain imaging pre- and postcontrast material injection, showing hypointense lesions and enhanced lesions, respectively, which correspond to hyperintense lesions on T2-weighted images (Barkhof et al. 1998; Paty and Li 1996; van Walderveen et al. 1995) (Fig. 16.5).

The hypointense lesions, also called black holes, reflect a destructive type of lesion, with complete demyelination and axonal loss (van Waesberghe et al. 1999; van Walderveen et al. 1998b). Enhanced MS lesions on T1-weighted MRI after Gd-DTPA injection reflect active MS plaques with macrophage infiltration. Extracellular contrast agents such as gadolinium-diethyl-enetriaminepentacetic acid (Gd-DTPA) produce enhancement in regions with an abnormal blood-brain barrier.

The paramagnetic effect of such agents produces a marked shortening of the T1 relaxation time of nearby water protons.

While the normal dose of gadolinium is 0.1 mmol Gd-DPTA per kilogram body weight, using a triple dose considerably increases the detection of

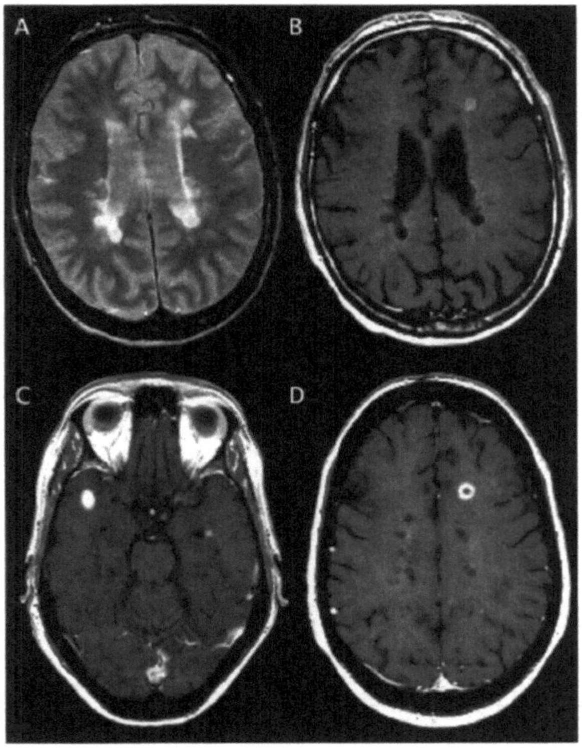

Fig. 16.5A–D. Illustration of **A** a proton density weighted axial image and **B** a T1-weighted axial image of an MS patient. There are several hypointense lesions (*black holes*) on the T1-weighted image corresponding to hyperintense lesions on the proton density weighted MR image. The location of the lesions is typically periventricular and characteristically the total number and volume of the black holes is lower than the proton density lesions. Black holes reflect the more destructive lesions with demyelination and axonal loss. **C** Axial T1-weighted MR image with clearly enhanced lesions and **D** an axial T1-weighted image with a ring enhancement of another MS patient. The enhanced lesions, due to an abnormal blood-brain barrier, reflect active MS lesions with macrophage infiltration. The ring enhancement on **D** is a reactivation of the edge of a black hole. Note also the other black holes on **D**

enhanced lesions (Filippi et al. 1997; Rovaris et al. 1998; Wolansky et al. 1994), being much more effective than the use of MT background suppression (Waesberghe et al. 1998a). Since the degree of leakage depends on the time after injection, a postinjection delay of 15–30 min should be employed. The lesions only detected with triple dose or delayed scanning have less severe damage to the blood-brain barrier. Magnetization transfer analysis of these lesions shows less tissue destruction indicating that less aggressive lesions are identified with this technique.

16.3.2 Spinal Cord

T1-weighted MRI of the spinal cord rarely shows focal enhancing lesions after administration of Gd-DTPA (Larsson et al. 1989). The use of a triple dose Gd-DTPA increases the sensitivity for detecting enhancing spinal cord lesions (Yousry et al. 1998), but still the occurrence of spinal cord enhancement is a rare phenomenon. Also the occurrence of hypointense lesions in the spinal cord is rare. Therefore, T1-weighted MRI is important to exclude other spinal cord pathology rather than to confirm the diagnosis of MS.

16.4 MRI Criteria for MS

16.4.1 Brain

White matter lesions are detected in 90%–97% of definite MS patients. Although MS lesions can be located anywhere in the white matter of the brain, typical locations are the periventricular region, corpus callosum, temporal lobes, and infratentorially. Classically, MS is considered to be a pure white matter disease, but lesions may also be observed at the border of the white and gray matter (juxtacortical) (Kidd et al. 1999) and in the basal ganglia. In some cases, tissue damage may start in the white matter and proceed into the gray matter, although the basal ganglia and the cortex contain myelin as well. Therefore, MS lesions can also start in the myelin of the gray matter. The occurrence of juxtacortical lesions can be well appreciated especially on heavily T2-weighted images and FLAIR, but on the proton density weighted images the connection with the gray matter is best observed.

The occurrence of juxtacortical lesions is of great diagnostic importance (Barkhof et al. 1997), since the subcortical u-fibres are characteristically spared in ischaemic white matter disorders.

The typical shape of MS lesions is ovoid, due to the perivenular localization of MS lesions. However, when lesions increase in size the ovoid shape may disappear and the lesions may follow for example the contour of the white matter or ventricles. Also, for very small lesions and for lesions with a long axis perpendicular to the imaging plane, the ovoid shape

Table 16.1. Standard and optional protocol for MRI of brain, optic nerves and spinal cord in MS patients

	TR	TE	TI	Flip angle	NEX	Slice thickness (mm)
Standard protocol						
Brain						
T2-weighted axial SE	2700	45/90	0	90	1	3
T1-weighted axial SE	700	15	0	90	2	3
Optic nerves						
STIR	2500	20	150	90	1	4
Spinal cord						
T2-weighted axial SE	2200	20/80	0	65	1	3
T1-weighted axial SE						
Option protocol						
Brain						
T1-weighted SE axial postgadolinium	700	15	0	90	2	3
Turboflair sagittal	9000	105	2200	180	1	3
GE axial (MTR measurement)	704	10	0	30	1	3
Spinal cord						
STIR	2200	30	110	90	1	3

TR, repetition time; TE, echo time; TI, inversion time; NEX, number of excitations.

may not be clearly present. Figure 16.6 shows examples of T2-weighted images with different types of focal MS lesions. MRI criteria (Table 16.2) for diagnostic purposes based on the location and number of lesions have been defined by Paty et al. 1988, Fazekas et al. 1988 and Barkhof et al. 1997.

With respect to T1-weighted imaging, some hyperintense lesions on T2-weighted MRI appear hypointense on the T1-weighted SE compared to the 'normal' white and gray matter (Fig. 16.5), with a signal intensity between CSF and gray matter. Usually, the number of hypointense lesions observed on the T1-weighted MRI is far less than the number observed on the T2-weighted MRI.

The pathological hallmark of persistent hypointense lesions is a chronic state of demyelination with axonal loss and gliosis (van Walderveen et al. 1998b; van Waesberghe et al. 1999) leading to an enlarged extracellular space with slowly relaxing CSF (Barkhof et al. 1998). Acute lesions may also be hypointense on T1-weighted MRI (without contrast administration) but these may recover.

Enhanced MS lesions on T1-weighted MRI after Gd-DTPA injection (Fig. 16.5) due to breakdown of the blood-brain barrier reflect active MS plaques with macrophage infiltration. Enhancement is a regular finding in new lesions and is strongly related to an exacerbation of MS (Miller et al. 1993a, 1998). Most of the enhanced lesions can be recognized as a hyperintense abnormality on T2-weighted images, although this is not universally true. Detection of enhanced lesions on T1-weighted images is specific for the diagnosis MS, since the presence of both enhancing and non-enhancing lesions indicates dissemination of the disease process in time, a prerequisite for the diagnosis MS.

Looking at the development of an MS lesion (Guttman et al. 1995), a small lesion initially enhances homogeneously, then if the lesion expands over the next few days to weeks, enhancement may be seen as an expanding ring at or near the edge of the lesion (Fig. 16.5). Enhancement usually ceases after about 1 month, and subsequently the T2-weighted lesion becomes smaller. Persistent enhancement beyond 1 month is unusual. Studies with monthly MRI showed that 73% of the enhanced lesions were observed on one scan, 21% on two consecutive scans and only 6% on three or four consecutive scans (Bastianello et al. 1990). Usually, a hyperintense T2-lesion remains visible, but may also recover and disappear.

When the inflammation is very aggressive a hypointense lesion may remain visible on the T1-weighted MRI immediately or after several active periods of that particular lesion.

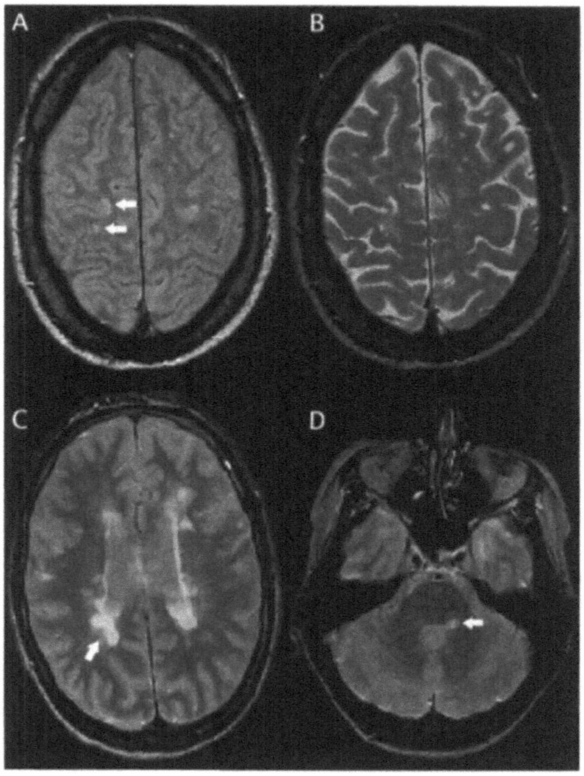

Fig. 16.6A–D. Illustration of hyperintense white matter lesions on T2-weighted CSE images. **A** A proton density weighted image and **B** a heavily T2-weighted image of an MS patient with juxtacortical lesions (located against the grey matter). *The arrows in* **A** show two examples of juxtacortical lesions, but *on the left side* there are more juxtacortical lesions observed. Theoretically, the lesions can begin in the white matter and proceed in the grey matter or the lesions start in the myelin of the grey matter. Note that these lesions can only be classified as juxtacortical on the proton density weighted images and that there is no white matter left between the lesion and the grey matter. However, the lesions are more appreciated on the heavily T2-weighted image (**C**), a proton density image of an MS patient with typically periventricular lesions showing so-called Dawson fingers (*arrow*) and **D** a proton density weighted image of another MS patient with an infratentorial lesion abutting the 4th ventricle (*arrow*). Both locations are typical for MS

16.4.2 Spinal Cord

Involvement of the spinal cord is a typical feature of MS and important with respect to the development of disability (Thielen et al. 1996). About 75–90% of MS patients have spinal cord abnormalities. There are two kinds of abnormalities observed on T2-weighted sagittal MR imaging, i.e., focal hyperintense lesions and diffuse hyperintensities in the whole or in a part of the spinal cord (Kidd et al. 1993; Lycklama et al. 1997, 1998). Focal hyperintense lesions are usually one to two vertebra in length, have a cigar shape on the sagittal image and are wedge-shaped on the axial image, and are usually located in the lateral and posterior column (Tartaglino et al. (1995). The diffuse hyperintense abnormality is only observed on the proton density weighted MRI and is not well demarcated.

This diffuse hyperintense signal is usually several segments in length, frequently up to the whole spinal cord and can be present in the whole diameter. Overall, MRI abnormalities are found more frequently in the cervical than in the thoracic or lumbal cord, which is in agreement with previous pathological observation (Fog 1950; Oppenheimer 1978). Focal or diffuse abnormalities of the spinal cord do not occur in healthy people including the older age groups with possible vascular disorders (Thorpe et al. 1993). Therefore, while many ischaemic disorders may interfere with the interpretation of white matter MS lesions in the brain, the spinal cord lesions are more specific for MS.

T1-weighted hypointensity and enhancement after contrast injection appear significantly less often in the spinal cord than in the brain and at present have less diagnostic and clinical impact. Figure 16.7 shows examples of focal and diffuse abnormalities on sagittal proton density weighted and heavily T2-weighted MR images in comparison to a spinal cord of a normal control.

Table 16.2. MRI criteria for the diagnosis of multiple sclerosis

Criteria	Description
Paty (1988)	Either four lesions or three lesions, one of which is periventricular
Fazekas (1988)	Three lesions, fulfilling two of the following criteria: A lesion larger than 6 mm A lesion abutting the ventricle An infratentorial lesion
Barkhof (1997)	a) Using only T2-weighted images Minimum of nine lesions b) Using T2- and T1-weighted images postgadolinium * 1 juxtacortical lesion * 1 gadolinium enhanced lesion * 1 infratentorial lesion * 1 periventrical lesion Cumulative change model: with more criteria fulfilled the chance of developing MS increases; when four criteria are fulfilled the change of clinical definite MS is 80%

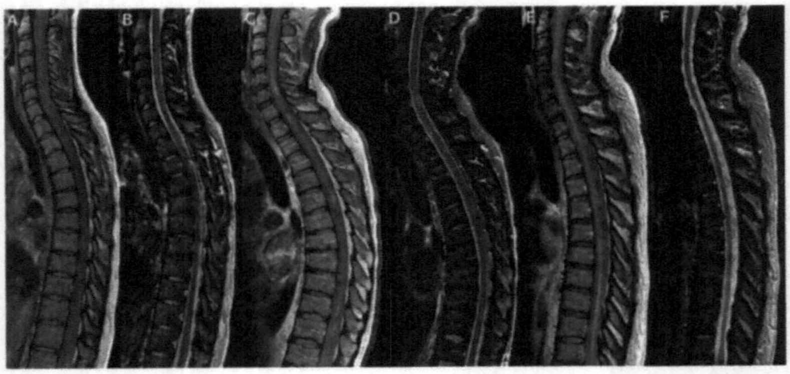

Fig. 16.7A–F. Illustration of proton density and heavily T2-weighted sagittal MR images of the spinal cord of **A,B** a normal control, **C,D** an MS patient with focal spinal cord lesions, and **E,F** an MS patient with diffuse abnormality of the spinal cord. On the proton density weighted image and heavily weighed T2-weighted images, the normal spinal cord has an isointense and hypointense signal intensity compared to CSF, respectively (**A,B**). The focal hyperintense lesions (**C,D**) can be observed on the proton density and on the heavily T2-weighted images. Note that in between these lesions the cord still has a normal low signal. The diffuse abnormality of the whole cord (**E,F**) is observed on the proton density weighted images with a hyperintense signal, while on the heavily T2-weighted images diffuse abnormalities cannot be detected. The diffuse spinal cord abnormalities correlate more with a primary progressive disease course. Note also that the spinal cord of the MS patient with the diffuse abnormality (**F**) is thinner than the spinal cord of the normal control (**B**) due to atrophy

The performance of axial spinal cord imaging can be important to confirm dubious lesions, and to determine which tract is involved, although the quality of the images is usually poorer than sagittal MR images.

16.5 Differential Diagnosis

Although T2-weighted brain MRI is very sensitive in detecting white matter lesions, the presence of hyperintense T2 lesions in the brain is a completely non-specific finding and occurs in the vast majority of white matter diseases. Table 16.3 shows a list of common disorders with possible white matter lesions.

Multifocal areas of high signal intensity within the cerebral white matter with or without altered signal in the immediate periventricular region may be seen on T2-weighted MRI in neurologically healthy people. The incidence of such abnormalities increases with age, and early studies reported a prevalence of more than 30% over the age of 60 years.

Additional criteria to differentiate MS lesions from ischaemic disorders are summarized in Table 16.4. Figure 16.8 shows an image of a typical ischaemic disorder with sparing of the u-fibres.

Furthermore, a high signal around the pole of the frontal ventricle horn (caps) is common and is due to an age-related focal loss of ependyma with subependymal gliosis, leading to an increased water content. Imaging of the spinal cord may in this respect be very helpful, since the presence of spinal cord abnormalities is more specific for MS (Thorpe et al. 1993).

The indications for spinal cord MRI in (suspected) MS are summarized in Table 16.5.

An often posed question is whether gadolinium should routinely be administered. In patients with two attacks already, an abnormal T2-weighted MR scan suffices to show dissemination in space. However, with only one clinical attack, gadolinium may additionally show dissemination in time (enhancing and non-enhancing lesions). Gadolinium is also indicated when other inflammatory disorders are suspected, for example, neurosarcoidosis or SLE.

16.6 Practical Guidelines

The diagnostic MR criteria of Paty, Fazekas and Barkhof (see above) differ; however, in this setting the most strict criteria of Barkhof are taken as a lead.

For brain imaging a T1-weighted SE pre- and post-gadolinium injection and a T2-weighted dual-echo SE should be obtained. In addition a (sagittal) FLAIR sequence can be employed to discover more easily jux-

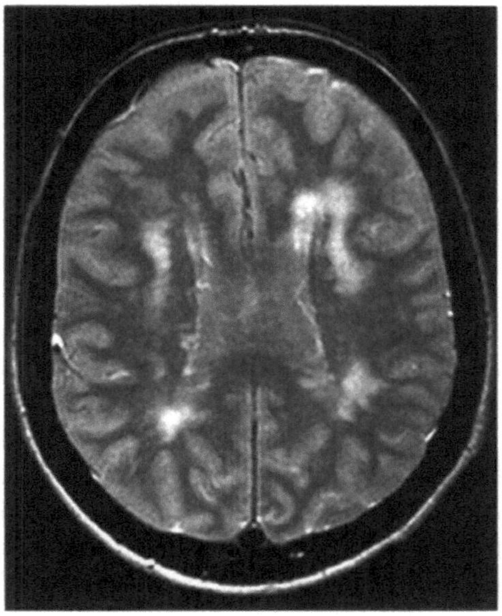

Fig. 16.8. Illustration of an axial proton density weighted brain image with typical ischaemic lesions in a patient with hypertension. The white matter lesions are symmetrical and confluating. The u-fibres are typically spared, in contrast to MS lesions, which are frequently juxtacortically located

Table 16.4. Criteria to differentiate MS lesions from hypoxic/ischaemic disorders

Criteria	MS	Hypoxic/ischaemic
Corpus callosum lesions	++	-
u-Fibre involvement	++	-
Basal ganglia lesions	+/-	++
Infratentorial lesions	++	+/-
Gadolinium enhancement	+	-
Temporal bone lesions	++	-
Arterial territory	-	+/-
Ovoid shape	++	-
Periventricular location	++	-

Table 16.5. Indications for spinal cord imaging

1. Clinically isolated syndrome with only spinal cord symptoms
2. Negative brain scan
3. Aspecific brain MRI findings
4. Atypical new spinal cord symptoms
5. Primary progressive MS

Table 16.3. Differential diagnosis of white matter lesions of the type observed in MS

Hypoxic/ischaemic

Macroangiopathy: atherosclerosis, hyperhomocysteinaemia, amyloid angiopathy
Microangiopathy: diabetic microangiopathy, hypertension
Systemic: perioperative hypotension, embolic
Unknown: depression, Alzheimer's, migraine

Inflammatory

MS variants: Charcot type (classic), Marburg type (fulminant), Balo type (concentric sclerosis)
Schilder type (diffuse sclerosis), Devic type (neuromyelitis optica)
Vasculitis: systemic lupus erythematodes (SLE), M. Behçet, M. Sjogren
Sarcoidosis
Inflammatory bowel disease

Infectious

Protozoal: cryptococcus, toxoplasmosis, cysticercosis
Spirochaetal: neurosyphilis, neuroborreliosis
Viral: HIV, progressive multifocal leucencephalopathy (PML)
Bacterial: tuberculosis, brucellosis
Postinfectious: acute demyelinating encephalomyelopathy (ADEM), subacute sclerosing
Postinfectious encephalitis (SSPE)

Toxic-metabolic

Central pontine myelinolysis (CPM), carbon monoxide (CO) intoxication, Methotrexate (MTX) treatment, Marchiafavi-Bignami, funicular myelinolysis (B_{12} deficiency)

Traumatic

Radiotherapy, postcontusion

tacortical lesions, in the corpus callosum and basal ganglia. When there are nine T2 lesions or more, the diagnosis MS is quite likely (Barkhof et al. 1997).

When the number of lesions is below nine, but are in the typical areas, additional information should be sought. Enhancing lesions or spinal cord lesions would strongly support MS.

Absence of white matter lesions in the typical brain areas or only brain lesions which spare the u-vessels and absence of spinal cord abnormalities argues against the diagnosis MS.

Furthermore, serial MRI can assist diagnosis of MS in those patients in whom the criteria of dissemination in time, a necessity for the clinical diagnosis of MS, has not been fulfilled by the presence of enhanced and non-enhanced T2-weighted lesions at the same time.

16.7 Clinical Correlations and Non-conventional MRI Parameters

16.7.1 The Clinicoradiological Paradox

Counting the number and measuring the volume of the MS brain lesions on T2- and T1-weighted images are used for the correlation with clinical parameters and for the evaluation of the effect of different drugs in clinical trials (Evans et al. 1997). The different types of MS (RR, SP, PP) tend to have their own typical MR pattern (Filippi et al. 1994; van Walderveen et al. 1998a). RR-MS patients have on average a lower volume of T2-weighted lesions than SP-MS patients. PP-MS patients on the other hand tend to have a volume of T2-weighted lesions close to or even lower than the RR-MS patients.

Correlation between T2-lesion volume and clinical disability is present, but weak (Filippi et al. 1995; Gasparini et al. 1996; Losseff et al. 1996a; Lycklama et al. 1998; Riahi et al. 1998; Tubridy et al. 1998). The highest predictive value is obtained at presentation (Morrissey et al. 1993), where the number of T2 lesions predicts (time to) conversion to MS and future disability. The volume of hypointense lesions on T1-weighted images correlates slightly stronger with disability (Truyen et al. 1996; van Walderveen et al. 1995, 1998a). Overall, T2-weighted hyperintense and T1-weighted hypointense lesions both reflect the past disease activity of MS, where black holes represent the more destructive MS lesions. Enhanced lesions represent present activity of the disease and correlate strongly with the occurrence of relapses (Barkhof et al. 1992; Gonzalez et al. 1987; Kappos et al. 1999; Katz et al. 1993; Miller et al. 1993a; Thorpe et al. 1996b). MRI is 5–10 times more sensitive than clinical relapses in detecting disease activity in RR-MS and SP-MS patients. This is why monthly MRI is used to monitor preliminary trials in these clinical subgroups of patients.

However, caution is necessary since the correlation between MRI activity and disease progression is not yet fully established (Kappos et al. 1999).

There is also a correlation between spinal cord abnormalities and clinical parameters. MS patients with spinal cord abnormalities are more disabled and PP-MS patients tend to have the most extensive spinal cord involvement for both focal lesions and diffuse abnormalities, SP-MS patients intermediate and RR-MS patients the smallest (Filippi et al. 1996a,b; Lycklama et al. 1997, 1998; Thorpe et al. 1996a). However, the clinicoradiological paradox urges us to find additional parameters that play a role in the disease development of MS.

Obviously, other pathological changes must be present outside the focal MS lesions, most likely in the normal appearing white matter.

16.7.2 Atrophy

Atrophy of the brain and spinal cord of MS patients is a possible marker of axonal loss in MS lesions but also in the normal appearing white matter. Brain atrophy can be determined by an increase of the volume of ventricles and peripheral CSF and a decrease of brain tissue. Clinical correlations with brain atrophy are relatively strong (Lycklama et al. 1998; Loseff et al. 1996b), and highly reproducible methods to measure brain atrophy are now presented, showing a yearly increase in atrophy over time in MS patients. Possibly, this parameter will be used in future treatment evaluation.

Atrophy of the spinal cord, determined by a decrease of the cross sectional area, has been noted focally at the site of a lesion, as well as for the whole spinal cord (Filippi et al. 1996b; Kidd et al. 1993, 1996; Losseff et al. 1996c, 1998; Stevenson et al. 1998; Thorpe et al. 1996a). The occurrence of atrophy correlates with the appearance of diffuse abnormalities on the sagittal MRI. Measurements in the axial plane of the cross sectional area show that MS patients with diffuse spinal cord abnormalities have a smaller cross sectional area and are more disabled than MS patients without diffuse abnormalities (LYCKLAMA et al. 1998). STEVENSON et al. 1998, 1999 demonstrated that it is possible to measure changes in cord cross sectional area over time. Serial measurement of spinal cord atrophy may be important to evaluate therapeutic efficacy, especially in PP-MS patients.

16.7.3 Magnetic Transfer Imaging

While conventional MRI measures signal primarily from the free water protons, magnetization transfer (MT) imaging indirectly detects macromolecular associated hydrogen nuclei via their interaction with the free protons. In normal adult CNS, white matter exhibits the largest MT effect due to the macromolecular content of the highly structured and lipid rich myelin (VAN WAESBERGHE et al. 1996a). MT can be applied in different ways. Firstly, MT can be used for background suppression to obtain higher sensitivity for detection of MS lesions (HIEHLE et al. 1995; VAN WAESBERGHE et al. 1998a,b). A second application is the MT ratio, which is lower in MS lesions than in the normal appearing white matter correlating with the amount of demyelination and axonal loss. MT ratios can be analysed using analysis of regions of interest or using whole brain MT histograms (FILIPPI et al. 1998b; GASS et al. 1994; SILVER et al. 1997; VAN WAESBERGHE et al. 1998a,b) (Fig. 16.9).

MT ratio (MTR) analysis constantly reveals abnormalities in the normal appearing white matter, indicating that non-focal pathology occurs in MS, especially in progressive patients. MTR may already be reduced prior to onset of new lesion formation, but becomes markedly reduced (indicating demyelination) after onset of enhancement. In some lesions MTR may recover after cessation of enhancement, which might indicate remyelination, while in others MTR will remain low and be associated with a persistent black hole indicating axonal loss (VAN WAESBERGHE et al. 1999).

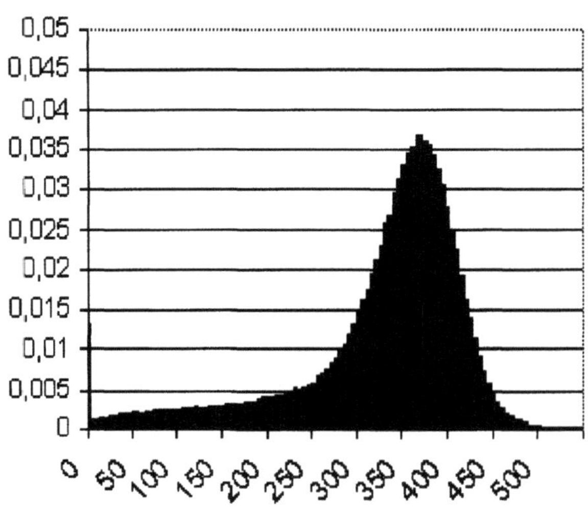

Fig. 16.9. Illustration of an MTR histogram with on the y-axis the percentage of brain pixels corrected for the size of the brain and on the x-axis the MTR values. Before an MTR histogram can be calculated postprocessing of the images with and without magnetic transfer contrast is needed. The equation (M0–Ms)/M0) is used, where M0 stands for signal intensity from an unprepared sequence and Ms for signal intensity from an MT-presaturated pulse sequence. The main MTR histogram parameters are the relative peak height, representing the percentage of the total number of brain pixels forming the highest bin, and the MTR value of the peak, representing the MTR value on the x-axis of the highest bin (normal appearing white matter). For MS patients, the peak shifts to the left and the relative peak height are lower indicating diffuse demyelination of the white and gray matter

16.7.4 Diffusion Weighted Imaging

Diffusion weighted imaging (DWI) is a novel technique, based on the application of MR gradients which result in dephasing of the signal intensity due to the Brownian motion of water protons. The water protons diffuse faster along myelinated fibres than across them and the apparent diffusion coefficient (ADC) is directionally restricted, or anisotropic. The anisotropy is marked in the white matter and minimal in the grey matter of the brain (LE BIHAN et al. 1995). With DWI a map of anisotropy of the white matter, related to the limited freedom of mobility of water along the direction of intact myelinated fibres, can be obtained. In MS lesions, increases and decreases in diffusion have been reported. An increase is thought to reflect edema and expanded extracellular space, a decrease acute demyelination. Possibly, this technique will provide more insight into the pathological substrate of different lesions and normal appearing white matter.

16.8 Conclusion

Although the diagnosis of MS is still mainly a clinical diagnosis, MRI plays an important role, and its value is still increasing. Especially, the use of gadolinium and spinal imaging are important. Different MRI techniques can be applied to obtain a higher sensitivity in the detection of MS lesions.

Another goal is to obtain additional information about the tissue characteristics, for example with magnetic transfer and diffuse imaging.

Further, the clinicoradiological paradox urges us to obtain more objective radiological and clinical parameters of MS lesions and normal appearing white matter of the brain and spinal cord.

Newer MR techniques, such as standardized atrophy measurements and MT measurement of the whole brain tissue, seem promising techniques to assess the degree of axonal loss. The use of 3D MR sequences gives the possibility of following changes in MS more reproducibly, facilitating the monitoring of drug effects.

References

Barkhof F, Scheltens P, Frequin ST et al. (1992) Relapsing-remitting multiple sclerosis: sequential enhanced MR imaging vs clinical findings in determining disease activity. Am J Roentgenol 159: 1041–1047

Barkhof F, Filippi M, Miller DH et al. (1997) Comparison of MRI criteria at first presentation to predict conversion to clinically definite multiple sclerosis. Brain 120: 2059–2069

Barkhof F, McGowan JC, van Waesberghe JH et al. (1998) Hypointense multiple sclerosis lesions on T1-weighted spin echo magnetic resonance images: their contribution in understanding multiple sclerosis evolution. J Neurol Neurosurg Psych 64: S77-S79

Baratti C, Barkhof F, Hoogenraad F et al. (1995) Partially saturated fluid attenuated inversion recovery (FLAIR) sequences in multiple sclerosis: comparison with fully relaxed FLAIR and conventional spin-echo. Magn Reson Imaging 13: 513–521

Bastianello S, Pozzilli C, Bernardi S et al. (1990) Serial study of gadolinium-DTPA MRI enhancement in multiple sclerosis. Neurology 40: 591–595

Bastionello S, Bozzao A, Paolillo A et al. (1997) Fast spin-echo and fast fluid-attenuated inversion-recovery versus conventional spin-echo sequences for MR quantificaiton of multiple sclerosis lesions. Am J Neuroradiol 18: 699–704

Bruck W, Bitsch A, Kolenda H et al (1997) Inflammatory central nervous system demyelination: correlation of magnetic resonance imaging findings with lesion pathology. Ann Neurol 42: 783–793

Evans AC, Frank JA, Antel J et al. (1997) The role of MRI in clinical trials of multiple sclerosis: comparison of image processing techniques. Ann Neurol 41: 125–132

Fazekaz F, Offenbacher H, Fuchs S et al. (1988) Criteria for an increased specificity of MRI interpretaion in elderly subjects with suspected multiple sclerosis. Neurology 38: 1822–1825

Filippi M, Barker GJ, Horsfield MA et al. (1994) Benign and secondary progressive multiple sclerosis: a preliminary quantitative MRI study. J Neurol 241: 246–251

Filippi M, Paty DW, Kappos L et al. (1995) Correlations between changes in disability and T2-weighted brain MRI activity in multiple sclerosis: a follow-up study. Neurology 45: 255–260

Filippi M, Campi A, Colombo B et al. (1996a) A spinal cord MRI study of benign and secondary progressive multiple sclerosis. J Neurol 243: 502–505

Filippi M, Campi A, Marinelli V et al. (1996b) Brain and spinal cord MR in benign multiple sclerosis: a follow-up study. J Neurol Science 143: 143–149

Filippi M, Barkhof F, Bressi S et al. (1997) Inter-rater variability in reporting enhancing lesions present on standard and triple dose gadolinium scans of patients with multiple sclerosis. Multiple Sclerosis 3: 226–230

Filippi M, Horsfield MA, Ader HJ et al. (1998a) Guidelines for using quantitative measures of brain magnetic resonance imaging abnormalities in monitoring the treatment of multiple sclerosis. Ann Neurol 43: 499–506

Filippi M, Rocca MA, Martino G et al. (1998b) Magnetization transfer changes in the normal appearing white matter precede the appearance of enhancing lesions in patients with multiple sclerosis. Ann Neurol 43: 809–814

Finelli DA, Hurst GC, Karaman BA et al. (1994) Use of magnetization transfer for improved contrast on gradient-echo MR images of the cervical spine. Radiology 193: 165–171

Fog T (1950) Topographic distribution of plaques in the spinal cord in multiple sclerosis. Arch Neurol Psychiatry 63: 382–414

Gass A, Barker GJ, Kidd D et al. (1994) Correlation of magnetization transfer ratio with clinical disability in multiple sclerosis. Ann Neurol 36: 62–67

Gass A, Moseley IF, Barker GJ et al. (1996) Lesion discrimination in optic neuritis using high-resolution fat-suppressed fast spin-echo MRI. Neuroradiology 38: 317–321

Gasperini C, Horsfield MA, Thorpe JW et al. (1996) Macroscopic and microscopic assessments of disease burden by MRI in multiple sclerosis: relationship to clinical parameters. J Magn Reson Imaging 6: 580–584

Gawne-Cain ML, O'Riordan JI, Thompson AJ et al. (1997a) Multiple sclerosis lesion detection in the brain: a comparison of fast fluid-attenuated inversion recovery and conventional T2-weighted dual spin echo. Neurology 49: 364–370

Gawne-Cain ML, Silver NC, Moseley IF et al. (1997b) Fast FLAIR of the brain: the range of appearances in normal subjects and its application to quantification of white-matter disease. Neuroradiology 39: 243–249

Gonzalez-Scarano F, Grossman RI, Galetta S et al. (1987) Multiple sclerosis disease activity correlates with gadolinium-enhanced magnetic resonance imaging. Ann Neurol 21: 300–306

Guttmann CR, Ahn SS, Hsu et al. (1995) The evolution of multiple sclerosis lesions on serial MR. AJNR 16: 1481–1491

Hajnal JV, Bryant DJ, Kasuboski L et al (1992) Use of fluid attenuated inversion recovery (FLAIR) pulse sequences in MRI of the brain. J Comput Assist Tomogr 16: 841–844

Hashemi RH, Bradley WG, Chen DY et al. (1995) Suspected multiple sclerosis: MR imaging with a thin-section fast FLAIR pulse sequence. Radiology 196: 505–510

Hiehle JF, Grossman RI, Ramer KN et al. (1995) Magnetization transfer effects in MR-detected multiple sclerosis lesions: comparison with gadolinium-enhanced spin-echo images and nonenhanced T1-weighted images. AJNR 16: 69–77

Hittmair K, Mallek R, Prayer D et al. (1996) Spinal cord lesions in patients with multiple sclerosis: comparison of MR pulse sequences. AJNR 17: 1555–1565

Kappos L, Moeri D, Radue EW et al. (1999) Predictive value of gadolinium-enhanced magnetic resonance imaging for relapse rate and changes in disability or impairment in multiple sclerosis: a meta-analysis. Lancet 353: 964–969

Katz D, Taubenberger JK, Cannella B et al. (1993) Correlation between magnetic resonance imaging findings and lesion development in chronic, active multiple sclerosis. Ann Neurol 34: 661–669

Keiper MD, Grossman RI, Brunson JC et al. (1997) The low sensitivity of fluid-attenuated inversion recovery (FLAIR) imaging in the detection of multiple sclerosis of the spinal cord. AJNR 18: 1035–1039

Kidd D, Thorpe JW, Thompson AJ et al. (1993) Spinal cord MRI using multi-array coils and fast spin echo. II. Findings in multiple sclerosis. Neurology 43: 2632–2637

Kidd D, Thorpe JW, Kendall BE et al. (1996) MRI dynamics of brain and spinal cord in progressive multiple sclerosis. J Neurol Neurosurg Psychiatry 60: 15–19

Kidd D, Barkhof F, McConnell R et al. (1999) Cortical lesions in multiple sclerosis. Brain 122: 17–26

Larsson EM, Holtas S, Nilsson O (1989) Gd-DTPA-enhanced MR of suspected spinal multiple sclerosis. AJNR 10: 1071–1076

LeBihan D, Turner R, Patronas N (1995) Diffusion MR imaging in normal brain and in brain tumors. In: LeBihanD (ed) Diffusion and perfusion magnetic resonance imaging. Applications to functional MRI. Raven Press, New York, pp 134–140

Losseff NA, Kingsley DP, McDonald WI et al. (1996a) Clinical and magnetic resonance imaging predictors of disability in primary and secondary progressive multiple sclerosis. Multiple Sclerosis 1: 218–222

Losseff NA, Wang L, Lai HM et al. (1996b) Progressive cerebral atrophy in multiple sclerosis. A serial MRI study. Brain 119: 2009–2019

Losseff NA, Webb SL, O'Riordan JI et al. (1996c) Spinal cord atrophy and disability in multiple sclerosis. A new reproducible and sensitive MRI method with potential to monitor disease progression. Brain 119: 701–708

Losseff NA, Miller DH (1998) Measures of brain and spinal cord atrophy in multiple sclerosis. J Neurol Neurosurg Psychiatry 64: S102–105

Lublin FD, Reingold SC (1996) Defining the clinical course of multiple sclerosis: results of an international survey. Neurology 46: 907–911

Lycklama a Nijeholt GJ, Barkhof F, Castelijns JA et al. (1996) Comparison of two MR sequences for the detection of multiple sclerosis lesions in the spinal cord. AJNR 17: 1533–1538

Lycklama a Nijeholt GJ, Barkhof F, Scheltens P et al. (1997) MR of the spinal cord in multiple sclerosis: relation to clinical subtype and disability. AJNR 18: 1041–1048

Lycklama a Nijeholt GJ, van Walderveen MA, Castelijns JA et al. (1998) Brain and spinal cord abnormalities in multiple sclerosis. Correlation between MRI parameters, clinical subtypes and symptoms. Brain 121: 687–697

Mascalchi M, Dal Pozzo G, Bartolozzi C (1993) Effectiveness of the short TI inversion recovery (STIR) sequence in MR imaging of intramedullary spinal lesions. Magn Reson Imaging 11: 17–25

McDonald WI, Miller DH, Barnes D (1992) The pathological evolution of multiple sclerosis. Neuropathol Appl Neurobiol 18: 319–334

Miller DH, Barkhof F, Nauta JJ (1993a) Gadolinium enhancement increases the sensitivity of MRI in detecting disease activity in multiple sclerosis. Brain 116: 1077–1094

Miller DH, McManus DG, Bartlett PA et al. (1993b) Detection of optic nerve lesions in optic neuritis using frequency-selective fat-saturation sequences. Neuroradiology 35: 156–158

Miller DH, Rudge P, Johnson G et al. (1998) Serial gadolinium enhanced magnetic resonance imaging in multiple sclerosis. Brain 111: 927–939

Morrissey SP, Miller DH, Kendall BE et al. (1993) The significance of brain magnetic resonance imaging abnormalities at presentation with clinically isolated syndromes suggestive of multiple sclerosis. A 5-year follow-up study. Brain 116: 135–146

Oppenheimer DR (1978) The cervical cord in multiple sclerosis. Neuropathol Appl Neurobiol 4: 151–162

Paty DW, Oger JJF, Kastrukoff LF (1988) MRI in the diagnosis of MS: a prospective study with comparison of clinical evaluation, evoked potentials, oligoclonal banding and CT. Neurology 38: 180–185

Paty DW, Li DK (1996) Importance of magnetic resonance imaging and gadolinium enhancement. Ann Neurol 40: 951–953

Poser CM, Paty DW, Scheinberg L et al. (1983) New diagnostic criteria for multiple sclerosis: guidlines for research protocols. Ann Neurol 13: 227–231

Riahi F, Zijdenbos A, Narayanan S et al. (1998) Improved correlation between scores on the expanded disability status scale and cerebral lesion load in relapsing-remitting multiple sclerosis. Results of the application of new imaging methods. Brain 121: 1305–1312

Rovaris M, Mastronardo G, Gasperini C et al. (1998) MRI evolution of new MS lesions enhancing after different doses of gadolinium. Act Neurol Scand 98: 90–93

Rydberg RN, Hammond CA, Grimm RC et al (1994) Initial experience in MR imaging of the brain with fast fluid-attenuated inversion-recovery pulse sequence. Radiology 193: 173–180

Silver NC, Barker GJ, McManus DG et al. (1997) Magnetisation transfer ratio of normal brain white matter: a normative database spanning four decades of life. J Neurol Neurosurg Psychiatry 62: 223–228

Stevenson VL, Gawne-Cain ML, Barker GJ et al. (1997) Imaging of the spinal cord and brain in multiple sclerosis: a comparative study between fast FLAIR and fast spin echo. J Neurol 244: 119–124

Stevenson VL, Leary SM, Losseff NA et al. (1998) Spinal cord atrophy and disability in MS: a longitudinal study. Neurology 51: 234–238

Stevenson VL, Miller DH, Rovaris M et al. (1999) Primary and transitional progressive MS. A clinical and MRI cross-sectional study. Neurology 52: 839–845

Tartaglino LM, Croul SE, Flanders AE et al. (1995) Multiple sclerosis in the spinal cord: MR appearance and correlation with clinical parameters. Radiology 195: 725–732

Thielen KR, Miller GM (1996) Multiple sclerosis of the spinal cord: magnetic resonance appearance. J Comput Assist Tomogr 20: 434–438

Thomas DJ, Pennock JM, Hajnal JV et al. (1993) Magnetic resonance imaging of spinal cord in multiple sclerosis by fluid-attenuated inversion recovery. Lancet 341: 593–594

Thorpe JW, Kidd D, Kendall BE et al. (1993) Spinal cord MRI using multi-array coils and fast spin echo. I. Technical aspects and findings in healthy adults. Neurology 43: 2625–2631

Thorpe JW, Halpin SF, McManus DG et al. (1994a) A comparison between fast and conventional spin-echo in the detection of multiple sclerosis lesions. Neuroradiology 36: 388–392

Thorpe JW, McManus DG, Kendall BE et al. (1994b) Short tau inversion recovery fast spin-echo (fast STIR) imaging of the spinal cord in multiple sclerosis. Magn Reson Imaging 12: 983–989

Thorpe JW, Kidd D, Moseley IF et al. (1996a) Spinal MRI in patients with suspected multiple sclerosis and negative brain MRI. Brain 119: 709–714

Thorpe JW, Kidd D, Moseley IF et al. (1996b) Serial gadolinium-enhanced MRI of the brain and spinal cord in early relapsing-remitting multiple sclerosis. Neurology 46: 373–378

Tien RD, Hesselink JR, Szumowski J (1991) MR fat suppression combined with Gd-DTPA enhancement in optic neuritis and perineuritis. J Comput Assist Tomogr 15: 223–227

Truyen L, van Waesberghe JH, van Walderveen MA et al. (1996) Accumulation of hypointense lesions ("black holes") on T1 spin-echo MRI correlates with disease progression in multiple sclerosis. Neurology 47: 1469–1476

Tubridy N, Coles AJ, Molyneux P et al. (1998) Secondary progressive multiple sclerosis: the relationship between short-term MRI activity and clinical features. Brain 121: 225–231

Van Waesberghe JH, Castelijns J, Barkhof F (1996a) Magnetization transfer imaging in multiple sclerosis. Int MS J 3: 47–57

Van Waesberghe JH, Castelijns JA, Weerts JG et al. (1996b) Disappearance of multiple sclerosis lesions with severely prolonged T1 on images obtained by a FLAIR pulse sequence. Magn Reson Imaging 14: 209–213

Van Waesberghe JH, Castelijns JA, Lazeron RH et al. (1998a) Magnetization transfer contrast (MTC) and long repetition time spin-echo MR imaging in multiple sclerosis. Magn Reson Imaging 16: 351–358

Van Waesberghe JHTM, Van Buchem MA, Filippi M et al. (1998b) MR outcome parameters in multiple sclerosis: comparison of surface-based thresholding segmentation and magnetization transfer ratio histographic analysis in relation to disability. AJNR 19: 1857–1862

Van Waesberghe JHTM, Kamphorst W, de Groot CJA et al. (1999) Axonal loss in MS lesions: MRI insights into substrated of disability. Ann Neurol (in press)

Van Walderveen MA, Barkhof F, Hommes OR et al. (1995) Correlating MRI and clinical disease activity in multiple sclerosis: relevance of hypointense lesions on short-TR/short-TE (T1-weighted) spin-echo images. Neurology 45: 1684–1690

Van Walderveen MA, Barkhof F, Tas MW et al. (1998a) Patterns of brain magnetic resonance abnormalities on T2-weighted spin echo images in clinical subgroups of multiple sclerosis: a large cross-sectional study. Eur Neurol 40: 91–98

Van Walderveen MA, Kamphorst W, Scheltens P et al. (1998b) Histopathologic correlate of hypointense lesions on T1-weighted spin-echo MRI in multiple sclerosis. Neurology 50: 1282–1288

White SJ, Hajnal JV, Young IR et al (1992) Use of fluid-attenuated inversion recovery pulse sequences for imaging the spinal cord. Magn Reson Medicine 28: 153–162

Wolansky LJ, Bardini JA, Cook SD et al. (1994) Triple-dose versus single-dose gadoteridol in multiple sclerosis patients. J Neuroimaging 4: 141–145

Yousry TA, Gunter F, Walther E et al. (1998) Triple dose of gadolinium-DTPA increases the sensitivity of spinal cord MRI in detecting enhancing lesions in multiple sclerosis. J Neurol Sciences 158: 221–225

17 Imaging in AIDS

KATHERINE A. MISZKIEL, ADAM D. WALDMAN

CONTENTS

17.1 Introduction

Infection with the human immunodeficiency virus-1 (HIV-1) has now been recognized for almost 2 decades. The World Health Organization estimated that, by early 1998, over 30 million people worldwide had been infected with this virus, and at least 11.7 million would have died as a result. The rampant spread of infection continues with nearly 16,000 new infections each day and, by the year 2000, the number of individuals affected will have increased to 40 million people (Joint United Nations Programme on HIV/AIDS World Health Organization report on the global HIV/AIDS epidemic. June 1998. UNAIDS and WHO, Geneva, 1998).

HIV-1 is a lymphotropic, neurotropic RNA retrovirus which infects human T-lymphocytes of the helper/ inducer subset as well as microglia, monocytes and macrophages. Neurological disease in HIV infection is relatively common and is the presenting illness in 10–20% of patients with AIDS (LEVY et al. 1985). However, although the central nervous system (CNS) probably becomes infected early in the course of HIV infection, as evidenced by early detection of HIV-1 antibodies and direct virus isolation from cerebrospinal fluid, the majority of neurological disease occurs in the later stages of infection on a background of profound immunosuppression (LEVY et al. 1985; RESNICK et al. 1985).

The spectrum of neurological diseases encountered in AIDS includes the effects of direct CNS infection by HIV-1 which results in the AIDS-dementia complex (ADC) in its most severe form, as well as opportunistic infection with a variety of parasites, fungi, viruses and bacteria. In addition, patients with AIDS have a significant increase in the incidence of both primary and secondary intracranial lymphomas.

Imaging plays an important role in the management of CNS disease associated with HIV infection. In some cases, imaging findings alone may be sufficiently characteristic to make a specific diagnosis and direct treatment. In many others, they are less specific, but allow an acceptable level of diagnostic confidence when taken in conjunction with clinical features and relevant microbiological investigations. However, there are a significant number of patients, particularly those with multiple coexistent pathologies, in whom the clinical features and structural imaging appearances are non-specific, complex or atypical. Although histological tissue analysis will usually establish a definitive diagnosis in such cases, brain biopsy in patients with AIDS is associated with a higher risk than in the non HIV-infected popula-

K.A. MISZKIEL, MRCP, FRCR
Lysholm Department of Radiology, The National Hospital for Neurology and Neurosurgery, Queen Square, London, WC1 3BG, UK
A.D. WALDMAN, MA, PhD, MRCP, FRCR
Lysholm Department of Radiology, The National Hospital for Neurology and Neurosurgery, Queen Square, London, WC1 3BG, UK

tion, with a morbidity of up to 12% and mortality of 2% (Levy et al. 1992; Antinori et al. 1997); non-invasive imaging techniques which can accurately differentiate between disease entities are therefore clearly desirable.

Both characteristic and atypical neuroradiological CT and MRI appearances in most of the disease processes encountered in HIV infection have been extensively described elsewhere in the literature and will not be reproduced in detail here. The purpose of this chapter is to concentrate on the use, role and impact of some of the non-invasive techniques which yield physiological and biochemical information in (1) advancing the understanding of these diseases and (2) as an adjunct to conventional structural imaging in clinical practice. The potential "added value" of these techniques is in augmenting the sensitivity and specificity of conventional imaging, allowing earlier diagnosis and refinement of the neuroradiological differential in problem cases, respectively. Some techniques also provide quantitative markers of disease progression and treatment response. The focus will be particularly on more recent studies using magnetic resonance spectroscopy, magnetization transfer, and diffusion and perfusion-weighted imaging methods, but will also include observations using more conventional imaging techniques.

17.2 Magnetic Resonance Spectroscopy

Localized magnetic resonance spectroscopy (MRS) allows the quantification of major neurochemicals from the amplitudes of assigned resonances in spectra acquired within a defined region of tissue. This provides a non-invasive method of gaining in vivo biochemical information on molecules which are present at around mM (millimoles/litre) concentrations.

To date, the vast majority of spectroscopic studies of HIV-related brain disease, and all of those related to structural lesions, have used single-voxel ^{1}H spectroscopy, and discussion will largely be limited to this technique which is rapid to perform and generally considered to be robust. It is worthwhile to discuss briefly the main methods for acquiring and analysing spectra, as these have a bearing on interpretation of data obtained.

For single-voxel ^{1}H MRS, two main types of pulse sequence have been used to select a voxel from which spectra are acquired: STEAM (stimulated echo acquisition mode) and PRESS (point resolved spectroscopy). Both allow satisfactory voxel localization. PRESS sequences offer the advantage of a twofold higher signal, and less susceptibility to motion, diffusion and homonuclear coupling effects. STEAM, however, allows shorter echo times, slightly better spatial definition of the voxel and more effective water suppression and allows metabolites with short T2 (such as *myo*-inositol [Mi]) or highly J-coupled (such as glutamate/glutamine [Glx]) to be detected.

STEAM has therefore traditionally been the method of choice to acquire spectra at short echo times TE 20–50 ms, and PRESS longer TE 135/270 ms. Technological advances now allow reliable acquisition of PRESS spectra at TE=35 ms and improved voxel definition; the twofold signal/noise ratio advantage which allows similar quality spectra to be obtained from a smaller voxel in a given time makes this the likely method of choice for future studies. It is, however, worthy of note that the current reference data at short echo times are mostly from STEAM, and caution must be exercised in comparing spectra acquired using the two different techniques; it may be some time before such data are established for short TE PRESS.

The main metabolites which are resolved at 1.5 T are outlined in Table 17.1/Fig. 17.1 (normal brain spectrum). Lactate (doublet at 1.35 ppm) is not seen in normal brain and overlaps the lipid resonances. If there is uncertainty as to the presence of lactate on short TE spectra, this can usually be resolved by performing long TE (130 ms/270 ms) where the lipid resonances have decayed.

It has previously been assumed that interpretation of MRS after the administration of i.v. gadolinium chelates is not possible, although recent studies show that although this results in some line-broadening, spectra may still be interpreted with confidence (Lin et al. 1999). This has important implications for voxel positioning in relation to focal lesions which may not be conspicuous on pre-contrast images. Potential pitfalls with single-voxel techniques in the evaluation of focal lesions are sampling error, partial volume effects or variation related to voxel positioning. Magnetic resonance spectroscopic imaging (MRSI), which allows spectra to be generated from a one-, two- or three-dimensional array of much smaller voxels, offers a potential solution to this but this technique is time-consuming, quantification of metabolite concentrations is difficult and, at the time of writing, commercially available programs only support acquisition of longer TE spectra, precluding evaluation of Mi and Glx.

Table 17.1. Summary of the metabolite peaks identified on ^{1}H spectroscopy and their significance

Metabolite	Chemical shift	Physiological and pathophysiological significance
NAA (*N*-acetyl aspartate)	2.02 ppm	Neuronal cell marker. Exact physiological role uncertain. Decreased in infiltrative processes and necrosis
Cr (creatine-containing compounds, including phosphocreatine) Other metabolites are often expressed as ratio to Cr	3.0 ppm	Compound related to energy storage; thought to be a marker of energetic status of cells
Cho (choline-containing compounds)	3.2 ppm	Detectable resonance is predominantly free choline and derivatives, a marker of membrane turnover. Elevated in neoplasms
Mi (myo-inositol and other inositol containing compounds)	3.56 ppm	Sugar metabolite in inositol triphosphate intracellular second messenger signalling pathway osmolyte; thought to be a glial marker. Elevated in Alzheimer's disease and hyperosmolar states
Glx (glutamate/glutamine)	2.1–2.4 ppm	Difficult to quantify reliably at moderate (1.5–3 T) field strength. Intermediary amino acid metabolites. Elevated in encephalopathies
Lactate doublet (separated by 7 Hz, 0.11 ppm)	1.33 ppm	Only observed in pathology. Increased in areas of ischaemia or necrosis. Also thought to be elevated in foamy macrophages at 1.5 T)
Lipids	0.9–1.3 ppm	Only observed in pathology. Elevated in tumours and necrotic tissue

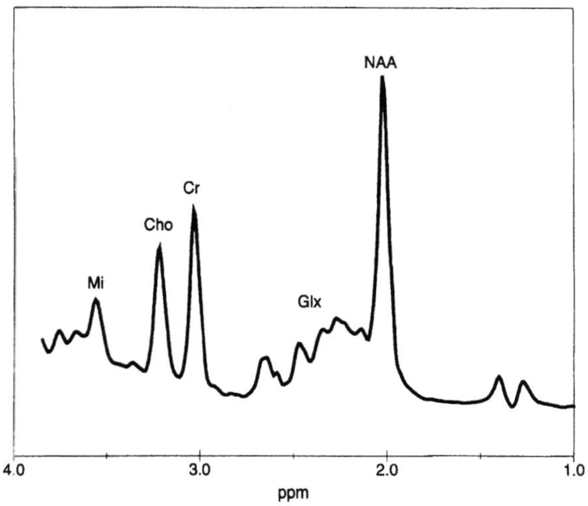

Fig. 17.1. Normal ^{1}H magnetic resonance spectrum from human frontal white matter (2.6 cm^3 voxel, PRESS, TE=30, TR=3000: 192 transients) showing resonances corresponding to *N*-acetylaspartate CH_3 (*NAA*), creatine/phosphocreatine (*Cr*), choline containing compounds (*Cho*) and Myo-inositols (*Mi*). The complex resonance downfield of NAA corresponds to overlapping resonances including glutamate/glutamine (*Glx*). (Courtesy of Mr. D. McManus, Institute of Neurology, London, UK)

The MRS examination can be performed in concert with structural MRI using a clinical scanner with the appropriate software, and takes approximately 15 min in total to acquire. Satisfactory automated systems for acquiring spectra are commercially available. Most data have been obtained at 1.5 T; however, lower field techniques have been demonstrated clinically in other diseases (Rai et al. 1999) and could also be applied to HIV-related disease; this increases the potential accessibility of MRS as a clinical tool in a greater number of hospitals.

Evaluation of spectra may be by semiquantitative inspection of the spectra by an experienced observer, or by a number of quantitative analyses. Most employ fitting of the peaks in the spectra to establish their area, and this can be performed either in the time domain or post Fourier transformation in the frequency domain. Automated peak assignment and measurement software is available on current versions of some proprietary instrument software. These are usually taken as a ratio to that of the creatine (Cr) resonance which is effectively used as an internal standard. However, the assumption that Cr is constant does not always hold and metabolite changes may be over- or underestimated if Cr falls. Quantification of individual metabolite concentrations circumvents this problem, but requires more involved calibration and correction processes. Whilst it is possible to quantify concentrations absolutely (in mM/ml or mM per gram of tissue), this is difficult to do reliably, and many centres prefer to quantify in terms of "institutional units".

17.3 MRS in Focal Lesions

17.3.1 Cerebral Toxoplasmosis and Primary Central Nervous System Lymphoma

Toxoplasma abscesses and lymphoma are the two most common destructive focal intracranial mass lesions seen in the AIDS population, the former being the more common of the two pathologies (Levy et al. 1990; Cornford et al. 1992). CNS toxoplasmosis results from reactivation of a previously acquired infection with the obligate intracellular protozoan, *Toxoplasma gondii*, and usually occurs in the late stages of HIV infection when the CD4+ lymphocyte count is markedly suppressed.

The incidence of cerebral toxoplasmosis ranges between 13.4–33% in the AIDS population (Anders et al. 1986; Levy et al. 1985). The typical imaging appearances in cerebral toxoplasmosis are of multiple intraparenchymal abscesses with a predilection for the basal ganglia, thalami and cerebral hemisphere white matter. The lesions are often necrotic, with thick irregular ring enhancement, much associated perilesional vasogenic oedema and mass effect (Ramsey and Dean 1997). Abscesses can also be haemorrhagic (Trenkwalder et al. 1992) and, although in the majority of cases they are multifocal, solitary lesions occur in up to 30% of cases (Dina 1991).

Primary CNS lymphoma in the AIDS population accounts for 2–10% of intracranial mass lesions (Bantz et al. 1989; So et al. 1986); it is usually of the high-grade B-cell type and pathogenesis is linked to infection with the Epstein-Barr virus (Bashir et al. 1993). T-cell lymphoma has also been reported (Iglesias-Rozas et al. 1991). Although at imaging up to 70% of lymphoma masses are solitary, they are often rapidly progressive and because of this, at autopsy, are nearly always multifocal (Morgello et al. 1990). Lymphoma mass lesions are often necrotic as they outgrow their blood supply and therefore are ring-enhancing, with a thick irregular rim or show more confluent enhancement. Spontaneous haemorrhage into the lesions is unusual but may occur on treatment with steroids or radiotherapy (Cordoliani et al. 1992). As with toxoplasma abscesses, there is often much associated vasogenic oedema and mass effect and lymphoma also has a predilection for the subcortical grey matter. A useful radiological discriminator between these two pathologies is the presence of periventricular spread with lymphoma, resulting in subependymal enhancement. Leptomeningeal involvement, however, is very unusual in this condition; therefore CSF cytology is rarely positive and, ideally, histological confirmation is required for definitive diagnosis (Ruiz et al. 1997).

The clinical and radiological differentiation between cerebral toxoplasmosis and lymphoma can be very difficult, and in addition the two pathologies may be synchronous. Either disease can present as single or multifocal mass lesions with a similar clinical presentation, with focal neurology depending on lesion site and size.

Serology for toxoplasmosis is often positive, but specificity is low and only approximately one-third of cases will demonstrate a rise in the antibody IgG titre. In addition intrathecal production of antibody occurs in 50% and detection of *T. gondii* in the plasma and CSF with PCR has been disappointing (Derouin et al. 1991; Cristina et al. 1993).

Cerebral toxoplasmosis accounts for nearly two-thirds of brain masses in the AIDS population. In most institutions, any such patient presenting with an intracranial mass which could be either of these two conditions is treated empirically for toxoplasmosis and re-evaluated at 2 weeks, with a view to proceeding to brain biopsy if there has been no clinical or radiological improvement (Porter et al. 1992). There are several problems with such a management strategy, which include drug-related toxicity and side effects with antimicrobial therapy, patient compliance and rapid growth of lymphoma whilst commencement of appropriate treatment with radiotherapy is delayed. In addition, inappropriate treatment with steroids may result in a misleading improvement in imaging appearances.

A number of studies have been performed to evaluate non-invasive imaging techniques which can accurately differentiate between these two disease entities and avoid the need for biopsy. Although initial results using positron emission tomography (PET) and single photon emission computed tomography (SPECT) were promising, due to various limitations associated with both techniques, interest has focused on MRS as a potential non-invasive method for distinguishing between intracranial mass lesions in AIDS on the basis of their biochemical profile.

In an important early series (Chang et al. 1995b), a combination of MRI and localized ^{1}H spectroscopy at 1.5 T using short TE STEAM and a long TE PRESS sequences were used to study patients with AIDS and intracranial mass lesions, and metabolite peaks in the lesions compared with those in the structurally normal contralateral hemisphere. Toxoplasmosis abscesses had reduced choline (Cho), creatine containing compounds (Cr) and *N*-acetyl aspartate (NAA) peaks, but a markedly elevated lactate and lipid peak when compared with the spectrum from the contralateral cerebral hemisphere. The Mi peak was absent. By comparison, in lymphoma mass lesions, the Cho was elevated and there was less reduction in the Cr and NAA peaks. Lactate and lipid peaks were elevated, but less so than in toxoplasma abscesses. The Mi peak was present in lymphoma, but reduced (Table 17.2, Fig. 17.2).

The NAA peak consists predominantly of *N*-acetyl aspartate, which is found in neurons and is reduced in neuronal loss and dysfunction; thus disease processes where tissue destruction is a feature, as occurs in abscesses, will have reduced NAA peaks; in lymphoma, the neoplastic tissue infiltrates through normal tissue; thus there is less reduction in the NAA peak. The increased Cho peak seen in lymphoma is probably the result of increased cell membrane synthesis and turnover with resultant cleavage of free choline and glycerophosphocholine from the membrane. In contrast, in an abscess cavity such as

Table 17.2. Summary of the different studies of ^{1}H spectroscopy in focal lesions in AIDS since 1995. *The number of arrows* gives some indication of the relative increase or decrease of metabolites measured (*Toxo* toxoplasmosis, *PML* progressive multifocal leukoencephalopathy, *Lymph* lymphoma)

Reference	Spectroscopy parameters	Lesions analysed	Voxel size	Findings					
				Mi	Cho	Cr	NAA	Lac/Lip	
Chang et al.	STEAM	PML: 12	Variable	↑ (2)	↑	↓	↓	↑ (3)	
(1995)	TE 30 ms	Toxo: 11	3–10 ml	↓	↓	↓↓↓	↓↓↓	↓↓↓ (7)	
	TE 270 ms	Lymph: 8		↓	↑↑	↓↓	↓↓	↑↑ (2)	
	TR 2000 ms	Crypto: 4		↓	↓	↓↓	↓↓↓	↑ (lip)	
				Mi	Cho	Cr	NAA	Lac/Lip	
Chang et al.	STEAM	Mixed toxo/	8 ml	↓	↑	↓	↓	↑↑	
(1995a)	TE 30 ms	Lymph: 1		Spectral pattern combination of that of toxoplasmosis and lymphoma					
	TE 270 ms								
	TR 2000 ms								
Chinn et al.	PRESS	Toxo: 18	Variable	Three spectral patterns identified					
(1995)	TE 135 ms	Lymph: 9	2.9–8 ml	1. ↑↑ lipid peaks – remainder ↓					
	TR 1600 ms			2. ↑↑ Cho/Cr with ↓ NAA					
				3. Features of patterns 1 and 2					
				Mi	Cho	Cr	NAA	Lac	Lip
Chang et al.	STEAM	PML: 20	Variable	↑/↓	↑	↓	↓	↑ (15)	↑ (18)
(1997)	TE 30 ms		2.05–8.5 ml						
	TE 270 ms								
	TR 2000 ms								
	PRESS								
	TE 30 ms								
	TE 270 ms								
	TR 300 ms								
				NAA/Cr	NAA/Cho	Cho/Cr	Lac	Lip	
Simone et al.	Spin echo	Toxo: 20	Variable	↓ (4)	↓ (13)	↑↑ (8)	↑ (4)	↑ (7)	
(1998)	TE 135 ms	PML: 8	3.37– 8 ml	↓↓ (7)	↓↓ (5)	↑ (2)	↑ (6)		
	TR 1500 ms	Lymph: 7		↓↓ (5)	↓↓↓ (6)	↑↑↑ (4)	↑ (2)	↑ (5)	
				NAA/Cr	Cho/Cr	Lip/Cr	Lac		
Iranzo et al.	STEAM	PML: 6	8 ml	↓	↑	↑	↑		
(1999)	TE 135 ms								
	TR 2000 ms								
	PRESS								
	TE 20 ms								
	TR 1600 ms								

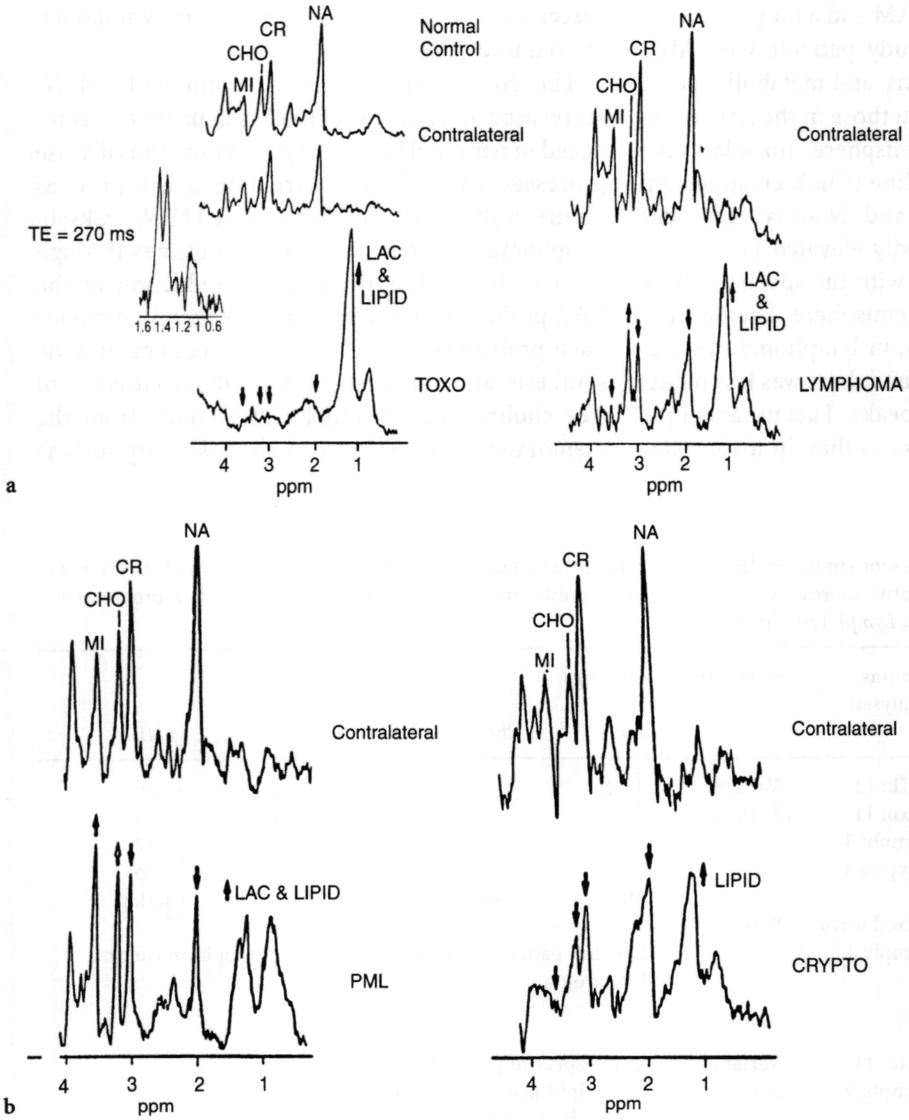

Fig. 17.2a,b. Representative ^{1}H spectra from toxoplasmosis lesion (*Toxo*) on the left and lymphoma lesion (*right*) are shown in a, and of a PML lesion (*left*) and cryptococcal abscess (*right*) in b. The spectra are compared with contralateral control spectra. (From: Chang L, Miller B, McBride D, Cornford M, Oropilla G, Buchthal S, Chiang F, Aronow H, Ernst T. Brain lesions in patients with AIDS: H-1 MR spectroscopy. Radiology 1995; 197: 525–531. With permission)

occurs in toxoplasmosis, there is cellular loss which probably accounts for the reduction in Cho. The lactate peak was high in toxoplasmosis and intermediately raised in lymphoma as a result of tissue ischaemia and anaerobic metabolism, which occurs to a greater extent in abscesses. Overall the five metabolite peaks helped predict the correct diagnosis with an accuracy of 84–94%, for all the intracranial masses evaluated in this study (including progressive multifocal leukoencephalopathy and cryptococcomas, discussed further below).

The same group of investigators also report on the spectrum obtained in a patient with a large intracranial mass which was histologically proven to be a mixture of lymphoma and toxoplasmosis; it had a mixture of spectroscopic features described for each of the two pathologies, with the high lipid and lactate peak seen in cerebral toxoplasmosis, decreased NAA, Cr and Mi peaks consistent with brain damage, but a preserved Cho peak which is a feature of lymphoma (Chang et al. 1995a).

Other MRS studies have, however, yielded less clear cut differentiation between toxoplasma and lymphoma. Chinn et al. (1995) obtained spectra from 15 *T. gondii* abscesses and 8 lymphomatous masses using a spin-echo technique (TE 135 ms) and calculated metabolite ratios for Cho, Cr, NAA, lactate and lipids. They found abnormal metabolite ratios in all the lesions with the spectra falling into three broad categories: one type showed very large lipid peaks with relative suppression of the other metabolites; the second type showed elevation of the Cho/Cr ratio with diminished NAA relative to the other peaks; the third type had features of the other two categories; examples of each of the three spectra were obtained from both *T. gondii* and lymphoma mass lesions. Lactate was not detected in any of the spectra and overall there were no significant differences in any of the metabolite ratios between these two pathologies (Table 17.2). They proposed that the reason for this overlap was that in AIDS, lymphomatous masses were often necrotic with a composition similar to necrotic abscesses, and this would explain the similarity between the MRI appearances and spectral profile, the latter also being dependent on lesion maturity (Chinn et al. 1995).

A more recent study (Simone et al. 1998) evaluated the metabolite ratios (NAA/Cho, NAA/ Cr and Cho/Cr) obtained from spin-echo spectra acquired at 1.5 T with an echo-time of 135 ms in 20 HIV-1 seropositive patients with toxoplasmosis and 7 with lymphoma. The spectra were compared to those from normal appearing white matter of the centrum semiovale obtained in normal controls. Although there was a significant difference in the means of the three metabolite ratios in toxoplasmosis compared with normal controls, with reduced NAA/Cr, NAA/ Cho and raised Cho/Cr, significant pathological differences in these three ratios were only recorded in 20%, 65%, and 40% of abscesses respectively. In contrast to the findings of Chang et al., a lactate peak was only seen in 20% and a lipid peak in 35% of toxoplasma abscesses.

In the seven patients with lymphoma studied, there was a significant reduction in the NAA/Cr, NAA/ Cho, and a significant increase in the Cho/Cr ratios compared with the control group. NAA/Cr and NAA/ Cho ratios were also significantly reduced compared with toxoplasmosis. Reduction in the NAA/Cr and NAA/Cho and increase in the Cho/Cr ratios was seen in 71%, 86% and 57% of lymphoma lesions respectively and a lactate peak was seen in 29% and a lipid peak in 71% (Table 17.2).

The authors also performed serial spectra on patients with toxoplasmosis while on appropriate antimicrobial therapy. The NAA/Cr ratios were lower in those patients with acute lesions than in those in remission, and in three cases the ratio returned to normal on treatment over the subsequent 8 months. A high Cho/Cr ratio found in four patients on their first study, recovered to within normal limits during follow-up, but increased further in another two cases, in accordance with clinical deterioration. In addition, a lactate peak, although seen infrequently, was only observed in acute toxoplasmosis lesions. Overall, the authors found that using the three metabolite ratios as a combined variable, lesion discrimination with ^{1}H MRS had a low overall diagnostic accuracy of only 30% for toxoplasmosis and 57.1% for lymphoma, a conclusion not dissimilar to that reached by Chinn et al.

There are several possible reasons for the disparity in the findings in these studies. The first is location of the voxel in relation to the lesion, and the parts of the lesion sampled. Regional variations in the chemistry of focal brain lesions are well recognized (Segebarth et al. 1990) and the spectral pattern of a central area of necrosis in a lymphomatous lesion may well resemble that of toxoplasma abscess, with depletion of normal metabolites and markedly increased lipid and lactate resonances. Indeed, spectroscopic sampling of necrotic areas of any lesion is, as with histological analysis, less likely to discriminate between different pathological causes; selection of the voxel to include areas of active pathology is clearly critical in this regard. For the single-voxel technique, the advent of short TE PRESS, which allows the use of smaller voxels to reduce partial-volume effects, and the use of intravenous gadolinium to define different regions of focal lesions and aid positioning, will make this process more reliable. The development of reliable short echo-time spectroscopic imaging is also likely to have a major impact in this area.

A second reason for these discrepant results may be the use of metabolite ratios rather than concentrations, as alteration in Cr concentration will influence metabolite levels as well as changes in the concentration of the metabolite itself. The observation that Cr levels themselves were highly discriminant lends weight to this argument (Chang et al. 1995). Comparison of metabolite ratios with apparently normal contralateral cerebral white matter has been advocated; however, the diffuse abnormalities in metabolite concentrations which have been reported in HIV-1 seropositive patients with varying degrees of clinical neurological problems and without structural imaging abnormalities (Paley et al. 1995) suggests that this approach may also be vulnerable to systematic errors.

Thirdly, the spectroscopic methods used by these investigators differed. Metabolites such as Mi and Glx are not visible at long TE. Moreover, the evaluation of resonances at 0.9–1.3 ppm at TE=135 ms alone is difficult as lipid signals overlap with those of lactate (which is in negative phase at this echo time and will subtract from the signal).

Comparison of measurements at short TE (30–35 ms) and long TE (270 ms) allows lactate to be detected. Spectra measured at longer echo times are also more sensitive to changes in metabolite relaxation time which are known to be associated with pathological processes (Wilkinson et al. 1995), and is a further potential source of systematic error in quantification. The repetition time (TR) will also influence signal intensity and hence quantification (particularly of species with long relaxation times) if the system is not at equilibrium (TR of 1500 ms should be considered a minimum at 1.5 T, and TR>2000 is generally recommended for quantitative studies).

Finally, differences in patient selection (particularly with regard to the chronicity of toxoplasma lesions) and ascertainment (not all lesions were confirmed histologically) may also contribute to the different conclusions drawn in the above studies.

It appears that MRS has the potential to distinguish between lymphoma and toxoplasma masses, although the reliability of this technique in a clinical context remains an unresolved issue. In order to validate the very promising results of Chang et al., further studies using short TE examinations (supplemented by longer TE where significant lipid or lactate resonances are present) with careful voxel positioning, rigorous quantification and comparison with matched normal subjects are required.

17.3.2 CNS Cryptococcosis

Infection with the ubiquitous saprophytic fungus *Cryptococcus neoformans* is the third most common opportunistic infection occurring in AIDS, usually when the CD4+ lymphocyte count is less than 200 (Zuger et al. 1986). CNS cryptococcosis occurs in up to 5% of patients with AIDS and usually presents with rather non-specific symptoms and signs, with focal neurology occurring relatively infrequently (Chuck et al. 1989). The diagnosis is primarily microbiological, and is based on India ink or mucicarmine staining of CSF, cryptococcal latex agglutination titres in blood and CSF and positive blood cultures. Although imaging may be normal or show the non-specific signs of atrophy or white matter hyperintensity of HIV encephalopathy (HIVE), several characteristic imaging appearances have been described. As the fungus spreads haematogenously to the CNS the earliest signs of infection include enlarged perivascular spaces mainly in the basal ganglia, thalamus and brainstem; this sign in itself is non-specific, being seen in normal individuals and with increased frequency in ageing and in atrophy (Heier et al. 1989). With disease progression the perivascular spaces enlarge due to accumulation of organisms and mucoid material, with the formation of the characteristic pseudocysts/cryptococcomas, the distribution of which reflects that of the enlarged perivascular spaces. Typically the cryptococcomas are hyperintense on T2, and of intermediate or low signal on T1-weighted sequences, exert only local mass effect, and show no associated surrounding oedema or enhancement (Miszkiel et al. 1996). There have been a few reports of enhancing intraparenchymal cryptococcomas, but this feature is rare, as is leptomeningeal enhancement (Tien et al. 1991; Andreula et al. 1993; Berkefeld et al. 1999) which probably reflects the combination of a protective polysaccharide capsule around the organism and the profoundly immunosuppressed state of the patients. Atypical imaging appearances described include multiple scattered non-enhancing white matter lesions, choroid plexus lesions and an acquired extra-axial collection of organisms and mucoid material resembling an arachnoid cyst. With treatment, the radiological improvement often lags significantly behind both the clinical improvement and the reduction in microbiological parameters of disease (Andreula et al. 1993; Miszkiel et al. 1996; Berkefeld et al. 1999).

The typical imaging appearances described in CNS cryptococcosis do not often cause diagnostic difficulty and thus there has been less impetus to apply advanced MR imaging techniques. However, Chang et al. performed MRS on cryptococcomas in four patients. MR spectra showed that these lesions were primarily lipid with reduction in the peaks of all of the normally detectable metabolites, NAA, Cho, Cr and Mi. The NAA and Cr peaks were significantly higher than in toxoplasmosis and the choline peak was significantly lower than the markedly elevated peak seen in lymphoma. There was no significant difference in the Mi peaks in cryptococcomas and the other three types of mass lesions evaluated (toxoplasmosis, lymphoma and PML). Thus, despite the crytococcomas being a type of fungal abscess there was less spectroscopic evidence of frank brain destruction than occurs in toxoplasma abscesses (Chang et al. 1995). Whilst these observations are interesting and may yield insight into the pathophysiology of cryptococcal infection, there is currently little clinical role for additional imaging techniques in this condition (Table 17.2, Fig. 17.2).

23.3.3 Progressive Multifocal Leukoencephalopathy

Progressive multifocal leukoencephalopathy, first described by Astrom et al. (1958), results from reactivation of opportunistic infection with the JC virus, a ubiquitous papova virus which is usually non-pathogenic in the immunocompetent host. In patients with impaired cell mediated immunity, however, the virus infects oligodendrocytes resulting in demyelination; PML was infrequently encountered in the days prior to the AIDS epidemic but is also seen in the context of immunosuppression associated with lymphoproliferative disorders, organ transplantation and autoimmune diseases. Neuropathological autopsy series have reported a prevalence of PML in AIDS patients as high as 11% (THURNHER et al. 1997); it usually develops in the late stages of disease when the patient is profoundly immunosuppressed and typically presents with focal neurological signs depending on the site of pathology (VON EINSIEDEL et al. 1993; SIMPSON and TAGLIATI 1994); prognosis is poor with average survival limited to 6–9 months (BERGER et al. 1988).

Lesions of PML have characteristic appearances on MRI; they can be solitary or multiple and most frequently develop in the periventricular and subcortical white matter of the parietal and frontal lobes although one-third of patients also have posterior fossa involvement. On MRI, lesions are hypointense on T1 and hyperintense on T2 with a typical scalloped appearance if subcortical fibres are involved. In a recent study (THURNHER et al. 1997) of 73 PML lesions in 21 patients, lesions in the occipital lobe, corpus callosum and thalami were more frequently seen than had been previously described. In addition the authors described a new radiological feature of a cystic area of varying size, within the lesions in 12/16 patients, which corresponded to an area of focal necrosis at autopsy (Fig. 17.3). Contrary to many other studies, in a third of their patients, lesions were associated with some mass effect and minimal compression of the ipsilateral ventricle. In agreement with most other studies, none of the lesions showed contrast enhancement; however, faint and peripheral lesion enhancement has been reported and the presence of enhancement cannot be considered to exclude the diagnosis (CHANG et al. 1997). Seventeen patients in this study had follow-up imaging and showed strikingly rapid radiological progression in both the number and size of lesions, a feature which had not been previously strongly emphasized in the literature as a frequent feature of this condition.

A more recent study of 48 patients with histologically proven PML showed that mild mass effect seen on MRI in 5 patients was associated with a significantly shorter survival period. Size, location, number or type of lesions, or presence of atrophy were not correlated with survival; interestingly a trend was observed between the number of discrete PML lesions and increasing survival rates, presumably explained by the fact that with disease progression lesions coalesce and become more confluent (DONOVAN et al. 1999).

Metabolite levels in PML were measured as part of the study of focal brain lesions in AIDS described above (Sect. 17.3.1; CHANG et al. 1995). Decreased NAA peaks, slightly reduced Cr and increased Cho peaks were seen in PML and overall the metabolite levels were significantly different to those in toxoplasmosis, but indistinguishable from lymphoma. The lipid peak was not analysed separately from the lactate peak in this study. The Mi levels in PML ranged from mildly decreased to greatly increased levels (Table 17.2, Fig. 17.2).

A subsequent study from the same group (CHANG et al. 1997) used a combination of MRI and single

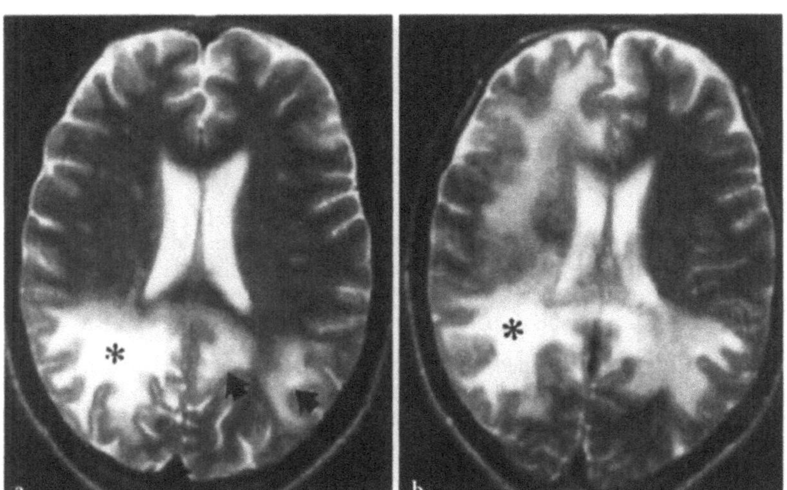

Fig. 17.3a,b. T2-weighted axial images showing a large right parietal lesion of PML (a) with marked central hyperintensity and a rim of moderate hyperintensity (*asterisk*). Note the two contralateral PML lesions (*arrows*). Repeat imaging 4 weeks later (b) demonstrates progressive disease in both cerebral hemispheres, though the right parietal lesion (*asterisk*) is unchanged. (From: Thurnher MM, Thurnher SA, Muhlbauer B, Hainfellner JA, Steuer A, Fleischmann D, Tratattnig S, Budka H, Schindler E. Progressive multifocal leukoencephalopathy in AIDS: Initial and follow-up CT and MRI. Neuroradiology 1997; 39: 611–618. With permission)

voxel MRS to evaluate a total of 68 PML lesions in 20 patients with AIDS. Fifty percent of the patients imaged had posterior fossa lesions with 61% of them originating at the pontocerebellar junction, a much higher proportion than described in many previous studies. The area postrema of the 4th ventricle lacks a blood-brain barrier and is highly vascularized and the high proportion of lesions in the posterior fossa in this study supports the hypothesis of haematogenous entry to the brain by the JC virus. Slight contrast enhancement was seen in four lesions, two of which underwent spontaneous remission; the implied local disruption of the blood-brain barrier suggests a more aggressive inflammatory response to the virus by perivascular T-lymphocytes, and is associated with a more favourable prognosis.

Spectra acquired from the PML lesions were compared with those obtained from normal-appearing white matter in the contralateral hemisphere and from 20 normal age-matched controls. Short TE (30 ms) STEAM or PRESS sequences were used (and where peaks were present in the 1.35 ppm region, these were supplemented by corresponding long TE=270 ms sequences to differentiate lactate and lipid resonances), and metabolite concentrations calculated. The NAA concentration in the PML lesions was markedly lower than in normal controls and a significant reduction in Cr and increase in Cho were also seen. However, in the structurally normal contralateral white matter, Cr levels were slightly elevated and Glx levels slightly, but significantly, depressed compared with normal controls. Lactate was detected in 75% and lipid in 90% of the lesion spectra, but neither was detected in contralateral white matter. Mi concentrations were variable, increased in some lesions, decreased in others and overall the group mean value was not significantly different to that of normals (Table 17.2). Six patients had serial MRS studies, and in most of these Mi decreased progressively with time, accompanied by clinical and radiological deterioration. However, two patients who had both clinical and radiological spontaneous remission of PML showed the highest Mi concentrations at early follow-up. This suggests that changes in Mi may also be a predictor of progression of PML (Chang et al. 1997).

A smaller recent study (Iranzo et al. 1999) measured metabolite ratios in spectra obtained from six patients with histologically confirmed PML with STEAM and PRESS sequences. They found a homogeneous pattern in all spectra obtained, with a significantly reduced NAA/Cr, significantly increased Cho/Cr and lipid /Cr ratios compared with spectra obtained from healthy controls. Lactate was also present in all the PML spectra (Table 17.2, Fig. 17.4).

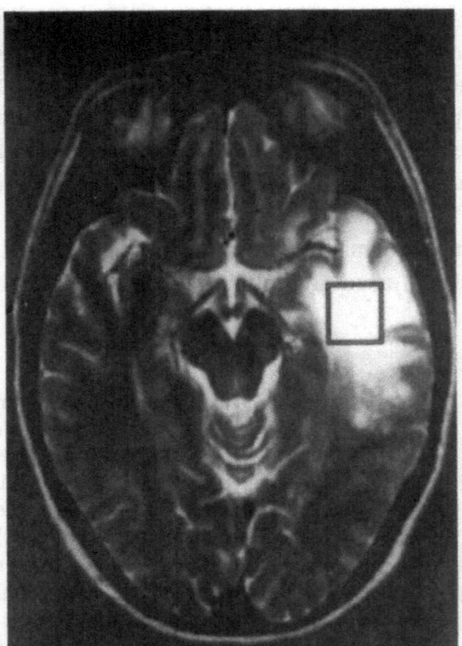
a

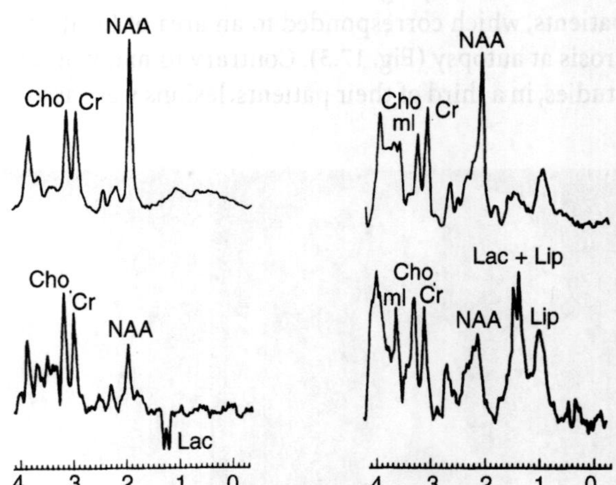

b

Fig. 17.4a,b. T2-weighted axial image showing a characteristic hyperintense lesion of PML in the left temporal lobe in (**a**) with voxel placement centrally within the lesion for MRS. Image (**b**) shows in vivo localized ^{1}H MRS (PRESS-135 and STEAM-20) spectra from white matter in control subjects (*control*) and PML in HIV-seropositive patients (*PML*). In comparison with the spectra of normal white matter, note the increase in lipids (*Lip*), lactate (*Lac*), the mild increase in choline (*Cho*) and myo-inositol (*mI*). (From: Iranzo A, Moreno A, Pujol J, Marti-Fabregas J, Domingo P, Molet J, Ris J, Cadafalch J. Proton magnetic resonance spectroscopy pattern of progressive multifocal leukoencephalopathy in AIDS. JNNP 1999; 66: 520–523. With permission)

These findings are in keeping with those of CHANG et al. (1997).

However, SIMONE et al. (1998), using spin echo sequences (TE 135 ms), did not detect a lipid peak in any of the eight patients with PML they evaluated, though lactate peaks were present in 75% of lesions. An increased Cho/Cr ratio was only found in 25%, with reduced NAA/Cr in 87.5% and reduced NAA/Cho in 62.5%; and the authors were able to classify PML lesions correctly according to spectral pattern in 75% of cases, with a significantly lower mean NAA/Cr in PML than in toxoplasmosis (Table 17.2). The differences between this study and those using short echo times may be attributed, at least in part, to differential change in relaxation times of these metabolites, which is emphasized at longer echo times.

The reduction in NAA, a marker of healthy neurons, can be used to evaluate the extent of neuronal and axonal loss and damage and the reduction in Cr reflects cell loss; elevated Cho is consistent with increased cell turnover with breakdown of cell membranes and myelin as part of the process of demyelination that occurs in PML.

The variable concentration of Mi in PML may be an indication of different stages in the natural history of the disease, with a higher levels reflecting a more fulminant process of glial activity and a more active repair process; this appears to be supported by the results of serial MRS. The increased lipid concentration is most probably due to the breakdown products of demyelination. Lactate is a product of anaerobic metabolism and associated with local tissue ischaemia, but it has been suggested from a study of acute stroke lesions that it may also be associated with the presence of certain cell types, such as foamy macrophages (which may respire anaerobically). The lactate in the demyelinating lesions of PML is thought to originate from a combination of enlarged abnormal oligodendrocytes, bizarre giant astrocytes, foamy macrophages and areas of necrosis. Another finding that emerged from this study was that abnormal metabolite concentrations were also found in normal appearing contralateral white matter with lower concentrations of NAA and Glx, reflecting neuronal loss and higher levels of Cr, Cho and Mi, suggesting possible subclinical infection with JC virus with or without the additional direct effects of infection with HIV-1.

It seems then that PML has consistent spectral features on short echo time MRS, and can be distinguished from toxoplasmosis but probably not lymphoma using this technique alone. The combination of improvement in the sensitivity of PCR analysis for the JC virus DNA, which approaches 86% (CHANG et al. 1997), and the use of ^{1}H MRS, may enable more accurate non-invasive diagnosis of PML, which will be particularly important if a successful therapeutic regimen becomes a reality. The prognostic use of monitoring metabolite levels (particularly Mi) and subtle peripheral contrast enhancement (see also Sect. 17.5.1) may also be of clinical importance.

17.4 MRS in Diffuse Processes

17.4.1 AIDS Dementia Complex

The dementia that occurs in AIDS (AIDS dementia complex, ADC) is a progressive subcortical dementia which increases in prevalence in the later stages of HIV infection and AIDS. It is the commonest neurological complication seen in AIDS, causes progressive neurocognitive, motor and behavioural deterioration and may ultimately affect up to 60% of sufferers. More than 90% of those with ADC will have histological evidence of HIV encephalitis characterized by myelin pallor, astrogliosis, microglial nodules, with multinucleate giant cells and perivascular macrophages. The cortex is also affected with resultant neuronal loss. Although most of the cells infected with the HIV-1 virus are macrophages and microglia, astrocytes can also be infected, but neurons are rarely so. The neuronal damage and loss that occurs is therefore thought to be a secondary effect of infection and is likely to be multifactorial, but as yet is incompletely understood. Effects on calcium and *N*-methyl-D-aspartate receptor operated channels causes a detrimental increase in intracellular calcium; viral replication in the monophage-macrophage cells results in the release of neurotoxic viral proteins such as tat, gp120 and nef and other locally released factors such as quinolinic acid, arachadonic acid catabolites, leukotrienes, glutamate and other excitatory amino acids are also likely to be involved in this process. The radiological manifestation of these microscopic changes can be seen on MRI as HIV encephalopathy (HIVE), the features of which are progressive generalized atrophy with ventricular and sulcal enlargement. Abnormal signal hyperintensity on T2-weighted images may also be seen in the cerebral white matter, with little if any corresponding signal change on T1-weighted images. In the early stages the white matter changes are patchy and seen most frequently in the periventricular regions and centrum semiovale, but become more confluent and symmetrical with time; the subcortical white matter is spared, which may be useful in differentiating from early lesions of PML. These white matter lesions are not associated with mass effect, nor do they show enhancement after contrast agent.

Studies in seropositive patients have shown that qualitative and semiautomated quantitative measurements of cerebral atrophy correlate with abnormal neurology, particularly encephalopathy (PALEY et al. 1994; HARRISON et al. 1998).

Single voxel MRS is particularly well-suited to the study of diffuse intracerebral processes, and this technique has been used in a number of series to relate metabolite changes with other markers of disease at different stages of the ADC. One of the larger earlier studies (CHONG et al. 1993) correlated the results of single voxel spectroscopy with CDC (Centres for Disease Control and Prevention) stage, immunological and clinical markers of disease, and with the findings on conventional MRI in a cohort of 103 HIV-1 seropositive patients and 23 normal controls. Long TE spin echo spectra obtained in white matter showed a reduction in the mean metabolite ratios of NAA/Cr, NAA/Cho and an increase in the Cho/Cr in seropositive patients compared with controls. The mean NAA/Cr was 9% lower in symptomatic (CDC IV) than asymptomatic (CDC II and III) patients. Significantly lower NAA/Cho, NAA/Cr ratios were seen in patients with CD4+ lymphocyte counts less than 200 and in those with an abnormal neurological examination. Not surprisingly, significant differences in metabolite ratios were also observed in patients with MRI changes of HIVE. Abnormal metabolite ratios were also seen in a proportion of patients (11/103) with a normal MRI and conversely 22 patients with abnormal imaging had normal spectra. What was clear from this study was that MRS in ADC provides complementary information to MRI about the extent and severity of cerebral involvement by HIV encephalitis; subtle changes in metabolite ratios may be detected before there is radiological evidence of HIVE and indeed spectroscopy correlated with the presence of abnormal neurology better than did MRI (CHONG et al. 1993).

Changes in the T2 relaxation time of NAA in patients with AIDS, particularly those with diffuse white matter hyperintensity on MRI, have been demonstrated (WILKINSON et al. 1994), and a number of more recent studies have been performed using short echo times in an attempt to minimize the potentially confounding effects of this on metabolite quantification. All have shown significantly decreased levels of NAA/Cr of between 20% and 30% in neurologically symptomatic AIDS patients when compared to healthy controls (JARVICK et al. 1993; PALEY et al. 1995; LAUBENBERGER et al. 1996). However, ratios of other metabolites measured in different studies varied; PALEY et al. found no differences in Cho/Cr or Mi/Cr, whereas LAUBENBERGER measured significantly higher levels of both in the ADC group. In the case of Mi/Cr variability was large, and there was considerable overlap. The ratio Mi/NAA showed no overlap between the normal subjects and ADC groups. The differences between these results may in part reflect differences in the subject populations. LAUBENBERGER also examined a group of asymptomatic patients with AIDS who showed more modest, but statistically significant, reductions in NAA/Cr but which overlapped considerably with the normal controls.

Proton MR spectroscopic imaging (MRSI) or chemical shift imaging (CSI) has provided information on the anatomical distribution of metabolic abnormalities in ADC (BARKER et al. 1995), and confirms the decreased NAA and increased Cho white matter levels seen in the single voxel studies, with more extensive metabolite changes in subjects with dementia (Fig. 17.5). Metabolite abnormalities were

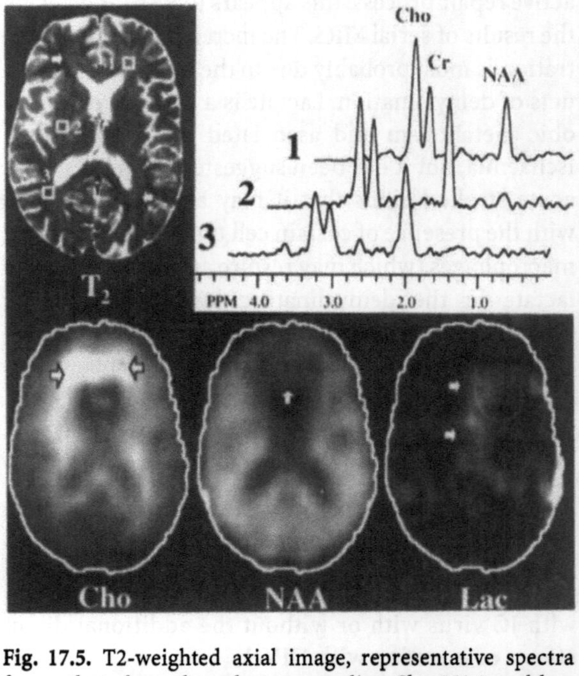

Fig. 17.5. T2-weighted axial image, representative spectra from selected voxels and corresponding Cho, NAA and lactate metabolite maps acquired in a patient with mild to moderate dementia. *The arrows* indicate areas of signal abnormality. (From: Barker PB, Lee RR, McArthur JC. AIDS dementia complex: evaluation with proton MR spectroscopic imaging. Radiology 1995; 195: 58–64. With permission)

again seen in areas of brain which appeared normal on MRI. Moreover, reduction in NAA was most pronounced in the frontal regions, which is in accord with the distribution of neuronal loss that has been documented at postmortem (EVERALL et al. 1991).

A separate series using CSI (MOLLER et al. 1999) demonstrated significant reductions in the NAA/Cr and NAA/Cho ratios and a significant increase in the Cho/Cr ratio in the grey matter of the insula and striatum in HIV-seropositive patients with AIDS, CD4+ lymphocyte counts <200, neurological signs and those with atrophy on MRI. The cortical reduction in NAA, assumed to be due to neuronal loss and/or dysfunction is consistent with the findings of several neuropathological studies (EVERALL et al. 1991,1993). It has also been shown that the basal ganglia in patients with AIDS carry the highest viral load and are reduced in volume (AYLWARD et al. 1993); the reduction in NAA in this region again reflects this. MRS has also been used to assess the effect and response of HIV-1 seropositive patients to antiretroviral drugs. WILKINSON et al. (1997) examined a group of HIV-seropositive but asymptomatic subjects and found no significant differences in the NAA/Cho, NAA/Cr and Cho/Cr ratios between those taking the antiretroviral agent, zidovudine, and those not taking it. Reductions in the NAA/Cho ratio have also been shown to be transiently reversible in patients with ADC when treated with anti-retroviral agents, such as zidovudine. In the small number of patients studied, the metabolite ratios on MRS mirrored clinical improvement on initiation of zidovudine therapy, with an initial increase in NAA/Cr and decrease in Cho/Cr, followed by decrease in NAA/Cr and increase in Cho/Cr. This chronological change in the metabolite ratios may be explained by the mechanism of action of zidovudine. After initiation of therapy there is an initial fall in the plasma concentration of viral RNA, which reaches maximum suppression at about 7 days; hence the initial improvement in metabolite ratios; this is followed by a return of the viral load to baseline levels over the subsequent weeks which parallels the clinical deterioration and the fall in NAA/Cr and increase in Cho/Cr. On initiation of zidovudine therapy, a reduction in white matter hyperintensity also often accompanied the transient clinical improvement, but atrophy progressed, suggesting that the latter process is irreversible and less closely correlated with clinical assessment (WILKINSON et al. 1997).

With the recent introduction of highly active antiretroviral therapy (HAART, namely simultaneous treatment with at least three combination antiretroviral drugs, one of which is a protease inhibitor) there has been a marked and significant change in the morbidity and mortality patterns in patients with HIV disease, including a reduction in neurological complications (SACKTOR et al. 1999). Studies have shown that within 3 months of starting HAART, the plasma viral load is suppressed to undetectable levels, although this may be a transient phenomenon since with prolonged therapy, plasma and CSF viral load levels may start to increase again after 6 months (MCARTHUR et al. 1999).

CHANG et al. studied a group of 16 patients with mild ADC before and at least 3 months after starting HAART, using ^{1}H-MRS, to ascertain the effect of this treatment regimen on measurable metabolite concentrations. Pre-treatment Cho/Cr and [Cho] were significantly elevated in the basal ganglia compared with controls. After treatment, Cho/Cr normalized and [Cho] showed a trend towards normalization. In the midfrontal cortex the Cho/Cr was not significantly elevated compared with controls, although it showed a significant decrease with treatment; these changes were due to trends towards a decrease in [Cho] and an increase in [Cr].

The [Mi] was also significantly elevated in the basal ganglia and frontal white matter at baseline and reduced significantly with treatment. The changes in [Mi] in the frontal white matter correlated with the improvement in CD4+ lymphocyte count and the clinical ADC stage, but only showed a trend towards correlation with the plasma viral load. No significant changes in [NAA] were observed at baseline or after treatment in the patients, although NAA/Cr was elevated in the basal ganglia at baseline due to a reduction in [Cr] (CHANG et al. 1999).

The most sensitive marker of early brain injury in HIV infection has recently shown to be the glial marker Mi (CHANG et al. 1999a) and the current study shows that it is more sensitive than [Cho] in monitoring the effects of HAART on HIV-associated brain injury. The reduction in [Cr] in the basal ganglia is likely to be due to cell loss and decreased metabolism. The lack of significant changes detected in [NAA] may be due to the early clinical stage of dementia in the patients studied and voxel localization. This preliminary study confirms the clinical efficacy of HAART, and establishes the important correlation between neurochemical levels, particularly Mi, and clinical and laboratory indices of treatment response.

What is apparent from all these studies is that MRS is a useful adjunct to MRI in evaluating patients with ADC. Metabolite abnormalities can be detected in asymptomatic patients and those with normal imaging, which may have important implications with regard to the timing of initiation of anti-retroviral therapy. Moreover, metabolite response to retroviral agents appears to reflect clinical response, suggesting another role for MRS in therapeutic monitoring; further longitudinal studies are required in patients on HAART to determine whether ^{1}H-MRS may be useful in detecting the development of drug resistance and the consequent HIV-related brain injury.

23.4.2 CMV Encephalitis

CNS infection with the herpes virus *cytomegalovirus* (CMV) in AIDS is secondary to reactivation of a previously acquired infection. It is the most common opportunistic infection diagnosed at autopsy though is less commonly diagnosed antemortem (Kure et al. 1991). CNS involvement usually occurs in the context of widespread systemic infection and the clinical presentation with neurocognitive deficits may be similar to that seen in HIV-associated dementia, although the course is often more rapidly progressive. The MR imaging appearances of CMV encephalitis can be identical to HIVE, with confluent and symmetrical areas of hyperintensity in the white matter on T2-weighted sequences without associated mass effect; these correspond pathologically to areas of infarction or necrosis, resulting from infection of the vascular endothelial cells by the virus and resultant vascular occlusion. CNS CMV infection can also present as a rapidly progressive necrotizing encephalitis, with destructive enhancing periventricular lesions, since the virus has a predilection for the ependymal and subependymal regions of the brain (Holland et al. 1994).

It is often difficult to differentiate between HIVE and CMV encephalitis on clinical and imaging grounds (Miller et al. 1996) and detection of viral DNA in CSF by polymerase chain reaction (PCR) has a variable sensitivity of 82%–95% (Cinque et al. 1995; Weinberg et al. 1998). Wilkinson et al. (1996) evaluated the potential of MRS to differentiate between these two clinical conditions. They measured metabolite ratios using a spin echo technique (TE 135 ms) in patients with diffuse white matter abnormalities; at autopsy CMV encephalitis was confirmed in seven and HIVE in six; none had the two conditions synchronously. Significantly higher NAA/Cho ratios were found in those with CMV encephalitis. Although the NAA/Cr ratio was higher and the Cho/Cr ratio lower in the group with CMV infection, these differences did not reach statistical significance. The authors made the assumption that the Cr peak was constant; thus patients with HIVE had higher Cho and smaller NAA peaks than those with CMV encephalitis. This was surprising considering CMV encephalitis is often associated with more extensive inflammation and necrosis than is seen in HIVE, and thus one would expect a higher Cho peak and a lower NAA peak in the former (Wilkinson et al. 1996).

Although the results from this small retrospective study are promising there do not appear to have been any further reports in the literature of larger or prospective studies of MRS in differentiating these two disease processes.

17.5 Magnetization Transfer Imaging

Magnetization transfer (MT) imaging exploits the variation in the interaction between protons in water with those bound to macromolecules in different tissues to generate contrast, and is a useful technique for characterizing structural changes in these tissues. The free water protons rotate freely in solution and yield a clearly defined MR signal (which is used to generate the MR image) whereas those bound to macromolecules, by virtue of their restricted rotational freedom and heterogeneous chemical shifts, produce an envelope of broad, overlapping signals which are effectively invisible. Magnetization, however, may be transferred from the bound to unbound proton pool. If the macromolecular proton pool is saturated by an off-resonance pulse (i.e. with a frequency away from the water resonance) prior to acquisition of an MR image, there is a resultant decrease in signal intensity from the mobile proton pool. The difference in signal intensity induced by MT is proportional to the degree of interaction between the two pools; this depends on a complex combination of dipole interactions, chemical exchange and other factors such as the relaxation times of the protons and their rotational freedom. Many of these, in turn, depend on the specific tissue characteristics, and particularly the microscopic architecture of membranes and their associated macromolecules. Although T2-weighted MRI is very sensitive for the detection of pathology, particularly in white matter, it is not always helpful in differentiating the processes of oedema, gliosis or demyelination, and assessing the degree of MT may be helpful.

The degree of magnetization transfer may be expressed, quantitatively, as the magnetization transfer ratio (MTR)=(M0+M1)/M0, where M1 and M0 are the pixel signal intensities with and without magnetization transfer-saturation, respectively.

In the brain, the MTR is highest for white matter (probably due to the macromolecular structure of myelin), intermediate for grey matter and lowest for CSF.

MT techniques have already proven useful in imaging of several neurological diseases such as multiple sclerosis (Gass et al. 1994), systemic lupus erythematosus (Campi et al. 1996) and primary and secondary tumours (Kurki et al. 1996; Finelli et al. 1998). They have also been applied to the problem of differentiating PML lesions from white matter lesions (WML) of HIVE in patients with AIDS.

17.5.1 Progressive Multifocal Leukoencephalopathy

Dousset et al. (1996) compared the MTR in lesions of PML and HIVE with that from the white matter of a group of normal controls. Diagnosis was made on the basis of clinical and imaging features, with histological confirmation only in equivocal cases.

They found a significant reduction in the MTR of PML (22%±2.3%) compared with HIVE (40%±3.8%), and an MTR in white matter of normal controls 47%±2.3%.

In addition, the MTR of normal-appearing white matter in both the PML and HIVE group showed a slight (1–2%), but statistically significant, reduction when compared with normal controls (Dousset et al. 1996).

A more recent study by Ernst et al. (1999), in which 42 lesions in 21 patients with AIDS and either PML or HIV related white matter lesions (HIV-WML) were evaluated prospectively with a combination of conventional MR imaging and T1-weighted spin-echo MT sequences, showed similar results. As the MTR was heterogeneous within the lesions, the authors calculated average and minimum MTRs for the lesions. They found that there was a highly significant difference between the average MTR in PML (26.1%±4.0%) and HIV-WML (38.0%±2.6%) (Fig. 17.6). This compares with the MTR of normal appearing white matter of 47.9%±2.2%. Moreover, there was no overlap between the minimum or average MTRs calculated in the two pathological groups, and the MTR was able to differentiate between lesions of PML and HIV-WML as small as 0.5 cm^2.

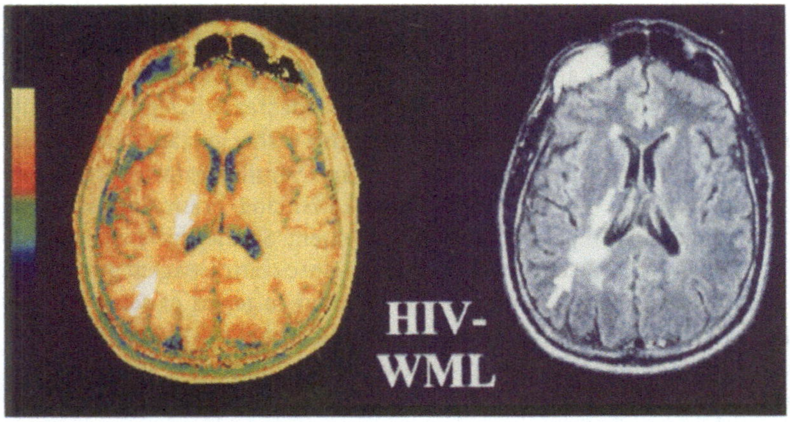

a

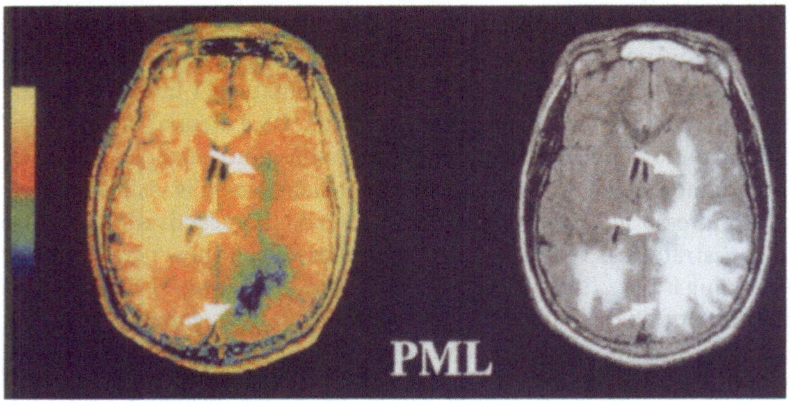

b

Fig. 17.6a,b. Magnetization transfer ratio maps (*left*) corresponding to the FLAIR images (*right*) of HIV-WML in (**a**) and PML in (**b**). Although the appearances are similar on the FLAIR images the MTRs of the two lesions are markedly different. The HIV-WML shows only moderate and relatively homogeneous reduction in MTR, whereas the PML lesion has areas of very low MTR consistent with the pathological process of demyelination. In HIV-WML the myelin is relatively intact. The same MTR colour ratio scale is used for both lesions, with bright yellow corresponding to the highest MTR value of 52%. (From: Ernst T, Chang L, Witt M, Walot I, Aronow H, Leonido-Yee M, Singer E. Progressive multifocal leukoencephalopathy and human immunodeficiency virus-associated white matter lesions in AIDS: magnetization transfer MR imaging. Radiology 1999; 210: 539–543. With permission)

In PML lesions, no correlation was found between the age of a lesion (determined according to duration of clinical symptoms) and MTR, but the minimum MTR was inversely related to lesion size. Most PML lesions had a lower MTR in the centre, with a progressive outward increase towards normal values. This radial distribution is not completely surprising as Thurnher et al. (1997) described imaging features of cystic/necrotic change in the PML lesions in his cohort. In contrast, for WML, the average MTR correlated with lesion size (Ernst et al. 1999).

The following are apparent from these early studies:

Distinct differences in MTR between PML and HIV-WML allow differentiation between the two processes with a diagnostic accuracy of greater than 90%, even in small lesions. The more extreme changes in MTR in PML are likely to reflect demyelination, tissue destruction and necrosis which are characteristic pathological features of PML; this parameter is particularly sensitive to demyelination, and the values obtained for PML lesions are similar to those found in multiple sclerosis (MS) plaques (Dousset et al. 1992; Grossman et al. 1994). In contrast, WML lesions tend to be non-demyelinating, and associated with an increased water content and inflammatory infiltrate of macrophages, multinucleate giant cells, perivascular lymphocytes and microglial nodules, leading to more modest reduction in MTR.

Abnormal MTR in structurally-normal white matter in AIDS patients suggests either subclinical involvement of more extensive areas of the brain either by HIV-1, or possibly also the JC virus in those with PML. The small absolute reduction in MTR, however, currently limits the use of this as a diagnostic tool in an individual patient.

The imaging and clinical features of PML are usually sufficiently characteristic to make a confident diagnosis and although HIV-WML can appear similar to PML on T2-weighted sequences, unlike PML, they often have little or no corresponding signal change on T1-weighted sequences. However, there are many reports in the literature of cases with atypical features and very early small lesions of PML, at a time when the patient is asymptomatic, may be indistinguishable from HIV-WML. Differentiation is important due to the very different prognosis in these two conditions and will become more so as new developments in drug treatment strategies emerge. It is in these cases where MT imaging is likely to play an important role. Further longitudinal studies are clearly required to evaluate the chronological changes in MTR that occur with disease progression, and whether it will play a role in monitoring response to therapy.

To the author's knowledge, to date there has not been any data about MTI in other opportunistic viral infections occurring in AIDS such as CMV, herpes simplex and h. zoster. These also cause white matter lesions, which in the case of CMV can look identical on conventional imaging to the white matter changes of HIVE (Miller et al. 1996).

17.5.2 Magnetization Transfer to Improve Tissue Contrast

MT techniques can also be used with T1, T2, time-of-flight MRA sequences and with Gd-enhanced T1-weighted sequences to augment tissue contrast.

There are two commonly used ways of improving the detection of enhancing lesions on postcontrast T1-weighted MR sequences: one is to increase the dose of contrast used and the other to increase the delay between contrast injection and image acquisition to coincide with maximum uptake of contrast in the extracellular space. The former has direct financial implications in terms of contrast consumption, and the latter may be unacceptable in claustrophobic or very ill patients and also has a detrimental effect on patient throughput. An alternative strategy is to apply the MT technique to post-contrast-weighted sequences. This causes a decrease in signal intensity of white and grey matter with a greater reduction in the latter, and thus an overall greater contrast between normal non-enhancing brain and areas of pathological enhancement. Studies have shown that sequences with triple-dose contrast agent and single dose with MT are similar in terms of sensitivity of lesion detection (Mathews et al. 1994). MRI with MT has proved useful in improving the detection rate of enhancing cerebral metastases, as in this condition, the number of lesions detected can have great implications with regard to treatment options (Peretti-Viton et al. 1998). There is, however, a paucity of information on post-contrast MT imaging in cerebral HIV infection and AIDS. Potential uses include differentiating lymphoma and toxoplasmosis in AIDS if only one enhancing lesion is visible on conventional sequences, predicting reactivation of treated toxoplasma abscesses, which show persistent but subtle enhancement and evaluating PML lesions in which the presence of contrast enhancement appears to have prognostic significance. This area has yet to be exploited.

17.6 Perfusion Weighted Imaging in AIDS

Perfusion-weighted imaging (pMRI) allows regional blood perfusion in tissues to be measured; this is achieved using either analysis of T2* weighted signal intensity to monitor the passage of paramagnetic contrast agent through the brain or using arterial spin-labelling techniques. Whilst the latter is entirely non-invasive and in theory allows more rigorous quantification of absolute blood flow, discussion will be limited to the former technique which is far more rapid to perform and analyse, and is currently more commonly used in a clinical environment. Echo planar imaging (EPI) techniques are used to allow rapid sequential image acquisition after the rapid bolus injection of a paramagnetic contrast agent into a peripheral vein. As the contrast medium travels through the vessels, it causes a localized loss in signal in the adjacent water protons due to susceptibility effects. The signal change with time in an area of interest is monitored, which allows derivation of perfusion parameters rCBV (regional cerebral blood volume) and rCBF (regional cerebral blood flow) from which perfusion can be calculated.

To date, there has been little published in the literature about perfusion MR imaging in HIV infection. An early study by LAISSY et al. (1994), using contrast-enhanced fast MRI (T1-weighted GE FLASH sequence), found that there was a significant difference in the enhancement of lymphoma and toxoplasmosis on both the spin-echo and FLASH sequences, with lymphoma exhibiting greater and earlier enhancement (LAISSY et al. 1994).

More recently ERNST et al. (1998) focussed on the differentiation of lymphoma and toxoplasma abscesses using perfusion-weighted imaging. They evaluated six patients with active lymphoma and five patients with toxoplasmosis using a combination of conventional MR imaging sequences and perfusion MR using a single-shot gradient echo-planar sequence with paramagnetic contrast agent. Regional cerebral blood volume (rCBV) maps were reconstructed and regions of interest included both the necrotic and enhancing portions of the masses, and these were compared to the corresponding contralateral area. They found that active portions of lymphoma consistently showed markedly elevated rCBV, with an average maximum rCBV of 258%±99%, compared with normal brain, though the average rCBV was only mildly elevated by 135%±48%, this latter value encompassing the areas of necrosis with reduced perfusion. The toxoplasmosis lesions had reduced perfusion in all areas, including the enhancing rims and surrounding vasogenic oedema, but particularly in the necrotic centres (Figs. 17.7, 17.8). Overall there was a statistically significant difference in the average and maximum rCBV values between the two groups expressed as a percentage of the values for the normal-appearing contralateral brain, and the maximum rCBV values were the most discriminatory. The reason behind the reduced perfusion in toxoplasmosis abscesses and in areas of necrosis in lymphomas is the relative lack of vasculature in these areas and the vasoconstriction caused by mass effect from vasogenic oedema; the active regions of lymphoma showed elevated perfusion due to the neovascularization. Perfusion weighted imaging was also useful in differentiating between recurrent lymphoma (which had previously been successfully treated) and an enhancing area of radiation necrosis (ERNST et al. 1998).

Although radioisotope PET and SPECT studies have also proven to be useful in differentiating lymphoma from toxoplasmosis, as the former lesion is hypermetabolic, perfusion MR imaging has several advantages over these nuclear medicine techniques; it allows better spatial and time resolution, is rapid and easy to perform at the same time as the structural MRI examination, does not require the use of additional contrast agent, and hence offers potential cost and time benefits. Further studies with larger numbers of patients are required, as well as longitudinal studies, to evaluate the full potential of perfusion MR imaging in differentiating between these two disease processes, but preliminary results appear promising.

Perfusion MRI has also recently been used in the evaluation of patients with early stage HIV-cognitive motor complex disorder/ADC to determine whether abnormalities of rCBF occur. When the results obtained in 19 affected patients were compared with those of 15 healthy seronegative controls, there was a statistically significant decrease bilaterally in the rCBF in the lateral frontal cortices and inferior medial parietal regions in seropositive patients compared with controls and a statistically significantly increase in the posterior inferior parietal white matter. The changes in the rCBF also correlated with several parameters of disease in the HIV patients; the CD4 and lymphocyte count correlated with rCBF in the temporo-parietal regions; the regional rCBF correlated inversely with viral load, positively with the Karnofsky score and inversely with the HIV dementia scale (CHANG et al. 2000).

The findings of regional variation in rCBF are in agreement with results from several nuclear medicine studies using SPECT and PET. SPECT studies

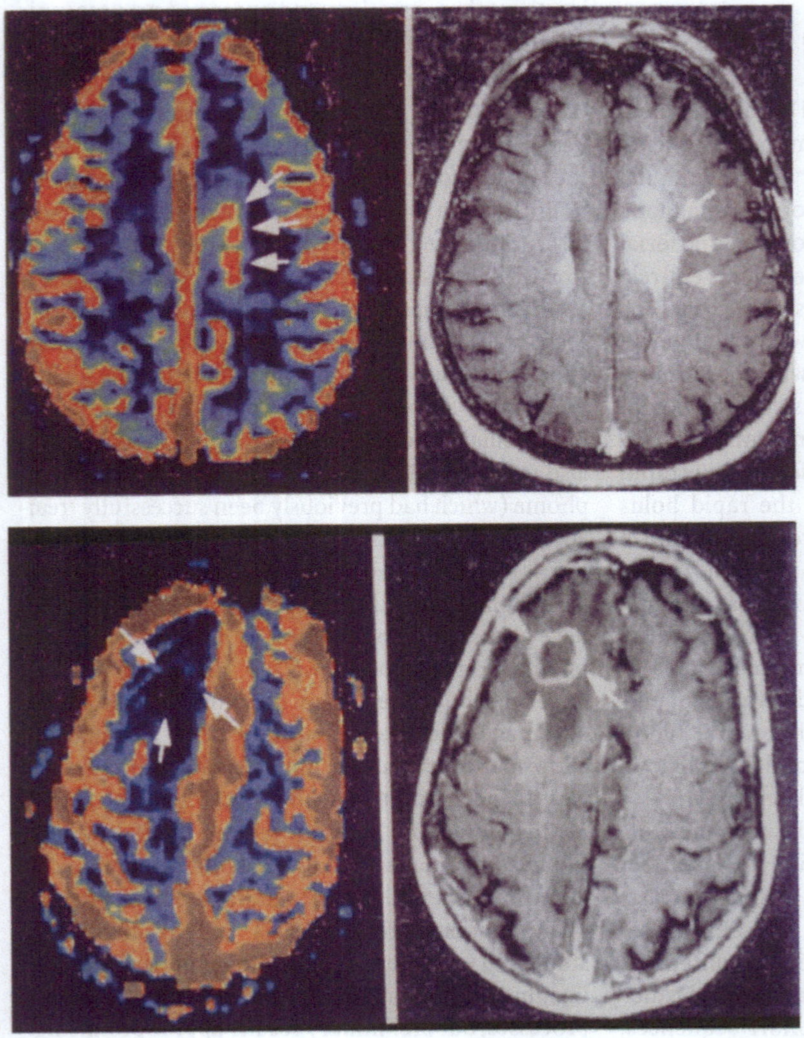

a

b

Fig. 17.7a,b. rCBV maps from perfusion MRI (2,500/30) *on the left* and gadolinium enhanced T1-weighted image (500/11) *on the right* showing a lymphoma lesion in the left centrum semiovale in **a** and a right frontal toxoplasma abscess in **b**, indicated by the *arrows*. The lymphoma lesion shows areas of greatly increased rCBV (*arrows*), and in the example shown was 270% of that of the contralateral brain region. In contrast to image **a** the rCBV in the toxoplasma abscess in consistently reduced in the central regions as well as in the enhancing rim and in the surrounding perilesional oedema (*arrows*). In this example the maximum rCBV was 94% of that in the contralateral region. (From: Ernst TM, Chang L, Witt M, Aronow HA, Walot I, Goldberg MA. Cerebral toxoplasmosis and lymphoma in AIDS: perfusion MR imaging experience in 13 patients. Radiology 1998; 208: 663–669. With permission)

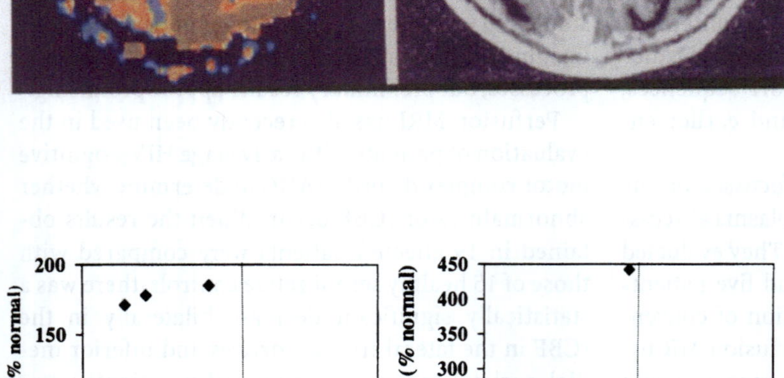

a b

Fig. 17.8a,b. Plots showing the average (**a**) and maximum (**b**) rCBV values for active toxoplasmosis (GG) and lymphoma (uu) lesions relative to the average rCBV values of the corresponding normal appearing contralateral regions. The difference between the toxoplasmosis and lymphoma lesions was statistically significant for both variables ($P<0.005$).The maximum rCBV shows greater separation between the two lesion types. (From: Ernst TM, Chang L, Witt M, Aronow HA, Walot I, Goldberg MA. Cerebral toxoplasmosis and lymphoma in AIDS: perfusion MR imaging experience in 13 patients. Radiology 1998; 208: 663–669. With permission) have shown multifocal perfusion defects in the cortex. Widespread decreased perfusion was also seen in the frontal cortex and to a lesser extent in the temporal and parietal cortex but also in the deep grey matter; many of these studies used qualitative visual analysis without quantitative evaluation (HOLMAN et al. 1992; HARRIS et al. 1994; ROSCI et al. 1996; COSTA et al. 1988). Some PET studies using ^{18}F-fluorodeoxyglucose have shown hypermetabolism in the basal ganglia and thalami in patients with early HIV dementia (ROTTENBERG et al. 1996; HINKIN et al. 1995), though in the later stages there was evidence of subcortical as well as cortical hypometabolism (ROTTENBERG et al. 1987).

The regions of the brain which had a reduction in rCBF (lateral frontal and medial parietal) in Chang's study (CHANG et al. 2000) showed positive correlation with viral load. It is postulated that the brain damage that occurs in HIV infection is not only caused directly by the HIV viral proteins (gp120 and Tat), but that secondary mediators such as cytokines, chemokines, free radicals and excitatory amino acids are also involved. If the increase in rCBF in the posterior lateral parietal white matter represents a true or absolute increase, this could be a reflection of the inflammatory component that is seen histologically in patients with HIV dementia. Quantitative pMRI may thus prove to be a useful additional imaging technique in monitoring disease severity in patients with HIV dementia and evaluating the effects of existing and new antiretroviral therapies.

17.7 Cerebrovascular Disease

Cerebral infarction is seen quite frequently in the paediatric HIV population, and is a recognized but somewhat forgotten neurological complication of CNS HIV infection in adults. Discussion here will be limited to disease in adults. The aetiology is multifactorial and infection with agents such as varicella zoster, CMV, tuberculosis and syphilis is an important contributory factor. Intravenous drug abuse and ingestion of other illicit drugs also plays an important role and may result in bacterial endocarditis, increased platelet aggregation and emboli as well as vasculitis. In adults, the quoted frequency of diagnosed infarcts of 0.5–7% (LEVY et al. 1985; ENGSTROM et al. 1989) was much lower than detected in autopsy series with infarcts seen in up to 34% of cases (MIZUSAWA et al. 1988; KIEBURTZ et al. 1993), suggesting that in this patient population many infarcts are clinically silent.

However, a recent study by GILLAMS et al. (1997) reviewing the frequency, aetiology and distribution of infarcts on MRI in a cohort of 71 HIV infected patients found a much higher frequency of infarcts with 22 infarcts occurring in 13/71 (18%) patients, six of whom had multiple infarcts. The two most common distributions for these ischaemic lesions were the lenticulostriate (15/22) and the vertebrobasilar (5/22) territories, with involvement of the middle cerebral artery (MCA) territory in the remaining two. Six of the patients were intravenous drug or cocaine users; concurrent opportunistic infection was seen in five patients, although this was found to be a causative factor at autopsy in only one patient. MRA, performed in eight patients, showed findings consistent with a vasculitis in two, complete or partial occlusion of the MCA in two, and in the remaining four was normal. In the two with vasculitis no other aetiological factor, apart from HIV-1 infection, was identified (GILLAMS et al. 1997).

There have been several reports of cerebral vasculitis occurring in association with HIV infection (BERGER et al. 1990; CALABRESE 1991; GHERARDI et al. 1993). It has been postulated that the HIV-1 virus itself can cause cerebral vasculitis and this may be an important contributor to ischaemic events in this patient group. Recent evidence in support of this hypothesis comes from measurements of cerebrovascular reserve capacity (CRC) in a cohort of 31 asymptomatic HIV-1 seropositive subjects, using transcranial Doppler ultrasound (BRILLA et al. 1999). The mean blood flow velocity (BFV) in the MCA and its increase (CRC) after systemic administration of the vasodilator, acetazolamide, was significantly reduced in HIV-positive patients compared with that in ten age-matched normal controls. Importantly, none of the patients had any evidence of a CNS opportunistic infection and, in 25 patients, the cranial CT or MR studies were normal (two patients had a few scattered white matter lesions, one an incidental haemangioma and another mild cerebral atrophy). The authors postulated that these observations are likely to reflect alterations of cerebral resistance at an arteriolar level, but the causative mechanisms remain uncertain. There was no correlation between the BFV and CRC and the duration of seropositivity or degree of haematological immunosuppression.

This is an area in which further study is clearly justified, and pMRI is in many ways ideal for studying regional perfusion and reserve and, in concert with diffusion imaging, for investigating acute cerebral events. However, despite the recent enthusiasm for the use of these techniques in studying cerebrovascular disease and informing acute management in the general population at the time of writing, they have yet to applied to cerebrovascular disease in the HIV-infected population.

17.8 Diffusion Weighted Imaging in AIDS

Diffusion weighted imaging (DWI) yields information on the microscopic random Brownian motion of water molecules in tissue; the average distance travelled by a molecule in a given time may be represented quantitatively by the diffusion coefficient (*D*). Calculation of *D* for each pixel of an MR image can be used to generate a map of the apparent diffusion coefficients (ADC map). Diffusion weighted images are usually represented by ADC maps (where free diffusion is depicted as high signal) or by qualitative diffusion weighted images (in which restricted diffusion shows as high signal). As DWI is highly motion sensitive, the MR images are again acquired rapidly using single-shot echoplanar imaging (EPI).

In normal brain the diffusion of free water is most restricted in white matter (it is anisotropic in this tissue, being greatest along the axis of the white matter tracts) and is least restricted in CSF. Thus DWI provides unique information about the diffusional properties of water in various pathological conditions; it allows vasogenic oedema, where extracellular volume and hence ADC is increased, to be distinguished from cytotoxic oedema, where swelling of the cells restricts interstitial space, and hence reduces ADC. It has already been applied with success in the imaging of tumours (Sugahara et al. 1999), demyelinating disorders (Werring et al. 1999), but most commonly in demonstrating signal changes corresponding to infarcts and ischaemic lesions before they are apparent on conventional T1- or T2-weighted images (Gonzales et al. 1999; Yamada et al. 1999; Sunshine et al. 1999).

However, there has been very little published in the literature to date of DWI in imaging intracranial disease in AIDS, with only a few preliminary reports of DWI in a toxoplasmosis ring-enhancing abscess and lesions of PML (Chang and Ernst 1997). In the toxoplasma abscess which had considerable surrounding vasogenic oedema, the ADC was much higher (350%) in the area of oedema than in normal contralateral white matter, whereas that in the lesion taken as a whole was higher (105%) than normal brain, but lower than in the oedema. The increased extracellular water content in the area of vasogenic oedema allows increased mobility of the water molecules and this explains the higher ADC (Fig. 17.9); similar observations have been made in studies of DWI in tumours (Brunberg et al. 1995; Tien et al. 1994). The relatively lower ADC in the centre of the abscess cavity can be explained by the viscous nature

a,b

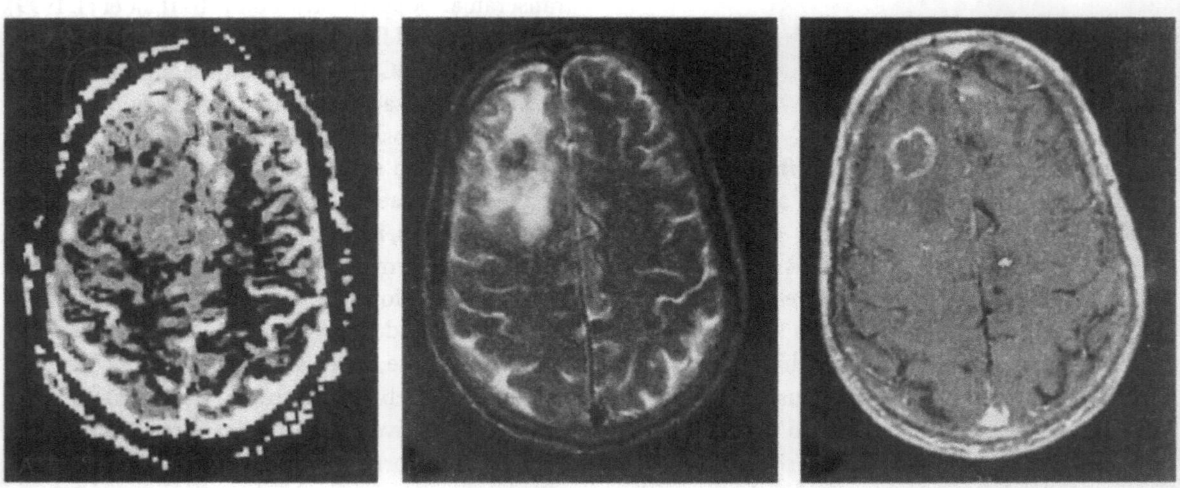

c

Fig. 17.9a–c. An apparent diffusion coefficient (ADC) map from DWI in a patient with a histologically proven toxoplasmosis lesion (**a**) in the right frontal lobe. Note the slightly decreased but heterogeneous ADC pattern in the lesion, and the relatively increased ADC in the surrounding oedema. The corresponding T2-weighted (**b**) and T1-postcontrast (**c**) images are shown. Note the heterogeneous signal within the lesion in image (**b**) and the hyperintense surrounding oedema corresponding to the region of increased ADC on DWI. (From: Chang L, Ernst T. MR spectroscopy and diffusion-weighted MR imaging in focal brain lesions in AIDS. Neuroimaging Clinics of North America 1997; 7 (3): 409–426. With permission) of the necrotic inflammatory contents, although there is still more free motion of water molecules here than in normal brain (CHANG and ERNST 1997).

ADC values in PML lesions are higher than those of normal white matter as there is greater free movement of water in these areas of demyelination and increased water content, and it seems likely that the ADC values increase with lesion progression as the degree of demyelination increases (Fig. 17.10); this has potential implications for longitudinal measurements but these preliminary observations need to be first confirmed with further larger studies (CHANG and ERNST 1997).

A recent study comparing the diffusion characteristics of brain abscesses and cystic brain tumours (gliomas) in the non-HIV population showed that the central contents of brain abscesses were hyperintense and those of cystic or necrotic tumours were hypointense to normal brain on diffusion maps (KIM et al. 1998), with corresponding higher or lower mean signal intensity ratios of 4.4±1.8 and 0.4±0.1 respectively.

The findings are consistent with the different physical properties of the cavity contents, with increased diffusion properties of cystic/necrotic tumours and decreased diffusion properties of abscess cavities containing viscous pus and a prominent inflammatory cellular component. Although ADC values were not calculated in this study, the findings were confirmed in a later study by DESPRECHINS et al. (1999) in which ADC values were calculated. These small series illustrate the potential role of DWI in differentiating between infective and neoplastic aetiologies with necrotic/cystic elements. Further research is required to determine the extent of variation of diffusion parameters in each of these pathologies before this can be extrapolated to toxoplasmosis and lymphoma in AIDS.

17.9 Conclusion

Recent advances in MR imaging techniques have been applied in the neuroradiological investigation of patients with HIV infection and AIDS but the clinical application of these techniques is still in its

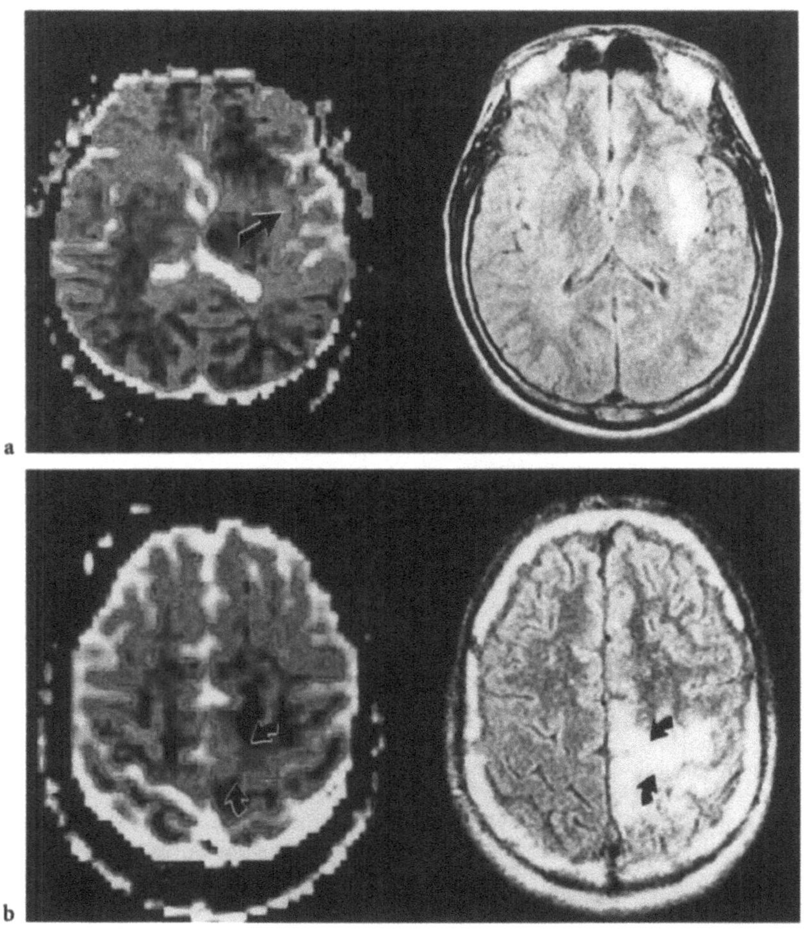

Fig. 17.10a,b. ADC maps (*left*) and FLAIR images (*right*) from a patient with a positive polymerase chain reaction for JCV and characteristic MR spectroscopy for PML. The ADC map in **a** shows slightly increased diffusion coefficients of +28% (*arrow*) in the region of the left external capsule region corresponding to the lesion seen on the FLAIR image. In image **b** the ADC map from another PML lesion (with the corresponding FLAIR image) shows variable (*arrows*) but increased diffusion coefficients (+63%) due to diffusion anisotropy due to differing fibre orientations. (From: Chang L, Ernst T. MR spectroscopy and diffusion-weighted MR imaging in focal brain lesions in AIDS. Neuroimaging Clinics of North America 1997; 7 (3): 409–426. With permission)

infancy. They yield information about neurochemistry (MRS), blood perfusion (PWI) and the behaviour of tissue water (DWI and MTI) which reflect pathophysiological changes on a cellular and subcellular level which are complementary to the relatively crude functional information from conventional structural MRI.

Although the main diagnostic problem in AIDS remains the differentiation of cerebral lymphoma from toxoplasmosis, MRS in combination with conventional MR imaging seems to increase diagnostic confidence and, importantly, may obviate the need for biopsy. It also seems likely that MR perfusion imaging may make a positive contribution to solving this diagnostic dilemma.

Many studies have demonstrated spectroscopic metabolite changes that occur in different stages of the AIDS-dementia complex and have shown that early changes are detectable in asymptomatic patients and those with normal imaging. This has important implications with regards to timing the introduction of anti-retroviral drug regimens and therapeutic monitoring of new treatments. The further development of proton CSI will circumvent many of the problems of sampling inherent in single voxel techniques and allow regional metabolite abnormalities to be evaluated.

MTI seems to have a high sensitivity in differentiating early PML lesions from the white matter lesions of HIVE, an important distinction to make because of the differing prognosis in these two disease processes. MTI in combination with MRS may have a useful role to play in longitudinal studies of patients with PML, as new drug therapies are introduced.

References

Anders KH, Guerra WF, Tomiyasu U et al. (1986) The neuropathology of AIDS: UCLA experience and review. Am J Pathol 124: 537–557

Andreula CF, Burdi N, Carella A (1993) CNS cryptococcosis in AIDS: spectrum of MR findings. J Comput Assist Tomogr 17: 731–734

Antinori A, Ammassari A, DeLuca A et al. (1997) Diagnosis of AIDS-related focal brain lesions. A decision making analysis based on clinical and neuroradiologic characteristics combined with polymerase chain reaction assays in CSF. Neurology 48: 687–694

Astrom KE, Mancall EL, Richardson EP (1958) Progressive multifocal leukoencephalopathy: hitherto unrecognised complication of chronic lymphatic leukemia and Hodgkin's disease. Brain 81: 93–111

Aylward EH, Henderer JD, McArthur JC et al. (1993) Reduced basal ganglia volume in HIV-1 associated dementia: results from quantitative neuroimaging. Neurology 43: 2099–2104

Bantz S, Iglesias-Rozas JR, Jautzke G, Adler T (1989) Cerebral lymphomas in AIDS. Clin Neuropathol 8: 219

Barker PB, Lee RR, McArthur JC (1995) AIDS dementia complex: evaluation with proton MR spectroscopic imaging. Radiology 195: 58–64

Bashir R, Luka J, Cheloha K, Chamberlain M, Hochberg F (1993) Expression of Epstein-barr virus proteins in primary CNS lymphoma in AIDS patients. Neurology 43: 2358–2362

Berger JR, Mucke L (1988) Prolonged survival and partial recovery in AIDS-associated progressive multifocal leukoencephalopathy. Neurology 38: 1060–1065

Berger JR, Harris JO, Gregorios J, Norenberg M (1990) Cerebrovascular disease in AIDS: a case control study. AIDS 4: 239–244

Berkefeld J, Enzenberger W, Lanfermann H (1999) Cryptococcus meningoencephalitis in AIDS: parenchymal and meningeal forms. Neuroradiology 41: 129–133

Brilla R, Nabavi DG, Schulte-Altedorneburg G et al. (1999) Cerebral vasculopathy in HIV infection revealed by transcranial doppler. Stroke 30: 811–813

Brunberg J, Chenevert T, McKeever P et al. (1995) In vivo MR determination of water diffusion co-efficients and diffusion anisotropy: correlation with structural alterations in gliomas of the cerebral hemisphere. AJNR 16: 361

Calabrese LH (1991) Vasculitis and infection with the human immunodeficiency virus. Rheum Dis Clin North Am 17: 131–147

Campi A, Filippi M, Gerevini S et al. (1996) Multiple white matter lesions of the brain: magnetization transfer ratios in systemic lupus erythematosus and multiple sclerosis. Int J Neuroradiol 2: 134

Chang L, Cornford ME, Chiang FL, Ernst TM, Sun NCJ, Miller BL (1995a) Radiologic- pathologic correlation. Cerebral Toxoplasmosis and lymphoma in AIDS. AJNR 16: 1653–1663

Chang L, Miller B, McBride D et al. (1995b) Brain lesions in patients with AIDS: H-1 MR spectroscopy. Radiology 197: 525–531

Chang L, Ernst T, Tornatore C et al. (1997) Metabolite abnormalities in progressive multifocal leukoencephalopathy by proton magnetic resonance spectroscopy. Neurology 48: 836–845

Chang L, Ernst T (1997) MR spectroscopy and diffusion-weighted MR imaging in focal brain lesions in AIDS. Neuroimaging Clin North Am 7: 409–426

Chang L, Ernst T, Leonido-Yee M, Walot I, Singer E (1999a) Cerebral metabolites correlate with clinical severity of HIV-cognitive motor complex. Neurology 52: 651–657

Chang L, Ernst T, Leonido-Yee M et al. (1999b) Highly active antiretroviral therapy reverses brain metabolite abnormalities in mild HIV dementia. Neurology 53: 782–789

Chang L, Ernst T, Leonido-Yee M, Speck O (2000) Perfusion MRI detects rCBF abnormalities in early stages of HIV-cognitive motor complex. Neurology 54: 389–396

Chinn R, Wilkinson ID, Hall-Craggs MA et al. (1995) Toxoplasmosis and primary central nervous system lymphoma in HIV infection: diagnosis with MR spectroscopy. Radiology 197: 649–654

Chong WK, Sweeney B, Wilkinson ID et al. (1993) Proton spectroscopy of the brain in HIV infection: correlation with clinical, immunologic, and MR imaging findings. Neuroradiology 188: 119–124

Chuck SL, Sande MA (1989) Infections with Cryptococcus neoformans in acquired immunodeficiency syndrome. New Engl J Med 321: 794–799

Cordoliani YS, Derosier C, Pharaboz C, Jeanbourquin D, Schill H, Cosnard G (1992) Primary cerebral lymphoma in patients with AIDS: MR findings in 17 cases. Am J Roentgenol 159: 841–847

Cinque P, Vago L, Terreni MR et al. (1995) Diagnosis of cytomegalovirus infection of the nervous system in AIDS by polymerase chain reaction analysis of cerebrospinal fluid. Scand J Infect Dis Suppl 99: 92–94

Cornford ME, Holden JK, Boyd MC, Berry K, Vinters HV (1992) Neuropathology of acquired immunodeficiency syndrome (AIDS): report of 39 autopsies from Vancouver, British Columbia. Can J Neurosci 19: 442–452

Costa DC, Ell PJ, Burns A, Philpot M, Levy R (1988) CBF tomograms with 99mTc-HMPAO in patients with dementia (Alzheimers type and HIV) and Parkinson's disease: initial results. J Cereb Blood Flow Metab 8: S109-S115

Cristina N, Pelloux H, Goulhot C, Brion JP, Leclercq P, Ambroise-Thomas P (1993) Detection of Toxoplasma gondii in AIDS patients by the polymerase chain reaction. Infection 21: 150–153

Derouin F, Thulliez Ph, Garin YJF (1991) Toxoplasma serology in HIV-infected patients values and limitations. Pathol Biol 39: 255–259

Desprechins B, Stadnik T, Koerts G, Shabana W, Breucq C, Osteaux M (1999) Use of diffusion-weighted MR imaging in differential diagnosis between intracerebral necrotic tumours and cerebral abscesses. AJNR 20: 1252–1257

Dina TS (1991) Primary central nervous system lymphoma versus toxoplasmosis in AIDS. Radiology 179: 823–828

Donovan Post MJ, Yiannoutsos C, Simpson D et al. (1999) Progressive multifocal leukoencephalopathy in AIDS: are there any MR findings useful to patient management and predictive of patient survival? AJNR 20: 1896–1906

Dousset V, Grossman R, Ramer K et al. (1992) Experimental allergic encephalomyelitis and multiple sclerosis: lesion characterization with magnetization transfer imaging. Radiology 182: 483–495

Dousset V, Armand J-P, Lacoste D et al. (1997) Magnetization transfer study of HIV encephalitis and progressive multifocal leukoencephalopathy. AJNR 18: 895–901

Engstrom JW, Lowenstein DH, Bredesden DE (1989) Cerebral infarctions and transient neurological deficits associated with acquired immunodeficiency syndrome. Am J Med 86: 528–532.

Ernst TM, Chang L, Witt M, Aronow HA, Walot I, Goldberg MA (1998) Cerebral toxoplasmosis and lymphoma in AIDS: perfusion MR imaging experience in 13 patients. Radiology 208: 663–669

Ernst T, Chang L, Witt M et al. (1999) Progressive multifocal leukoencephalopathy and human immunodeficiency virus-associated white matter lesions in AIDS: magnetization transfer MR imaging. Radiology 210: 539–543

Everall IP, Luthbert PJ, Lantos PL (1991) Neuronal loss in the frontal cortex in HIV infection. Lancet 337: 1119–1121

Everall IP, Luthbert PJ, Lantos PL (1993) Neuronal number and volume alterations in the neocortex of HIV-infected individuals. J Neurol Neurosurg Psychiatry 56; 481–486

Finelli DA, Hurst GC, Gullapalli RP (1998) T1-weighted three-dimensional magnetization transfer MR of the brain: improved lesion contrast enhancement. AJNR 19: 59–64

Gass A, Barker GJ, Kidd D et al. (1994) Correlation of magnetization transfer ratio with clinical disability in multiple sclerosis. Ann Neurol 36: 62

Gherardi R, Belec L, Mhiri C et al. (1993) The spectrum of vasculitis in human immunodeficiency virus-infected patients. Arthritis Rheum 36: 1164–1173

Gillams AR, Allen E, Hrieb K, Venna N, Craven D, Carter AP (1997) Cerebral infarction in patients with AIDS. AJNR 18: 1581–1585

Gonzalez RG, Schaefer PW, Buonanno FS et al. (1999) Diffusion-weighted MR imaging : diagnostic accuracy in patients imaged within 6 hours of stroke symptom onset. Radiology 210: 155–162

Gossman RI (1994) Magnetization transfer in multiple sclerosis. Ann Neurol 36: S97-S99

Harris GJ, Pearlson GD, McArthur JC, Zefer S, LaFrance LD (1994) Altered cortical blood flow in HIV-seropositive individuals with and without dementia: a single photon emission computed tomography study. AIDS 8: 495–499

Harrison MJG, Newman SP, Hall-Craggs MA et al. (1998) Evidence of CNS impairment in HIV infection: clinical, neurophysiological, EEG, and MRI/ MRS study. J Neurol Neurosurg Psychiatry 65: 301–307

Heier LA, Bauer CJ, Schwartz L et al. (1989) Large Virchow-Robin spaces: MR-clinical correlation. AJNR 10: 929–936

Hinkin C, vanGorp W, Mandelkern M et al. (1995) Cerebral metabolic change in patients with AIDS: report of a six-month follow-up using positron- emission tomography. J Neuropsychiatr Clin Neurosci 7: 180–187

Holland NR, Power C, Mathews VP, Glass JD, Forman M, McArthur JC (1994) Cytomegalovirus encephalitis in acquired immunodeficiency syndrome (AIDS). Neurology 44: 507–514

Holman BL, Garada B, Johnson KA et al. (1992) A comparison of brain perfusion SPECT in cocaine abuse and AIDS dementia complex. J Nucl Med 33: 1312–1315

Iglesias-Rozas JR, Bantz B, Adler T et al. (1991) Cerebral lymphoma in AIDS; clinical radiological, neuropathological and immunopathological study. Clin Neuropathol 10: 65–72

Iranzo A, Moreno A, Pujol J et al. (1999) Proton magnetic resonance spectroscopy pattern of progressive multifocal leukoencepahlopathy in AIDS. JNNP 66: 520–523

Jarvick JG, Lenkinski RE, Grossman RI, Frank I, Ramer KN (1993) Proton MR spectroscopy in HIV infected patients; characterization of abnormalities with imaging and clinical correlation. Radiology 186: 739–744

Kim YJ, Chang K-H, Song IC (1998) Brain abscess and necrotic or cystic brain tumor: discrimination with signal intensity on diffusion-weighted MR imaging. AJR 171: 1487–1490

Kure IC, Llena JF, Lyman WD et al. (1991) Human immunodeficiency virus-1 infection of the nervous system; an autopsy study of 268 adult, paediatric and fetal brains. Hum Pathol 22: 700–710

Kurki T, Lundbom N, Komu M et al. (1996) Tissue characterisation of intracranial tumours by magnetization transfer and spin-lattice relaxation parameters in vivo. J Magn Reson Imaging 6: 573

Laissy J-P, Soyer P, Tebboune J et al. (1994) Contrast-enhanced fast MRI in differentiating brain toxoplasmosis and lymphoma in AIDS patients. J Comput Assist Tomogr 18: 714–718

Laubenberger J, Haussinger D, Bayer S et al. (1996) HIV-related metabolic abnormalities in the brain: depiction with proton MR spectroscopy with short echo times. Radiology 199: 805–810

Levy JA, Shinabukuro J, Hollander H et al. (1985) Isolation of AIDS. related retroviruses from the cerebrospinal fluid and brain of patients with neurologic symptoms. Lancet 2: 586–588

Levy RM, Bredesden DE, Rosenblum ML (1985) Neurological manifestations of acquired immunodeficiency syndrome (AIDS): experience at UCSF and review of the literature. J Neurosurg 62: 475–495

Levy RM, Mills CM, Posin JP, Moore SG, Rosenblum ML, Bredesen DE (1990) The efficacy and clinical impact of brain imaging in neurologically symptomatic AIDS patients: a prospective CT/MRI study. J Acquir Immune Def Syndr 3: 461–471

Levy RM, Russel E, Yungbluth M, Frais-Hidvegi D, Brody BA, Dal Canto MC (1992) The efficacy of image-guided stereotactic brain biopsy in neurologically symptomatic acquired immunodeficiency syndrome. Neurosurgery 30: 186–190

Lieburtz KD, Eskin TA, Ketonen L, Tuite MJ (1993) Opportunistic cerebral vasculopathy and stroke in patients with AIDS. Arch Neurol 50: 430–432

Lin AP, Moreno A, Norfray JF, Ross BD (1999) No impact of Gd-DTPA on quantitative MRS (QMRS) of human brain tumors. Radiology 213(P): 355

McArthur JC, Nance-Sproson T, Childs E et al. (1998) Virologic response in cerebrospinal fluid after initiation of antiretroviral therapy. J Neurovirol 4: 359

Miller RF, Lucas SB, Hall-Craggs MA et al. (1996) A comparison of MR imaging and CSF analysis with neuropathological findings in the diagnosis of HIV and CMV associated CNS disease in AIDS. J Neurovirol 2: 44

Miszkiel KA, Hall-Craggs MA, Miller RF et al. (1996) The spectrum of MRI findings in CNS cryptococcosis in AIDS. Clin Radiol 51: 842–850

Mizusawa H, Hirano A, Llena JF, Shintaku M (1988) Cerebrovascular lesions of AIDS. Acta Neuropathol (Berl) 76: 451–457

Moller HE, Vermathen P, Lentschig MG (1999) Metabolic characterization of AIDS dementia complex by spectroscopic imaging. J Magn Reson Imaging 9: 10–18

Morgello S, Petito CK, Mouradian JA (1990) Central nervous lymphoma in the acquired immune deficiency syndrome. Clin Neuropathol 9: 205–215

Paley MNJ, Chong WK, Wilkinson ID et al. (1994) Cerebrospinal fluid-intracranial volume ratio measurements in patients with HIV infection: CLASS image analysis technique. Radiology 190: 879–886

Paley M, Wilkinson ID, Hall-Craggs MA, Chong WK, Chinn RSJ, Harrison MJG (1995) Short echo time proton spectroscopy in the brain in HIV infection/AIDS. Magn Reson Imaging 13: 871–875.

Pallella FJ Jr, Delaney KM, Moorman AC et al. (1998) Declining morbidity and mortality among patients with advanced human immunodeficiency virus infection. HIV outpatient study investigators. N Engl J Med 338: 853–860

Peretti-Viton P, Taieb D, Viton JM et al. (1998) Contrast-enhanced magnetisation transfer MRI in metastatic lesions of the brain. Neuroradiology 40: 783–878

Porter SB, Sande MA (1992) Toxoplasmosis of the central nervous system in the acquired immunodeficiency syndrome. N Engl J Med 7: 1643–1648

Rai GS, McConnell JR, Waldman AD, Chaudry M, Grant D (1999) Automated proton MR spectroscopy in Alzheimer's disease. Lancet 353: 1063–1064

Ramsey RG, Dean AD (1997) Central nervous system toxoplasmosis. Neuroimaging Clin North Am 7: 171–186

Resnick L, diMarzo-Veronese F et al. (1985) Intrablood-brain barrier synthesis of HTLV-III IgG in patients with neurologic symptoms associated with AIDS or AIDS related complex. N Engl J Med 313: 1498–1504

Rosci MA, Pignorini F, Bernabei A et al. (1996) Methods for detection of early signs of AIDS dementia complex in asymptomatic subjects: a quantitative tomography study in 18 cases. AIDS 6: 1309–1316

Rottenberg DA, Moeller JR, Strother SC et al. (1987) The metabolite pathology of the AIDS dementia complex. Ann Neurol 22: 700–706

Rottenberg DA, Sidtis JJ, Strother SC et al. (1996) Abnormal cerebral glucose metabolism in HIV-1 seropositive subjects with and without dementia. J Nucl Med 37: 1133–1141

Ruiz A, Donovan Post JM, Bundschu C, Ganz WI, Georgiou M (1997) Primary central nervous system lymphoma in patients with AIDS. Neuroimaging Clin North Am 7: 281–296

Sacktor N, Lyes R, McFarlane G et al. (1999) HIV-1 related neurological disease incidence changes in the era of highly active antiretroviral therapy. Neurology 52: A252-A253

Segebarth CM, Baleriaux DF, Luyton PR, denHollander JA (1990) Detection of metabolic heterogeneity of human intracranial tumours in vivo by ^{1}H NMR spectroscopic imaging. Magn Res Med 13: 62–76

Simone IL, Frederico F, Tortorella C et al. (1998) Localised 1-H spectroscopy for metabolic characterisation of diffuse and focal brain lesions in patients infected with HIV. JNNP 64: 516–523

Simpson D, Tagliati M (1994) Neurologic manifestations of HIV infection. Ann Intern Med 121: 769–785.

So YT, Beckstead JH, Davis RL (1986) Primary central nervous lymphoma in acquired immunodeficiency syndrome: clinical and pathologic study. Ann Neurol 20; 566–572

Sugahara T, Korogi Y, Kochi M et al. (1999) Usefulness of diffusion-weighted MRI with echo-planar technique in the evaluation of cellularity of gliomas. J Magn Reson Imaging 9: 53–60

Sunshine JL, Tarr RW, Lanzieri CF, Landis MD, Selman R, Lewin JS (1999) Hyperacute stroke: ultrafast MR imaging to triage patients prior to therapy. Radiology 212: 325–332

Thurnher MM, Thurnher SA, Muhlbauer B et al. (1997) Progressive multifocal leukoencephalopathy in AIDS: initial and follow-up CT and MRI. Neuroradiology 39: 611–618

Tien RD, Chu K, Hesselink JR et al. (1991) Intracranial cryptococcosis in immunocompromised patients: CT and MR findings in 29 cases. AJNR 12: 283–289

Tien RD, Felsberg GJ, Friedman H et al. (1994) MR imaging of high-grade cerebral gliomas: value of diffusion weighted echoplanar pulse sequences. Am J Roentgenol 162: 671

VonEinsiedel RW, Fife TD, Aksamit AJ et al. (1993) Progressive multifocal leukoencephalopathy in AIDS: a clinicopathologic study and review of the literature. J Neurol 240: 391–406

Weinberg A, Spiers D, Cai GY, Long CM, Sun R, Tevere V

(1998) Evaluation of a commercial PCR kit for diagnosis of cytomegalovirus infection of the central nervous system. J Clin Microbiol 36: 3382–3384
Wilkinson ID, Paley M, Chong WK et al. (1994) Proton spectroscopy in HIV infection: relaxation times of cerebral metabolites. Magn Reson Imaging 12: 951–957
Wilkinson ID, Miller RFD, Paley MNJ et al. (1996) Cerebral proton magnetic resonance spectroscopy in cytomegalovirus encephalitis and HIV leucoencephalopathy/encephalitis. AIDS 10: 1443–1444
Wilkinson ID, Miller RF, Miszkiel KA et al. (1997) Cerebral proton magnetic resonance spectroscopy in asymptomatic HIV infection. AIDS 11: 289–295
Yamada N, Imakita S, Sakuma T (1999) Value of diffusion-weighted imaging and apparent diffusion coefficient in recent cerebral infarctions: a correlative study with contrast T1-weighted imaging. AJNR 20: 193–198
Zuger A, Louie E, Holzman RS et al. (1986) Cryptococcal disease in patients with the acquired immunodeficiency syndrome. Ann Intern Med 104: 234–240

18 Imaging of Intracranial Abnormalities in Neurofibromatosis Types 1 and 2

WILLIAM MUKONOWESHURO, PAUL D. GRIFFITHS

CONTENTS

18.1 Introduction

The neurofibromatoses form the largest group of the neurocutaneous disorders. These are autosomal dominant gene disorders characterised by a propensity to dysplasia or neoplasia of the central and peripheral nervous system, skin and eyes. They were first recognised as a pathologic entity in the nineteenth century although case reports of patients with illnesses very much like neurofibromatosis existed in the literature from as early as the 13th century (MULVIHILL et al. 1988). Considerable confusion exists in the literature between the two main types of neurofibromatosis and a multitude of terms has been used to describe them. A National Institute of Health consensus development conference enumerated the clinical diagnostic criteria for each of the forms of neurofibromatosis (Tables 18.1, 18.2) and introduced the now widely accepted nomenclature neurofibromatosis 1 (NF1) and neurofibromatosis 2 (NF2) (NATIONAL INSTITUTE OF HEALTH CONSENSUS DEVELOPMENT CONFERENCE 1987). The recent identification of the NF1 gene and gene product *neu-*

W. MUKONOWESHURO
Specialist Registrar in Radiology, Radiology Department, Floor C, Royal Hallamshire Hospital, Glossop Road, Sheffield, South Yorkshire, S10 2JF, UK
P.D. GRIFFITHS, MD
Schering Professor of Radiology, Section of Academic Radiology, The University of Sheffield, Floor C, Royal Hallamshire Hospital, Glossop Road, Sheffield, South Yorkshire, S10 2JF, UK

Table 18.1. Diagnostic criteria for NF1 (NIH) (Adapted from NIH Conference Report 1988)

Two or more of the following define NF1:
1. Six or more café-au-lait macules over 5 mm in greatest diameter in prepubertal individuals and over 15 mm in postpubertal individuals
2. Two or more neurofibromas of any type or one plexiform neurofibroma
3. Freckling in the axillary or inguinal regions
4. Optic glioma
5. Two or more Lisch nodules (iris harmatomas)
6. A distinctive osseous lesion such as sphenoid dysplasia or thinning of long bone cortex with or without pseudoarthrosis
7. A first degree relative (parent, sibling or offspring) with NF-1 by the above criteria

Table 18.2. Modified diagnostic criteria for NF2 (NIH) (Adapted from Gutmann et al. 1997)

Definite (confirmed) NF2 is diagnosed by:
1. Bilateral vestibular schwannomas or
2. First degree relative with NF2 and
   a) Unilateral vestibular schwannoma aged <30 years or
   b) Any two of the following:
      Meningioma, glioma, schwannoma, neurofibroma, juvenile posterior subcapsular lenticular opacities/juvenile cortical cataract

Probable NF2 requiring further investigation is suggested by:
1. Unilateral vestibular schwannoma at age <30 years and at least one of: meningioma, glioma, schwannoma, juvenile posterior subcapsular lenticular opacities/juvenile corti cal cataract
2. Multiple meningiomas (two or more) plus: unilateral vestibular schwannoma, juvenile posterior subcapsular lenticular opacities/juvenile cortical cataract

rofibromin in 1990 and 1991 respectively and the NF2 gene and gene product *merlin* or *schwannomin* in 1993 (Martin et al. 1990; Rouleau et al. 1993; McCollin et al. 1993) have confirmed the separate nature of these disease processes and enabled accurate distinctions to be made between them (Gutmann et al. 1997). In this chapter we will review the pathological and neuroimaging findings of the two disorders.

18.2 Neurofibromatosis 1

18.2.1 Epidemiology and Genetics

NF1 accounts for approximately 90% of cases of neurofibromatosis. It affects 1 in 3000–4000 individuals and is inherited as an autosomal dominant condition with a high degree of penetrance though 30–50% of cases result from fresh mutations (Huson and Hughes 1994). There appears to be preferential mutation of the paternally derived chromosomes in cases of fresh mutations (Stephens et al. 1992). The NF1 gene has been localised to locus 17q 11.2 (Ledbetter et al. 1989). Its gene product *neurofibromin* has a central domain that bears sequence similarities with a family of proteins that regulate proto-oncogene p21-ras and therefore acts as a tumour suppressor agent. These proteins are also known as GTPase-activating proteins (GAP) because they stimulate the intrinsic GTPase activity of Ras. Inactivation of both NF1 GAP alleles has been shown in some malignancies and probably accounts for the development of most tumours in NF1 (Cappione et al. 1997; Guha et al. 1996; Sawada et al. 1996). A specific form of neurofibromin may be important in the development of the nervous system, which would account for the learning disabilities that occur in NF1 sufferers.

18.2.2 Clinical Features

The diagnosis of NF1 is usually made on clinical grounds using the NIH criteria (Table 18.1).

18.2.2.1 Cutaneous Manifestations

The cutaneous manifestations of NF1 disease are usually the most obvious clinically. Café au lait spots are hyperpigmented macules, which may be present at birth though they usually develop within the first 2 years of life. They tend to increase in size with age until adulthood when they become static or even regress. They are characteristic of NF1 if they are numerous (>6) and large. Skinfold freckling develops later and is typically seen in the axillary and inguinal regions as well as in the submammary folds in women. Dermal neurofibromas do not usually develop until preadolescence. They also increase in size and number with age and have been reported to progress with pregnancy in some patients. Dermal neurofibromas are always benign and are not associated with any symptoms other than the cosmetic deformity although some patients experience pruritis and some subcutaneous fibromas are associated with paraesthesia (Gutmann et al. 1997; Huson et al. 1988).

Plexiform neurofibromas (PNF) are almost always congenital lesions. They are most commonly large diffuse tumours associated with hypertrophy of adjacent soft tissues although a localised nodular variety occurs. They tend to grow along nerve fascicles and have a 5% lifetime risk of malignant transformation (Gutmann 1998; Huson 1988). PNF do not metastasise but have a tendency for centripetal growth along the nerve of origin and may cause compression of brain and spinal cord occasionally with fatal consequences. Head and neck PNF are relatively common and most frequently involve the V1 portion of the trigeminal nerve (Fig. 18.1).

Orbital PNF may be associated with buphthalmos (approximately 50%), osseous dysplasia (thought to be due to mesodermal dysplasia) and central nervous system dysplasias including dural ectasia and aqueduct stenosis (Braffmann et al. 1990).

Sphenoid dysplasia is often associated with plexiform neurofibroma although it may occur in the absence of a mass lesion (Fig. 18.1). It occurs in 1–7% of NF1 patients although some series report an incidence as high as 18.4% (Cnossen et al. 1998; Harkens and Dolan 1990; McFarlane et al. 1995). Patients usually present with pulsating exophthalmos and facial asymmetry. Pulsatile exophthalmos may be present at birth before the bony abnormality has fully developed. A minority of patients with sphenoid dysplasia develop enophthalmos secondary to microphthalmia or to associated dysplasia of the lateral wall of the orbit which enables orbital contents to prolapse into the temporal fossa (McFarlane et al. 1995). Sphenoid dysplasia may also be associated with non-correctable loss of vision.

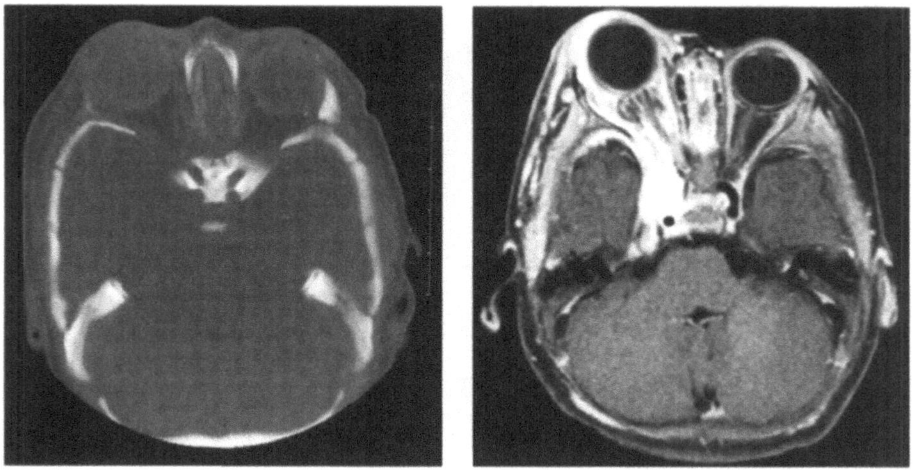

a b

Fig. 18.1a,b. Sphenoid dysplasia with adjacent plexiform neurofibroma (**a**). Axial CT on bone windows demonstrates expansion of the anterior portion of the right middle cranial fossa due to dysplasia and thinning of the right sphenoid bone. Mild proptosis is demonstrated (**b**). Axial postcontrast T1 W imaging through the orbits demonstrates extensive enhancement within the soft tissues on the lateral aspect of the right globe and scalp which extends through the orbital fissure into the region of the right cavernous sinus. This is a typical plexiform neurofibroma involving the V1 distribution of the trigeminal nerve which is commonly associated with sphenoid dysplasia (reproduced with permission of the editor, *Neuropediatrics*)

18.2.2.2 Ocular Manifestations

Lisch nodules (harmatomas of the iris) are the commonest ocular manifestation of NF1. They increase in size and number with age and are best detected by slit lamp biomicroscopy. Discrete areas of hyperpigmentation on the choroid are the second commonest ocular manifestation and further orbital manifestations of NF1 include intraaorbital neurofibromas, exopthalmos related to bony abnormalities such as sphenoid dysplasia or to retro-orbital tumours and optic gliomas, buphthalmos and astrocytic harmatomas (Huson et al. 1988; Mulvihill et al. 1990). Intraocular tumours can predispose to retinal and/or choroidal detachment (Fig. 18.2).

Optic pathway gliomas occur in 5–15% of NF1 patients (Lewis et al. 1984; Listernick et al. 1989). About 90% are diagnosed between 1 and 7 years of age. The majority of optic pathway gliomas in childhood are pilocytic astrocytomas with higher-grade gliomas occurring in older patients. Twenty per cent of childhood optic pathway gliomas behave aggressively resulting in early patient death with the median time of death being 4 years from diagnosis (Elster 1992; Mulvihill et al. 1988). Nearly 50% of optic gliomas are symptomatic at presentation but the majority do not progress to cause further visual loss or other complications (Gutmann 1998). Chiasmatic and optic tract gliomas may have a more aggressive course and therefore poorer prognosis. Gliomas that involve the third ventricle and hypothalamus may result in hypopituitarism, obesity, dwarfism, or diabetes insipidus (Pomeranz 1987). Treatment of optic gliomas with surgery, radiotherapy or chemotherapy is reserved for cases of rapidly progressive optic pathway gliomas or gliomas presenting with metastases or evidence of raised intracranial pressure (Cappelli et al. 1998; Listernick et al. 1994).

18.2.2.3 Endocrine Manifestations

Endocrine disorders occur in 1–3% of NF1 patients. Central precocious puberty occurs in 3% of children with NF1 while phaechromocytomas tend to be a disorder of adults with NF1. While earlier studies reported precocious puberty only in association with optic chiasm glioma (Habiby et al. 1995), other studies have found some children with NF1 developing precocious puberty in the absence of optic chiasm glioma suggesting that the disease itself predisposes to this complication (Listernick et al. 1995).

18.2.2.4 Neuropsychological and Brain Manifestations

Forty to 60% of NF1 patients have some degree of mental disability that interferes with school perfor-

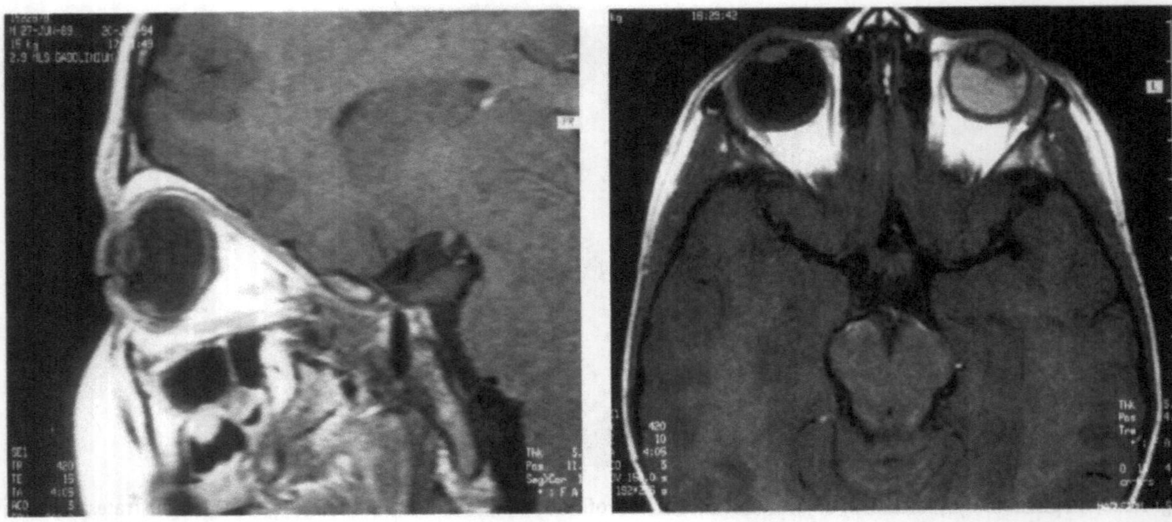

a b

Fig. 18.2. a Sagittal oblique T1 W images with gadolinium DTPA through the orbit in a 5-year-old child with neurofibromatosis. There is a 5-mm mass lesion related to the inferior portion of the globe which protrudes into the vitreous body. This is likely to represent an astrocytic hamartoma or a retinal neurofibroma (**b**). Axial T1 W images through the orbits 2 years later, after loss of vision in the left eye, demonstrate the result of chorioretinal detachment, presumably secondary to the intraocular mass (reproduced with permission of the editor, *Neuropediatrics*)

mance. The majority have an IQ in the low average range and most have specific learning disorders such as attention deficit, visual-spatial and reading difficulties. The type and severity of mental impediment does not correlate with the type or number of brain lesions seen on MR although some investigators have found a correlation between neurofibromatosis bright objects (NBO) in the thalamus and specific learning disabilities (Moore et al. 1996; Duffner et al. 1989; Ferner et al. 1993).

NF1 sufferers are also prone to headaches, seizures, speech and hearing impediments. Huson et al. report epilepsy in 8% of adult NF1 sufferers and affected relatives (Huson et al. 1988; Gutmann et al. 1997).

Relative macrocephaly is common in children and adults with NF1. It is thought to be due to a generalised increase in the size of the brain and is not always associated with hydrocephalus or structural brain abnormalities. There is no correlation between macrocephaly and intellectual handicap (North et al. 1993; Van Es et al. 1996).

Hydrocephalus may occur secondary to aqueduct stenosis, which may be due to an identifiable cause such as an associated glioma or an aqueductal web. No obvious cause may be evident, in which case the aqueduct is thought to be obstructed by a proliferation of subependymal glial cells, which do not behave in a progressive manner. However, clinically significant hydrocephalus is uncommon (Huson and Hughes 1994) (Fig. 18.3).

High signal intensity areas on long TR sequences – (NBO) – are found in 43–93% of NF1 sufferers. They show age related change in their frequency showing maximum prevalence and volume in children aged 4–10 years and occurring less frequently before 4 and after 10 years of age (Griffiths et al. 1999). They do not usually cause clinical symptoms although a link has been established for thalamic NBO and certain types of learning impairment (Moore et al. 1996).

Brain gliomas occur with increased frequency in NF1 (1–3%), occur at an earlier age than the non-NF1 population and are frequently multicentric (Huson and Hughes 1994). Most gliomas seen in NF1 are pilocytic astrocytomas but more aggressive gliomas such as glioblastoma multiforme have also been described. The cerebellum and brainstem are the most frequently affected sites (Braffmann et al. 1990). Cerebellum tumours have been reported to have a poor prognosis in NF1; however, the increasing discovery of 'incidental' cerebellar tumours on MR challenges this assertion (Elster 1992). Recent studies have shown a relatively benign course for most brainstem gliomas. In one paper only 11/21 tumours showed radiological or clinical progression and in seven of those the tumour went on to stabilise or even regress (Pollack et al. 1996).

Other intracranial neoplasms such as acoustic schwannomas, medulloblastomas and meningiomas

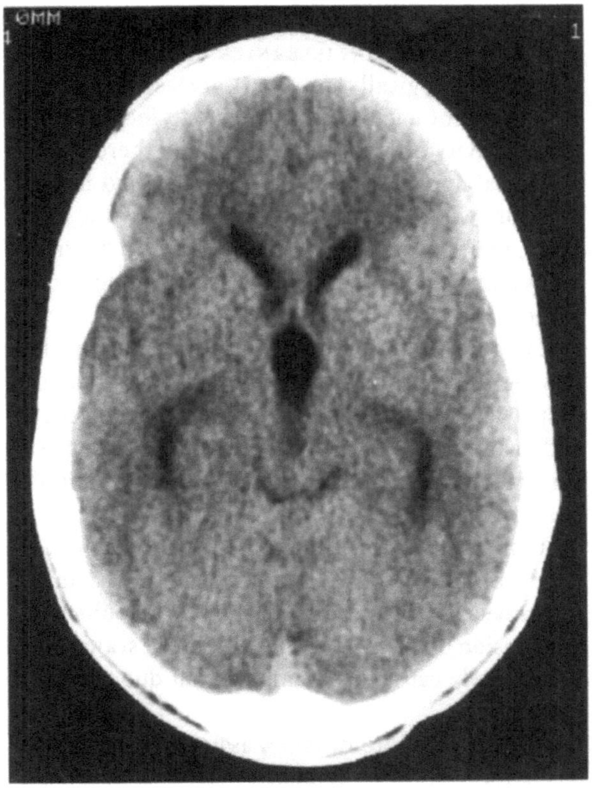
a

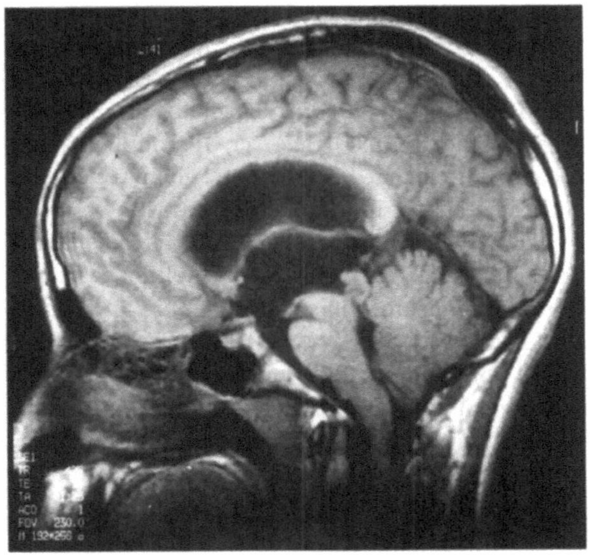
b

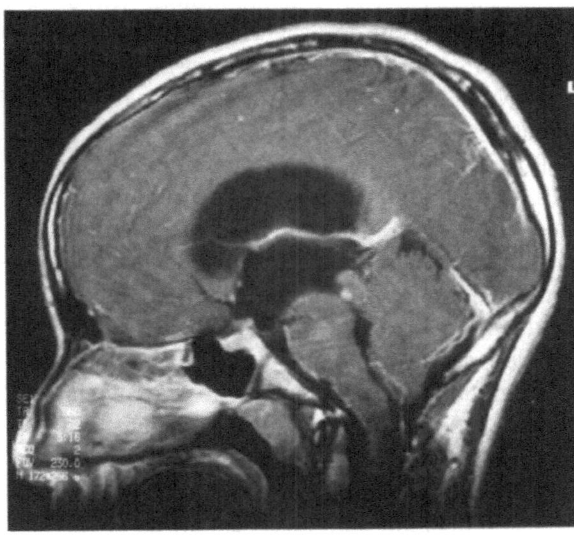
c

Fig. 18.3a–c. A 13-year-old child with neurofibromatosis showing a small asymptomatic tumour within the tectum of the mid brain (**a**). Axial non-enhanced CT demonstrates triventricular hydrocephalus which was attributed to aqueduct stenosis (**b,c**). However, sagittal T1 W images before (**b**) and after gadolinium DTPA (**c**) show a small enhancing nodule within the mid brain tectum. The child remained asymptomatic and a presumptive diagnosis of low grade astrocytoma was made (reproduced with permission of the editor, *Neuropediatrics*)

are not seen any more commonly in NF1 than in the general population contrary to reports from earlier major clinical series which did not make a distinction between NF1 and NF2 and therefore tended to overestimate the prevalence of other intracranial neoplasms in NF1 (Huson and Hughes 1994).

Other central nervous system abnormalities occurring with increased frequency in NF1 include meningocoeles, arachnoid cysts, dural ectasia and cerebrovascular disease including arteriovenous malformations, aneurysms and vascular stenoses (Van Es et al. 1996; Westacott et al. 1988; Zachos et al. 1997). Cases of NF1 associated with agenesis of the corpus callosum have been described (Atlas et al. 1988).

18.2.3 Neuroimaging

18.2.3.1 Optic Nerve and Eye

Optic pathway gliomas are the commonest tumour in NF1 and are most commonly pilocytic astrocytomas. The tumours either cause diffuse expansion resulting in a fusiform mass and obscuration of the optic nerve without extensive subarachnoid spread or predominantly infiltrate the subarachnoid space with minimal involvement of the optic nerve.

On CT optic nerve gliomas appear as fusiform swelling of the optic nerves which may enhance with intravenous iodinated contrast media and sometimes produce enlargement of the optic foramina. Bilateral tubular expansion of the optic nerves was considered pathognomonic of NF1 (Listernick et al. 1989; Huson and Hughes 1994). However, CT scanning cannot reliably differentiate between optic glioma and dural ectasia because of its poor tissue contrast.

Magnetic resonance (MR) imaging is the imaging modality of choice because of its multiplanar capabilities and lack of ionising radiation. Appearances on T2 weighted scans are typical with a compact low signal core and a higher intensity circumferential component. Involved optic chiasm and optic tracts or radiation are usually isointense with brain on T1 and hyperintense with brain on T2 weighted images (Braffmann et al. 1990). They usually enhance with gadolinium DTPA (Fig. 18.4).

The appearance of chiasmal tumour with diffuse enlargement of the optic chiasm and nerves is diagnostic for optic glioma and obviates the need for biopsy (Van Es et al. 1996). Dural ectasia is reliably differentiated from optic glioma on MR.

Routine screening of asymptomatic children with NF1 for optic glioma does not affect clinical outcome since most optic gliomas do not progress to visual loss and although up to 52% are associated with an abnormal visual examination, the visual impairment rarely progresses (Listernick et al. 1995). However, detailed serial ophthalmological examinations at least annually are recommended in young children (Listernick et al. 1994). Most clinicians will perform imaging if and when the child becomes symptomatic. When imaging is considered MR should be used and the minimum investigation should include T1 and T2 weighted images in the axial and coronal planes followed by postgadolinium sagittal and axial images. It is vitally important to give gadolinium on the first MR examination. If optic glioma is suspected clinically or shown on the MR sequences listed above, postgadolinium T1 weighted images with spectral fat saturation should be performed in the coronal plane from globes to brainstem. Postgadolinium imaging in the sagittal oblique plane along the course of the optic nerves shows the extent of the optic glioma elegantly but usually does not give extra information.

A small proportion of optic gliomas behave aggressively. Earlier studies quoted a figure of 20% although this has been shown to be an overestimate on more recent studies. However, the proportion of aggressive tumours is still significant particularly in the 1st year of diagnosis (Elster et al. 1992). Some authorities have suggested repeat MR examinations at 3, 9, 15, 24 and 36 months after diagnosis to look for volume changes (Listernick et al. 1994). However, a radiologically detected increase in tumour bulk does not necessarily correlate to increased tumour activity or clinical deterioration; therefore radiological appearances must be interpreted in conjunction with clinical findings (Gutmann et al. 1997). Other groups rely on the follow up by visual fields and evoked potentials in cases of optic glioma without mass effect.

CT is not indicated in the routine situation but may be used in two situations: to assess sphenoid dysplasia with thin sections and 3D reconstructions and in any acute neurological presentations suggesting raised intracranial pressure or intracranial haemorrhage.

Retinal astrocytic harmatomas occur in a minority of NF1 patients. The tumours usually arise in the retina near the optic disc and show as an enhancing mass lesion on post Gd-DTPA enhanced scans. They occasionally cause visual impairment due to retinal detachment.

Ocular neurofibromas show as hypointense masses on T1 and slightly hyperintense masses on T2 weighted scans, which enhance with Gd DTPA. They may also be complicated by retinal detachment (Fig. 18.2).

18.2.3.2 Plexiform Neurofibroma

Plexiform neurofibromas (PNF) occur almost exclusively in NF1 and contain Schwann cells and perineural fibroblasts. They arise from major nerve plexi and tend to grow along nerve fascicles.

MR is the imaging modality of choice for PNF, which shows them to be slightly hyperintense to muscle on short TR sequences and markedly hyperintense to muscle on long TR sequences. There may be a variable area of central hypointensity on T2 weighted MR sequences possibly due to fibrous components with surrounding myxoid matrix (Braffman et al. 1990). Enhancement with Gd-DTPA is common and is usually intense (Fig. 18.1).

18.2.3.3 Sphenoid Dysplasia

Sphenoid dysplasia is an uncommon manifestation of NF1 thought to occur as a result of a mesodermal dysplasia resulting in abnormal ossification and development of the greater wing of the sphenoid bone. It is invariably a unilateral abnormality affecting the left side more commonly than the right. The typical

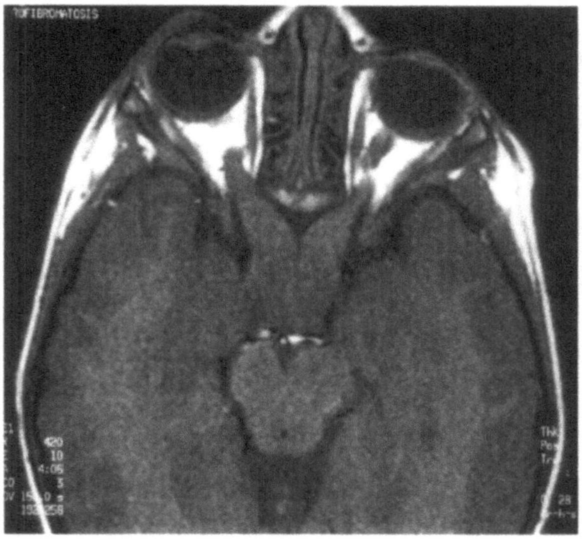

a

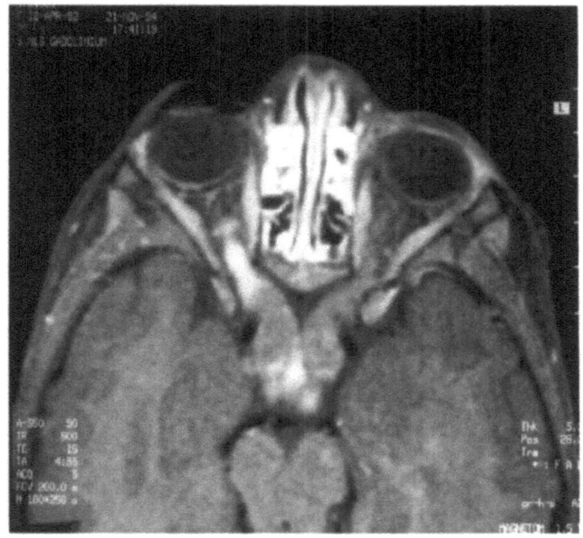

b

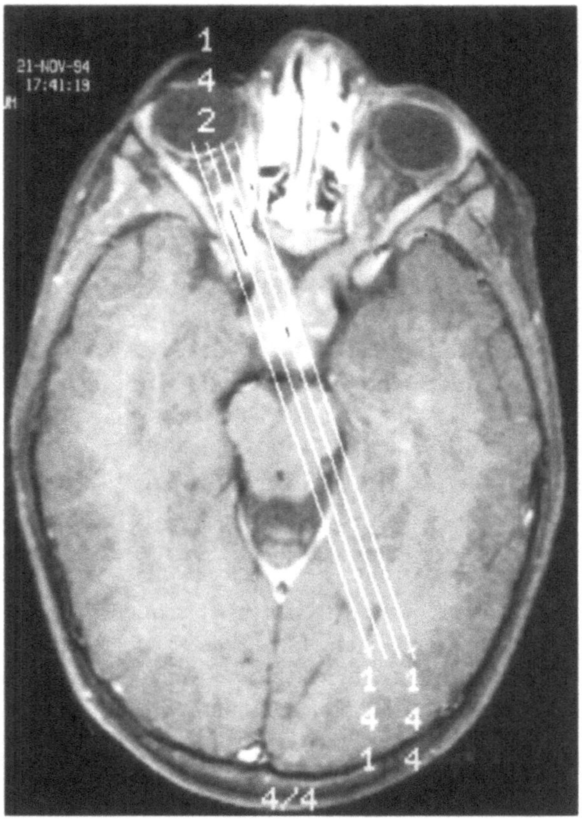

c

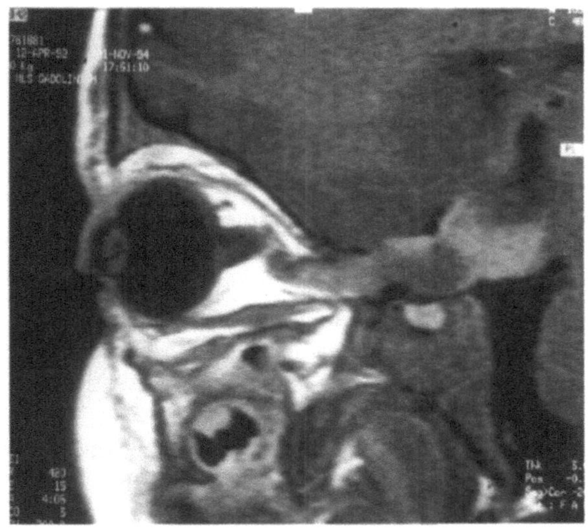

d

Fig. 18.4a–d. Child aged 2 years with bilateral optic glioma (**a,b**). Axial T1 W images before (**a**) and after gadolinium DTPA (**b**). All portions of the optic nerves and the optic chiasm are bulky. There is enhancement of both optic nerves particularly of the orbital and canalicular portion of the right optic nerve (**c,d**). Postgadolinium imaging in the plane of the optic nerve shows patchy enhancement along the course of the right optic nerve as far back as the optic chiasm (reproduced with permission of the editor, *Neuropediatrics*)

radiological features are a defect involving part or all of the greater wing of the sphenoid bone, elevation of the lesser wing of the sphenoid, enlargement of the ipsilateral orbit and distortion of the sella turcica (Fig. 18.1). The ipsilateral temporal lobe is usually enlarged resulting in enlargement of the middle cranial fossa. The floor of the orbit is occasionally involved in the disease process and hypoplasia of the ethmoid and maxillary sinuses may occur secondary to the orbital changes. A thick sheet of fibrous tissue usually covers the bone defect and the superior orbital fissure is usually protected by thickened dura. Occasionally this is absent and a meningocoele projects into the retrobulbar region (McFarlane et al. 1995).

Plain radiographs demonstrate the enlargement of the orbit and the superior orbital fissure as well as the secondary hypoplasia of the ethmoid and maxillary sinuses.

CT demonstrates the bone defects well particularly on 3D reconstructions (Zimmermann et al. 1983). In addition enlargement of the middle cranial fossa and any associated soft tissue abnormalities such as meningocoeles, temporal arachnoid cysts, or neurofibromatous tissues are also demonstrated.

MR imaging is inferior to CT and plain radiography in evaluation of the bony defects; however, it is the preferred modality for demonstrating the associated soft tissue abnormalities. T1 weighted Gd-DTPA enhanced scans with spectral fat saturation show enhancement of any abnormal neurofibromatous tissues in the retrobulbar region well.

18.2.3.4 Brain in NF1

18.2.3.4.1 Neurofibromatosis Bright Objects

MR imaging defined a pathology in NF1 that had not been described previously by CT or pathological investigation. These abnormalities have been called NBO and are isointense with gray matter on T1 weighted sequences and hyperintense on T2 weighted sequences. NBO occasionally have high signal characteristics on T1 weighted scans but they do not enhance with gadolinium DTPA, show no evidence of mass effect neither are they associated with neurological deficits (Aoki et al. 1989; Ferner et al. 1993; Mirowitz et al. 1989; Moore et al. 1996) (Fig. 18.5).

Subsequent reports have described NBO on CT as well defined hypodense foci but MR is considerably more sensitive (Menor and Marti-Bonmati 1992).

NBO are found most frequently in the globus pallidus, brainstem and cerebellum and occasionally subcortical white matter and dentate nuclei (Griffiths et al. 1999). Itoh et al. (1994) reported NBO in 93% of their patients younger than 15 years of age, 57% of 16–30 year olds and 29% of those older than 30 years. While basal ganglia, internal capsule and brainstem NBO were seen in all age groups in this study, cerebellar and dentate nucleus lesions were rare after the 3rd decade (Itoh et al. 1994). NBO have only been described in NF1, leading some authors to believe they are pathognomonic of NF1 and it has been suggested that they may be useful as an additional imaging diagnostic criterion for NF1 particularly when present in young patients with no or subtle clinical stigmata (Di Mario et al. 1993; Duffner et al. 1989; Itoh et al. 1994). However, data on their specificity for NF1 is scarce and their clinical significance is still debated, so current recommendations do not recognise them as a diagnostic criterion for NF1 (Gutmann et al. 1997).

The exact nature of NBO is unclear. Many pathologies have been postulated such as harmatomas, heterotopia, dysplasias or areas of gliosis; but these do not explain the signal characteristics and age related behaviour of NBO (Griffiths et al. 1999; Itoh et al. 1994; Mautner et al. 1991). Further hypotheses suggest that NBO are areas of dysmyelination (Di Paolo et al. 1995; Sevick et al. 1992). Postmortem studies are sparse but three children who had died from complications of NF1 showed intramyelinic vacuoles 5–100 μm in diameter suggestive of intramyelinic spongiosis (Di Paolo et al. 1995). A proliferative or neoplastic potential in NBO has been suspected by some investigators who suggest that NBO could be low-grade tumours (Itoh et al. 1994; Mukonoweshuro et al. 1999). Some NBO have been shown to have mass effect and others occurred in conjunction with gliomas further strengthening possibilities of a malignant potential (Di Mario et al. 1998; Ferner et al. 1993; Sevick et al. 1992). Our group has documented the evolution of five tumours in areas of previously recognised NBO (Griffiths et al. 1999) on serial scans (Fig. 18.6).

Functional studies with 18F-2-fluoro-2-deoxy-D-glucose and PET showed diffuse cerebral hypometabolism with normal metabolic activity in areas of T2 hyperintensity suggesting that NBO have normal blood supply (Balestri et al. 1994). Proton spectroscopy studies have shown NBO to have spectra similar to normal brain and different from gliomas (Castillo et al. 1995). It is possible that proton spectroscopy may be a useful clinical tool in distinguishing atypical NBO from glioma (Fig. 18.5).

18.2.3.4.2 Brain Gliomas

Brain gliomas occur with increased frequency in NF1 patients and are usually low-grade astrocytomas although approximately 50% became malignant gliomas in one study. The preferred method of imaging is MR, which is superior to CT scanning particularly at imaging brain stem lesions. Gliomas in NF1 are radiologically no different to those seen in non-NF1 cases, appearing as masses which are isointense or slightly hypointense to normal brain on T1-weighted and high signal on long TR sequences and often enhance with gadolinium DTPA (Braffmann et al. 1990).

The cerebellum and brainstem are the most commonly affected regions although diffuse gliomas of the cerebral hemispheres have been reported. Cerebellar tumours have previously been regarded as having a particularly poor prognosis in NF1 but the increasing discovery of 'incidental' tumours on MR challenges this finding (Elster 1992). Recent work

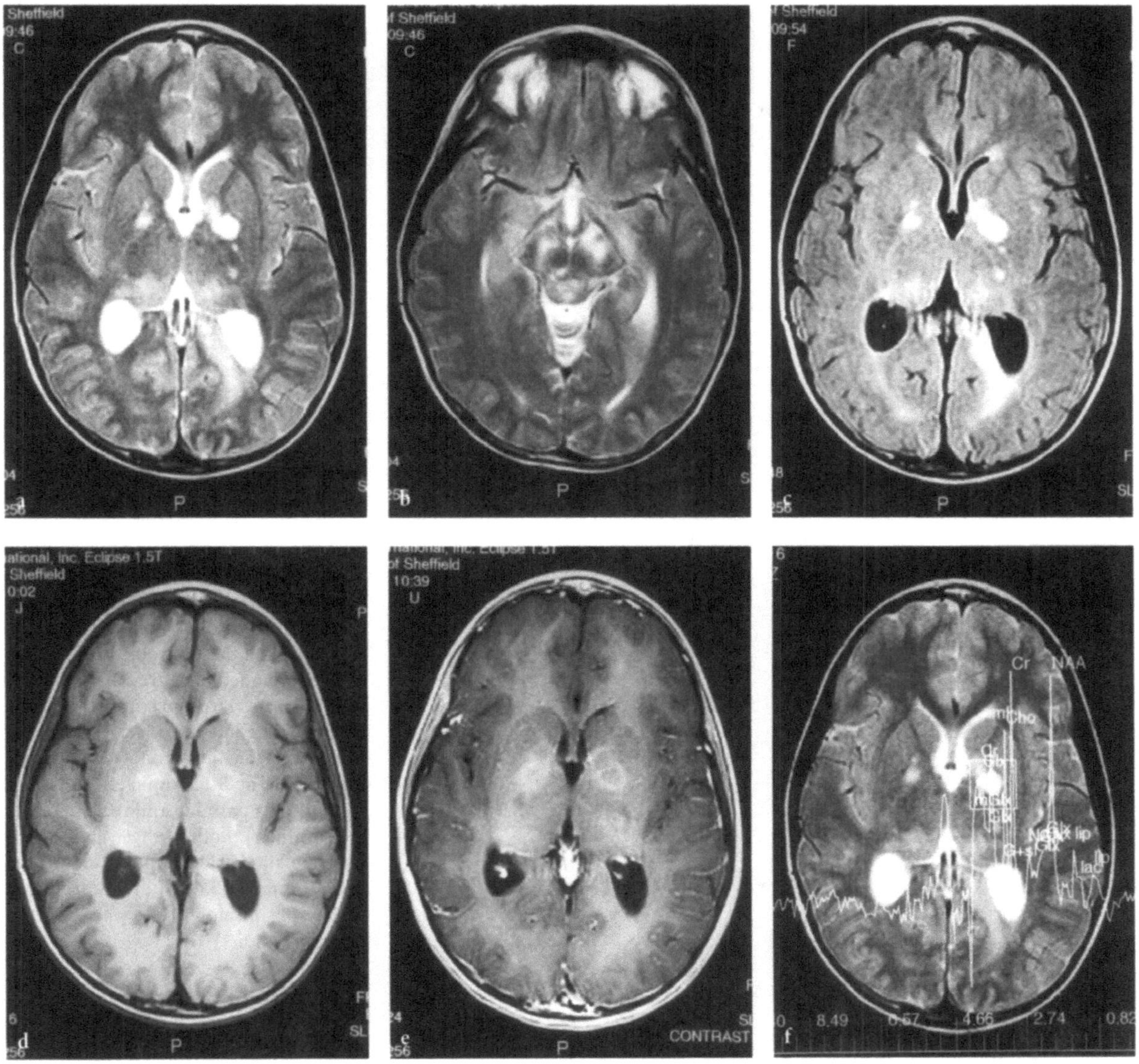

Fig. 18.5a–f. Neurofibromatosis bright objects (NBO) (**a,b**). T2 weighted scans. There are typical NBO in both globus pallidi and both cerebral peduncles of the mid brain. **c** FLAIR image demonstrates the lesions well and confirms the absence of oedema or mass effect associated with the lesions (**d**). Pre-contrast T1 W image shows a high signal rim around the globus pallidi lesions which are otherwise isointense with grey matter (**e**). However, as is typical of these lesions they do not enhance on the post Gd DTPA enhanced images. **f** MR spectroscopy shows reduced NAA peaks in this case

has shown a relatively benign course of most brainstem glioma in NF1. Most of the tumours show slow radiological progression with a tendency to stabilise or even regress (Pollack et al. 1996; Leisti et al. 1996; Morris et al. 1997).

The frequency of follow up for children with known brain tumours will vary with local policies depending on the tumour grade, biological activity and treatment. Guidelines for the technique of assessing children with brain tumours have been put forward by the United Kingdom Childhood Cancer Study Group and their French counterparts Societe Francais Oncologie Pediatrique [United Kingdom Children's Cancer Study Group (UKCCSG) and Société d'Oncologie Pédiatrique (SFOP) Panelists (in press) and we use those guidelines to assess children with NF1 and brain glioma.

18.2.3.5
Other Pathology

Other parenchymal abnormalities that may simulate neoplasia but show spontaneous regression are seen

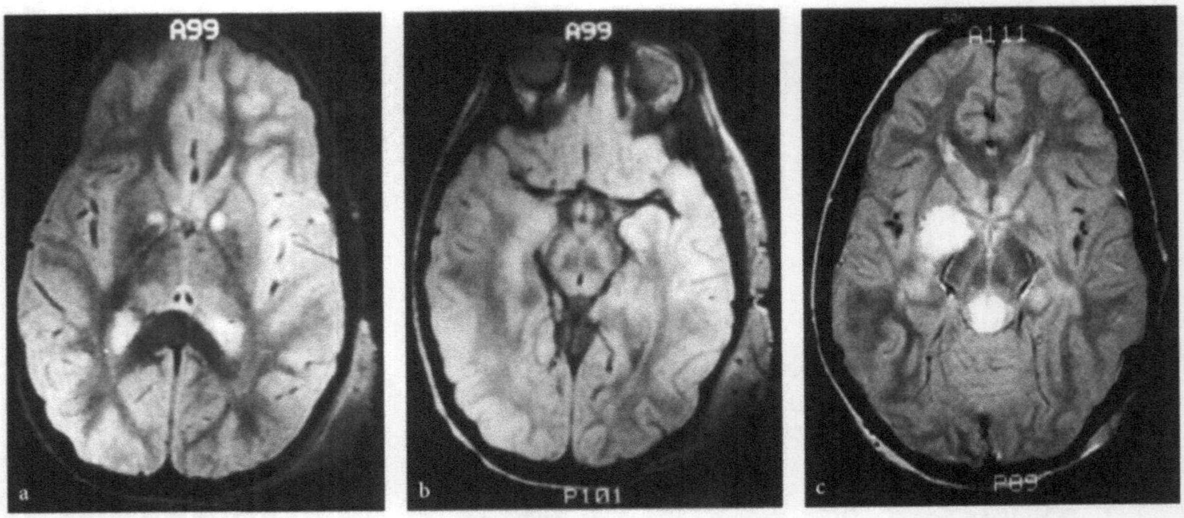

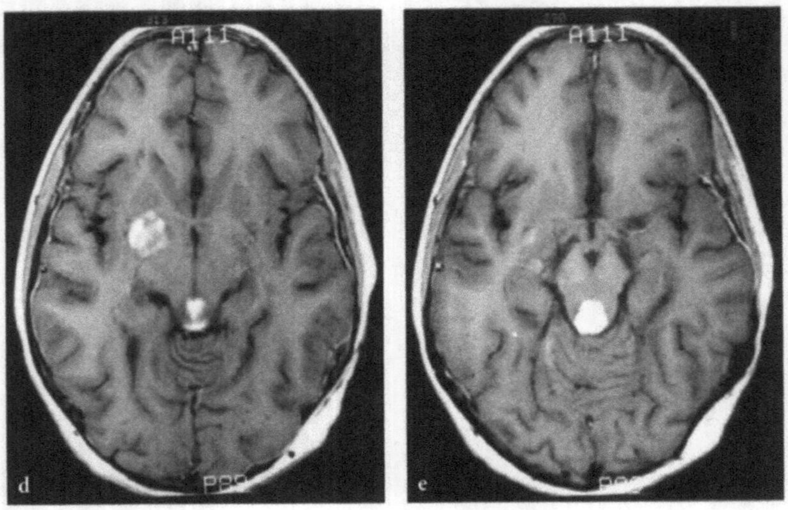

Fig. 18.6a–e. Demonstration of evolution of tumour in a child with neurofibromatosis **(a,b)**. Axial long TR sequences show neurofibromatosis bright objects in the globus pallidi bilaterally. Note also that there is some prominence of the periaqueductal grey matter of the mid brain. A large plexiform neurofibroma of the left scalp is present **(c–e)**. Five years later there is now evidence of mass effect on T2 W images within the right globus pallidus and tectum of the mid brain **(c)**. Both of these areas demonstrate significant enhancement with gadolinium DTPA **(d,e)** (reproduced with permission of the editor, *Neuropediatrics*)

in NF1. Morris et al. (1997) describe an enhancing brain lesion which regressed spontaneously without treatment. We recently had a patient with a large area of abnormality in the left frontal lobe, which had appearances highly suggestive of a glioma. The child presented with a stroke-like event and seizures 3 weeks after a viral illness. A repeat MR 4 weeks later showed complete resolution of the abnormality. A presumptive diagnosis of acute disseminated encephalomyelitis was made (Fig. 18.7).

An association between NF1 and arachnoid cysts particularly in the temporal regions is recognised. The cysts are usually unilateral although a few cases of bilateral temporal arachnoid cysts have been described (Martinez-Lage et al. 1993).

Optic nerve dural ectasia occurs in NF1 and may result in enlargement of the optic canal. On CT dural ectasia and optic nerve glioma cannot be readily differentiated since they both appear as diffuse enlargement of the anterior optic pathways. Serial CT scanning would, however, show non-progressive enlargement in the case of dural ectasia whereas optic glioma would increase in size with time. MR is the imaging modality of choice, however, because of its superior soft tissue resolution, which enables reliable differentiation between dural ectasia and optic nerve glioma; dural ectasia appearing as widening of the perioptic dural sheath whereas optic glioma is shown as a solid tumour (Lovblad et al. 1994).

Certain cerebrovascular lesions such as aneurysms, arteriovenous malformations and vascular occlusions occur with increased frequency in NF1 (Norton et al. 1995; Van Es et al. 1996). Vascular stenoses may produce a *moyamoya* appearance on catheter angiography which has typical appearances on MR angiography and imaging (Fig. 18.8).

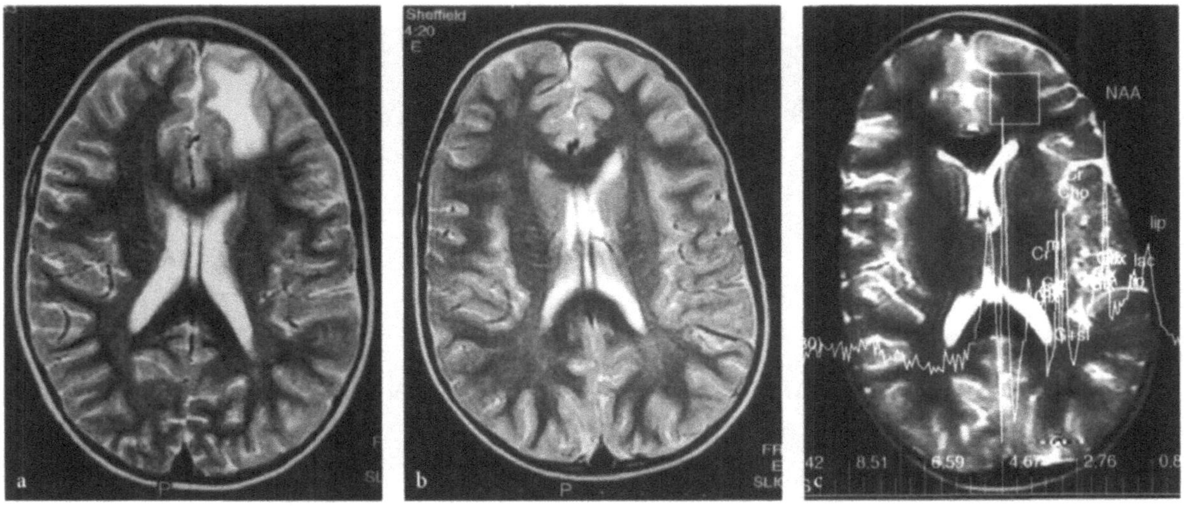

Fig. 18.7. a Patient with bilateral basal ganglia NBO and an abnormal area in left frontal lobe initially thought to represent glioma (**b**). A repeat MR a few weeks later shows complete resolution of the frontal lobe lesion. The patient had recovered from a viral illness 4 weeks prior to presentation. A presumptive diagnosis of ADEM was made for the frontal lobe lesion (**c**). MR spectroscopy shows normal choline, creatinine and NAA but high levels of lipid, presumably from increased myelin metabolism

18.3 Neurofibromatosis 2

18.3.1 Epidemiology and Genetics

Neurofibromatosis 2 (NF2) is much less common than NF1 with an incidence of 1/37,000 (Tos and Thomsen 1984). It is an autosomal dominant disorder with the abnormal gene located on chromosome 22. There is considerable clinical variability in NF2 patients with mild and severe forms being recognised. There is accumulating evidence linking the more severe clinical forms to truncating mutations (Evans et al. 1998) although there is still considerable variability of clinical severity of the disease even within families identified as having these truncating mutations and so caution must still be exercised in attempts at prognostication on the basis of this finding alone (Scoles et al. 1996; Evans et al. 1998).

18.3.2 Clinical Features

NF2 predisposes patients to the development of cranial and peripheral nerve schwannomas, cranial and spinal meningiomas, gliomas (particularly ependymoma) and a variety of ocular abnormalities. The age of onset of the disease is variable but is usually later than NF1. Some studies have described ages of onset ranging from 11 to 70 years (Parry et al. 1994; Mautner et al. 1996). Ten per cent of NF2 sufferers present before the age of 10 years. Early onset of symptoms is usually associated with more severe disease (Gutmann et al. 1997). The diagnostic criteria for NF2 are summarised in Table 18.2.

18.3.2.1 Cutaneous Manifestations

Skin tumours occur in up to 64% of affected individuals and are associated with more severe disease (Parry et al. 1994). They are usually schwannomas and not neurofibromas although neurofibromas and mixed tumours may also be found. Though they may predate other manifestations of NF2 by several years they rarely contribute to disease severity (Evans et al. 1997). A proportion of NF2 patients have café-au-lait spots [33% in Mautner et al.'s series (1997), 43% in Evans et al.'s series (1992)] but the café-au-lait spots are usually small and sparse, i.e., less than six in number. The diagnosis of NF1 or NF1 mosaicism should be considered in any patient found to have numerous or large café-au-lait spots (Mautner et al. 1997; Evans et al. 1992).

18.3.2.2 Ocular Manifestations

Ocular abnormalities are common and include developmental abnormalities such as epiretinal mem-

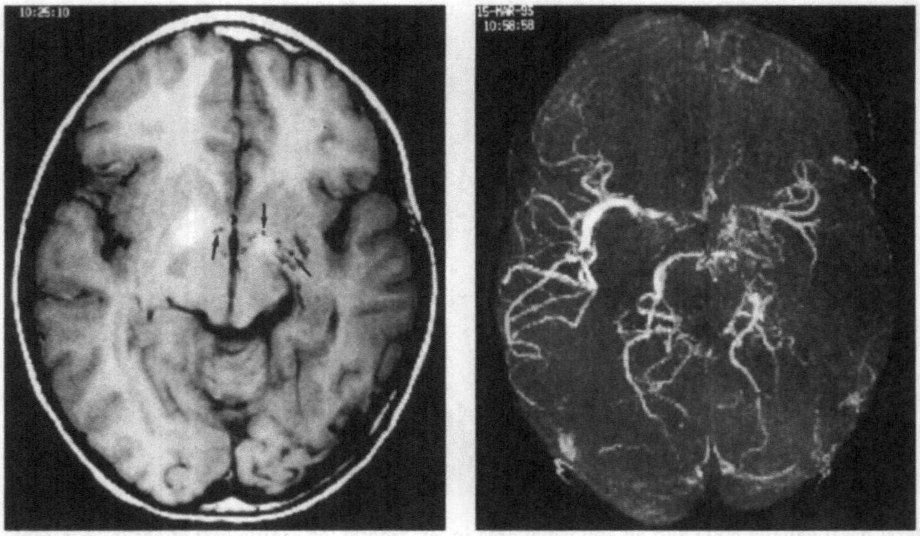

a b

Fig. 18.8a,b. Eight-year-old child with neurofibromatosis showing vascular occlusion and a "moyamoya" appearance. The child has a history of recurrent transient ischaemic attacks and small strokes (**a**). Axial T1 through the basal ganglia demonstrates enlargement of the perforating vessels in the left basal ganglia bilaterally (*arrows*). There is a marked loss of volume within the left hemisphere, particularly posteriorly due to previous ischaemia and infarctions. Note the bright objects of neurofibromatosis within the globus pallidus bilaterally (**b**). 3D time-of-flight MR angiography through the circle of Willis demonstrates occlusion of the terminal internal carotid artery on the left and its immediate branches as well as attenuation of the left posterior cerebral artery. The distal portions of the left middle cerebral artery and posterior cerebral artery are fed by perforating collaterals. Similar but less severe changes are demonstrated along the course of the terminal portion of right carotid artery and its immediate branches (reproduced with permission of the editor, *Neuropediatrics*)

branes, retinal harmatomas and cataracts. Retinal and epiretinal abnormalities affect 9–22% of NF2 patients. Lens abnormalities include juvenile posterior subcapsular cataracts (incidence 32.8–72.4%), cortical wedge cataracts (14.2–26.5%) and mixed cataracts (12.5–27.1%) (Gutmann et al. 1997). Cataracts were found to cause significant reduction of visual acuity in 54% in Mautner's study while Parry et al. (1994) found this in 33% (Mautner et al. 1996; Parry et al. 1994). Where congenital or juvenile cataracts are found in a person with a first-degree relative with NF2 detailed evaluation for NF2 should be performed.

18.3.2.3
Brain

Intracranial tumours are common in NF2 and are responsible for most of the morbidity and mortality associated with the disease. Vestibular schwannomas particularly if they are bilateral are the hallmark of the disease (Fig. 18.9).

Schwannomas may also involve any of the other cranial nerves. Other tumours occurring with increased frequency in NF2 include meningiomas, astrocytomas and ependymomas (Evans et al. 1992).

The development of tumours is age related. Patients presenting in the 1st decade are more likely to have meningiomas or spinal tumours than vestibular schwannomas. Presentation with vestibular schwannomas becomes more common from the 2nd decade. Patients with the severe form of NF2 present early with multiple intracranial and spinal tumours.

Patients with tumour present with effects directly related to the tumour or symptoms of raised intracranial pressure. Presentation is with hearing loss or tinnitus, headaches and other symptoms of raised intracranial pressure and epileptic convulsions. Loss of balance occurs commonly in patients with vestibular schwannomas and may even occur after the tumours have been excised. Swimming difficulties due to disorientation under water occur in some NF2 patients. Visual impairment may occur secondary to corneal disease due to bilateral facial nerve palsy complicating vestibular schwannoma excision or may be a result of papilloedema, frontal tumours or optic nerve sheath meningiomas (Evans et al. 1992).

There is no gender difference in tumour behaviour and there is no proven effect of pregnancy on vestibular schwannoma growth (Evans et al. 1992).

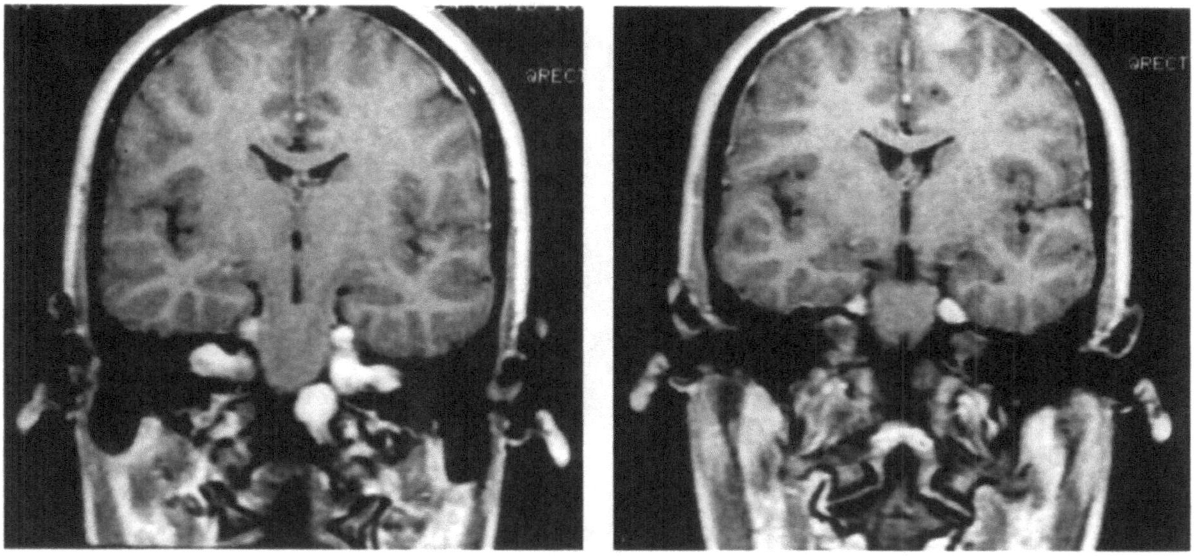

a b

Fig. 18.9a,b. NF2 patient with bilateral deafness. Coronal postgadolinium T1 W images (**a**). Bilateral vestibular schwannomas and unilateral glossopharyngeal nerve schwannoma (**b**). Bilateral trigeminal nerve schwannomas. (Courtesy of Dr. C.A.J. Romanowski, consultant neuroradiologist, Royal Hallamshire Hospital, Sheffield, UK)

18.3.3 Neuroimaging

MR imaging is the preferred modality for investigating intracranial and spinal abnormalities. There is no role for plain film radiography or CT in the routine imaging of NF2 patients although both these modalities may demonstrate calcification and hyperostosis associated with meningiomas. Large intracranial tumours will also be demonstrated on CT.

Vestibular schwannomas arise from the glial-schwann cell interface of the vestibular portion of the vestibulocochlear nerve. The tumours may arise within the internal auditory canal or at the cerebellopontine angle with intracanalicular tumour extension if large. Whereas in non-NF2 vestibular schwannomas the tumours tend to be well encapsulated and displace the cochlear nerve, those occurring in NF2 tend to form grape-like clusters that often infiltrate and engulf the cochlear nerve (Subach et al. 1999). Large tumours may develop areas of cystic degeneration within or adjacent to the tumour. The tumours are iso-/hypodense to brain on CT and show dense uniform enhancement; or ring enhancement in the case of cystic tumours, following intravenous contrast administration. On MR they are iso-/ slightly hypointense to grey matter on T1 weighted sequences and hyperintense to grey matter on T2 weighted sequences. They show intense, uniform enhancement following administration of Gd-DTPA (Figs. 18.9, 18.10).

Contrast enhanced MR scans demonstrate vestibular schwannomas with a sensitivity approaching 100%. However, false positive scans occur due to enhancing benign conditions such as arteriovenous malformations, arachnoiditis and the Ramsay-Hunt syndrome (Hermans et al. 1997).

Currently recommendations suggest that the minimum investigation for vestibular schwannomas should consist of fat saturated (suppressed) images acquired in 3-mm sections through the internal auditory canals in axial and coronal planes pre- and postenhancement with gadolinium DTPA if small intracanalicular lesions are to be demonstrated (Gutmann et al. 1997). However, recent work with high resolution 3D spin echo or gradient echo MR sequences that stress T2 weighted information and produce images where CSF retains a high signal and appears very bright and the nerves and brain appear very dark has shown a high sensitivity for the detection of vestibular schwannomas without the need for intravenous Gd-DTPA. Vestibular schwannomas are seen on these sequences as low signal nodular abnormalities distorting the contour of the nerve. Multiplanar reformatting of the three dimensional data allows visualisation of the nerves along the entire length of the internal auditory canal. Diagnostic difficulties on these techniques usually arise because of partial voluming particularly where the nerves are closely related to bony structures/spurs within the canal which produce small areas of low signal within the CSF in

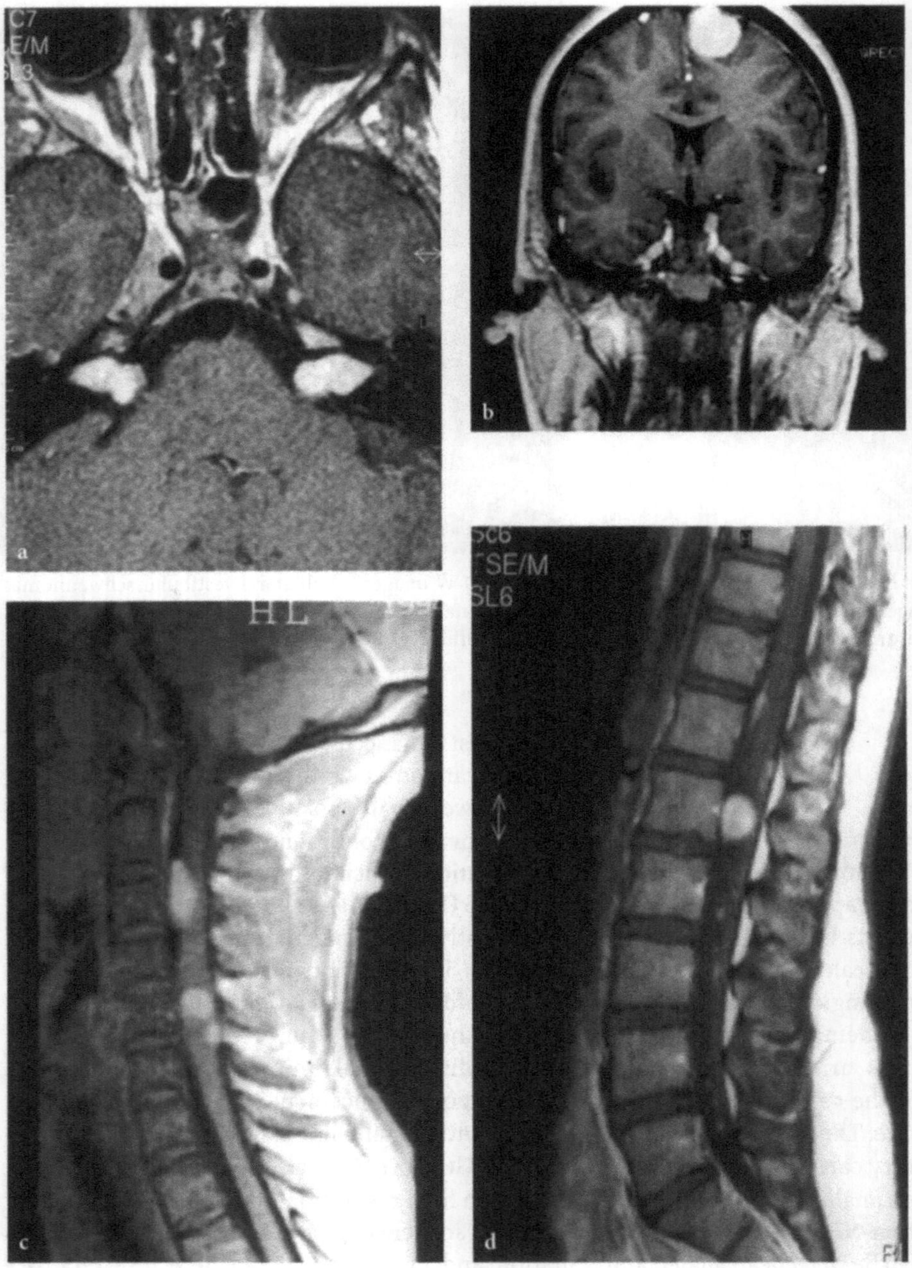

Fig. 18.10a–d. Twenty-seven-year-old man with NF2. **a** Axial post-gadolinium image showing bilateral vestibular schwannomas **(b)**. Coronal enhanced T1 W image showing left parafalcine meningioma. Note the characteristic intense uniform enhancement of the tumour **(c,d)**. Enhanced sagittal MR images of the cervical and lumbar spine showing multiple intradural spinal meningiomas. (Courtesy of Dr. C.A.J. Romanowski, consultant neuroradiologist, Royal Hallamshire Hospital, Sheffield, UK)

the canal (Hermans et al. 1997; Curtin 1997). Three-dimensional constructive interference in steady state (3D-CISS) sequence – a T_2* weighted refocusing three-dimensional gradient echo sequence may be useful. This uses a fast imaging with a steady precession (FISP) sequence that is performed once with alternating radiofrequency pulses and repeated with non-alternating radiofrequency pulses thereby compensating for flow irregularities in CSF, endolymph or perilymph. Hermans et al. (1997) found the sequence to be up to 98.6% sensitive and 68.9% specific for the detection of vestibular schwannomas (Held et al. 1997; Hermans et al. 1997). There is a role for these heavily T2-weighted sequences in screening investigations for vestibular schwannomas as long as the referring clinicians and radiologist are aware of the risk of missing a small number of small tumours and are prepared to carry out contrast enhanced MR scans, or follow up examinations in cases of uncertainty (Curtin 1997; Held et al. 1997). Other pathologies that could contribute to the vestibular symptoms and would have been detected as enhancing lesions on postgadolinium scans such as leukaemia; lymphoma and sarcoid will also not be detected on these non-contrast enhanced sequences.

Schwannomas of the other cranial nerves occur in a significant proportion of patients with NF2 (Fig. 18.9). MAUTNER et al. (1996) found schwannomas of the Xth and XIIth cranial nerves in 17% of patients in their study. Imaging of the head in NF2 patients should therefore include sections to demonstrate these nerves (MAUTNER et al. 1996). Pre- and postcontrast (Gd-DTPA) scans are necessary to demonstrate other intracranial tumours in NF2. Meningiomas, cranial nerve schwannomas, and ependymomas in NF2 should be monitored, since they are not always slow growing (GUTMANN et al. 1997).

Meningiomas are well-circumscribed extra-axial tumours with a wide attachment to the adjacent dura. They are usually slow growing and may contain calcifications within them, which may be visible on plain films if extensive; however, more aggressive tumours may occur in NF2. Some meningiomas have cystic components associated with them. The tumours may be associated with peritumoral oedema, which is usually minimal but may occasionally be extensive. There is no relationship between the size of the tumour and the amount of associated peritumoral cerebral oedema. The tumours enhance avidly and homogeneously postcontrast injection on MR and CT (Fig. 18.10). MR imaging is superior to CT in defining the anatomical location, vascularity, arterial encasement and venous sinus invasion of the meningiomas. On MR meningiomas are homogeneous or heterogeneous in echotexture depending on tumour vascularity, calcification and/or cystic components; and are iso/or hypointense to grey matter on T1 weighted scans and iso- to hyperintense to grey matter on T2 weighted scans (SPAGNOLI et al. 1986).

A high proportion of patients have spinal tumours (Fig. 18.10). The majority of these are schwannomas although neurofibromas, meningiomas and intramedullary tumours (mainly ependymomas but also astrocytomas) also occur. Full spinal MR imaging with and without gadolinium enhancement should be performed on all newly diagnosed NF2 patients to aid in prognostication. Where intramedullary lesions are demonstrated annual follow-up MR should be performed. However, patients with dumbbell tumours, spinal meningiomas, and cauda equina tumours can undergo imaging again if symptoms change or appear. If tumours are found, follow-up MR imaging should be performed every 6–12 months (MAUTNER et al. 1996; GUTMANN et al. 1997).

18.3.4 Stereotactic Radiosurgery Treatment of Vestibular Schwannomas

The management of vestibular schwannomas in NF2 is complicated and should probably be carried out by a multidisciplinary team of experts at specialist centres. Not only are NF2 patients at increased risk of complete deafness from bilateral vestibular schwannomas but they also commonly have associated intracranial neoplasms complicating their management. In addition, vestibular schwannomas in NF2 often encase the cochlear nerve making auditory nerve damage more likely at surgery.

The treatment options available include conservative management with close observation of the tumours and intervention on demonstration of continued tumour growth or progression of symptoms; surgical excision of the tumour and stereotactic radiosurgery. Small (<1.5 cm) intracanalicular vestibular schwannomas should probably be surgically excised since complete microsurgical removal with preservation of hearing and facial nerve function is feasible. Large tumours (>3 cm) at the cerebellopontine angle should be managed conservatively and debulked or excised when brainstem compression or loss of facial and/or hearing function develops (LINSKEY et al. 1992; GUTMANN et al. 1997).

Stereotactic radiosurgery has been shown to be effective in the treatment of vestibular schwannomas less than 3 cm in diameter (Fig. 18.11).

In their experience of 40 patients with 45 vestibular schwannomas, SUBACH et al. (1999) report tumour regression in 36%, tumour growth arrest in 62% and postradiosurgery tumour growth in 2%. With modern treatment planning methods using MR for localisation, and the reduction of surface radiation dose to the tumour while using an increased number of radiosurgical isocentres, cranial nerve damage and hearing loss have been reduced. Cranial nerve damage usually occurs within the first 2–3 years post-treatment. Hearing preservation is probably better than with surgery and even in cases where hearing loss occurs, it has a gradual onset postradiosurgery which allows the patient time to adapt psychologically to the handicap and to learn other ways of communicating such as lip reading and sign language, whereas postsurgery deafness occurs immediately. Radiosurgery induces a fibrotic reaction within the treated area; however, most reports show that this does not appear to hamper subsequent surgery in most patients. In the rare instances of tumour regrowth, it usually occurs within the first 2–3

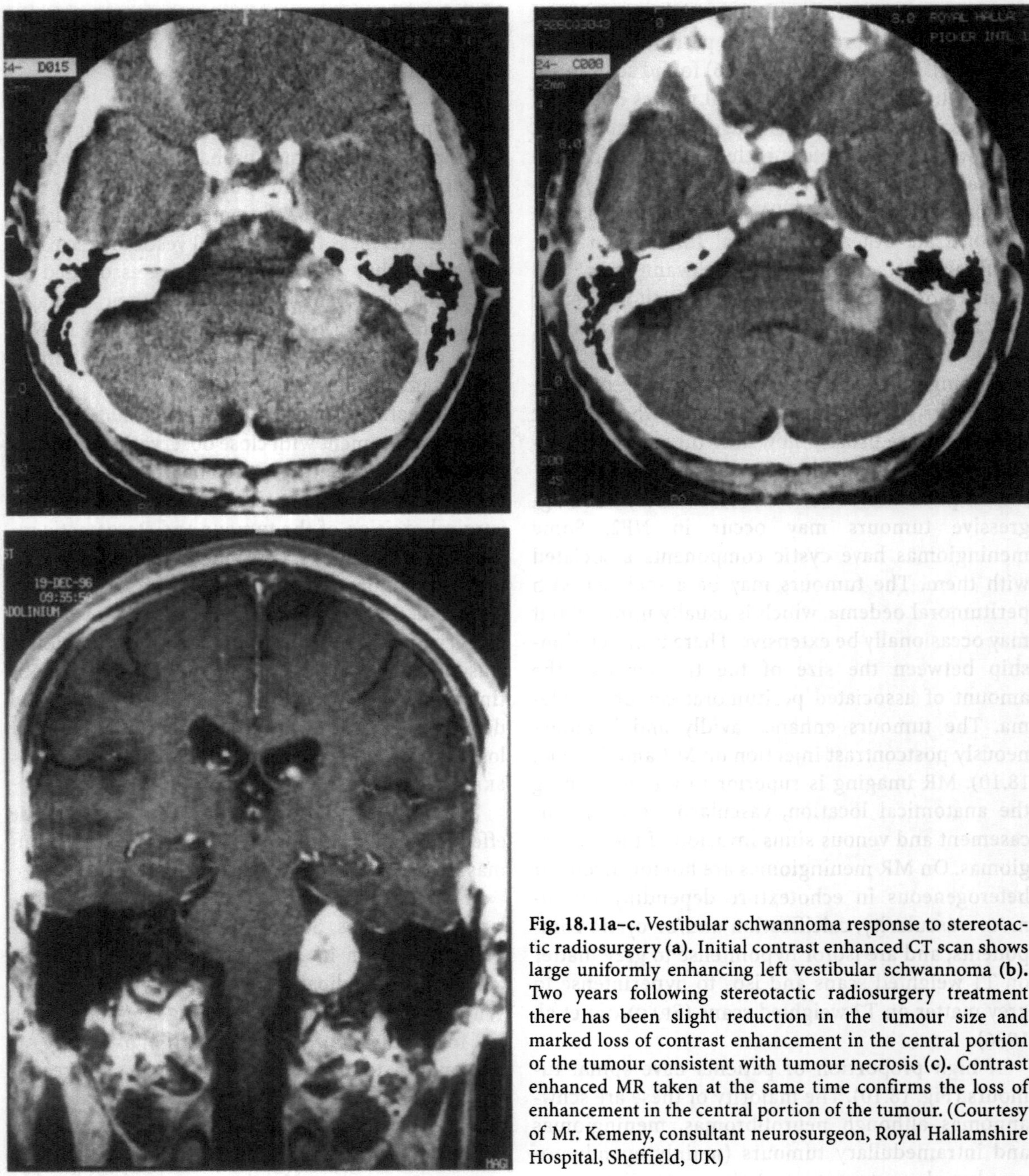

Fig. 18.11a–c. Vestibular schwannoma response to stereotactic radiosurgery (**a**). Initial contrast enhanced CT scan shows large uniformly enhancing left vestibular schwannoma (**b**). Two years following stereotactic radiosurgery treatment there has been slight reduction in the tumour size and marked loss of contrast enhancement in the central portion of the tumour consistent with tumour necrosis (**c**). Contrast enhanced MR taken at the same time confirms the loss of enhancement in the central portion of the tumour. (Courtesy of Mr. Kemeny, consultant neurosurgeon, Royal Hallamshire Hospital, Sheffield, UK)

years post-treatment (Kodziolka et al. 1998; Subach et al. 1999; Linskey et al. 1992). In view of all these factors and the fact that radiosurgery is extremely well tolerated by patients because of the significantly lower morbidity associated with it compared to surgery, stereotactic radiosurgery should probably be offered as the primary treatment modality for vestibular schwannomas less than 3 cm in diameter in NF2 patients. If the patients are followed up closely, the small number whose tumours continue to grow and those at risk of developing hydrocephalus can be identified and offered surgery (Kodziolka et al. 1998; Subach et al. 1999).

Other intracranial neoplasms in NF2 should probably not be treated by radiotherapy because of the high risk of inducing malignant transformation in the tumours in these patients who have an inactivated tumour suppressor gene (Gutmann et al. 1997).

18.4 Other Forms of Neurofibromatosis

NF1 and NF2 have considerable variability in their clinical expression but the non-classical presentations are still classified as either NF1 or NF2 and are not recognised as separate disease entities. Non-generalized forms of NF1 such as segmental distribution of neurofibromas and pigmentary lesions (café-au-lait spots, freckling, or Lisch nodules) and NF2 such as spinal neurofibromatosis occur. These are referred to as mosaic NF1 or NF2 and occur due to somatic mosaicism in which some of the cells in an affected individual harbour an NF1 or NF2 gene mutation while other cells in the same individual lack alterations in either the NF1 or NF2 gene. The genetic concern in these patients is the transmissibility of the disorder because if their germ cells are also mosaic for NF1 or NF2 then their offspring could develop classical NF1 or NF2; therefore individuals with mosaic forms of neurofibromatosis probably require more detailed genetic counselling than individuals with classic forms of NF1 or NF2 (Sloan et al. 1990).

Several families with multiple café-au-lait spots but no other clinical manifestations of NF1 have been described in the literature. Genetic analysis of these families has shown linkage to chromosome 17q where the NF1 gene resides in some families whereas other families showed no linkage to NF1 and probably represented a rare but separate disorder (Charrow et al. 1993; Abelovich et al. 1995). Because of the rarity of isolated multiple café-au-lait spots all patients with multiple café-au-lait spots should be treated as evolving NF1 (Gutmann et al. 1997).

Patients with multiple central and peripheral nervous system schwannomas (multiple schwannomatosis) but without bilateral vestibular schwannomas and do not meet diagnostic criteria for NF2 have been described. These individuals do not develop the other tumors seen in NF2 nor do they show any manifestations of NF1. Only 1 in 14 of these patients has a family history of schwannomatosis and they carry a less than 50% genetic risk of transmitting the disorder to their offspring. Genetic analysis in some of these families has failed to demonstrate consistent linkage to the NF2 gene locus. Clinically these patients are afflicted with pain arising from their schwannomas to a greater extent than is seen with either NF1 or NF2 (McCollin et al. 1996).

Families with multiple meningiomas have been reported, but this syndrome is not linked to chromosome 22q (Pulst et al. 1993). The disorder probably results from alterations in other negative growth regulators important for meningeal cell growth and differentiation.

18.5 Conclusion

Understanding of the genetic basis of the neurofibromatoses and their clinical manifestations continues to improve and it is also now possible to make confident diagnoses of NF1 or NF2 in most patients using the combination of clinical, genetic and radiological findings. Modern imaging techniques can now confidently detect intracranial lesions associated with NF1 and NF2 at their earliest and often pre-symptomatic stages. However, as treatment options available to these patients continue to improve the challenge for cheaper, faster, safer and more accurate imaging modalities for screening in these patients remains.

References

Abeliovich D, Gelman-Kohan Z, Silverstein et al. (1995) Familial café-au-lait spots: a variant of neurofibromatosis type 1. J Med Genet 32: 985–986

Aoki SA, Barkovich AJ, Nishimura K et al. (1989) Neurofibromatosis types 1 and 2: cranial MR findings. Radiology 172: 527–534

Atlas SW, Zimmerman RA, Bruce D et al. (1988) Neurofibromatosis and agenesis of the corpus callosum in identical twins: MR diagnosis. Am J Neuroradiol 9: 598–601

Balestri P, Lucignani G, Fois A et al. (1994) Cerebral glucose metabolism in neurofibromatosis type 1 assessed with [18F]-2-fluoro-2-deoxy-D-glucose and PET. J Neurol Neurosurg Psychiatry 57: 1479–1483

Braffman BH, Bilaniuk LT, Zimmerman RA (1990) MR of central nervous system neoplasia in the phakomatoses. Semin Roentgenol XXV (2): 198–217

Cappelli C, Grill J, Raquin M et al. (1998) Long term follow up of 69 patients treated for optic pathway tumours before the chemotherapy era. Arch Dis Child 79: 334–338

Cappione AJ, French BL, Skuse GR (1997) A potential role for NF1 mRNA editing in the pathogenesis of NF1 tumors [see comments]. Am J Hum Genet 60: 305–312

Castillo M, Green C, Kwock L et al. (1995) Proton MR spectroscopy in patients with neurofibromatosis type 1: evaluation of harmatomas and clinical correlation. Am J Neuroradiol 16: 141–147

Charrow J, Listernick R, Ward K (1993) Autosomal dominant multiple cafe-au-lait spots and neurofibromatosis-1: evidence of non-linkage. Am J Med Genet 45: 606–608

Cnossen MH, De Goede-Bolder A, Van den Broek KM et al. (1998) A prospective 10-year follow-up study of patients with neurofibromatosis type 1. Arch Dis Child 78: 408–412

Curtin HD (1997) Rule out eighth nerve tumor: contrast-enhanced T1-weighted or high-resolution T2-weighted MR? Am J Neuroradiol 18: 1834–1838

DiMario FJ jr, Ramsby G, Greenstein R et al. (1993) Neurofibromatosis type 1: magnetic resonance imaging findings. J Child Neurol 8: 32–39

DiMario FJ, Ramsby G (1998) Magnetic resonance imaging lesion analysis in neurofibromatosis type 1. Arch Neurol 55: 500–505

DiPaolo DP, Zimmerman RA, Rorke LB et al. (1995) Neurofibromatosis type 1: pathologic substrate of high-signal-intensity foci in the brain. Radiology 195: 721–724

Duffner PK, Cohen ME, Seidel FG et al. (1989) The significance of MRI abnormalities in children with neurofibromatosis. Neurology 39: 373–378

Elster AD (1992) Radiologic screening in the neurocutaneous syndromes: strategies and controversies. Am J Neuroradiol 13: 1078–1082

Evans DGR, Huson SM, Donnai D et al. (1992) A clinical study of type 2 neurofibromatosis. QJM 84: 603–618

Evans DGR, Trueman L, Wallace A et al. (1998) Genotype/phenotype correlations in type 2 neurofibromatosis (NF2): evidence for more severe disease associated with truncating mutations. J Med Genet 35: 450–455

Ferner RE, Chaudhuri R, Bingham J et al. (1993) MRI in neurofibromatosis 1. The nature and evolution of increased intensity T2 weighted lesions and their relationship to intellectual impairment. J Neurol Neurosurg Psychiatry 56: 492–495

Griffiths PD, Blaser S, Mukonoweshuro W, et al. (1999) T2-weighted hyperintensities in NF1 – a proliferative potential. Pediatrics (*in press*)

Guha A, Lau N, Huvar I et al. (1996) Ras-GTP levels are elevated in human NF1 peripheral nerve tumors. Oncogene 12: 507–513

Gutmann DH (1998) Recent insights into neurofibromatosis type 1: clear genetic progress. Arch Neurol 55: 778–780

Gutmann DH, Aylsworth A, Carey JC et al. (1997) The diagnostic evaluation and multidisciplinary management of neurofibromatosis 1 and neurofibromatosis 2. JAMA 278: 51–57

Habiby R, Silverman B, Listernick R et al. (1995) Precocious puberty in children with neurofibromatosis type 1. J Pediatr 126: 364–367

Harkens KH, Dolan D (1990) Correlative imaging of sphenoid dysplasia accompanying neurofibromatosis. Ann Otol Rhinol Laryngol 99: 137–141

Held P, Fellner C, Fellner F et al. (1997) MRI of inner ear and facial nerve pathology using 3D MP-RAGE and 3D-CISS sequences. BJR 70: 558–566

Hermans R, Van der Goten A, De Foer B et al. (1997) MRI screening for acoustic neuroma without gadolinium: value of 3DFT-CISS sequence. Neuroradiology 39: 593–598

Huson S, Harper PS, Compston DAS (1988) Von Recklinghausen neurofibromatosis, a clinical and population study in South East Wales. Brain 111: 1355–1381

Huson SM, Hughes RAC (1994) The neurofibromatoses. A pathogenetic and clinical overview. Chapman and Hall, London, pp 160–232

Itoh T, Magnaldi S, White RM et al. (1994) Neurofibromatosis type 1: the evolution of deep gray and white matter abnormalities. Am J Neuroradiol 15: 1513–1519

Leisti EL, Pyhtinen J, Poyhonen M (1996) Spontaneous decrease of a pilocytic astrocytoma in neurofibromatosis type 1. Am J Neuroradiol 17: 1691–1694

Lewis RA, Gerson LP, Axelson KA et al. (1984) Von Recklinghausen neurofibromatosis. Incidence of optic gliomata. Ophthalmology 91: 929–935

Listernick R, Charrow J, Greenwald M et al. (1994) Natural history of optic pathway tumours in children with neurofibromatosis type 1: a longitudinal study. J Pediatr 125: 63–66

Listernick R, Charrow J, Greenwald MJ et al. (1989) Optic gliomas in children with neurofibromatosis type 1. J Pediatr 114: 788–792

Listernick R, Darling C, Greenwald M et al. (1995) Optic pathway tumors in children: the effect of neurofibromatosis type 1 on clinical manifestations and natural history. J Pediatr 127: 718–722

Listernick R, Louis DN, Packer RJ et al. (1997) Optic pathway gliomas in children with neurofibromatosis 1: consensus statement from the NF1 optic pathway glioma task force. Ann Neurol 41: 143--149

Lovblad KO, Remonda L, Ozdoba C et al. (1994) Dural ectasia of the optic nerve sheath in neurofibromatosis type 1: CT and MR features. J Comput Assist Tomogr 18: 728–730

Martin GA, Viskochil D, Bollag G et al. (1990) The GAP-related domain of the neurofibromatosis type 1 gene product interacts with ras p21. Cell 63: 843–849

Martinez-Lage JF, Poza M, Rodriguez Costa T (1993) Bilateral temporal arachnoid cysts in neurofibromatosis. J Child Neurol 8: 383–385

Mautner VF, Lindenau M, Baser ME et al. (1996) The neuroimaging and clinical spectrum of neurofibromatosis 2. Neurosurgery 38: 880–886

Mautner VF, Lindenau M, Baser ME et al. (1997) Skin abnormalities in neurofibromatosis 2. Arch Dermatol 133: 1539–1543

Mautner VF, Schneider E, Fabra M et al. (1991) Klinische Bedeutung signalintenser Herde in der zerebralen Magnetresonanztomographie bei Neurofibromatose [Clinical relevance of signal- intense foci in cerebral magnetic resonance tomography in neurofibromatosis.(German)] Fortschr Neurol Psychiatr 59: 25–30

McCollin M, Mohney T, Trofatter J et al. (1993) DNA diagnosis of neurofibromatosis 2: altered coding sequence of the merlin tumor suppressor in an extended pedigree. JAMA 270: 2316–2320

McCollin M, Woodfin W, Kronn D et al. (1996) Schwannomatosis: a clinical and pathologic study. Neurology 46: 1072–1079

McFarlane R, Levin AV, Weksberg R et al. (1995) Absence of the greater sphenoid wing in neurofibromatosis type I: congenital or acquired: case report. Neurosurgery 37: 129–133

Menor F, Marti-Bonmati I (1992) CT detection of basal ganglion lesions in neurofibromatosis type 1: correlation with MRI. Neuroradiology 34: 305–307

Mirowitz SA, Sartor K, Gado M (1989) High-intensity basal ganglia lesions on T1- weighted MR images in neurofibromatosis. Am J Neuroradiol 10: 1159–1163

Moore BD, Slopis MD, Schomer D et al. (1996) Neuropsychological significance of high signal intensity on brain MRIs of children with neurofibromatosis. Neurology 46: 1660–1668

Morris PW, Glasier CM, Smirnioptopoulos JG et al. (1997) Disappearing enhancing brain lesion in a child with neurofibromatosis type 1. Pediatr Radiol 27: 260–261

Mukonoweshuro W, Griffiths PG, Blaser S (1999) Neurofibromatosis type 1: the role of neuroradiology. Neuropediatrics (*in press*)
Mulvihill JJ (moderator) Neurofibromatosis 1 (Recklinghausen disease) and Neurofibromatosis 2 (bilateral acoustic neurofibromatosis). An update (1990). Ann Intern Med 113: 39–52
National Institutes of Health Consensus Development Conference (1988) Neurofibromatosis conference statement. Arch Neurol 45: 575–578
North K, Joy P, Yuille D et al. (1994) Specific learning disability in children with neurofibromatosis type 1: significance of MRI abnormalities. Neurology 44: 878–883
Norton KK, Xu J, Gutmann DH (1995) Expression of the neurofibromatosis 1 gene product, neurofibromin, in blood vessel endothelial cells and smooth muscle. Neurobiol Dis 2: 13–21
Parry DM, Eldridge R, Kaiser-Kupfer MI et al. (1994) Neurofibromatosis 2 (NF2): clinical characteristics of 63 affected individuals and clinical evidence for heterogeneity. Am J Med Genet 52: 450–461
Pollack IF, Mulvihill JJ (1997) Neurofibrmatosis 1 and 2. Brain Pathol 7: 823–836
Pollack IF, Schultz B, Mulvihill JJ (1996) The management of brainstem gliomas in patients with neurofibromatosis 1. Neurology 46: 1652–1660
Pomeranz SJ, Shelton JJ, Tobias J et al (1987) MR of visual pathways in patients with neurofibromatosis. Am J Neuroradiol 8: 831–836
Rouleau GA, Merel P, Lutchman M et al. (1993) Alteration in gene encoding a putative membrane-organizing protein causes neurofibromatosis type 2. Nature 363: 515–521
Sawada S, Florell S, Purandare SM et al. (1996) Identification of NF1 mutations in both alleles of a dermal neurofibroma. Nat Genet 14: 110–112
Scoles DR, Baser ME, Pulst SM (1996) A missense mutation in the neurofibromatosis 2 gene occurs in patients with mild and severe phenotypes. Neurology 47: 544–546
Sevick RJ, Barkovich AJ, Edwards MSB et al. (1992) Evolution of white matter lesions in neurofibromatosis type 1: MR findings. Am J Roentgenol 159: 171–175
Sloan JB, Fretzin DF, Bovenmyer DA (1990) Genetic counseling in segmental neurofibromatosis. J Am Acad Dermatol 22: 461–467
Spagnoli MV, Goldberg HI, Grossman RI et al. (1986) Intracranial meningiomas: high-field MR imaging. Radiology 161: 369–375
Stephens K, Kayes L, Riccardi VM et al. (1992) Preferential mutation of the neurofibromatosis type 1 gene in paternally derived chromosomes. Hum Genet 88: 279–282
Subach BR, Kodziolka D, Lunsford LD et al. (1999) Stereotactic radiosurgery in the management of acoustic neuromas associated with neurofibromatosis type 2. J Neurosurg 90: 815–822
Tos M, Thomsen J (1984) Epidemiology of acoustic neuromas. J Laryngol Otol 98: 685–692
United Kingdom Children's Cancer Study Group (UKCCSG) and Societe d'Oncologie Pediatrique (SFOP) Panelists (1998) A protocol for imaging paediatric brain tumours. Clin Radiol *(in press)*
Van Es S, North KN, McHugh K et al. (1996) MRI findings in children with neurofibromatosis type 1: a prospective study. Pediatr Radiol 26: 478–487
Westacott S, Mohan D, Norman PF et al. (1988) MRI of vertebral arteriovenous malformations in neurofibromatosis. Br J Neurosurgery 2: 385–389
Zachos M, Parkin PC, Babyn PS et al. (1997) Neurofibromatosis type 1 vasculopathy associated with lower limb hypoplasia. Pediatrics 100: 395–398

19 Neuroradiology for Endocrine Disease

James Byrne

CONTENTS

19.1 Introduction

Patients with endocrine diseases are referred for neuroradiological investigation in order to demonstrate possible lesions of the hypothalamic-pituitary axis. Patients may also be suspected of harbouring pathology of the pituitary because of neurological symptoms and signs (such as headache, visual disturbance and bitemporal hemianopia) without evidence of an endocrine disturbance, at least initially. The imaging strategies of both types of patient are generally the same and will be covered in this chapter. In addition the diagnostic problem posed by a patient with biochemical evidence of endocrine disease includes patients with ectopic hormone production, due to a variety of causes. These will be discussed and exemplified by the investigation of patients presenting with Cushing's syndrome. Imaging is therefore directed at the sella turcica and parasellar regions but may involve sampling of the pituitary venous effluent for functional evaluation.

19.2 Imaging of Pituitary

19.2.1 Techniques

Magnetic resonance imaging (MRI) is the optimum imaging method with high quality computer tomography (CT) an acceptable alternative. The advantages of MRI are: (a) direct multiplanar scanning, (b) lack of ionising radiation and (c) good anatomical tissue discrimination, without the need for pharmaceutical contrast agents. The axial plane is a relatively poor technique for demonstrating the vertical relationships of structures lying between the floor of the IIIrd ventricle and sella turcica; therefore assessment of the pituitary and hypothalamus is easiest in the sagittal and coronal planes. MRI in these planes provides the optimum demonstration of the pituitary stalk and the relationships of intrasellar contents with the cavernous and sphenoid sinuses as well as the contents of the chiasmatic cistern. The disadvantage of MRI (apart from logistical difficulties of its availability and cost) is its relative insensitivity to pathological calcification and lack of signal from corticated bone. CT may be required to demonstrate or exclude pathological calcification and is more sensitive than plain film radiography. The only remaining role for the latter in pituitary imaging is to exclude metallic implants that might be contraindications to MRI.

Apart from its complementary role to MRI for detecting pathological calcification, CT scanning remains the primary imaging modality for a small pro-

J. Byrne, MD
Department of Neuroradiology, The Radcliffe Infirmary, Woodstock Road, Oxford, OX2 6HE, UK

portion of patients who are unable to undergo MRI because of extreme claustrophobia, cardiac pacemakers or other implants such as intracranial aneurysms, clips and traumatic metallic fragments. CT is then best performed to obtain direct coronal plane images by scanning the patient prone or supine with their neck extended. Scans acquired in this way are generally superior in quality to axial images subsequently reformatted into the coronal or sagittal planes by computer post-processing. They expose the patient and their eyes to lower doses of ionising radiation but depend on patients being able to lie still with their neck extended.

Various technical refinements to pituitary MRI have been advocated but given the enormous number of potentially useful MRI sequence protocols basic scanning methods are remarkably similar between centres. It is agreed that the structures of the sella region are best imaged using T_1-weighted (T_1W) sequences, since cerebrospinal fluid provides inherent tissue contrast with the surrounding structures. The anatomical relationships of the hypophysis, infundibulum and hypothalmus are easily identified. Using T_1W sequences the nuclei of the hypothalmus cannot be distinguished, but if phospholipid vesicles are present in the neurohypophysis they are visible as high signal areas (Kucharczyk et al. 1990). Physiological bright signal in the stalk and posterior pituitary is evident in up to 50% of T_1W head scans; its frequency declines with increasing age (Brooks et al. 1989; Wolpert et al. 1988). Temporal variations in bright signal from the neurohypophysis and its reduction in patients with diabetes insipidus suggest that it is derived from neurosecretory granules (Fujisawa et al. 1987; Mark et al. 1991). It is usually not possible to distinguish the anterior from the posterior lobes of the gland without the benefit of this specific change in magnetic property.

In practice T_1W spin echo sequences are performed with repetition times (TR) of 500–600 ms, echo times (TE) of 15 ms and two or more excitations. Scanning is performed in coronal and sagittal planes using matrix size 256×256, to give 3-mm-thick contiguous slices. Typically scanning takes 5–8 min at 1.5 T for each sequence. An alternative approach is to use a T_1W gradient echo technique with a three-dimensional (3D) Fourier synthesis so that subsequent computer manipulation allows the imaged sample to be viewed in any plane. Some centres perform both sequence types because image clarity is superior in the former but the 3D sequence allows post-processing to review and clarify any suspicious areas.

The power of MRI to resolve different structures depends on the signal-to-noise ratio (SNR) of the acquired signal. A high signal-to-noise ratio is required to detect small abnormalities and small anatomic structures. Simply increasing the matrix size, i.e. the number of pixel (or voxel) elements, won't improve the SNR, though decreasing the pixel size will improve the spatial resolution of the image. To improve the SNR and spatial resolution, it is necessary to increase the magnet gradient strengths and to acquire more data by lengthening the scan time (Kucharczyk et al. 1990). Pituitary MRI is therefore best performance in high field strength imagers using longer echo-time (TE) sequences (Scott 1996).

The need for routine intra-venous administration of paramagnetic agents, such as gadolinium, is controversial. The pituitary gland and stalk enhance whilst the hypothalamus and optic chiasm don't if the blood-brain barrier is intact. Surrounding blood vessels, meninges and the mucosa of the paranasal sinuses all enhance. On T1 W MRI it is normally easy to identify these structures. The same is not true of CT and intravenous injection of iodinated contrast media has been advocated to improve tissue contrast. CT, unlike MRI, can't distinguish blood flow without contrast agents, nor intracranial arteries and veins. After contrast enhancement, intra-dural arteries can be differentiated on CT but similar enhancement levels of arterial and venous blood within the cavernous sinus prevent demonstration of the intracavernous carotid arteries as separate structures. Fast MRI sequences have been used to study the timing of intravenously administered gadolinium uptake by the hypophysis. So called dynamic scans are obtained at 20–30 s intervals and have been used to demonstrate that the stalk and posterior lobe enhance 20 s after gadolinium injection and that enhancement extends into the anterior portion of the gland within 80 s (Sakamoto et al. 1991). Dynamic scanning has been developed as a means of increasing detection rates of microadenomas. Its role and that of gadolinium enhanced MRI in the investigation of different pathologies will be considered below.

The disadvantages of CT over MRI should not be exaggerated. Radiation exposure is a definite concern when an individual undergoes multiple follow-up scans but the accuracy of CT is similar to MRI for diagnosis of macroadenoma (Buchfelder et al. 1992). It will provide virtually all the pre-operative data for transphenoidal hypophysectomy, including the bony structure of the ethmoid and sphenoid sinuses, though not an accurate assessment of the position of the carotid arteries. Pre-operative angiography may then be necessary and angiography should always be considered when CT raises the possibility of a thrombosed aneurysm (RICHMOND et al. 1980). Intra-arterial angiography is now virtually obsolete since MR and CT angiography (MRA, CTA) are capable of identifying the positions of the intracavernous and supra-clinoid carotid arteries and differentiate pituitary mass lesions from aneurysms. Very rarely the diagnoses of a substantially thrombosed aneurysm requires intra-arterial digital subtraction angiography (IA-DSA). Angiography continues to have a role during catheter navigation for venous sampling in patients being investigated for causes of Cushing's syndrome (see below).

19.2.2 Macroadenoma

Adenoma larger than 1 cm in maximum diameter are conventionally classified as macroadenomas irrespective of their endocrine characteristics. The role of imaging is to identify the cause of an endocrine disturbance, to accurately localise the tumour for surgical or radiotherapy planning and to assist in the decision to treat by surgical or medical means. It is therefore directed at identifying tumour and its extent. In cases of non-functioning adenoma, patients may present with symptoms of hypopituitarism with signs of a parasellar mass lesion, and the differential diagnosis includes other causes of sella region masses.

The imaging features of pituitary tumours producing different hormones are similar. On CT adenomas are isodense or hypodense relative to brain tissue and show variable patterns of enhancement after radiographic contrast media administration (DAVIS et al. 1985). On MRI signal return is typically similar to that of brain on both T_1W and T_2W sequences. Cysts or areas of necrosis cause foci of moderate hypointensity on T_1W and hyperintensity on T_2W sequences and heterogeneous enhancement with gadolinium. They can't be distinguished on CT (DAVIS et al. 1985) or MRI (LUNDIN et al. 1992b). Signal due to haemorrhage is more specific but temporally variable because the magnetic effects of iron within red blood cells change as they break up and haemoglobin degrades. In general these are best appreciated on T_1W MRI since within days of haemorrhage concentrations of methaemoglobin increase in areas of haemorrhage causing T_1 recovery time shortening and bright signal on this sequence (DOOMS et al. 1986). In the acute period after haemorrhage (less than 3 days) MRI changes are non-specific but acute haemorrhage is hyperdense on CT. As haematomas liquidify in the next 2–3 weeks, their density reduces and they become hypodense on CT. Methaemoglobin and haemosiderin can persist for months in the brain so that chronic haemorrhage is easily identified but the temporal evolution of haemorrhage within pituitary adenomas is unknown because bleeding may be asymptomatic (WAKAI et al. 1981) (Fig. 19.1). KURIHARA et al. (1998) recently studied the MRI characteristics of intratumoural cavities identified pre-operatively and correlated these with operative findings. Repeat haemorrhage was demonstrated in some tumours and 12 of 14 cysts judged as non-haemorrhagic on MRI contained haemorrhagic components. The incidence of intratumoural haemorrhage is therefore probably underestimated on imaging. Fluid levels, with high signal supernatant, were evident on T_1W MRI in the pituitary haemorrhages studied by LENTHALL et al. (1999), who attributed this finding to extracellular methaemoglobin. These patients were therefore scanned in the subacute or chronic phase after bleeding and rarely gave a history of pituitary apoplexy. The T_1 shortening or paramagnetic effect of methaemoglobin is simulated by fat and some tumour products secreted by lesions such as craniopharyngioma, with which it may be confused, though the scan appearances of tumours in patients presenting acutely with pituitary apoplexy will usually reflect the extent of haemorrhage and/or necrosis and gadolinium enhancement will occur at the margins of necrotic areas.

There have been attempts to correlate the imaging features of pituitary tumours with hormonal activity. Features such as tumour size, evidence of local invasion, CT density and MRI signal have been studied. LUNDIN et al. (1992b) found signal intensity in non-haemorrhagic and non-cystic areas of tumour to be similar for prolactin (PRL) and growth hormone (GH) secreting tumours. In this series of 115 patients, haemorrhage and invasion of the skull base was more common with PRL secreting tumours (Fig. 19.2). MR spectroscopy is capable of measuring fundamental chemical characteristics but does not give hormone specific information (ARNOLD et al. 1991). Though given the accuracy of biochemical assays and the frequency of mixed hormone adenomas the need to make the distinction on imaging is debatable. Its more important contribution to patient management is accurate delineation of tumour extent and effect on adjacent structures.

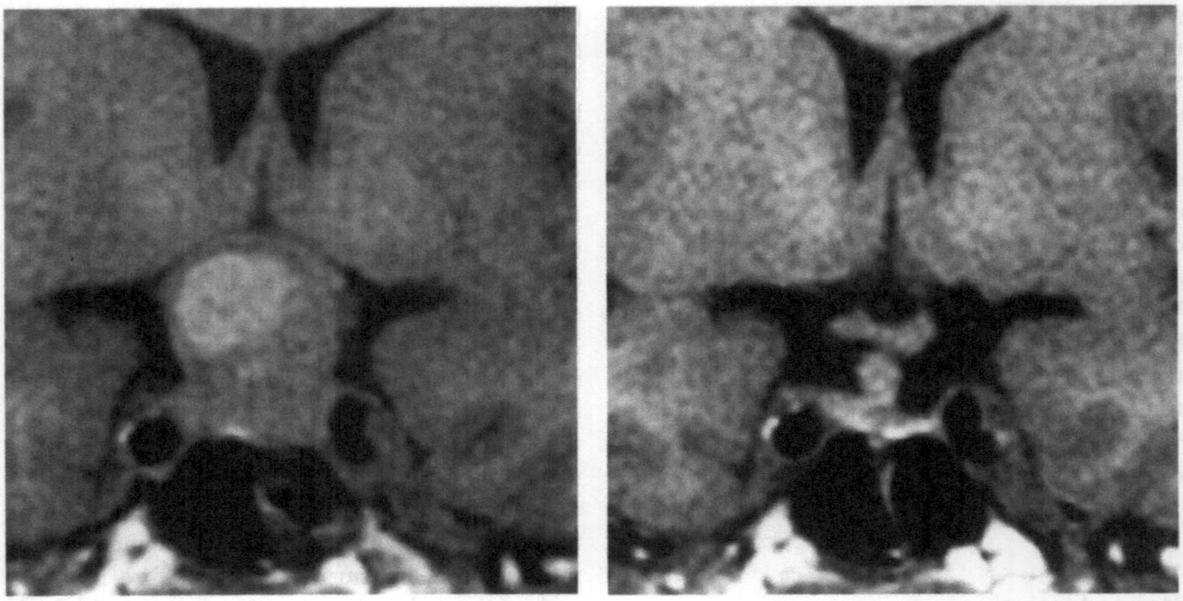

Fig. 19.1a,b. Coronal TIW MRI, showing a large prolactinoma before (a) and after surgical resection (b). The tumour returned mixed signal due to a haemorrhagic component. In this case intratumoural haemorrhage was asymptomatic

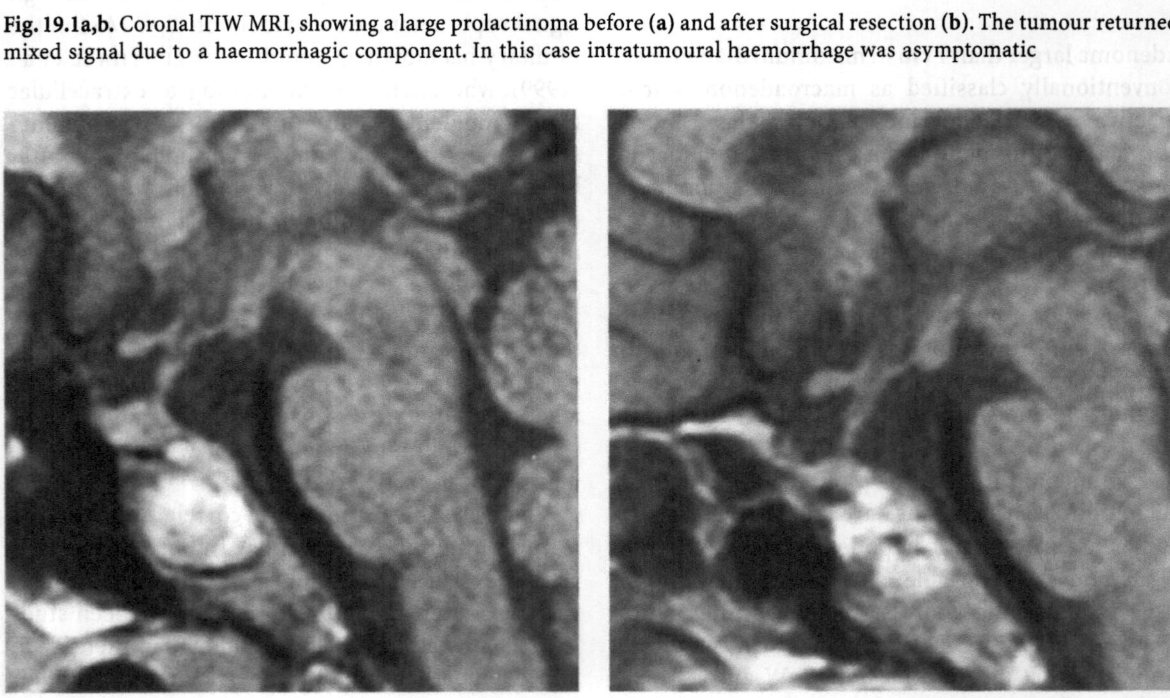

Fig. 19.2a,b. Sagittal TIW MRI before (a) and after (b) transphenoidal tumour resection. At surgery a prolactin secreting adenoma was found to have invaded the clivus

Pre-operative MRI should help the surgeon by differentiating tumour from normal gland and by identifying likely areas of local invasion. Tumour invasion of the cavernous sinus, sphenoid bone and extension into the chiasmatic cistern are evident on MRI. Such behaviour has been identified surgically and histologically in all tumour types (Scheithauer et al. 1986). Local invasion is evident on surgical examination in 35–40% of tumours (Scheithauer et al. 1986) but is found nearly twice as frequently on microscopic examination (Selman et al. 1986). It is more likely with increasing tumour size (Selman et al. 1986) and has obvious implications for the patient's prognosis. Scotti et al. (1988) studied the MRI features useful in the pre-operative diagnosis of cavernous sinus invasion. Encasement of the carotid artery was the most specific sign of cavernous sinus invasion. They correctly identified cavernous sinus involvement in 10 of 11 macroadenomas but in only 2 of 13 microadenomas. Asymmetry of the cavernous sinuses, displacement of their lateral walls and of the carotid arteries were inconsistent features of invasion. They found an indistinct medial sinus wall an unreliable sign, being common in controls. Administration of gadolinium is helpful in identifying normal pituitary gland and distinguishing it from tumour (STEINER et al. 1994).

How effective is imaging in defining residual or recurrent tumour after hypophysectomy? The timing of post-operative scanning is important since early post-surgical changes due to local swelling (in the first 1–2 weeks) and surgical packing materials, used in the transphenoidal exposure, may show little reduction in the mass of a pituitary tumour (DINA et al. 1993). Gelfoam packing material returns hypointense or hyperintense signal and enhances on early post-operative MRI after gadolinium. Its reabsorption takes 4–15 months and can be monitored on serial scans (STEINER et al. 1992). Biological packing material returns mixed signal with fat being hyperintense and muscle isointense on T_1W MRI. Re-expansion of the normal pituitary gland and reabsorption of packing material is usually evident on follow-up scans at 3 months. Early scanning is therefore only useful to investigate possible surgical complications and scanning to identify residual tumour is best delayed for at least 3 months. The signal returned by residual tumour is usually the same as that of tumour at presentation but gadolinium enhancement is less helpful at distinguishing it from normal gland after operation (DINA et al. 1993). In the longer term downward herniation of the chiasm and optic recess of the third ventricle may be evident but this finding does not correlate with the severity of any visual symptoms (KAUFMAN et al. 1989).

Imaging has a continuing role in follow-up of treated patients. Demonstration of tumour regression or recurrence relies on comparisons between follow-up scans. The protocol for post-operative follow-up imaging in Oxford is for a baseline study to be obtained 4 months after hypophysectomy followed by interval MRI 12 months and 5 years later. More frequent scans are obtained if the patient's visual fields change or histological examination of the resected tumour suggests local invasiveness. Patients treated medically for functional macroadenomas are also monitored by serial imaging, in combination with biochemical and clinical follow up assessments. A reduction in the size of prolactin secreting macroadenomas after treatment with dopamine agonists may be accompanied by haemorrhage and therefore changes in signal returned by the tumour on MRI (LUNDIN et al. 1992a). Growth hormone secreting tumours may also shrink in response to treatment with somatostatin analogues but this is less consistent and changes of necrosis or haemorrhage are infrequent. Reductions in tumour size can be demonstrated within weeks (LUCAS-MORANTE et al. 1994) but continued shrinkage has been documented up to 3 years after starting treatment (LUNDIN et al. 1997). Early follow up imaging is therefore useful to document tumour response. A base-line study is obtained when the patient starts treatment and is then repeated 3 and 12 months later. Subsequent imaging is performed with regard to the response to therapy and dictated by the clinical and biochemical findings.

19.2.3 Microadenomas

In most patients the presence of a microadenoma is assumed from biochemical testing and imaging is undertaken to confirm an intrasella source and to guide its transphenoidal excision. To identify adenomas less than 10 mm in size demands the highest standards of imaging technique and interpretation. Microadenomas show little inherent contrast to normal pituitary tissue on CT and scanning requires intravenous radiographic contrast agents to demonstrate non-enhancement of the microadenoma against a background of normal gland enhancement. On MRI, microadenomas are typically hypointense relative to normal gland on T_1W sequences and this inherent contrast may or may not be amplified by scanning after enhancement with intravenous gadolinium (Fig. 19.3).

It is generally accepted that scanning is best performed in the coronal plane and largely accepted that MRI is the modality of choice. JOHNSON et al. (1992) prospectively evaluated CT and MRI in a group of patients with suspected microadenomas and clearly showed that MRI was more accurate. The strength of their conclusion lies in the study's methodology which was designed to answer the clinical question: which modality should be used to investigate the suspected microadenoma patient? Whereas most other studies compare detection rates on MRI and CT retrospectively against surgical or histological diagnoses. However, it is wrong to conclude that CT is markedly inferior to MRI and it continues to have advocates (WU and THUOMAS 1995) since cur-

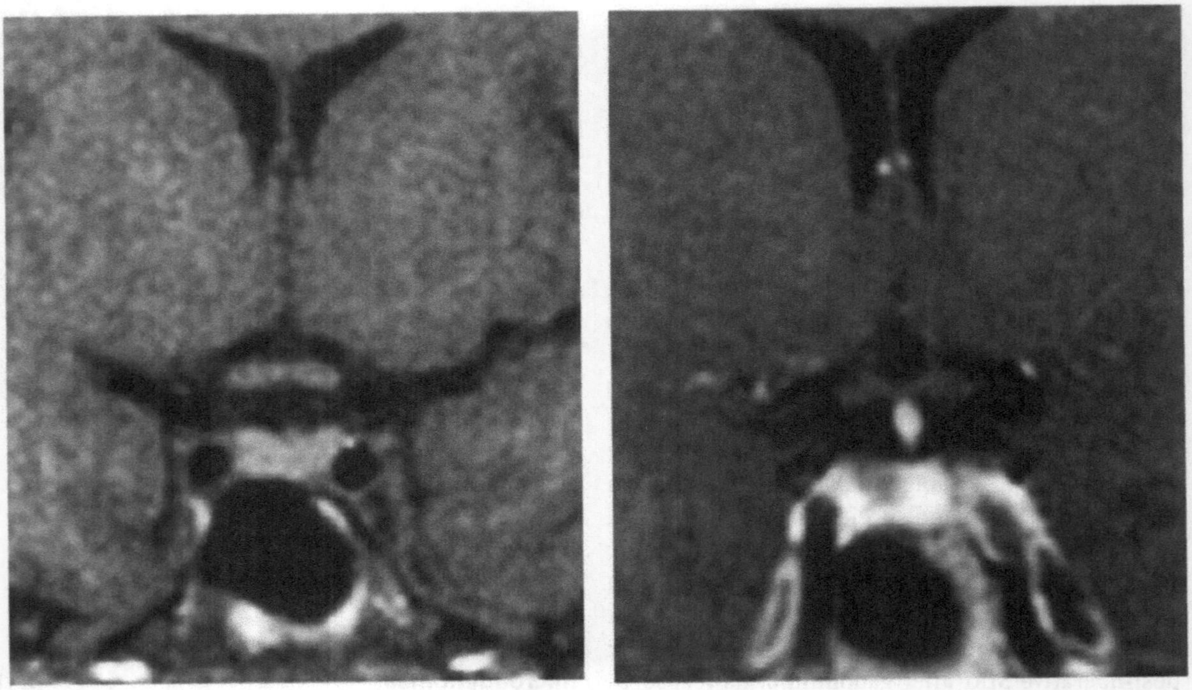

a b

Fig. 19.3a,b. Coronal T1 W MRI before (**a**) and after (**b**) gadolinium enhancement (T1W-GD). A microadenoma in the right side of the sella is isointense with normal gland before gadolinium administration but is evident as a hypointense fucus surrounded by hyperintense tissue after enhancement

rent scanners are capable of 1.5 mm scan planes and it remains superior to MRI at delineating bone.

The need for high precision scanning has stimulated research to develop better MRI techniques. A coronal T_1W sequence with gadolinium, performed at 1.5 Tesla, has a sensitivity of 80% or better (Kucharczyk et al. 1986; Peck et al. 1989). Most centres perform scans in the coronal and sagittal planes with or without gadolinium enhancement. A 3D volume scan has the theoretical advantage of allowing post-processing of images in different planes, higher resolutions and better signal to noise ratios but adds to the overall scan time. Techniques such as 3D-SPGR (Wu and Thuomas 1995) and 3D-FLASH (Stadnik et al. 1990) have demonstrated the utility of this approach. The value of conventional intravenous gadolinium enhancement is controversial; there are reports of improved sensitivity (Doppman et al. 1988; Davis et al. 1987) and the converse (Dwyer et al. 1987). Davis et al. (1987) found gadolinium useful when scanning patients at 0.5 Tesla but the benefit is less apparent when scanning on higher field strength imagers (Stadnik et al. 1990).

An alternative approach to increase the detection rate for microadenoma is dynamic MRI. This technique employs rapid sequential imaging to show temporal differences in gadolinium uptake between adenoma and normal gland. In this way microadenomas which enhance shortly after normal gland enhancement can be identified. Early studies showed that normal pituitary enhanced before adenomas (Miki et al. 1990), and, using region of interest analysis, that enhancement of the posterior lobe preceded the anterior lobe (Sakamoto et al. 1991). Recently using faster acquisition times (5–10 s per image) Yuh et al. (1994) found that macroadenoma enhanced at the same time as the posterior lobe and before the anterior lobe suggesting that they have a direct blood supply. Dynamic scanning with various fast imaging techniques has been used to identify microadenomas not detected on conventional MRI (Kucharcayk et al. 1994; Davis et al. 1994). Kucharczyk et al. (1994) identified 3 microadenomas in 18 patients on dynamic imaging, which had not been evident on conventional imaging. However they also reported false positive results in 4 of 13 controls. A similar experience was reported by Tabarin et al. (1998) for the detection of microadenomas in patients with Cushing's disease. However, the improved sensitivity (67% compared with 52%) enjoyed by dynamic MRI was offset by reduced specificity (80% versus 100%) compared to conventional MRI (Tabarin et al. 1998). The sensitivity of unenhanced high resolution MRI for pituitary microadenoma is in the order of 60–80%. Conventional scanning with contrast enhancement detects 5–10% more lesions and dynamic scanning a further 5–10% of lesions (Elster 1994). Detection rate can thus be improved but at the expense of a higher false positive rate.

The problems associated with imaging at this level are both technical and biological. Technically dynamic MRI demands the maximum of man and machine, and both can be frustrated by the occurrence of small co-incidental pituitary lesions, so-called incidentalomas (Elster 1994). An autopsy study found asymptomatic small lesions in 27% of normal glands (Burrow et al. 1981) but a more recent report estimated their incidence at only 6% (Teramoto et al. 1994). Such lesions may cause imaging features that are interpreted as microadenomas, for example, Chong et al. (1994) found focal hypointensities in the pituitary glands of 38% of normal volunteers using unenhanced MRI and Ahmadi et al. (1992) found stalk deviation on MRI in 46% of normal subjects. That such "lesions" exist, whatever their incidence, means that we are unlikely to ever achieve 100% specificity rates on imaging alone.

Furthermore it can be argued that there is no need to expend imaging resources in the search for a microadenoma when patients will be treated without surgery. In such patients the role of imaging is simply to exclude a macroadenoma which has the potential to cause compression symptoms, though it is logical to attempt to identify the cause of a patient's endocrine disturbance. MRI may therefore not be the best method of screening patients with hyperprolactinaemia. Sawers et al. (1997) compared the usefulness of imaging by MRI to functional testing using a dopamine antagonist (domperidone). The incidence of MRI detectable microadenomas in hyperprolactinaemic patients with a normal PRL response was only 10%, whilst microadenomas were detected in 63% of patients with abnormal responses. Since a quarter of their patients had normal responses to this test and most patients with hyperprolactinaemia are treated without surgery they proposed that MRI be reserved for patients who showed an abnormal response to domperidone. Furthermore larger tumours are associated with higher levels of PRL. Rand et al. (1996) found that detection rates by MRI and the size of PRL secreting adenomas was proportional to serum PRL levels. It is therefore important that imaging protocols should be designed as part of an overall management strategy for patients presenting with endocrine disease.

19.3 Imaging of Other Intracranial Causes of Endocrine Diseases

The pituitary fossa and suprasella regions are sites of a gamut of non-pituitary tumours that may cause endocrine disturbances by virtue of being located within or close to the hypothalamic-pituitary axis. The differential diagnosis of such tumours will be discussed and then craniopharyngioma and Rathke's cleft cyst considered in further detail.

19.3.1 Non-Pituitary Tumours of the Suprasellar and Parasellar Regions

The pre-operative differentiation of sellar and parasellar masses relies principally on imaging. The most common problem is to distinguish pituitary macroadenomas from craniopharyngiomas, meningioma and rarer causes of tumour in this region, since clinical symptoms and signs may be unhelpful, with the exceptions of diabetes insipidus and precocious puberty which suggest hypothalmic involvement. The imaging differential is best considered by study of the effect of a mass lesion on the optic chiasm. Thus lesions that arise above the chiasm include ependymoma, craniopharyngioma, haemangioblastoma, glioma (usually astrocytoma), hamartoma of the hypothalamus and lipoma. Ependymoma and haemangioblastoma may arise within the anterior part of the IIIrd venticle (Black et al. 1991) and Morrison et al. (1984) reported 5 intraventricular craniopharyngiomas in a series of 73 intraventricular tumours. Involvement of the hypothalmus by hamartoma, glioma, terratoma or lipoma causes precocious puberty (Taveras 1996). Local pressure effects from optic chiasm tumour or an arachnoid cyst may also cause precocious puberty (Reith et al. 1987). In children with precocious puberty hypothalamic hamartoma will be the cause in a third of cases though paradoxically larger hamartomas are less likely to cause this endocrine disturbance (Hubbard and Egelhoff 1989). Unlike other tumours in the region of the hypothalamus, hamartomas are isodense on CT and isointense on MRI relative to grey matter (Fig. 19.4). They also don't calcify or enhance after administration of intravenous contrast media and thereby can usually be distinguished from craniopharyngioma and glioma.

The optic chiasm will be depressed by lesions arising in the floor of the third ventricle and elevated

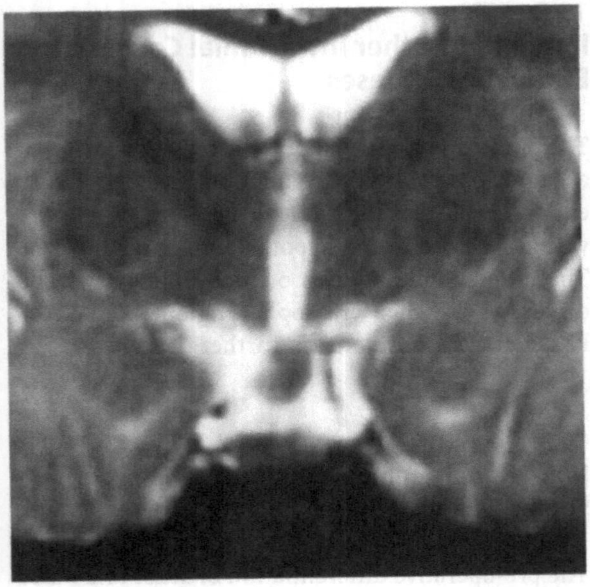

Fig. 19.4. Coronal T2 W MRI showing a mass arising from the hypothalamus and extending into chiasmatic cistern. This child presented with precocious puberty and a hamartoma of the hypothalamus was diagnosed

by suprasellar extension of intrasellar or parasellar tumours. The latter include meningioma, aneurysm, schwannoma (particularly of the trigeminal nerve), chordoma, chondrosarcoma, lymphoma and metastases. These lesions should be considered in the differential diagnosis of pituitary macroadenomas as well as the rarer tumours of the neurohypophysis: pilocystic astrocytoma and granular cell tumour (also known as choristoma). Imaging must distinguish intracranial aneurysm and the possibility of this diagnosis was, prior to MRI, an indication for pre-operative intra-arterial angiography. Blood flow in an aneurysm sac should be evident on MRI which can be supplemented by MR angiography. However if doubt remains, and this may be the case if an aneurysm if substantially thrombosed, intra-arterial angiography should be performed. Meningioma in this region may be parasella and invade the cavernous sinus or arises from the tuberculum sellae (Fig. 19.5). CT may show calcification but MRI is best at defining tumour extent. Meningiomas typically enhance homogeneously after gadolinium administration (Cappabianca et al. 1999). Primary tumours arising in the sphenoid bone and clivus, such as chordoma, giant cell tumour and chondrosarcoma, or carcinomas arising in the nasopharynx, are associated with bone destruction, calcification and a variable degree of enhancement. They may simulate bone invasion by pituitary macroadenoma. Imaging by CT and MRI is helpful, since the former will demonstrate bone erosion and the latter the effect of tumour mass on adjacent tissues. Intrasellar or suprasellar metastases should always be considered in the differential since their CT and MRI appearance is variable and they can be indistinguishable from other tumour types (Fig. 19.6). They may cause symptoms due to diabetes insipidus, or hypopituitarism, and the most common primary tumours are breast and lung (Akio et al. 1998).

Finally, tumours may arise in the chiasmatic cistern and simulate suprasellar extension of a macroadenoma. The differential diagnosis includes: optic nerve glioma, meningioma, craniopharyngioma, aneurysm and metastasis. Again MRI has made a substantial contribution to refining the pre-operative diagnosis in this region. The key lies in its ability

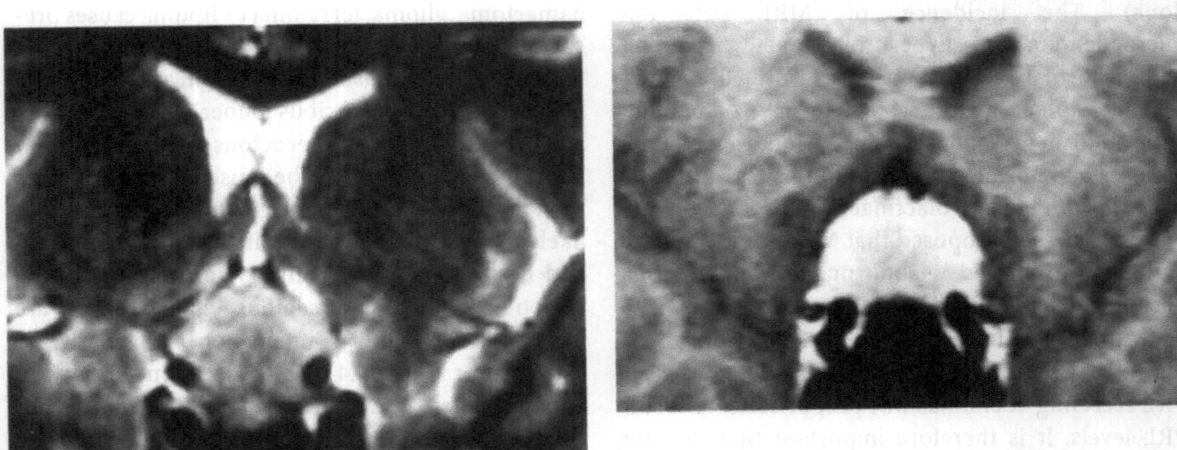

a b

Fig. 19.5a,b. Coronal T2 W (**a**) and T1W-GD (**b**) MRI showing an intensely enhancing meningioma arising from the planum sphenoidale. The tumour is elevating the anterior communicating artery and extends over the diaphragma sella (**a**) to identify the anterior optic pathway and thereby distinguish optic nerve glioma from extra-axial tumour. This largely depends on using T_1W coronal images to follow the pathway from optic nerves to tracts. SUMIDA et al. (1998) found that the optic nerves, chiasm and tracts could be visualised in over 84% of patients with pituitary adenoma, craniopharyngioma or Rathke's cleft cyst. The chiasm and tracts could be identified in 85% of 14 patients with meningioma but in only 50% were the optic nerves visible, reflecting the frequent anterior location of this tumour (Fig. 19.6). Contrast media is useful for the identification of meningioma and metastases. Optic nerve glioma involving the chiasm rarely enhances and the imaging diagnosis depends on identifying enlargement of the optic pathway since this tumour spreads transneurally. Other features of neurofibromatosis type I are evident in a quarter of patients with optic nerve gliomas, so imaging should include the whole cranium (PONT and ELSTER 1992). Optic nerve and chiasm gliomas are usually isointense to grey matter on T_1W and isointense or hyperintense on T_2W sequences. Involvement of the optic tracts and tumour extension into brain parenchyma is often associated with hyperintense signal on T_2W sequences. Unless tumours are large it is usually possible to identify CSF separating chiasm tumours from the diaphragma sella and so exclude there being suprasellar extensions of an intrasellar mass (Fig. 19.7).

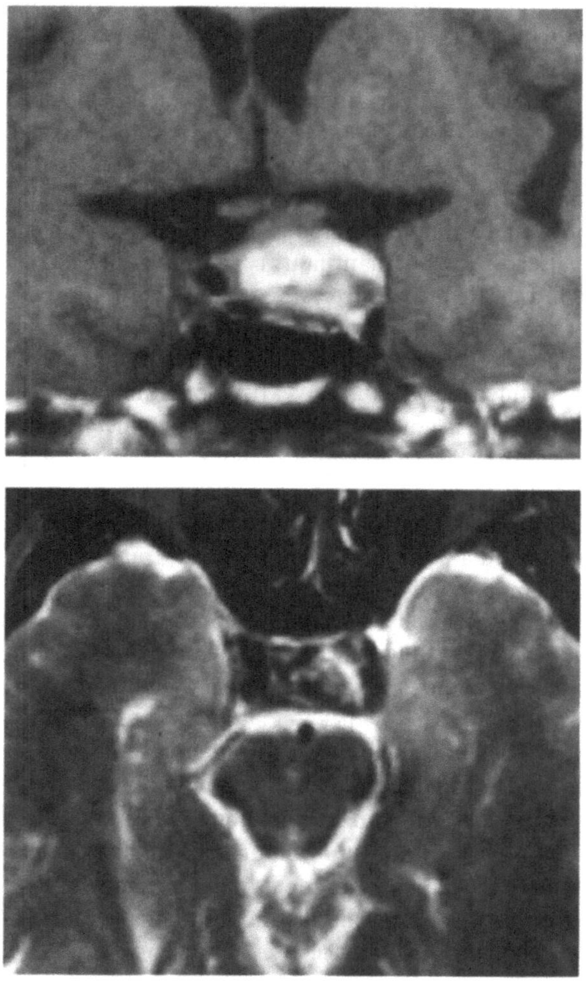

a

b

Fig. 19.6a,b. Coronal T1 W (a) and axial T2 W (b) MRI of an intrasella melanoma metastasis. The tumour contains paramagnetic melanin that causes its hyperintense signal on T1 W MRI. Normal pituitary gland is seen displaced superiorly and lying against the optic chiasm (a)

Nuclear medicine techniques such as positron emission tomography (PET) or single-photon emission tomography (SPECT) have been used to obtain in vivo characterisation of pituitary tissue and to differentiate it from other neoplasms. The presence of octreotide-binding somatostatin receptors in non-functioning adenomas cause them to take up ^{111}In-DTPA-octreotide (KRENNING et al. 1993) but meningiomas may also express somatostatin receptors and take up somatostatin receptor specific isotopes (LAMBERTS et al. 1991). However, tracers that bind to the enzyme monoamino oxidase b have been used to differentiate meningioma from pituitary adenoma using PET (BERGSTRÖM et al. 1992) and more recently a D_2 dopamine receptor specific isotope, [^{18}F]fluoroethyl-spiperone, to differentiate non-functioning adenomas from craniopharyngioma and meningioma (LUCIGNANI et al. 1997). PET using tracers such as [^{18}F]fluorodeoxyglucose and [^{11}C]methionine can be used to study rates of glucose metabolism and protein synthesis. It can be used to assess tumours after treatment by differentiating viable tumour from scar and monitoring pharmacological treatments (MUHR et al. 1988). However, the current availability of scanners limits the use of PET to selected patients and research.

19.3.2 Craniopharyngioma

Craniopharyngioma arise from remnants of Rathke's pouch. The pouch forms part of the intermediate part of the anterior lobe and pars tuberalis anterior to the pituitary stalk (TAVERAS 1996). They represent approximately 3% of all intracranial tumours, with an incidence of 0.13/100,000 person years in the USA (BUNIN et al. 1998). A modest male predominance (1.3:1) has been reported in the UK (RAJAN et al. 1993) but equal incidences between the sexes have been reported from the USA and Finland (BUNIN et

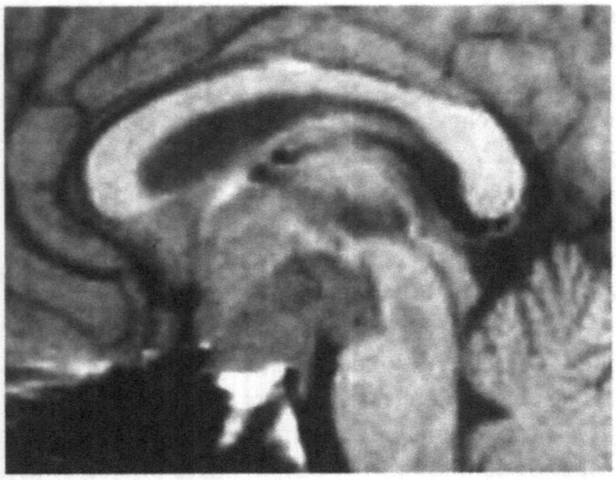

Fig. 19.7. Sagittal T1 W MRI showing a large optic nerve glioma filling the chiasmatic cistern, elevating the brain and extending posteriorly to displace the brain stem. This indolent tumour has eroded the planum sphenoidale and the dorsum sella

al. 1998). The peak age at diagnosis is 5–15 years with a second peak in late middle age (55–75 years). This bimodal age distribution of incidence has been linked to histological tumour variants: an adamantinuous type being commoner in children and young adults and a squamous-papillary type in older patients (KAHN et al. 1973; ADAMSON et al. 1990). Approximately 50% of patients present under the age of 20 years and calcification is commoner in younger patients; being demonstrable in 70% of tumours (TAVERAS 1996). Tumour usually occurs above the sella, with 5% purely intrasellar, 20% purely suprasellar and 75% both intra and extrasellar (HARWOOD-NASH 1994). The 5-year survival reported in a recent study of their epidemiology was 80% (BUNIN et al. 1998).

The imaging appearance of craniopharyngioma depends on how much of the tumour is cystic and how much solid (Fig. 19.8). Typically tumours have a relatively circumscribed outline, cystic areas don't enhance but they may be septated with thick enhancing walls whereas solid elements do enhance. Calcification patterns vary from solid lumps to popcorn-like foci or less commonly an eggshell pattern lining the wall of a cyst. In addition to calcification these tumours may contain paramagnetic substances which shorten T1 recovery time. Craniopharyngioma cysts contain, variously, cholesterol, triglycerides, methaemoglobin and desquamated epithelium. High concentrations of protein or methaemoglobin affect the MRI signal and produce the characteristic T_1W hyperintensity of a paramagnetic substance.

Imaging protocols therefore need to include both CT and MR scanning. Craniopharyngiomas on CT are typically of mixed alternatively with or without calcification. Routine enhancement with intravenous contrast media is not recommended, unless MRI is contraindicated, since areas of enhancement are best interpreted on MRI performed in multiple planes. Contrast enhancement improves tumour definition from normal structures (HALD et al. 1994). The signal of solid tumour is isointense or hypointense relative to brain on pre-contrast T_1W sequences and enhances after gadolinium. On T_2W sequences it is usually of mixed hypo- or hyperintensity. Larger areas of calcification are usually hypointense on both T_1W and T_2W sequences. Cysts are hyperintense on T_2W and hypointense on T_1W sequences but if they contain paramagnetic substances, particularly breakdown products of haemoglobin, this pattern will be reversed or they appear hyperintense on both T_2W and T_1W sequences.

There have been attempts to correlate the heterogeneous MRI appearances with the two histological variants. SARTORETTI-SCHEFER et al. (1997) compared the scans of 42 patients with histologically proven craniopharyngioma and described typical patterns. The adamantinous type were either mixed solid-cystic or mainly cystic tumours with hyperintense cysts on T_1W MRI. The squamous-papillary type was solid or mixed solid-cystic tumours with hypointense cysts on T_1W MRI. Some imaging features were useful to distinguish the two histological variants. These were: encasement of vessels, a lobulated shape and hyperintense cyst signal for the adamantinous type and a round shape, hypointense cysts and a predominantly solid appearance for the squamous-papillary type. Calcification was commoner in the adamantinous tumour but not discriminatory. However, others have not found such imaging features to correlate with the patient's age, or tumour type (WEINER et al. 1994; ELDEVIK et al. 1996). Though apparently contradictory reports may be due to some series containing higher proportions of tumours with mixed histology (ELDEVIK et al. 1996). Furthermore the importance of histological type to the patients prognosis remains controversial (PETITO 1996) and the distinction is not related to the chance of recurrence after surgical excision.

MRI with and without contrast enhancement is the modality of choice for patient follow-up after treatment with surgery and/or radiotherapy. The timing of examinations should be dictated by the

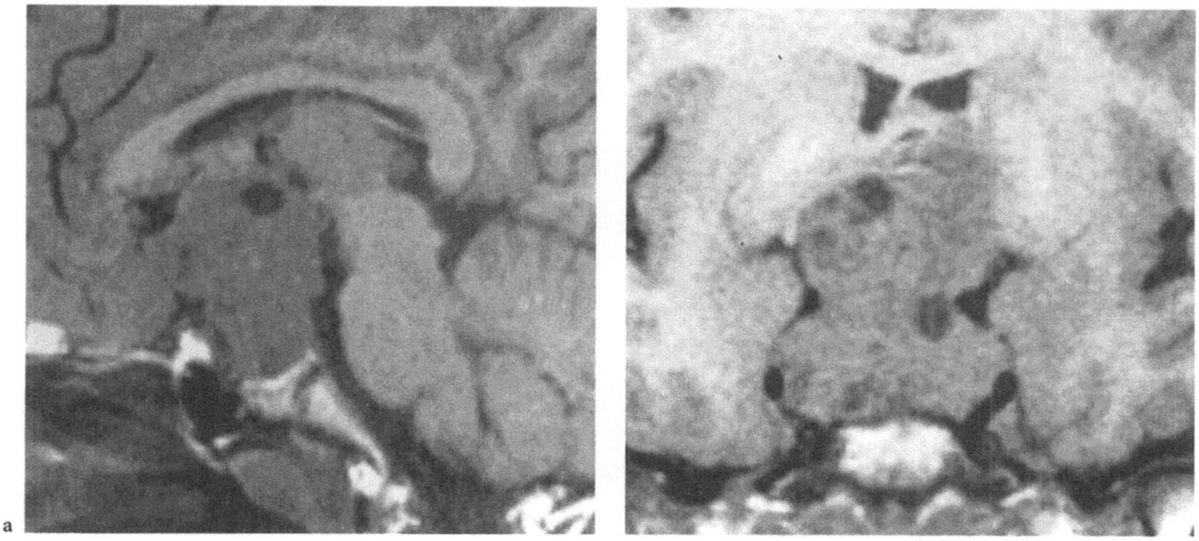

Fig. 19.8a,b. Sagittal (**a**) and coronal (**b**) TIW MRI showing a large dumbbell shaped tumour enlarging the pituitary fossa and filling the chiasmatic cistern. The tumour is generally of similar signal to that of brain but contains areas of hypointense which resemble cysts rather than areas of necrosis. Fluid filled cysts were found at surgery. The histological diagnosis was craniopharyngioma

extent of surgical resection and clinical findings. MRI may show unsuspected residual tumour elements and early post-operative scanning is useful in establishing a baseline for follow-up imaging (HALD et al. 1996). Similarly after radiotherapy tumour response can be documented on MRI 5% (ELDEVIC et al. 1998).

19.3.3 Rathke's Cleft Cysts

Symptomatic Rathke's cleft cysts are pathological enlargements of remnant of Rathke's pouch which typically arise between the two lobes of the pituitary. Small intrasellar cysts are benign incidental autopsy findings (SHANKLIN 1951) but enlargement of a cyst within the sella may cause symptoms due to compression of the pituitary gland, or if they expand into the chiasmatic cistern, compression of the anterior optic pathways. Cysts are lined by cuboidal or columnar epithelium and contain a variety of fluid types, which at surgery has the consistency of CSF, "motor-oil" or a milky fluid (SUMIDA et al. 1994).

The imaging characteristics of Rathke's cleft cysts depend on their location and contents. They can be similar to those of non-calcified craniopharyngiomas (KUCHARCZYK et al. 1987) or a suprasellar arachnoid cyst (HOFFMAN et al. 1982; ONDA et al. 1989). The CT appearance is typically of a non-calcified intrasellar cystic mass. On MRI signal returned by the cyst is variable (Fig. 19.9). It may follow that of CSF (i.e. hypointense on T_1W and hyperintense on T_2W sequences) or be characteristic of a protein rich fluid (i.e. hyperintense on both T_1W and T_2W sequences) or altered haemorrhage (i.e. hyperintense on T_1W and hypointense on T_2W sequences) (ASARI et al. 1990; MIZE et al. 1989). Though the cyst wall does not enhance, administration of intravenous gadolinium is useful in order to exclude craniopharyngioma and to show the position of normal pituitary (SUMIDA et al. 1994). Rathke's cleft cysts in atypical locations may make differentiation from an arachnoid cyst of the chiasmatic cistern difficult. They have, like craniopharyngioma, rarely been found in the nasopharynx associated with persistent remnants of the craniopharyngeal duct (ROTTENBERG et al. 1994). Another atypical feature is the occasional finding of a central hypo- or isointense focus within the cyst (Fig. 19.10). This is presumed to be due to desquamatised epithelium forming a "waxy nodule" (KUCHARCZYK et al. 1987).

The pre-operative diagnosis is important since simple surgical excision or cyst aspiration is usually curative, unlike craniopharyngioma. Differentiation from cystic craniopharyngiomas, despite the advan-

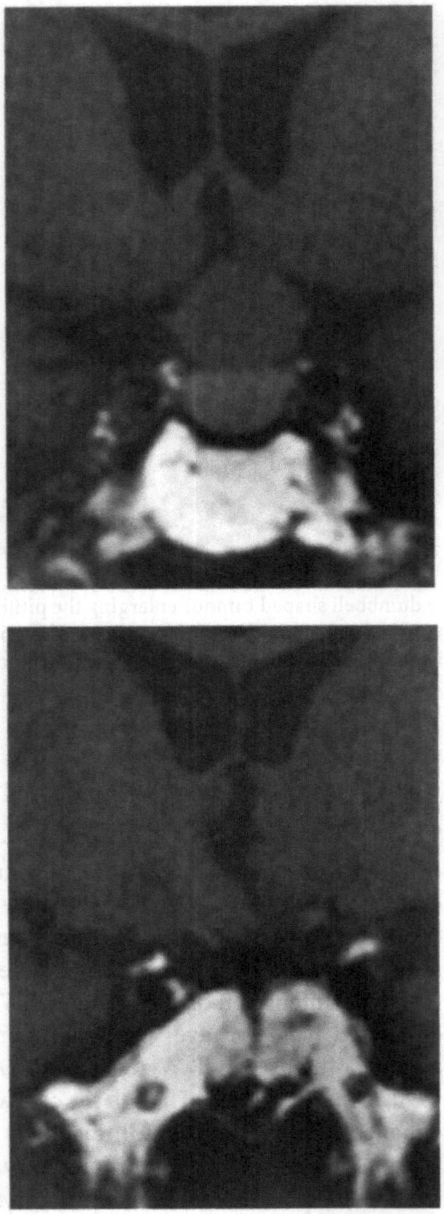

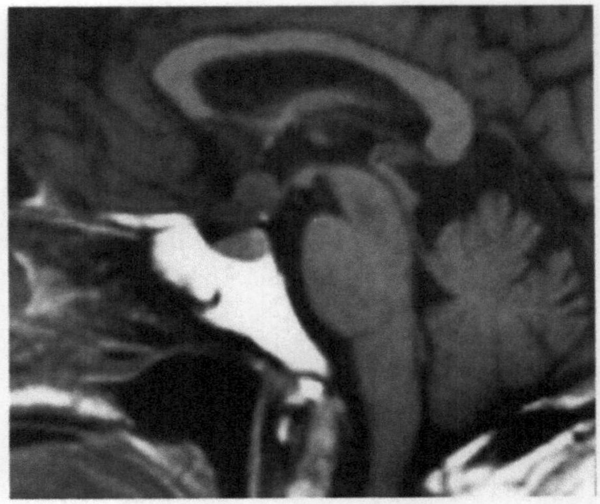

a b c

Fig. 19.9a–c. Unenhanced T1 W MRI showing a Rathke's cleft cyst. Coronal (a) and sagittal (b) scans performed before operation show a lobulated outline to the lesion which returns homogeneous signal of two intensities. A defect in the sphenoid bone is evident on b and c due to persistence of the craniopharyngeal duct. This is best seen on the coronal image (c) performed after surgical confirmation of the diagnosis

tages of MRI, can still be difficult, particularly in children (Christophe et al. 1993). High quality imaging is therefore mandatory.

19.4 Inflammatory Lesions of the Pituitary and Parasellar Regions

Several inflammatory conditions may affect the sellar and parasellar tissues causing symptoms and signs similar to pituitary neoplasms.

19.4.1 Pituitary Abscess

Abscesses of the pituitary may be secondary to infections of the paranasal sinuses, meningitis or they may occur spontaneously. Isolated pituitary abscesses usually do not cause systemic signs of infection and unlike most abscesses they may develop slowly, thus simulating chronic pituitary enlargement due to tumours. Imaging may show enlargement of the pituitary fossa with erosion of its margins due to a cystic pituitary mass. On CT abscesses resemble necrotic or cystic tumours with prominent marginal enhancement after

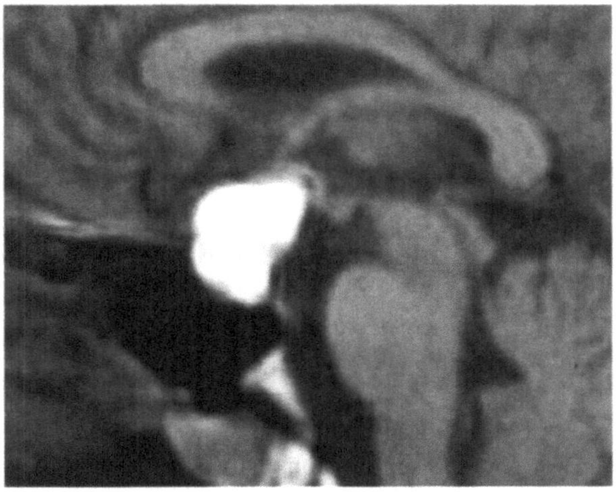

Fig. 19.10. Sagittal T1 W MRI of another patient with a Rathke's cleft cyst. The cyst contains paramagnetic material and returns hyperintense signal. A small focus of hypointense signal at the posterior wall is probably due to desquamatised epithelium

intravenous contrast administration. On MRI hyperintense signal on both T_1W and T_2W sequences suggests a haemorrhagic pituitary adenoma; gadolinium enhancement is similar to that evident on CT.

The pre-operative diagnosis of abscess is therefore difficult and since they are best treated by transphenoidal drainage often the diagnosis is made at surgery. It is important to consider abscess in the differential diagnosis of cystic or necrotic pituitary tumours, particularly those with avid contrast media enhancement, since surgical exploration by craniotomy risks intracranial spread of infection.

19.4.2 Lymphocytic Adenohypophysitis

This rare autoimmune disorder occurs due to diffuse infiltration of the anterior lobe by lymphocytes (Quencer 1980). The adenohypophysitis does not normally contain lymphocytes and the inflammatory process causes its enlargement and destruction. It is more common in women and occurs in late pregnancy or in the post-partum period. Hypopituitarism and diabetes insipidus are common and suprasellar extension of the swollen gland may cause symptoms of chiasm compression. Hyperprolactinaemia may also occur (Hungerford et al. 1983). Antipituitary antibodies have been demonstrated in some patients (Mayfield et al. 1980) but they have also been identified in 18% of post-partum women (Pouplard 1982).

Typical appearances on MRI are an enlarged gland, which is intensely enhancing and thickening of the pituitary stalk (Fig. 19.11). Dural enhancement and enhancement along the infundibulum was seen in four of five patients reported by Ahmadi et al. (1995). Similar findings have been described in the rare patients with Wegener's granulomatosis and pituitary involvement who may also present with diabetes insipidus (Katzman et al. 1999). On T_1W MRI the gland was isointense or minimally hyperintense relative to grey matter. After intravenous gadolinium administration enhancement was either homogeneous or heterogeneous which therefore simulated necrotic or haemorrhagic pituitary adenomas. The diagnosis should be considered since treatment is with corticosteroids and surgical exploration can be avoided for patients without visual symptoms. Sato et al. (1998) recently reported delayed dynamic enhancement of the pituitary in patients with lymphocytic hypophysitis which they attributed to decreased vasculature. This study illustrates how in vivo imaging can be used to extend our understanding of pathological processes.

19.4.3 Inflammatory Diseases of the Chiasmatic Cistern

Involvement of the suprasellar region by sarcoidosis, Langerhans cell histiocytosis or tuberculous meningitis may cause endocrine symptoms such as diabetes insipidus and abnormalities on imaging. In Langerhans cell histiocytosis (also called eosinophic granulomatosis) patients present with diabetes insipidus and bone lesions. The former frequently leads to imaging of the hypothalamic-pituitary axis and MRI shows thickening of the pituitary stalk (Tien et al. 1990). Normal posterior pituitary high signal is typically absent. The diagnosis may be made by recognition of bone lesions which often occur in the skull; one of the rare situations when plain skull radiographs may be helpful.

Granulomatous leptomeningitis is more frequently evident in the basal cisterns than elsewhere in the cranium but this may reflect their size, rather than a predisposition of the disease for this location. Involvement of the chiasmatic cistern is more likely to be diagnosed because patients present with visual or endocrine symptoms (Post et al. 1982; Engelken et al. 1992). Sarcoid granulomas may be identified as meningeal masses isodense on CT and isointense on MRI, relative to grey matter. They are best demonstrated on T_1W MRI with gadolinium enhancement.

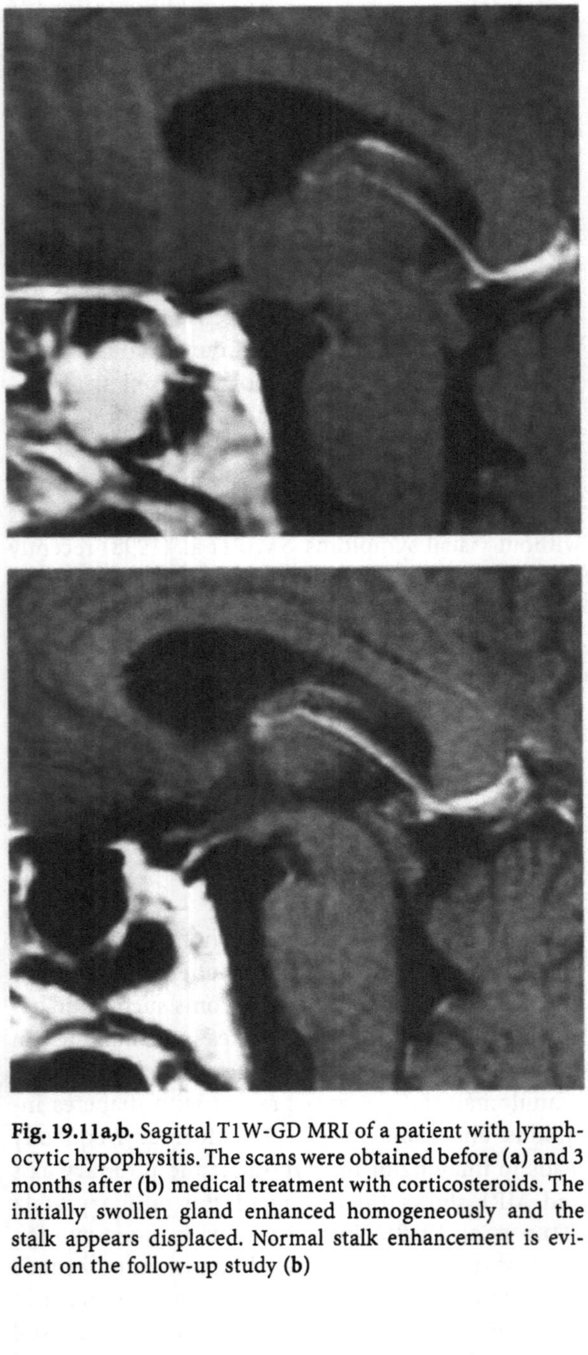

a

b

Fig. 19.11a,b. Sagittal T1W-GD MRI of a patient with lymphocytic hypophysitis. The scans were obtained before (**a**) and 3 months after (**b**) medical treatment with corticosteroids. The initially swollen gland enhanced homogeneously and the stalk appears displaced. Normal stalk enhancement is evident on the follow-up study (**b**)

Other foci of meningeal enhancement should be sought since it may be necessary to resort to biopsy to confirm the diagnosis (WILLIAMS et al. 1990) and a superficial focus would be more accessible. The differential for pathological meningeal enhancement in the suprasellar region includes metastastic tumour and it is important to keep this possibility in mind. In a recent report of two patients, initial imaging performed for idiopathic diabetes insipidus was negative, but 1–2 years later metastatic germinoma was demonstrated in the hypothalamus (APPIGNANI et al. 1993). Interval imaging and a high degree of suspicion is therefore warranted.

19.5 Assessment of Patients with Cushing's Syndrome

Imaging is the cornerstone of the diagnostic assessment of patients with Cushing's syndrome. The diagnosis is based on clinical examination and biochemical tests, including corticosteroid estimations and dexamethasone suppression tests. Investigation then becomes a search for the source of adrenocorticotrophin (ACTH) overproduction, since surgical excision of such a lesion is curative. MRI will demonstrate a pituitary ACTH-producing tumour, i.e. Cushing's disease, in 70%–80% of patients (TABARIN et al. 1998; ESCOUROLLE et al. 1993). Cushing's syndrome, in patients without evidence of a pituitary lesion, may be due to an ectopic source of ACTH and most centres advocate inferior petrosal sinus (IPS) sampling to distinguish between pituitary and ectopic ACTH-producing lesions. The test may also help when the results of other biochemical tests and MRI are equivocal, since there remains the small possibility of false positive MRI findings (TABARIN et al. 1998). Sampling from the IPS or cavernous sinuses is primarily intended to measure the ratio of central to peripheral plasma ACTH levels (Fig. 19.12). The reliability of the test can be improved by administering corticotrophin-releasing hormone (CRH), which amplifies the ratio by up to 5 times (LOPEZ et al. 1996). A secondary benefit, if bilateral sampling is performed, is that the levels of ACTH between the two sides can be compared and the source of excessive production lateralised. Bilateral sampling can be sequential or simultaneous. The test can accurately distinguish Cushing's disease in approximately 90% of patients (OLDFIELD et al. 1991; KALTSAS et al. 1999; LOPEZ et al. 1996). Based on intersinus gradients greater than 1.4, KALTAS et al (1999) reported sensitivity rates for tumour lateralisation of 83% (compared to 72% for MRI).

Inferior petrosal sinus sampling has been the subject of two recent reports of complications causing brain stem strokes (MILLER et al. 1993; STURROCK et al. 1997). The risk of a complication causing a permanent neurological complication has been estimated at 0.0001% by DOPPMAN (1999) and can be minimised by sampling from the internal jugular veins rather than in the proximal (superior) portion of the IPS or cavernous sinuses. Its use remains controversial and

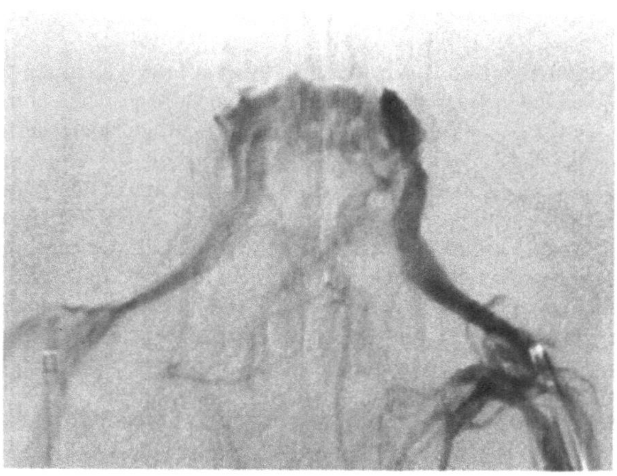

Fig. 19.12. Frontal digital subtraction angiography of the cavernous and inferior petrosal sinuses. This venogram was performed following contrast media injection of the left inferior petrosal sinus and shows extensive communications between the two cavernous sinuses. Sampling catheters have been positioned in the distal portions of both inferior petrosal sinuses in preparation for venous sampling after corticotrophin-releasing hormone administration

the extent to which it is employed varies from centre to centre. A recently described alternative is to sample after metyrapone rather than CRH stimulation (CUNEO et al. 1997), though it has yet to be proven whether this test is safer. Intraoperative tumour localisation using ultrasound has been found to aid surgery for patients with biochemical evidence of Cushing's disease but negative MRI. WATSON et al. (1998) reported being able to localise 69% of tumour in such patients.

The search for the source of ectopic ACTH production presents a further challenge in patients with Cushing's syndrome and may involve extensive imaging by planar scanning and nuclear medicine techniques (TABARIN et al. 1999). These are unlikely to involve the neuroradiology department and are therefore beyond the scope of this review.

19.6 Conclusion

Imaging makes a major contribution in the investigation of patients with endocrine disease. The neuroradiologist has a central role in this process but does so as part of a team. The mainstay of imaging is currently MRI but a range of modalities can be employed and diagnostic strategies continue to evolve.

References

Adamson TE, Wiestler OD, Kleihues P et al. (1990) Correlation of clinical and pathological features in surgically treated craniopharyngiomas. J Neurosurg 73: 12–17

Ahmadi H, Larsson EM, Jinkins JR (1992) Normal pituitary gland: coronal MR imaging of infundibular tilt. Radiology 171: 389–392

Ahmadi J, Meyers GS, Segall HD et al. (1995) Lymphocytic adenohypophysitis: contrast-enhanced MR imaging in five Ccases. Radiology 195: 30–34

Akio M, Meyer FB, Laws ER (1998) Symptomatic pituitary metastases. J Neurosurg 89: 69–73

Appignani B, Landy H, Barnes P (1993) MR in central idiopathic diabetes insipidus in children. AJNR 14: 1407–1410

Arnold DL, Emrich JF, Shoubridge EA et al. (1991) Characterization of astrocytomas, meningiomas, and pituitary adenomas by phosphorus magnetic resonance spectroscopy. J Neurosurg 74: 447–453

Asari S, Ito T, Tsuchida S, Tsutsai T (1990) MR appearance and cyst contents of Rathke's cleft cysts. J Comput Assist Tomogr 14: 532–535

Bergström M, Muhr C, Jossan S et al. (1992) Differentiation of pituitary adenoma and meningioma; visualization with positron emission tomography and [^{11}C]-L-deprenyl. Neurosurgery 30: 855–861

Black ML, Tien RD, Hesselink JR (1991) Third ventricular hemangioblastoma: MR appearance. AJNR 12: 553

Brooks BS, El Gammal T, Allison JD et al. (1989) Frequency and variation of the posterior pituitary bright signal on MR images. AJNR 10: 943–948

Buchfelder M, Nistor R, Fahlbusch R et al. (1992) The accuracy of CT and MR evaluation of the sella turcica for detection of adrenocorticotropic hormone - secreting adenomas in Cushing disease. AJNR 14: 1183–1190

Bunin GR, Surawicz, TS, Witman PA et al. (1998) The descriptive epidemiology of craniopharyngioma. J Neurosurg 89: 547–551

Burrow G, Wortzman G, Rewcastle N (1981) Microadenomas of the pituitary and abnormal sellar tomograms in an unselected autopsy series. N Eng J Med 301: 156–158

Cappabianca P, Cirillo S, Alfieri A et al. (1999) Pituitary macroadenoma and diaphragma sellae meningioma: differential diagnosis on MRI. Neuroradiology 41: 22–26

Chong BW, Kucharczyk W, Singer W et al. (1994) Pituitary gland MR: a comparative study of healthy volunteers and patients with microadenomas. AJNR 15: 675–679

Christophe C, Flamant-Durand J, Hanquinet S et al. (1993) MRI in seven cases of Rathke's cleft cyst in infants and children. Pediatr Radiol 23: 79–82

Cuneo RC, Lee W, Harper J et al. (1997) Metyrapone pretreated inferior petrosal sinus sampling in the differential diagnosis of ACTH-dependent Cushing's syndrome. Clin Endocrinol 46: 607–618

Davis PC, Hoffman JC Jr., Tindall GT et al. (1985) CT-surgical correlation in pituitary adenomas: evaluation in 113 patients. AJNR 6: 711–716

Davis PC, Hoffman JC, Malko JA et al. (1987) Gadolinium-DTPA and MR imaging of pituitary adenoma: a preliminary report. AJNR 8: 817–823

Davis WL, Lee JN, King BD et al. (1994) Dynamic contrast-enhanced MR imaging of the pituitary gland with fast spin-echo technique. JMRI 4: 509–511

Dina TS, Feater SH, Laws ER et al. (1993) MR of the pituitary gland

postsurgery: serial MR studies following transsphenoidal resection. AJNR 14: 763–769
Dooms GC, Uske A, Brant-Zawadzki M et al. (1986) Spin-echo MR imaging of intracranial hemorrhage. Neuroradiology 28: 132–138
Doppman JL (1999) There is no simple answer to rare complication of inferior petrosal sinus sampling. AJNR 20: 191–192
Doppman JL, Frank JA, Dwyer AJ et al. (1988) Gadolinium DTPA enhanced MR imaging of ACTH-secreting microadenomas of the pituitary gland. J Comput Assist Tomogr 12: 728–735
Dwyer AJ, Frank JA, Doppman JL et al. (1987) Pituitary adenomas in patients with Cushing disease: initial experience with Gd-DTPA-enhanced MR imaging. Radiology 163: 421–426
Eldevik OP, Blaivas M, Gabrielsen TO et al. (1996) Craniopharyngioma: radiologic and histologic findings and recurrence. AJNR 17: 1427–1439
Eldevic OP, Gabrielsen TO, Altinok D (1998) Contrast enhancement in the craniopharyngioma cyst wall caused by irradiation. Acta Radiologica 39: 180–182
Elster AD (1994) High-resolution, dynamic pituitary MR imaging: standard of care or academic pastime? AJR 163: 680–682
Engelken JD, Yuh WTC, Carter KD et al. (1992) Optic nerve sarcoidosis. MR findings. AJNR 13: 228–230
Escourolle H, Abecassis JP, Bertagna X et al. (1993) Comparison of computerized tomography and magnetic resonance imaging for the examination of the pituitary gland in patients with Cushing's disease. Clin Endocrinol 39: 307–313
Fujisawa I, Asato R, Nishimura K et al. (1987) Anterior and posterior lobes of the pituitary gland: assessment by 1.5 T MR imaging. J Comput Assist Tomogr 11: 214–220
Hald JK, Eldevik OP, Brunberg JA et al. (1994) Craniopharyngiomas – the utility of contrast medium enhancement for MR imaging at 1.5 T. Acta Radiologica 35: 520–525
Hald JK, Eldevik OP, Quint DJ et al. (1996) Pre- and postoperative MR imaging of craniopharyngiomas. Acta Radiologica 37: 806–812
Harwood-Nash DC (1994) Neuroimaging of childhood craniopharyngioma. Pediatr Neurosurg 21: 2–10
Hoffman HJ, Hendricks B, Humphries RP et al. (1982) Investigations and management of suprasellar arachnoid cysts. J Neurosurg 57: 597–602
Hubbard AM, Egelhoff JC (1989) MR imaging of large hypothalamic hamartomas in two infants. AJNR 10: 1277–1279
Hungerford GD, Biggs PJ, Levine JH et al. (1983) Lymphoid adenohypophysitis with radiologic and clinical findings resembling pituitary tumour. AJNR 3: 444–446
Johnson MR, Hoare RD, Cox T et al. (1992) The evaluation of patients with a suspected pituitary microadenoma: computer tomography compared to magnetic resonance imaging. Clin Endocrinol 36: 335–338
Kahn EA, Gosch HH, Seeger JF et al. (1973) Forty-five years experience with craniopharyngiomas. Surg Neurol 1: 5–12
Kaltsas GA, Giannulis MG, Newell-Price JD et al. (1999) A critical analysis of the value of simultaneous inferior petrosal sinus sampling in Cushing's disease and the occult ectopic adrenocorticotropin syndrome. J Clin Endocrinol Metab 84: 487--492
Katzman GL, Langford CA, Sneller MC et al. (1999) Pituitary involvement by Wegener's granulomatosis: a report of two cases. AJNR 20: 519–523
Kaufman B, Tomsak RL, Kaufman BA et al. (1989) Herniation of the suprasellar visual system and third ventricle into empty sellae: morphologic and clinical considerations. AJNR 10: 65–76
Krenning EP, Kwekkeboom DJ, Bakker WH et al. (1993) Somatostatin receptor scintigraphy with ^{111}In-DTPA-D-Pne and ^{123}I-Tyr3-octeotride: the Rotterdam experience in more than 1000 patients. Eur J Nucl Med 20: 716–721
Kucharczyk W, Bishop JE, Plewes DB et al. (1994) Detection of pituitary microadenomas: comparison of dynamic keyhole fast spin-echo, unenhanced, and conventional contrast-enhanced MR imaging. AJR 163: 671–679
Kucharczyk W, Davis DO, Kelly WM et al. (1986) Pituitary adenomas: high-resolution MR imaging at 1.5 T. Radiology 161: 761–765
Kucharczyk W, Lenkinski RE, Kucharczyk J et al. (1990) The effect of phospholipid vesicles on the NMR relaxation of water: an explanation for the MR appearance of the neurohypophysis? AJNR 11: 693–700
Kucharczyk W, Peck WW, Kelly WM et al. (1987) Rathke cleft cysts: CT, MR imaging and pathological features. Radiology 165: 491–495
Kurihara N, Takahashi S, Higano S et al. (1998) Hemorrhage in pituitary adenoma: correlation of MR imaging with operative findings. Eur Radiol 8: 971–976
Lamberts SW, Krenning EP, Renbi JC (1991) The role of somatostatin and its analogs in the diagnosis and treatment of tumours. Endocr Rev 12: 450–482
Lenthall RK, Dean JR, Bartlett MR et al. (1999) Intrapituitary fluid levels following haemorrhage: MRI appearances in 13 cases. Neuroradiology 41: 167–170
Lopez J, Barcelo B, Lucas T et al. (1996) Petrosal sinus sampling for diagnosis of Cushing's disease: evidence of false negative results. Clin Endocrinol 45: 147–156
Lucas-Morante T, Garcia-Uria J, Estrada J et al. (1994) Treatment of invasive growth hormone pituitary adenomas with long-acting somatostatin analog SMS 201–995 before transsphenoidal surgery. J Neurosurg 81: 10–14
Lucignani G, Losa M, Moresco RM et al. (1997) Differentiation of clinically non-functioning pituitary adenomas from meningiomas and craniopharyngiomas by positron emission tomography with [^{18}F]fluoro-ethyl-spiperone. Eur J Nucl Med 24: 1149–1155
Lundin P, Bergström K, Nyman R et al. (1992) Macroprolactinomas: serial MR imaging in long-term bromocriptine therapy. AJNR 13: 1279–1291
Lundin P, Engström BE, Karlsson FA et al. (1997) Long-term octreotide therapy in growth hormone-secreting pituitary adenomas: evaluation with serial MR. AJNR 18: 765–772
Lundin P, Nyman R, Burman P et al. (1992) MRI of pituitary macroadenomas with reference to hormonal activity. Neuroradiology 34: 43–51
Mark LP, Haughton VM, Hendrix LE et al. (1991) High-intensity signals within the posterior pituitary fossa: a study with fat-suppression MR techniques. AJNR 12: 529–532
Mayfield RK, Levine JH, Gordon L et al. (1980) Lymphoid adenohypophysitis presenting as a pituitary tumour. Am J Med 69: 619–623
Miki Y, Matsuo M, Sadahiko N et al. (1990) Pituitary adenomas and normal pituitary tissue: enhancement pat-

terns on gadopentetate-enhanced MR imaging. Radiology 177: 35–38
Miller DL, Doppman JL, Peterman SB et al. (1993) Neurologic complications of petrosal sinus sampling. Radiology 185: 143–147
Mize W, Ball WS, Towbin RB et al. (1989) Atypical CT and MR appearances of a Rathke's cleft cyst. AJNR 10: 583–584
Morrison G, Sobel DF, Kelley WM et al. (1984) Intraventricular mass lesions. Radiology 153: 435–442
Muhr C, Bergstrom L, Lundberg PO et al. (1988) Malignant prolactinomas with multiple intracranial metastases studied with positron emission tomography. Neurosurgery 22: 374–349
Oldfield EH, Doppman JL, Nieman LK et al. (1991) Petrosal sinus sampling with and without corticotrophin-releasing hormone for differential diagnosis of Cushing's syndrome. N Eng J Med 325: 897–905
Onda K, Tanaka K, Takeda N et al. (1989) Symptomatic Rathke's cleft cyst simulating arachnoid cyst. Neurol Med Chir 29: 1039–1043
Peck WW, Dillon WP, Norman D et al. (1989) High resolution MR imaging of pituitary microadenomas at 1.5 T: experience with Cushing's disease. AJR 152: 145–151
Petito CK (1996) Craniopharyngiomas: prognostic importance of histologic features. AJNR 17: 1441–1442
Pont MS, Elster AD (1992) Lesions of skin and brain: modern imaging of the neurocutaneous syndromes. AJR 158: 1193–1203
Post MJD, Quencer RM, Tabei SI (1982) CT demonstration of sarcoidosis of the optic nerve, frontal lobes and falx cerebri: case report and literature review. AJNR 3: 523–526
Pouplard A (1982) Pituitary autoimmunity. Horm Res 16: 289–297
Quencer RM (1980) Lymphocytic adenohypophysitis: autoimmune disorder of the pituitary gland. AJNR 1: 343–345
Rajan B, Ashley S, Gorman G et al. (1993) Craniopharyngioma: long-term results following limited surgery and radiotherapy. Radiother Oncol 26: 1–10
Rand T, Kink E, Sator M et al. (1996) MRI of microadenomas in parients with hyperprolactinaemia.. Neuroradiology 38: 744–746
Reith KG, Comite F, Dwyer AJ et al. (1987) CT of cerebral abnormalities in precocious puberty. AJNR 8: 283–290
Richmond IL, Newton TH, Wilson CB (1980) Indications for angiography in the preoperative evaluation of patients with prolactin - secreting pituitary adenomas. J Neurosurg 52: 378–380
Rottenberg GT, Chong WK, Powell M et al. (1994) Cyst formation of the craniopharyngeal duct. Clin Radiol 49: 126–129
Sakamoto Y, Takahashi M, Korogi Y et al. (1991) Normal and abnormal pituitary glands: gadopentetate dimeglumine-enhanced MR imaging. Radiology 178: 441–445
Sartoretti-Schefer S, Wichmann W, Aguzzi A et al. (1997) MR differentiation of adamantinous and squamous-papillary craniopharyngiomas. AJNR 18: 77–87
Sato N, Sze G, Endo K (1998) Hypophysitis: endocrinologic and dynamic MR findings. AJNR 19: 439–444
Sawers HA, Robb OJ, Walmsley D et al. (1997) An audit of the diagnostic usefulness of PRL and TSH responses to domperidone and high resolution magnetic resonance imaging of the pituitary in the evaluation of hyperprolactinaemia. Clin Endocrinol 46: 321–326
Scheithauer BW, Kovacs KT, Laws ER et al. (1986) Pathology of invasive pituitary tumors with special reference to functional classification. J Neurosurg 65: 733–744
Scott WA (1996) Magnetic resonance imaging of the brain and spine. Lippincott-Raven, Philadelphia, New York, pp 59–63
Scotti G, Yu CY, Dillon WP et al. (1988) MR imaging of cavernous sinus involvement by pituitary adenomas. AJNR 9: 657–664
Selman WR, Laws ER, Scheithauer BW et al. (1986) The occurrence of dural invasion in pituitary adenomas. J Neurosurg 64: 402–407
Shanklin WM (1951) The incidence and distribution of cilia in the human pituitary with a description of micro-follicular cyst derived from Rathke's cleft. Acta Anat 11: 361–382
Stadnik T, Stevenaert A, Beckers A et al. (1990) Pituitary microadenomas: diagnosis with two- and three-dimensional MR imaging at 1.5 T before and after injection of gadolinium. Radiology 176: 419–428
Steiner E, Knosp E, Herold CJ et al. (1992) Pituitary adenomas: findings of postoperative MR imaging. Radiology 185: 521–527
Steiner E, Math G, Knosp E et al. (1994) MR-appearance of the pituitary gland before and after resection of pituitary macroadenomas. Clin Radiol 49: 524–530
Sturrock ND, Jeffcoate WJ (1997) A neurological complication of inferior petrosal sinus sampling during investigation for Cushing's disease: a case report. J Neurol Neurosurg Psychiatry 62: 527–528
Sumida M, Arita K, Migita K et al. (1998) Demonstration of the optic pathway in sellar/juxtasellar tumours with visual disturbance on MR imaging. Acta Neurochir (Wien) 140: 541–548
Sumida M, Uozumi T, Mukada K et al. (1994) Rathke cleft cysts: correlation of enhanced MR and surgical findings. AJNR 15: 525–532
Tabarin A, Laurent F, Catargi B et al. (1998) Comparative evaluation of conventional and dynamic magnetic resonance imaging of the pituitary gland for the diagnosis of Cushing's disease. Clin Endocrinol 49: 293–300
Tabarin A, Valli N, Chason P et al. (1999) Usefulness of somatostatin receptor scintigraphy in patients with occult ectopic adrenocorticotropin syndrome. J Clin Endocrinol Metab 84: 1184–1185
Taveras JM (1996) Neuroradiology, 3rd ed. Williams & Wilkins, Baltimore, pp 639–641
Teramoto A, Hirakawa K, Sanno N, Osamura J (1994) Incidental pituitary lesions in unselected 1000 autopsy specimens. Radiology 193: 161–164
Tien RD, Naston TH, McDermott MW et al. (1990) Thickened pituitary stalk on MR images in patients with diabetes insipidus and Langerhaus cell histiocytosis. AJNR 11: 703–708
Wakai S, Fukushima T, Teramoto A et al. (1981) Pituitary apoplexy: its incidence and clinical significance. J Neurosurg 55: 187–193
Watson JC, Shawker TH, Nieman LK et al. (1998) Localization of pituitary adenomas by using intraoperative ultrasound in patients with Cushing's disease and no demonstrable pituitary tumor on magnetic resonance imaging. J Neurosurg 89: 927–932
Weiner HL, Wisoff JH, Rosenberg ME et al. (1994) Cran-

iopharyngiomas: a clinicopathological analysis of factors predictive of recurrence and functional outcome. Neurosurgery 35: 1001–1011
Williams DW III, Elster AD, Kramer SI (1990) Neurosarcoidosis: gadolinium-enhanced MR images. J Comput Assist Tomogr 14: 704–707
Wolpert SM, Osborne M, Anderson M et al. (1988) The bright pituitary gland – a normal MR appearance in infancy. AJNR 9: 1–3
Wu W, Thuomas KA (1995) Pituitary microadenoma MR appearance and correlation with CT. Acta Radiologica 36: 529–535
Yuh WTC, Fisher DJ, Nguyen HD et al. (1994) Sequential MR enhancement pattern in normal pituitary gland and pituitary adenoma. AJNR 15: 101–108

20 Imaging in Ophthalmology

Abdelouhab Abanou, Marie-Thérèse Iba-Zizen, Mohammed Jidal, Luc Bellinger, Emmanuel A. Cabanis

CONTENTS

20.1 Introduction

The optic pathway extends from the cornea to the visual cortex. It exhibits features that deserve specific neuroradiological investigation. The first characteristic is the anatomical and functional unity of the visual pathway. The second is the differences between child and adult disorders (Ball 1997). In addition, the small size of visual pathways necessitates high-resolution imaging. In children, the presence of leucocoria, an acute or subacute exophthalmia associated with inflammatory signs, may lead to the discovery of retinoblastoma or rhabdomyosarcoma. In adults, lesions of the eyeball may reveal a melanoma or a malignant tumour of the lacrimal gland.

A. Abanou, MD; M.T. Iba-Zizen, MD; M. Jidal, MD; L. Bellinger, MD
Centre Hospitalier National d'Ophthalmologie des Quinze-Vingts, Service de Neuro-imagerie et radiologie, Rue de Charenton 28, 75571 Paris Cedex 12, France
E.A. Cabanis, MD
Professor, Centre Hospitalier National d'Ophthalmologie des Quinze-Vingts, Service de Neuro-imagerie et radiologie, Rue de Charenton 28, 75571 Paris Cedex 12, France

The other situations are more or less common to child and adult diseases. Various lesions can be investigated by CT scans and magnetic resonance imaging (MRI). Techniques based on ultrasound are essentially used by the ophthalmologist in the early stage of the diagnosis. MRI and CT scans are complementary techniques. CT is used for oculo-orbito-facial biometry. CT can easily distinguish between the density of the intraorbital fat tissue, and bone lyses or condensation. MRI is more useful for establishing the precise anatomical lesion location and its extension. Furthermore, this technique is superior to CT as it offers more precise tissue characterisation (fat, water, necrosis, haemoglobin catabolism). In addition it may be repeated as often as needed, being a non-invasive procedure (Cabanis et al. 1996).

The anatomical and functional unity is the principle reason for avoiding routine use of surface antennas, which limit the investigation to the orbital apex. In our department cephalic and facial MRI are exclusively achieved by using head antennas. Thus imaging of the complete visual pathway is homogeneous from the cornea to the visual cortex. For this, we use the neuro-ocular plane (NOP) and the oblique transhemispheric neuro-ocular plane (OTNOP). In paediatrics, intravenous sedation is used on a routine and ambulatory basis with drugs such as midazolam and propofol. Using MRI thin slices and a matrix with a sufficient number of acquisitions, more anatomical details can be shown. Surface and volume reformatting is also possible, as for CT scans. Fast MRI sequences are now possible. Small details need high resolution: 3-mm slices with less than a 10% gap, and a 512/384 matrix. These details are now accessible in a reasonable acquisition time.

20.2 Anatomy and Biometrics

The fundamental plane for all neurophthalmological investigations is the NOP (Cabanis 1983). It is a horizontal cephalic orientation where the patient gazes forward, revealing both lenses, the head of the optic nerves and the optic canals. This plane allows a precise anatomical reference (misdiagnosis between optical canal and orbital fissure) and exact biometric measurements to be obtained. The OTNP shows the lens, the optic nerve, the homolateral canal and the foramen magnum. In the NOP, drawing a horizontal line allows two segments to be defined: the pre- and retrobicanthal segments. Thus exophthalmia can be graded from I to III. Similarly the transverse diameter of the orbital segment of the optic nerve and extraocular rectus muscles can be measured.

20.3 Ocular and Orbitofacial Traumatology

In a first step, X-rays and CT are undertaken to eliminate the presence of metallic intraorbital objects. Secondly, it is necessary to define the traumatic lesions of the eyeball, the orbit and the face. Eye lesions can exist solely or be associated with orbitofacial or encephalic injury.

20.3.1 Intraocular Foreign Body and Eyeball Lesion

Metallic objects are the more frequently encountered lesions of the eyeball. The incidence of windscreen related injuries has decreased in the last few years. Foreign objects are now easily seen with X-rays and CT (Girardot et al. 1994).

However, some locations remain difficult to investigate: this is the case for parascleral objects and objects along the medial orbital wall. In this context, the orbital apex, the optical canal and the encephalon must be investigated. Post-traumatic vascular or encephalic lesions can be observed. CT is useful in distinguishing the hyperdensity of a hyphema, or that of an intravitreous haemorrhage. Rupture of the eyeball is diagnosed by the loss of its normal morphology. Retinal or choroidal detachment (RD, CD) can also be suspected (Fig. 20.1a). MRI can detect ocular, muscular, and cerebral injuries. Nevertheless it cannot be used unless ferromagnetic objects are excluded.

20.3.2 Orbital Fractures

Emphysema and periorbital haematoma diplopia are the major signs of orbital fractures. In this context CT is the method of choice to show a direct fracture. The MRI can also show a fracture as an interruption of cortical bone hyposignal. If a woody foreign body is suspected, MRI must performed.

Fracture of the ethmoidal planum is frequent because of its fragile structure, often creating a pneumo-orbit and an ethmoidal haemosinus. Fracture of the orbital floor (central by the infraorbital canal) may be responsible for suborbital anaesthesia and vertical diplopia. CT and MRI can identify a simple defect or a defect with intermediate fragments, and incarceration of orbital fat tissue and less frequently of the inferior rectus muscle.

Fracture of the orbital roof is much less frequently observed. It may lead to meningocerebral infection beginning in the frontal lobe. This complication implies the use of both CT and MRI.

With optic nerve trauma both CT and MRI need to be performed. Thin slices allow the optical canal to be studied. In the Hartman-Gilles orientation on standard X-rays, the integrity of the cortical optic canal and the continuity of the jugo-opticoclinoid line must be respected. MRI scans in another step using a T2 short inversion time (STIR) may detect signal abnormalities of the optic nerve and eventually haematic modifications of the optic canal.

Haematomas of the inferior rectus muscle are not exceptional. Subperiostal haematoma (below the roof of the orbit) and orbital haematoma are well delineated by MRI and their signal in this acute stage is the signal of acute haemorrhage.

The Silverman syndrome deserves special attention as ocular cerebral and osseous lesions may coexist.

20.4 Eye and Orbit Malformations

Three eyeball malformations can be distinguished: osseous orbital malformations and craniofacial dysraphism.

20.4.1 Eyeball Malformations (Goddé-Jolly and Dufier 1992)

Coloboma is a result of incomplete closure of the embryonic fissure (Fig. 20.1c). It lies on the head of the optic nerve, chorioretina or iris. On imaging the characteristic aspect is a glove-finger deformation

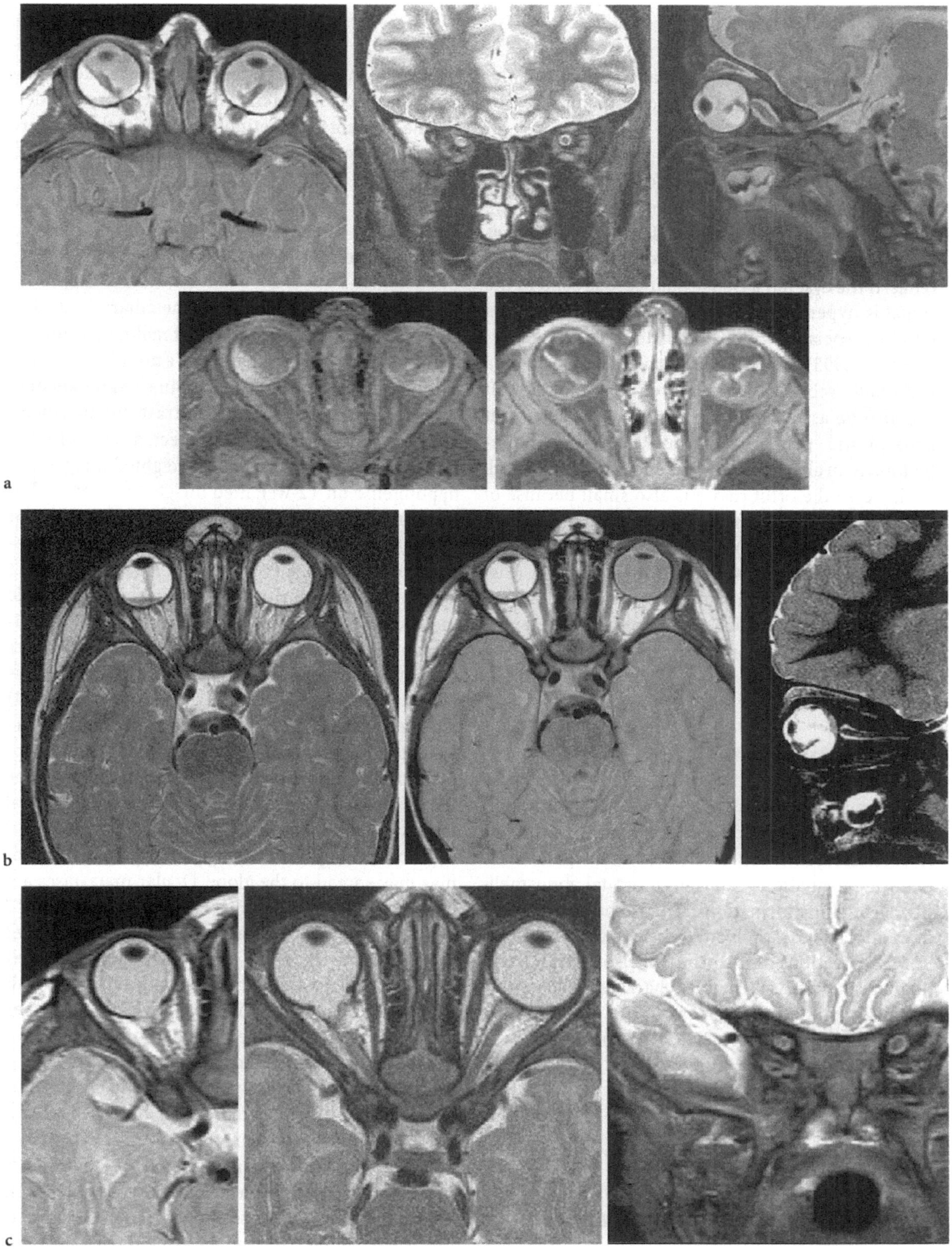

Fig. 20.1. **a** Bilateral retinal detachment with haemorrhagic subretinal fluid, and choroidal detachment in the left eye. Hypersignal of the right optic nerve. Thickening and postcontrast enhancement in the detached retina. Coats' disease is the diagnosis which was made (axial T2 WI, coronal T2 WI, OTNOP T2 WI, axial T1 WI with fat saturation before and after Gd administration). **b** PHPV of the right eye. Small globe, retinal detachment with fluid-fluid level (serohaemorrhagic subretinal fluid). Persistent hyaloid, deep less anterior chamber (axial T2 WI plane heavy and short weighted, and T2 WI OTNOP). **c** Right optic nerve coloboma. The defect of the orbit posterior rim (glove finger) is pathognomonic. Note the colobomatous cyst on the nasal sector and optic nerve atrophy with small optic canal (axial and coronal T2 WI)

with a dehiscence of the papillary segment of the optic nerve. Uni- or bilateral locations may be observed.

Microphthalmia (decrease of the eyeball length) can be associated with cystic coloboma, which is located at the inferior part of the orbit. The cyst is hypodense on CT, and intense on T1-weighted images and on T2-weighted images as compared to the vitreous. If the cyst has a rich proteinaceous content the signal is hyperintense. Osseous or fibrous dysplasia may be associated with colobomatous cyst (De Potter et al. 1995). Non-colobomatous microphthalmia is a small eyeball easily measured with biometry. It can also be associated with cataract and persistent hyperplastic primary vitreous (PHPV). Anophthalmia is an absence of the eye and is often bilateral. In this case the orbit cavity is also small because of the absence of its growth induction by the eyeball (Albernaz et al. 1997).

PHPV is clinically suggested by leucocoria (Fig. 20.1b). Microphthalmia and persistent hyaloid are observed on MRI, which also eliminates the existence of a tumoral lesion.

20.4.2 Orbital Malformations

Orbital malformations are observed in trigonocephaly, scaphocephaly and brachycephaly. Crouzon's or Apert's disease with sphenoidal ethmoidal and maxillary malformations can lead to orbital abnormalities. Orbital malformations can also be encountered in craniofacial dysraphism (Tessier's classification).

Malformations of the orbit are also seen in Recklinghausen's disease. They are characterised by sphenoidal dysplasia, enlargement of the orbital fissure and scalloping of the spinal bodies. Corpus callosum agenesis and septo-optic dysplasia are possible associated findings.

20.5 Tumoral and Vascular Orbitopathies

In these cases biometric measurements and 2D and 3D reconstructions should be performed. MRI protocols include several weighted sequences: T1-weighted images, T2-weighted images, STIR, T-weighted images with fat suppression pre- and postgadolinium-DTPA (Gd-DTPA) injection. It is only when these sequences are done that the diagnosis of ocular, orbital tumours as well as their local regional effect and extension can be confirmed. Melanoma in adults and retinoblastoma in children are the two most frequently encountered tumours.

20.5.1 Ocular Tumours (Reese 1976)

The melanoma develops from the ciliary body and choroids and is the most frequent malignant tumour of the globe. Two types may exist: a nodular form and a diffuse form. Choroidal melanoma is spontaneously hyperdense on CT, with contrast enhancement, and associated RD may be detected. On MRI the tumour is hyperintense on T1-weighted images and hypointense on T2-weighted images as compared to the vitreous (Fig. 20.2). Post-Gd-DTPA enhancement of the lesion contrasts with the absence of enhancement of the RD (De Potter et al. 1995). This aspect is found in the majority of melanomas. The amelanic melanoma may exhibit different signal abnormalities and is often difficult to differentiate from other benign lesions or metastases. The aspect of RD is characteristic as a V shape (Girardot et al. 1994) attached to the papilla and hyperintense on both T1-weighted images and T2-weighted images. Fat suppression and Gd differentiate the melanoma from the RD. Melanomas may spread to surrounding orbital structures and metastases in the lung and the liver.

Primary lung, breast and gastrointestinal carcinomas may spread to the globe. Ocular metastases are bilateral multifocal and display hyperdensity on CT and enhance with contrast material (De Potter et al. 1995; Cabanis et al. 1996). T1-weighted images show a hypersignal as compared to the vitreous, with minimal Gd enhancement. On T2-weighted images the lesion is intense. The diagnosis of metastases is not difficult if the primary tumour is known.

Occasionally ocular lymphoma can be encountered in patients with cerebral lymphoma (Fig. 20.3). On CT, choroidal and haemangioma are as hyperdense and postcontrast highly enhanced. On MRI the lesion is hyperintense on T1-weighted images and isointense on T2-weighted images. In von Hippel-Lindau disease, retinal haemangiomas display the same signal as choroidal haemangioma with moderate postcontrast enhancement (Stroszczynski 1998).

In children leucocoria is suggestive of retinoblastoma, Coats' disease, PHPV, retrolental fibrosis or *Toxocara canis*-induced endophthalmia (Fig. 20.2). As the melanoma is the most common intraocular malignant tumour, retinoblastoma can be either sporadic or hereditary (Ball 1997; Reese 1976). CT shows hyperdense lesion with irregular contours and often calcifications. After injection moderate postcontrast enhancement is observed. The eyeball is of normal shape. Extension towards the optic nerve, orbit and brain is possible. Three distinct forms are observed: exophytic, endophytic and a form with diffuse and subtle spread to the retina with no evident mass. The latter is not easy to diagnose. On T1- and T2-weighted images the lesion is heterogeneous with slight postcontrast enhancement (Fig. 20.2). This heterogeneity is due to the components of the tumours as the calcifications, necrosis and associated RD. RD is frequently associated with the exophytic form. The "pseudoglioma" is the principal differential diagnosis. On MRI, a small eyeball and persistent hyaloid in PHPV are found. The T1-weighted images and T2-weighted images hypersignal of RD, and the post-Gd-DTPA enhancement of the retina, allow the diagnosis of Coats' disease to be established (Ball 1997) with RD. The subretinal fluid on hypersignal is on both T1-weighted images and T2-weighted images without postcontrast enhancement. In retrolental fibrosis the principal features are small eyeball and RD.

20.5.2 Orbital Tumours (Bilaniuk et al. 1990; Mafee et al. 1987)

CT and MRI are the methods of choice for investigating orbital tumours, allowing an early diagnosis. Orbital tumours can be classified as primary intra- or extracoronal or secondary tumours spreading from the eyelid conjunctiva or sinus (Fig. 20.3). The metastases extend to the eyeball or to the structures of the orbit.

The most typical orbital tumour is the optic glioma or juvenile pilocytic astrocytoma (Ball 1997). This lesion is observed in the context of Recklinghausen's neurofibromatosis in 12–38% of cases. A visual loss and proptosis are the principal signs. It spreads into the optic chiasm through the canalar and cisternal segments of the optic nerve and optic tract. On CT the tumour appears as a fusiform or global enlargement of the optic nerve and of the optic canal. The aspect of postcontrast enhancement is variable. On MRI it appears as an isosignal as compared to the gray matter on T1-weighted images and a hypersignal on T2-weighted images with a possible postcontrast enhancement. It is essential to identify the spread of these diseases towards the brain (Linder et al. 1987). In Recklinghausen's neurofibromatosis, proliferation of arachnoids and dural cells may be seen as an enlargement of the perioptic spaces. The trapping of CSF at the anterior section of the optic nerve is also a characteristic sign of glioma. MRI shows an area of abnormal signal in the midbrain, thalamus cerebellar hemispheres and diencephalic peduncles. This abnormality may resolve spontaneously.

Plexiform neurofibroma is a benign tumour seen in type I neurofibromatosis. It has a typical aspect and may be associated with sphenoidal dysplasia and widening of the orbital fissure. On CT the lesion is homogeneously enhanced by contrast material and bone modifications. MRI reveals a diffuse homogeneous and infiltrating tumour at the anterior section (eyelid) of the orbit. Compared to the muscles, the lesion is always post-Gd enhanced on T1-weighted images, and hyperintense on T2-weighted images.

Meningiomas of the optic nerve sheath are observed in both adults and children (Fig. 20.4). In the latter group these tumours are observed in type II neurofibromatosis. Slow growing and progressive visual loss are the clinical characteristics. Meningiomas are tumours originating from arachnoid cells. The development from the optic nerve sheath is frequent. The encephalic location may spread to perioptic sheaths. A meningiomatous reaction may be observed near the optic glioma. A standard X-ray shows condensation of the optical canal or sphenoid bone. On CT there is an enlargement of the neuro-optic complex which is spontaneously hyperdense with or without calcifications. The lesion is highly postcontrast enhanced, forming a typical "tram-track" aspect. On MRI the aspect is isointense or hypointense on T1-weighted images as compared to muscles. The meningiomas show iso- or hyperintense signals on T2-weighted images with intense T1-weighted images post-Gd enhancement. T1-weighted images must be performed with fat suppression (De Potter et al. 1995; Cabanis et al. 1996).

Osteomeningioma of the external wall of the orbit is in both intraorbital and intracephalic positions, and extends towards the external temporal fossa. On CT the lesion is spontaneously hyperdense with a mass effect on the external rectus muscle. Osteocondensation of the sphenoid is also observed. MRI shows the thickening of the dura and delineates the osteocondensation.

Fibrous dysplasia is a bone disease characterised by the spread of the fibrous tissue within the diploë.

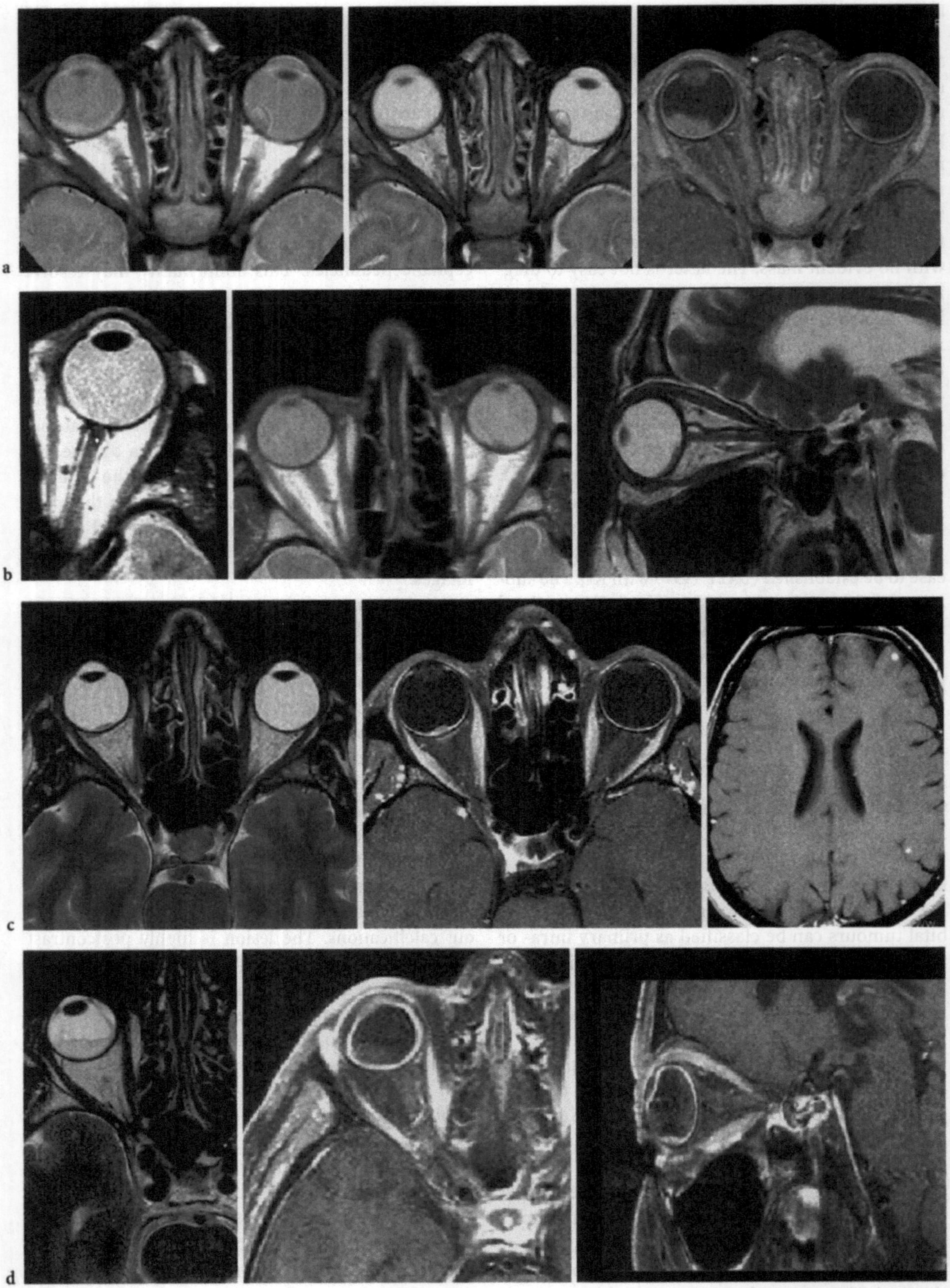

Fig. 20.2. **a** Bilateral endophytic retinoblastoma on PD. Temporal location of the tumour in the right eye with a minimal RD. Nasal location on the left, without RD. Moderate postcontrast enhancement (axial short and heavy T2 WI, axial T1 WI with fat saturation after Gd administration). **b** Small uveal melanoma of the left eye in a T2 WI axial plane, arciform and well delineated on T2 WI in the left OTNOP. **c** Ocular metastasis of the right eye on PD WI, and postcontrast T WI in axial planes. Brain metastases are shown. **d** Choroidal detachment with fluid-fluid level on T2 WI, postcontrast enhancement on axial plane and OTNOP

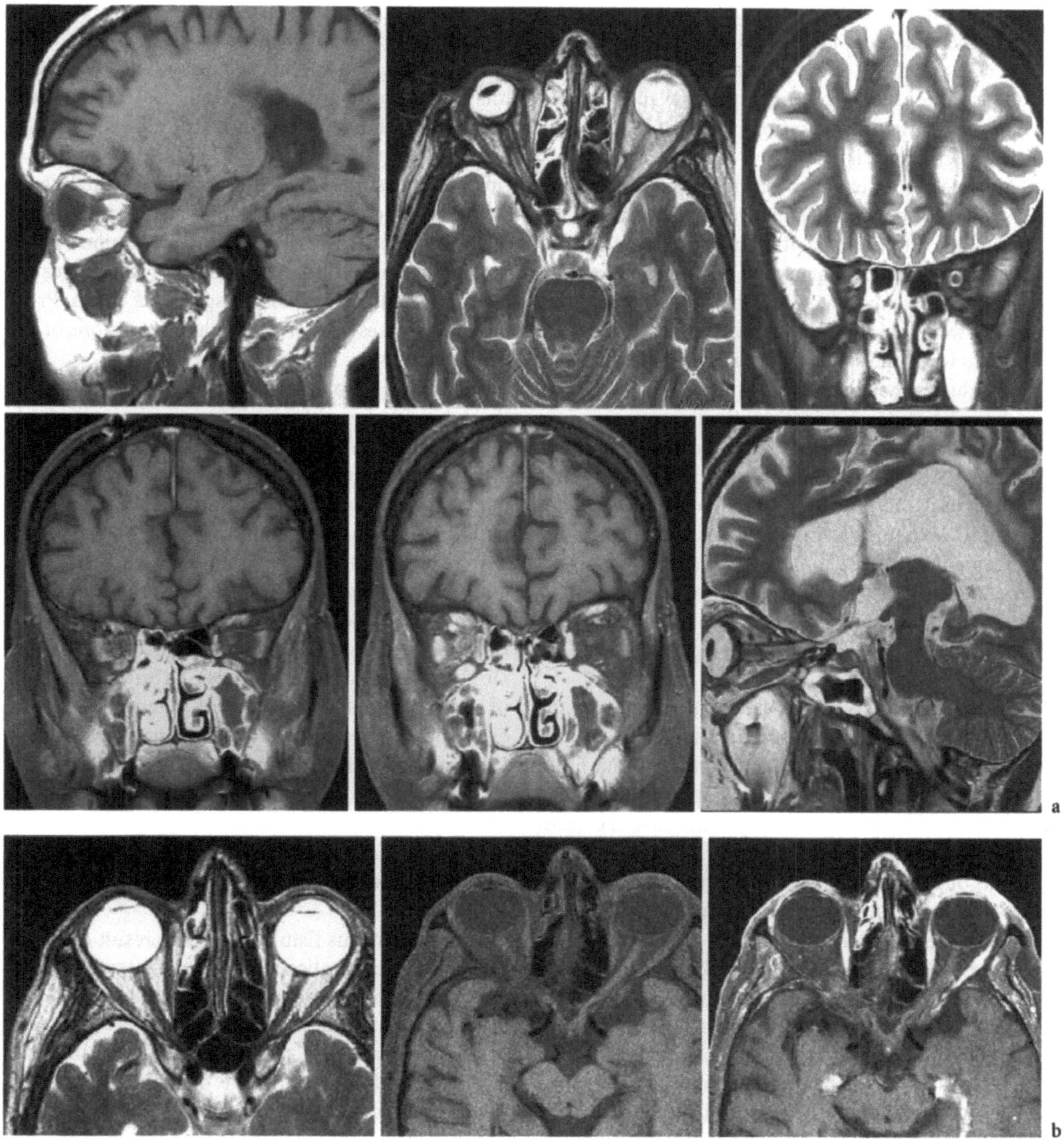

Fig. 20.3. a A late stage of a right ocular lymphoma with an atrophic globe with atrophic optic nerve and perioptic space enlargement (sagittal T1 WI, axial and coronal T2 WI). Perioptic and orbital fat enhancement of the apex (coronal T1 WI with fat saturation). Primitive cerebral lymphoma exhibiting a hypersignal in the periventricular white matter (T2 WI, OTNOP). **b** Spinocellular tumour of the left conjunctiva, possibly ignored on T2 WI, and well detected after contrast administration and

It involves the base skull or facial bone. Exophthalmia and mass effect at the orbital apex may be important. CT and MRI show a heterogeneous and hypodense/intense thickening aspect of the affected bone. Contrast administration is useless because the aspect is characteristic.

Mucocele is an expansive intrasinusal lesion, with erosion of the bone of the involved sinus. It causes exophthalmia and diplopia. It homogeneous or not, hyperdense and not enhanced by contrast material on CT. Its signal is increased on both T1-weighted images and T2-weighted images. Ethmoidal location is very frequent while the sphenoid is rarely invaded. This lesion is due to the obstruction of sinusal ostia leading to chronic haemorrhagic and inflammatory reaction.

Dermoid cysts are frequently located at the base of the eyebrow. Their aspect is typical and their diagnosis is easy. On CT, cyst is hypodense and well delineated without osteolysis and postcontrast enhancement. On MRI the T1-weighted image signal depends on the presence of the proteinaceous and water content (hypersignal) and the sebaceous product gland (hyposignal). On T2-weighted images the signal increases heterogeneously.

Haemangioma is a very frequent tumour of the orbit with a cavernous aspect in adults and a capillary one in children. Capillary haemangioma has a proliferative phase followed by an involutive one with an infiltrative tendency. In this case the most common location is a nasal sector. It is poorly delineated. On T1-weighted images there is either a hypo- or isosignal as compared to the muscles with post-Gd enhancement, but without post-Gd enhancement of nutritive vessels. T2-weighted images reveal hyperintensity as compared to the muscles. Cavernous haemangioma and intraconal lesion is often encountered in females. It is more homogeneous, well delineated than capillary haemangioma, iso- or hypointense on T1-weighted images and hyperintense on T2-weighted images. The lymphangioma develops from lymphatic vessels. It is also an infiltrating lesion poorly encapsulated with a hypersignal on T1-weighted images; and on T2-weighted images is enhanced heterogeneously after contrast. Relapses and worsening are often observed and haemorrhagic foci can occur. The signal depends on the age of haemorrhage (Adenis and Morax 1998; Cabanis et al. 1996; Ball 1997).

Malignant tumours of the lacrimal gland (cystic adenocarcinoma) are frequently observed in females. They exhibit an extraconal and posteroseptal development (Adenis and Morax 1998). CT shows an isodense lesion to the muscles with a variable enhancement after contrast administration. On MRI the tumour is isointense or hyperintense on T1-weighted imaging and hyperintense on T2-weighted imaging as compared to the muscles. T1-weighted images with fat suppression reveal a highly intense lesion after administration of Gd. Bone modifications are possible. Infiltration of the lacrimal gland can also be observed in lymphoproliferative syndromes. In this case MRI aspects are similar to primary cancers. Secondary lesions of breast cancer are characterised by lyses of the sphenoid wings. Prostatic metastases present as condensing lesions of the sphenoid wing.

In children, malignant rhabdomyosarcomas of the orbit develop either in situ or by secondary extension. Three forms are observed. One of these forms developing very fast from the embryonic remnants may be mistaken with an infectious or idiopathic pseudotumoral lesion. T1-weighted imaging may reveal an isointense tumour which is hyperintense on T2-weighted imaging. It is enhanced by Gd and may be osteolytic on CT. If any doubt persists, a biopsy of the lesion is indicated (Goddé-Jolly and Dufier 1992; Kodsi et al. 1994). Orbital metastases of neuroblastomas present with haemorrhage and ecchymosis. They reveal 10% of all neuroblastomas. Perioptic extension is typical of leukaemia.

20.5.3 Vascular Disorders

Carotidocavernous fistula (CCF) is a result of an abnormal communication between the internal carotid artery and the cavernous sinus (Fig. 20.4). Blood flow is decreased in spontaneous CCF, which is observed in the elderly, and it is increased in traumatism-induced CCF, which is observed more often in younger patients. The consequences are exophthalmia, swelling of muscles, increased volume of cavernous sinus and dilatation of superior ophthalmic vein (SOV). Low flow fistula might cause isolated conjunctive hyperaemia. In this case, MRI reveals abnormal vessels within the cavernoma sinus with clinically a mild exophthalmia. MRA (3DTOF and 2DPC) may show an abnormal hypersignal corresponding to dilated vessels with a possible large hyposignal in SOV topography related to increased flow in this structure. In post-traumatic CCF, exophthalmia is more severe and there is rectus muscle swelling, a large hyposignal of SOV, and enlargement of the cavernomatous sinus. In this case, MRA in addition shows a very large SOV with an inversion of its flow direction on 2DPC sequences.

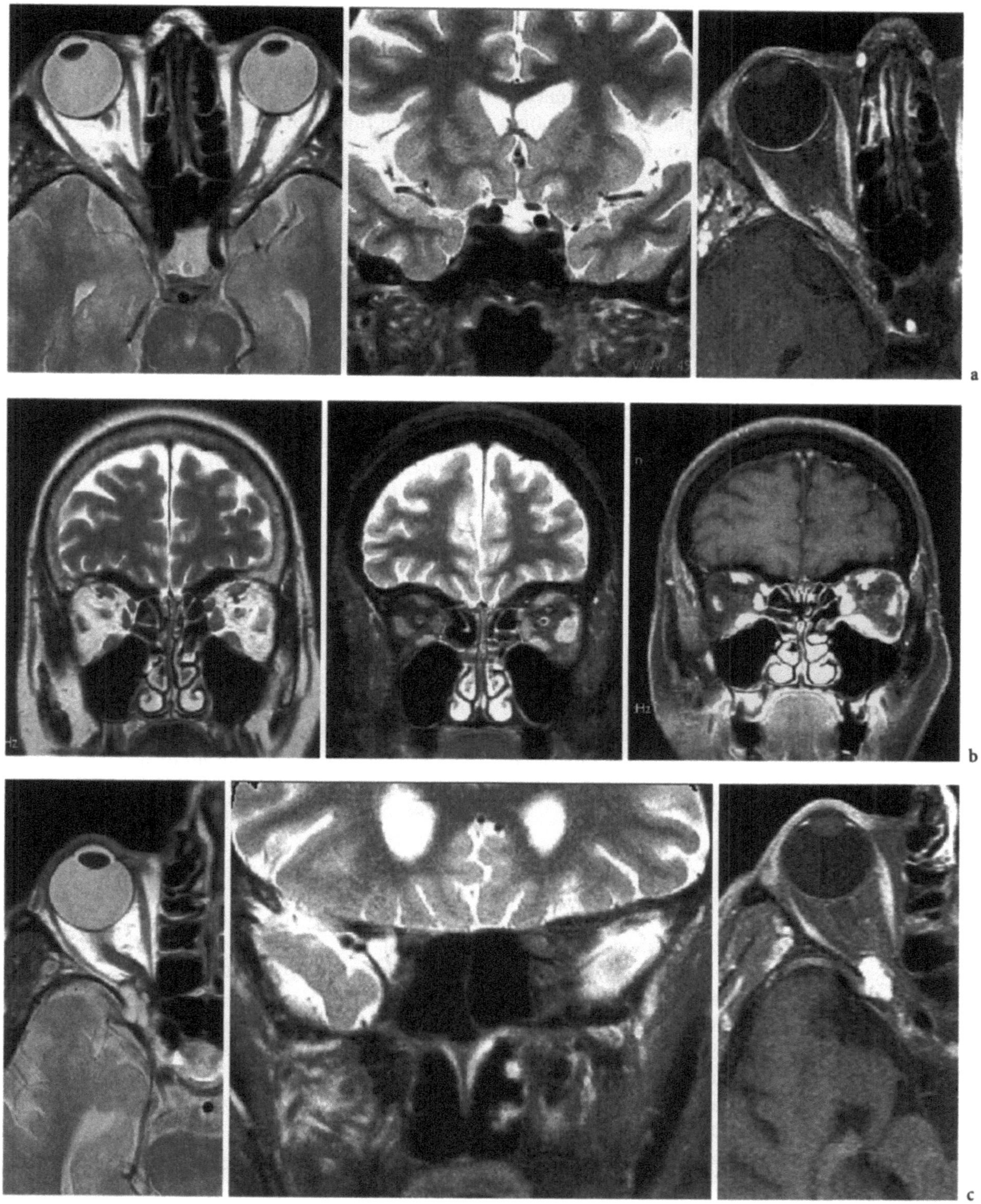

Fig. 20.4. a Meningioma as a right paraoptic nerve mass in the apex shown on T2 WI and postcontrast T1 WI. Note on coronal T2 WI the atrophy of the cisternal portion of the right optic nerve, as compared to the opposite side. **b** Carotidocavernous fistula observed as a swelling of the left rectus muscles. Intense postcontrast T1 WI enhancement. Enlargement of the SOV due to the increased blood flow. **c** Non-thrombosed orbital varicosity at the right apex near the optic canal with a mass effect on the optic nerve. T2 WI hypersignal on the axial and coronal planes, and postcontrast enhancement on T1 WI

Conventional angiography may be needed if a treatment is to be proposed.

Orbital varicose is responsible for positional exophthalmia. It is diagnosed with CT, which may reveal and exacerbate the exophthalmia in procubitus or with Valsalva's manoeuvre. The iodine contrast is necessary. The MRI shows hyperintense on both T1-weighted images and T2-weighted images with a hypersignal after contrast. An acute thrombosis lesion is a hyposignal on both T1-weighted images and T2-weighted images.

20.6 Inflammatory and Infectious Disorders

20.6.1 Basedow's Ophthalmopathy

Basedow's disease is responsible for 10% of exophthalmia. Thirty percent of patients exhibit eyelid oedema, exophthalmia and inflammatory changes within the orbit, leading to a decreased motility of the ocular globe. CT and MRI reveal muscular and fat tissue hypertrophy. Furthermore the muscular signal is decreased on T1-weighted images and increased on T2-weighted images. In severe cases, CT and MRI may show deformation of the internal orbital walls. Biometric measurements help to monitor the disease (Cabanis et al. 1996).

20.6.2 Cellulitis and Abscess (Hoffmann et al. 1998)

Orbital cellulitis provokes pain, palpebral oedema and chemosis (Fig. 20.5). Preseptal and retroseptal cellulitis must be distinguished. Subperiostic abscess may develop from this infectious process (Adenis and Morax 1998). CT scan shows palpebral and subcutaneous tissue swelling. Sinusitis is a frequent associated finding. Subperiostic abscess is a space occupying lesion, hypodense on CT with peripheral postcontrast enhancement. On MRI it is an intraorbital mass, hypointense on T1-weighted images and hyperintense on T2-weighted images. The outcome of orbital cellulitis is favourable with antibiotics. Subperiostic abscess may need drainage. In children it is necessary to differentiate these two lesions from rhabdomyosarcoma and rule out the presence of a foreign body (wood).

20.6.3 Inflammatory Idiopathic Pseudotumour and Lymphoproliferative Disorders

There are four subtypes of idiopathic pseudotumour (IPT): pseudo-lymphoma, reactive lymphoid hyperplasia, atypical lymphoid hyperplasia and lymphocytic lymphoma. IPTs cause pain, exophthalmia and low visual acuity (Adenis and Morax 1998). Their topography may be anterior, posterior, in the lacrimal fossa, or muscular (myositis). On CT these lesions are hyperdense with a slight postcontrast enhancement. MRI reveals a mass infiltrating the intraorbital tissue or the sheath of the optic nerve. On T1-weighted images and T2-weighted images, IPT appears isointense as compared to muscles (De Potter et al. 1995; Bencherif et al. 1993). In the chronic stage it can display low signal intensity. After Gd administration, homogeneous enhancement is usual. This process may involve sclera, Tenon's capsule, and the lacrimal gland. It is important to distinguish an IPT-induced myositis from Basedow's disease myopathy. In IPT, involvement of the tendon is possible.

The lymphoma is usually located on the superior, anterior or temporal part of the orbit. It is a spontaneously hyperdense tumour on CT adjacent to the globe extending towards the lacrimal gland. MRI reveals an iso- or hypointense lesion on T2-weighted images and T1-weighted images with postcontrast enhancement (Fig. 20.5).

20.7 Optic Neuritis and Papilledema

CT and MRI have had an enormous impact in investigating optic nerve diseases: tumours, inflammation, optic atrophy. In multiple sclerosis a hypersignal within the optic nerve is observed on STIR sequences (Cabanis et al. 1996; Ball 1997; Tourbah et al. 1999). A postcontrast enhancement is possible. A decreased size of the opticoperioptic complex confirms the clinically observed optic atrophy. Besides MRI helps to exclude mass lesion. In paediatrics, the origin of optic neuritis may be inflammatory as in juvenile multiple sclerosis, or infectious. Bilateral papilledema is caused by intracranial hypertension thrombophlebitis, rarely by cauda equina tumour. On CT optic nerve size is

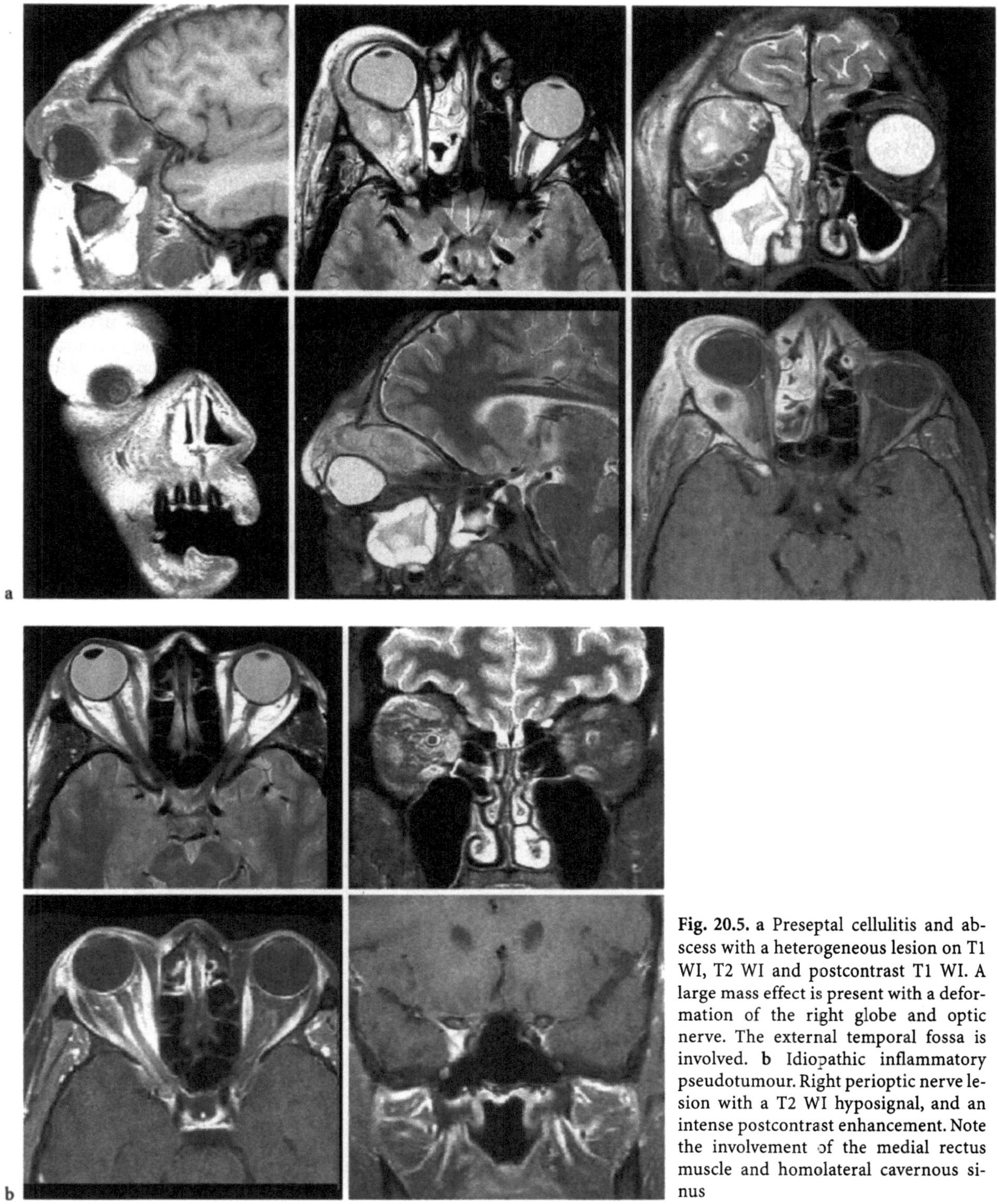

Fig. 20.5. a Preseptal cellulitis and abscess with a heterogeneous lesion on T1 WI, T2 WI and postcontrast T1 WI. A large mass effect is present with a deformation of the right globe and optic nerve. The external temporal fossa is involved. b Idiopathic inflammatory pseudotumour. Right perioptic nerve lesion with a T2 WI hyposignal, and an intense postcontrast enhancement. Note the involvement of the medial rectus muscle and homolateral cavernous sinus

enlarged. MRI shows the enlargement involves particularly perioptic spaces. Besides CT can reveal calcifications due to drusen. Idiopathic (benign) intracranial hypertension (pseudo tumour cerebri) is more frequently observed in females with overweight. Lumbar puncture confirms the diagnosis and allows improvement of the symptomatology, which can be monitored with MRI.

References

Adenis JP, Morax S (1998) Pathologie orbito-palpébrale. Masson, Paris

Albernaz VS, Castillo M, Hudgins PA, Mukherdji SK (1997) Imaging findings in patients with clinical anophthalmos. AJNR 18: 555–561

Ball WS Jr (1997) Pediatric Neuroradiology. Lippincott Raven, Philadelphia New York

Bencherif B, Zouaoui A, Chedid G, Kujas M, Van Effenterre R, Marsault C (1993) Intracranial extension of an idiopathic orbital inflammatory pseudotumor. AJNR 14: 181–184

Bilaniuk LT, Zimmerman RA, Newton TH (1990) Magnetic resonance imaging: orbital pathology. In: Newton TH, Bilaniuk LT (eds) Radiology of the Eye and Orbit. Raven Press, New York, p 5

Cabanis EA (1983) Détermination par tomodensitométrie d'un "nouveau" plan de référence céphalique orienté selon les voies visuelles: le Plan Neuro-Oculaire (PNO). Mémoire pour le D.E.R.B.H. mention Anatomie Université Paris V René Descartes, Paris

Cabanis EA, Bourgeois H, Iba-Zizen MT et al. (1996) L'imagerie en ophtalmologie. Masson, Paris

Carmody RF, Mafee MF, Goodwin JA, Small K, Haery C (1994) Orbital and optic pathway sarcoidosis: MR findings. AJNR 15: 775–783

De Potter P, Shields JA, Shields CL (1995) MRI of the eye and orbit. Lippincott, Philadelphia

Girardot C, Hazebroucq VG, Fery-Lemonnier E et al. (1994) MR imaging and CT of surgical materials currently used in ophthalmology: in vitro and in vivo study. Radiology 191: 433–439

Goddé-Jolly D, Dufier JL (1992) Ophtalmologie Pédiatrique. Masson, Paris

Hoffmann KT, Hosten N, Lemke AJ, Sander B, Zwicker C, Felix R (1998) Septum orbitale: high-resolution MR in orbital anatomy. AJNR 19: 91–94

Kodsi SR, Shetlar DJ, Campbell RJ, Garrity JA, Bartley GB (1994) A review of 340 orbital tumors in children during a 60-year period. Am J Ophthalmol 117: 177–182

Linder R, Campos M, Schafer M (1987) CT and MRI of orbital abnormalities in neurofibromatosis and selected craniofacial anomalies. Radiol Clin North Am 25: 787–802

Mafee MF, Putterman A, Valvassori GE, Campos M, Capek V (1987) Orbital space-occupying lesions: role of computed tomography and magnetic resonance imaging. Radiol Clin North Am 25: 529–559

Newman NJ, Miller NR (1998) Clinical Neuro-ophthalmology. Williams and Wilkinns, Baltimore

Reese AB (1976) Tumors of the eye. Harper and Row Publisher, Hagerstown

Stroszczynski C, Hosten N, Bornfeld N et al (1998) Choroidal hemangioma: MR findings and differentiation from uveal melanoma. AJNR 19: 1441–1447

Tourbah A, Gout O, Liblau R, Lyon-Caen O, Bougniot C, Iba-Zizen MT, Cabanis EA (1999) Encephalitis after hepatitis B vaccination. Recurrent disseminated encephalitis or MS? Neurology 53: 386–401

21 Pediatric Neuroimaging: Cortical Developmental Malformations

PHILIPPE DEMAEREL

CONTENTS

21.1 Introduction

Although malformations of cortical development are as old as mankind, paradoxically they are a fast evolving subject in the field of pediatric neuroradiology. The superiority of magnetic resonance (MR) imaging allowed the description of sometimes very subtle abnormalities that remained undetected on cranial computed tomography and has improved our understanding of malformations of the cerebral neocortex.

Traditionally the proposed classifications were based on the pathological findings but there remained problems with the terminology and classifications because the link with the embryology and symptomatology was missing.

With the improved insight in genetics, embryology, imaging and pathology, a new classification has been proposed. Neuronal migration disorders constitute only one part of this classification and should be reserved for disorders of brain development thought to result from abnormal neuronal migration. Two other major groups of cortical developmental malformations are those caused by disorders of cell proliferation and those resulting from disorders of cortical organization.

The spectrum of cortical developmental malformations has recently been studied (LEVENTER at al. 1999). The main malformations observed were heterotopic gray matter (19%), cortical tubers (17%), focal cortical dysplasia (16%), polymicrogyria (16%) and agyria/pachygyria (15%).

New observations will be discussed as well as the changes in approach that are caused by the new classification.

The prenatal detection of cortical developmental malformations will be discussed in Chap. 23.

21.2 Technical Aspects

Both T1- and T2-weighted images must be obtained at the same time. Due to the myelination of the white matter, its signal closely resembles that of gray matter at some time during the 1st year of life. Therefore T1-weighted images are mandatory between 9 and 18 months of age while T2-weighted images are most useful in the first 6 months of life to analyze the gyration.

One should be careful when analyzing routine T2-weighted sequences with 5 or 6 mm slice thickness (Fig. 21.1). This often results in averaging of the undulating cortical gyri with the white matter and the CSF. This may result in the false impression of increased thickness of the cortex when oblique to the plane of section. Routine (fast) spin-echo T2-weighted images are not recommended in the search for cortical developmental malformations. Our department uses a double echo short time inversion recovery (DESTIR) sequence which offers an excellent differentiation between gray and white matter (TR/TE/TI = 5100/23,85/145 ms). Others have suggested the use of a T2-weighted fast multiplanar inversion recovery sequence (CHAN et al. 1998). The inversion

PH. DEMAEREL, MD, PhD
Consultant Neuroradiologist, Department of Radiology, University Hospitals, Herestraat 49, Leuven 3000, Belgium

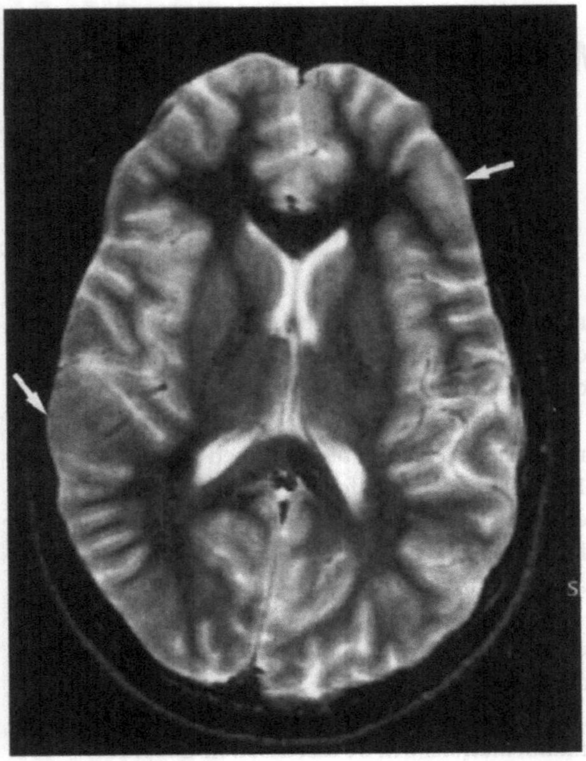

Fig. 21.1. Axial DESTIR T2-weighted MR image showing the false impression of increased thickness of the cortex on a 5 mm slide (*arrow*)

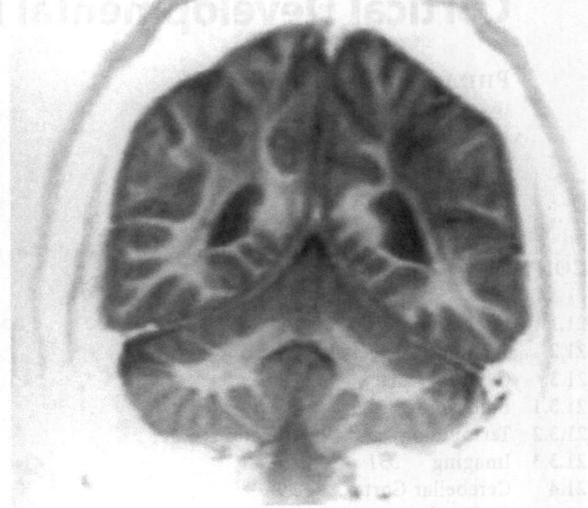

Fig. 21.2. Coronal T1-weighted IR MR image providing an optimal gray-white contrast

time of 200 ms results in an additive effect of T1 and T2 prolongation and a maximal discrimination of the gray and white matter. The images of these T2-weighted sequences look like the histopathological myelin stain. Heavily T1-weighted inversion recovery sequences are also characterized by an optimal gray/white contrast (Fig. 21.2). A three-dimensional T2-weighted volumetric sequence may prove to be useful but is not routinely available at this moment.

The use of three-dimensional Fourier transform T1-weighted volumetric imaging of the brain was an important step forward in the analysis of subtle cortical malformations. In approximately 9 min 160, usually sagittal, slices of 1 mm are obtained with a voxel size of 1×1×1 mm^3. These settings guarantee high resolution multiplanar reformations. Reformations are extremely useful to correct for asymmetrical positioning of the head. Postprocessing allows an analysis of the entire frontal and parietal cortex on one axial slice (Fig. 21.3). Using such 3D data, surface rendering can be performed to demonstrate the topographic delineation of the cortical abnormalities and their relation to adjacent gyri and sulci (Lee et al. 1997) (Fig. 21.4).

The use of a phased-array head coil offers an increased signal-to-noise ratio that can be used to improve both signal and contrast resolution (Fig. 21.5). These surface coils are not yet routinely available but they will become an important technical improvement in our search for small cortical abnormalities (Grant et al. 1997).

Multimodal image coregistration techniques that allow visualization of the relationship between structural lesions and cellular metabolism or function may offer new dimensions for surgical planning of cortical malformations (Fig. 21.6).

Other useful postprocessing techniques consist of a mathematical analysis of the brain such as analysis of the gray-white junction, the gray and white matter volume and the brain surface. Contralateral abnormalities have been found in patients with apparent unilateral changes and abnormalities extending beyond the visualized MR changes (Sisodiya et al. 1995).

21.3 Cerebral Cortex

21.3.1 Embryology

The mechanism of neuronal migration is still not completely elucidated (Rakic 1988; Sidman and a 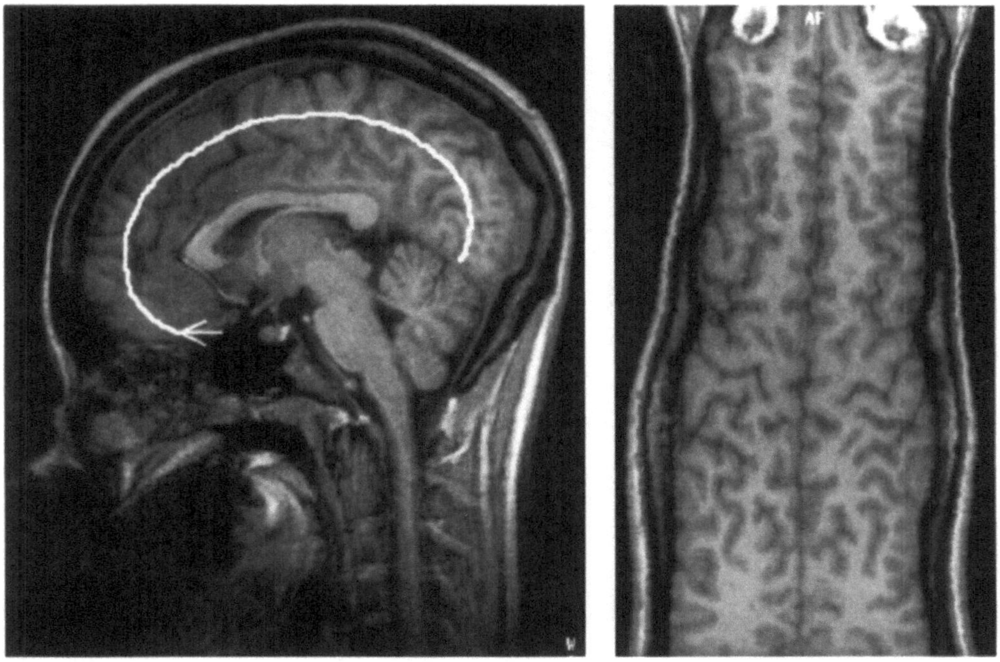 b

Fig. 21.3a,b. Reformatted image after a postprocessing procedure consisting of cutting a curved slice through the 3D data set (a) to display the frontal, parietal and occipital cortex in the axial plane (b)

Rakic 1973). During the 7th fetal week, germinal layers begin to form in the vesicle walls of telencephalic outpouchings (vesicles) at the foramina of Monro. At that time, the ventricular zone, intermediate zone (future white matter) and marginal zone can be appreciated as distinct. This is the period of neuronal and glial proliferation. The onset of neuronal migration to the cortex occurs during the 8th fetal week. Cells in the germinal zone elongate with the nucleus further from the ventricular surface. The migration process is fed by active proliferation of cells from the germinal matrix. After mitosis, the newly formed neuroblasts are distant from the ventricular surface. Later, as the distance increases, migration occurs along the radial glial fibers which span the distance from the ventricular surface to the pia. The migration continues until the 24th week of gestation and may continue up to a few months after birth. Neurons of the deepest cortical layers are the first to radially migrate, while the neuroblasts destined for the more superficial cortical layers (layers 6, 5, 4, 3 and 2) migrate past them. The cells of layer 1 are the exception by arriving first at their final superficial cortical destination. The initial cortical plate is noted at 7–10 weeks of gestation. A progressive condensation occurs and by the 16th week a six-layered cortex can be observed. The normal cortex is not thicker than 4.5 mm.

A tangential neuronal migration, complementary and orthogonally to the radial migration, has been observed and forms complex three-dimensional neural structures (Rakic 1990).

Abnormal tissue is sometimes seen extending from the ventricle to the pia. This may suggest an abnormality of the radial glial-neuronal unit along which stem cells differentiate and migrate. Following the completion of neuronal migration and early cortical organization, the glial cells that are dispersed transform into mature astrocytes. The sulcation is most pronounced between 26 and 28 weeks of gestation, but continuous until shortly after birth. Particular attention has been paid to the opercular formation (Chen et al. 1996). The first sulcus to form at approximately 14–16 weeks is the circular sulcus of the sylvian fissure. Around 20 weeks the posterior operculum is formed and around 19–22 weeks the insular cortex can be observed and the opercular formation proceeds from posterior to anterior. The insular gyri are observed at 32–34 weeks of gestation. The anterior portion of the insula remains exposed until 38 weeks. The rolandic fissure, the parieto-occipital and superior temporal sulcus develop later. A large number of sulci can be observed at 32–33 weeks of gestation. The sulci have an adult appearance at birth but continue to deepen over the next weeks.

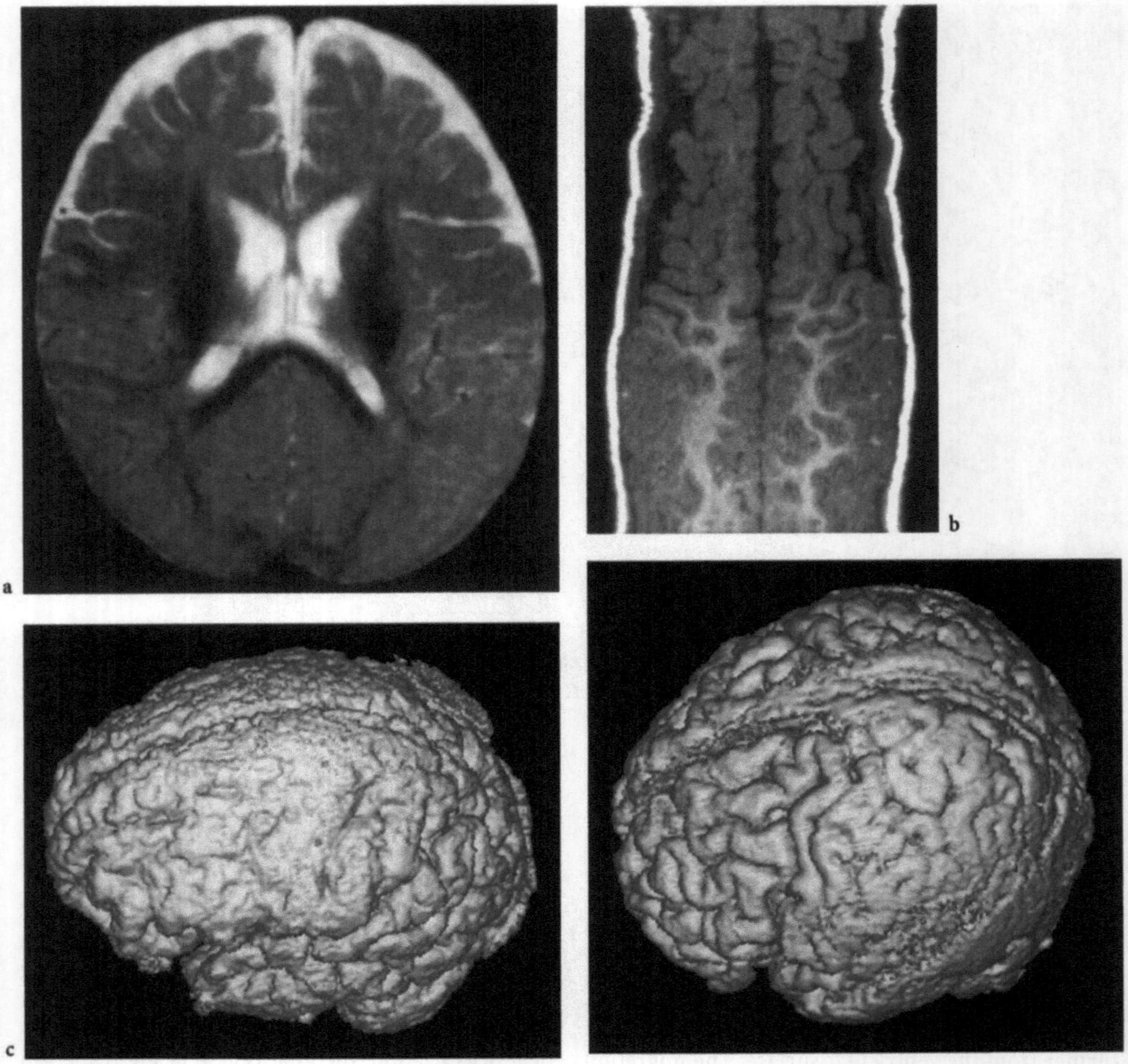

Fig. 21.4a–d. Axial DESTIR T2-weighted (**a**) and reformatted curved gradient-echo T1-weighted (**b**) MR images. Note that the abnormalities are clearly seen on the curved axial slice (**b**) compared to the T2-weighted image (**a**). Surface reconstruction from a 3D data set in a 6-month-old child with bilateral cortical developmental abnormalities in the parietal lobe (**c**). For comparison, a normal 3D data set is shown (**d**)

21.3.2 Terminology and Classification

Although terms such as lissencephaly, pachygyria, schizencephaly, polymicrogyria, cortical dysplasia and heterotopia all sound familiar, it is very difficult to find a reliable and exact definition for each of these terms. Clinicians, radiologists and pathologists all have their own definitions to explain the abnormalities. It is accepted now these different cortical malformations are not well defined separate entities and that there are overlaps. Cortical dysplasia was being used to cover different cortical developmental abnormalities. Indeed, it had been suggested to use the term cortical dysplasia instead of polymicrogyria (Ball 1997). Schizencephaly has been referred to as an extreme form of cortical dysplasia. Subpial heterotopia and focal subcortical heterotopia have been considered as cortical dysplasia too. Cortical dysplasia is a general term which only refers to a malformative lesion of the neocortex which exhibits a spectrum of pathological changes reflecting a disturbance in the process of its development and should rather be reserved for cases with a proved

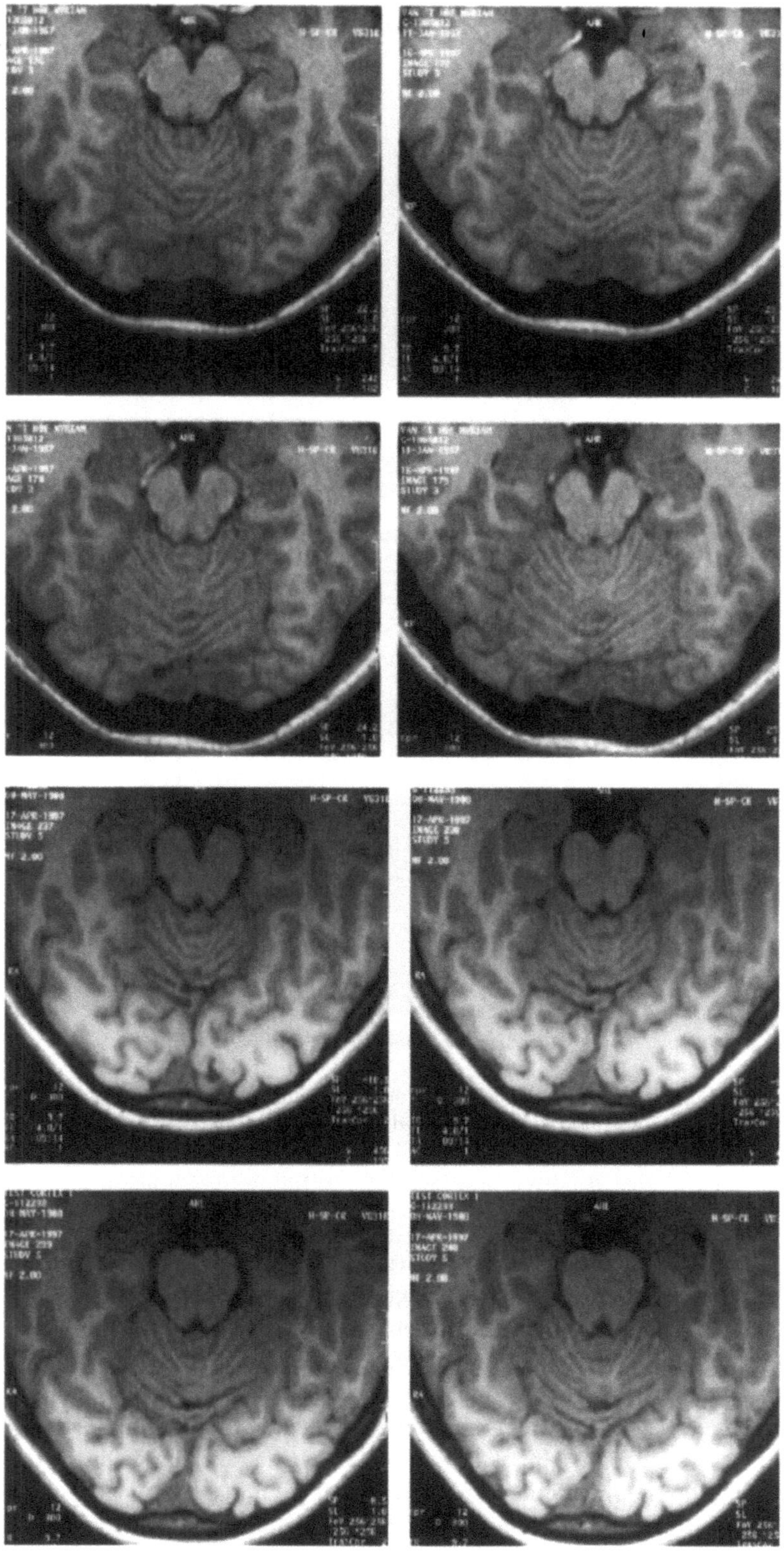

a

b

Fig. 21.5a,b. T1-weighted 3D volumetric imaging with axial reformatted slices obtained with a circularly-polarized head coil (**a**) and with a phased-array head coil (**b**) in a volunteer demonstrating the improved contrast resolution when using the passed-array head coil

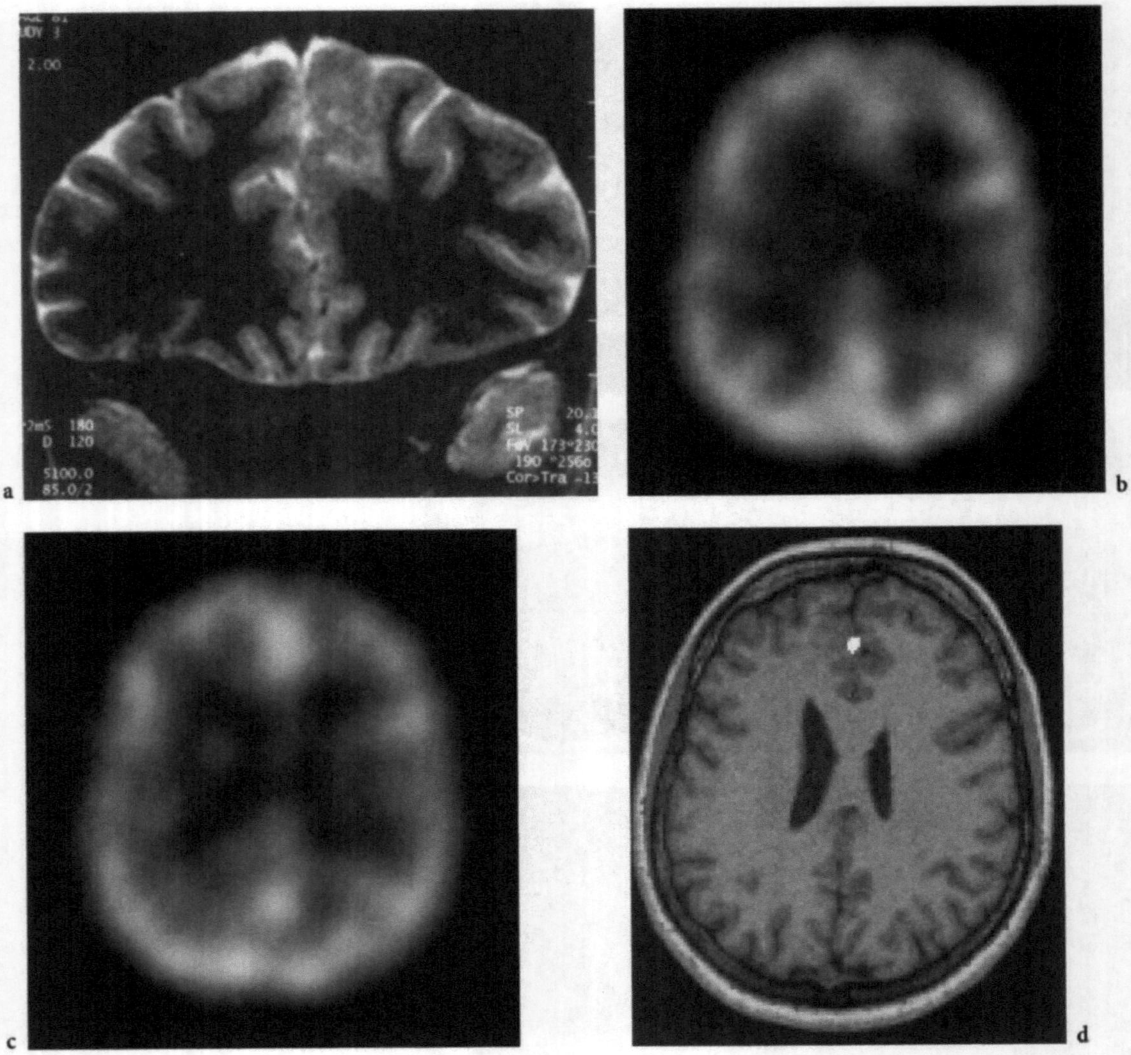

Fig. 21.6a–d. Coronal T2-weighted MR image showing focal cortical dysplasia in the left frontal lobe (**a**). ^{99m}Tc-ECD SPECT images of brain perfusion were coregistered and (after normalization) subtracted (ital ?????-interidal ???? SPECT) (**b,c**). A fusion image was continuted showing ???? the differences between the two SPECT images overlayed on a T1-weighted MR image (**d**). (Courtery of Dr. Sc. Dupont, Department of Nuclear Medicine, Catholic University of Leuven, Belgien)

neuropathological proof. The term is misleading too because of the existence of a well defined entity called focal cortical dysplasia of Taylor. Cortical dysgenesis would therefore be a better term because dysgenesis refers to "defective development," and thus has neither histological nor pathogenetic connotations. But this term resembles cortical dysplasia and we do not advocate its use. Cortical developmental malformation is the best general term to cover all these abnormalities.

There is no consensus on the classification of cortical developmental malformations, due to our incomplete understanding of the mechanisms underlying their pathophysiology. Confusion exists regarding the terminology and different names are used for malformations that appear identical on clinical, radiological and pathological examination. Moreover, two or more cortical developmental malformations may coexist and it is likely that several morphological subcategories form parts of a spectrum of the same disease (Raymond et al. 1994).

In 1986, textbooks classified dysplasias of the cerebral cortex as agyria, polymicrogyria, pachygyria and cortical heterotopias (Naidich and Zimmerman 1986). In the recent textbooks of pediatric neuroradiology, the classifications were still based on the pathological classification but had become more detailed (Barkovich 1996; Ball 1997).

Another classification aiming at standardization and uniformity has been suggested which is based on morphology alone, using both neuroimaging and pathological criteria (RAYMOND et al. 1994). In this classification the following types of cortical dysgenesis presenting with epilepsy are distinguished in patients presenting with epilepsy: (1) abnormalities of gyration, (2) heterotopias, (3) (hemi) megalencephaly, (4) focal cortical dysplasia/microdysgenesis, (5) tuberous sclerosis, (6) cortical dysgenesis associated with neoplasia and (7) dysgenesis of the archicortex. This results in a completely different classification compared to what had been used before. For instance, polymicrogyria is classified in the same group as agyria, focal cortical dysplasia is considered a one separate entity. A particular subcategory of cortical dysgenesis may share several MR features with other subcategories. Cortical dysgenesis is most frequently seen in the frontal lobe. The exceptions are subependymal heterotopia, often located along the posterior hors of the lateral ventricles and macrogyria/polymicrogyria with clefts, located in the region of the central sulcus and the sylvian fissure (RAYMOND et al. 1994).

More recently there has been a reclassification of the disorders of cortical malformation according to the embryological stages of brain cortex development at which these malformations are proposed to have occurred (BARKOVICH et al. 1996). Neuroimaging, pathological aspects as well as modern insights in genetics play a role in this classification. The framework consists of four major groups which are always divided into generalized and focal abnormalities. The flexibility of this classification is its major advantage.

The first group, the malformations due to abnormal neuronal and glial proliferation, includes microlissencephaly, focal cortical dysplasia with balloon cells, hemimegalencephaly, focal transmantle dysplasia, tuberous sclerosis and neoplasias such as dysembryoplastic neurectodermal tumor, gangliocytoma and ganglioglioma.

The second group consists of the different types of lissencephaly and heterotopia and the focal agyria/pachygyria complex. These malformations result from an abnormal neuronal migration.

The third group, due to abnormal cortical organization, includes polymicrogyria, schizencephaly and focal cortical dysplasia without balloon cells. These abnormalities are associated with disruption of the process of gyral formation and subsequent cellular organization of the cortex.

The fourth group consists of cortical malformations not classified in the previous groups.

This classification is to be considered as a very important step forward because for the first time the different malformations are classified in a flexible system. The classification has been used to label cortical developmental malformations in a series of 109 patients (LEVENTER et al. 1999). All malformations were analyzed in detail on the different imaging sequences. This approach is important in order to further elucidate the developmental basis of malformations and their underlying cause. Polymicrogyria is now separately classified as a malformation due to abnormal cortical organization. Schizencephaly, considered as an extreme form of polymicrogyria, is listed in this category too, because of the known associated areas of polymicrogyria. Focal cortical dysplasia belongs to a different category and there is no longer any confusion.

It has been proposed that cortical malformations result from a complex disarray of functional interactions of specific genes, trophic factors, adhesion molecules and other surface factors involved during the formation of the cortex (RORKE 1994).

Recently the term microlissencephaly has been questioned. This will be discussed in Sect. 21.3.3.1

21.3.3 Imaging

New observations will be discussed in relationship to the newly proposed classification (BARKOVICH et al. 1996).

21.3.3.1 Abnormalities of Neuronal and Glial Proliferation

Focal Cortical Dysplasia. As we have mentioned earlier cortical dysplasia is an extremely confusing term, which is used frequently to describe malformations of cortical development. Focal cortical dysplasia (FCD) is a separate entity, first described by Taylor, consisting of cortical disorganization with abnormal giant neurons (TAYLOR et al. 1971). In the meantime it is accepted that FCD may range from minimal cortical laminar changes (possibly not always visible on MR imaging) to extensive changes (LEE et al. 1998). FCD is considered as a localized disruption of the cortical lamination and a failure of the myelin arborization. Two different types are distinguished pathologically: type II differs from type I by the occurrence of balloon cells and neuronal cytomegaly. On imaging this is reflected in the T2 prolongation of subcortical white matter. The high signal may partly be due to gliosis (YAGISHITA et al. 1997) (Fig. 21.7).

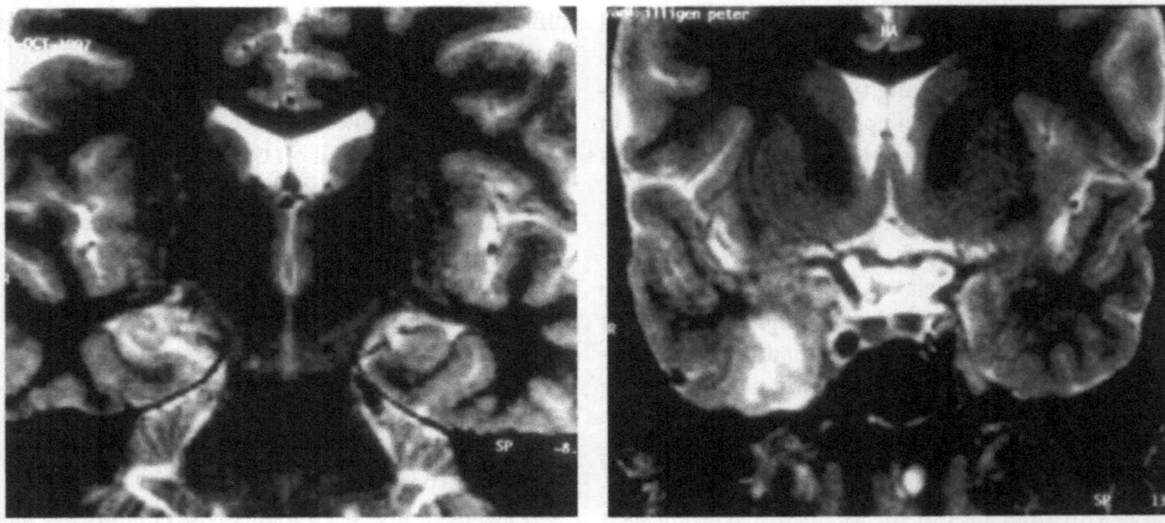

a b

Fig. 21.7a,b. Coronal DESTIR T2-weighted MR images of dual pathology. Hippocampal sclerosis (**a**) is seen in the presence of focal cortical dysplasia (**b**)

The resemblance between the microscopic appearance of FCD and cortical tubers suggests an overlap between FCD and tuberous sclerosis. FCD has also been called a form fruste of tuberous sclerosis.

Blurring of the gray-white matter interface (probably due to a reduction in the number of myelinated fibers) and a variability of cortical thickness are characteristic of type I cortical dysplasia. It has been demonstrated that the signal of the affected cortex is higher than normal on highly T1-weighted images. Contrast enhancement has been reported occasionally (Lee et al. 1998). FCD is usually not associated with abnormalities of gyration (Yagishita et al. 1997) but may coexist with mesial temporal sclerosis (Ho et al. 1998) (Fig. 21.7). Sometimes FCD cannot be differentiated from polymicrogyria. The blurring of the gray-white matter junction is usually not seen in polymicrogyria.

Signal alteration and cortical thickening are statistically helpful in differentiating FCD from tumors. FCD are rarely seen in the medial temporal lobe (Bronen et al. 1997).

Focal Transmantle Dysplasia. This malformation strongly resembles focal cortical dysplasia, described by Taylor in 1971: abnormal organization of the cortex, neuronal cytomegaly, balloon cells, blurring of the gray-white junction and astrogliosis. The main difference is the extension of the abnormality from the wall of the ventricle to the cortex (Fig. 21.8). Focal transmantle dysplasia is distinguishable from focal subcortical heterotopia by the demonstration of abnormal cortical lamination and the presence of balloon cells. On imaging the so-called "transmantle sign," an area returning an abnormal signal, is thought to be characteristic (Barkovich et al. 1997).

It is very likely that focal transmantle dysplasia is part of the spectrum of focal cortical dysplasias to which the next entity also belongs.

Sublobar Dysplasia. This rare abnormality was recently described in five patients (Barkovich et al. 1998). It consists of a sublobar region of dysplastic brain, separated from the normal brain tissue (Fig. 21.9). The ventricle appears abnormal too and the cortex is involved over its entire thickness. It cannot be excluded that this entity may represent a less severe form of hemimegalencephaly (Fig. 21.10).

Microlissencephaly. Incomplete microlissencephaly is characterized by microcephaly and a decreased cortical thickness with diminished and shallow sulci (Barkovich et al. 1997). These patients are divided into five groups based upon a clinicoradiological correlation. These cortical developmental malformations are different from classical and cobblestone lissencephalies which belong to the group of abnormalities of neuronal migration. Microlissencephaly could reflect a diminished number of neurons but the underlying reason of impairment of proliferation remains unknown. The simplified gyral pattern with too few, abnormally shallow sulci is a common feature in the five groups (Fig. 21.11). The proposed classification may become a first useful tool in establishing a prognosis for these patients. This classification too is to be

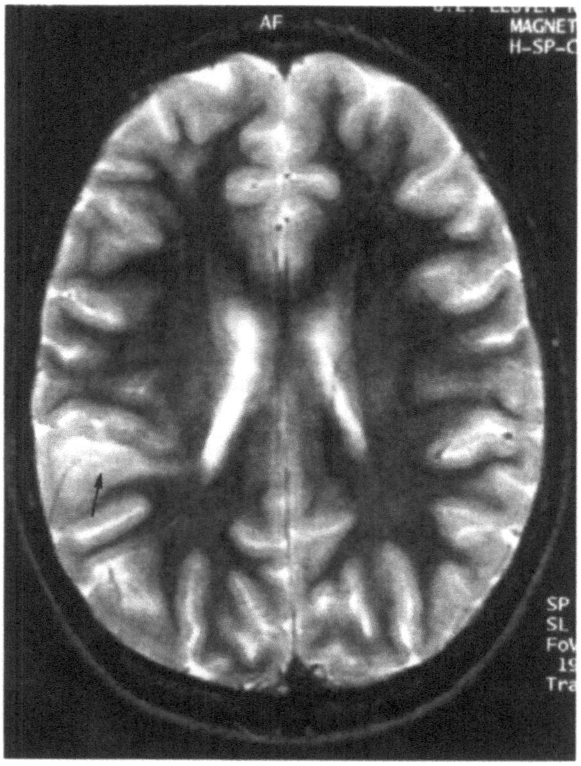

a

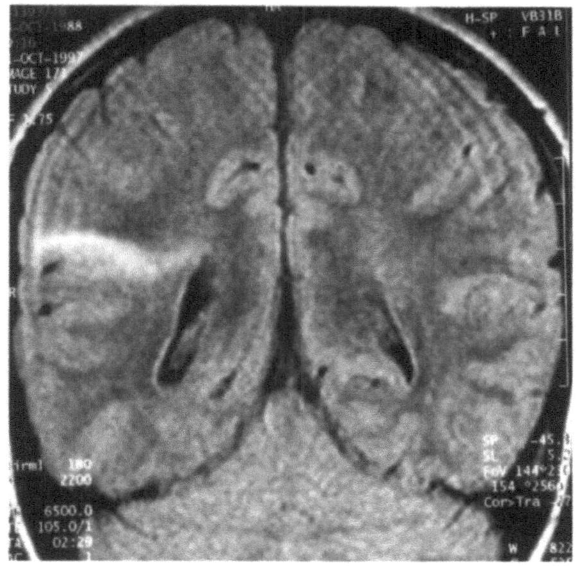

b

Fig. 21.8a,b. Axial DESTIR T2-weighted (**a**) and coronal fast FLAIR (**b**) images in transmantle dysplasia. Poorly defined gray-white matter junction with subcortical T2 prolongation and extension radially towards the lateral ventricle. The extension is best seen on the FLAIR image

regarded as an initial framework. Because these patients do not have the typical MR findings in lissencephaly and the term microlissencephaly can therefore be confusing, the term oligogyric microcephaly was proposed (Hanefeld 1998). Recently this classification was extended to ten groups and the term microlissencephaly was reserved for groups 5 to 8. Groups 1 to 4 are now called microcephaly with simplified gyral pattern and groups 9 and 10 are called "micro"polymicrogyria (Dobyns and Barkovich 1999). It is clear that this is not the end of the discussion and that MR imaging is likely to contribute to the classification of these malformations.

Tumours. Lesions of proliferation following an abnormal induction event during brain development may be malformative, hamartomatous, neoplastic or a combination of a malformative disorder consisting of neoplasias on a background of disordered cortex. Some of these tumours are discussed in Chap. 9.

More and more evidence exists that some tumors may have a dysplastic or dysgenetic origin. A possible hypothesis would be that these tumors are lesions that arise from a preexisting cortical developmental malformation. Sometimes it may be difficult to classify a lesion as a tumour or a developmental malformation, e.g., Lhermitte-Duclos and dysplastic gangliocytoma.

Gangliogliomas have been found in association with a cortical developmental malformation and an anaplastic ganglioglioma arising from a preexisting subependymal heterotopia has been reported too (Demaerel et al. 1996) (Fig. 21.12).

Tuberous Sclerosis Complex. Tuberous sclerosis (TS) is a phakomatosis with dysplasias frequently affecting the brain, skin, eyes, kidneys and heart. Cortical tubers, white matter lesions, subependymal nodules and subependymal giant cell astrocytoma can be observed on brain imaging. In addition to these structural abnormalities, cystlike white matter lesions or inclusions have been reported in almost 50% of patients with TS (Van Tassel et al. 1997). The underlying pathogenesis remains unknown and it may concern degeneration as well as dysplasia.

Two types of cortical tubers are distinguished, those with a smooth surface (type 1) and those with a central depression (type 2) (Fig. 21.13). The expansion of a gyrus, the location in the frontal lobe, the high signal in the cortex and in the subcortical white matter suggest a cortical tuber rather than a ganglioglioma or an oligodendroglioma (Yagishita et al. 1999). Cortical tubers without other stigmata of TS are distinct from focal cortical dysplasia, but there are overlaps and similarities. There is no evidence of gyral expansion or central depression in fo-

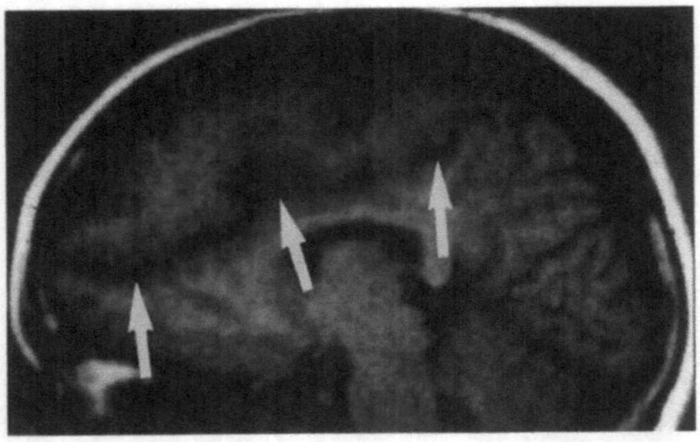

Fig. 21.9. Sagittal T1-weighted image of frontal sublobar dysplasia shows the abnormal gyration and sulcation. The abnormal region is separated from normal brain by a large sulcus. Note the thinning of the anterior part of the corpus callosum (courtesy of A.J. Barkovich UCSF Medical Center, San Francisco)

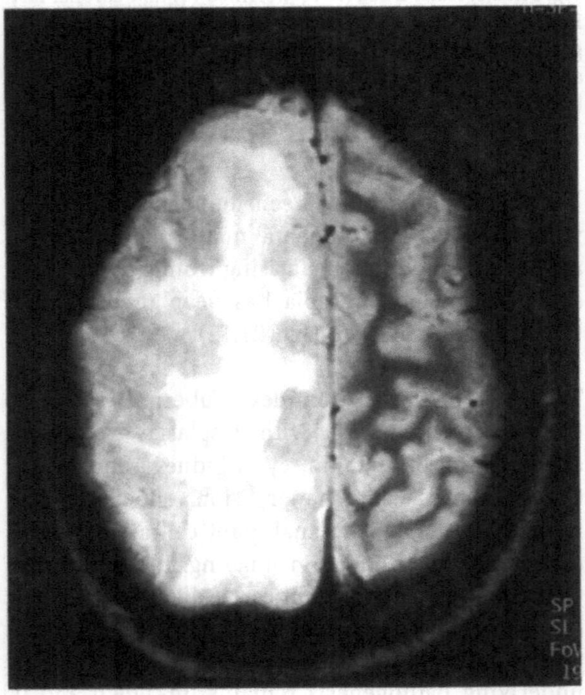

Fig. 21.10. Axial proton density weighted MR image in a boy with unilateral megalencephaly demonstrating cortical developmental abnormalities as well as diffuse white matter involvement

cal cortical dysplasia. Calcification is more common in cortical tubers. There are numerous abnormal neurons in focal cortical dysplasia. The cytoarchitectural abnormalities are more extensive in cortical tubers.

In infants under 3 months of age all these lesions can be easily identified except the cortical tubers and the cystlike white matter lesions (Baron and Barkovich 1999). Extensive focal megalencephaly and hemimegalencephaly have been described in association with TS (Griffiths et al. 1998). The appearance of the tubers changes as the white matter myelinates. The tubers may return a low T2 signal compared to the immature brain (Fig. 21.14).

21.3.3.2 Abnormalities of Neuronal Migration

Bilateral Periventricular Nodular Heterotopia and Bilateral Laminar Heterotopia. An ever increasing number of genetic syndromes are being identified with cortical developmental malformations as one of the major abnormalities. Bilateral periventricular nodular heterotopia has been observed in at least seven syndromes including at least four that are inherited as X-linked traits (Fig. 21.15). Three of them have been mapped to the same region in chromosome Xq28. They may all be caused by different mutations of the BPNH gene (Guerrini et al. 1998).

It is interesting to note that patients with BPNH can present clinically and electrographically with temporal lobe epilepsy and that temporal lobe resection not always results in cessation of seizures. This observation stresses the potential role of techniques such as MR spectroscopy in the presurgical work-up of cortical developmental malformations. It has been demonstrated that metabolic changes can extend to normal appearing regions adjacent to the visible abnormalities.

Mutations in the X-linked gene double cortin have been found in females with bilateral laminar heterotopia (also called double cortex or subcortical band heterotopia) and confirm the underlying genetic abnormality in some cortical developmental malformations (Fig. 21.16). This gene would code a protein involved in the adhesion of neurons to the radial glial fibers during the migration from the ventricular wall to the cortex.

Cobblestone Lissencephalies. Several important reports have been published on congenital muscular dystrophy (CMD), an entity that has been classified as one of the cobblestone lissencephaly syndromes. Two types of cerebral cortical dysgenesis that correspond to known pathological types of cortical dysplasia have been observed in Fukuyama CMD (Aida 1998). Unlayered polymicrogyria (type 2 dysplasia) was seen predominantly in the frontal lobes and ap-

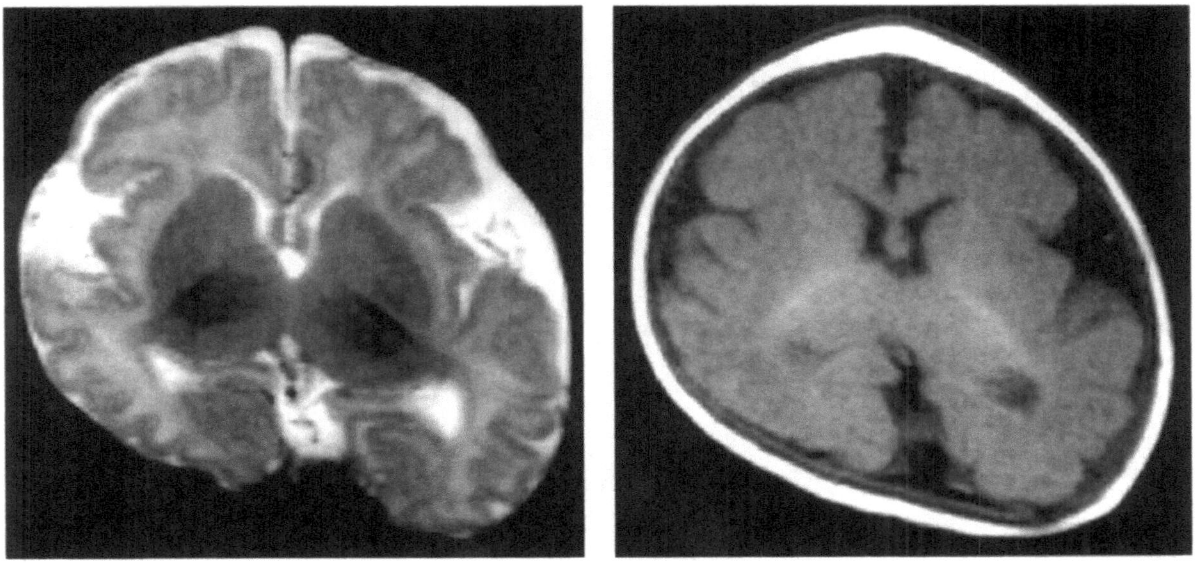

a b

Fig. 21.11a,b. Axial DESTIR T2-weighted (**a**) and T1-weighted (**b**) images in a 3-month-old boy with microlissencephaly. Note the diminished number of gyri and the superficial sulcation

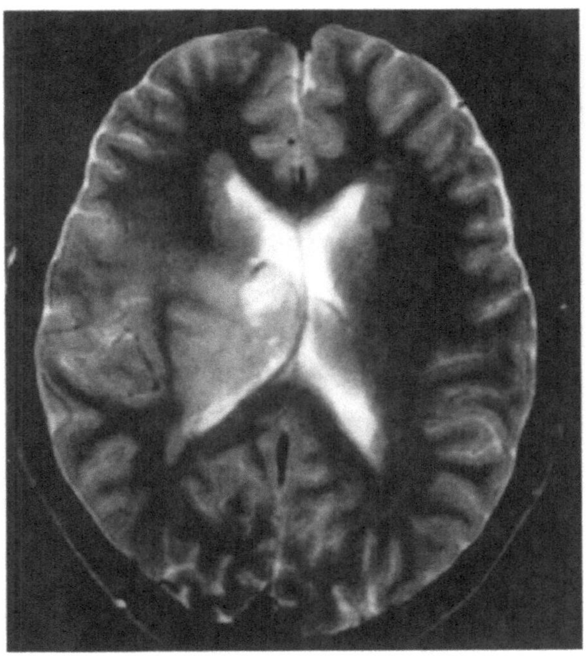

Fig. 21.12. Axial T2-weighted image of subependymal gray matter heterotopia with additional anaplastic ganglioglioma

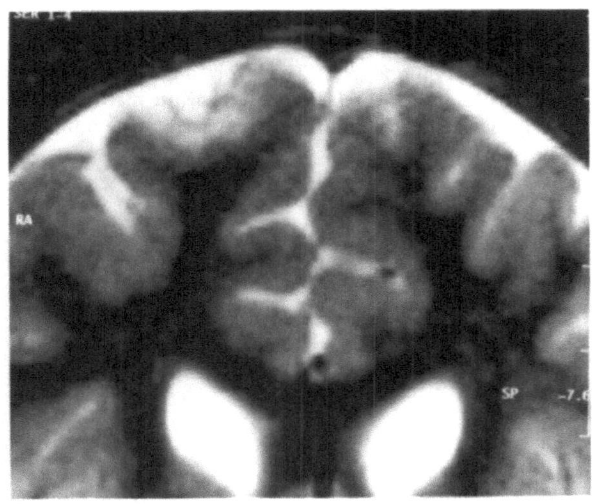

Fig. 21.13. Coronal DESTIR T2-weighted MR image in a patient with so-called form fruste of tuberous sclerosis. Note the central depression in the cortical tuber (*arrow*)

pears as thickened cortex with a bumpy gray-white matter interface (Fig. 21.17). The second pattern (type 3 dysplasia pathologically) was found in the temporo-occipital lobes and appeared as cortical thickening with a smooth surface. Other abnormalities included white matter dysmyelination, brain stem hypoplasia, dilated ventricles and cerebellar abnormalities. These findings are characteristic and allow the diagnosis of Fukuyama CMD in the appropriate clinical setting.

MR imaging allowed the distinction of four distinct types of CMD (Barkovich 1998). In pure or merosin deficient CMD there are no cerebral or cerebellar cortical malformations but pontine hypopla-

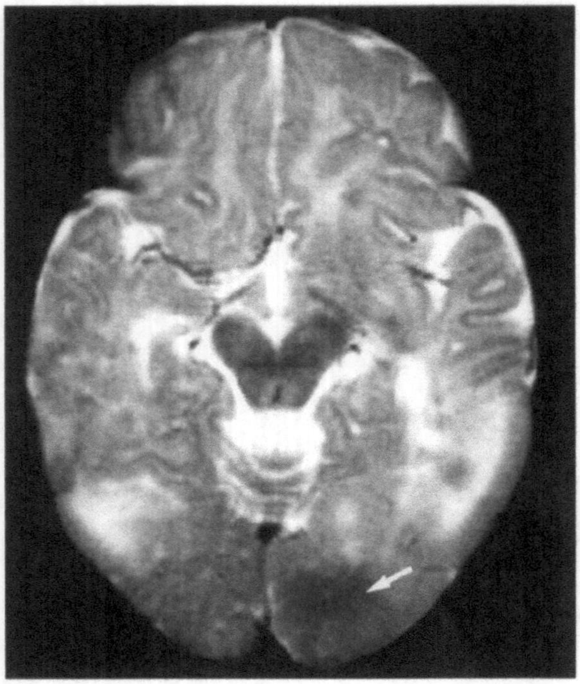

Fig. 21.14. Axial DESTIR T2-weighted MR image in a 6-month-old girl with tuberous sclerosis. Cortical tubers are seen in both temporal lobes. The involved gyri are enlarged. Note the prolonged T2 relaxation in the white matter and the low signal of the occipital tuber compared to the immature brain substance (*arrow*)

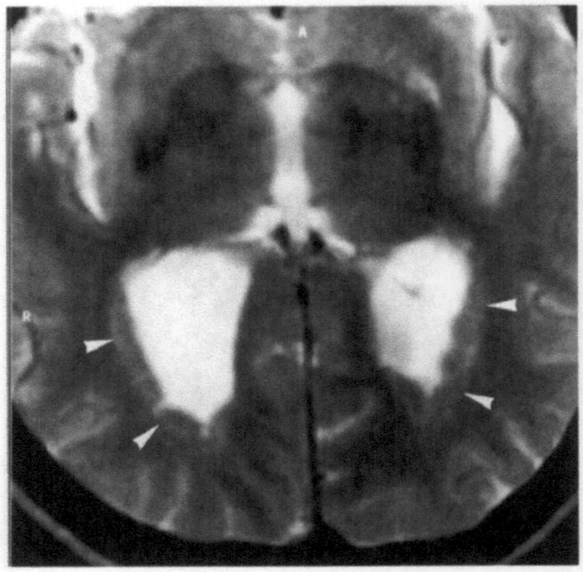

Fig. 21.15. Axial DESTIR T2-weighted MR image of bilateral periventricular nodular heterotopia (*arrowhead*)

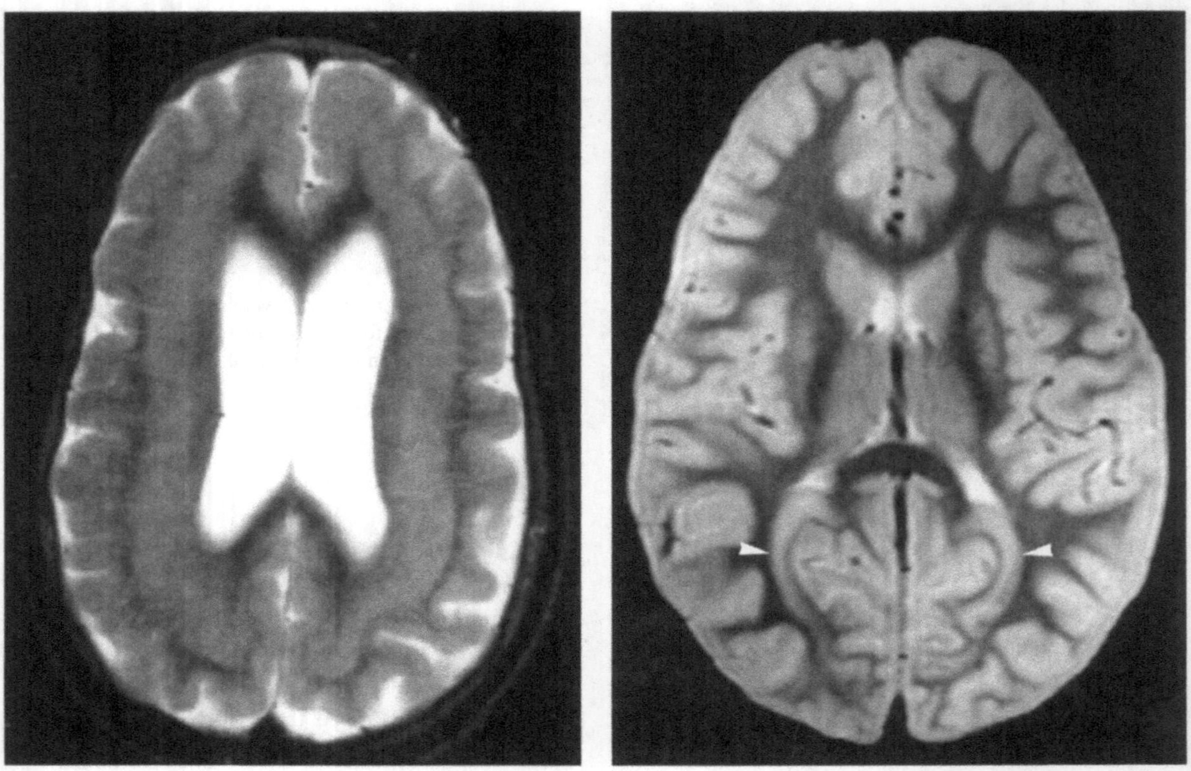

a b

Fig. 21.16a,b. Axial DESTIR T2-weighted (**a**) and proton density weighted (**b**) MR images in diffuse band heterotopia or double cortex (**a**) and in localized bilateral laminar heterotopia (**b**) (*arrowhead*)

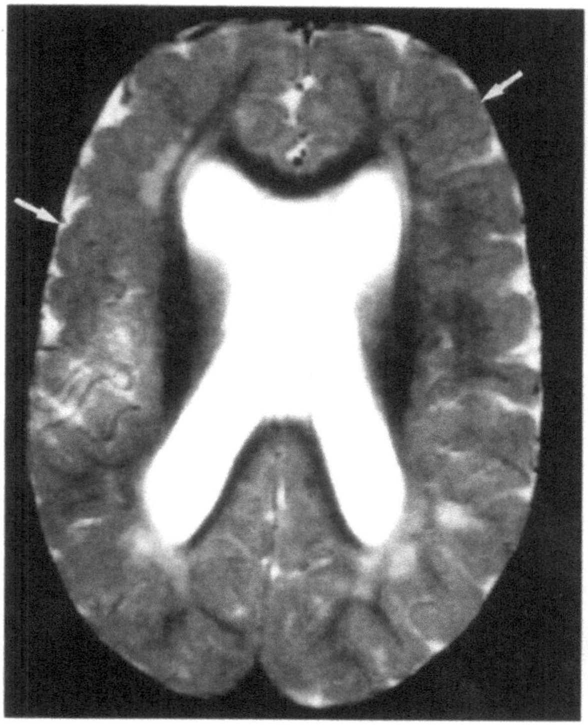

Fig. 21.17. Axial DESTIR T2-weighted MR image in unlayered polymicrogyria demonstrating the thickened frontoparietal cortex, the bumpy gray-white matter interface and the subcortical T2 prolongation

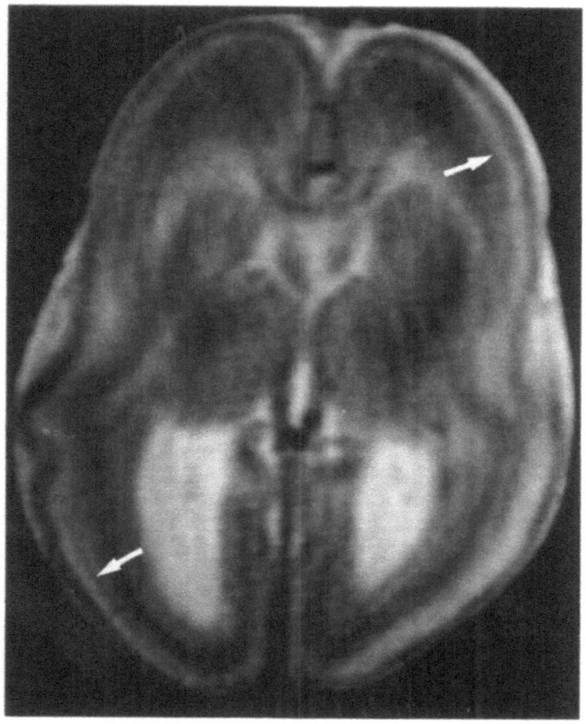

Fig. 21.18. Axial DESTIR T2-weighted MR image in type 1 lissencephaly. Note the pathologically identified paucicellular band between the superficial cortex and the heterotopic neurons (*arrow*)

sia and white matter abnormalities are seen. In the three other disorders, Fukuyama CMD, Walker-Warburg syndrome and muscle-eye-brain disease, there are cerebral and cerebellar cortical malformations in addition to the formerly described abnormalities. In another study, Fukuyama CMD was not included in this classification while CMD with occipital agyria was included as a separate disorder (van der Knaap et al. 1997). Cerebral and cerebellar dysplasia was lacking in this group.

Type 1 lissencephaly is characterized by agyria and cortical thickening (Fig. 21.18). Neuropathological correlation revealed a new feature (Landrieu et al. 1998). It concerns a thin, paucicellular myelinated band between the true superficial cortex and the large band of heterotopic neurons. On MR imaging this band is recognizable as a high signal area.

Subcortical Heterotopia. Subcortical heterotopia is considered as a well-defined clinicoradiological entity (Barkovich 1996). It consists of an irregularly lobulated mass of gray matter, primarily located in the white matter of the cerebrum (Figs. 21.19, 21.20). The size of the hemisphere is diminished, the cortex thinned and the sulci shallow. Associated dysplasia of the basal ganglia and abnormalities of the corpus callosum are often associated.

21.3.3.3 Abnormalities of Cortical Organization

Bilateral Perisylvian Polymicrogyria. Polymicrogyria (or non-lissencephalic cortical dysgenesis) refers to an abnormal gyration characterized by an excessive number of small gyri. Most authors accept that this malformation may result from a postmigration vascular insult in layer 5 of the cortex, between 20 and 24 weeks of gestation. But in some cases association with gene mutation has been reported, suggesting a possible genetic cause.

Recently several reports have been published on bilateral perisylvian polymicrogyria, which is due to an abnormal cortical organization (Rolland et al. 1995; Gropman et al. 1997; Miller et al. 1998) (Fig. 21.21). Clinically congenital hemiplegia, dysarthria, facial-lingual diplegia with childhood-onset seizures, pseudobulbar palsy and variable mental retardation have been reported. MR imaging shows the polymicrogyria involving a variable part of the opercular cortex and part of the corticospinal tracts. This clinico-

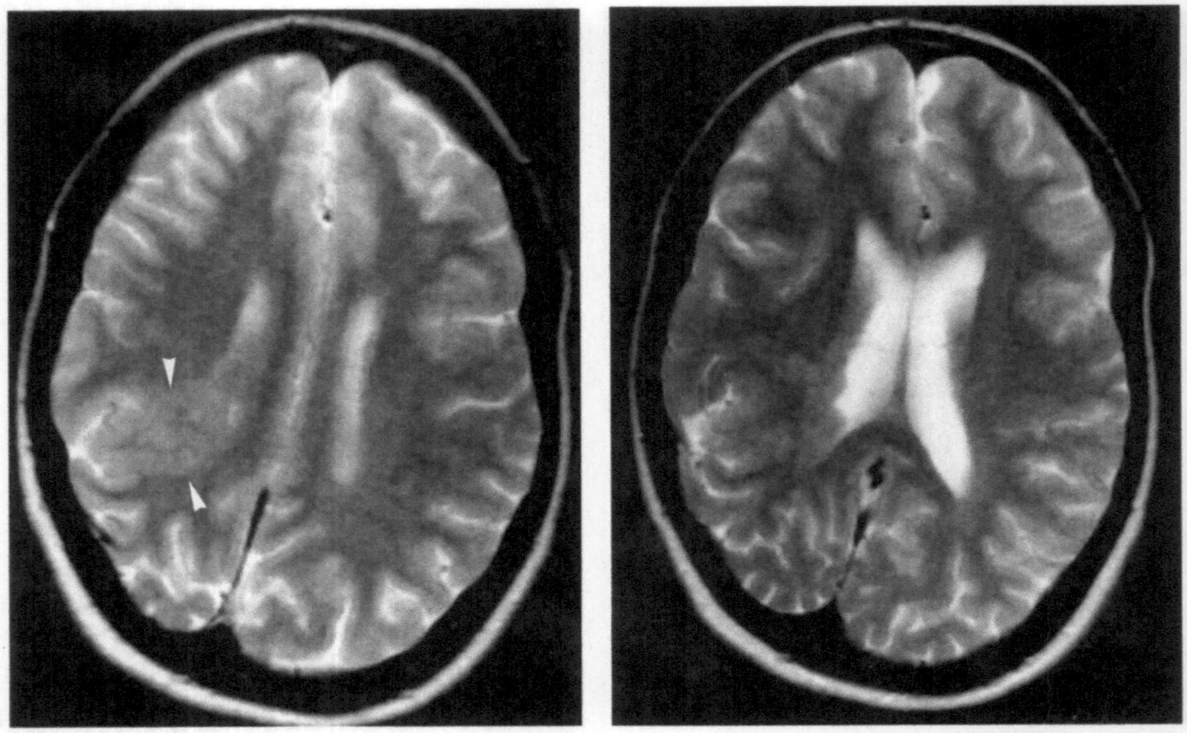

Fig. 21.19a,b. Axial DESTIR T2-weighted MR images of subcortical heterotopia in the right frontal lobe (*arrow*). There were associated abnormalities in the corpus callosum and in the basal ganglia. The size of the right hemisphere was diminished

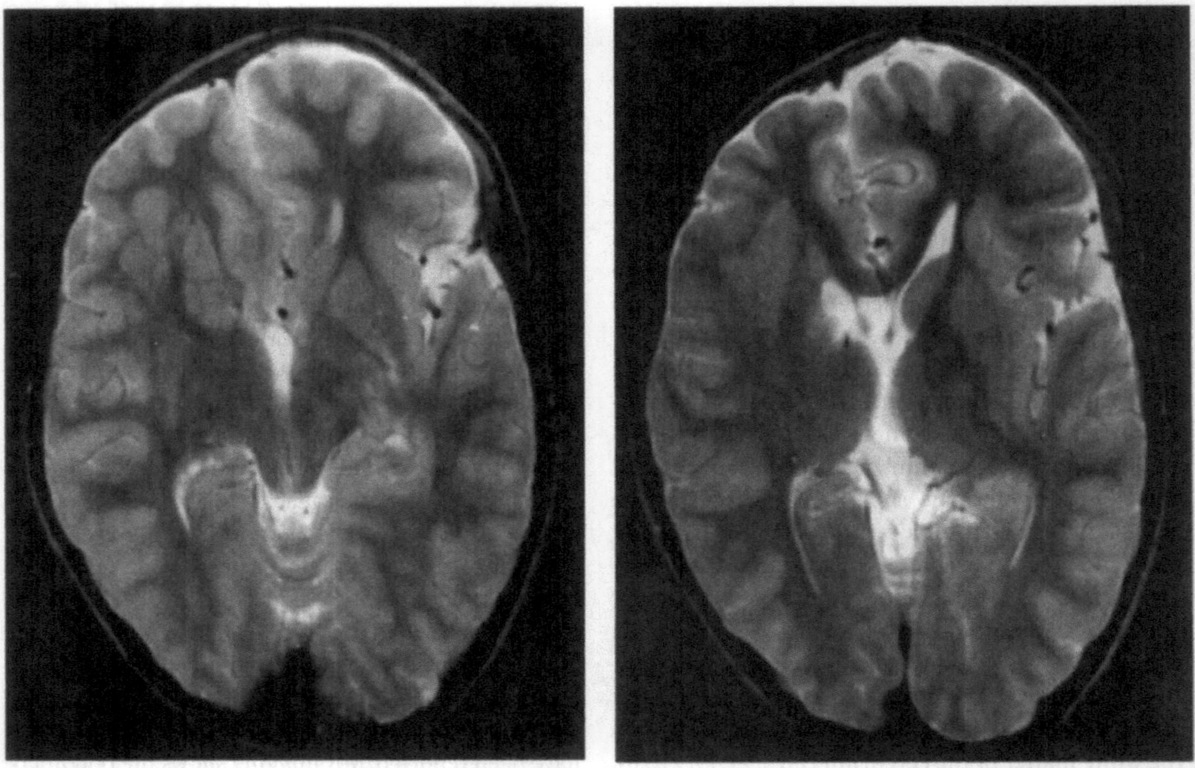

Fig. 21.20a,b. Axial DESTIR T2-weighted MR images of subcortical heterotopia and subependymal heterotopia. Note the abnormal formation of the sulcus and adjacent cortex (*arrowhead*)

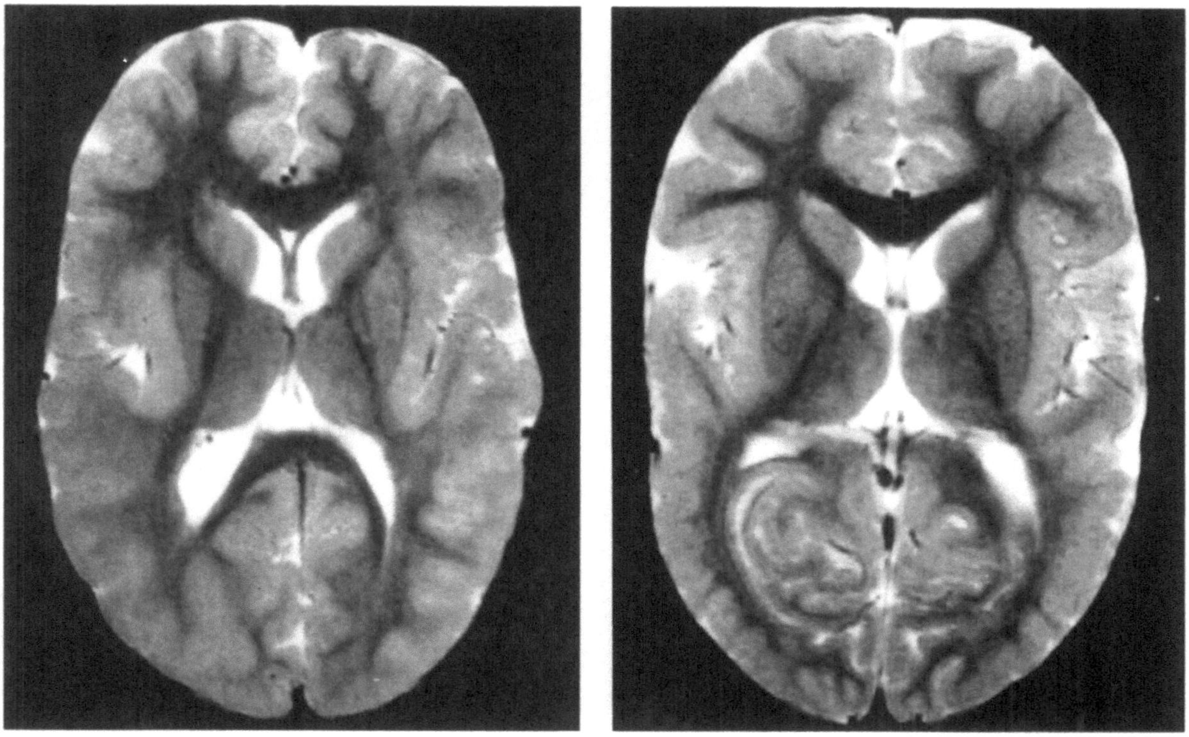

Fig. 21.21a,b. Axial DESTIR T2-weighted MR images in two children with bilateral perisylvian polymicrogyria. Note the abnormal development of the temporal and occipital cortex in both patients and the presence of subgerdymal ??? heterotopic modules (a)

morphological syndrome is now called "congenital bilateral perisylvian syndrome." Usually the sylvian fissure and the perisylvian cortex are involved, but the thickness of the abnormal cortex may be within the normal range. A reliable criterion to decide about this disorder is an assessment of the degree of depth of the sylvian fissure on a sagittal image and to compare this with normal subjects on a normalized image in the same anatomical space (Van Bogaert et al. 1998). The opercular malformations have been grouped into five types according their embryogenesis, type 1 displaying the most severe abnormalities. The first three types are characterized by thickened cortex and absent or incompletely formed opercular formation (with abnormal insular gyri). Types 4 and 5 occur later in the embryogenesis (at 30–34 weeks of gestation) and the insular lobes, circular sulcus, temporal and frontoparietal opercula can be recognized. Type 2 is often observed in bilateral perisylvian polymicrogyria.

Schizencephaly is almost always associated with polymicrogyria of the cortex lining the cleft and therefore congenital bilateral perisylvian polymicrogyria should be considered as part of the spectrum (Fig. 21.22). It has been suggested to stop using the term schizencephaly as it only describes the presence of a cleft.

Two types of polymicrogyria exist: brain injury occurring during the early second trimester of pregnancy has been associated with unlayered polymicrogyria, lacking any cortical organization; injury occurring later (18–24 weeks of gestation) may result in layered polymicrogyria, consisting of a four-layered cortex with associated laminar necrosis. Associated anomalous venous drainage is commonly seen when there is an infolding of dysplastic cortex. These anomalous veins are probably caused by lack of condensation of the veins. This term refers to persistence of the tributaries of the embryonic dural plexus, which will later coalesce to form the normal superficial cortical veins and dural sinuses.

21.4 Cerebellar Cortex

21.4.1 Embryology

The development of the cerebellum begins with the fusion of the rhombic lips in the midline. Fusion starts rostrally to form the flocculi of the hemi-

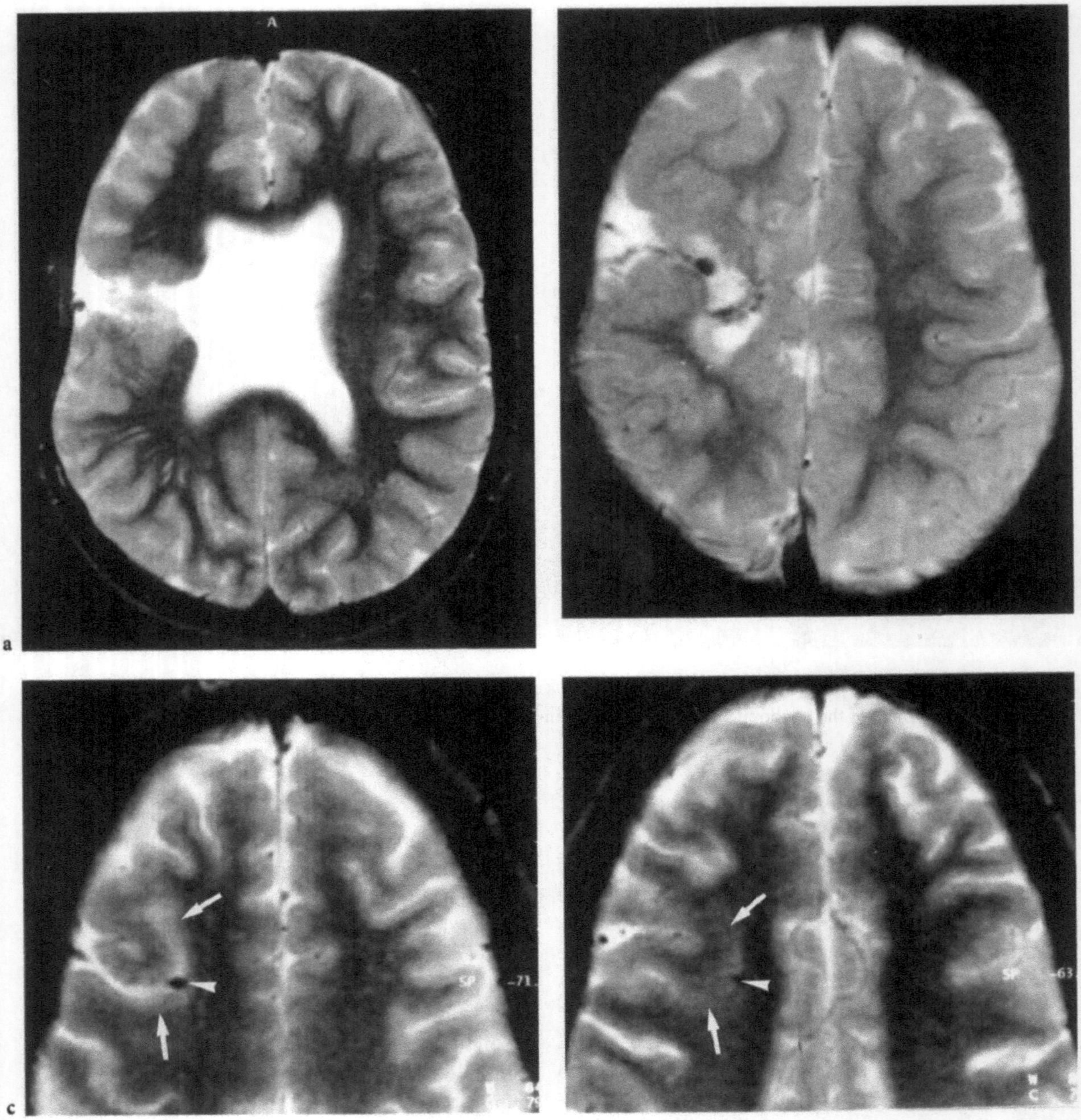

Fig. 21.22a–d. Axial DESTIR T2-weighted MR images in open lip (**a**) and closed lip (**b**) right sided schizencephaly. A less severe form is shown in **c,d**. Note the presence of an abnormal draining vein (**c**, *arrowhead*)

spheres and the nodulus of the vermis (archicerebellum). The anterior lobe forms next followed by the posterior lobe. It extends caudally and by the 15th week of gestation the cerebellum is completely formed. The vermis is formed before the hemispheres.

A different concept has been suggested in which the cerebellum arises from one embryonic primordium or rhombic lip (Sidman and Rakic 1982).

The flocculi of the hemispheres and the vermis are called paleocerebellum while the remainder of the hemispheres is called neocerebellum.

The first fissure to appear at about 12 weeks of gestation is the posterolateral fissure, which separates the flocculonodular lobe from the remainder of the cerebellum.

By 13 weeks, the anterior lobe is separated from the posterior lobe by the primary fissure and consists of the three lobules of the vermis: lingula, central lobule and culmen. The second and third lobules have hemispheric extensions. Vermian differentiation occurs first in the most posterior part of the primordium and develops toward the anterior part.

The cerebellar cortex consists of three layers: the outer molecular layer, the intermediate Purkinje cell layer and the inner granular cell layer. In the foetus and until the end of the first postnatal life an external granular cell layer is present external to the molecular layer. Two pathways are followed for the outward migration of the cells between 9 and 13 weeks of gestation. An inward migration, at approximately 16 weeks of gestation, forms part of the molecular and inner granular cell layer. Meningeal cells seem to play a role in the foliation and lamination of the cerebellar cortex.

21.4.2 Terminology and Classification

Cerebellar malformations of cortical development are less well-known. These, sometimes subtle, changes are usually not visualized on computed tomography. Most of these malformations were only reported in the beginning of the nineties. Gyri and sulci are called folia and fissures in the cerebellum. Similar to the cerebrum, the cerebellum consists of two hemispheres, but in addition a midline structure, the vermis, is present. Malformations can be present in the vermis and/or in the hemispheres.

The developmental abnormalities of the cerebellum are classified into three categories: dysgenesis of the paleocerebellum, dysgenesis of the neocerebellum and cystic or cystlike malformations. Cerebellar neuronal migration disorders were not mentioned until the early nineties.

Dandy-Walker complex and Joubert's syndrome are the best known examples of paleocerebellar dysgenesis and will not be discussed here further.

Rhombencephalosynapsis and tectocerebellar dysraphia were reported in the early nineties. More recently rostral vermian dysplasia has been described.

In the category of neocerebellar dysgenesis, cerebellar dysplasia has been described in absence of any syndrome. Neocerebellar dysgenesis include abnormalities of the folia such as allogyria, microgyria, macrogyria, agyria and polygyria.

Lhermitte-Duclos syndrome is a diffuse hypertrophy of the cerebellar cortex and is classified with the cerebellar dysplasias although it has been reported confusingly as dysplastic gangliocytoma. Part of a hemisphere is affected but the vermis and the contralateral hemisphere can be involved. The folia are broadened and firm, the molecular layer is thickened and a thick layer of abnormal neurons is present.

The cyst or cystlike malformations include the megacisterna magna and the arachnoid cyst.

21.4.3 Imaging

Rhombencephalosynapsis. This malformation consists of absence of the vermis and fusion of the cerebellar hemispheres (Fig. 21.23). Embryologically there seems to be a failure to form the vermis and a lack of normal cellular proliferation, migration and differentiation. It is probably due to maldevelopment of the rhombic lip in the early fetal period. The complexity of this process explains the occurrence of associated developmental abnormalities as well as the occurrence of complete or partial rhombencephalosynapsis.

As the anomaly most likely occurs between 5 and 6 weeks of gestation, metencephalosynapsis would be a better term than rhombencephalosynapsis.

Another possible explanation could be the failure of vermian differentiation in the more rostral part of the midline rhombic lip at about 12 weeks. The fused cerebellar hemispheres may be explained by the unpaired cerebellar primordium. Rhombencephalosynapsis could therefore represent a failure of vermian differentiation rather than maldevelopment. Undivided cerebellar hemispheres would therefore be more correct than fused (Utsunomiya et al. 1998).

Cortical Dysgenesis. For the same reason as in the cerebral cortical developmental malformations, dysgenesis is preferable to dysplasia.

This abnormality has been seen in patients with Fukuyama congenital muscular dystrophy but has also been described in association with an intrauterine infection. It has recently been described in the absence of these syndromes (Demaerel et al. 1998). There were supratentorial cortical developmental anomalies but these were different from the cobblestone lissencephaly, seen in Fukuyama congenital muscular dystrophy and related syndromes. The abnormality consists of disorderly alignment of the folia with sometimes intraparenchymal cystlike abnormalities, possibly reflecting a more severely affected cerebellum (Fig. 21.24). These cystlike inclu-

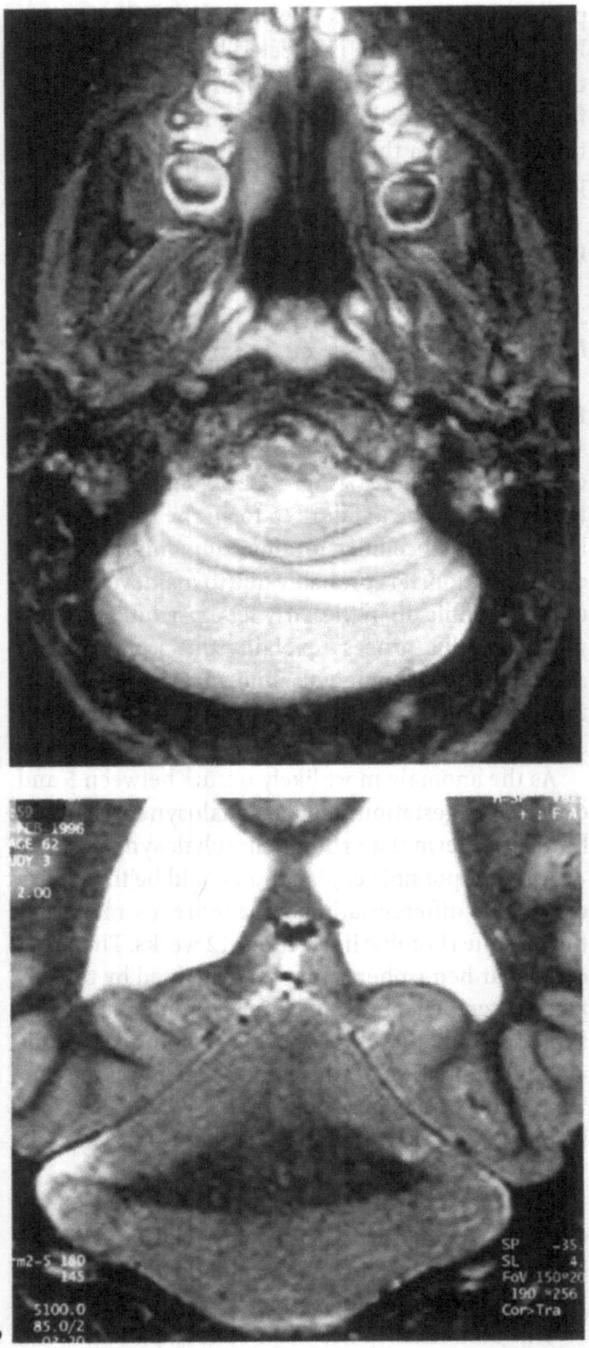

Fig. 21.23a,b. Axial (a) and coronal (b) DESTIR T2-weighted MR images in rhombencephalosynopsis. The cerebellar hemispheres are fused. Note the dilated ventricles

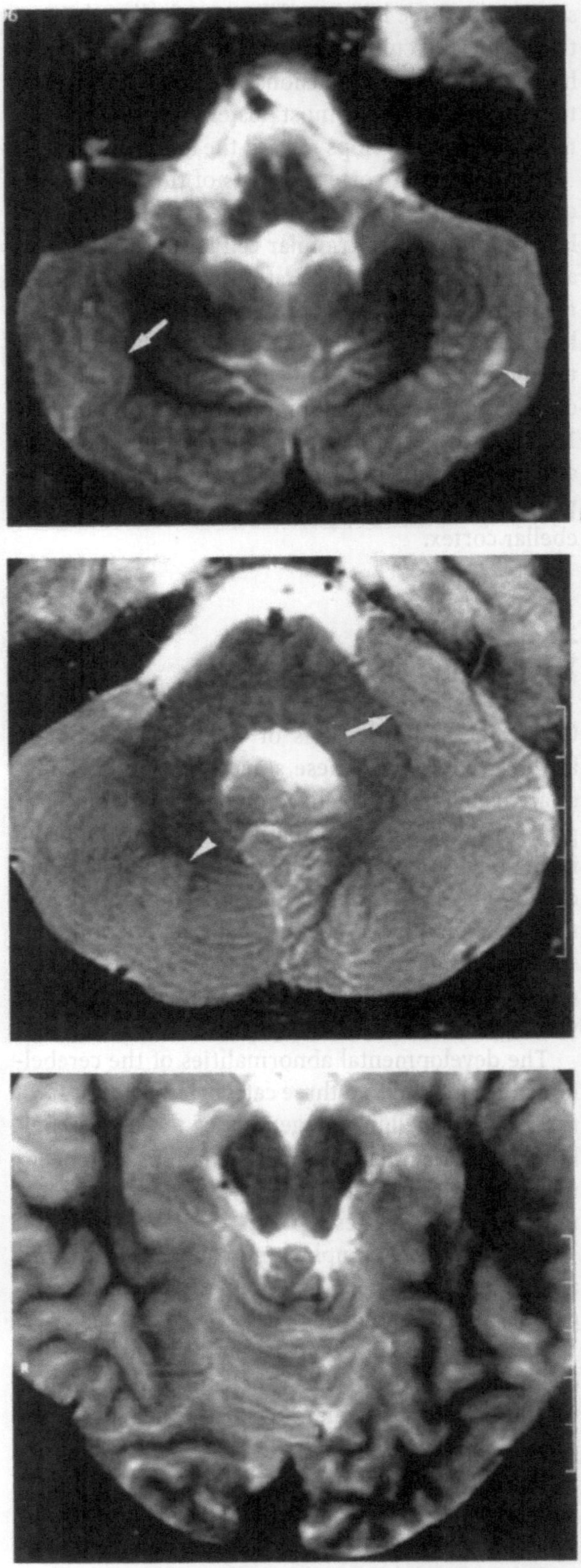

Fig. 21.24a–c. Axial DESTIR T2-weighted MR images in cerebellar cortical dysgenesis. Note the bumpy gray-white matter interface and the cyst-like abnormalities within the cortex (a, *arrowhead*). There is an additional hypertrophy of the left cerebellar hemisphere suggesting a partial Lhermitte-Duclos syndrome (b, *arrowhead*) and there is abnormal fissuration of the vermis (c, *arrow*)

sions may represent remnants or sequelae of the migration of neurons. The nodulus, flocculus and the tonsils are common sites of cortical dysplasia. Histologically, there is a fusion of the molecular layers, a granular layer deficit and Purkinje cells are scattered at the boundaries of these layers.

Cerebellar cortical dysgenesis probably represents a spectrum of abnormalities ranging from minimal to extensive.

Lhermitte-Duclos Syndrome. Lhermitte-Duclos syndrome or focal/diffuse hypertrophy of the cerebellar cortex is usually reported between the 3rd and 6th decades of life but has been described in children too (Fig. 21.25). Pathologically the folia are broadened and firm and the molecular layer is thickened. A thick layer of abnormal large neurons replaces the inner granular layer. The white matter digitations are thinner and there is a disorder of the migration of cerebellar neurons (Demaerel et al. 1995). More recently a new entity called "macrocerebellum" has been introduced (Bodensteiner et al. 1997). The abnormality consists of an enlarged cerebellum with normal imaging features. Compared with the cerebellar volume of an age-matched control group, the volumes in four children were above normal. A delayed myelination of the cerebrum was observed and clinically the children were hypotonic and had a delayed motor and cognitive development and oculomotor apraxia. The authors also report two patients with an enlarged vermis and normal hemispheric volumes.

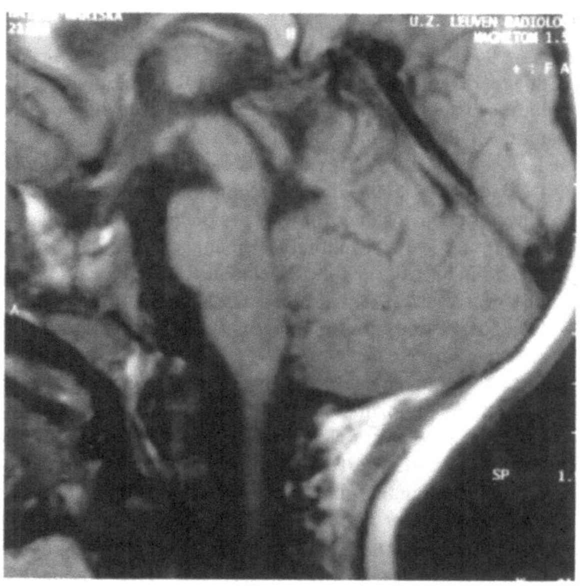

Fig. 21.25. Sagittal T1-weighted MR image in Lhermitte-Duclos syndrome or diffuse hypertrophy of the cerebellar cortex. Note the abnormal foliation and fissuration and the tumour-like appearance

Rostral Vermian Dysplasia. These malformations seemed to involve the paleocerebellum but the term rostral vermian was preferred in agreement with the experimental studies. The abnormalities consist of a more or less extensive defective foliation and abnormal fissuration in the anterior lobe (culmen and central lobule) of the vermis and its hemispheric extensions (Fig. 21.26).

The imaging findings can be very subtle on axial images but are usually well seen on coronal images (Demaerel et al. 1999). This may explain why the abnormality has not been described before. Coronal sections through the cerebellum are not routinely obtained.

A hypothesis that may explain these changes was found in experiments on rats and hamsters (von Knebel Doeberitz 1986). Treatment with 6-hydroxydopamine led to a defective foliation in rats by fusion of neighboring folia. Meningeal cells, which play a role in foliation and lamination of the cerebellar cortex, are destroyed by this treatment and the vermis is more severely affected. It remains unclear why the posterior vermis appears less affected but possibly meningeal cells more rapidly in this part of the cerebellum.

The clinical correlation between the imaging findings and the symptomatology remains unclear. A mild degree of rostral vermian dysplasia may certainly represent an incidental imaging finding.

Abnormalities of the inferior portion of the vermis have been described in patients with ocular motor apraxia (Sargent et al. 1997). The superior portion of the vermis appeared irregular and asymmetrical in two patients and a destructive etiology was suggested.

A partial fusion of the cerebellar hemispheres together with vertical foliation, vermian hypoplasia and small cystic inclusions has been described (Takanashi et al. 1999). At present the underlying cause of this abnormality is not fully understood but the authors speculate that a gene expressed in cerebellar development is mutated and that this mutation disrupts the process of migration.

21.5 Conclusion

The classification of cerebral cortical developmental malformations, proposed by Barkovich, is an excel-

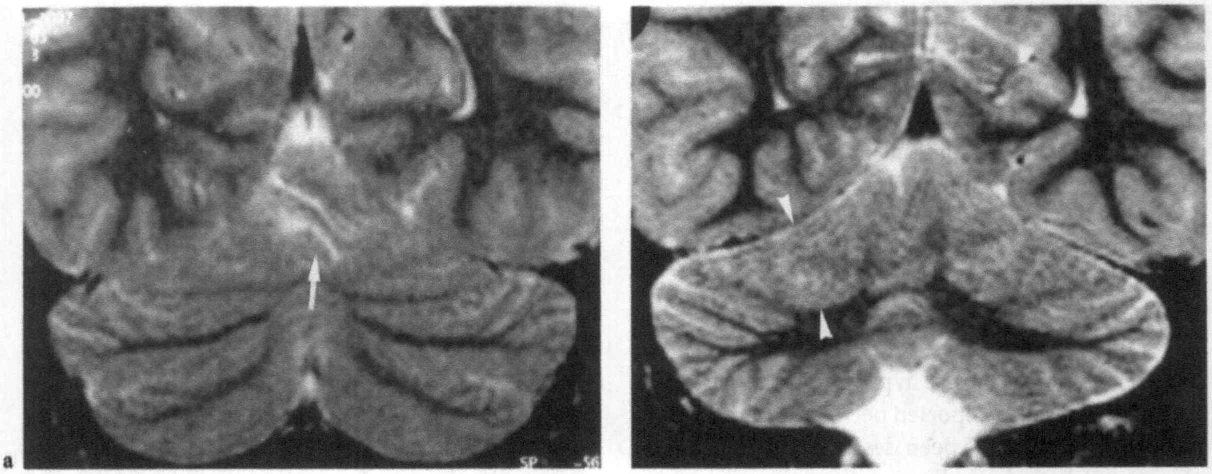

Fig. 21.26a,b. Coronal DESTIR T2-weighted MR images in rostral vermian dysplasia. The abnormal fissuration limited to the vermis is shown in a. Hemispheric extension and cortical thickening are shown in b

lent working tool for all interested disciplines. With our increasing insight in developmental neurobiology it is likely that this classification will mature which will allow a better identification of their incidence and modes of inheritance of these malformations. Magnetic resonance imaging will certainly lead to the detection of more subtle abnormalities. A rigorous analysis of the images is necessary for accurate genetic counseling and possible preoperative lesion localization.

There is a renewed interest in cerebellar cortical malformations which can be recognized on MR images. Many of these abnormalities remain incompletely understood but improved insights in genetics, embryology and pathology are likely to increase our knowledge of these cortical malformations.

References

Aida N (1998) Fukuyama congenital muscular dystrophy: a neuroradiologic review. J Magn Res Imaging 8: 317–326

Ball WS (1997) Congenital malformations of the brain. In: Ball WS, Pediatric neuroradiology. Lippincott-Raven Publishers, Philadelphia, pp 91–174

Barkovich AJ (1996) Congenital malformations of the brain and skull. In: Barkovich AJ, Pediatric neuroimaging, 2nd ed, Lippincott-Raven Publishers, Philadelphia, pp 177–276

Barkovich AJ, Kuzniecky RI, Dobyns WB, Jackson GD, Becker LE, Evrard P (1996) A classification scheme for malformations of cortical development. Neuropediatrics 27: 59–63

Barkovich AJ (1996) Subcortical heterotopia: a distinct clinicoradiological entity. Am J Neuroradiol 17: 1315–1322

Barkovich AJ, Kuzniecky RI, Bollen AW, Grant PE (1997) Focal transmantle dysplasia: a specific malformation of cortical development. Neurology 49: 1148–1152

Barkovich AJ, Peacock W (1998) Sublobar dysplasia. A new malformation of cortical development. Neurology 50: 1383–1387

Barkovich AJ (1998) Neuroimaging manifestations and classification of congenital muscular dystrophies. AJNR Am J Neuroradiol 19: 1389–1396

Baron Y, Barkovich AJ (1999) MR imaging of tuberous sclerosis in neonates and young infants. AJNR Am J Neuroradiol 20: 907–916

Bodensteiner JB, Schaefer GB, Keller GM, Thompson JN, Bowen MK (1997) Macrocerebellum: neuroimaging and clinical features of a newly recognized condition. J Child Neurol 12: 365–368

Bronen RA, Vives KP, Kim JH, Fulbright RK, Spencer SS, Spencer DD (1997) Focal cortical dysplasia of Taylor, balloon cell subtype: MR differentiation from low-grade tumor. AJNR Am J Neuroradiol 18: 1141–1151

Casteels I, Demaerel Ph, De Cock P, Casaer P, Spileers W, Wilms G, Baert AL (1995) Leber's congenital amaurosis and Lhermitte-Duclos syndrome: a previously unreported association. J Pediatr Ophthal Strabismus 32: 117–119

Chan S, Chin SS, Goodman RR, DeLaPaz RL, Pedley TA (1998) Prospective magnetic resonance imaging identification of focal cortical dysplasia including the non-balloon cell subtype. Ann Neurol 44: 749–757

Chen C-Y, Zimmerman RA, Faro S et al. (1996) MR of the operculum: abnormal opercular formation in infants and children. AJNR Am J Neuroradiol 17: 1303–1311

Demaerel Ph, Droessaert M, Lammens M et al. (1996) Anaplastic (malignant ganglioglioma arising from heterotopic grey matter nodules. J Neuro-oncol 30: 237–242

Demaerel P, Lagae L, Casaer P, Baert AL (1998) MR imaging in cerebellar cortical dysplasia. AJNR Am J Neuroradiol 19: 984–986

Demaerel P, Wilms G, Marchal G (1999) Rostral vermian cortical dysplasia: MRI. Neuroradiology 41: 190–194

Dobyns WB, Patton MA, Stratton RF, Mastrobattista JM, Blanton SH, Northrup H (1997) Cobblestone lissencephaly

with normal eyes and muscle. Neuropediatrics 27: 70–75
Dobyns WB, Barkovich AJ (1999) Microcephaly with simplified gyral pattern (oligogyric microcephaly) and microlissencephaly: reply. Neuropediatrics 30: 104–106
Grant PE, Barkovich AJ, Wald LL, Dillon WP, Laxer KD, Vigneron DB (1997) High-resolution surface-coil MR of cortical lesions in medically refractory epilepsy: a prospective study. AJNR Am J Neuroradiol 18: 291–301
Griffiths PD, Gardner S-A, Smith M, Rittey C, Powell T (1998) Hemimegalencephaly and focal megalencephaly in tuberous sclerosis complex. AJNR Am J Neuroradiol 19: 1935–1938
Gropman AL, Barkovich AJ, Vezina LG, Conry JA, Dubovsky EC, Packer RJ (1997) Pediatric congenital bilateral perisylvian syndrome: clinical and MRI features in 12 patients. Neuropediatrics 28: 198–203
Guerrini R, Dobyns WB (1998) Bilateral periventricular nodular heterotopia with mental retardation and frontonasal malformation. Neurology 51: 499–503
Hanefeld F, Kruse B, Holzbach U et al. (1995) Hemimegalencephaly: localized proton magnetic resonance spectroscopy in vivo. Epilepsia 36: 1215–122
Hanefeld FA (1998) Oligogyric microcephaly. Neuropediatrics 30: 102–103
Iannetti P, Spalice A, Atzei G, Boemi S, Trasimeni G (1996) Neuronal migrational disorders in children with epilepsy: MRI, interictal SPECT and EEG comparisons. Brain Develop 18: 269–279
Landrieu P, Husson B, Pariente D, Lacroix C (1998) MRI-neuropathological correlations in type 1 lissencephaly. Neuroradiology 40: 173–176
Lee BCP, Hatfield G, Park TS, Kaufman BA (1997) MR imaging surface display of the cerebral cortex in children. Pediatr Radiol 27: 199–206
Lee BCP, Schmidt RE, Hatfield GA, Bourgeois B, Park TS (1998) MRI of focal cortical dysplasia. Neuroradiology 40: 675–683
Leventer RJ, Phelan EM, Coleman LT, Kean MJ, Jackson GD, Harvey AS (1999) Clinical and imaging features of cortical malformations in childhood. Neurology 53: 715–722
Li LM, Cendes F, Cunha Bastos A, Andermann F, Dubeau F, Arnold DL (1998) Neuronal metabolic dysfunction in patients with cortical developmental malformations. A proton magnetic resonance spectroscopic imaging study. Neurology 50: 755–759
Miller SP, Shevell M, Rosenblatt B, Silver K, O'Gorman A, Andermann F (1998) Congenital bilateral perisylvian polymicrogyria presenting as congenital hemiplegia. Neurology 50: 1866–1869
Naidich TP, Zimmerman RA (1986) Congenital malformations of the brain. In: Brant-Zawadzki M, Norman D (eds) Magnetic resonance imaging of the central nervous system. Raven Press, New York, pp 131–150
Rakic P (1988) Specification of cerebral cortical areas. Science 241: 170–176
Rakic P (1990) Principles of neural cell migration. Experientia 46: 882–891
Raymond AA, Fish DR, Sisodiya SM, Alsanjari N, Stevens JM, Shorvon SD (1995) Abnormalities of gyration, heterotopias, tuberous sclerosis, focal cortical dysplasia, microdysgnesis, dysembryoplastic neuroepithelial tumour and dysgenesis of the archicortex in epilepsy. Brain 118: 629–660
Rolland Y, Adamsbaum C, Sellier N, Robain O, Ponsot G, Kalifa G (1995) Opercular malformations: clinical and MRI features in 11 children. Pediatr Radiol 25: S2-S8
Rorke LB (1994) A perspective: The role of disordered genetic control of neurogenesis in the pathogenesis of migration disorders. J Neuropathol Exp Neurol 53: 105–117
Sargent MA, Poskitt KJ, Jan JE (1997) Congenital ocular motor apraxia: imaging findings. AJNR Am J Neuroradiol 18: 1915–1922
Sidman RL, Rakic P (1973) Neuronal migration, with special reference to developing human brain: a review. Brain Research 62: 1–35
Sidman RL, Rakic P (1982) Development of the human central nervous system. In: Haymaker W, Adams RD (eds) Histology and Histopathology of the Central Nervous System. Thomas, Springfield, pp 3–145
Sisodiya SM, Free SL, Stevens JM, Fish DR, Shorvon SD (1995) Widespread cerebral structural changes in patients with cortical dysgenesis and epilepsy. Brain 118: 1039–1050
Spreafico AC, Battaglia G, Arcelli P et al. (1998) Cortical dysplasia. An immunocytochemical study of three patients. Neurology 50: 27–36
Takanashi J, Sugita K, Barkovich AJ, Takano H, Kohno Y (1999) Partial midline fusion of the cerebellar hemispheres with vertical foliation: a new cerebellar malformation AJNR Am J Neuroradiol 20: 1151–1153
Taylor DC, Falconer MA, Bruton CJ, Corsellis J (1971) Focal dysplasia of the cerebral cortex in epilepsy. J Neurol Neurosurg Psychiatry 34: 369–387
Utsunomiya H, Takano K, Ogasawara T, Hashimoto T, Fukushima T, Okazaki M (1998) Rhombencephalosynapsis: cerebellar embryogenesis. AJNR Am J Neuroradiology 19: 547–549
Van Bogaert P, David P, Gillain CA et al. (1998) Perisylvian dysgenesis: clinical, EEG, MRI and glucose metabolism features in 10 patients. Brain 121: 2229–2238
van der Knaap MS, Smit LME, Barth PG et al. (1997) Magnetic resonance imaging in classification of congenital muscular dystrophies with brain abnormalities. Ann Neurol 42: 50–59
Van Tassel P, Curé JK, Holden KR (1997) Cystlike white matter lesions in tuberous sclerosis. AJNR Am J Neuroradiol 18: 1367–1373
von Knebel Doeberitz C, Sievers J, Sadler M, Pehleman FW, Berry M, Halliwell P (1986) Destruction of meningeal cells of the newborn hamster cerebellum with 6-hydroxydopamine prevents foliation and lamination in the rostral cerebellum. Neuroscience 17: 409–426
Yagishita A, Arai N, Maehara T, Shimizu H, Tokumaru AM, Oda M (1997) Focal cortical dysplasia: appearance on MR images. Radiology 203: 553–559
Yagishita A, Arai N (1999) Cortical tubers without other stigmata of tuberous sclerosis: imaging and pathological findings. Neuroradiology 41: 428–432

22 Pediatric Neuroimaging: Metabolic Diseases

Zoltán Patay

Contents

22.1 Introduction

Metabolic diseases may be divided into two main groups: inborn errors of metabolism and acquired metabolic diseases.

Inborn errors of metabolism include genetic disorders which may involve the central nervous system to varying degrees. Many of them are seen in the pediatric age group although late onset forms are also well-known.

Z. Patay, MD, PhD
Consultant Neuroradiologist, Department of Radiology, MBC 28, King Faisal Specialist Hospital and Research Centre, PO Box 3354, 11211 Riyadh, Kingdom of Saudi Arabia

Acquired neurometabolic diseases include common and uncommon conditions, such as ketoacidosis in diabetes mellitus, various hypovitaminoses (Wernicke's encephalopathy, subacute combined degeneration of the spinal cord) and toxic (alcohol, lead, drug and chemotherapy induced) encephalopathies, most of which are encountered in specific clinical contexts and in adults.

Several misconceptions are traditionally linked to the inherited neurometabolic diseases in the medical imaging community:

1. Inborn errors of metabolism are rare diseases.
2. Inborn errors of metabolism are difficult to diagnose by neuroimaging.
3. Inborn errors of metabolism are therapy resistant, relentlessly devastating diseases.

The introduction of improved diagnostic methods (advanced imaging, sophisticated laboratory, histopathological and molecular genetic investigational tools) and promising new therapeutic options necessitates revision of these misconceptions.

Many of the individual inborn errors of metabolism are rare. However, the whole group of neurometabolic disorders, when taken together, accounts for a considerable percentage of diseases of the central nervous system, especially in the pediatric population. Furthermore, since many of the inborn errors of metabolism are of autosomal recessive inheritance, in communities where consanguinity is frequent (Amish family, some Jewish communities, North-American Indian and Saudi tribes) the occurrence of certain, otherwise uncommon or even exceptional diseases may be relatively high.

22.2 The Problems of Classification of Inborn Errors of Metabolism

Several attempts have been made to classify the inborn errors of metabolism. Some of them are very complex but none of them is universally applicable, for reasons of failing to fulfill the distinctly specific practical criteria of use in clinical, pathological or radiological settings.

22.2.1
Cellular Organelle and Biochemical Classification

According to the principal cellular organelle or biochemical abnormality neurometabolic diseases may be classified as organic acidurias, amino acidemias, lysosomal storage diseases, peroxisomal diseases, mitochondrial diseases and diseases of vitamin and metal metabolism. This is probably the most complex but still a somewhat inconsistent classification since overlapping between the subgroups exists (e.g. some of the organic acidurias are related to mitochondrial enzyme deficiency). Furthermore, several entities, especially leukodystrophies (Alexander's disease, van der Knaap's disease, vanishing white matter disease, Aicardi-Goutieres syndrome) do not fit into this classification. Its rather frequent use is, however, justified by the advantage of highlighting the common denominator in many of the clinically or radiologically different entities.

22.2.1.1
Organic Acidurias

Some of the organic acidurias, such as L-2-hydroxyglutaric aciduria, glutaric aciduria type 1, 4-hydroxybutyric aciduria, a-ketoglutaric aciduria (Al Aqeel et al. 1994), mevalonic aciduria and *N*-acetylaspartic aciduria (Canavan's disease) present with central nervous system manifestations only (i.e., without systemic metabolic derangements). Others have systemic manifestations too, such as acidosis, ketosis or ketoacidosis.

22.2.1.2
Amino Acidemias

The best known in this group are phenylketonuria, non-ketotic hyperglycinemia, maple syrup urine disease (MSUD), hyperhomocystinemia, tyrosinemia, and a group of diseases referred to as urea-cycle defects.

22.2.1.3
Lysosomal Disorders

Lysosomes are intracellular organelles containing enzymes, the primary role of which is the breaking down of macromolecules (proteins, nucleic acids, lipids, polysaccharides) in normal (physiological cell constituent turnover) and abnormal (inflammation) conditions. Macromolecules to be eliminated enter the lysosomes where the hydrolytic process takes place and the end products may be eliminated thereafter. Deficiency of lysosomal enzymes leads to abnormal intralysosomal accumulation of specific macromolecules. This progressively interferes with the normal function of the lysosomes and the entire cell and a "storage" disease develops. Depending on the function of the deficient enzyme and the stored macromolecules, several types and subtypes of lysosomal storage diseases are known. Some of them present with central and/or peripheral nervous system involvement (leukodystrophy, polyneuropathy), others have skeletal (dysostosis), visceral (hepatosplenomegaly, renal cardiac and pulmonary disease) or cutaneous manifestations.

22.2.1.3.1
Mucopolysaccharidoses

Mucopolysaccharidoses are caused by the impaired degradation of acid mucopolysaccharides. They include the so-called Hurler's, Scheie's, Hurler-Scheie, Sanfilippo's, Morquio's, Maroteaux-Lamy and Sly's diseases. Skeletal (dysostosis multiplex) and visceral (hepatosplenomegaly) abnormalities are the most common clinical and imaging features of these diseases. They are followed by the clinical manifestations of central nervous system involvement, related to the intraneuronal and perivascular storage of mucopolysaccharides. Another potentially relevant manifestation of some of these diseases (Hurler-Scheie, Scheie's, Morquio's, Maroteaux-Lamy) is the compression of the spinal cord with cranio-cervical junction predilection due to dural thickening and subsequent narrowing of the foramen magnum and the upper cervical spinal canal.

22.2.1.3.2
Glycoproteinoses

This group consists of several neurovisceral storage disorders including a-mannosidosis, a-fucosidosis and aspartylglycosaminuria, which share many similarities with the mucopolysaccharidoses from both the clinical and the imaging points of view.

22.2.1.3.3
Mucolipidoses

These diseases are characterized by the storage of mucopolysaccharides and glycolipids and, hence, the clinical manifestations are often reminiscent of those in mucopolysaccharidoses and sphingolipidoses. This group comprises such rare diseases as sialidoses, galactosialidosis, and mucolipidoses type II, III and IV.

22.2.1.3.4
Sphingolipidoses

This is a rather heterogeneous group including cerebrosidoses, gangliosidoses and a few other mixed or individual entities.

Cerebrosidoses. This group includes metachromatic leukodystrophy (MLD) and globoid cell leukodystrophy, better known as Krabbe's disease.

Gangliosidoses. GM_1 gangliosidosis typically presents with prominent visceral involvement and variable neurological manifestations. In GM_2 gangliosidosis neurological signs dominate.

Other Mixed or Individual Entities. Multiple sulfatase deficiency is due to several deficient sulfatase enzymes which individually cause various cerebrosidoses and mucopolysaccharidoses and, therefore, the resultant mixed storage disorder due to accumulation of mucopolysaccharides and sulfatides.

In Niemann-Pick disease intraneuronal accumulation of sphingomyelin, in Gaucher's disease that of glucocerebroside, occurs.

Other rare individual entities include Fabry's disease and Farber's disease.

A special form of lysosomal disorder is the so-called Chédiak-Higashi syndrome (Ballard et al. 1994), which is related to a peculiar structural abnormality (i.e., fusion disorder of the primary lysosomes) and may present with white matter disease.

22.2.1.4 Peroxisomal Diseases

Peroxisomes are cellular organelles which contain several dozens of enzymes involved in different metabolic pathways, including lipid metabolism and, therefore, are indispensable in the normal myelination process. The number of peroxisomes and their enzymatic activity is variable as a function of the actual tissue metabolic requirements. For example, they are more abundant in the oligodendrocytes in neonates and infants during the active myelination process than later in life. Peroxisomal diseases typically present with involvement of the central nervous system with predilection of the white matter.

Peroxisomal disorders are caused by total or partial absence of peroxisomal activity and represent a real continuum of diseases. The most severe forms (Zellweger's disease, neonatal adrenoleukodystrophy, rhizomelic chondrodysplasia punctata) are characterized by generalized absence of peroxisomal activity and hence present with pre- or immediate postnatal onset. These are generalized systemic diseases, in which involvement of the central nervous system is always severe but not exclusive. They typically lead to death within the first few months or years of life. Other forms with multiple peroxisomal dysfunctions are of infantile or childhood onset (infantile Refsum's disease, Zellweger-like syndrome) and the disease course is more prolonged. If the metabolic abnormality is limited to the loss of a single peroxisomal function – e.g., metabolism of phytanic acid in Refsum's disease or degradation of very long chain fatty acids in X-linked adrenoleukodystrophy (X-ALD) – the resultant disease may be of childhood, juvenile or adult onset. Some of them may be compatible with life (adrenomyeloneuropathy, Refsum's disease), others (X-ALD) are not.

22.2.1.5 Mitochondrial Diseases

This group includes various clinical entities, the common biochemical feature of which is impairment of the cellular energy production. Although the mitochondrial dysfunction is generalized, the clinical manifestations typically involve muscle and brain, because of their high energy requirements. The best known entities in this group are MELAS (mitochondrial myopathy, encephalopathy, lactic acidosis and stroke-like episodes), MERRF (myoclonic epilepsy with ragged red fibers), Kearns-Sayre syndrome, Leigh's disease and Leber's hereditary optic neuropathy (LHON). In mitochondrial diseases both white and gray matter lesions are common.

22.2.1.6 Diseases of Metal or Vitamin Metabolism

Defect in the copper metabolism may cause Menkes' disease (intracellular copper transport abnormality) or Wilson's disease (extracellular copper transport abnormality). Disorders of the B_{12} vitamin metabolism are known to be associated with various neurological disorders (hyperhomocystinemia, subacute combined degeneration of the spinal cord).

22.2.2 Leukodystrophies and Poliodystrophies

Classification of inherited neurometabolic diseases – according to the primarily involved substance – into leukodystrophies and poliodystrophies is a helpful diagnostic imaging concept, because of the inherently high sensitivity of MRI in the demonstration of signal differences between normal and abnormal gray and white matter, based on their different T1 and T2 relaxation properties.

Primary leukodystrophies are degenerative diseases that involve primarily or preferentially the cerebral white matter, due to an enzymatic disturbance leading to abnormal myelin synthesis or myelin breakdown. The best known of these diseases are MLD, Krabbe's disease, Canavan's disease, Pelizaeus-Merzbacher disease, multiple sulfatase deficiency, X-ALD, Alexander's disease, Aicardi-Goutieres syndrome, Zellweger syndrome.

Poliodystrophies are less frequently encountered and include neuronal ceroid lipofuscinosis, fucosidosis, neurovisceral storage disorders (GM1 and GM2 gangliosidosis, mucopolysaccharidoses, mucolipidosis) Alper's disease, Menkes' disease, etc.

However, many of the primary leukodystrophies present with clinical or imaging evidence of gray matter involvement. In Canavan's disease pallidal lesions, in Krabbe's disease putaminal lesions are typical imaging findings. Conversely, poliodystrophies (e.g., neuronal ceroid lipofuscinosis, mucopolysaccharidoses) and systemic neurometabolic diseases (e.g., mitochondrial diseases) may also show signs of extensive white matter disease and mimic leukodystrophy. In organic acidurias both gray and white matter involvement is common. Amino acidemias present with preferentially white matter disease; however, clinical (seizures) and electrophysiological (EEG) signs often suggest some degree of gray matter involvement. Most of the lysosomal storage disorders are characterized by gray matter disease, but involvement of the white matter is not unusual and some of them present with leukodystrophy exclusively. These observations render this classification sometimes difficult to use in neuroimaging.

22.2.3 Clinical Features

22.2.3.1 Age at Onset

Depending on the age at onset of the clinical disease the following categories may be used: neonatal (from birth to 1 month), early and late infantile (1–6 months and 6 months to 3 years), early and late juvenile (3–6 and 6–16 years) and adult (16 and over).

As clear manifestation of their considerable phenotypic variations, almost all neurometabolic diseases have several clinical forms depending on the age of onset. As a general rule, within the same disease category, earlier onsets usually suggest a more profound metabolic derangement whereas later onset forms represent clinically milder but not necessarily benign variants. The differences in the onset and clinical course among the various peroxisomal disease entities, as a function of the severity of the underlying enzymatic abnormality, well illustrate this concept.

Lysosomal storage disorders are rarely apparent at birth. Most of them present in early (Tay-Sachs, Sandhoff's, Hunter's disease) or late (fucosidosis, Hurler's, Maroteaux-Lamy syndromes) infancy. Hurler-Scheie and Scheie's syndromes have late infantile or juvenile forms. Fabry's disease is of juvenile or adult onset. Many of the lysosomal storage diseases have various – neonatal, infantile, juvenile and adult – forms (Gaucher's disease, MLD, multiple sulfatase deficiency, Krabbe's disease, GM_1 and GM_2 gangliosidoses, neuronal ceroid lipofuscinoses).

Most organic acidemias present either during the first few days of life (primary lactic acidosis, urea-cycle defects, propionic acidemia, methylmalonic aciduria, isovaleric acidemia) or infancy (glutaric aciduria type 1, biotinidase deficiency).

In mitochondrial diseases the age of onset shows significant variations. MELAS may appear from early infancy to adulthood, LHON is of late juvenile or adult onset and Kearns-Sayre syndrome is typically seen in the juvenile age group.

Significant, sometimes extreme, deviations from the above outlined forms presenting especially with unusual late onset are increasingly identified. The term of late onset, however, is relative and hence it may be appropriately assigned to propionic aciduria developing in a 5-year-old child (Perez Cerda et al. 1998), as well as to Krabbe's disease in a 39-year-old (Turazzini et al. 1997), MELAS in a 60-year-old (Kimata et al. 1998) or neuronal ceroid lipofuscinosis in a 64-year-old patient (Hammersen et al. 1998).

22.2.3.2 Clinical Presentation

Neurometabolic diseases may manifest as acute or chronic encephalopathy. However, mixed forms characterized by progressive encephalopathy and occasional metabolic deteriorations are also common.

Metabolic disorders with lactic acidosis (pyruvate carboxylase, pyruvate dehydrogenase deficiency), ketosis (isovaleric acidemia, propionic acidemia, methylmalonic acidemia) or ketoacidosis (multiple carboxylase deficiency, ethylmalonic aciduria) are most likely to present with acute metabolic decompensation (coma, hypotonia, seizures, metabolic stroke with rapid onset of extrapyramidal movement disorders). Amino acidemias (neonatal MSUD, non-ketotic hyperglycinemia), neonatal peroxisomal disorders (Zellweger syndrome, neonatal adrenoleukodystrophy) are also frequently associated with deleterious acute metabolic crisis. Respiratory alkalosis in the neonate is felt to be pathognomonic for urea-cycle defects (Maestri et al. 1999).

Lysosomal storage diseases, late onset peroxisomal diseases, some of the organic acidurias (glutaric aciduria type 1, 4-hydroxybutyric aciduria, biotinidase deficiency), and a few of the amino acidemias (phenylketonuria, homocystinuria) and mitochondrial diseases exhibit a more insidious course and result in chronic progressive encephalopathy.

Leukodystrophies are typically associated with progressive neurological manifestations (Aicardi 1993). Schematically, in leukodystrophies pyramidal signs, whereas in basal ganglia diseases extrapyramidal movement disorders (dyskinesia, choreoathetosis, tremor), predominate.

22.3 The Concept of Selective Vulnerability and Pattern Recognition

22.3.1 Selective Vulnerability

One of the most striking imaging features of the neurometabolic diseases is the highly variable pattern of involvement of the central nervous system. This is to a great extent explained by the selective vulnerability of the different structures to different noxa, especially in the developing brain. The exact nature of the metabolic disorder, in particular the type and quantity of the specific lacking or excess metabolites (biochemical phenotype), as determined by the underlying molecular genetic disorder (genotype) and the degree of the resultant enzymatic dysfunction, the age of onset (maturity of the brain), the distinct histobiochemical properties (neurotransmitters) of the different anatomical and functional systems, all have a significant impact on the clinical manifestations (clinical phenotype) and the magnitude and topographic distribution of imaging abnormalities (radiological phenotype).

The specific energy and nutrient requirements of certain structures (myelinating white matter, basal ganglia), as a function of age, have a definite influence on selective vulnerability. The cerebral white matter is particularly vulnerable before 32 weeks of gestation, whereas the basal ganglia are most prone to metabolic derangements during the last 3 gestational months and during the first 3 years of life. This is believed to explain why hypoxic-anoxic episodes lead to periventricular leukoencephalomalacia in the preterm and to basal ganglia disease in the term infants (Menkes and Curran 1994). Similarly, organic acidurias with postnatal onset are characterized by disturbances of the amino and fatty acid supply to the citric acid cycle, and therefore preferentially present with basal ganglia disease.

In the neonatal MSUD elective involvement of the myelinating white matter is a strikingly distinct pathological-radiological finding. Conversely, in the late onset (or intermittent) form of MSUD pallidal and thalamic changes are conspicuous.

It is noteworthy that isomers of the same abnormal metabolite (L-2-hydroxyglutaric aciduria and D-2-hydroxyglutaric aciduria) may result in distinctly different clinical and imaging phenotypes (Baker et al. 1997; D'Incerti et al. 1998; Barth et al. 1993).

Intrauterine onset of the metabolic disorder may lead to malformation or disturbed development of the central nervous system, as it is demonstrated by the very characteristic bilateral polymicrogyria within the Sylvian fissures in Zellweger disease. Pachygyria has been observed in non-ketotic hyperglycinemia (Fletcher et al. 1995) and cortical dysplasia is one of the hallmark imaging findings in some of the congenital muscular dystrophies (Fukuyama, Santavuori, Walker-Warburg and Fowler types). Agenesis of the cerebellar vermis may occur in glutaric aciduria type 2 (Tanakashi et al. 1999). Callosal dysgenesis may be seen in mucolipidosis type IV (Frei et al. 1998). In glutaric aciduria type 1 the almost invariably present bilateral open Sylvian fissures (disturbed opercularization) suggest a prenatal disease onset. In siblings with ethylmalonic aciduria, Chiari type 1 malformation and tethered cord have been described (Nowaczyk et al. 1998).

22.3.2 Pattern Recognition

Pattern recognition in neuroimaging means the recognition of the imaging manifestations of selective vulnerability. It requires experience, but more importantly, meticulous image analysis.

Evaluation of the white matter structures should always include the cerebellar white matter, the brain stem tracts, and the cerebral white matter. Special attention should be paid to the possible involvement of the cortical-spinal tracts, the internal capsules, the corpus callosum and the subcortical U-fibers, since involvement or sparing of these structures has significant differential diagnostic value. Assessment of the gray matter structures includes the dentate nuclei, the thalami, the globi pallidi, the putamina, the caudate nuclei and the cortex.

All of these structures are evaluated for both volume changes (atrophy, swelling) and signal abnormalities (T1 and T2 shortening or prolongation). The presence or absence of signal enhancement within the lesion areas after intravenous gadolinium injection may also provide a helpful clue to differential diagnosis.

The systematic application of this concept in the diagnostic imaging evaluation of neurometabolic diseases (van der Knaap et al. 1991) has resulted in a more accurate description of distinct lesion patterns in many of the known neurometabolic disorders and also led to the identification of new clinical-radiological entities during the past 1 or 2 decades, such as L-2-hydroxyglutaric aciduria (Barth et al. 1992), infantile onset encephalopathy with swelling and discrepantly mild clinical course (van der Knaap et al. 1995), familial leukodystrophy with adult onset dementia and abnormal glycolipid storage (Simon et al. 1998), and leukodystrophy with ovarian dysgenesis (Schiffmann et al. 1997). The emergence of further entities may also be anticipated.

The concept of pattern recognition may be further expanded to involve data from other imaging modalities (CT, diffusion-weighted imaging) and MR spectroscopy. This approach helped to identify and characterize such new diseases as the vanishing white matter disease (Hanefeld et al. 1993; van der Knaap et al. 1997), and creatine deficiency in the brain (Stoeckler et al. 1994). The application of the concept, however, is not exclusive to neuroimaging. Clinical diagnosis in neurometabolic diseases is typically based on the recognition of specific clinical signs and symptoms characterizing more or less distinct phenotypes. Hence, a clinical-radiological pattern recognition may be advocated, where the integration of clinical data (gender, onset and type of the clinical manifestations, clinical evolution, physical or ophthalmological stigmata), imaging abnormalities (lesion types and patterns), and MR spectroscopic findings may significantly enhance the specificity of the entire diagnostic work-up.

The positive and specific diagnosis may be established or confirmed by laboratory and/or histological examinations. Biochemical work-up of urine or blood samples is sometimes simple and straightforward, but may occasionally require sophisticated and costly equipment. Enzyme activity determinations are possible from fibroblast or peripheral blood cell cultures. Histological diagnosis may be obtained by peripheral nerve (MLD, Krabbe's disease), muscle (mitochondrial disease), skin, mucosa or liver biopsy (storage diseases, Wilson's disease) in some cases. In others, brain biopsy or autopsy may confirm the correct diagnosis (Alexander's disease). However, narrowing the spectrum of possible differential diagnostic options in suspected neurometabolic diseases based on clinical-radiological pattern recognition may significantly reduce the amount and hence the cost of additional diagnostic investigations. The specific diagnosis is therefore reached faster and in a more cost-effective way.

22.4 Diagnostic Imaging in Neurometabolic Diseases

In centers which specialize in the management of neurometabolic diseases, and hence benefit from a considerable expertise (Ozand et al. 1992), the specific diagnosis is often established or strongly suggested based on clinical manifestations and sophisticated laboratory screening studies, such as tandem mass spectrometry (Rashed et al. 1995, 1997). The role of neuroimaging in such settings is not infrequently limited to providing an initial baseline "inventory" of the lesions and then occasional follow-ups in order to monitor the disease progress and possible response to therapy.

Somewhat paradoxically, the diagnostic burden is often heavier on radiologists working in general neuroimaging practices. These centers are more likely to be involved in primary screening and the referring diagnoses may not be suggestive of neurometabolic diseases. A high index of suspicion, knowledge of the basic MRI semiology of neurometabolic diseases and a systematic approach to image analysis and interpretation are indispensable. More importantly, as an absolute prerequisite, an appropriately performed MRI study, taking full advantage of available technical options, is mandatory in order to enhance sensitivity and specificity and identify definite, probable and possible neurometabolic disease and hence warrant further, targeted investigations.

22.4.1
Computer Tomography and Ultrasound

In clinically suspected neurometabolic diseases, the role of CT in the imaging work-up is secondary to that of MRI. In rare situations, however, performed as a complementary study, CT can enhance diagnostic specificity. The demonstration of the rather typical hyperdense basal ganglia in Krabbe's disease and hyperdense thalami in GM_2 gangliosidoses (Brismar et al. 1990) by CT has definite diagnostic value, if a previous MRI study suggested such diagnoses. The demonstration of basal ganglia calcifications is straightforward by CT in Cockayne's syndrome, Aicardi-Goutieres syndrome and some of the mitochondrial encephalopathies (Sue et al. 1998). In the malignant, biopterin dependent form of phenylketonuria, the CT presentation with extensive subcortical calcifications may be almost pathognomonic. This is important because calcifications are not always conspicuous on MR images and their appearance is inconsistent. Theoretically, calcifications present with hyposignal on both T1- and T2-weighted images; however, due to variations of the crystalline structure, they may occasionally be hyperintense on the T1-weighted images.

In some of the neurometabolic diseases, especially those which are associated with morphological abnormalities of the brain, such as glutaric aciduria type 1, cerebral ultrasound may be suggestive even before the appearance of clinical signs and symptoms (Forstner et al. 1999). In infantile leukodystrophies presenting with macrocephaly ultrasound may have an important role in ruling out hydrocephalus and orienting the diagnosis towards a possible neurometabolic disease.

22.4.2
Magnetic Resonance Imaging and Spectroscopy

22.4.2.1
MR Imaging Protocols and Aspects of Evaluation in Neurometabolic Diseases

In the conventional MRI evaluation high spatial and contrast resolution are equally important. High resolution MRI (512×512 matrix) in conjunction with conventional (T1-, proton density- and T2-weighted) and special purpose sequences (inversion recovery, FLAIR) enhance lesion conspicuity, allowing more accurate structure-related lesion depiction, which constitutes the foundation of the pattern recognition-based imaging work-up.

22.4.2.1.1
Sagittal T1-Weighted (Spin-Echo) Images

The sagittal T1-weighted images allow accurate assessment of the possible morphological changes of the corpus callosum and of the cerebellar vermis (Fig. 22.1).

Segmental or diffuse atrophy of the corpus callosum may reflect focal or diffuse loss of white matter in the hemispheres. Abnormally thin corpus callosum is a characteristic finding in non-ketotic hyperglycinemia (Press et al. 1989) and in the advanced stages of leukodystrophies. Direct callosal involvement is typically seen in MLD, X-ALD, Krabbe's disease, in the advanced stage of Canavan's disease and often but not always in Alexander's disease. The gradient of the disease process (postero-anterior or antero-posterior) is usually well demonstrated, too. Sparing of the corpus callosum is characteristically seen in van der Knaap's disease, in GM_1 (Chen et al. 1998) and GM_2 gangliosidosis and in the early stages of Canavan's disease and Cockayne's syndrome. Assessment of the corpus callosum is, therefore, an important element in the pattern recognition process and is particularly helpful in the differential diagnosis of leukodystrophies.

Cerebellar atrophy with vermian predominance is a rather typical feature of 3-methylglutaconic aciduria and Cockayne's syndrome.

22.4.2.1.2
Axial T1-Weighted (Inversion Recovery or Spin-Echo) Images

The axial inversion recovery sequence provides T1-weighted images with exquisite contrast resolution between white and gray matter structures. It allows assessment of the normal or abnormal myelination process. It accurately demonstrates the involvement (Canavan's disease, Alexander's disease) or sparing (X-ALD, MLD) of the subcortical U-fibers in leukodystrophies (Fig. 22.2).

Conventional T1-weighted spin-echo images may also be used for the same purposes, but in most cases the abnormalities are less conspicuous. Conversely, abnormal hyperintensity of the basal ganglia, e.g., in cases of hepatic encephalopathy, is often more conspicuous on T1-weighted spin-echo than on inversion recovery images.

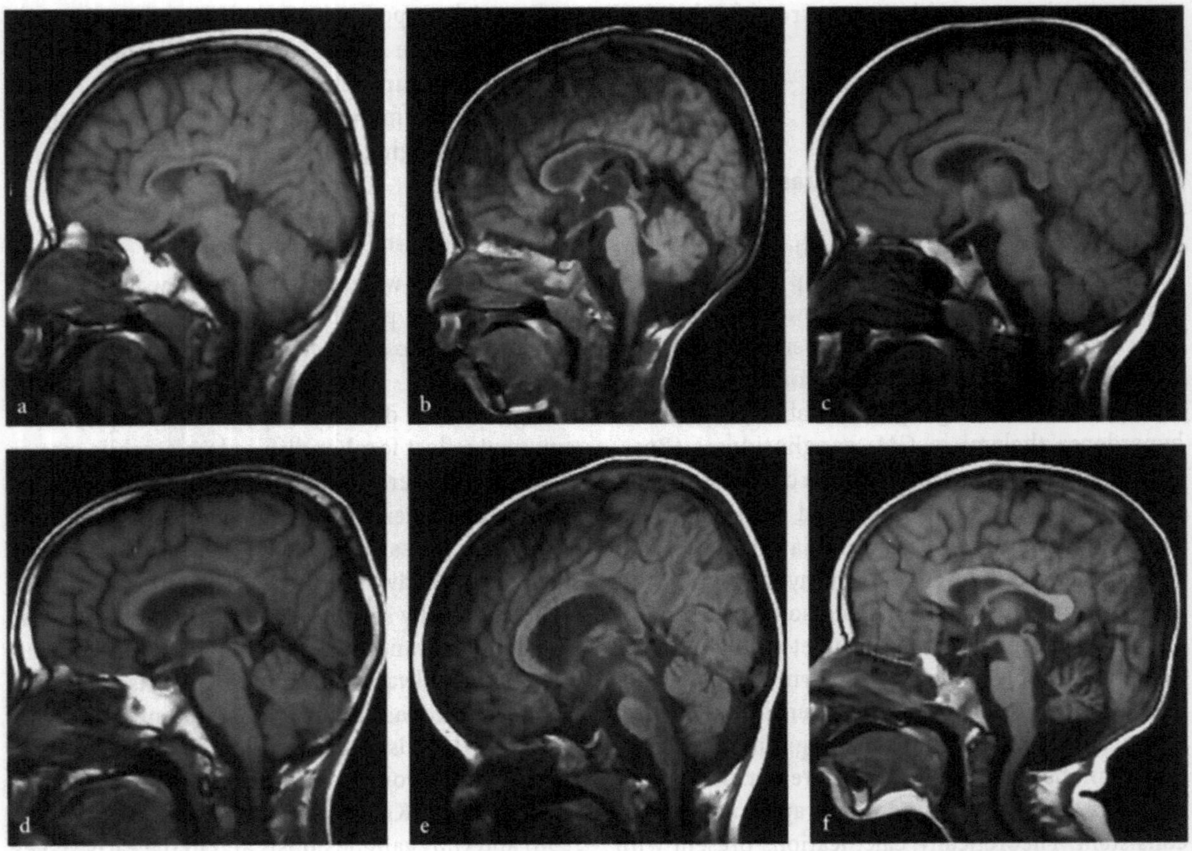

Fig. 22.1a–f. Sagittal images of the midline structures of the brain in various neurometabolic diseases. In non-ketotic hyperglycinemia (**a**) hypoplasia, in Krabbe's disease (**b**) atrophy of the corpus callosum is demonstrated. In MLD (**c**) and Canavan's disease (**d**) the signal changes suggest involvement of the entire corpus callosum. In X-ALD (**e**) the splenium is abnormal but the rostral components are spared. Prominent atrophy of the cerebellar vermis in 3-methylglutaconic aciduria (**f**)

22.4.2.1.3
Axial Proton Density and T2-Weighted
(Fast Spin-Echo or Spin-Echo) Images

Axial long TR (proton density and T2-weighted) images are considered to be the gold standard for the depiction of parenchymal lesions characterized by T2 prolongation. The T2-weighted images are essential in the assessment of the myelination pattern, especially in the 10–18 months age range, where T1-weighted (and inversion recovery) images may already be insensitive. The U-fibers are also well assessed with this technique, allowing double-checking of findings on the T1-weighted images. In the neonate and young infant the T2-weighted images often allow better assessment of the cortex and more accurate depiction of cortical abnormalities than the T1-weighted images. Using a high resolution matrix, accurate topographical localization of focal lesions within the basal ganglia or the brainstem is further facilitated, which provides useful information for disease specific pattern recognition. Lesions to the subthalamic nuclei, the tails of the caudate nuclei, the globi pallidi and the peripheral cerebellar areas are, however, often more conspicuous on coronal images (Fig. 22.3).

The value of the recently available fluid-attenuated inversion recovery (FLAIR), turbo gradient spin-echo (TGSE) and ultrafast echo-planar techniques is not established yet. The FLAIR technique may be helpful in demonstrating cystic-necrotic lesions within a markedly abnormal white matter, for instance in Alexander's, Canavan's or Krabbe's disease (Fig. 22.4).

22.4.2.2
Anatomical Structure-related Lesion Identification and Pattern Recognition on Conventional MR Images

Detection and identification of lesions within specific anatomical structures is a key element in pattern recognition. As mentioned earlier, neurometabolic diseases may involve white or gray matter structures

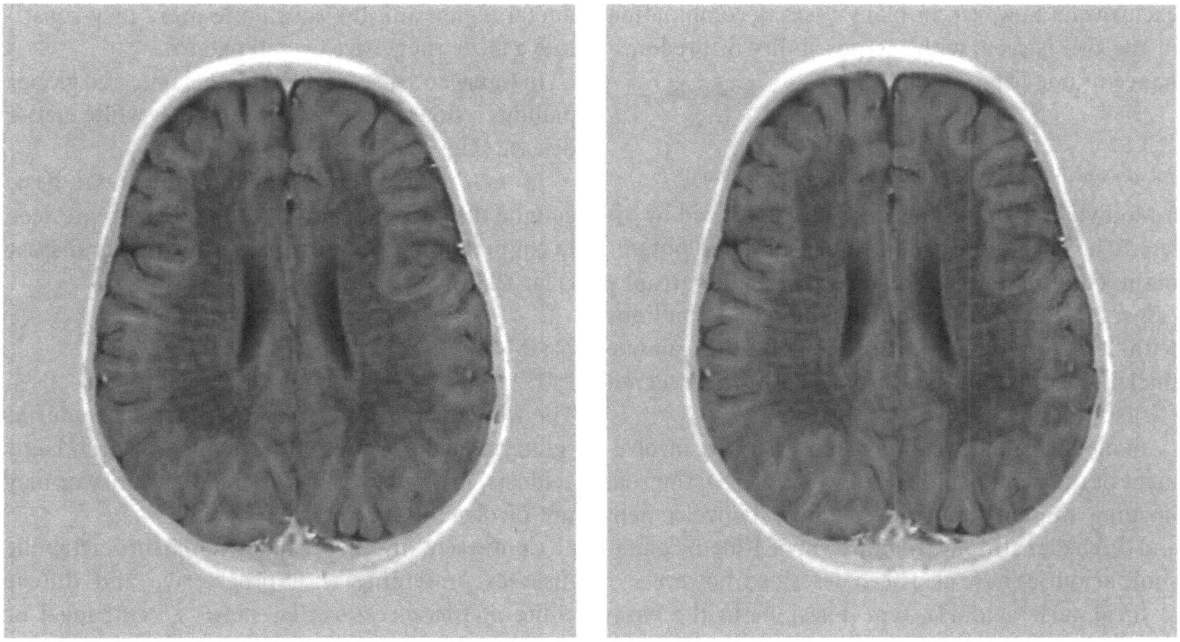

a b

Fig. 22.2a,b. Axial inversion recovery images in Canavan's disease and in MLD. In Canavan's disease (**a**) involvement of the cerebral white matter is diffuse, in MLD the subcortical U-fibers are relatively, but not entirely, spared (**b**)

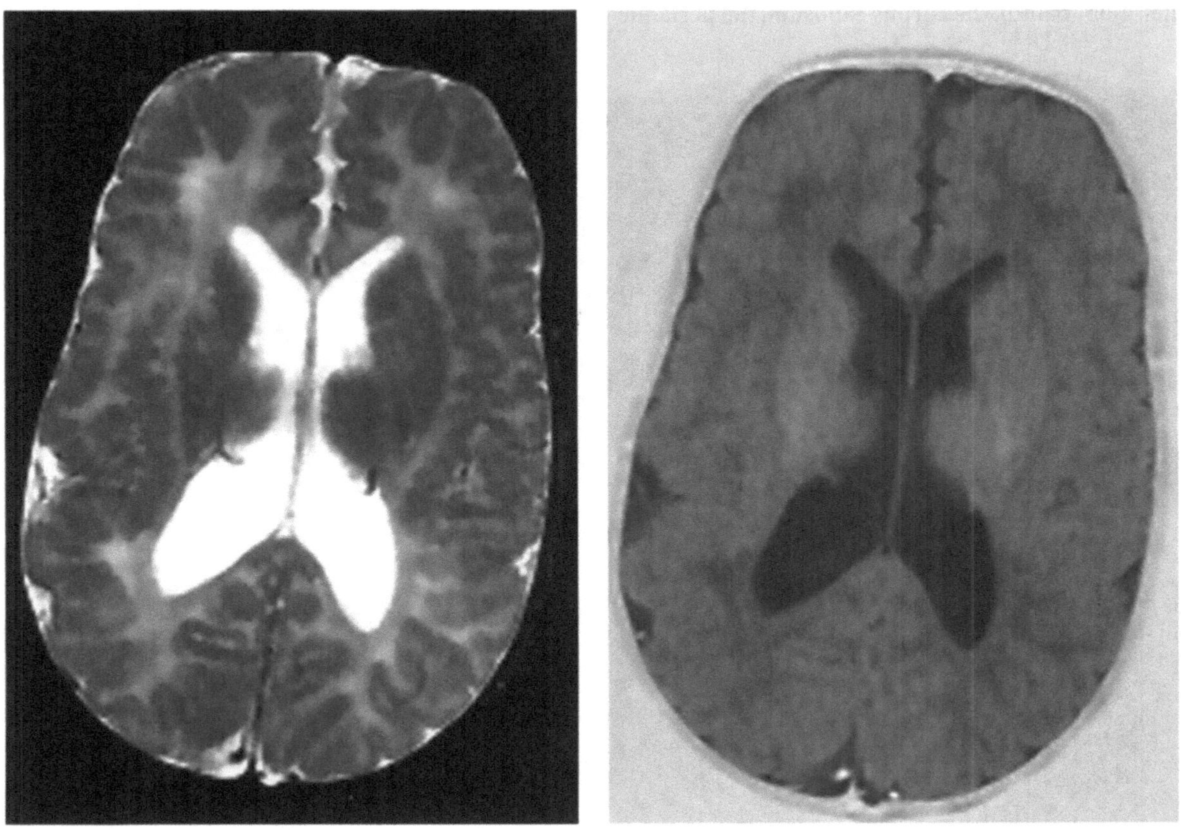

a b

Fig. 22.3a,b. Cortical dysplasia (polymicrogyria) in the Sylvian fissures bilaterally in a 3-month-old girl with Zellweger disease. The lesions are easier to identify on the axial T2-weighted (**a**) than on the inversion recovery (**b**) image exclusively; however, in many cases, a combination of the two is seen, with the possibility of predominance of one over the other.

22.4.2.2.1
Patterns of Basal Ganglia and Thalamic Involvement

3-Methylglutaconic aciduria is characterized by bilateral lesions to the caudate nuclei and the putamina in conjunction with marked cerebellar atrophy (Figs. 22.1f, 22.5a). Lesions to the globus pallidus with less prominent involvement of the caudate nuclei and the putamina have also been observed (Gibson et al. 1999).

In methylmalonic aciduria almost selective involvement of the globi pallidi is seen (Fig. 22.5b). Unusual imaging presentation with putaminal involvement and cerebellar atrophy (reminiscent of 3-methylglutaconic aciduria) have also been described, however.

In glutaric aciduria, type 1 lesions to the basal ganglia involve the caudate nuclei, the putamina and the globi pallidi (Fig. 22.5c).

In Leigh's disease involvement of the putamina (Medina et al. 1990; Valvanne et al. 1998) and of the subthalamic nuclei (Savoiardo and Uziel 1991) with or without associated lesions in the caudate nuclei, globi pallidi, the corpus callosum, the periaqueductal region and the substantia nigra may constitute a fairly suggestive overall pattern.

In Canavan's disease bilateral thalamic and globus pallidus lesions are present with diffuse white matter disease (Fig. 22.8b).

In L-2-hydroxyglutaric aciduria bilateral basal ganglia disease and sparing of the thalami are seen in conjunction with centripetal white matter disease (Fig. 22.5d).

22.4.2.2.2
Patterns of White Matter Involvement

The white matter lesions in some organic acidurias (glutaric aciduria type I, propionic aciduria, lactic acidosis) are patchy and scattered. They may or may not involve the subcortical U-fibers.

Conversely, myelin breakdown in neurometabolic diseases presenting with progressive and diffuse white matter disease often shows a centrifugal or centripetal pattern.

In X-ALD (Fig. 22.6) and in MLD (Fig. 22.7) the white matter disease is characteristically centrifugal but at the same time a postero-anterior or antero-posterior gradient may also be present. In both diseases the subcortical U-fibers are spared until the advanced stage. In X-ALD symmetrical involve-

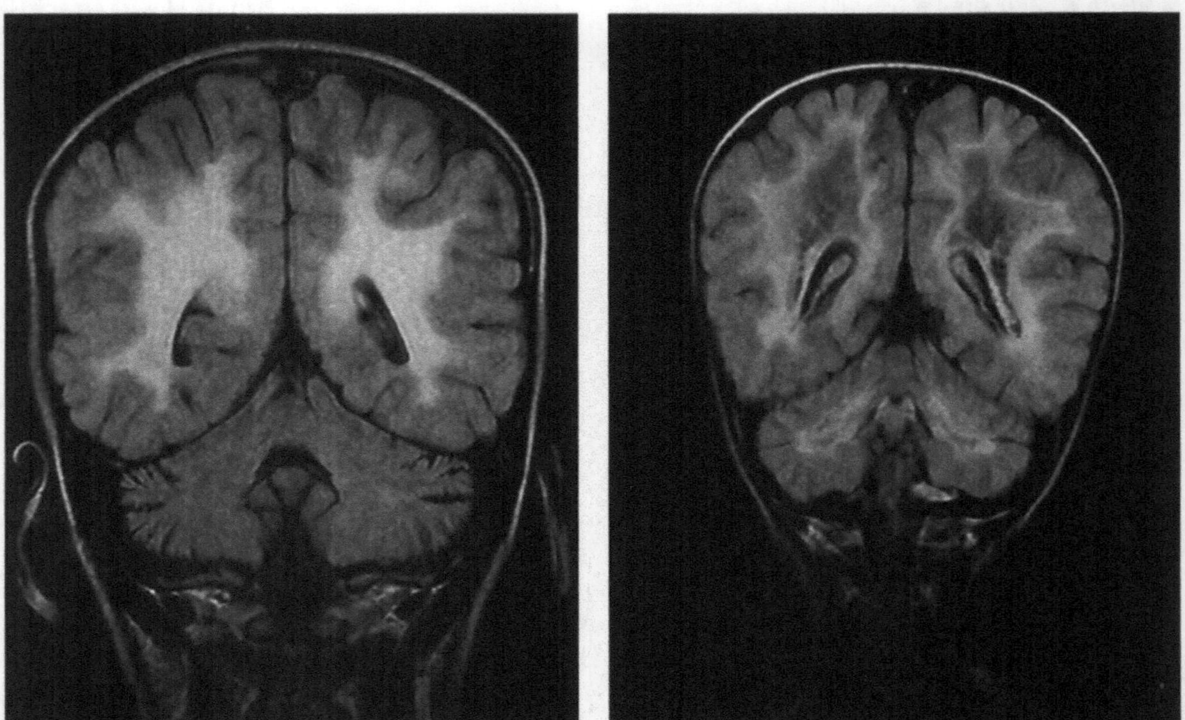

a b

Fig. 22.4a,b. White matter disease in MLD (**a**) and Krabbe's disease (**b**) demonstrated by FLAIR sequences. In Krabbe's disease the periventricular cystic-necrotic areas are well appreciated. Similar changes may be seen in Canavan's disease too (Fig. 22.8c)

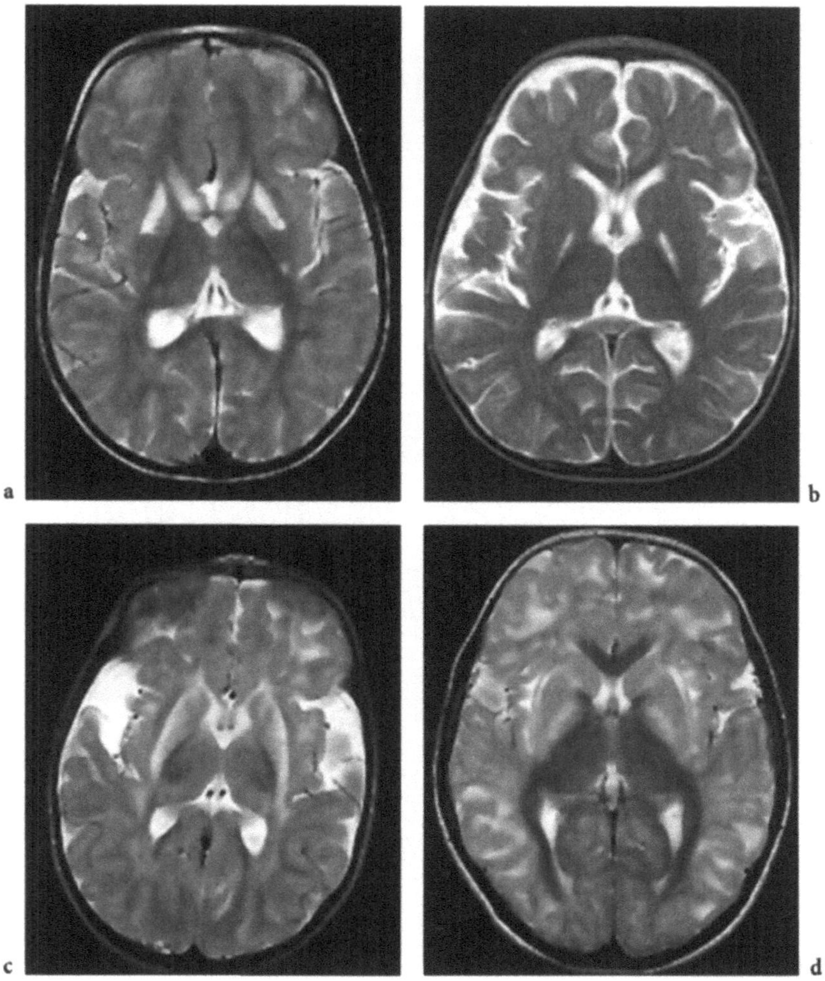

Fig. 22.5a–d. Axial T2-weighted fast spin-echo images, showing different patterns of involvement of the basal ganglia in 3-methylglutaconic aciduria (**a**), in methylmalonic aciduria (**b**), in glutaric aciduria type 1 (**c**) and in L-2-hydroxyglutaric aciduria (**d**)

ment of the pontomedullary corticospinal tracts has been found to be highly characteristic (BARKOVICH et al. 1997). In MLD relative preservation of the perivascular white matter areas may lend a tigroid appearance to the centrum semiovale on both T1- and T2-weighted images (KIM et al. 1997). With other characteristic elements (involvement of the corpus callosum, the posterior limbs of the internal capsules) this is highly suggestive, but non-specific to MLD, since a similar pattern has been found in other diseases, such as Pelizaeus-Merzbacher disease, Cockayne's disease and even in neuronal ceroid lipofuscinosis.

A typical centripetal disease progress is seen in 2-L-hydroxyglutaric aciduria (Fig. 22.5d) and Canavan's disease (Fig. 22.8). Involvement of the subcortical U-fibers is always present.

22.4.2.2.3
Involvement of the Spinal Cord, of the Cauda Equina and of the Peripheral Nervous System

Literature data on the imaging findings of spinal cord and cauda equina lesions in inherited neurometabolic diseases are sparse (BEWERMEYER et al. 1985). This may be partially explained by technical reasons, the small size of the anatomical structures rendering accurate evaluation difficult by the currently available MRI techniques. Histopathological data, however, suggest that both white matter tracts and gray matter structures are prone to involvement in a series of diseases, including Canavan's disease, Cockayne' syndrome, Krabbe's disease, GM2 gangliosidosis, non-ketotic hyperglycinemia, cerebrotendinous xanthomatosis, carbohydrate-deficient glycoprotein syndrome, glutaric aciduria type 2, cobalamin

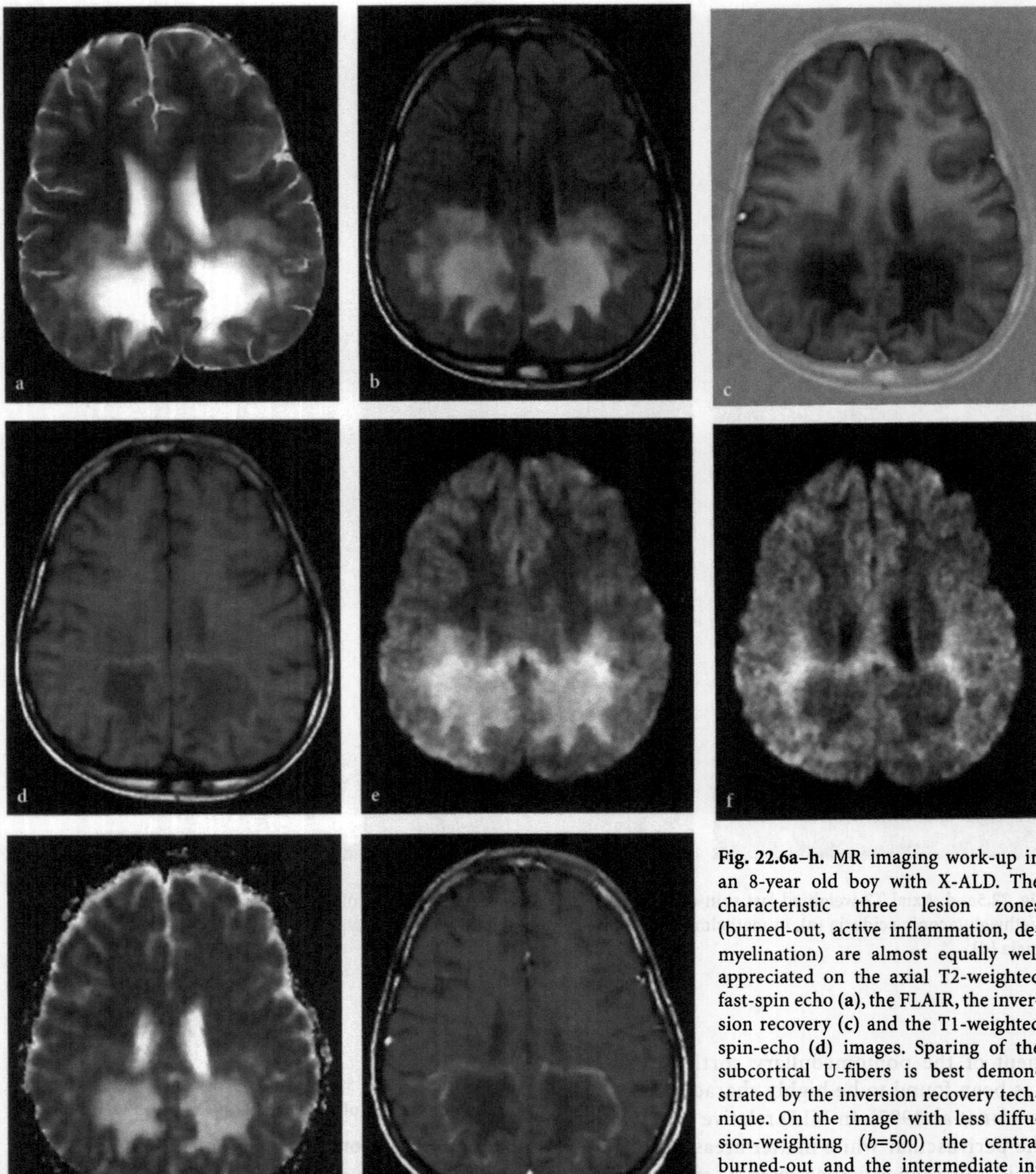

Fig. 22.6a–h. MR imaging work-up in an 8-year old boy with X-ALD. The characteristic three lesion zones (burned-out, active inflammation, demyelination) are almost equally well appreciated on the axial T2-weighted fast-spin echo (**a**), the FLAIR, the inversion recovery (**c**) and the T1-weighted spin-echo (**d**) images. Sparing of the subcortical U-fibers is best demonstrated by the inversion recovery technique. On the image with less diffusion-weighting (b=500) the central burned-out and the intermediate inflammation zones are not clearly differentiated from each other, due to T2 shine-through artifact (**e**). Using a stronger diffusion gradient setting (b=1000) the zone of inflammation maintains its increased signal intensity appearance, consistent with isotropically restricted water diffusion, whereas the burned-out zone is hypointense suggestive of isotropically increased water diffusion (**f**). The validity of these observations is confirmed by the apparent diffusion coefficient (ADC) map (**g**), where the zone of inflammation is clearly identified as a hypointense (decreased apparent diffusion coefficient) area between the hyperintense (increased apparent diffusion coefficient) burned-out and the demyelination zones. On the gadolinium-enhanced T1-weighted spin-echo image (**h**) the signal enhancement is limited to the area of inflammation

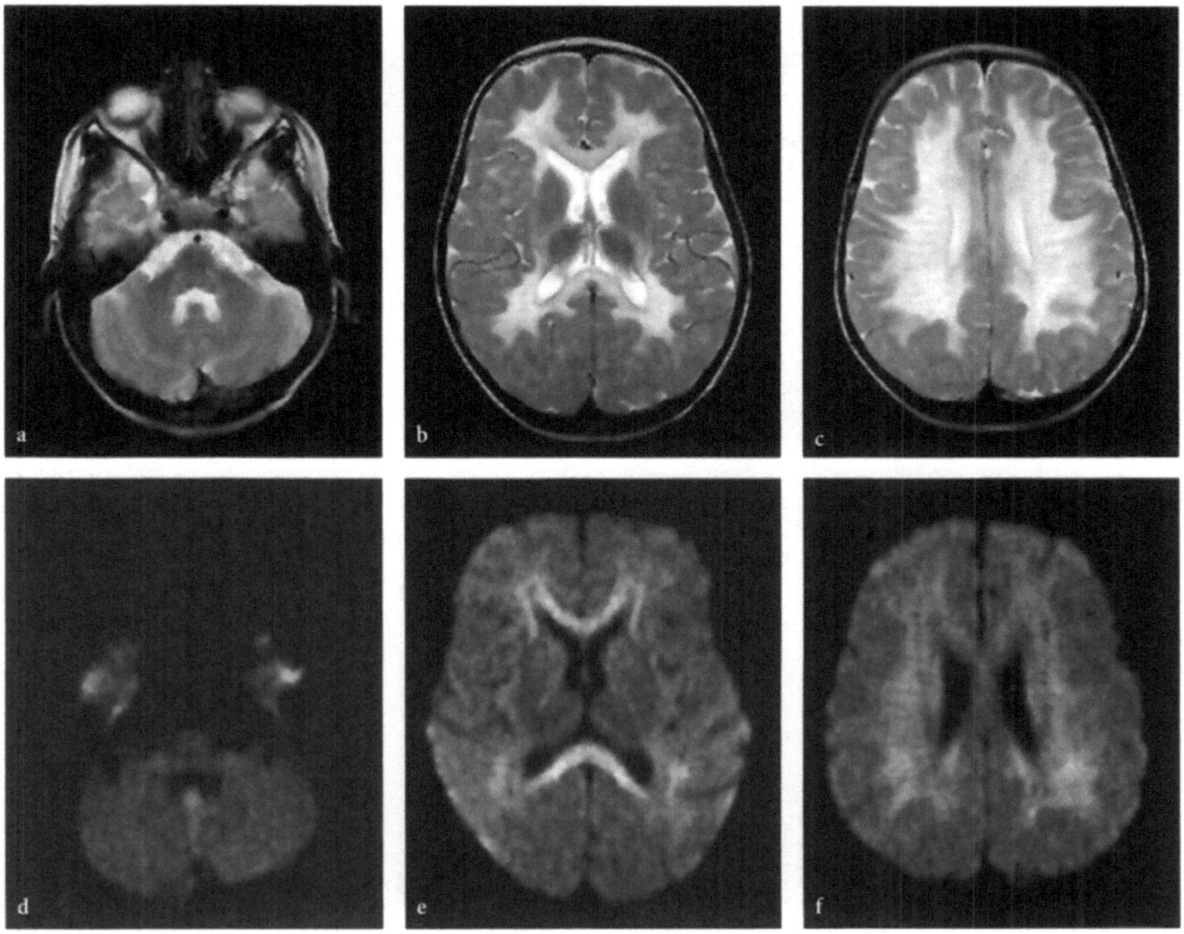

Fig. 22.7a–f. Axial MR images of the brain in a 3-year-old boy with MLD. Sparing of the brainstem structures (**a**), involvement of the corpus callosum and of the posterior limbs of the internal capsules (**b**) as well as the "tigroid" pattern of the white matter disease at the level of the centrum semiovale (**c**) are well demonstrated on the axial T2-weighted fast spin-echo images. Active disease within the corpus callosum (**e**) and a centrifugal disease progression are suggested by the signal abnormalities (isotropically restricted water diffusion) on the diffusion-weighted echo planar image (**e**). The "tigroid" pattern is also conspicuous with the DWI technique (**f**)

and methyltetrahydrofolate deficiency (hyperhomocystinemia). The spinal cord may, however, be spared in cases of apparent involvement of the brain, for example, in L-2-hydroxyglutaric aciduria (Larnaout et al. 1994).

Peripheral nerves are known to be involved in MLD, Krabbe's disease and adrenomyeloneuropathy (Aicardi 1993; Solders et al. 1998; Marks et al. 1997). Imaging of possible peripheral nerve lesions in neurometabolic disorders is, however, not a domain for MRI.

22.4.2.2.4
Contrast Enhancement

Enhancement after intravenous contrast injection in X-ALD, limited to the zone of active inflammation, is a characteristic feature (Fig. 22.6 h). It is never observed in MLD. In Krabbe's disease patchy enhancement may occasionally be present within the periventricular white matter. Enhancement of the cauda equina roots has also been described in Krabbe's disease (Vasconcellos and Smith 1998).

22.4.2.3
Unusual or Misleading Imaging Presentations and Differential Diagnostic Problems

Some of the imaging findings may be misleading. Prominent bilateral subdural hematomas, for example, are not infrequent in glutaric aciduria type 1 and Menkes' disease and may be interpreted as signs of child abuse (Osaka et al. 1993). Awareness of this possible complication and recognition of the other

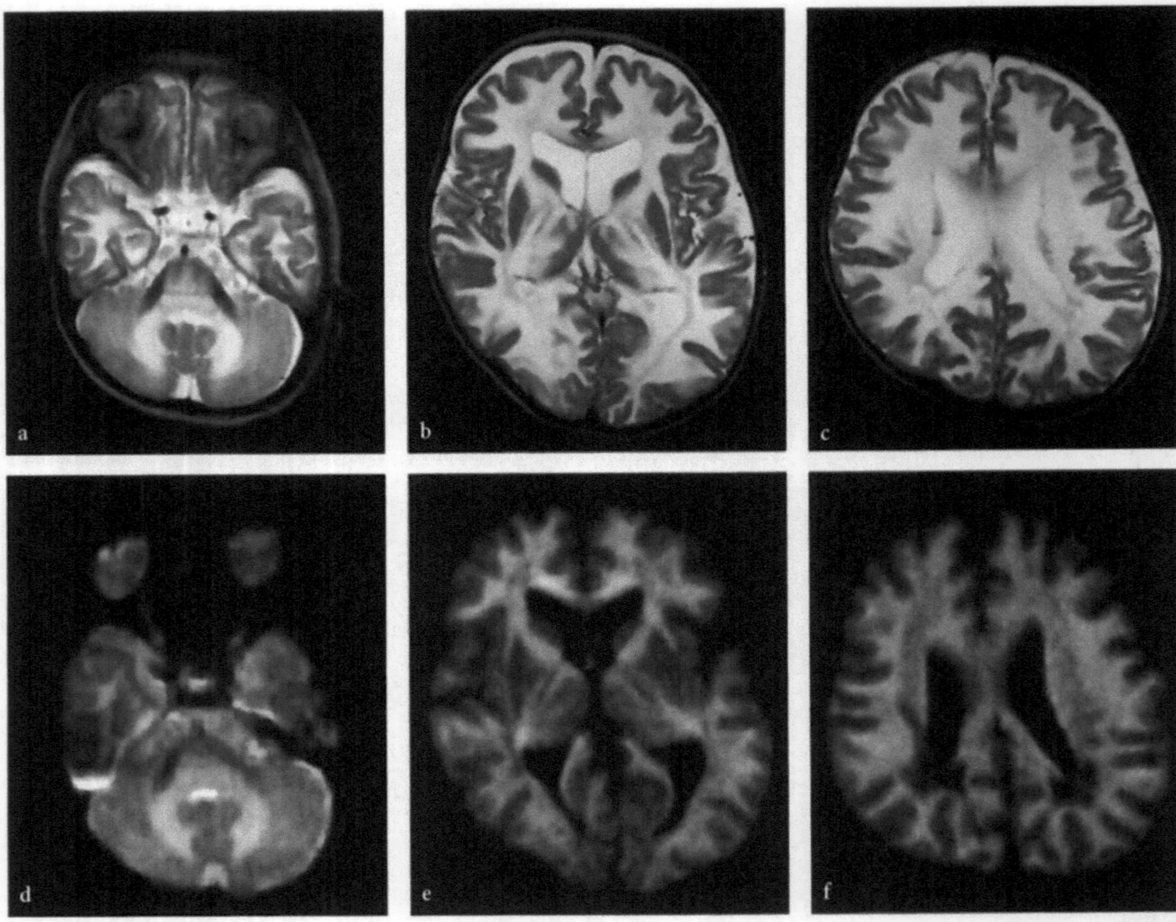

Fig. 22.8a–f. Axial MR images of the brain in a 7-month-old boy with Canavan's disease. The peculiar involvement pattern of the brainstem and the cerebellum (**a**), lesion to the globi pallidi and the thalami (**b**) and extensive cerebral white matter disease (**c**) are demonstrated by the axial T2-weighted fast spin-echo images. The corresponding diffusion-weighted images (**d–f**) show diffuse and homogeneous signal abnormalities within all of the lesion areas (isotropically restricted water diffusion, most probably related to vacuolating myelinopathy)

imaging or clinical hallmarks of the respective diseases helps to avoid misdiagnosis.

Symmetrical involvement of cerebellar, brainstem and cerebral structures is often an important element and diagnostic clue in neurometabolic diseases. Nevertheless, asymmetrical or scattered lesions by no means rule out the possibility of an essentially systemic metabolic disease, especially in the early stages.

Differentiation of metabolic brain lesions from acquired ones is important and sometimes difficult (Hoon et al. 1997). Differential diagnosis in neurometabolic disorders presenting with essentially white matter diseases includes periventricular leukoencephalomalacia, vasculitis, progressive multifocal leukoencephalitis, demyelinating diseases (e.g. Schilder's disease), HIV encephalitis, brucellosis, and toxic and post-irradiation encephalopathy. Basal ganglia involvement in inherited metabolic diseases may be difficult to differentiate from subacute sclerosing panencephalitis, extrapontine myelinolysis, carbon monoxide intoxication and the sequel of prolonged hypoxemia or anoxia (Ho et al. 1993).

22.4.2.3 Magnetic Resonance Spectroscopy

Due to its ability to non-invasively demonstrate normal and abnormal metabolites in vivo within the brain parenchyma and measure their concentrations, MR spectroscopy is a potentially valuable investigational tool in the inborn errors of metabolism. Depending on the employed resonance frequency range, MR spectroscopy may rely on signal obtained from non-water ^{1}H, ^{13}C or ^{31}P atoms. Illustrations of the use of 1H MR spectroscopy are shown in Figs. 22.9 and 22.10.

We refer to Chap. 5 for a review of this technique in metabolic diseases.

22.5 Classification of Inherited Neurometabolic Diseases According to the MR Imaging Appearance

Depending on the consistency of the imaging presentation (relative homogeneity or heterogeneity of the imaging phenotype) of the inherited neurometabolic disorders, pathognomonic, suggestive and non-specific patterns may be distinguished.

Pathognomonic lesion patterns include those seen in X-ALD, L-2-hydroxyglutaric aciduria, Canavan's disease, Alexander's disease, Zellweger disease, neonatal MSUD and mucopolysaccharidoses (when presenting with perivascular depositions).

The MRI findings in 3-methylglutaconic aciduria, glutaric aciduria type 1, phenylketonuria, MLD, Krabbe's disease, Pelizaeus-Merzbacher disease, van der Knaap's disease, and most of the mitochondrial diseases (Kearns-Sayre, Leigh's disease) are often so characteristic that a specific diagnosis may be proposed with a high degree of confidence.

Rather consistent MRI findings have been described in mucolipidosis type IV, including hypo- or dysplasia of the corpus callosum, cerebellar atrophy, periventricular and subcortical white matter as well as a markedly hypointense appearance of the basal ganglia and thalami on the T2-weighted images due to iron depositions (Frei et al. 1998).

Clinical data are also important and may "upgrade" a suggestive imaging pattern. In glutaric aciduria type 1 the combination of bilateral open Sylvian fissures and basal ganglia disease (Fig. 22.5c) seen in a macrocephalic infant or child presenting with progressive dystonia and choreoathetosis is almost pathognomonic for the disease (Martinez-Lage et al. 1994; Brismar and Ozand 1995; Liebel et al. 1980).

Some diseases inherently exhibit a non-specific imaging pattern. As a general rule, most inborn errors of metabolism may present with an unusual or non-specific pattern as a manifestation of their phenotypic heterogeneity.

22.6 Diffusion-Weighted MR Imaging in the Diagnostic Work-up of Neurometabolic Diseases

Diffusion-weighted imaging (DWI) is a special form of functional imaging at the cellular level. Recent improvements in MR gradient technology (faster and stronger gradient subsystems) allowing the routine use of the echo planar technique have made DWI feasible in clinical settings, due to dramatically reduced acquisition times (20–50 s).

In the non-myelinated white matter, no significant water diffusion anisotropy is present and the diffusion coefficient is higher than in the mature brain. After birth, as the myelination process progresses, diffusion anisotropy develops (completed within 6 months), leading to relatively free water diffusion along the fiber tracts and restricted diffusion across the myelin sheaths (Nomura et al. 1994). Besides the presence of extra- or intracellular barriers (myelin layers, cell or organelle membranes, fibers), other possible causes of water diffusion restriction in the brain parenchyma include increased extra- or intracellular microviscosity, which is induced by the presence of macromolecules.

Schematically, in cytotoxic (intracellular) edema, water accumulates within the cells (due to intracellular retention of sodium), where its diffusion is restricted in all directions (isotropically restricted water diffusion characterized by hypersignal on the diffusion-weighted images). In vasogenic edema excess water moves into the extracellular space. As a result, the apparent tissular water diffusion is increased, in the gray matter isotropically and in the white matter with a preferential direction along the fiber tracts.

In vivo demonstration of pathological water diffusion alterations is clinically important because with conventional MRI techniques, in particular on the long TR images, dys- or demyelination and all types of brain edema present with hypersignal; therefore differentiation between them based on T2 relaxation properties is impossible. By demonstrating abnormal water shifts between the extra- and intracellular spaces and the resultant apparent water diffusion changes, DWI has the unique potential to differentiate between cytotoxic and vasogenic edema (Ebisu et al. 1993), or dys- and demyelination (Ono et al. 1997) within the central nervous system. Hence, the pattern of diffusion abnormalities may enhance specificity.

Dysmyelination (Pelizaeus-Merzbacher disease) was found to be characterized by preserved diffusion anisotropy.

In some demyelinating diseases diffusion-weighted images suggest isotropically increased water diffusion (Alexander's disease), in some others isotropically restricted water diffusion (Canavan's disease); therefore different types and different stages of myelin breakdown may be identified based on water diffusion properties (Fig. 22.8). In other leu-

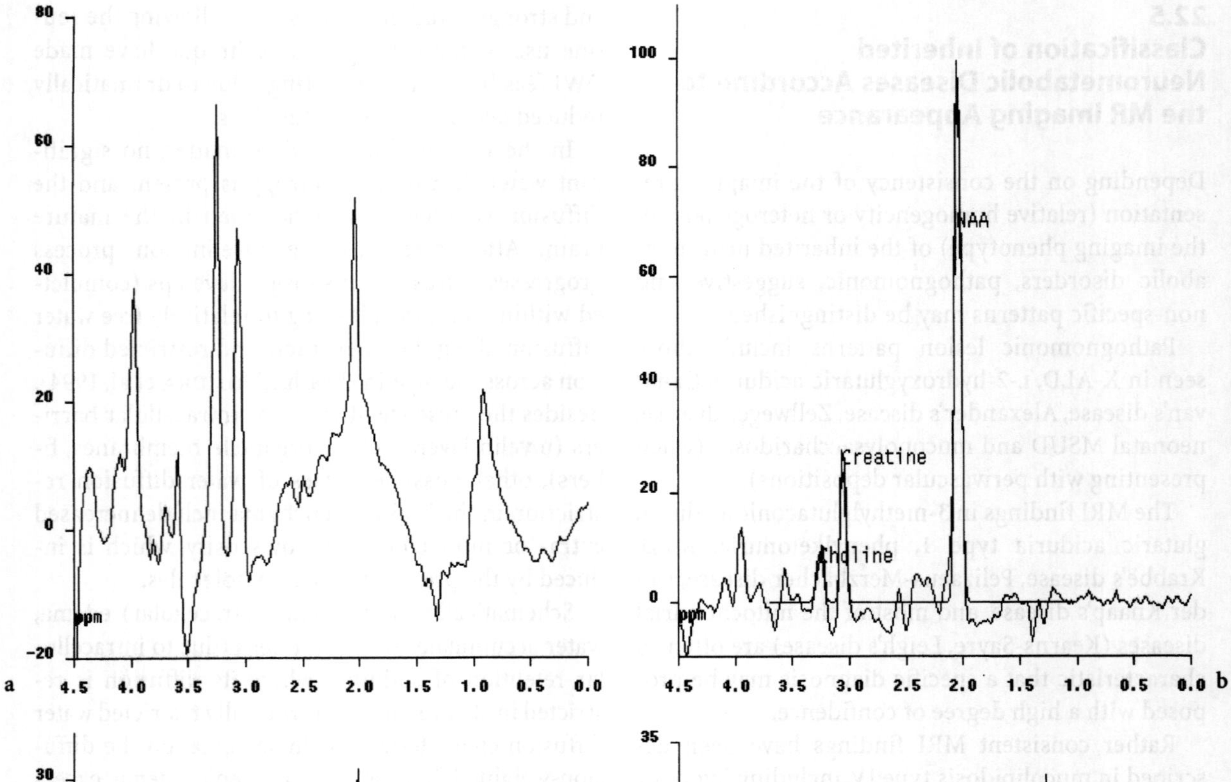

Fig. 22.9a–d. Proton MR spectra in various neurometabolic diseases. In MSUD using a STEAM sequence with 20 ms echo time (a), an abnormal peak is demonstrated at the 0.9 ppm level (corresponding to branched chain amino acids, notably leucin). In Canavan's disease (b) a markedly increased NAA peak is seen at the 2.02 ppm level of the spectrum obtained by the PRESS technique, using 135 ms echo time. In Krabbe's disease (c,d) very prominent lactate doublets are detected at the 1.3 ppm level using the PRESS technique. The peaks are negative with 135 ms echo time and positive with 270 ms (J-coupling)

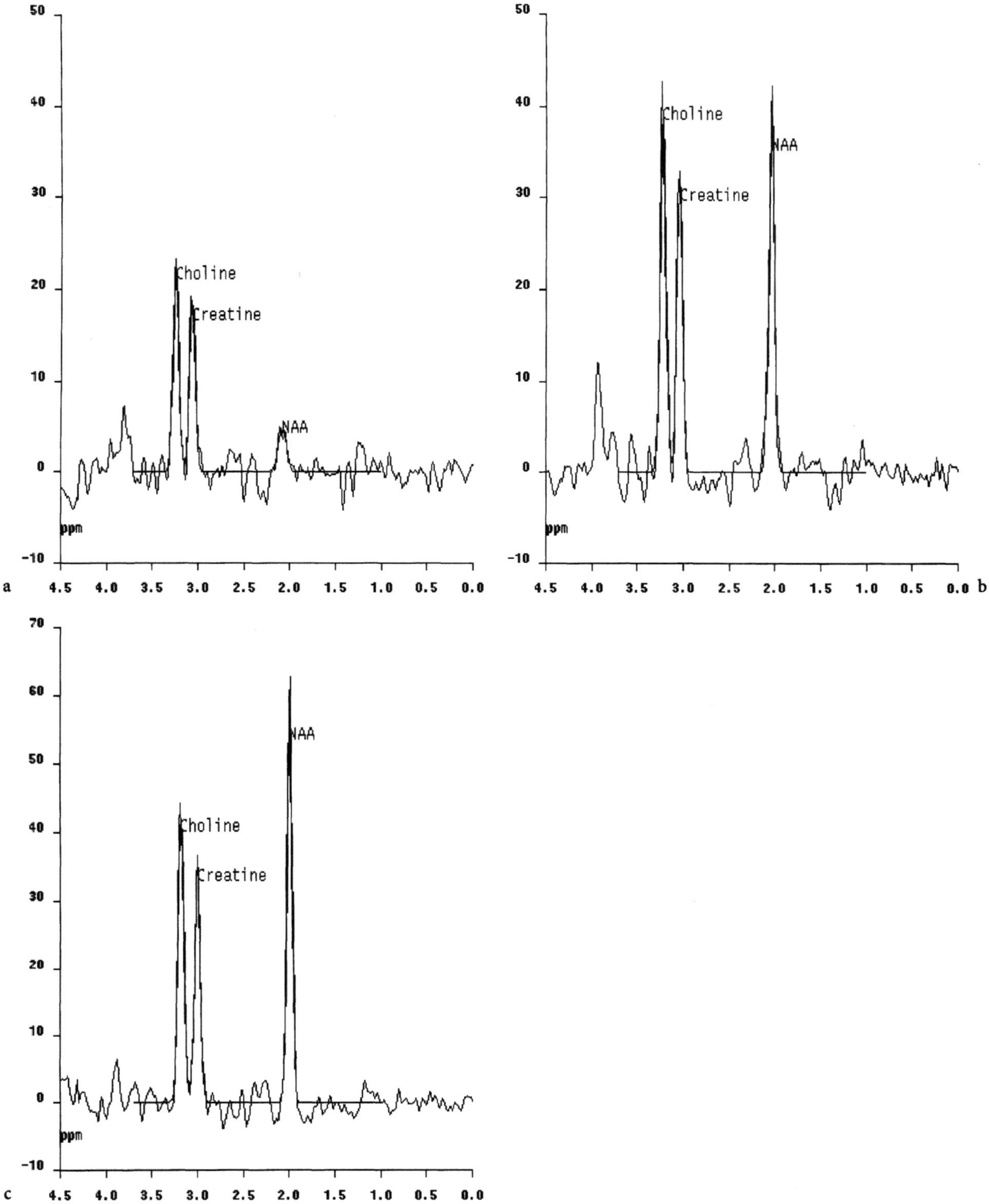

Fig. 22.10a–c. Multivoxel proton MR spectroscopic findings in X-ALD (same patient as Fig. 22.6) using the PRESS technique with 135 ms echo time. The sampling voxels were placed on the burned out zone (**a**), the intermediate (inflammation and demyelination) zones (**b**) and on the apparently normal frontal centrum semiovale (**c**). In the burned out zone, abnormal lactate is seen at the 1.3 ppm level, in conjunction with severely decreased NAA and less markedly decreased creatine and choline peaks at the 3.04 and 3.21 ppm levels. In the intermediate zone lactate is again noted. NAA is decreased, and choline is somewhat increased with respect to creatine. In the frontal centrum semiovale, choline is increased with respect to creatine and the NAA/choline ratio is somewhat decreased too, suggesting increased membrane turnover and impaired neuronal integrity in the apparently "normal" frontal white matter

kodystrophies (X-ALD, MLD, Krabbe's disease), diffusion abnormalities within the lesion area follow a more complex pattern and reflect the underlying pathological processes (Figs. 22.6, 22.7, 22.11).

It seems that a special type of brain edema ("myelin edema") related to vacuolating (or spongiform) myelinopathy has a peculiar appearance on the diffusion-weighted images. Vacuolating myelinopathy is a typical histopathological finding in neurometabolic diseases, such as Canavan's disease, van der Knaap's disease (VAN DER KNAAP et al. 1996) and neonatal MSUD. In vacuolating myelinopathy water is probably entrapped within vacuoles between the myelin sheet layers; therefore the resultant abnormality is an isotropically restricted water diffusion, similar to what happens in cytotoxic edema. This explains the markedly increased signal intensities in areas of vacuolating myelinopathy on diffusion-weighted images. The neonatal form of MSUD appears to be a model disease for this condition, since myelinopathy involves only myelinated structures and the resultant "myelin edema" – first described as "MSUD edema" (CAMPISTOL et al. 1992) – is exquisitely well demonstrated by diffusion weighted imaging (Fig. 22.12).

Another unique potential value of diffusion weighted imaging is the delineation of the active zone of the disease and the monitoring of disease progression.

It has also become evident, however, that DWI is not free from artifacts and diagnostic pitfalls. Since the echo planar technique is particularly sensitive to magnetic field inhomogeneity, susceptibility artifacts may significantly decrease image quality in proximity to the skull base. Motion artifacts may also be prominent, but the likelihood of this is somewhat counterbalanced by the very short acquisition times. Furthermore, any normal or abnormal tissue

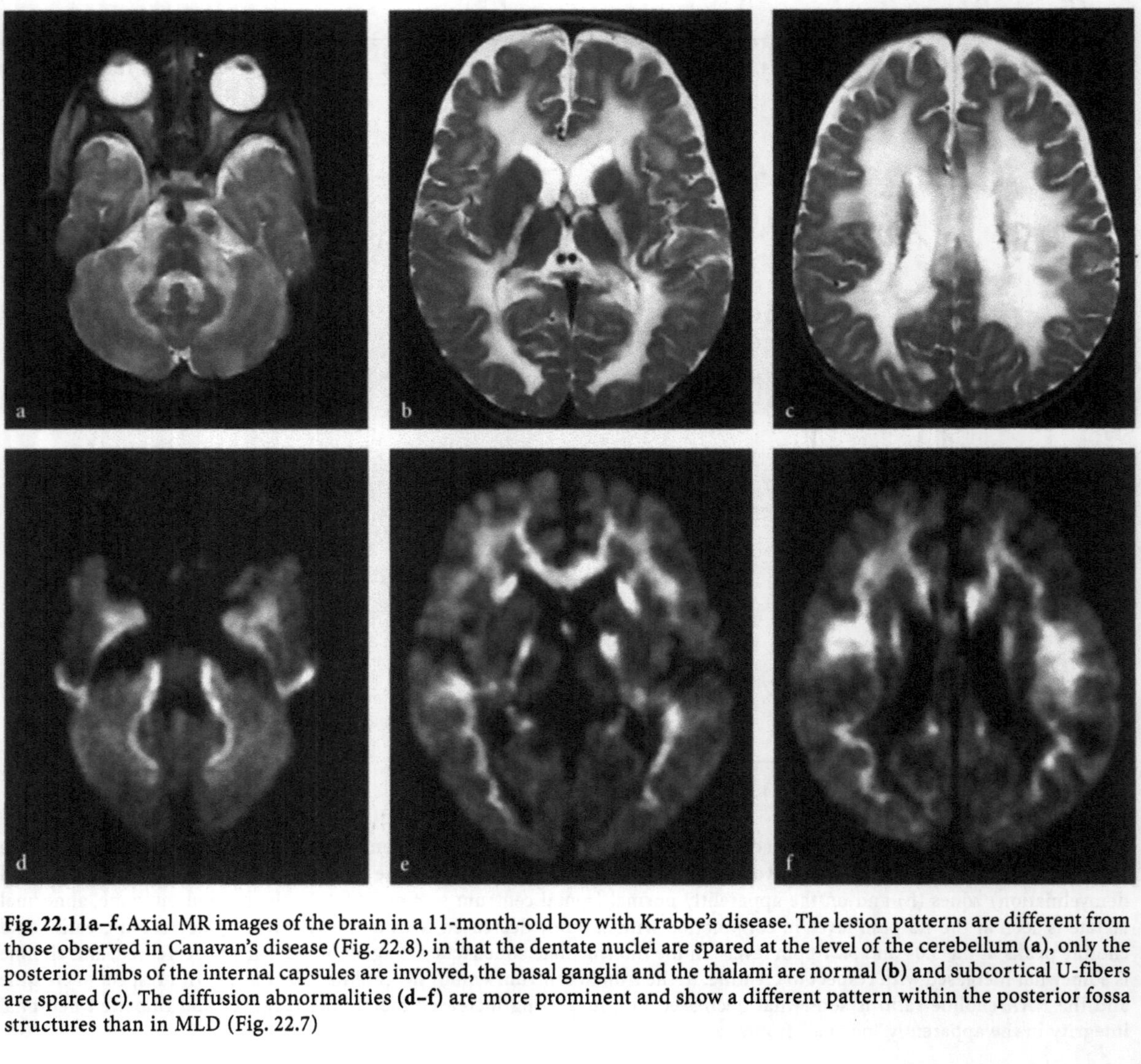

Fig. 22.11a–f. Axial MR images of the brain in a 11-month-old boy with Krabbe's disease. The lesion patterns are different from those observed in Canavan's disease (Fig. 22.8), in that the dentate nuclei are spared at the level of the cerebellum (**a**), only the posterior limbs of the internal capsules are involved, the basal ganglia and the thalami are normal (**b**) and subcortical U-fibers are spared (**c**). The diffusion abnormalities (**d–f**) are more prominent and show a different pattern within the posterior fossa structures than in MLD (Fig. 22.7)

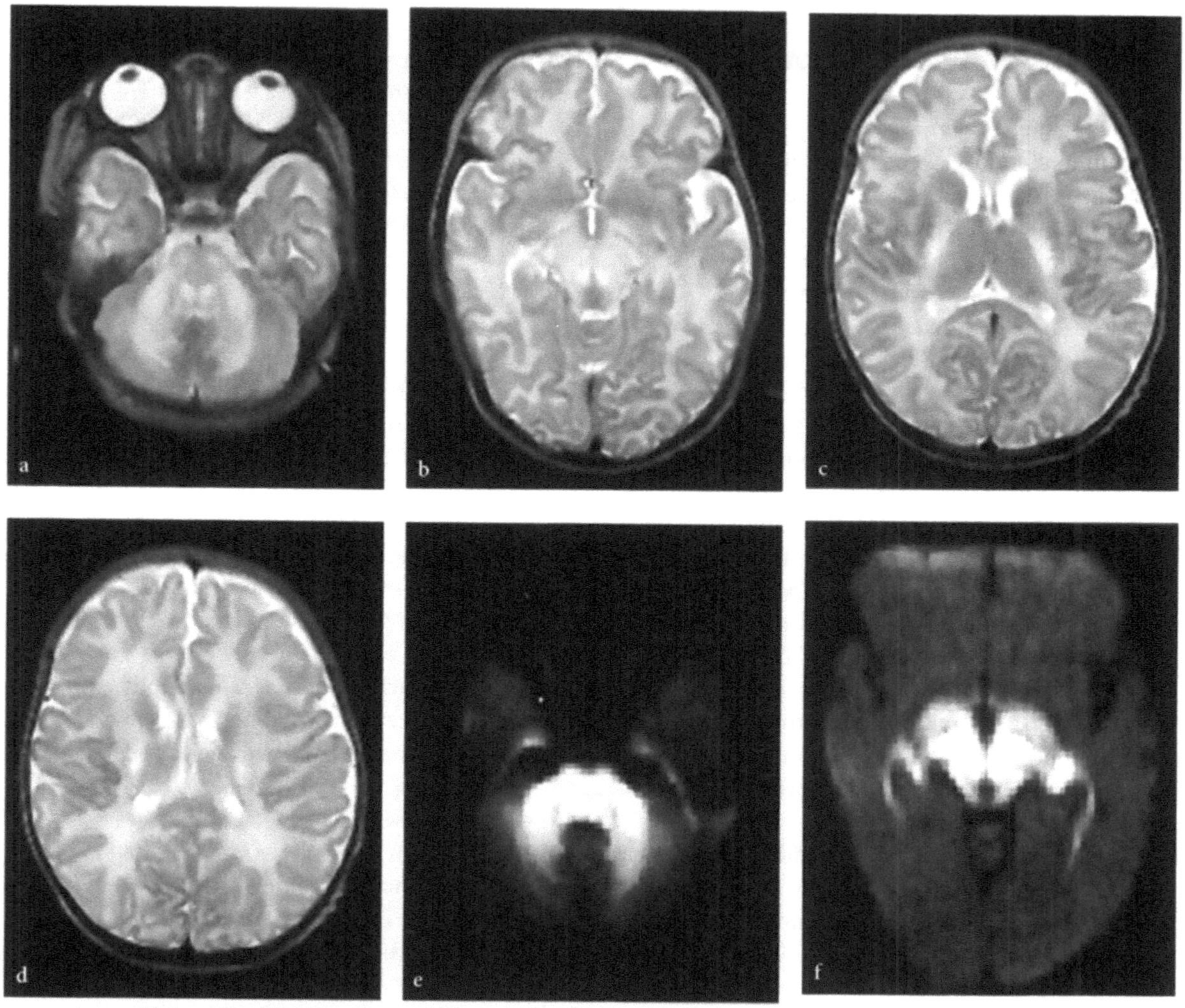

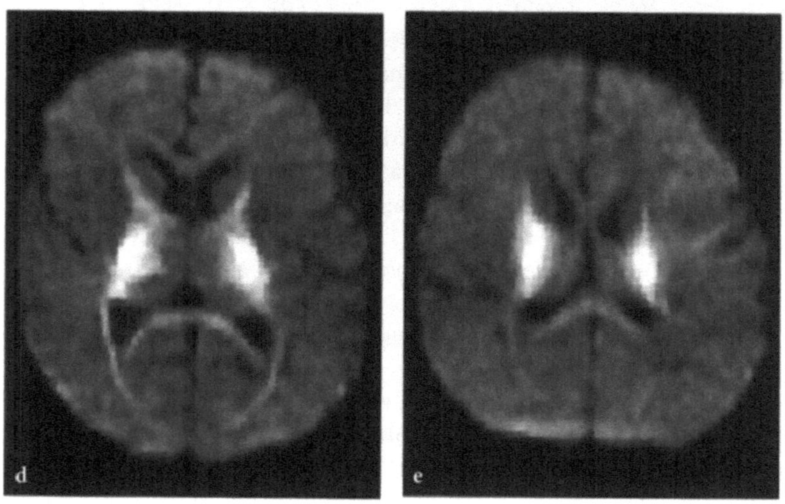

Fig. 22.12. Axial T2-weighted fast spin-echo (*upper row*) and diffusion weighted echo planar (*lower row*) images in a 1-month-old girl with MSUD. On the T2-weighted images the lesion areas are well appreciated at the level of the brainstem (where the myelination is relatively advanced already) but are poorly delineated supratentorially, where the non-myelinated white matter also shows an abnormal increased signal intensity appearance. On the diffusion-weighted images the lesions (corresponding to vacuolating myelinopathy) appear to be clearly limited to the myelinated or actively myelinating white matter structures and are clearly identified throughout the entire brain

with a long T2 relaxation time may "shine-through" the diffusion information and contaminate the images, potentially leading to erroneous interpretation. Correlation with apparent diffusion coefficient (ADC) maps – which are free of T2 information and show structures with increased water diffusion as hyperintense and with decreased water diffusion as hypointense areas – help to differentiate high signal related to true water diffusion restriction from T2 shine-through artifacts (Fig. 22.6e–g).

22.7 Molecular Genetic Considerations

Molecular genetics is most probably the missing link in our understanding of the remarkable heterogeneity of the clinical and imaging phenotypes within biochemically identical or similar entities.

The vast majority of the inborn errors of metabolism exhibit an autosomal recessive inheritance. A few diseases are characterized by an X-linked recessive transmission (X-ALD, Pelizaeus-Merzbacher disease, Hunter's disease, Fabry's disease). Interestingly, symptomatic female carriers of X-ALD have also been identified indicating a possible heterozygous state. Autosomal dominant inheritance has been described in a few rare, typically adult-onset leukodystrophies, such as the adult form of Pelizaeus-Merzbacher disease and MLD, in pigmentary orthochromatic leukodystrophy and a yet unlabeled white matter disease (Bergui et al. 1997).

In a group of mitochondrial diseases the genetic abnormality is encoded in the mitochondrial DNA and since the spermatocytes do not contain mitochondria, these diseases show a peculiar maternal transmission pattern.

The molecular genetic background of various neurometabolic diseases is progressively revealed. The location of the genes on specific chromosomes has been identified in many disorders (biotinidase deficiency, 4-hydroxybutyric aciduria, galactosemia, classical phenylketonuria, homocystinuria, tyrosinemia etc.) and an ever increasing number of mutations are recognized. At least 20 different mutations are known in glutaric aciduria type 1 (Biery et al. 1996) and 30 in methylmalonic aciduria (Adjalla et al. 1998).

Metachromatic leukodystrophy is caused by deficiency of the arylsulfatase A (ASA) enzyme. It is coded by a gene on chromosome 22. At least three distinct types of arylsulfatase A deficiency have been identified, related to the allelic heterogeneity of the arylsulfatase A locus. Depending on the type of mutation, inactive (ASA^-) or altered activity (the so-called pseudodeficiency allele, ASAp) enzymes may be synthesized. The enzyme coded by the pseudodeficiency allele has a decreased but sufficient residual activity. Homozygosity for alleles coding inactive enzymes (ASA^-) leads to manifest MLD. Conversely, homozygosity for the pseudodeficiency allele (ASAp) and compound heterozygosity for a pseudodeficiency allele and an allele coding inactive enzyme ($ASAp/ASA^-$) are not associated with clinically symptomatic disease, despite the significantly reduced enzyme activity (Kappler et al. 1991; Hohenschutz et al. 1989). It has been shown that an arylsulfatase A activity of approximately 10% of normal or higher prevents the development of the clinical disease. The different clinical phenotypes of MLD, infantile, juvenile and adult, are related to the actual percentage of residual enzyme activity. Schematically, between 2–5% of the disease is of late (juvenile or adult), below 2% it is of early (infantile) onset (Kappler et al. 1991, 1992; Polten et al. 1991).

Significant clinical phenotypic variations have been reported in several other inherited neurometabolic diseases, including glutaric aciduria type 1 (Kyllerman et al. 1994), 3-methylglutaconic aciduria (Gibson et al. 1999), 3-hydroxy-3-methylglutaryl-coenzyme A lyase deficiency (Gordon et al. 1994; Ferris and Tien 1993; Ozand et al. 1991) and in the vanishing white matter disease (van der Knaap et al. 1998), possibly related to different mutations. It is interesting to note that the same clinical entity such as Leigh's disease may have several causes (e.g., cytochrome *c* oxidase deficiency, pyruvate dehydrogenase deficiency and various mitochondrial DNA mutations) and, conversely, the same enzymatic abnormality (cytochrome *c* oxidase deficiency) may present with fundamentally different imaging phenotypes, i.e., with basal ganglia disease in the classical form of Leigh's disease or with leukodystrophy in others (Harpey et al. 1998).

The importance of residual enzyme activity has been advocated in other neurometabolic diseases, such as propionic aciduria (Perez Cerda et al. 1998), Canavan's disease (van Moers et al. 1991), Refsum's disease (Poll-The et al. 1989) and mitochondrial diseases (Mak et al. 1998) to explain significant differences of the onset and clinical course of the disease. Similarly to the observations with MLD, higher residual enzyme activities are typically associated with a later onset, milder clinical course or may be clinically asymptomatic as well. Catabolic stress situations (infection, excessive protein intake), however, are known to potentially lead to acute decompensation in previously asymptomatic neurometabolic diseases. This may be explained by mutations leading to borderline residual enzyme activities. Other, yet poorly understood factors may also intervene, since the variability in the clinical and radiological phenotypes is not always correlated with biochemical abnormalities (demonstrated by blood, urine or CSF tests), as it was shown in siblings with L-2-hydroxyglutaric aciduria presenting with clinical heterogeneity despite a remarkable biochemical homogeneity (de Klerk et al. 1997). Furthermore, patients with definite biochemical abnormalities and lesions to the brain may be clinically asymptomatic (Stoeckler et al. 1992).

A remarkable correlation between different mutations, clinical phenotypes (naturally mild, leaky, riboflavin dependent, therapy resistant), MRI findings and 18-FDG PET findings was also found in glutaric aciduria type 1 (Patay et al. 1999). The identification of the various mutation types of the glutaryl-coenzyme A dehydrogenase gene (Biery et al. 1996), leading to different structural and functional abnormalities of the coded enzyme tetramer, shed new light on the causes of the variability of enzymatic dysfunction and the resultant biochemical derangements. Mutations affecting the association of the enzyme subunits or the cofactor binding site are typically associated with relatively mild clinical presentations, whereas changes at the catalytic site of the subunits result in severe disease. Other investigators, however, found undetectable glutaryl CoA dehydrogenase activity in fibroblasts (homogeneity of the biochemical phenotypes) in patients presenting with clinically symptomatic or asymptomatic disease (heterogeneity of the clinical phenotypes) (Amir et al. 1987); therefore even the biochemical and the clinical phenotypes may differ from each other, addressing the highly multifactorial nature of the disease manifestations and the possible compensatory role of alternative metabolic subsystems in inherited neurometabolic disorders.

Understanding the molecular genetic background, the inheritance pattern and the possible other factors determining the clinical phenotypes constitutes the foundations of genetic counseling, which is a key element in the complex clinical management of the inherited neurometabolic diseases.

22.8 Clinical Considerations

22.8.1 Clinical Aspects

The clinical phenotypes (age of onset, neurological, ophthalmological, visceral abnormalities) of inherited neurometabolic diseases are often, but not always, characteristic (Aicardi 1993; Hoffmann et al. 1994; Rashed et al. 1994; Gascon et al. 1994).

Coarse, dysmorphic features as well as macrocephaly in leukodystrophies (Canavan's and Alexander's disease) or in organic acidurias (glutaric aciduria type 1,3-methylglutaconic aciduria, L-2-hydroxyglutaric aciduria), often apparent to the radiologist, may be indicators of a possible neurometabolic disease. Irritability, lethargy, behavioral changes, seizures, and failure to thrive are common but non-specific clinical presentations in inherited neurometabolic diseases.

The clinical phenotypes are sometimes atypical. Misleading clinical pictures suggestive of encephalitis, sequel of perinatal hypoxemia, occlusive arterial or dural venous sinus disease or even intracranial space occupying lesions are also well known (Williams et al. 1998; Hammersen et al. 1998). Environmental factors, such as minor head injury, have been suggested as possible initial triggering factor of leukodystrophies, such as X-ALD (Wilkinson et al. 1987; Carmant et al. 1998; Williams et al. 1998) and the vanishing white matter disease (van der Knaap et al. 1997) and may cause further confusion.

Diseases that typically or occasionally present with strokes or stroke-like episodes, such as homocystinuria (Ruano et al. 1998), MELAS, ornithine transcarbamylase deficiency (de Grauw et al. 1990; Mamourian and du Plessis 1991), propionic aciduria (Shigematsu et al. 1990) and ethylmalonic aciduria (Ozand et al. 1994), may represent a particularly challenging problem. Metabolic "stroke" with acute onset of an extrapyramidal syndrome occurs in organic acidurias, such as glutaric aciduria type 1 and methylmalonic acidemia (Heidenreich et al. 1988). These underscore the importance of careful analysis of the clinical history and awareness of the typical lesion patterns.

22.8.2 Therapeutic Aspects

The social and economic burden of neurometabolic diseases is considerable. Some of them respond well to treatment (Wilson's disease, the naturally mild and the riboflavin dependent forms of glutaric aciduria type 1, phenylketonuria, etc.), although subtle neurological or imaging abnormalities are often seen in clinically stable patients (Pietz et al. 1998). In many others, current therapeutic efforts are limited to symptomatic treatment (dietary control, medical treatment of movement disorders and epilepsy, etc). In the therapy resistant cases, the pathological process relentlessly progresses. In others, the disease progress may be arrested or slowed down. If damage to the central nervous system has already occurred, it can rarely be reverted. MRI and MR spectroscopy have a definite role in monitoring of therapeutic trials and identifying clinically useful or ineffective treatment protocols (Connelly et al. 1993; Schulze et al. 1998; Engelbrecht et al. 1997; Heindell et al. 1993; Pavlakis et al. 1998; Rajanayagam et al. 1996).

A more causal management of inborn errors of metabolism may be anticipated from new emerging therapeutic options, including bone marrow transplantation, somatic gene therapy and fetal neuronal transplants (Ozand and Gascon 1992).

The role of bone marrow transplantation in lysosomal storage diseases (MLD, Krabbe's disease, mucopolysaccharidoses) is the most confirmed of all and is increasingly used in humans. By repopulating the bone marrow of the patient by healthy pluripotential donor cells, normal lysosomal enzymes will be transferred into enzyme-deficient peripheral cells (fibroblasts, macrophages, monocytes) and perhaps even into glial cells. These cells may eventually be even replaced by donor-derived cells exhibiting normal enzyme activity. This may lead to stabilization of the disease or in some cases to improvement in clinically symptomatic patients (Solders et al. 1998). In MLD it has been also shown that results are significantly better in younger recipients and if the disease is diagnosed and treated before the appearance of clinical symptoms when damage to the brain parenchyma is minimal or absent. In Krabbe's disease, reversal of clinical and MRI abnormalities even in the late juvenile form was achieved and the development of clinically symptomatic disease could be prevented in a patient with the infantile form (Krivit et al. 1998). MRI and MR spectroscopy have, therefore, a significant role in the screening of affected families and in identifying prospective candidates for bone marrow transplantation as well as in the post-procedural follow-up.

22.9 Conclusion

Inborn errors of metabolism represent a particular area in neuroimaging, in that the boundaries between the genetic, biochemical, clinical and imaging domains are less well defined than in other pathological groups of the central nervous system. Therefore a complex approach to the problems is indispensable.

In the inherited neurometabolic diseases the questions certainly outnumber the answers. Conventional and advanced MRI techniques have had a major impact on our better understanding of the pathophysiological phenomena involved in neurometabolic diseases by providing valuable morphological, structural and even functional information of the central nervous system in affected patients. Molecular genetic, histopathology and biochemical data further broaden the radiologist's view in this particularly challenging field.

Acknowledgements. The author wishes to acknowledge and thank the support, guidance and stimulating collaboration of Mohammed Al-Essa MD, Zuheir Al-Rahbeeni MD, Jehad Al-Watban MD, Enrique Chaves-Carballo MD, Sarwat Hussain MD, Pinar Ozand MD, PhD, and Jaap Valk MD, PhD, before and during the preparation of this paper. Special credit is given to Jennifer Bryant, Christine Corcoran, Ghadheer Al-Thali, Angela Westlake and Edgardo Martinez for their help in putting together the photographic material and to Vivienne Kynoch for scientific secretarial assistance.

References

Adjalla CE, Hosack AR, Gilfix BM et al (1998) Seven novel mutations in mut methylmalonic aciduria. Hum Mutat 11: 270–274

Aicardi J (1993) The inherited leukodystrophies: a clinical overview. J Inherit Metab Dis 16: 733–743

Amir N, el-Peleg O, Shalev RS, Christensen E (1987) Glutaric aciduria type I: clinical heterogeneity and neuroradiologic features. Neurology 37: 1654–1657

Aqeel A, Rashed M, Ozand PT et al (1994) A new patient with alpha-ketoglutaric aciduria and progressive extrapyramidal tract disease. Brain Dev 16: S33-S37

Baker NS, Sarnat HB, Jack RM, Patterson K, Shaw DW, Herndon SP (1997) D-2-hydroxyglutaric aciduria: hypotonia, cortical blindness, seizures, cardiomyopathy and cylindrical spirals in sceletal muscle. J Child Neurol 12: 31–36

Ballard R, Tien RD, Nohria V, Juel V (1994) The Chédiak-Higashi syndrome: CT and MR findings. Pediatr Radiol 24: 266–267

Barkovich AJ, Ferriero DM, Bass N, Boyer R (1997) Involvement of the pontomedullary corticospinal tracts: A useful finding in the diagnosis of X-linked adrenoleukodystrophy. Am J Neuroradiol 18: 95–100

Barth PG, Hoffmann GF, Jaeken J et al. (1992) L-2-hydroxyglutaric acidemia: a novel inherited neurometabolic disease. Ann Neurol 32: 66–71

Barth PG, Hoffmann GF, Jaeken J et al. (1993) L-2-hydroxyglutaric acidaemia: clinical and biochemical findings in 12 patients and preliminary report on L-2-hydroxyacid dehydrogenase. J Inherit Metab Dis 16: 753–761

Bergui M, Bradac GB, Leombruni S, Vaula G, Quattrocolo G (1997) MRI and CT in an autosomal-dominant adult-onset leukodystrophy. Neuroradiology 39: 423–426

Bewermeyer H, Bamborschke S, Ebhardt G, Hünermann B, Heiss WD (1985) MR imaging in adrenoleukodystrophy. J Comput Assist Tomogr 9: 793–796

Biery BJ, Stein DE, Morton DH, Goodman SI (1996) Gene structure and mutations of glutaryl-coenzyme A dehydrogenase: impaired association of enzyme subunits that is due to an A421 V substitution causes glutaric acidemia type 1 in the Amish. Am J Hum Genet 59: 1006–1011

Brismar J, Brismar G, Coates R, Ozand PT (1990) Increased density of the thalamus on CT scans in patients with GM2 gangliosidosis. Am J Neuroradiol 11: 125–130

Brismar J, Ozand PT (1995) CT and MRI of the brain in glutaric acidemia type 1: A review of 59 published cases and report of 5 new patients. Am J Neuroradiol 16: 675–683

Campistol J, Ribes A, Alvarez L, Christensen E, Millington DS (1992) Glutaric aciduria type I: unusual biochemical presentation. J Pediatr 121: 83–86

Carmant L, Décarie JC, Fon E, Shevell MI (1998) Transient visual symptoms as the initial manifestation of childhood leukodystrophy. Pediatr Neurol 19: 62–64

Chen CY, Zimmerman RA, Lee CC, Yuh YS, Hsiao HS (1998) Neuroimaging findings in late infantile GM1 gangliosidosis. Am J Neuroradiol 19: 1628–1630

D'Incerti L, Farina L, Moroni I, Uziel G, Savoiardo M (1998) L-2-Hydroxyglutaric aciduria: MRI in seven cases. Neuroradiology 40: 727–733

de Grauw TJ, Smit LM, Brockstedt M, Meijer Y, vd Klei-von Moorsel J, Jakobs C (1990) Acute hemiparesis as the presenting sign in a heterozygote for ornithine transcarbamylase deficiency. Neuropediatrics 21: 133–135

de Klerk JBC, Huijmans JGM, Stroink H, Robben SGF, Jakobs C, Duran M (1997) L-2-hydroxyglutaric aciduria: clinical heterogeneity versus biochemical homogeneity in a sibship. Neuropediatrics 28: 314–317

Ebisu T, Naruse S, Horikawa Y et al. (1993) Discrimination between different types of white matter edema with diffusion-weighted MR imaging. JMRI 3: 863–868

Engelbrecht V, Rassek M, Huismann J, Wendel U (1997) MR and proton MR spectroscopy of the brain in hyperhomocysteinemia caused by methylenetetrahydrofolate reductase deficiency. Am J Neuroradiol 18: 536–539

Ferris NJ, Tien RD (1993) Cerebral MRI in 3-hydroxy-3-methylglutaryl-coenzyme A lyase deficiency: case report. Neuroradiology 35: 559–560

Fletcher JM, Bye AME, Nayanar V, Wilcken B (1995) Non-ketotic hyperglycinemia presenting as pachygyria. J Inher Metab Dis 19: 665–668

Forstner R, Hoffmann GF, Gassner I et al. (1999) Glutaric aciduria type 1: ultrasonographic demonstration of early signs. Pediatr Radiol 29: 138–143

Frei KP, Patronas NJ, Crutchfield KE, Altarescu G, Schiffmann R (1998) Mucolipidosis type IV. Characteristic MRI findings. Neurology 51: 565–569

Gascon GG, Ozand PT, Brismar J (1994) Movement disorders in childhood organic acidurias. Clinical, neuroimaging, and biochemical correlations. Brain Dev 16: S94-S103

Gibson KM, Wappner RS, Jooste S et al. (1999) Variable clinical presentation in three patients with 3-methylglutaconyl-coenzyme A hydratase deficiency. J Inher Metab Dis 21: 631–638

Gordon K, Riding M, Camfield P, Bawden H, Ludman M, Bagnell P (1994) CT and MR of 3-hydroxy-3-methylglutaryl-coenzyme A lyase deficiency. Am J Neuroradiol 15: 1474–1476

Hammersen S, Brock M, Cervos-Navarro J (1998) Adult onset ceroid lipofuscidosis with clinical findings consistent with a butterfly glioma. J Neurosurg 88: 314–318

Hanefeld F, Holzbach U, Kruse B, Wilichowski E, Christen HJ, Frahm J (1993) Diffuse white matter disease in three children: an encephalopathy with unique features on magnetic resonance imaging and proton magnetic resonance spectroscopy. Neuropediatrics 24: 244–248

Harpey JP, Heron D, Prudent M et al. (1998) Diffuse leukodystrophy in an infant with cytochrome-c oxidase deficiency. J Inher Metab Dis 21: 748–752

Heidenreich R, Natpwicz M, Hainline BE et al. (1988) Acute extrapyramidal syndrome in methylmalonic acidemia: "metabolic stroke" involving the globus pallidus. J Pediatr 113: 1022–1027

Heindel W, Kugel H, Roth B (1993) Noninvasive detection of increased glycine content by proton MR spectroscopy in the brains of two infants with nonketotic hyperglycinemia. Am J Neuroradiol 14: 629–635

Ho VB, Fitz CR, Chuang SH, Geyer CA (1993) Bilateral basal ganglia lesions: pediatric differential considerations. RadioGraphics 13: 269–292

Hoffmann GF, Gibson KM, Trefz FK, Nyhan WL, Bremer HJ, Rating D (1994) Neurological manifestations of organic acid disorders. Eur J Pediatr 153: S94-S100

Hohenschutz C, Eich P, Friedl W, Waheed A, Conzelmann E, Propping P (1989) Pseudodeficiency of arylsulphatase A: a common genetic polymorphism with possible disease inplications. Hum Genet 82: 45–48

Hoon AH, Reinhardt EM, Kelley RI et al. (1997) Brain magnetic resonance imaging in suspected extrapyramidal cerebral palsy: observations in distinguishing genetic-metabolic from acquired causes. J Pediatr 131: 240–245

Kappler J, Leinekugel P, Conzelmann E et al. (1991) Genotype-phenotype relationship in various degrees of arylsulphatase A deficiency. Hum Genet 86: 463–470

Kappler J, von Figura K, Gieselmann V (1992) Late-onset metachromatic leukodystrophy: molecular pathology in two siblings. Ann Neurol 31: 256–261

Kappler J, Watts RWE, Conzelmann E, Gibbs DA, Propping P, Gieselmann V (1991) Low arylsulphatase A activity and choreoathetotic syndrome in three siblings: differentiation of pseudodeficiency from metachromatic leukodystrophy. Eur J Pediatr 150: 287–290

Kim TS, Kim IO, Kim WS et al. (1997) MR of childhood metachromatic leukodystrophy. Am J Neuroradiol 18: 733–738

Kimata KG, Gordan L, Ajax T, Davis PH, Grabowski T (1998) A case of late-onset MELAS. Arch Neurol 55: 722–725

Krivit W, Shapiro EG, Peters C et al. (1998) Hematopoietic stem-cell transplantation in globoid-cell leukodystrophy. N Eng J Med 338: 1119–1126

Kyllerman M, Skjeldal OH, Lundberg M et al. (1994) Dystonia and dyskinesia in glutaric aciduria type I: clinical heterogeneity and therapeutic considerations. Mov Disord 9: 22–30

Larnaout A, Hentati F, Belal S, Ben Hamida C, Kaabachi N, Ben Hamida M (1994) Clinical and pathological study of three Tunisian siblings with L-2-hydroxyglutaric aciduria. Acta Neuropathol (Berl) 88: 367–370

Liebel RL, Shih VE, Goodman SI et al. (1980) Glutaric acidemia: a metabolic disorder causing progressive choreoathetosis. Neurology 30: 1163–1168

Maestri NE, Clissold D, Brusilow SW (1999) Neonatal onset ornithine transcarbamylase deficiency: a retrospective analysis. J Pediatr 134: 268–272

Mak SC, Chi CS, Tsai CR (1998) Mitochondrial DNA 8993 T-C mutation presenting as juvenile Leigh syndrome with respiratory failure. J Child Neurol 13: 349–351

Mamourian AC, du Plessis A (1991) Urea cycle defect: a case with MR and CT findings resembling infarct. Pediatr Radiol 21: 594–595
Marks HG, Scavina MT, Kolodny EH, Palmieri M, Childs J (1997) Krabbe's disease presenting as a peripheral neuropathy. Muscle Nerve 20: 1024–1028
Martinez-Lage JF, Casas C, Fernandez MA, Puche A, Rodriguez Costa T, Poza M (1994) Macrocephaly, dystonia, and bilateral temporal arachnoid cysts: glutaric aciduria type 1. Childs Nerv Syst 10: |8–203
Medina L, Chi TL, DeVivo DC, Hilal SK (1990) MR findings in patients with subacute necrotizing encephalomyelopathy (Leigh syndrome): correlation with biochemical defect. Am J Neuroradiol 11: 379–384
Menkes JH, Curran J (1994) Clinical and MR correlates in children with extrapyramidal cerebral palsy. Am J Neuroradiol 15: 451–457
Nomura Y, Sakuma H, Takeda K, Tagami T, Okuda Y, Nakagawa T (1994) Diffusional anisotropy of the human brain assessed with diffusion-weighted MR: relation with normal brain development and aging. Am J Neuroradiol 15: 231–238
Nowaczyk MJM, Blaser SI, Clarke JTR (1998) Central nervous system malformations in ethylmalonic encephalopathy. Am J Med Genet 75: 292–296
Ono J, Harada K, Sakurai K, Okada S (1997) Differentiation of dys- and demyelination using diffusional anisotropy. Pediatr Neurol 16: 63–66
Osaka H, Kimura S, Nezu A, Yamazaki S, Saitoh K, Yamaguchi S (1993) Chronic subdural hematoma, as an initial manifestation of glutaric aciduria type-1. Brain Dev 15: 125–127
Ozand PT, Aqeel A, Gascon G, Brismar J, Thomas E, Gleispach H (1991) 3-Hydroxy-3-methylglutaryl-coenzyme A (HMG-CoA) lyase deficiency in Saudi Arabia. J Inher Metab Dis 14: 174–188
Ozand PT, Devol EB, Gascon GG (1992) Neurometabolic diseases at a national referral center: five years experience at the King Faisal Specialist Hospital and Research Centre. J Child Neurol 7: S4-S11
Ozand PT, Gascon GG (1992) Treatment of inherited neurometabolic diseases: the future. J Child Neurol 7: S132-S140
Ozand PT, Rashed M, Millington DS et al. (1994) Ethylmalonic aciduria: an organic acidemia with CNS involvement and vasculopathy. Brain Dev 16: S12-S22
Patay Z, Ozand P, Al-Watban J et al. (1999) Glutaric aciduria type 1: MR Imaging and 18-FDG PET findings with clinical and genetic correlations. Eur Radiol (in press)
Pavlakis SG, Kingsley PB, Kaplan GP, Stacpoole PW, O'Shea M, Lustbader D (1998) Magnetic resonance spectroscopy. Use in monitoring MELAS treatment. Arch Neurol 55: 849–852
Pérez Cerdá C, Merinero B, Martí M et al. (1998) An unusual late-onset case of propionic acidaemia: biochemical investigations, neroradiological findings and mutation analysis. Eur J Pediatr 157: 50–52
Pietz J, Dunckelmann R, Rupp A et al. (1998) Neurological outcome in adult patients with early-treated phenylketonuria. Eur J Pediatr 157: 824–830
Poll-The BT, Skjeldal OH, Stokke O, Poulos A, Demaugre F, Saudubray JM (1989) Phytanic acid alpha-oxidation and complementation analysis of classical Refsum and peroxisomal disorders. Hum Genet 81: 175–181
Polten A, Fluharty AL, Fluharty CB, Kappler J, von Figura K, Gieselmann V (1991) Molecular basis of different forms of metachromatic leukodystrophy. N Eng J Med 324: 18–22
Press GA, Barshop BA, Haas RH, Nyhan WL, Glass RF, Hesselink JR (1989) Abnormalities of the brain in nonketotic hyperglycinemia: MR manifestations. Am J Neuroradiol 10: 315–321
Rajanayagam V, Grad J, Krivit W et al. (1996) Proton MR spectroscopy of childhood adrenoleukodystrophy. Am J Neuroradiol 17: 1013–1024
Rashed M, Ozand PT, al Aqeel A, Gascon GG (1994) Experience of King Faisal specialist hospital and research centre with Saudi organic acid disorders. Brain Dev 16: S1-S6
Rashed MS, Bucknall MP, Little D et al. (1997) Screening blood spots for inborn errors of metabolism by electrospray tandem mass spectrometry with a microplate batch process and a computer algorithm for automated flagging of abnormal profiles. Clin Chem 43: 1129–1141
Rashed MS, Ozand PT, Bucknall MP, Little D (1995) Diagnosis of inborn errors of metabolism from blood spots by acylcarnitines and amino acids profiling using automated electrospray tandem mass spectrometry. Pediatr Res 38: 324–331
Ruano MM, Castillo M, Thompson JE (1998) MR imaging in a patient with homocystinuria. AJR 171: 1147–1149
Savoiardo M, Uziel G (1991) MRI findings in Leigh's disease with cytochrome-c-oxidase deficiency. Neuroradiology 33: S507-S508
Schiffmann R, Tedeschi G, Kinkel P et al. (1997) Leukodystrophy in patients with ovarian dysgenesis. Ann Neurol 41: 654–661
Schulze A, Mayatepek E, Langhans CD, Bachert P, Ruitenbeek W, Rating D (1998) In vivo methods for therapy monitoring in lactic acidosis. J Inher Metab Dis 21: 691–692
Shigematsu Y, Mori I, Nakai A et al. (1990) Acute infantile hemiplegia in a patient with propionic acidaemia. Eur J Pediatr 149: 659–660
Simon DK, Rodriguez ML, Frosch MP, Quackenbush EJ, Feske SK, Natowicz MR (1998) A unique familial leukodystrophy with adult onset dementia and abnormal glycolipid storage: a new lysosomal disease? J Neurol Neurosurg Psychiatry 65: 251–254
Solders G, Celsing G, Hagenfeldt L, Ljungman P, Isberg B, Ringdén O (1998) Improved peripheral nerve conduction, EEG and verbal IQ after bone marrow transplantation for adult metachromatic leukodystrophy. Bone Marrow Transplant 22: 1119–1122
Stöckler S, Slavc I, Ebner F, Baumgartner R (1992) Asymptomatic lesions of the basal ganglia in a patient with methylmalonic aciduria [letter]. Eur J Pediatr 151: 920
Sue CM, Crimmins DS, Soo YS et al (1998) Neuroradiological features of six kindreds with MELAS tRNA Leu A3243G point mutation: implications for pathogenesis. J Neurol Neurosurg Psychiatry 65: 233–240
Tanakashi J, Sugita K, Kohno Y (1999) Neuroradiologic findings in glutaric aciduria type II. Pediatr Neurol 20: 142–145
Turazzini M, Beltramello A, Bassi R, Del Colle R, Silvestri M (1997) Adult onset Krabbe's leukodystrophy: a report of 2 cases. Acta Neurol Scand 96: 413–415
van der Knaap MS, Barth PG, Stroink H et al. (1995) Leukoencephalopathy with swelling and a discrepantly mild clinical course in eight children. Ann Neurol 37: 324–334
van der Knaap MS, Barth PG, Vrensen GFJM, Valk J (1996) Histopathology of an infantile-onset spongiform leukoen-

cephalopathy with a discrepantly mild clinical course. Acta Neuropathol 92: 206–212
van der Knaap MS, Kamphorst W, Barth PG, Kraaijeveld CL, Gut E, Valk J (1998) Phenotypic variation in leukoencephalopathy with vanishing white matter. Neurology 51: 540–547
van der Knaap MS, Valk J, de Neeling N, Nauta JJP (1991) Pattern recognition in magnetic resonance imaging of white matter disorders in children and young adults. Neuroradiology 33: 478–493
van Moers A, Sperner J, Michael T, Scheffner D, Schutgens RHB (1991) Variable course of Canavan disease in two boys with early infantile aspartoacylase deficiency. Dev Med Child Neurol 33: 824–828
Vasconcellos E, Smith M (1998) MRI nerve root enhancement in Krabbe Disease. Pediatr Neurol 19: 151–152
Wilkinson IA, Hopkins IJ, Pollard AC (1987) Can head injury influence the site of demyelination in adrenoleukodystrophy? Dev Med Child Neurol 29: 797–800
Williams GA, Pearl GS, Pollak MA, Anderson RE (1998) Adrenoleukodystrophy: unusual clinical and radiographic manifestation. South Med J 91: 770–774

23 Pediatric Neuroimaging: Fetal MR Imaging

NADINE GIRARD, CHARLES RAYBAUD, DANIELLE GAMBARELLI

Contents

23.1 Introduction

Ultrasonography (US) is currently the primary imaging method for routine examination of the fetal brain (MONTEAGUDO and TIMOR-TRITSCH 1997; ECONOMIDES and BRAITHWAITE 1998; ECONOMIDES et al. 1998; LEVI 1998; ISAKSEN 1998) and specially by using three-dimensional ultrasonography (KELLY et al. 1994; HATA et al. 1998; KURJAK et al. 1998). However, magnetic resonance imaging (MRI) constitutes a useful procedure when ultrasonography is inadequate or equivocal and is also a powerful tool to illustrate the morphological changes of the developing brain as well as fetal abnormalities (GIRARD and RAYBAUD 1992; GIRARD et al. 1992, 1993, 1995, 1996; SONIGO et al. 1996). Fetal MRI is becoming a valuable adjunct to the evaluation of an abnormal fetus because of the developments in fast imaging and in fetal surgery (FARMER 1998). MRI is also becoming a potential and contributive tool in perinatal autopsy (LANGER et al. 1998), for in vitro study (BRISSE et al. 1997; WOODWARD et al. 1997) as well as in fetal volume estimations (GARDEN and ROBERTS 1996).

The safety of MRI is now well documented. Many studies have shown that neither magnetic fields, regardless of their strength, nor radio frequency waves pose a proven risk for the fetus. In experimental studies MRI has been applied to various living organs (THOMAS and MORRIS 1981; COOKE and MORRIS 1981; SCHWARTZ and CROOKS 1982). When uterine cervix cells, lymphocytes, bacteria and hamster ovary cells were submitted to the same magnetic resonance conditions as in vivo MRI examinations, no observable mutations or toxic effects were observed, thus suggesting the absence of side effects for the embryo. In a study of 181 women, albeit not pregnant, REID (REID et al. 1982) did not observe any side effects due to MRI. JOHNSON (JOHNSON et al. 1984) noted no effect on fetal heart rate or umbilical artery flow in 15 women whose pregnancy dated 13–40 weeks after amenorrhea. No deleterious effects were found from fetal MRI in a long term study of children who had undergone fetal MRI between 21 weeks of gestation and term (BAKER et al. 1994).

23.2 MRI Techniques

23.2.1 Sedation

At the beginning of our experience (in the mid 80s), the most important factor in obtaining good quality

N. GIRARD, MD
Department of Radiology, Hôpital Nord, Université de la Méditerranée, Chemin des Bourrelly, 13915 Marseille Cédex 20, France
C. RAYBAUD, MD
Department of Neuroradiology, Hôpital Timone, Université de la Méditerranée, 13915 Marseille Cedex 20, France
D. GAMBARELLI, MD, MCU-PH
Department of Neuropathology, Hôpital Timone, Université de la Méditerranée, 13915 Marseille Cédex 20, France

images was adequate sedation. Thus MRI at that time was performed only in cases in which fetal blood sample had already been previously scheduled to achieve caryotyping and laboratory testing (GIRARD et al. 1992a,b, 1993, 1995; D'ERCOLE et al. 1993, 1998). MRI was done after fetal curarization achieved by injecting vecuronium bromide into the umbilical vein, following fetal blood samplings, leading to fetal paralysis. The estimated risk of fetal mortality during blood sampling is between 1% and 2% (DAFFOS et al. 1985; DAFFOS 1990). This factor was not taken into account by the obstetricians in making the decision to perform MRI since a fetal blood sample had already been scheduled. Complications of umbilical cord puncture occurred in 3 cases of 56 procedures: suspected umbilical cord hematoma, staphylococcus epidermis septicemia, bradycardia. Fetal curarization is also used for invasive antenatal procedures, particularly intravascular transfusion (DECRESPIGNY et al. 1985; MOISE et al. 1987). Vecuronium bromide was administered because the effects of this substance which has a short half-life are almost immediate and last about 2 h.

From 1991 on, because of improvements in MRI sequences, sedating the mother with flunitrazepam (Rohypnol) ensured sufficient immobility in most cases. However, MR examination is always easier when the fetus is in cephalic presentation: in breech presentation or transverse lie position, the fetal head moves with the mother's breathing.

23.2.2 MR Sequences

The MRI technique is related to the stage of development of the central nervous system that is due to the morphological and maturational changes including histogenesis and myelination. MR images obtained at different stages of development result from changes in brain tissue water content, from the multiplication of glial cells which precedes myelination (the so-called myelination gliosis) (LARROCHE and AMAKAWA 1973), and from the accumulation of lipid myelin precursors, specially the galactocerebrosides, contained in cells (HOLMES 1986; BRODY et al. 1987; BARKOVICH et al. 1988; GIRARD et al. 1991; VAN DER KNAAP and VALK 1995; RAYBAUD and GIRARD 1998b). The optimal imaging parameters have thence to be used and adapted to the brain composition. T1 and T2 weighted sequences are routinely used and reliable. Indeed, the T1 value in a neonate on a 1 Tesla magnet varies from 1800 to 3000 ms depending on the brain structure being examined (personal data). The repetition time (TR) of an adequate T2 weighted sequence should be at least threefold the T1 value, resulting in a TR close to 10 s which is not routinely acceptable. However, a good compromise was achieved until recently by using turbo spin echo (TSE) sequences with an acceptable acquisition time (from 2 to 3 min). Currently HASTE sequence provides heavily T2 weighted images with low susceptibility weighting (YAMASHITA et al. 1997) in seconds only.

23.2.2.1 T1 Weighted Images

Spin Echo (SE), Turbo Spin Echo (TSE), or gradient echo sequence may be run.

Gradient echo images (FLASH sequence, i.e., fast low angle shot) are used in our experience because of excellent differentiation between the cortical ribbon, the white matter, and the ventricular walls as opposed to TSE images (compare Fig. 23.2 and Fig. 23.24). The sequence parameters are as follow: TR=300 ms, TE=8 ms to 11 ms, flip angle=90 degrees, this last parameter being the most important. Indeed a flip angle of 60 or 70 does not give such a high contrast as opposed to the Flash sequence with a flip angle of 90. The acquisition time ranges from 1 min 49 s to 2 min 39 s respectively on a 1.5 Tesla and 1 Tesla magnet, allowing 17 slices. On a 1.5 Tesla magnet the sequence is run with at least two bands of saturation that are positioned on the maternal subcutaneous fat of the abdominal wall and of the back in order to improve fetal head contrast.

Additional gradient echo images with fat saturation can be used on a 1.5 Tesla magnet to suppress the signal from peritoneal fat in order to obtain a better delineation of the fetal head as well as a good contrast between gray and white matter (Fig. 23.2, Fig. 23.22a). The signal of brain regions with developing myelination is not affected by the fat saturation since the composition of lipid myelin precursors is different from that of peritoneal and subcutaneous fat. The acquisition time of the fat saturation sequence is 1 min 49 s, allowing 9 slices.

Additional inversion recovery images can also be used, allowing a very good delineation of the cortical ribbon, and of extracerebral spaces or lesion (Fig. 23.2). The time of inversion recovery has obviously to be adapted to the developing brain; the sequence parameters are as followed: TR=5773 ms, TE=60 ms, TI=350, 1 acquisition, allowing 12 slices with 2 min 30 s of acquisition time.

23.2.2.2
T2 Weighted Images

TSE and/or HASTE sequence may be run depending on the equipment used.

T2 weighted TSE sequence needs a long TR and TE as in neonates to be adapted to the brain composition. The sequence parameters of the TSE sequence with phase coding (TPSE) are as followed: TR=5000 ms, TE=160 ms, matrix=198×256, acquisition time of 2 min 54 s for up to 17 slices.

More adequate and shorter is the TSE sequence with no phase coding consisting of a TR of 5302 ms, TE of 90 ms, 2 acquisitions, matrix of 208×256, an acquisition time of 2 min 36 s for up to 11 slices. The contrast obtained by this last sequence is closed to the one from HASTE images (compare Fig. 23.2 k,l,m,n,o and Fig. 23.3 s,t,u).

HASTE (Half-Fourier Single Shot Turbo Spin-Echo) images are available only with magnets of high gradient strength and are acquired much quicker: about 2 s for each slice, that is 30 s for 15 slices. The sequence parameters are as follows: TR=1800 ms, TE=90 ms. Images obtained from HASTE sequence are true T2 weighted images with low susceptibility weighting and sequential slice capability. This last advantage improves the management of fetal movement.

23.2.2.3
Other

Angiographic images can also be obtained with 1.5 Tesla magnet. We use in our institution a sequential 2D FLASH sequence, the parameters being a TR of 25 ms, TE of 9.8 ms, flip angle of 30, with an acquisition time of 2 min 11 s, that allows a good compromise between vascular and tissular contrast (Fig. 23.22e,f).

Images are obtained routinely in sagittal, coronal and axial planes relative to the fetal head with both T1 and T2 weighted sequences.

Either body phased array coil in combination with surface coil positioned on the mother abdomen or body coil alone can be used depending on the MR device used.

MRI of spine and spinal cord is not performed as commonly as brain MRI in the prenatal period. Indeed, ultrasonography is much more demonstrative than MRI in depicting spinal abnormalities. However MRI can be an additional procedure in some cases as will be shown later. Prenatal spine and spinal cord MRI is not quite as easy to perform since it is very difficult to obtain a good alignment of the spinal cord specially in the sagittal plane. This is related to the fetal position, the fetus being possibly tilted following the three planes of the space. Moreover, although 3 mm thick slices can be obtained with T1 and Turbo spin echo T2 weighted sequences, the HASTE sequence allows a 4 mm thick section only that is quite large specially in young fetuses.

No contrast media is used in utero. The gadolinium contrast agents are of low molecular weight and cross the placental barrier. These agents have been shown, in experimental animals, to cause fetal loss, retarded development, hyperactivity, skeletal and visceral abnormalities. Contrast agents thence have to be reserved for specific medical and surgical indications in which the mother outcome is affected (Coletti and Sylvestre 1994). However, published cases of gadolinium administration in pregnant women, either inadvertently or to demonstrate severity and extent of maternal disease, did not show adverse effects in the fetuses (Barkhof et al. 1992; Shoenut et al. 1993).

23.3
Illustration of the Normal Developing Fetal Brain Anatomy

As already mentioned, the brain development is related to morphological changes and maturation including histogenesis and myelination. MRI may illustrate these changes; this is achieved through a careful analysis of the cortical ribbon, the migrant cells layer, the ventricular and CSF spaces morphology, the developing gyration, and the maturation.

23.3.1
Histogenesis and Morphological Changes

Morphological changes include changes in brain weight and volume, in surface configuration (that is the developing sulcation) and in internal configuration (that is ventricular morphology, depth of sulci, basal ganglia and thalamus) (Larroche 1977; Fees-Higgins and Larroche 1987).

Histogenesis includes neurogenesis and gliogenesis (Mickel and Gilles 1970; Berry 1986). Neuroblasts and glial cells originate from the germinal matrix. This is a layer of cells that completely surrounds the ventricular walls until week 30 of gestation; only the anterior subependymal matrix is still prominent by week 32–34; it persists in the form of a cluster of cells up to week 36–39. The neuroblast proliferation develops first, beginning at 7 weeks of gestation. The neural cells migrate toward the surface of the brain and form the cortex through a process of layering (the more recent layer being the more superficial), from week 6–7 to week 23, at which time the six layered cortex is fully achieved. The white matter is interposed between the cortex and the germinal matrix. From week 20 to birth, glial proliferation develops within the germinal matrix to form astroglia and oligodendroglia (the so-called "myelination gliosis") and the consequent migrating cells form an intermediate layer within the white matter.

These changes can be depicted by MRI (Girard et al. 1995; Chong et al. 1996).

- Ventricular morphology (Figs. 23.1, 23.2 and 23.3):
  The cerebral ventricles are large in young fetuses, from 20 to 25 weeks, corresponding to the normal so called "fetal hydrocephalus", specially the posterior horns; it is also known as the so-called colpocephaly. Later on the ventricles become smaller and are almost not visible by week 35. We know from the ultrasound literature that the measurements of the size of the atrium of the fetal lateral ventricle range from 3 to 11 mm on axial sections (Hipert et al. 1995). From our experience the measurements at the trigone are up to 12 mm from 20 to 26 weeks, are 10 mm by week 28, and do not exceed 9.5 mm beyond 32 weeks.
- Subarachnoid spaces morphology (Figs. 23.1, 23.2 and 23.3):
  The subarachnoid spaces are also prominent in young fetuses. Decrease in volume of the subarachnoid spaces can be seen from week 29 on, so that the delineation of the cortical ribbon is not easy on T1 WI only, and T2 WI are thence needed to distinguish the cortex and consequently the gyration from the overlying subarachnoid spaces and the underlying white matter.
- Sulcation and commissures (Table 23.1, Figs. 23.1, 23.2 and 23.3):
  From 20 to 25 weeks the brain is agyric with a widely opened and underdeveloped sylvian (lateral) fissures (Fig. 23.1) and the more significant sulci marking appear as follows: The parieto-occipital fissure is well shaped and achieved by week 23. The calcarine fissure is slightly deep by week 24 and is well depicted by week 28 with its typical "Y" shape. The central sulcus can be depicted as early as 24 weeks at the surface of the brain but is not yet very deep; it is well seen and deep by week 35. The pre- and post-central sulci infold by week 28 and become deep by week 37. The callosomarginal-paracentral fissure is well apparent by week 27–28; this is of great importance because it is the witness of corpus callosum normal development. The posterior portion of the superior temporal (parallel) sulcus is observed by week 28. From 28–29 weeks on the gyration develops but it is not possible to name accurately the secondary sulci. The corpus callosum can be seen on sagittal images as early as 20 weeks. However it is so thin in young fetuses that adequate morphology of the midline is a more reliable tool consisting of the presence of the septum, the morphology of the lateral ventricles and of the interhemispheric fissure, the depiction of a connection between the cerebral hemispheres.
- Migrating glial cells:
  A typical multilayered pattern is observed within the cerebral parenchyma from week 23 to week 28 on both T1 and T2 weighted images (Fig. 23.1). The cortical ribbon, the intermediate layer (corresponding to the migrating glial cells), and the periventricular area (corresponding to the germinal matrix) are of high signal and low signal intensity respectively on T1 WI and T2 WI. These signal changes are correlated, according to the histopathological data from the literature, to the high cellularity in those areas. The two layers of white matter, respectively overlying and underlying the intermediate layer of migrating cells, display low signal intensity on T1 WI and high signal intensity on T2 WI, since the immature unmyelinated white matter is extremely rich in water (900 mg/g). This multilayered pattern is only temporary because of the dispersion in migrant cells after 28 weeks. This multilayered appearance of the cerebral mantle constitutes a very important normal hallmark and its absence is highly suggestive of white matter lesion.
- Basal ganglia:
  Basal ganglia show high signal and low signal intensity respectively on T1 WI and T2 WI as early as 21 weeks that is again related to an increase in cellularity since myelination is known to appear later by week 28 (Fig. 23.1).

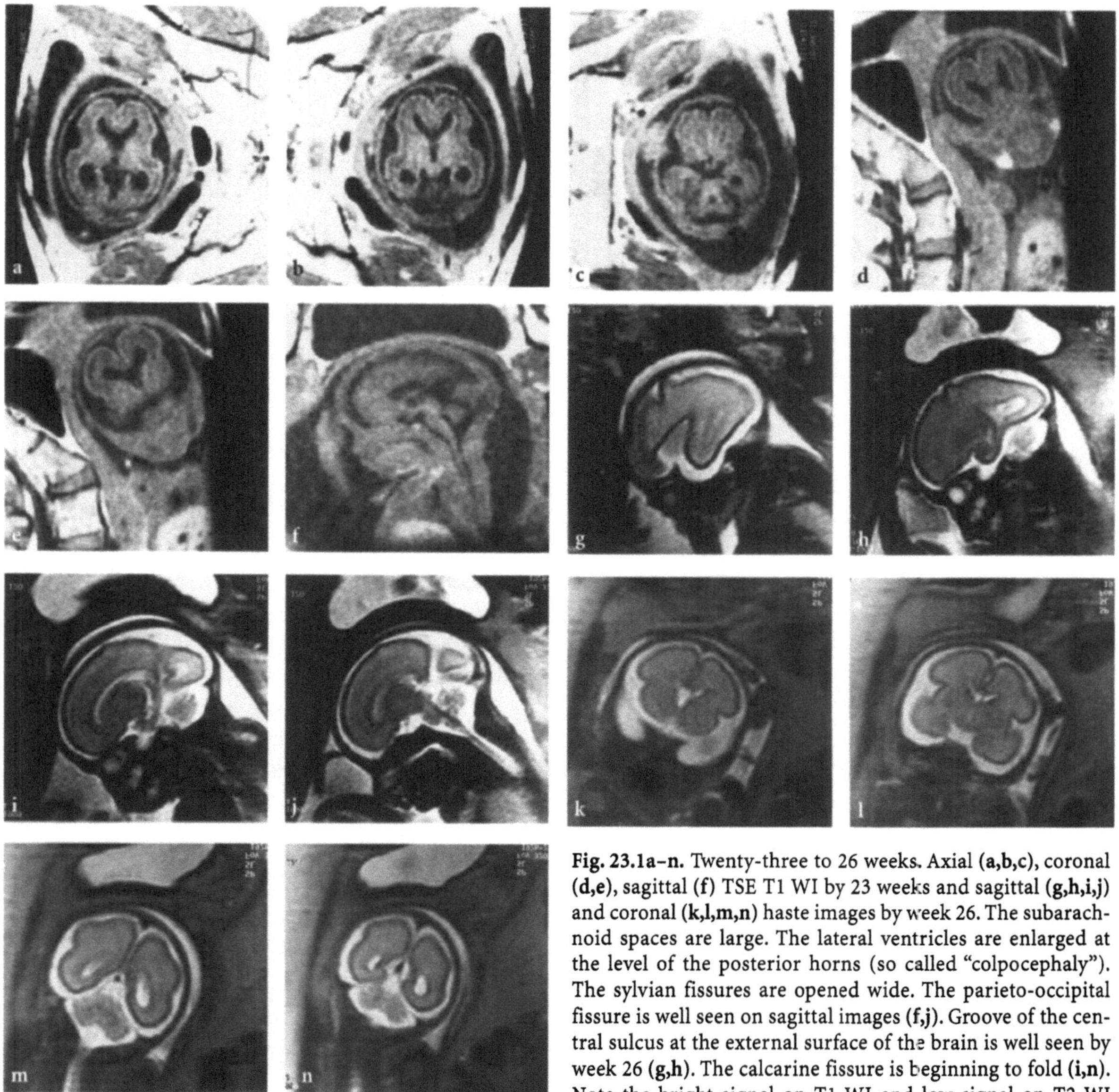

Fig. 23.1a–n. Twenty-three to 26 weeks. Axial (**a,b,c**), coronal (**d,e**), sagittal (**f**) TSE T1 WI by 23 weeks and sagittal (**g,h,i,j**) and coronal (**k,l,m,n**) haste images by week 26. The subarachnoid spaces are large. The lateral ventricles are enlarged at the level of the posterior horns (so called "colpocephaly"). The sylvian fissures are opened wide. The parieto-occipital fissure is well seen on sagittal images (**f,j**). Groove of the central sulcus at the external surface of the brain is well seen by week 26 (**g,h**). The calcarine fissure is beginning to fold (**i,n**). Note the bright signal on T1 WI and low signal on T2 WI within the posterior part of the brainstem (**c,f,j**) and within the middle cerebellar peduncle (**c,i,m**). Note the multilayered pattern on T1 and T2 WI: the cortical ribbon and the germinal matrix display bright signal on T1 WI (**a,b,d,e**) and low signal on T2 WI (**h,i,k,l,m,n**). The migrant cells appear as a layer of bright signal on T1 WI (**a,b,d,e**) and low signal intensity on T2 WI (**h,i,j,k,l,m**). The basal ganglia show high signal on T1 WI (**a,b,e**) and low signal on T2 WI (**h,i,l**)

Table 23.1. Landmarks in developing sulcation

Sulcus/fissure	Gestational age
Parieto-occipital fissure	20 weeks
Calcarine fissure	Folding by 24 weeks Achieved by 28 weeks
Calloso-marginal sulcus	Achieved by 27–28 weeks
Central sulcus	Folding by 24 weeks Achieved by 35 weeks
Superior temporal sulcus (middle and posterior portions)	27–28 weeks

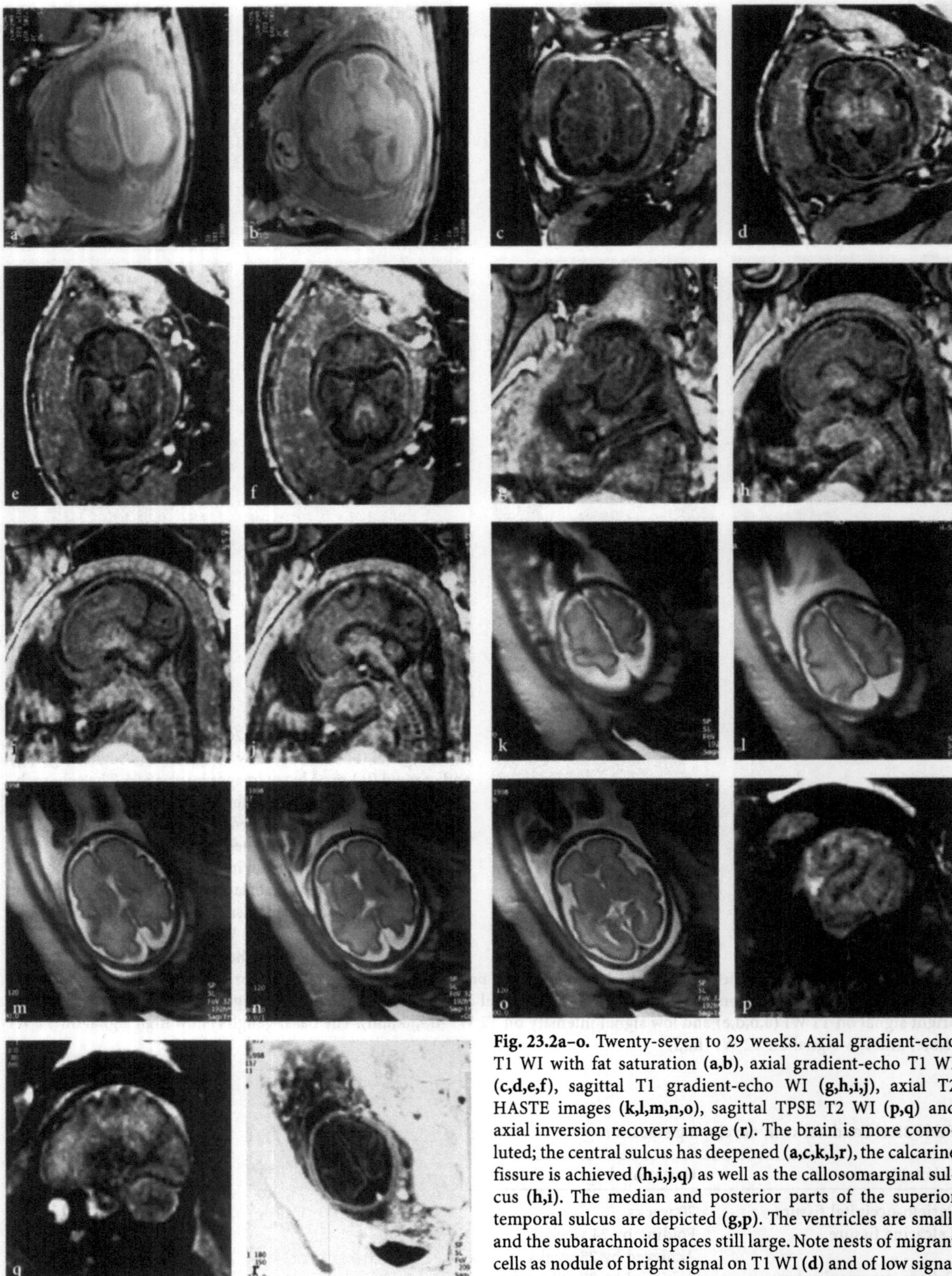

Fig. 23.2a–o. Twenty-seven to 29 weeks. Axial gradient-echo T1 WI with fat saturation (**a,b**), axial gradient-echo T1 WI (**c,d,e,f**), sagittal T1 gradient-echo WI (**g,h,i,j**), axial T2 HASTE images (**k,l,m,n,o**), sagittal TPSE T2 WI (**p,q**) and axial inversion recovery image (**r**). The brain is more convoluted; the central sulcus has deepened (**a,c,k,l,r**), the calcarine fissure is achieved (**h,i,j,q**) as well as the callosomarginal sulcus (**h,i**). The median and posterior parts of the superior temporal sulcus are depicted (**g,p**). The ventricles are small, and the subarachnoid spaces still large. Note nests of migrant cells as nodule of bright signal on T1 WI (**d**) and of low signal on Haste images in front of the frontal horns (**m,n,o**). Note that the fat saturation does not affect the signal from the cortical ribbon and basal ganglia (**a,b**). The bright signal on T1 WI within the basal ganglia (**d,h**) and the brain stem (**e,f,i,j**) is more conspicuous. The germinal matrix is becoming thinner and still shows bright signal on T1 WI (**b,d**) and low signal on T2 WI (**m,n,o**)

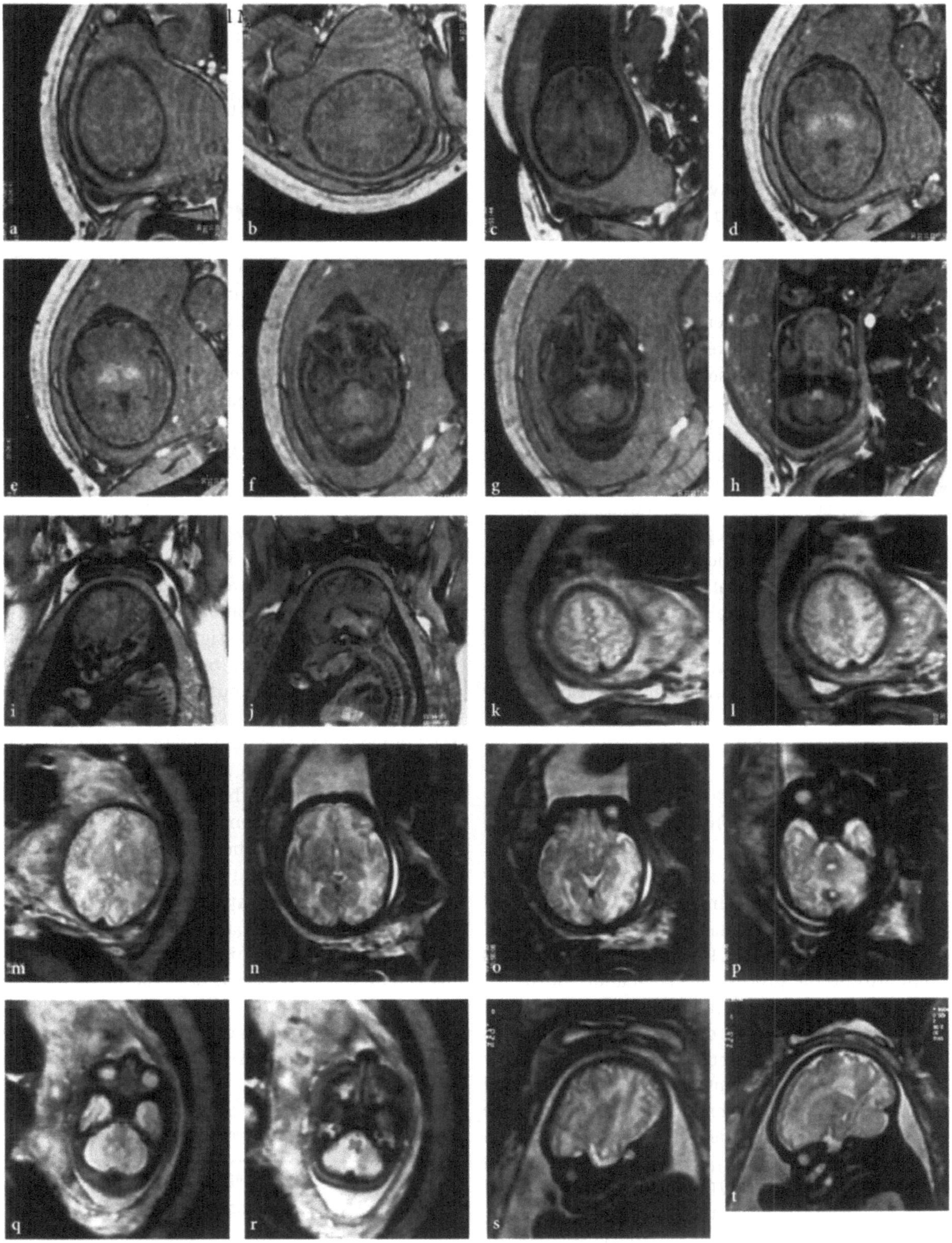

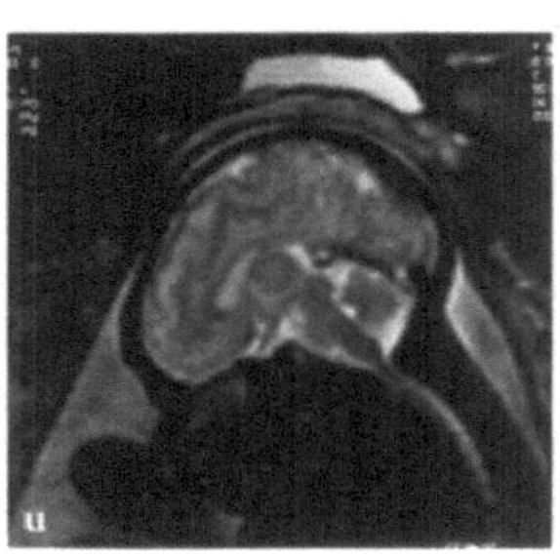

Fig. 23.3a–u. Thirty-five weeks. Axial gradient-echo T1 WI (**a,b,c,d,e,f,g,h**), sagittal gradient-echo T1 WI (**i,j**), axial TSE T2 WI (**k,l,m,n,o,p,q,r**), sagittal TSE T2 WI (**s,t,u**). The brain is now well convoluted. The lateral ventricles are almost not visible. The subarachnoid spaces have decreased in size. Note that gradient echo T1 WI still permit to differentiate the cortical ribbon from the underlying white matter. However the cortex is better analyzed on T2 WI. The sylvian fissures are almost developed because of development of the frontal and temporal opercula (**i,k**). The cortex in the central area displays high signal on T1 WI as well as the underlying white matter (**a,b,c,i**). Bright signal on T1 WI is seen within the posterior limbs of the internal capsule (**d**), the optic tracts (**e**) and the cerebral peduncles (**e**). The medulla shows bright signal on T1 WI (**g,h,j**) and low signal on T2 WI (**r,u**). The posterior part of the pons shows bright signal on T1 WI (**f,j**) and low signal on T2 WI (**p,q,u**)

23.3.2 Myelination

23.3.2.1 General Rules (Yakovlev and Lecours 1967; Gilles 1985; Kinney and Amstrong 1997)

The development of the myelination in the white matter is sequential, precisely determined, identical in all individuals, and has been well demonstrated by histologists. Myelination proceeds from the spinal cord to the brain, myelinated sensory tracts appear before the motor tracts, and the projection fibers before the associative fibers. In vivo MRI shows myelination in infants as the same precise sequence but with time delay when compared to the histological sequence. The myelination process takes place at different times and different speeds in different brain regions, and for a given structure the speed of myelination varies in relation to time. MRI demonstrates cortical myelination as well: myelination within the cortical areas proceeds gradually from place to place while white matter myelination jumps from one tract to the other following white matter tract bundles. Cortical myelination develops earlier than that of the corresponding white matter tracts and is not continuous with it.

23.3.2.2 MRI Signal and its Origin

Myelination is characterized by high signal intensity on T1 WI and low signal intensity on T2 WI. It is well known through postnatal studies that the signal changes appear first on T1 WI since those sequences demonstrate the process of myelination gliosis. T2 WI show signal changes later and thence depict the myelination proper. The origin of the MR signal is related to several parameters. One hypothesis is that the reduction of water content accounts for the signal changes, but this is not enough to explain the time difference in depicting these changes respectively on T1 and T2 WI. Another hypothesis is that the high signal intensity on T1 WI is due to cholesterol and galactolipids (Wolff and Balaban 1989; Koenig et al. 1990; Koenig 1991; Fralix et al. 1991) while the low signal intensity on T2 WI is caused by the presence of hydrophobic phospholipids. Cholesterol and cerebrosides are responsible for the signal changes because of a magnetization transfer effect (Kucharczyk et al. 1994): the stronger effect is obtained with the galactocerebrosides leading to shortening of T1 and T2 values resulting in high signal intensity on T1 WI and low signal intensity on T2 WI; the galactocerebrosides are the last to be incorporated in the myelin sheath so that signal changes on T2 WI occur later than on T1 WI.

23.3.2.3 Prenatal Depiction by MRI (Table 23.2)

From week 23 on, a high signal intensity on T1 WI and low signal intensity on T2 WI is observed in the brainstem, predominantly dorsally, corresponding to the sensory tracts (Fig. 23.1). This is related to the evolving process of myelination according to the histopathological studies that show that oligodendrogliosis is present as early as week 22 in the acoustic system of the brainstem. Microscopic myelination is already seen by week 20 in the medial longitudinal fasciculus of the medulla and pons, by week 23 in the medial lemniscus (Gilles 1985). High signal intensity is then observed on T1 WI in the posterior limb of the internal capsule by week 33, in the optic tracts and subcortical white matter of the central area by week 35 (Fig. 23.3). Those signal changes are due to myelination since histological studies (Gilles 1985) show myelination in the posterior limb of the internal capsules as early as 32 weeks, in the corticospinal tract of the mesencephalum and in the central corona radiata by week 34, in the optic tract by week 29, in the anterior limbs of the internal capsules and in the rostral optic radiations by week 38.

MRI detects a number of simple anatomical structures which appear at determined periods, thereby providing an easy and reliable approach to the morphological evaluation of the brain development and maturation. Signal changes can be explained by several phenomena including increase in cellularity, myelination gliosis and myelination proper. Potential benefits of prenatal MRI are thence the confirmation of brain abnormalities suspected

Table 23.2. Landmarks in developing myelination

Brain area	Gestational age	Signal on T1 WI	Signal on T2 WI
Brainstem (posterior area)	From 20–21 weeks on	Bright	Low
Basal ganglia	From 21–23 weeks on	Bright	Low
Migrant cells	From 20 to 28 weeks	Bright	Low
Internal capsule (posterior limb)	From 31–33 weeks on	Bright	–
Optic tracts	From 35 weeks on	Bright	–
Projection fibers (central area)	From 35 weeks on	Bright	–

by ultrasound, the follow up of the fetal brain when imaging is not conclusive, and the recognition of disorders of the brain histogenesis as early as possible.

23.4 Why is Fetal Brain MRI Performed?

In most cases MRI is performed because of abnormal ultrasonographic findings: ventricular dilatation is the most frequent appealing abnormality (in 38% of cases) followed by suspicion of a central nervous system (CNS) malformation in 31% of cases. Obviously those two conditions can overlap. Indeed ventricular dilatation may be of destructive origin, malformative origin, hydrocephalic origin, destructive and hydrocephalic origin, malformative and destructive origin. Malformative origin is easy to depict because of the specific abnormalities. A destructive origin is more difficult to depict but the diagnosis can be achieved by a careful analysis of the cortical ribbon, the ventricular wall as well as of the migrant cells in young fetuses (from 20 to 28 weeks). The most difficult problem is to achieve the analysis of hydrocephalus since post-natal criteria are not available in utero. Indeed prenatal hydrocephalus may be compatible with normal head circumference, with patent subarachnoid spaces, and even with normal ventricular size (see Sect. 23.5.5).

MRI is also used as a routine evaluation in cases with normal brain ultrasound because of:

- Pregnancy with potential destructive brain lesions in 12% consisting of: carbon monoxide poisoning; twin pregnancy ruling out hypoxic-ischemic brain lesion which are difficult to evaluate by ultrasonography only; maternal coagulation disorders such as cytothrombopenia.
- Maternal infection in 7% with potential fetal brain involvement consisting in most cases of toxoplasmosis seroconversion, followed by cytomegalovirus infection, and less commonly HIV, chicken pox, measles, hepatitis infections
- Fetuses presenting with extracerebral multiple malformations (in 3%), some extra-CNS lesion being associated with brain lesion (i.e., thoracic lymphangioma and megalencephaly, cardiac malformation and leukomalacia)
- Known CNS malformation or chromosomal aberration in the siblings (in 5%)
- Family history of genetic disorders involving the CNS (in 1%) (i.e., X-linked hydrocephalus, tuberous sclerosis)

Less commonly (3%) MRI is performed to evaluate cerebral, cervico-facial or pelvic masses, vertebral body malformation and suspected lymphangioma.

In a few cases MRI is used as an additional procedure because the sonographic examination is technically difficult specially when oligohydramnios is present (Levine et al. 1997).

23.5 Illustration of Brain Abnormalities

23.5.1 Malformations

According to the neuropathological literature (Norman et al. 1995; Harding and Copp 1997; Pinar et al. 1998) congenital malformations of the central nervous system (CNS) are among the most common anomalies, neural tube defects being the most frequent anomalies. In contrast, our experience of in vivo prenatal MRI of the CNS shows that commissural agenesis is the most frequent malformation (39%) probably because the neural tube defects are now easily depicted by US (Conoglio et al. 1996), MRI thereby becoming not worthwhile. Moreover the birth prevalence of neural tube defects has probably decreased as the result of early termination of the pregnancy following prenatal diagnosis, and of the preventive treatment (folate).

23.5.1.1 Commissural Disorders

23.5.1.1.1 Commissural Agenesis (CA)

This is the most common brain malformation (35 cases) in our experience (D'Ercole et al. 1998) and is quite easy to depict by MRI in utero through its specific morphological abnormalities (Fig. 23.4) consisting of ventricular dilatation predominantly of the posterior horns, parallel course of the lateral ventricles that appear widely apart, lack of the callosal and the hippocampal commissures (usually well depicted on the coronal views), absence of the callosomarginal fissure beyond 28 weeks. MRI is useful at demonstrating associated neuronal migration disorders as heterotopia. However it may be very difficult to achieve the overall evaluation of CA as opposed to post-natal MR examination (Raybaud and Girard 1998a), specially when it is partial and associated

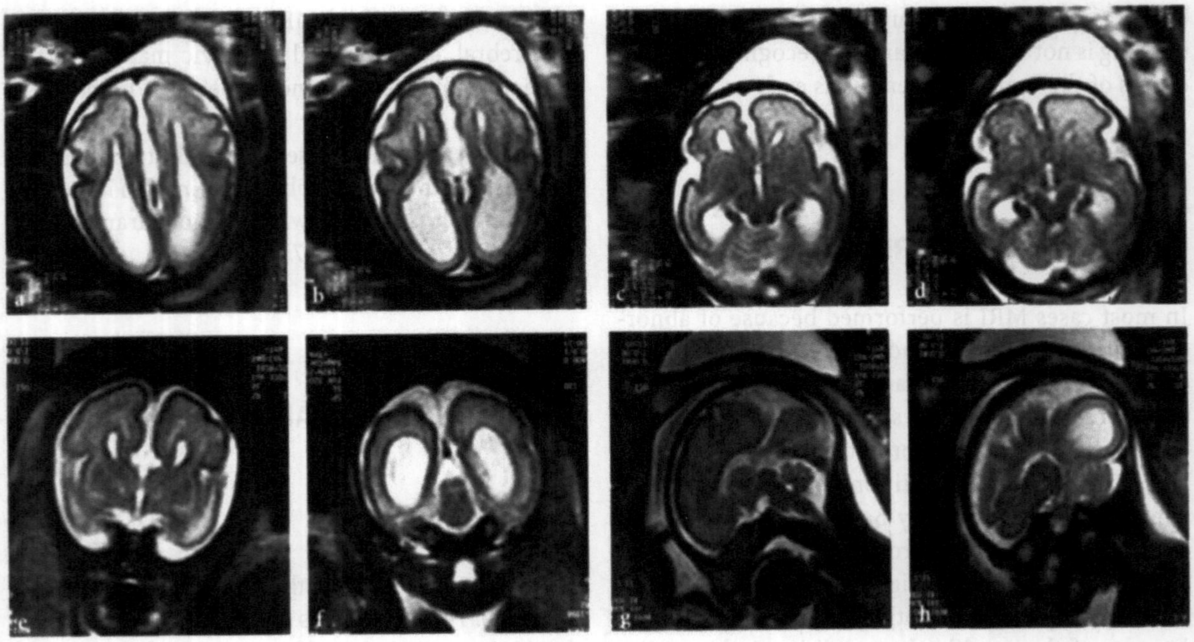

Fig. 23.4a–h. Twenty-six weeks, CA. Axial (**a,b,c,d**), coronal (**e,f**), sagittal (**g,h**) HASTE images. Parallel course of the lateral ventricles (**a,b**), ventricular dilatation specially of the posterior horns (**a,b,f,h**), lack of the interhemispheric commissure (**e**), enlarged temporal horns because of abnormal hippocampus (**c,d**). Note that the midsagittal section can be very confusing (**g**) since the midline structure of low signal corresponds to the commissure formed by the fornices

with cortical abnormalities. Commissural agenesis can be total, partial, or segmental. Agenesis may be related to an interhemispheric cyst. Isolated partial CA is uncommonly seen (1 case in our experience) and atrophy of the corpus callosum has to be ruled out before considering partial commissural agenesis as a malformation.

23.5.1.1.2
Septo-Optic Dysplasia

This malformation is not frequent (5 cases in our experience) but is quite easy to depict by MRI as compared to US examination. MR imaging shows (Fig. 23.5) moderate ventricular dilatation, absence of the septum, and deformation of the temporal horns; the anterior portions of the fornices can be present; heterotopia can be seen within the third ventricle.

23.5.1.2 Neural Tube Defects

In most cases MRI is not necessary since malformations such as anencephaly, iniencephaly, most myelomeningoceles, Chiari type 3 malformation, are well depicted by prenatal US. MRI is occasionally performed to evaluate anatomical parts that have herniated in the meningo-encephalocele, sometimes to describe brain changes in myelomeningocele by showing the Chiari type 2 deformation and hydrocephalus, in order to plan neonatal surgery when the pregnancy is continued.

On the other hand MRI is very helpful in the so called closed neural tube defect in the occipital area at differentiating encephalocele in which the subcutaneous fat is absent (Fig. 23.6) from simple meningocele in which the subcutaneous fat is present (Fig. 23.7).

MRI is also useful in evaluating lumbar abnormalities in which the spinal cord malformation is not associated with a meningocele (flat myelocele) and thereby difficult to depict by US, as opposed to myelo-meningocele in which the meningeal cyst is easy to detect on US.

23.5.1.3 Diverticulation Disorders

23.5.1.3.1
Holoprosencephaly

MRI is not necessary in alobar or semilobar holoprosencephaly since this malformation is quite well depicted by US. MRI is however performed when the abnormality is depicted late in pregnancy during the third trimester in order to rule out other malformation presenting with important ventricular dilata-

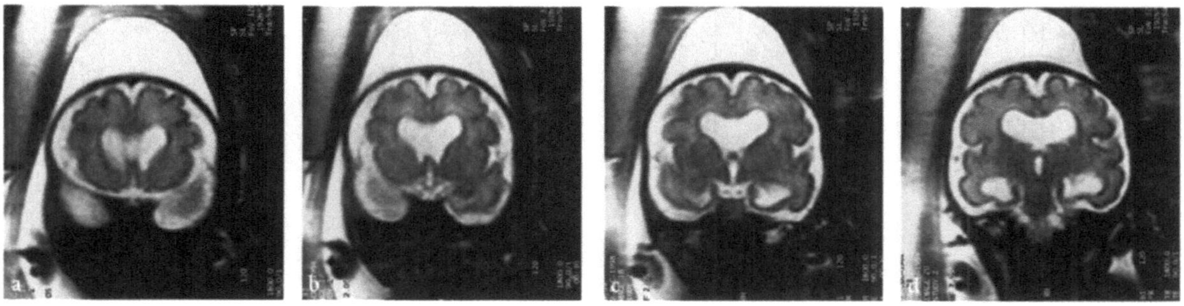

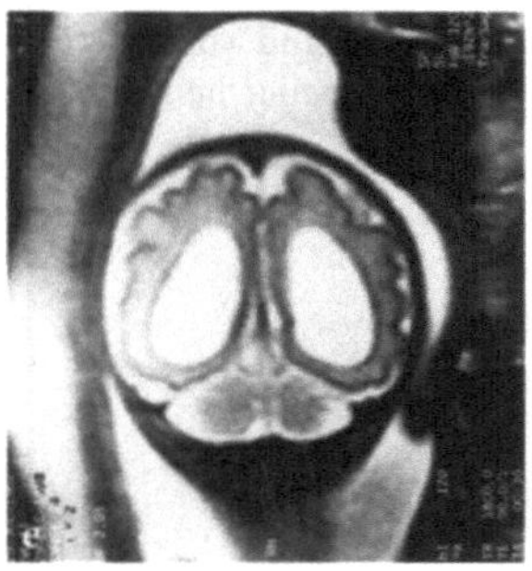

Fig. 23.5a–e. Thirty weeks, septo-optic dysplasia. Coronal (**a,b,c,d,e**) HASTE images. Important ventricular dilatation (**e**). Sharp edged shape of the floor of the frontal horns (**b**). The septum is absent (**b,c,d**). The anterior parts of the fornices are present (**a**) but then the abnormal commissure appear as an intraventricular nodule (**c,d**). The interhemispheric commissure is present but very thin. Note also the abnormal hippocampus bilaterally (**c,d**)

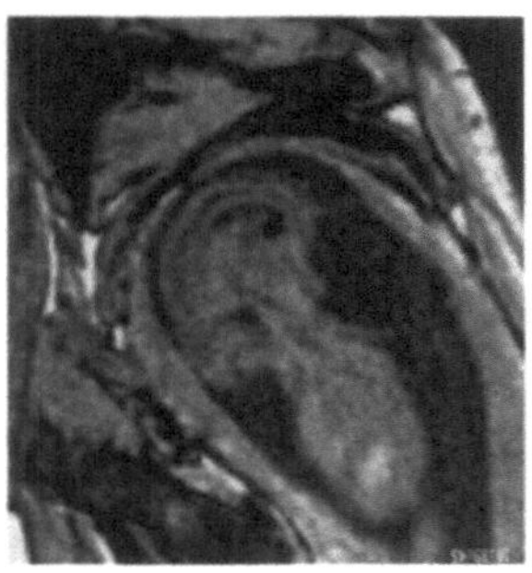

Fig. 23.6. Twenty weeks, Chiari type malformation, sagittal T1 WI. Posterior large meningoencephalocele. Note that the subcutaneous fat is absent

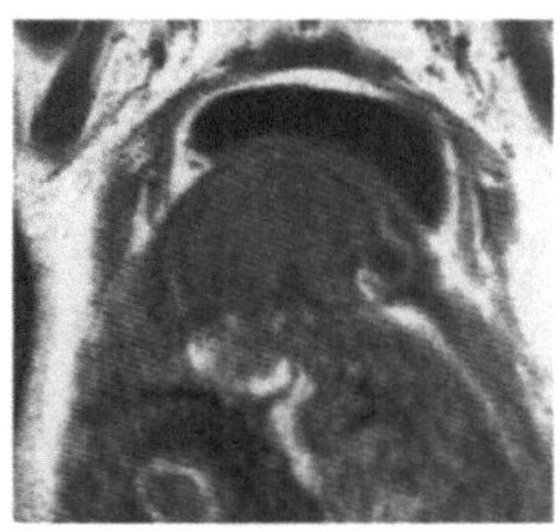

Fig. 23.7. Thirty-one weeks, occipital meningocele. Sagittal TSE T1 WI. Note that the subcutaneous fat is present

tion. MRI illustrates nicely the single vesicle with absence of the corpus callosum and lack of development of the interhemispheric fissure (Fig. 23.8).

MRI, in contrast, is very adequate in demonstrating lobar holoprosencephaly that is constantly miss by US. A careful analysis of the midline shows fused frontal lobes and continuity of the cortex across the midline (Fig. 23.9). A "splenium like" commissure can be seen posteriorly (Oba and Barkovich 1995).

23.5.1.3.2
Posterior Fossa Cystic Malformations

Severe forms of Dandy Walker malformation consisting of a huge posterior fossa cyst in combination to vermian agenesis and hydrocephalus is usually easy to depict by US and MRI is not thereby necessary. However MRI is very helpful at depicting the abnormalities (Dandy-Walker variant malformation, Blake's pouch), in which associated mild ventricular dilatation can be seen. Several MR examinations are usually performed in these conditions in order to detect late hydrocephalus and to plan delivery and consequently neonatal neurosurgery (Fig. 23.10). Enlarged retrocerebellar subarachnoid/subdural spaces is quite frequent and is reported here in our table as retrocerebellar cysts (although "cyst" is a misnomer). MRI shows better than US whether the dural structures, mostly the tentorium, are normally positioned or not.

23.5.1.4
Histogenetic Disorders *(*Robain *1996)*

These disorders are uncommonly suspected on US and thereby MRI is the most adequate technique to pick up such malformations. This is of utmost importance since most of these malformations are genetic disorders with consequent genetic counseling at least for future pregnancies (Andermann and Andermann 1996; Puche et al. 1998; Barkovich 1996; DesPortes et al. 1998).

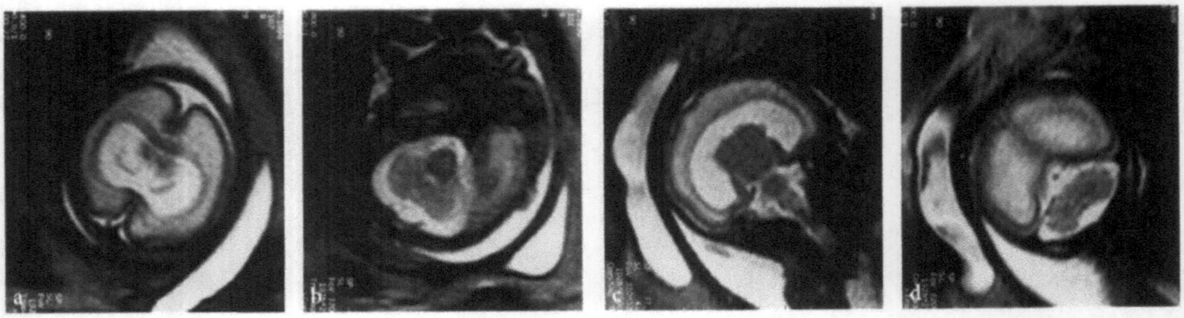

Fig. 23.8a–d. Twenty-four weeks, alobar holoprosencephaly and rhombencephalosynapsis. Axial (**a,b**) and coronal (**c,d**) HASTE images. Single vesicle (**a,c**), with groove of the interhemispheric fissure (**a**). Note the fused cerebellar hemispheres (**b,d**) compatible with rhombencephalosynapsis

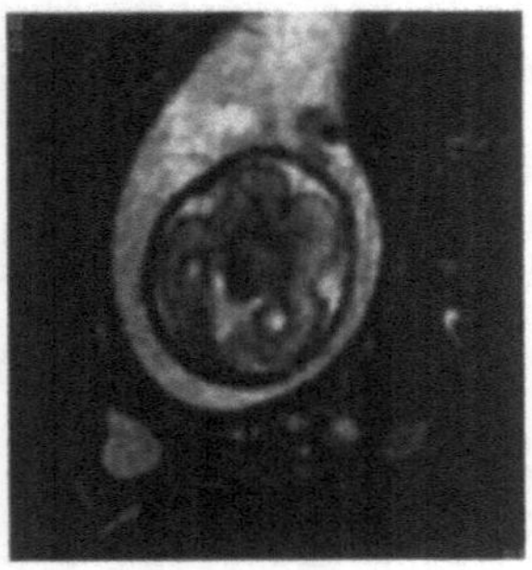

Fig. 23.9. Twenty-two weeks, lobar holoprosencephaly, axial TPSE T2 WI. Note the fused frontal lobes

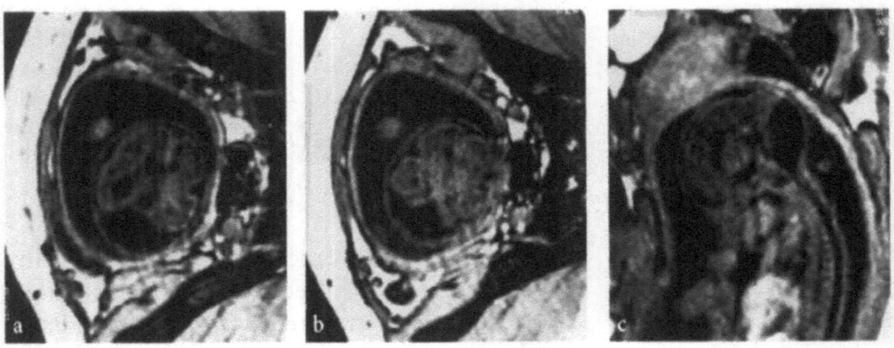

Fig. 23.10. Twenty-four weeks, Dandy-Walker malformation. Axial (**a,b**) and sagittal (**c**) gradient-echo T1 WI. Retrocerebellar cyst, with vermian agenesis and mild unilateral left-sided ventricular dilatation. MRI by week 31 did not show hydrocephalus. However ventricular shunt and shunt of the posterior fossa were performed in the neonatal period because of hydrocephalus

23.5.1.4.1 Abnormalities of Cell Proliferation

Premigratory disorders produce abnormal cell morphology that can involve neuronal and glial cell lines as giant neurons and bizarre glial cells, and include focal cortical dysplasia (Taylor's dysplasia and cortical tuber of tuberous sclerosis), diffuse cortical dysplasia as hemimegalencephaly (Robain 1996).

Hemimegalencephaly can be recognized as an enlarged cerebral hemisphere and possible cortical dysplasia. The case we observed in our series displayed a commissural agenesis, a disorganized cortex, and a Dandy-Walker malformation. However this case is far more complicated since the baby showed cytomegalovirus infection postnatally.

23.5.1.4.2 Abnormalities of Neuronal Migration

Disorders that begin during migration are characterized by disturbance of the normal neuronal arrangement. This group consists of lissencephaly (including type 1 agyria-pachygyria, type 2 or Walker-Warburg syndrome), some cases of micropolygyria (unlayered micropolygyria), gray matter heterotopia (nodular and laminar neuronal heterotopia) and micrencephaly.

The Walker-Warburg lissencephaly usually manifests as an important ventricular dilatation (Dobyns et al. 1989), associated with multiple cortical indentations, as on postnatal MR examinations, at least when prenatal MR is performed beyond 30 weeks of gestation when the developing gyration is supposed to show some determined landmarks (Fig. 23.11).

Although we did not experience lissencephaly type 1, this abnormality may be detected as a thickening of the cortical ribbon. Indeed the cortical ribbon is well recognizable as early as 20 weeks on MR.

Periventricular nodular gray matter heterotopia may be depicted by MRI as nodular lesions displaying a similar signal as the cortical ribbon (Fig. 23.12). Although no case was referred for suspected subcortical laminar heterotopia in our experience, the diagnosis could be achieved through a careful analysis of the signal of the subcortical white matter.

Micrencephaly may be very confusing in utero. Indeed, microcephalia vera might be compatible with a normal morphology, at least during the second trimester and early third trimester, since the primary disorder is of histogenetic origin and depicted on histological sections only. In late pregnancy MRI can depict the underdeveloped frontal lobes associated with the simplified gyral pattern with shallow sulci and too few sulci (Fig. 23.13). In most cases loss of white mater and mild or moderate ventricular dilatation is also seen. Nevertheless this type of diagnosis is difficult to achieve in utero (Persutte 1998) since a wide range of features can be described (Barkovich et al. 1998). Moreover abnormal frontal lobe development is very difficult to depict in early pregnancy since the normal frontal lobe development is achieved by term. Note that microcephaly and micrencephaly are two different entities, the former being a small head and the later being a small brain. From a histological point of view, developmental microcephalies consist of disturbances of neuronal-glial production, the representative examples being the radial microbrains related to severe reduction in neuronal-glial units and the microcephalia vera related to severe neuronal depletion (Evrard et al. 1989). However intrauterine fetal growth restriction (FGR) with prominent microcephaly is highly suggestive of microcephalia vera in our experience. We have also to keep in mind that FGR can be caused by numerous factors including fetal, placental and maternal factors (Lin and Santolaya-Forgas 1998; Burke et al. 1997).

Posterior fossa histogenetic disorders include cerebellar cortical dysplasia, heterotopias, cerebellar hypoplasia, rhombencephaloschisis, rhombencephalosynapsis. Cerebellar hypoplasias are difficult to assess since the cerebellar development is quite slow and cellular migration continues until 1 year of age. However severe hypoplasia (Fig. 23.14) and rhombencephalosynapsis (Fig. 23.8) are easy to depict.

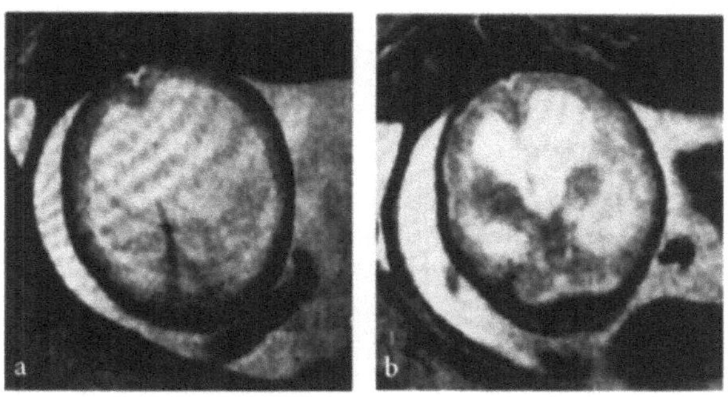

Fig. 23.11a,b. Thirty-two weeks, Walker-Warburg lissencephaly, axial TPSE T2 WI (**a,b**). Huge ventricular dilatation, multiple indentations in the subcortical areas, specially within the frontal lobes. Note that, although the interhemispheric is present and the meningeal thickening is not visible on MRI, there is a "fusion-like" aspect in the frontal areas (that is supposed to be related to the thickening of the meninges)

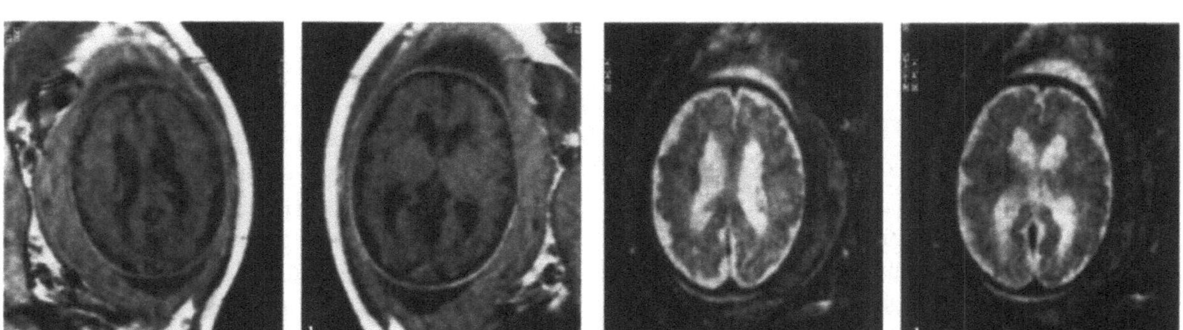

Fig. 23.12a–d. Thirty weeks, periventricular heterotopia and polymicrogyria, axial TSE T1 (**a,b**) and TPSE T2 (**c,d**) WI. The germinal matrix appears irregular and shows nodules isointense to the gray matter compatible with periventricular nodular heterotopia. Note the ventricular dilatation and the enlargement of the subarachnoid spaces. Note also too many and small sulci suggestive of polymicrogyria

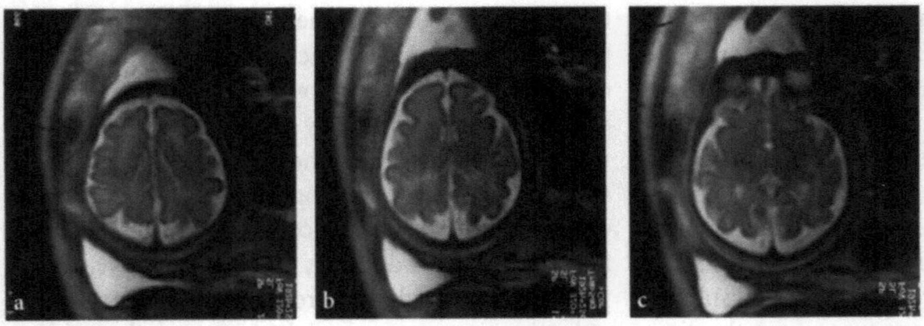

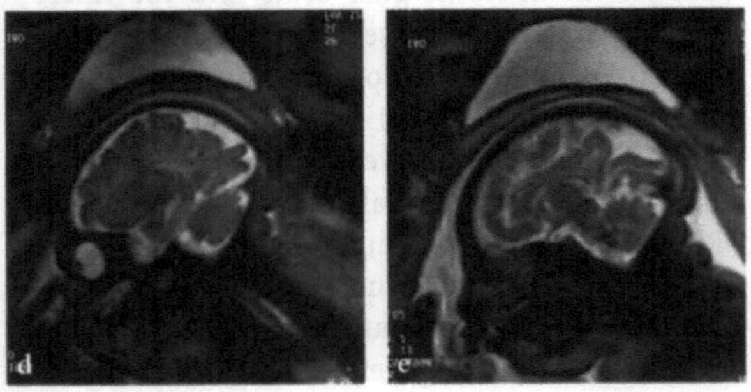

Fig. 23.13a–e. Thirty-six weeks, micrencephaly. Axial **(a,b,c)** and sagittal **(d,e)** haste images. The subarachnoid spaces are large. The frontal lobes appear underdeveloped. Note the broad and shallow gyri in the frontal regions characteristic of micrencephaly

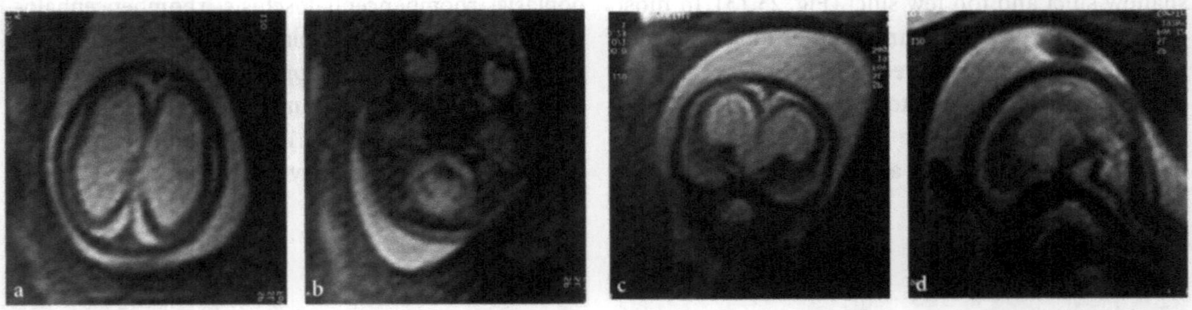

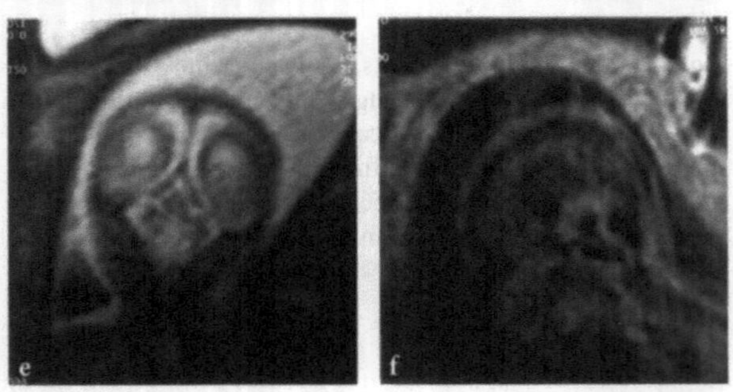

Fig. 23.14a–f. Twenty weeks, cerebellar hypoplasia, axial **(a,b)**, coronal **(c,d)**, sagittal **(e)** haste images and sagittal gradient-echo T1 WI **(f)**. Important hydrocephalus **(a,c,e)**. The cerebellar hemispheres are not developed **(b,d,e,f)**, since the lateral cerebellar masses are only recognizable. Note the curved aspect of the underdeveloped brainstem **(e,f)** as shown in the embryonic period. Also note that, although important hydrocephalus, the subarachnoid spaces are still patent and that the head circumference is not enlarged

23.5.1.4.3
Abnormalities of Cortical Organization

Four-layered micropolygyria is considered to represent the main postmigratory disorder. Micropolygyria (MPG) is the most common abnormality in our experience among histogenetic disorders. In late pregnancy MR shows the typical features of MPG as known in postnatal evaluation as multiple small and irregular sulci associated with enlarged overlying subarachnoid spaces (Raybaud et al. 1995, 1996) (Fig. 23.15). The diagnosis of cortical abnormalities can even be achieved earlier before 26 weeks of gestation specially in cases of destructive origin (the usual postmigratory MPG) (Larroche et al. 1994) by a careful analysis of the signal of the cortical ribbon (Fig. 23.16). Indeed two cases of PMG were of viral origin (cytomegalovirus) that could not be suspected on fetal samplings, the diagnosis of infection being achieved by histology.

MPG can also be related to migratory disorders (that is the so called unlayered MPG). The case we observed displays unilateral ventricular dilatation

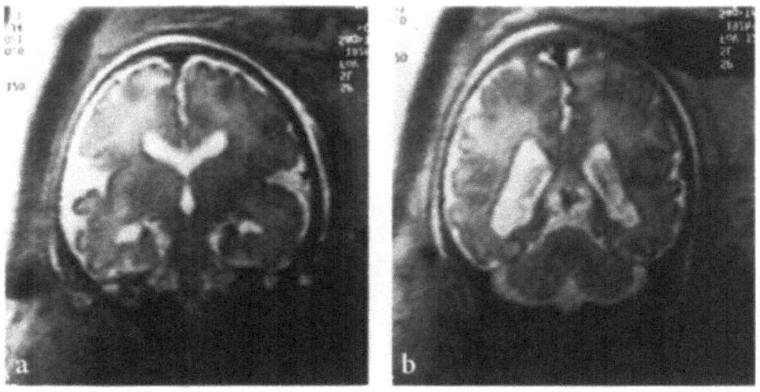

Fig. 23.15a,b. Thirty-five weeks, polymicrogyria, coronal haste images (a,b). The lateral ventricles are large and not compatible with the gestational age (a,b). Typical features of polymicrogyria in the left frontal and temporal opercula (a) associated enlargement of the subarachnoid spaces bilaterally

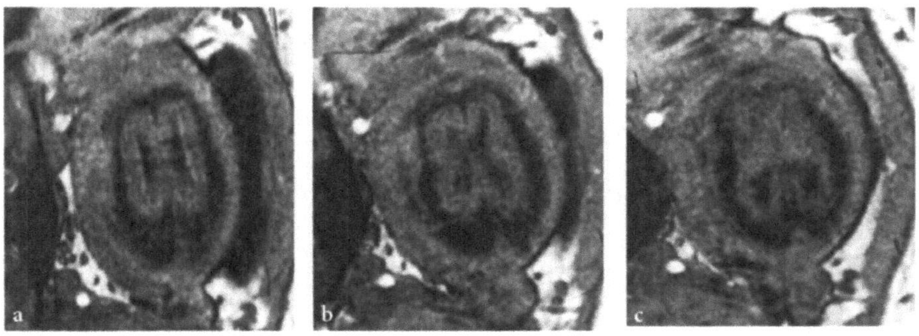

Fig. 23.16a–c. Twenty-three weeks, micropolygyria and destructive brain, axial TSE T1 WI (a,b,c). The lateral ventricles appear mildly enlarged (c). The multilayered pattern is not visible: the normal signal of the cortical ribbon and the intermediate layer of migrating cells are not recognizable (a,b). Note that the germinal matrix is recognizable only on the upper section (a) while its normal signal is missing elsewhere (b,c). Histology demonstrated micropolygyria, periventricular necrosis, ependymal destruction and cytomegalovirus inclusions

and a gyration not compatible with the gestational age (Fig. 23.17).

Schizencephaly is considered as part of the group of postmigratory disorders since most schizencephalies are of destructive origin. Although no cases have been referred to our institution, the diagnosis could be achieved by detecting the parenchymal cleft in combination with an abnormal cortical ribbon lining the cleft (pial-ependymal seam) as irregular surface identical to that of PMG.

23.5.2 Destructive (or Clastic) Lesions

Clastic lesions consist of hemorrhage, leukomalacia, gliosis, necrosis, ischemia, atrophy, abscess, these lesions being possibly associated (i.e., atrophy and leukomalacia, necrosis and atrophy) (Raybaud 1983). The diagnosis can be achieved through the analysis of the signal of the cortical ribbon, of the layer of migrant cells, of the germinal matrix, the morphology of the ventricles, of the subarachnoid spaces.

Any abnormality, such as loss of the normal signal of the cortical ribbon, loss of the visibility of the layer of migrating cells, loss of the normal signal or abnormal signal of the germinal matrix, irregular aspect of the germinal matrix, is highly suggestive of destructive lesion.

The frequency of such lesions is quite high in our experience since most cases of ventricular dilatation or hydrocephalus end up in destructive origin.

23.5.2.1 Hemorrhage

Hemorrhagic lesions can be easily depicted as high signal intensity on T1 WI (Fig. 23.18) and low signal intensity on T2 WI within the parenchyma, the ventricles, the germinal matrix, either alone or in combination. Ventricular dilatation or hydrocephalus can be associated.

More difficult to achieve is the depiction of old hemorrhage usually of the germinal matrix that appears irregular and of highly low signal intensity on T2 WI (Fig. 23.19). Mild or moderate ventricular dilatation is also seen in most cases.

Worth noting is that the cause of hemorrhage is not found, from the clinical history, in most cases. Trauma was the suspected mechanism in one case. In other cases, histological studies demonstrated ependymal abrasion alone or in combination with periventricular gliosis which is consistent with hypoxic-ischemic mechanism.

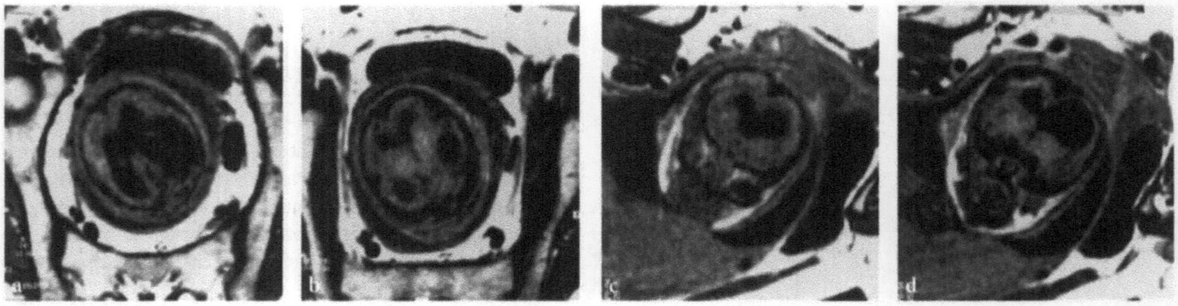

Fig. 23.17a–d. Thirty-one weeks, unlayered PMG, axial (**a,b**) and coronal (**c,d**) TSE T1 WI. Ventricular dilatation and unilateral hydrocephalus on the left side. The cortical ribbon is highly abnormal on the right side (**b,c**) with loss of its normal signal. Gyration is not consistent with the gestational age (**a,b**). Histology demonstrated unlayered MPG

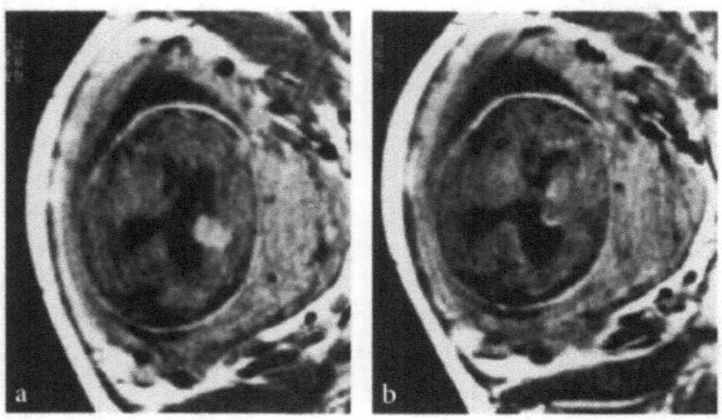

Fig. 23.18a,b. Thirty-one weeks, hemorrhage, axial (**a,b**) TSE T1 WI. Ventricular dilatation, hemorrhage as high signal intensity within the left lateral ventricle and the periventricular parenchyma (**a**), within the germinal matrix and the left basal ganglia (**b**)

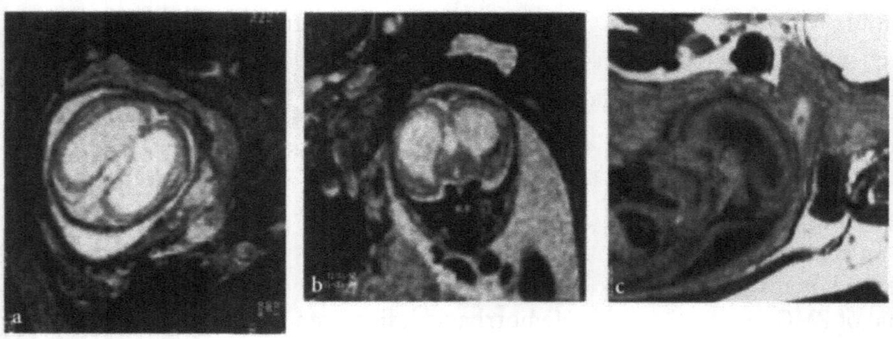

Fig. 23.19a–c. Twenty-one weeks, ventricular dilatation, old hemorrhage. Axial (**a**) and coronal (**b**) TPSE T2 WI, sagittal TSE T1 WI (**c**). The head circumference was normal. Important ventricular dilatation (hydrocephalus), with an old hemorrhage appearing as a highly hypointense localized thickening of the germinal matrix (**b**) on the left side. Note that the subarachnoid spaces are still patent. Note that the aqueduct is not visible (**c**)

Hemorrhage is known to cause porencephaly and hydranencephaly. Porencephaly can be depicted as localized enlargement of a lateral ventricle with loss of the normal signal of the germinal matrix, loss of the adjacent layer of migrating cells, and sometimes loss of the normal basal ganglia (caudate nucleus and lentiform nucleus either alone or in combination) in extensive damage.

In the chronic stage of hemorrhage, T2 weighted gradient echo imaging is obtained only through relatively long sequences, too long for good fetal imaging.

23.5.2.2
Ischemia, White Matter Vulnerability, Atrophy

The classical ischemia of arterial distribution, as known in the neonate, is not common in utero. MRI shows the lesion as low signal intensity on T1 WI, high signal intensity on T2 WI, involving either the cortical ribbon and the white matter (Fig. 23.20) or the white matter alone. This latter condition usually displays high signal intensity on T2 WI and normal signal intensity on T1 WI. Hemorrhagic infarction can also be seen. The cause responsible for ischemia was of placental origin in one case. In the other case of hemorrhagic infarction the cause is still controversial: a bichorial twin pregnancy was uneventful until cerebral infarction was found in one fetus which ended stillborn; the co-twin was born alive but died shortly after birth because of a suspected renal disease that is not yet characterized.

Venous thrombosis is not that uncommon and is well depicted as high signal intensity on T1 WI within dural sinuses (Fig. 23.21). In most cases associated brain lesions are seen. However in a recent case of torcular and unilateral lateral sinus thrombosis no parenchymal lesion was found (Fig. 23.22). The neonate was born at term and is currently doing well at 3 months of age. Post-natal MRI at 2 months of age did not show parenchymal abnormality.

Ischemic cerebral changes in utero consist most commonly in white matter necrosis or astrocytosis, alone or in combination, known as leukomalacia/gliosis (MARRET et al. 1998a, 1998b). These lesions are not easy to depict in utero. Post-natal criteria of leukomalacia as nodules of high signal on T1 WI and low signal on T2 WI are not a rule in the prenatal period (at least in our experience) (Fig. 23.22). In most cases white matter lesions are suspected on MRI through the loss of the layer of migrant cells in young fetuses (Fig. 23.16), alone or in combination with loss of the normal signal of the germinal matrix and/or of the cortical ribbon, irregular aspect of the germinal matrix (Fig. 23.23), with ventriculomegaly. In contrast, beyond 30 weeks of gestation ventriculomegaly and irregular ventricular walls (Fig. 23.24) can be seen as a similar feature as described on postnatal imaging examinations (LEVITON and GILLES 1996) for periventricular leukomalacia.

In contrast diffuse necrosis is easy to depict by MR through the loss of the normal signal of the cor-

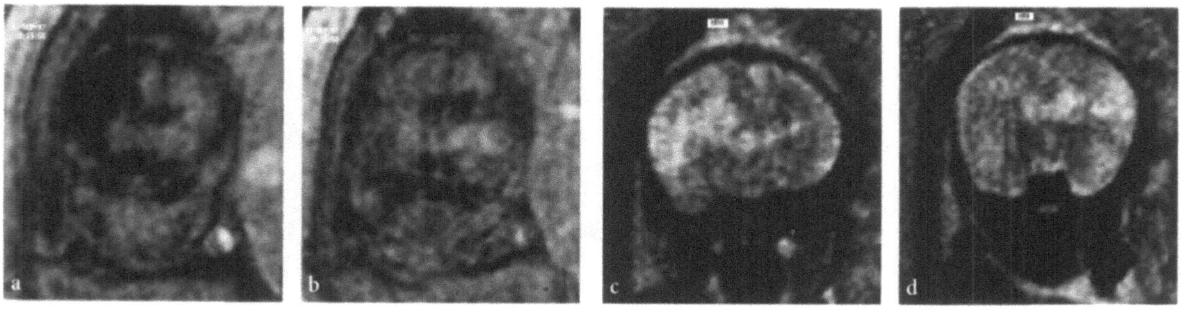

Fig. 23.20a–d. Thirty-six weeks, ischemic infarction, coronal gradient-echo T1 (**a,b**) and TPSE T2 (**c,d**) WI. Bilateral infarction in the frontal areas appear as low signal on T1 WI (**a,b**) and high signal on T2 WI (**c,d**)

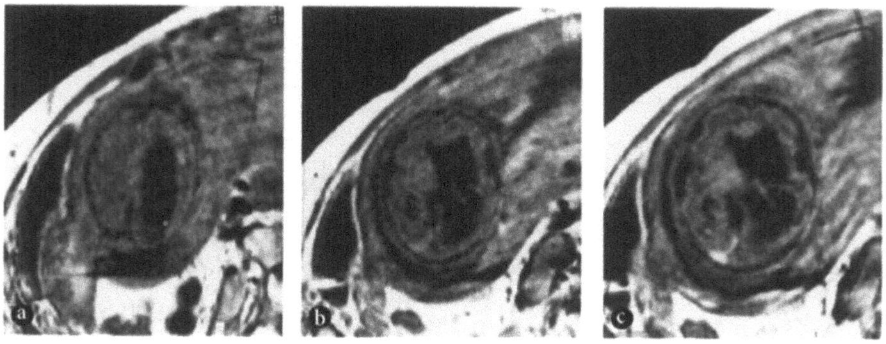

Fig. 23.21a–c. Twenty-seven weeks, venous thrombosis, leukomalacia, unilateral hydrocephalus, axial TSE T1 WI (**a,b,c**). Nodule of high signal intensity in the left periventricular frontal area (**a**). Note the bright signal within the straight sinus and the right lateral sinus suggestive of venous thrombosis (**b,c**). The basal ganglia on the left side are not visible (**b**) probably because of necrosis

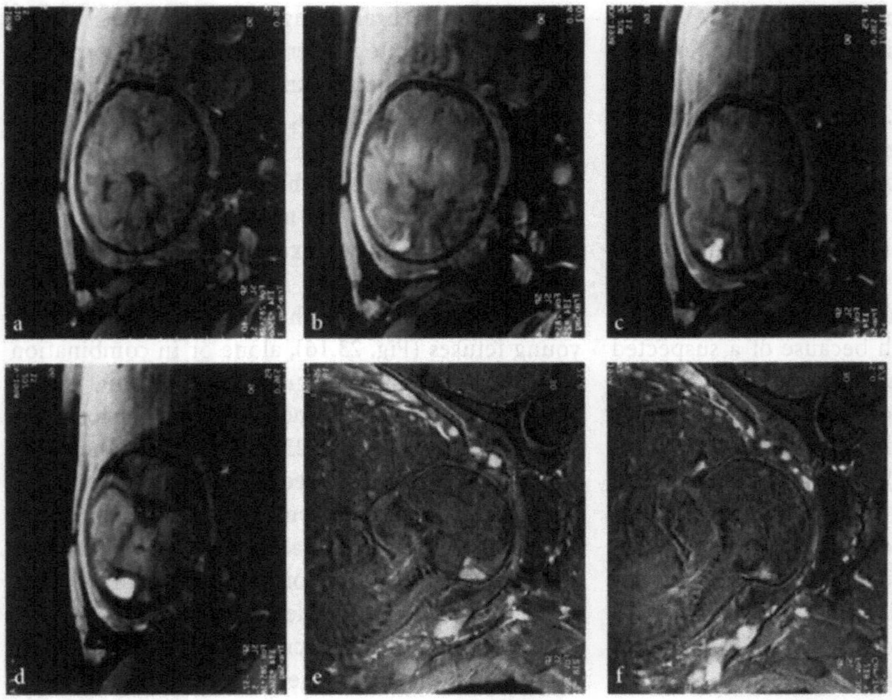

Fig. 23.22a–f. Thirty-one weeks, venous thrombosis. Axial (**a,b,c,d**) gradient-echo T1 WI with fat saturation, and sagittal (**e,f**) angiographic images (flip angle of 30). Spontaneous bright signal within the torcular (**b,c,d**) related to venous thrombosis with no brain abnormality (**a,b**) or abnormal vessels (**e,f**). Note that the signal from the cortex and basal ganglia is not affected by the fat saturation

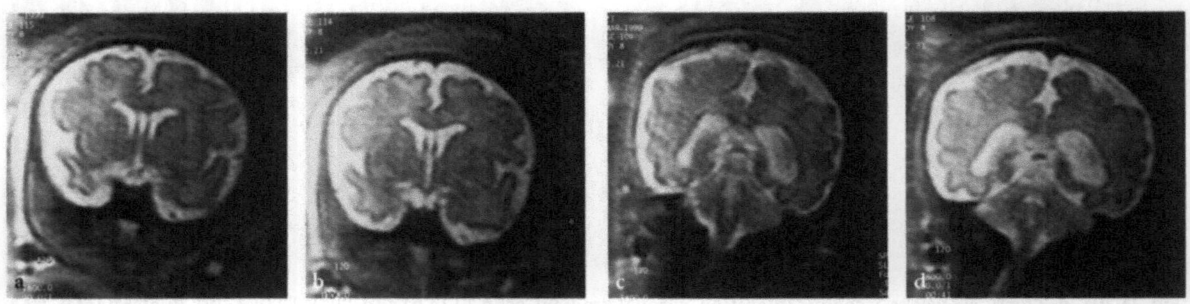

Fig. 23.23a–d. Thirty-one weeks, ependymal destruction, coronal haste images (**a,b,c,d**). Ventricular dilatation predominantly on the left side. The germinal matrix is thickened on the left side (**a**); its signal from is not homogeneous (**b**); the germinative zone shows an irregular aspect posteriorly and on the left side (**c,d**). Gross pathology demonstrated leukomalacia and ependymal destruction

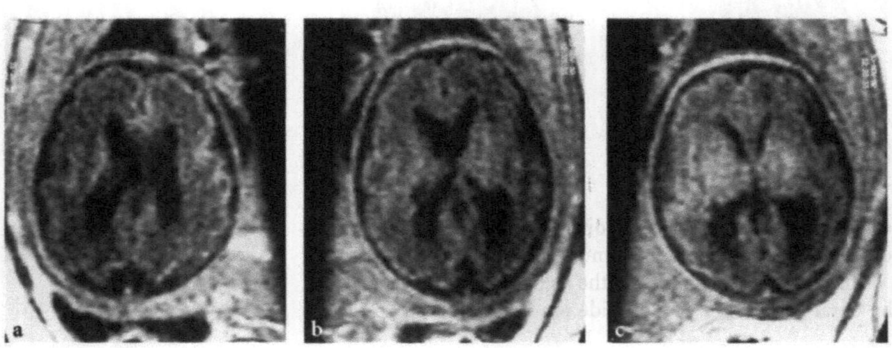

Fig. 23.24a–c. Thirty weeks, leukomalacia, axial TSE T1 WI (**a,b,c**). Ventricular dilatation (**a,b,c**) and irregular walls of the lateral ventricles predominantly on the right side (**b,c**)

tex and white matter on both T1 and T2 WI (Fig. 23.25) in a diffuse way.

Atrophy consists of a loss of white and/or gray matter. MRI shows a ventricular dilatation, enlarged subarachnoid spaces in late pregnancy, a thin cerebral mantle not consistent with the gestational age, alone or in combination with loss of the normal signal of the cortical ribbon, of the white matter in cases of gray and/or white matter lesions. White matter anomaly can be detected very early by MRI, as early as 20–21 weeks, the intermediate layer of migrant cells not being recognizable. Note that all cases diagnosed as atrophy on MR (Figs. 23.20, 23.23, 23.24 and 23.25) did show ependymal destruction and/or leukomalacia, and/or necrosis on histological studies.

Several important remarks about brain lesion of destructive origin have to be kept in mind:

(1) The mechanism for brain damage is rarely found either by in vivo imaging or clinical history and is thereby only suspected; the implication is that placental histological examination is necessary in order to detect placental origin to the brain damage with no recurrence and no consequence for future pregnancies.

(2) Moreover histological studies are not always possible in cases of termination of the pregnancy because of the tissular lysis with no correlation between MRI findings and pathology and thereby loss of expertise specially in cases of subtle lesions; in other cases a discrepancy can be seen between MR findings and histological data because of the time delay between MRI and medical termination of the pregnancy that can be up to 2–3 weeks (brain lesions being possibly strikingly severe on pathology as opposed to MRI data); the disadvantage of such a condition is the loss in self-confidence; in contrast, the dramatic advantage is the illustration of the evolving process of destruction (brain damage being possibly highly extensive in a short period of time).

(3) Prenatal US and/or MRI by identifying brain damage such as subtle ependymal destruction, foci of old hemorrhage of the germinal matrix, may help identify pathological conditions of fetal onset that contribute to neurological abnormalities (Scher et al. 1991); the so called group of congenital cerebral palsy can be now illustrated, thanks to MRI; cases of subtle damage with continuation of the pregnancy should permit the identification of prognosis factors on prenatal brain imaging.

23.5.2.3
Maternal Infection

Infective causes can be part of clastic lesions or of neuronal migration disorders, depending on the time of occurrence during pregnancy. The deleterious effects of maternal infection have been well recognized since the initial description of the adverse effects of rubella (Wolinsky 1998).

Toxoplasmosis is the most frequent infection in our experience. Toxoplasmosis can cause necrotizing meningoencephalitis with consequent hydrocephalus, calcifications, microcephaly, severe porencephaly and hydranencephaly (Friede 1989). Calcifications are better depicted by US (Drose et al. 1991). However macroscopic calcifications are a rare feature in the prenatal period. MRI is performed in our institution as a routine procedure in toxoplasmosis seroconversion in order to rule out brain lesion since the clinical outcome is quite good with medical treatment in cases with no parenchymal abnormalities. Subependymal cysts and ventricular dilatation can be seen in some cases. Although of potential benefit, MR effectiveness is limited since no gadolinium injection should be used in utero, to depict meningoencephalitis.

Cytomegalovirus (CMV) infection is considered as the most common and serious congenital infec-

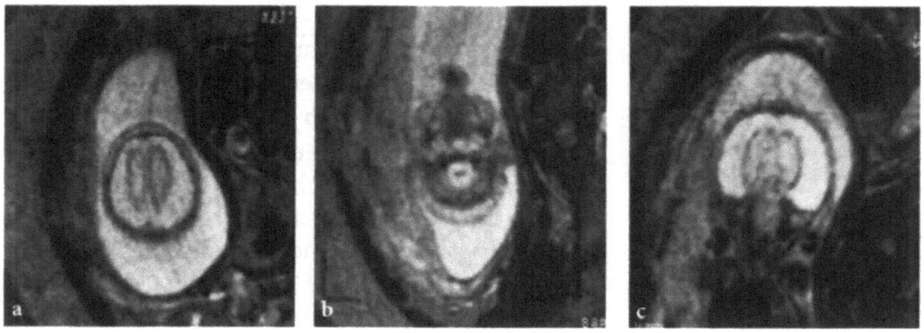

Fig. 23.25a–c. Twenty-one weeks, diffuse necrosis. Axial **(a,b)** and coronal **(c)** TPSE T2 WI. The cortical ribbon and migrant cells are not recognizable. Brain parenchyma displays high signal. The germinal matrix is thick and of low signal. Note that the 4th ventricle is enlarged and that the cerebellar are not recognizable **(b)**

tion (VOLPE 1995; STEINLIN et al. 1996; LIPITZ et al. 1997). Neuropathologically evidence for inflammation and destruction can be observed as micrencephaly, meningoencephalitis, calcifications (periventricular, cortical, or both), MPG, lissencephaly, cerebellar hypoplasia, periventricular leukomalacia or porencephaly, ventriculomegaly. US is the primary method to depict calcifications (TASSIN et al. 1991). MRI shows in our experience evidence for destruction as ventricular dilatation, subependymal cysts probably related to necrotizing lesions of the ependyma, periventricular necrosis (Fig. 23.26), MPG (Fig. 23.16). Malformation was also observed in one case as commissural agenesis in combination with disorganized cortex and heterotopia. Evidence for CMV infection was found postnatally.

Other infection can be observed such as varicella-zoster infection (LALLEMAND 1997; ONG and DANIEL 1998), hepatitis C virus (HCV), parvovirus B, HIV infections. Parvovirus B infection increases the risk of fetal loss (MILLER et al. 1998; HARGER et al. 1998), with no evidence of increased risk of developmental delay compared with any unselected group of children (MILLER et al. 1998). Vertical transmission of HCV is well recognized, most patients exhibiting chronic hepatitis (HUNT et al. 1997). Vertical transmission of HIV is also well known (ENCHA-RAZAVI et al. 1997) with very few fetuses showing evidence of brain lesions directly related to HIV infection consisting of edema, decrease in cellularity, proliferation of microglial cells. However the evaluation of cerebral changes in infants with maternal HIV infection shows other adverse effects related to drug addiction, vitamin deficiency, and other infections that interfere with brain development during pregnancy.

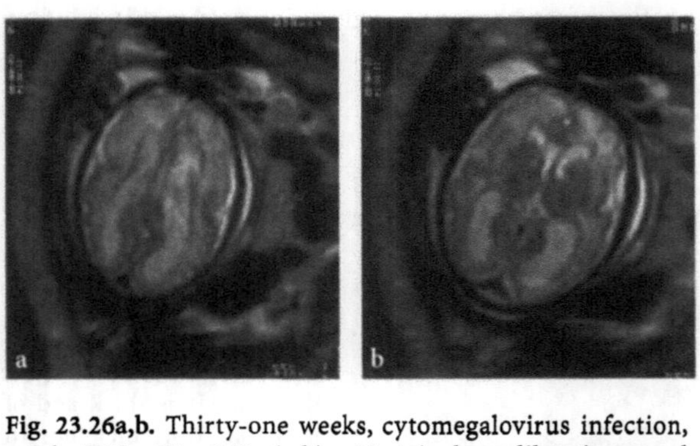

Fig. 23.26a,b. Thirty-one weeks, cytomegalovirus infection, axial TSE T2 WI (**a,b**). Ventricular dilatation and periventricular cysts in the white matter located close to the frontal horns

23.5.3 Tumours

The so called congenital CNS tumors are a rare group of tumors since the reported incidence ranges from 0.5% to 1.5% of all pediatric CNS tumours (FORT and RUSHING 1997). A tumour is considered to be congenital because it is present at the time of birth or because its onset or genesis has taken place in utero. Teratomas represent 1/3, gliomas (astrocytomas, glioblastomas, ependymomas and papillomas of the choroid plexus) 1/3 and others (PNET, meningiomas, craniopharyngiomas, lipomas and hamartomas) the last 1/3. Some hamartomas can have genetic implications such as tuberous sclerosis or Bourneville's disease, hypothalamic hamartoma (ENCHA-RAZAVI et al. 1992). Our series consists of intracranial teratomas in 3 (Fig. 23.27), malignant cerebral tumor in 1, saccrococcygeal teratoma in 1 (Fig. 23.28), facial angioma in 2. Note that among the 4 cases of intracranial brain tumours, US suspected a cerebral mass in one case only, the three remaining cases being referred for suspected arachnoid cysts in 2, ventricular dilatation in 1. Our cases of routine evaluation of familial tuberous sclerosis did not show evidence of brain lesions. However, normal fetal brain MRI does not exclude Bourneville's disease at all since the brain lesions can develop late after birth. Note that gadolinium injection is not allowed in utero even to evaluate brain tumours.

23.5.4 Vascular Malformations

According to the literature, cerebral arteriovenous malformations in the fetus consist in most cases of the vein of Galen aneurysm (COMSTOCK and KIRK 1991) which can be depicted as a pseudocystic, non-echogenic or poorly echogenic lesion on prenatal US. Intracranial arteriovenous shunts at fetal age consist of either a vein of Galen aneurysmal malformation (VGAM) or a dural sinus malformation (DSM) (LASJAUNIAS 1997). VGAM is now well recognized as the embryonic vascular malformation (RAYBAUD et al. 1989). Pial or non-galenic arteriovenous malformation are mostly seen in neonates. Several diseases are known to be hereditary such as Rendu-Osler-Weber disease linked to chromosome 9, neurofibromatosis type 1 linked to chromosome 17.

Our experience does not include cases of VGAM or DSM. The only case of supposedly vascular malformation consists of thrombosis of the torcular and

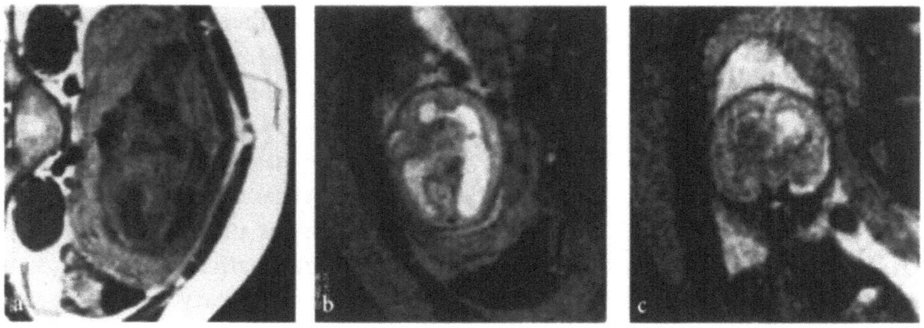

Fig. 23.27a–c. Twenty weeks, supratentorial teratoma. Axial TSE T1 WI (a), axial (b) and coronal (c) TPSE T2 WI. Unilateral ventricular dilatation; the heterogeneous midline mass displays isointense and bright signal on T1 WI (a) and low and high signal on T2 WI (b,c) that ended up as teratoma on histological sections

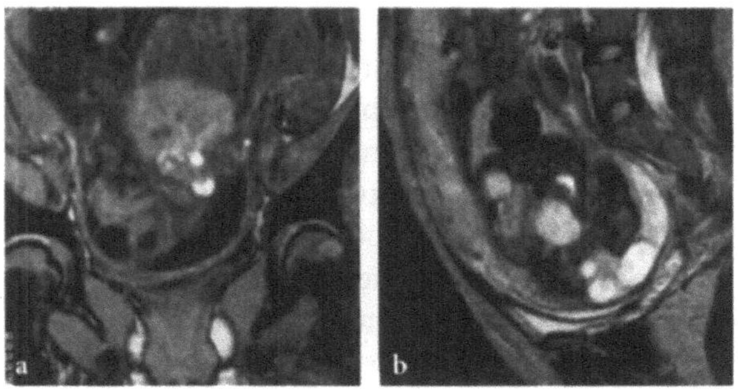

Fig. 23.28a,b. Thirty weeks, saccrococcygeal teratoma, sagittal gradient-echo T1 WI (a) and coronal TPSE T2 WI (b). The mass appears heterogeneous with cystic components as low signal intensity on T1WI and high signal intensity on T2 WI

of the right lateral sinus with no familial history of vascular disease and no coagulation disorders (Fig. 23.22).

23.5.5 Hydrocephalus versus Ventricular Dilatation

Ventricular dilatation is one of the most common clinical conditions (38% of cases in our experience) (Filly et al. 1991). As already mentioned ventricular dilatation may be of destructive origin, malformative origin, hydrocephalic origin, destructive and hydrocephalic origin, malformative and destructive origin. Malformative origin is easy to depict because of the specific morphological features as already seen above. A destructive origin is more difficult to depict but is still achieved through the ventricular morphology, the loss of the migrant cell layer visibility, the loss of the normal signal contrast, and loss of the maturation milestone.

The most difficult problem to solve is the analysis of hydrocephalus since post-natal criteria are not available in utero. Postnatal criteria of hydrocephalus are well known, consisting of global ventricular dilatation, obliteration of the pericerebral spaces, macrocephaly, and an apparent explanatory mechanism. Prenatal criteria of hydrocephalus are not that obvious since prenatal hydrocephalus may be compatible with normal head circumference (Figs. 23.14 and 23.19), with patent subarachnoid spaces (Figs. 23.14 and 23.19), and even with near-to-normal ventricular size. This is probably related to the fetal brain morphology and to the fetal cerebrospinal fluid (CSF) physiology with a peculiar role of the amniotic pressure (acting as a counterpressure), and of the pressure gradient between the ventricular and peripheral CSF. An apparent mechanism for ventricular dilatation can be found, but not as a rule. Our experience shows no apparent cause in 40% of the cases. Moreover almost similar images can be due to completely different causes (i.e., clastic versus malformative lesion) (compare Figs. 23.21 and 23.17). Nevertheless, the prognosis for ventricular dilatation found in utero is poor (Pretorius et al. 1985; Oi et al. 1990; Hilpert et al. 1995; Levitsky et al. 1995), the least unfavorable criteria consisting of isolated ventriculomegaly, late diagnosis (third trimester), slow evolution and a ratio between the ventricles and the hemispheres no more than 50% of normal value (Anhoury et al. 1991). Moreover, the outcome of isolated mild fetal cerebral ventriculomegaly (axial distance at the atrial level from 10 to 15 mm) shows neurologic developmental abnormalities in up to 19% (Vergani et al. 1998).

The last point about ventricular dilatation is the remarkable power of MRI in illustrating subarachnoid space development. The so called benign external hydrocephalus is characterized postnatally by macrocephaly, enlarged ventricles (at the level of the frontal horns in a symmetric way), enlarged subarachnoid spaces due to accumulation of CSF in the anterior parts of the hemispheres, and the square shape of the forehead (Maytal et al. 1987). The pathophysiology of benign enlargement of the ventricles includes prematurity (and intraventricular hemorrhage with its consequences in diminishing the ability of arachnoid granulations to absorb CSF), an osseous origin (skull base dysplasia), a vascular origin (arteriovenous malformation), and metabolic disease such as mucopolysaccharidoses. However in most cases the cause remains unknown and is probably constitutional. Our experience consists of four documented cases of benign external hydrocephalus. These children underwent in utero MRI that showed a mild ventriculomegaly (as asymmetric dilatation at the atria level) associated with an enlargement of the subarachnoid spaces *posteriorly* at the parieto-occipital levels. These neonates were born at term with no intrapartum history. Postnatal MRI from 2 to 4 months of age depicted the typical features of begnin external hydrocephalus as frontal accumulation of CSF. Here again the postnatal criteria are not available in utero: the accumulation of CSF displays a more posterior distribution as opposed to the postnatal period (Fig. 23.29). These antenatal features may reflect the development of CSF pathway that is known to spread from the ventral portion of the mes- and rhombencephalon caudally to the spinal cord, and cranially to the prosencephalon, the arachnoid granulations being seen by week 39 (Osaka et al. 1980; Gomez et al. 1981).

23.6 Illustration of Spine Abnormalities

MRI of spine and spinal cord is not performed as commonly as brain MRI in the prenatal period. Indeed, ultrasonography (Meizner 1997) is much more demonstrative than MRI in depicting spinal abnormalities as well as in the assessment of ossification of the fetal spine (Budorick et al. 1991) specially by the introduction of three-dimensional US. Moreover skeletal dysplasias are not frequent, the incidence being approximately 0.024% of births (Spirt et al. 1990). However MRI can be an additional procedure in some cases either by depicting signal abnormalities of the vertebral bodies as in cases of osteogenesis abnormalities or in cases of spine deformity related to vertebral malformation (i.e., kyphosis and dislocation in segmentary vertebral body agenesis) (Fig. 23.30).

23.7 Conclusions and Summary

MRI is extremely sensitive to parenchymal changes in the brain and is thence a powerful additional procedure in the prenatal diagnosis by illustrating nicely the normal developing brain as well as the pathological conditions that cannot be dissociated from the pathological, and sometimes the histological, studies. An understanding of the normal developing brain is known from gross pathology and histology as well as from the postnatal experience, and MRI is thereby the most effective imaging in vivo technique in detecting the normal hallmarks of brain development; these normal markings include the developing gyration and sulcation, and above all the signal changes on both T1 and T2 weighted sequences. Particular attention has to be given to the thickness and normal signal of the cortical ribbon, to the visibility of the layer of the migrating glial cells, to the thickness, regularity and normal signal of the germinal matrix, to the ventricular and subarachnoid space morphology, and to the maturation milestones. With this potential benefit of MRI, the diagnosis of destructive lesion may be achieved through the loss of the normal signal of the cortical ribbon, the loss of visibility of the migrant cell layer, the loss of normal thickness and signal of the germinal matrix, either alone or in combination; clastic lesion may thereby be depicted as early as 20 weeks; subtle damage such as localized ependymal destruction, known to interfere with the neurological and cognitive development, can also be identified. In contrast, brain malformations can be detected through their specific abnormalities; more to the point, histogenetic disorders such type 1 lissencephaly will probably be diagnosed more easily by abnormal thickened cortical ribbon, since in utero MRI is now a reliable method for differentiating the cortex from the underlying white matter.

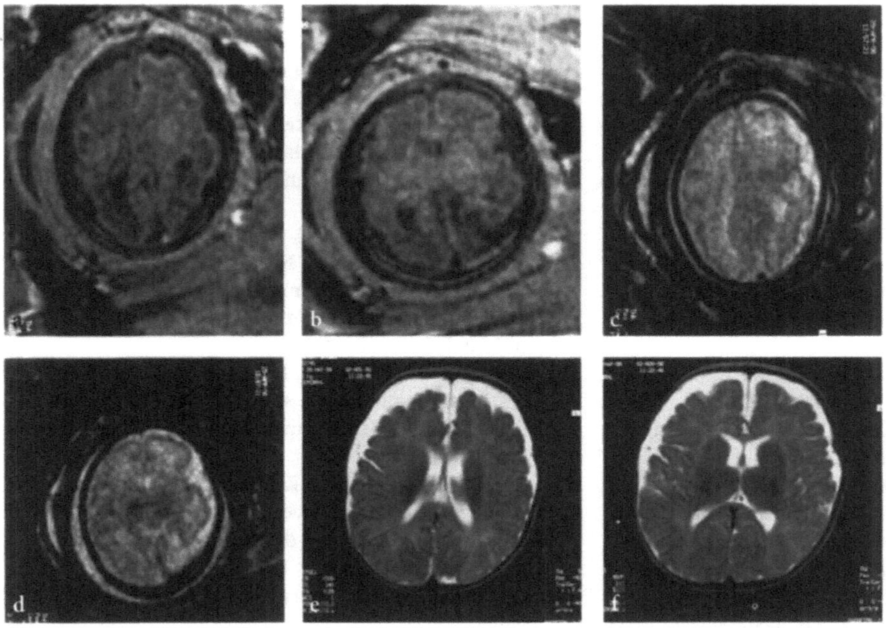

Fig. 23.29a–f. Thirty-one weeks, benign ventricular dilatation. Axial gradient-echo T1 WI (**a,b**) and axial TPSE T2 WI (**c,d**), axial T2 WI at 6 months of age (**e,f**). Mild ventricular dilatation at the level of the posterior horn on the right side (**a,b**). Enlarged subarachnoid spaces contralaterally (**c,d**) and accumulation of CSF posteriorly on the left side (**d**). The postnatal MRI shows typical features of the so-called benign external hydrocephalus (**e,f**)

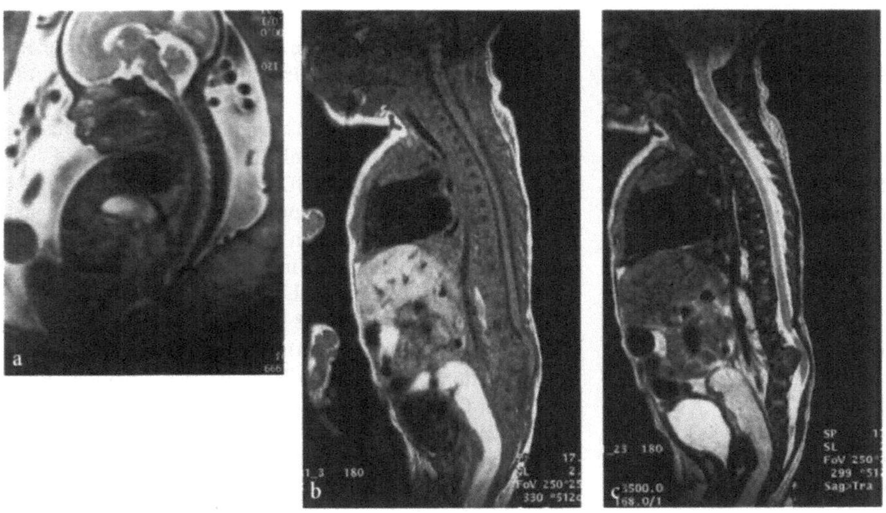

Fig. 23.30a–c. Twenty-six weeks, congenital lumbar luxation. Sagittal Haste image (**a**), postnatal sagittal T1 (**b**) and T2 (**c**) images by week 2. Lumbar kyphosis (**a**) as found in vertebral body agenesis. Post natal MRI shows additional spinal cord malformation as segmented agenesis of the spinal cord

References

Andermann E, Andermann F (1996) Genetic aspects of neuronal migration disorders. In: Guerrini R, Andermann F, Canapicchi R, Roger J, Zifkin BG, Pfanner P (eds) Dysplasia of cerebral cortex and epilepsy. Lippincot-Raven, Philadelphia, pp 11–15

Anhoury P, Andre M, Droullle P, Czorny A, Gilgenkrantz S, Schweitzer M, Leheup B (1991) Dilatation of the cerebral ventricles diagnosed in utero. 85 case histories. J Gynecol Obstet Biol Reprod 20: 191–197 (in French)

Baker PN, Johnson DM, Harvey PR, Gowland PA, Mansfield P (1994) A three year follow up of children imaged in utero with echo-planar magnetic resonance. Am J Obstet Gynecol 170: 32–33

Barkovich AJ, Kyos HC, Jackson DE, Norman D (1988) Normal maturation of the neonatal and infant brains: MR imaging at 1.5 T. Radiology 166: 173–180

Barkovich AJ (1996) Magnetic resonance imaging of lissencephaly, polymicrogyria, schizencephaly, hemimegalencephaly, and band heterotopia. In: Guerrini R, Andermann F, Canapicchi R, Roger J, Zifkin BG, Pfanner P (eds) Dysplasia of cerebral cortex and epilepsy. Lippincot-Raven, Philadelphia, pp 115–129

Barkovich AJ, Ferriero DM, Barr RM, Gressens P, Dobyns WB, Truwit ChL, Evrard Ph (1998) Microlissencephaly: a heterogeneous malformation of cortical development. Neuropediatrics 29: 113–119

Barkhof F, Heijboer RJJ, Algra PR (1992) Inadvertent IV administration of gadopentate dimeglumine during early pregnancy. AJR 158: 1171

Berry M (1986) Neurogenesis and gliogenesis in the human brain. Fd Chem Toxic 24: 79–89

Brisse H, Fallet C, Sebag G, Nessmann C, Blot P, Hassan M (1997) Supratentorial parenchyma in the developing fetal brain: in vitro MR study with histologic comparison. Am J Neuroradiol 18: 1491–1497

Brody BA, Kinney HC, Kloman AS, Gilles FH (1987) Sequence of central nervous system myelination in human infancy I: an autopsy study of myelination. J Neuropathol Exp Neurol 46: 283–301

Budorick NE, Pretorius DH, Grafe MR, Lou KV (1991) Ossification of the fetal spine. Radiology 181: 561–565

Burke CJ, Tannenberg AE, Payton DJ (1997) Ischemic cerebral injury, intrauterine growth retardation, and placental infarction. Dev Med Child Neurol 39: 726–730

Chong BW, Babcook CJ, Salamat MS, Nemzek W, Kroeker D, Ellis WG (1996) A magnetic resonance template for normal neuronal migration in the fetus. Neurosurgery 39: 110–116

Coletti PM, Sylvestre PB (1994) Magnetic resonance imaging in pregnancy. MRI Clinics North America 2: 291–307

Comstock CH, Kirk JS (1991) Arteriovenous malformations. Locations and evolution in the fetal brain. J Ultrasound Med 10: 361–365

Coniglio SJ, Anderson SM, Ferguson JE (1996) Functional motor outcome in children with myelomeningocele: correlation with anatomic level on prenatal ultrasound. Dev Med Child Neurol 38: 675–680

Cooke P, Morris P (1981) The effects of NMR on living organisms. II. A genetic study of human lymphocytes. Br J Radiol 54: 850

Daffos F, Capella-Pavlovsky M, Forestier F (1985) Fetal blood sampling during pregnancy with use of a needle guided by ultrasound: a study of 606 consecutive cases. Am J Obstet Gynecol 153: 655–660

Daffos F (1990) Acces to the fetus. Nouv Rev Fr Hematol 32: 431–433

De Crespigny LC, Robinson HP, Quinn M, Doyle I, Ross A, Cauchi M (1985) Ultrasound-guided fetal blood transfusion for severe rhesus isoimmunization. Obstet Gynecol 66: 529–532

D'Ercole C, Girard N, Boubli L, Potier A, Chagnon C, Raybaud C, Blanc B (1993) Prenatal diagnosis of fetal cerebral abnormalities by ultrasonography and resonance imaging. Eur J Obstet Gynecol Reprod Biol 50: 177–184

D'Ercole C, Girard N, Cravello L, Boubli L, Potier A, Raybaud C, Blanc B (1998) Prenatal diagnosis of fetal corpus callosum agenesis by ultrasonography and magnetic resonance imaging. Prenat Diagn 18: 247–253

Des Portes V, Pinard JM, Francis F, Chelly J (1998) Doublecortine, un nouveau gène exprimé dans le cerveau foetal, est impliqué dans les hétérotopies laminaires souscorticales et les lissencéphalies liées au chromosome X. Médecine/Sciences 14: 241–243

Dobyns WB, Pagon RA, Armstrong D, Curry CJR, Greenberg F, Grix A, Holmes LB, Laxova R, Michels VV, Robinow M, Zimmerman RL (1989) Diagnostic criteria for Walker-Warburg syndrome. Am J Med Genet 32: 195–210

Drose JA, Dennis MA, Thickman D (1991) Infection in utero: US findings in 19 cases. Radiology 178: 369–374

Economides DL, Whitlow BJ, Kadir R, Lazanakis M, Verdin SM (1998) First trimester sonographic detection of chromosomal abnormalities in an unselected population. Br J Obstet Gynaecol 105: 58–62

Economides DL, Braithwaite JM (1998) First trimester ultrasonographic diagnosis of fetal structural abnormalities in a low risk population. Br J Obstet Gynaecol 105: 53–57

Encha-Razavi F, Larroche JC, Roume J, Migne G, Delezoide AL, Gonzales M, Mulliez N (1992) Congenital hypothalamic hamartoma syndrome: nosological discussion and minimum diagnostic criteria of a possibly familial form. Am J Med Genet 42: 44–50

Encha-Razavi F, Larroche JC, Roume J, Mulliez N, Lescs MC (1997) Neuropathological study in 134 fetuses from HIV infected mother (in French). Arch Anat Cytol Path 45: 118–120

Evrard P, De Saint-Georges P, Kadhim HJ, Gadisseux JF (1989) Pathology of prenatal encephalopathies. In: Brookes PH (ed) Child neurology and developmental disabilities. Baltimore, pp 153–176

Farmer DL (1998) Fetal surgery: a brief review. Pediatr Radiol 28: 409–413

Fees-Higgins A, Larroche JC (1987) Development of the human fetal brain. An anatomical atlas. INSERM (ed) Masson, Paris

Filly RA, Goldstein RB, Callen PW (1991) Fetal ventricle: importance in routine obstetric sonography. Radiology 181: 1–7

Fort DW, Rushing EJ (1997) Congenital central nervous system tumors. J Child Neurol 12: 157–164

Fralix TA, Ceckler TL, Wolff SD, Simon SA, Balaban RS (1991) Lipid bilayer and water proton magnetization transfer: effect of cholesterol. Magn Reson Medicine 18: 214–223

Friede RL (1989) Infections in the fetus. In: Friede RL (ed) Developmental neuropathology 2nd edition. Springer-Verlag, Berlin, pp 156–168

Garden AS, Roberts N (1996) Fetal and fetal organ volume estimations with magnetic resonance imaging. Am J Obstet Gynecol 175: 442–448

Gilles FH (1985) Perinatal neuropathology. In: Davis RL, Robertson DM (eds) Textbook of neuropathology. Williams & Wilkins, Baltimore, pp 243–283

Girard N, Raybaud C, DuLac P (1991) MRI study of brain myelination. J Neuroradiol 18: 291–307

Girard N, Raybaud C, Boubli L, Cahen S, Potier A, Gamerre M (1992) Exploration par IRM du cerveau foetal in utero. Rev Im Med 4: 391–399

Girard NJ, Raybaud CA (1992) In vivo MRI of fetal brain cellular migration. J Comput Assist Tomogr 16: 265–267

Girard N, Raybaud C, DÍErcole C, Boubli L, Chau C, Cahen S, Potier A, Gamerre A (1993) In vivo MRI of the fetal brain. Neuroradiology 35: 431–436

Girard N, Raybaud C, Poncet M (1995) In vivo MR study of brain maturation in normal fetuses. Am J Neuroradiol 16: 407–413

Girard N, Raybaud C, Poncet M (1996) In vivo magnetic resonance imaging of the fetal brain. In: Guerrini R, Andermann F, Canapicchi R, Roger J, Zifkin BG, Pfanner P (eds) Dysplasia of cerebral cortex and epilepsy. Lippincot-Raven, Philadelphia, pp 101–103

Gomez DG, DiBenedetto AT, Pavese AM, Firpo A, Hershoan DB, Potts DG (1981) Development of arachnoid villi and

granulations in man. Acta Anat 111: 247–258
Harding B, Copp AJ (1997) Malformations. In: Graham DI, Lantos PL (eds) Greenfield's neuropathology, sixth edition. Arnold, London, pp 397–533
Harger JH, Adler SP, Koch WC, Harger GF (1998) Prospective evaluation of 618 pregnant women exposed to Parvovirus B19: risks and symptoms. Obstet Gynecol 91: 413–420
Hata T, Aoki S, Hata K, Miyazaki K, Akahane M, Mochizuki T (1998) Three-dimensional ultrasonographic assessments of fetal development, Obstet Gynecol 91: 218–223
Hilpert PL, Hall BE, Kurtz AB (1995) The atria of the fetal lateral ventricles: a sonographic study of normal atrial size and chroid plexus volume. AJR 164: 731–734
Holms GL (1986) Morphological and physiological maturation of the brain in the neonate and young child. J Clin Neurophysiol 3: 209–238
Hunt CM, Carson KL, Sharara AI (1997) Hepatitis C in pregnancy. Obstet Gynecol 89: 883–890
Isaksen CV, Eik-Nes SH, Blaas HG, Torp SH (1998) Comparison of prenatal ultrasound and postmortem findings in fetuses and infants with central nervous system anomalies. Ultrasound Obstet Gynecol 11: 246–253
Johnson IR, Symonds EM, Kean DM, Worthington BS, Broughton Pipkin F, Hawkes RC, Gyngell M (1984) Imaging of the pregnant human uterus with nuclear magnetic resonance. Am J Obstet Gynecol 148: 1136–1139
Kelly IMG, Gardener JE, Brett AD, Richards R, Lees WR (1994) Three-dimensional US of the fetus. Work in progress. Radiology 192: 253–259
Kenwrick S, Jouet M, Donnai D (1996) X linked hydrocephalus and MASA syndrome. J Med Genet 33: 59–65
Kinney HC, Armstrong DD (1997) Perinatal neuropathology. In: Graham DI, Lantos PL (eds) Greenfield's neuropathology, sixth edition. Arnold, London, pp 537–599
Koenig SH, Brown III RD, Spiller M, Lundbom N (1990) Relaxometry of brain: why white matter appears bright in MRI. Magn Reson Medecine 14: 482–495
Koenig SH (1991) Cholesterol of myelin is the determinant of gray-white contrast in MRI of brain. Magn Reson Medecine 20: 285–291
Koga Y, Tahara Y, Kida T, Matumoto Y, Negishi H, Fujimoto S (1997) Prenatal diagnosis of congenital unilateral hydrocephalus. Pediatr Radiol 27: 319–320
Kucharczyk W, MacDonald PM, Stanisz GH, Henkelman RM (1994) Relaxivity and magnetization transfer of white matter lipids at MR imaging: importance of cerebrosides and pH. Radiology 192: 521–529
Kurjak A, Kupesic S, Di Renzo GC, Pooh R, Kos M, Hafner T (1998) Recent advances in perinatal sonography. Prenat Neonat Med 3: 194–207
Lallemand AV (1997) The pathologist confronted by a hydrops fetalis management and review of the most frequent etiologies. Ann Pathol 17: 251–256 (in French)
Langer B, Choquet P, Ravier S, Gasser B, Schlaeder G, Constantinesco A (1998) Low-field dedicated magnetic resonance imaging: a potential tool for assisting perinatal autopsy. Ultrasound Obstet Gynecol 12: 271–275
Larroche JC, Amakawa H (1973) Glia of myelination and fat deposit during early myelogenesis. Biol Neonate 22: 421–435
Larroche JC (1977) Development of the central nervous system. In: Larroche JC (ed) Developmental pathology of the neonate. Elsevier/North-Holland Biomedical Press, Amsterdam, pp 319–353
Larroche JC, Girard N, Narcy F, Fallet C (1994) Abnormal cortical plate (polymicrogyria), heterotopias and brain damage in monozygous twins. Biol Neonate 65: 343–352
Lasjaunias P (1997) (ed) Vascular diseases in neonates, infants and children. Interventional neuroradiology management. Springer-Verlag, Berlin
Levi S (1998) Is antenatal screening for congenital defects feasible in average-risk populations? The Eurofetus Study. Prenat Neonat Med 3: 191–193
Levine D, Goldstein RB, Callen PW, Damato N, Kilpatrick S (1997) The effect of oligohydramnios on detection of fetal anomalies with sonography. AJR 168: 1609–1611
Leviton A, Gilles F (1996) Ventriculomegaly, delayed myelination, white matter hypoplasia, and "periventricular" leukomalacia: how are they related? Pediatr Neurol 15: 127–136
Levitsky DB, Mack LA, Nyberg DAA, Shurtleff DB, Shields LA, Nghiem HV, Cyr DR (1995) Fetal aqueductal stenosis diagnosed sonographically: how grave is the prognosis? AJR 164: 725–730
Lin CC, Santolaya-Forgas J (1998) Current concepts of fetal growth restriction: Part I. Causes, classification, and pathophysiology. Obstet Gynecol 92: 1044–1055
Lipitz S, Yagel S, Shalev E, Achiron R, Mashiach S, Schiff E (1997) Prenatal diagnosis of fetal primary cytomegalovirus infection. Obstet Gynecol 89: 763–767
Marret S, Zupan V, Gressens P, Lagercrantz H, Evrard P (1998a) Les leucomalacies périventriculaires. I. Aspects histologiques et étiopathogéniques. Arch Pédiatr 5: 525–537
Marret S, Zupan V, Gressens P, Lagercrantz H, Evrard P (1998b) Les leucomalacies périventriculaires. II. Diagnostic, séquelles et neuroprotection. Arch Pédiatr 5: 538–545
Maytal J, Alvarez LA, Elkin CM, Shinnar S (1987) External hydrocephalus: radiologic spectrum and differentiation from cerebral atrophy. AJNR 8: 271–278
Meizner I (1997) Fetal skeletal malformations revisited: steps in the diagnostic approach. Ultrasound Obstet Gynecol 10: 303–306
Miller E, Fairley CK, Cohen BJ, Seng C (1998) Immediate and long term outcome of human parvovirus B19 infection in pregnancy. Br J Obstet Gynaecol 105: 174–178
Moise KJ, Carpenter RJ, Deter RL, Kirshon B, Diaz SF (1987) The use of fetal neuromuscular blockade during intrauterine procedures. Am J Obstet Gynecol 157: 874–879
Monteagudo A, Timor-Tritsch IE (1997) Development of fetal gyri, sulci and fissures: a transvaginal sonographic study. Ultrasound Obstet Gynecol 9: 222–228
Norman MG, McGillivray, Kallouseek DK, Hill A, Poskitt KJ (1995) Congenital malformations of the brain. Pathological, embryological, clinical, radiological and genetics aspects, Oxford University Press, New York
Oba H, Barkovich AJ (1995) Holoprosencephaly: an analysis of callosal formation and its relation to development of the interhemispheric fissure. AJNR 16: 453–460
Oi S, Matsumoto S, Katayama K, Mochizuki M (1990) Pathophysiology and postnatal outcome of fetal hydrocephalus. Chid's Nerv Syst 6: 338–345
Okamura K, Murotsuki J, Sakai T, Matsumoto K, Shirane R, Yajima A (1993) Prenatal diagnosis of lissencephaly by magnetic resonance image. Fetal Diagn Ther 8: 56–59
Ong CL, Daniel ML (1998) Antenatal diagnosis of a porencephalic cyst in congenital varicella-zoster virus infection. Pediatr Radiol 28: 94

Osaka K, Handa H, Matsumoto S, Yasuda M (1980) Development of the cerebrospinal fluid pathways in the normal and abnormal embryos. Child's Brain 6: 26–38

Persutte WH (1998) Opinion. Microcephaly – no small deal. Ultrasound Obstet Gynecol 11: 317–318

Pinar H, Tatevosyants N, Singer DB (1998) Central nervous system malformations in a perinatal/neonatal autopsy series. Pediatr Dev Pathol 1: 42–48

Pretorius DH, Davis K, Manco-Johnson ML, Manchester D, Meier PR, Clewell WH (1985) Clinical course of fetal hydrocephalus: 40 cases. AJR 144: 827–831

Puche A, Rodriguez T, Domingo R, Casas C, Vicente T, Martinez-Lage JF (1998) X-linked subcortical laminar heterotopia and lissenceohaly: a new family. Neuropediatrics 29: 276–278

Raybaud C (1983) Destructive lesion of the brain. Neuroradiology 25: 265–291

Raybaud C, Strother CM, Hald JK (1989) Aneurysms of the vein of Galen: embryonic considerations and anatomical features relating to the pathogensis of the malformation. Neuroradiology 31: 109–128

Raybaud C, Canto-Moreira N, Girard N, Poncet M. Polymicrogyria (1995) MR appearance and its relationship to the fetal development of the cortex and its microvasculature. Int J Neuroradiol 1: 161–170

Raybaud C, Girard N, Canto-Moreira N, Poncet M (1996) High-definition magnetic resonance imaging identification of cortical dysplasias: micropolygyria versus lissencephaly. In: Guerrini R, Andermann F, Canapicchi R, Roger J, Zifkin BG, Pfanner P (eds) Dysplasia of cerebral cortex and epilepsy. Lippincot-Raven, Philadelphia, pp 131–143

Raybaud C, Girard N (1998) MRI anatomical study of telencephalic commissural agenesis and dysplasia (in French). Neurochirurgie 44(S1): 38–60

Raybaud C, Girard N (1998) Cerebral development and MRI. In: Garreau B (ed) Neuroimaging in child neuropsychiatric disorders. Springer-Verlag, Berlin, pp 59–88

Reid A, Smith FW, Hutchinson JMS (1982) Nuclear magnetic resonance imaging and its safety implications: follow up of 181 patients. Br J Radiol 55: 784–786

Robain O (1996) Introduction to the pathology of cerebral cortical dysplasia. In: Guerrini R, Andermann F, Canapicchi R, Roger J, Zifkin BG, Pfanner P (eds) Dysplasia of cerebral cortex and epilepsy. Lippincot-Raven, Philadelphia, pp 1–9

Scher MS, Belfar H, Martin J, Painter MJ (1991) Destructive brain lesions of presumed fetal onset: antepartum causes of cerebral palsy. Pediatrics 88: 898–906

Schwartz JL, Crooks LE (1982) NMR imaging produces no observable mutations or cytotoxicity in mammalians cells. Am J Roentgenol 139: 583–585

Shoenut JP, Semelka RC, Silverman R, Yaffe CS, Micflikier AB (1993) MRI in the diagnosis of Chrhn's disease in two pregnant women. J Clin Gastroenterol 17: 244–247

Sonigo P, Elmaleh A, Fermont L, Delezoide AL, Mirlesse V, Brunelle F (1996) Prenatal MRI diagnosis of fetal cerebral tuberous sclerosis. Pediatr Radiol 26: 1–4

Spirt BA, Oliphant M, Gottlieb RH, Gordon L¨P (1990) Prenatal sonographic evaluation of short-limbed dwarfism: an algorithmic approach. Radiographics 10: 217–236

Steilin M, Blaser S, Boltshauser E (1998) Cerebellar involvement in metabolic disorders: a pattern-recognition approach. Neuroradiology 40: 347–354

Steilin MI, Nadal D, Eich GF, Martin E, Boltshauer EJ (1996) Late intrauterine cytomegalovirus infection: clinical and neuroimaging findings. Pediatr Neurol 15: 249–253

Tassin GB, Maklad NF, Stewart RR, Bell ME (1991) Cytomegalic inclusion disease: Intrauterine sonographic diagnosis using findings involving the brain. AJNR 12: 117–122

Thomas A, Morris PG (1981) The effects of NMR exposure on living organisms. I. A microbiol assay. Br J Radiol 54: 615–621

Toti P, De Felice C, Palmeri MLD, Villanova M, Martin JJ, Buonocore G (1998) Inflammatory pathogenesis of cortical polymicrogyria: an autopsy study. Pediatr Res 44: 291–296

van der Knaap MS, Valk J (1995) (eds) Magnetic resonance of myelin, myelination and myelin disorders, 2nd edition. Springer-Verlag, Heidelberg

Vergani P, Locatelli A, Strobelt N, Cavallone M, Ceruti P, Paterlini G, Ghidini A (1998) Clinical outcome of mild fetal ventriculomegaly. Am J Obstet Gynecol 178: 218–222

Volpe JJ (1995) Intracranial infections. Viral, protozoan, and related intracranial infections. In: Volpe JJ (ed) Neurology of the newborn, third edition. Saunders Company, Philadelphia, pp 675–729

Wilhelm C, Keck C, Hess S, Korinthenberg R, Breckwoldt M (1998) Ventriculomegaly diagnosed by prenatal ultrasound and mental development of the children. Fetal Diagn Ther 13: 162–166

Wolff SD, Balaban RS (1989) Magnetization transfer contrast (MTC) and tissue water proton relaxation in vivo. Magn Reson Medecine 10: 135–144

Wolinsky JS (1998) Rubella virus and its effects on the developing nervous system. In: Johnson RT, Lyon G (eds) Virus infections and the developing nervous system. Kluwer Academic Publishers, Dordrecht, pp 125–142

Woodward PJ, Sohaey R, Harris DP, Jackson GM, Klatt EC, Alexander AL, Kennedy A (1997) Postmortem fetal MR imaging: comparison with findings at autopsy. AJR 168: 41–46

Yakovlev PI, Lecours AR (1967) The myelogenetic cycles of regional maturation of the brain. In: Minkowski A (ed) Regional development of the brain in early life. Blackwell Scientific Publications, Oxford, pp 3–70

Yamashita Y, Namimoto T, Abe Y, Takahashi M, Iwamasa J, Miyazaki K, Okamura H (1997) MR imaging of the fetus by a HASTE sequence. AJR 168: 513–519

24 Post-therapeutic Imaging

ROLF H. JÄGER

CONTENTS

24.1 Introduction

Monitoring the effects of medical or surgical treatment form an important part of routine neuroradiological practice. This chapter gives an update of recent developments in post-therapeutic imaging. It does not attempt to be an encyclopaedic description of post-therapeutic imaging appearances but focuses on the application of new imaging techniques and/or imaging findings following relatively new forms of treatment. The structure of this chapter is disease-based rather than technology-based and new imaging techniques are discussed under the heading of particular diseases to which they can be applied.

24.2 Imaging Following Therapy for Vascular Disease

Non-invasive imaging of the blood vessels of the brain with CT and MR angiography is gradually replacing intra-arterial catheter angiography for diagnostic purposes. This is a rapidly developing field and further refinement of these techniques can be expected with the introduction of multidetector spiral CT scanners and contrast-enhanced MR angiography using systems with high performance gradients.

CT and MR angiography are likely to play an increasing role in the follow-up of patients who have undergone endovascular or surgical treatment. This would obviate the need for repeated intra-arterial studies, and contribute towards a decrease of the overall morbidity by eliminating the small but not negligible risk of stroke, which is associated with conventional catheter angiography and lies between 1–4% (HEISERMAN et al. 1994).

In addition to advances in the structural imaging of large and medium-sized blood vessels, it is now possible to study cerebral haemodynamics at a microvascular level with MR and CT perfusion imaging. In the near future these methods will enable us to measure tissue perfusion and will be more widely available than positron emission (PET) or single proton emission tomography (SPECT), which have been used in the past for this purpose.

Physiological information can also be obtained from the assessment of molecular motion with diffusion-weighted MR imaging and the quantification of blood flow velocity with phase contrast MRA.

R. H. JÄGER, MD
Consultant Neuroradiologist, Lysholm Radiological Department, The National Hospital of Neurology and Neurosurgery, and Clinical Senior Lecturer, Institute of Neurology, Queen Square, London, WC1N 3BG, UK

To assess the effects of treatment, the ability to document changes in physiological parameters might be just as important as the documentation of structural change.

MR perfusion imaging has so far been mainly used to assess the haemodynamic repercussions of steno-occlusive disease (Sorensen et al. 1996). There is scope for an extended application of this method to assess haemodynamic disturbances caused by other cerebrovascular diseases such as vasospasm in subarachnoid haemorrhage and cerebral AVMs.

Established and potential applications of post-treatment MR and CT angiography and perfusion imaging are discussed below.

24.2.1 Steno-occlusive Disease

MR angiography has been shown to be useful in the diagnosis of stenosis or occlusion of intracranial arteries. 3D TOF MRA appears to be superior to phase-contrast MRA (Oelerich et al. 1998). Ohue et al. (1998) used 3D TOF MR angiography in patients treated with intra-arterial thrombolysis for acute stroke. They found an excellent correlation between intra-arterial DSA and MRA in the demonstration of the site of occlusion before treatment with thrombolysis and subsequent recanalisation. In one patient MRA had also correctly identified a residual MCA artery stenosis after thrombolytic treatment. MRA could have a major impact on the management of patients with acute stroke particularly for those receiving intravenous thrombolysis should its accuracy in demonstrating occlusion and recanalisation of intracranial arteries be confirmed by further studies.

CT scanning frequently represents the first-line investigation of patients with a "brain attack". In many units it is more accessible for emergency investigations than MRI. CT angiography has been shown to identify the site of intracranial occlusion in acute stroke. It could represent a good and practicable alternative to MRA for planning and monitoring thrombolysis, if future studies show it to be equally sensitive in detecting recanalisation and residual stenosis.

In patients with an acute stroke, MR perfusion and diffusion imaging are increasingly used in an effort to distinguish potentially salvageable from irreversibly damaged tissue (see chapter 10). Recently there has been a report on the use of MR perfusion and diffusion imaging following intra-arterial thrombolysis (Lansberg et al. 1999). The authors suggest that these techniques might have a role in assessing the success of thrombolytic therapy, which is backed up by the results of animal studies (Takano et al. 1998). These methods can also be used in chronic steno-occlusive disease of the carotid arteries to assess the haemodynamic repercussions of stenoses and the functioning of autoregulatory mechanisms. Gillard et al. (1998) studied patients before and after carotid endarterectomy with MR perfusion imaging. They found a shortening of bolus arrival time in five out of eight patients on the operated side compared to the contralateral circulation. The bolus arrival returned to normal within 3–5 months after surgery and the authors postulated that the early postoperative findings may reflect postoperative hyperaemia. Perfusion imaging may have the potential of identifying patients at risk of postcarotid endarterectomy perfusion syndrome, which carries an increased risk of cerebral haemorrhage.

Hyperperfusion was also the presumed mechanism for unilateral leptomeningeal enhancement, which was observed by Wilkinson et al. (1999) immediately following stenting of carotid artery stenoses (Fig. 24.1).

24.2.2 Aneurysms

The usefulness of both CTA and MRA in demonstrating untreated aneurysms larger than 3–5 mm is well established (Atlas et al.1997; Velthuis et al. 1997). Current treatment of cerebral aneurysms includes surgical clipping and endovascular coiling. Both methods introduce a metallic foreign body into the patient's brain, which has implications for subsequent CT and MR scanning.

The presence of aneurysm clips precluded the patients from entering an MR scanner in the past, but modern titanium clips no longer represent a contraindication for MR scanning (local safety policies may, however, vary according to experience). Titanium is not ferromagnetic, which is why modern clips are not deflected and do not cause geometric field distortion. We have shown (Grieve et al. 1999) that there is nevertheless a small focal signal dropout around titanium clips due to magnetic susceptibility effects. This makes MRA unsuitable for screening for a residual neck of the clipped aneurysm. It can, however, still be used for non-invasive follow-up of coincidental unruptured aneurysms (Fig. 24.2).

There are no safety concerns for using CTA in patients with aneurysm clips. It can therefore also be

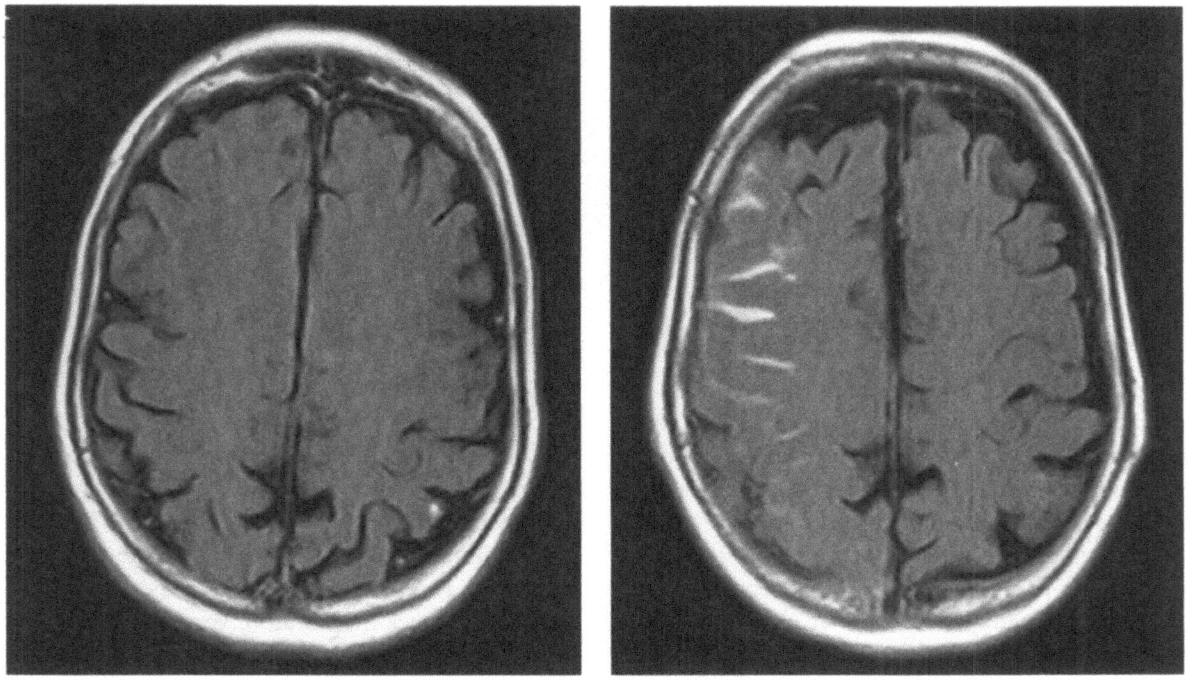

a b

Fig. 24.1a,b. Axial FLAIR sequence following injection of 20 ml Gd-DTPA prior to stenting of a right sided carotid artery stenosis (**a**) with no evidence of leptomeningeal enhancement. Axial FLAIR sequence immediately after stenting (**b**) without further contrast medium injection shows marked leptomeningeal enhancement ipsilateral to the stented carotid artery. Courtesy of Dr. Iain Wilkinson, Royal Hallamshire Hospital, Sheffield, UK

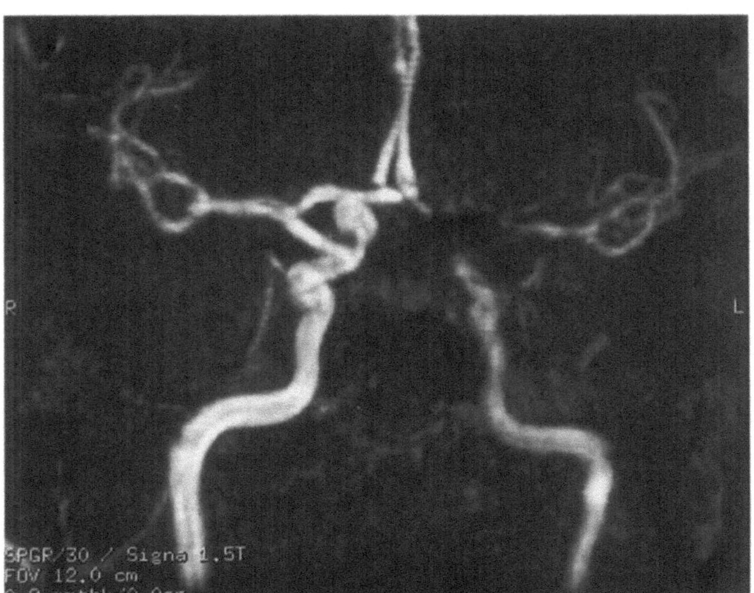

Fig. 24.2. 3D time-of-flight MR angiogram of the anterior cerebral circulation after clipping of a left terminal carotid artery aneurysm. Signal dropout around the titanium clip does not allow the assessment of the bifurcation from which the clipped aneurysm originated. The MRA shows, however, vasospasm of the distal left middle cerebral artery and a contralateral non-ruptured carotid-ophthalmic artery aneurysm

used in patients with old-fashioned aneurysm clips which are not MR compatible. Aneurysm clips cause beam-hardening artefacts on CT scans but the narrow collimation of the beam used in CTA reduces this artefact without completely eliminating it. The extent of this artefact is often difficult to predict in each individual case. Brown et al. (1999) described a technique to minimise beam-hardening artefact by tilting the patient's head, using an anteroposterior digital scout view as the reference image. The patient's head is subsequently tilted in such a way that the axial scanning plane through the aneurysm clip projects away from the circle of Willis. This maximises the image quality and allows follow-up of concomitant aneurysms or elucidation of equivocal findings on conventional angiograms. CTA can also demonstrate a residual neck of the clipped aneurysm when combined with subtraction and superimposition techniques (Vieco et al. 1996). In our own experience we have found the beam-hardening artefacts to be much less apparent on the 3D surface shaded images than on MIP images.

CTA is less useful in patients who have undergone endovascular coiling of aneurysms. GDC coils, which are composed of platinum, produce a much more marked beam-hardening artefact than aneurysm clips (Fig. 24.3a–c). Patients with platinum coils can, however, safely enter an MRI scanner (Hartman et al. 1997) and MR angiography can be used in the follow-up of coiled aneurysms (Derdeyn et al. 1997; Kähärä et al. 1999). Platinum coils still cause some susceptibility artefact on MRI, which is, however, less detrimental to the image quality than the beam-hardening artefact on CTA (Fig. 24.3d,e). Initial reports of using MRA for the follow-up of coiled aneurysms were encouraging: Derdeyn et al. (1997) reported a 100% sensitivity in detecting residual necks and were also able to show incomplete coiling with flow signal in the interstices between loops of coils. More recently, Kähärä et al. (1999) performed a blinded prospective study comparing DSA and MRA in the follow-up of coiled aneurysms and highlighted a few problems. Although they still found a 90% sensitivity in detecting remnant cavities with MRA, 6 out of 20 patients showed susceptibility artefact leading to false positive diagnoses of encroachment or occlusion of adjacent vascular segments in five patients. They also described one case where thrombus within a coiled giant aneurysm caused T1 shortening mimicking flow signal in the dome of the aneurysm. The authors conclude that MRA may be useful in the long-term follow-up of GDC-coiled small and medium-sized aneurysms, provided that the initial MRA is complemented by a DSA. They also point out the need for further prospective studies with a larger sample size.

24.2.3 AVMs

We showed in a prospective comparative study that the demonstration of feeding vessels, AVM nidus and draining veins on CT angiography correlates well with intraarterial DSA (Jäger et al. 1999). Multiple overlying vessels and the simultaneous demonstration of arteries and veins can become a problem in the interpretation of CTAs of very large AVMs.

Conventional 3D TOF MRA shows the AVM nidus and draining veins often incompletely because of saturation and spin dephasing effects. Phase-contrast MRA shows the draining veins better but the study might have to be repeated with a number of different velocity encoding steps, which lengthens the procedure.

Our own group and other investigators have shown that contrast-enhanced MR angiography can improve the delineation of the nidus and draining veins (Jäger et al. 1999).

CTA and contrast-enhanced MRA are likely to play a significant role in the imaging of AVMs after endovascular, radiosurgical and microsurgical treatment. Prospective comparison with conventional angiography is necessary to assess whether these new techniques can detect small residual nidi after endovascular, surgical or radiosurgical treatment.

CTA angiography can be used to show glue casts following endovascular treatment, provided the source data are reconstructed as maximum intensity projections since glue is indistinguishable from vessels on surface-shaded reconstructions (Fig. 24.4).

Both CTA and MRA use a volumetric data acquisition, which provides the potential for calculation of nidus volumes. This could be used for quantification of partial nidus obliteration. CTA may be particularly useful for quantification of partial embolisation procedures, because of its ability to visualise glue-casts.

Following treatment of AVMs with radiosurgery a number of specific complications can occur. These consist of leukoencephalopathy, radiation necrosis and radiation cysts (Fig. 24.5). Details of radiation injury to the brain and its imaging appearances are discussed below (see Sect. 24.3.1). The incidence of imaging changes following radiosurgery of AVMs is strongly dependent on the initial size of the AVM.

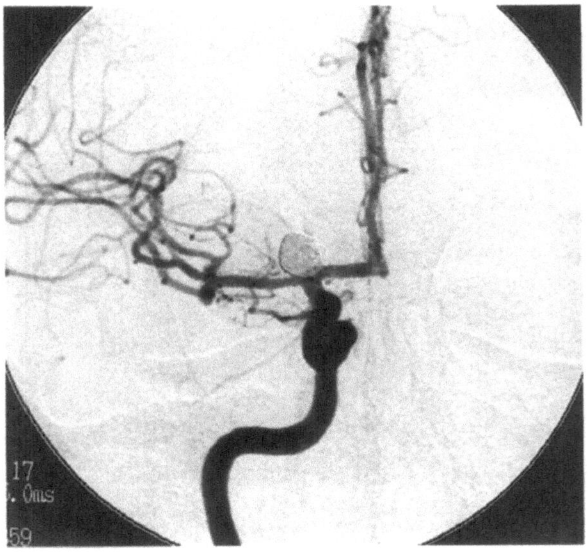

a

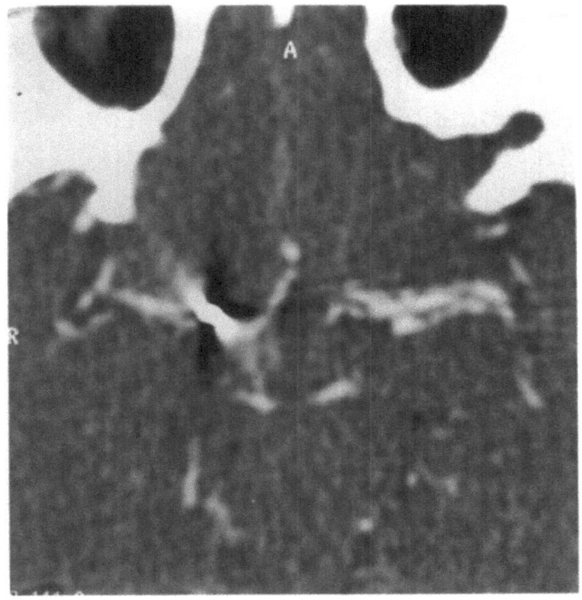

b

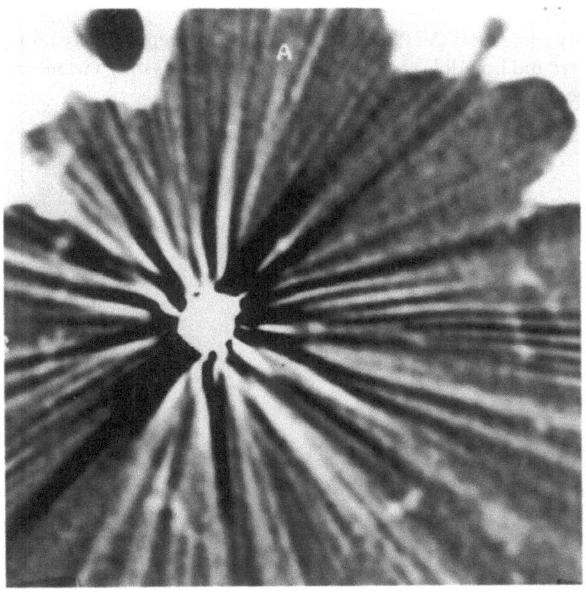

c

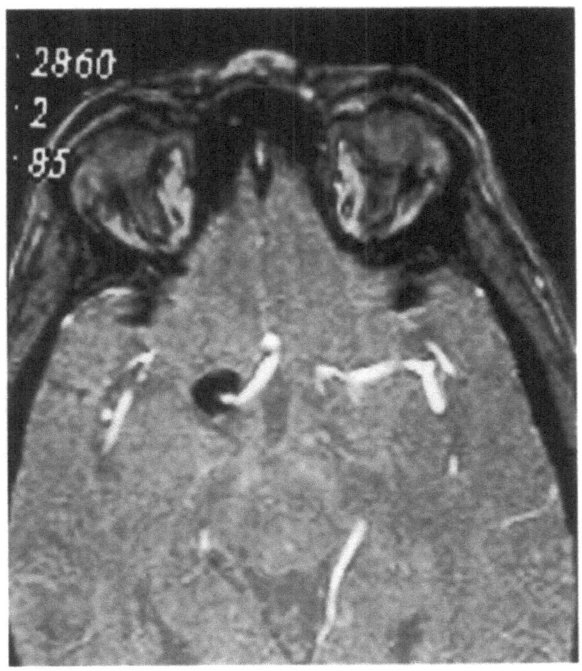

d

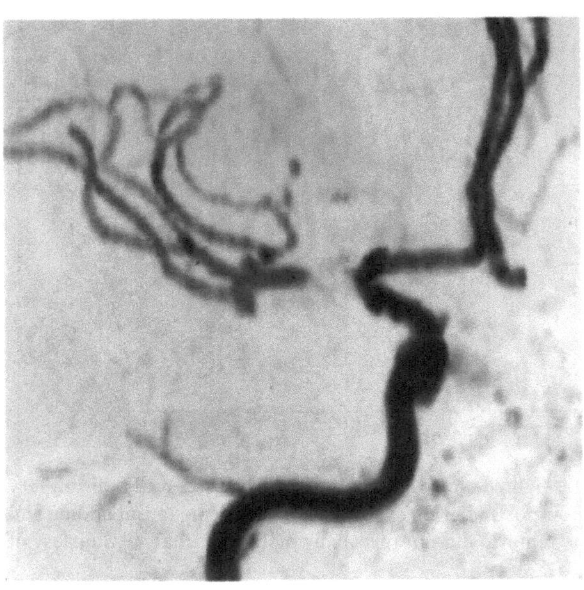

e

Fig. 24.3a–e. Fifty-year-old patient who had undergone coiling of an aneurysm at the terminal bifurcation of the right internal carotid artery. The DSA (**a**) shows complete obliteration of the coiled aneurysms and two additional small aneurysms arising from the trifurcation of the middle cerebral artery. Source images of a CT angiogram in this patient at the level of the neck (**b**) and fundus (**c**) of the coiled aneurysm demonstrate beam hardening artefact rendering the study non-diagnostic. Source data (**d**) and MIP image (**e**) of a 3D TOF MRA show less artefact than the CTA but there is still some loss of signal in the proximal portion of the MI segment. The coincidental MCA aneurysms are, however, well seen on the MIP image (**e**)

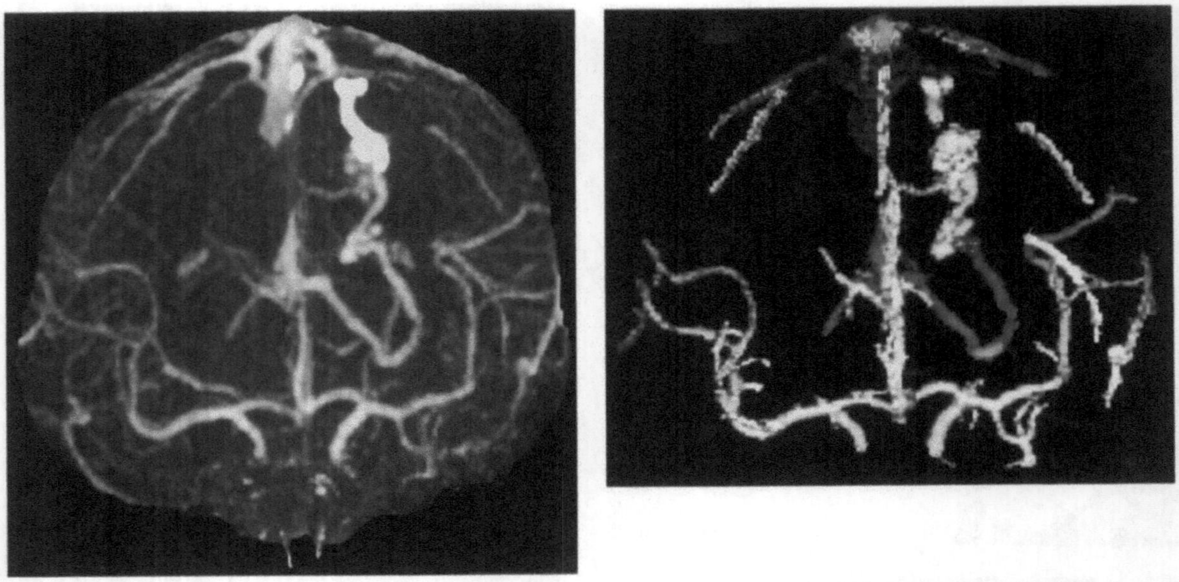

a b

Fig. 24.4a,b. Surface-shaded display (SSD) and maximum-intensity projection (MIP) of a small AVM with deep venous drainage, which had been partially embolised with mixture of histoacryl and lipiodol. The high-density glue cast is only visible on the MIP image (**a**) and remains undetected on the 3D SSD image (**b**)

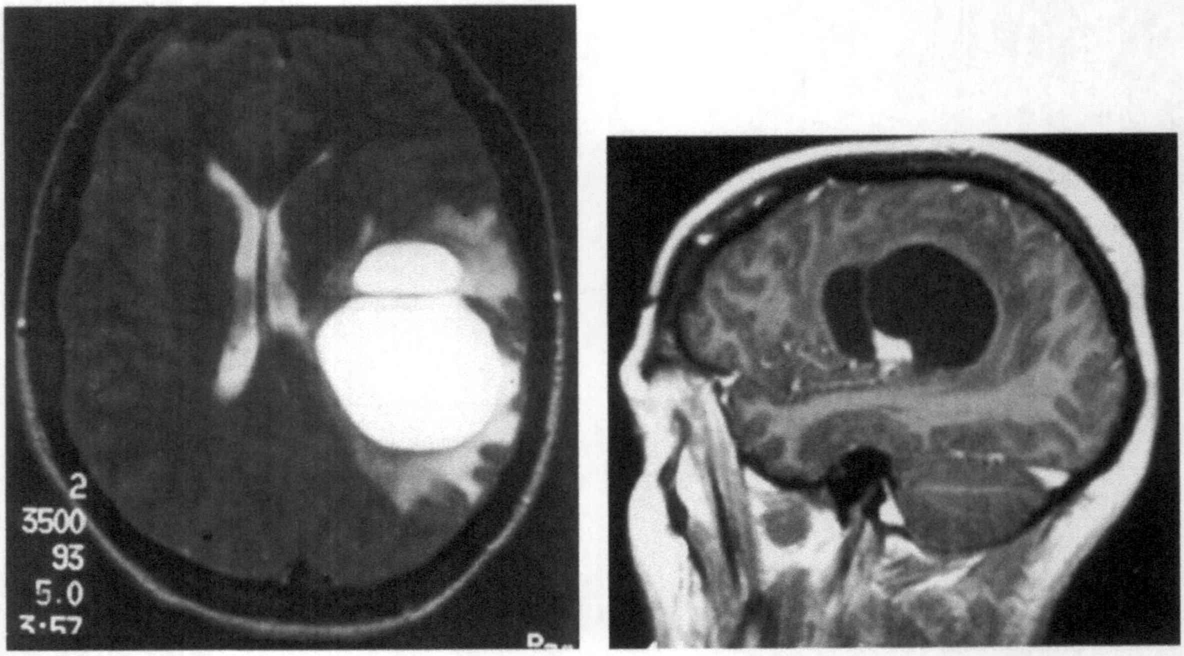

a b

Fig. 24.5a,b. Axial T2-weighted and sagittal contrast-enhanced T1 weighted images in a patient who had received radiosurgery for a frontoparietal AVM 15 years prior to the scan. The images show postradiation cysts with an enhancing mural nodule and surrounding vasogenic oedema. Histology following surgical cyst removal did not reveal any malignant change. Courtesy of Dr. Charles Romanowski, Royal Hallamshire Hospital, Sheffield, UK

Flickinger et al. (1992) found MR imaging changes at 2 years with a frequency of 0%, 6% and 46% for lesion volumes of 0–0.5 ml, 0.5–3.5 ml and 3.5–14.5 ml respectively. A recent paper by Miyawaki et al. (1999) looked at the results of large AVMs treated with a LINAC system and found at 5 years a 78% incidence of postradiosurgical MR imaging abnormalities in patients with AVMs larger than 30 ml. This was in contrast to an only 12.5% incidence of such abnormalities for AVMs smaller than 1 ml. The authors concluded that with increasing AVM size the dose-volume range for optimal balance between successful obliteration and the risk of complication narrows. Yamamoto et al. (1998) followed patients from 3 to 10 years after radiosurgery and found that adverse effects can occur at a late stage, long after obliteration of the AVM. They found a stenosis of the M1 segment of the middle cerebral artery appearing on serial MRA studies at 3 years, a delayed radionecrosis at 6 years, a dural AVM at 7 years and delayed cyst formation in three patients at 5, 7, and 10 years after radiosurgery. Two of these cysts had to be treated surgically; one regressed spontaneously.

We have recently used MR perfusion imaging to investigate perfusion abnormalities in patients with AVMs. These patients have a characteristic double negative peak on the time-signal intensity curves, due to recirculation (Jäger et al. 1999). In some patients with large AVMs we detected perfusion changes outside the AVM nidus, in the ipsilateral hemisphere. We have also been able to show changes on MR perfusion imaging following endovascular embolisation.

24.2.4 Caroticocavernous Fistulae

The treatment of choice for caroticocavernous fistulae is endovascular balloon occlusion. Gold valve balloons (Nycomed) are perfectly safe for MR scanning. We have used MRI with thin sections through the cavernous sinus to localise occlusion balloons and 3D TOF MR angiography to confirm patency of the internal carotid arteries in a number of patients. In patients where only subtotal occlusion could be achieved, 3D TOF MRA demonstrated residual venous drainage of the fistula (Fig. 24.6).

MRI scanning can also be useful to detect the cause of late complications of this procedure. Sencer et al. (1999) reported a patient who developed diplopia 1 year after endovascular balloon occlusion of a caroticocavernous fistula. An MRI scan revealed the migration of one of the multiple occlusion balloons into the superior ophthalmic vein, associated with impingement on the muscle cone in the orbital apex. The authors subsequently performed a CT guided puncture and deflation of the balloon, which resulted in immediate resolution of the symptoms.

24.3 Imaging Following Therapy for Neoplastic Disease

This section deals with the role of imaging following surgical and non-surgical treatment of benign and malignant brain tumours and following conditioning for bone marrow transplantation (BMT). The discussion of post-therapeutic imaging in specific tumours is preceded by a general description of the effects of radiotherapy and chemotherapy detectable on imaging.

24.3.1 Imaging Findings Following Radiotherapy and Chemotherapy

24.3.1.1 Radiotherapy

Radiotherapy can be given either as external beam therapy or as interstitial radiation by implantation of radioactive seeds (brachytherapy) (Hildebrand et al. 1997). There are two forms of external beam radiation: conventional fractionated radiotherapy and radiosurgery, which is a high precision localised, single fraction therapy, usually for lesions less than 3.5–4 cm in diameter (Brada 1999). The effect of radiation on the brain has a classic time dependent course, with the distinction of acute, early delayed and late radiation injury. Its severity depends on the total radiation dose, individual fraction size and volume of brain irradiated.

MR imaging is more sensitive than CT in detecting radiation induced damage to the brain such as diffuse white matter change, focal necrosis, CNS atrophy, teleangiectasia, optic neuritis and large vessel angiopathy and radiation induced neoplasias (Rabin et al. 1996) (Fig. 24.7). The only instance where CT is more sensitive is mineralising microangiopathy, which is found in a significant number of children after cranial radiation treatment and is associated with punctate calcification in the basal ganglia, cortex and brainstem.

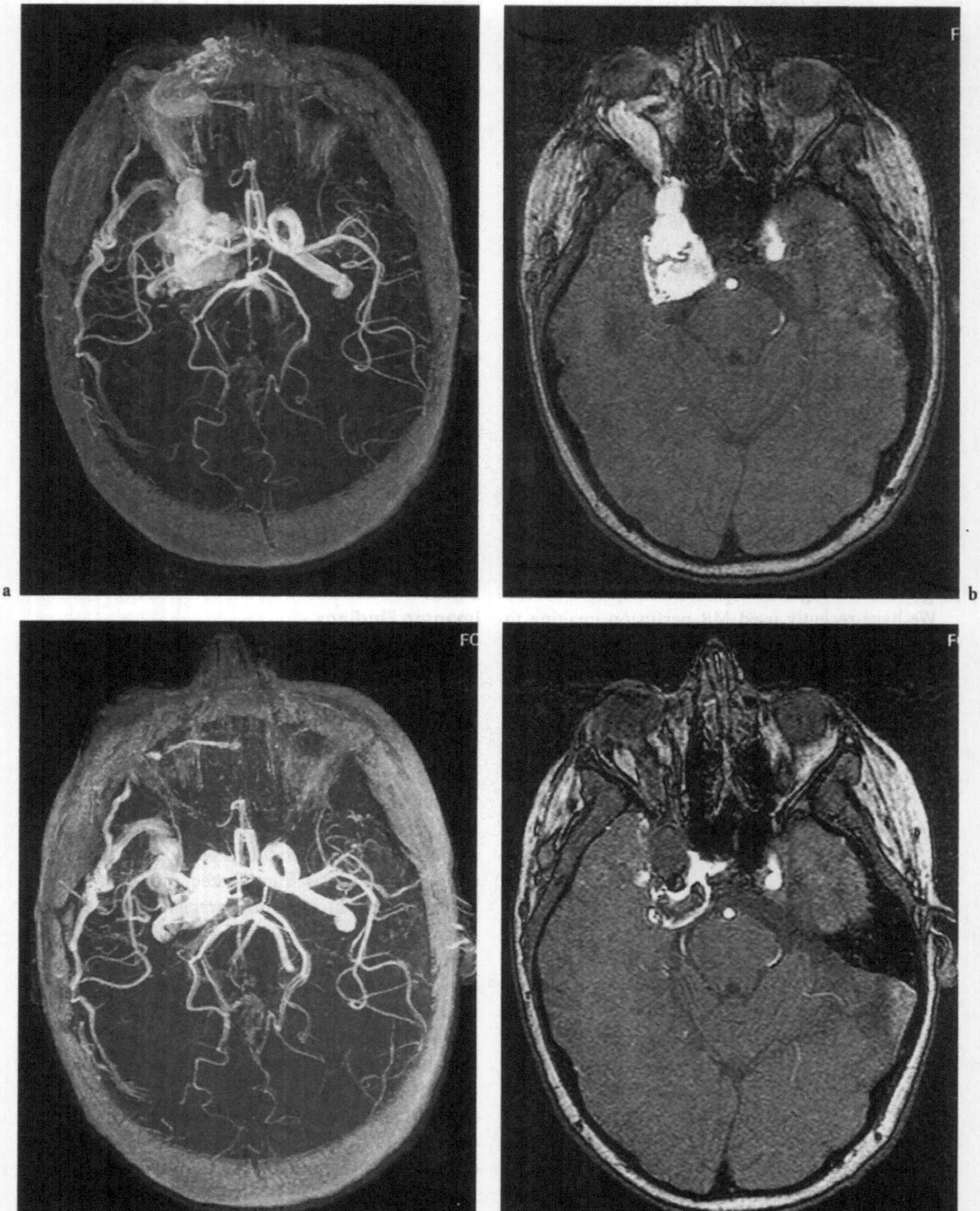

Fig. 24.6a–d. Axial MIP (**a,c**) and source images (**b,d**) of 3D TOF MR angiograms in a 14-year-old patient with a caroticocavernous fistula before (**a,b**) and after (**c,d**) occlusion with a gold valve balloon. The initial MRA shows a large caroticocavernous fistula draining into the ophthalmic and superficial cerebral veins. Complete balloon occlusion of the fistula was technically not possible. The post-treatment MRA shows a decrease in size of the fistula. Anterior drainage through ophthalmic veins in no longer visible but there remains some posterior drainage via the superficial cerebral vein (**c**). The axial source image (**d**) shows the position of the occlusion balloon, which is of low signal intensity. A further low-intensity structure posterior to it is likely to represent fresh clot. Note also the regression of the left proptosis

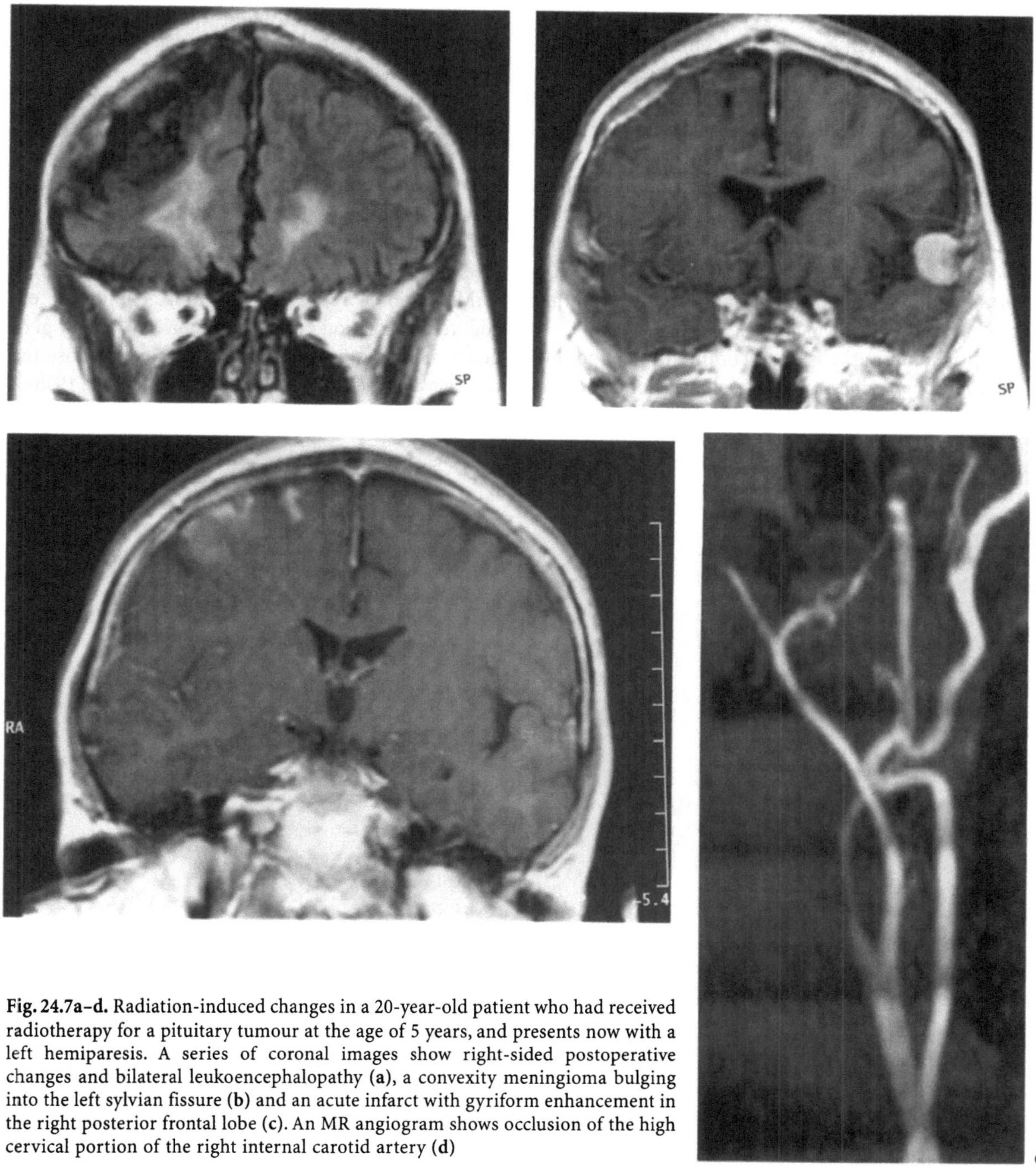

Fig. 24.7a–d. Radiation-induced changes in a 20-year-old patient who had received radiotherapy for a pituitary tumour at the age of 5 years, and presents now with a left hemiparesis. A series of coronal images show right-sided postoperative changes and bilateral leukoencephalopathy (**a**), a convexity meningioma bulging into the left sylvian fissure (**b**) and an acute infarct with gyriform enhancement in the right posterior frontal lobe (**c**). An MR angiogram shows occlusion of the high cervical portion of the right internal carotid artery (**d**)

Focal radiation necrosis is the most dreaded late complication and represents the single most dose-limiting factor. Necrosis occurs most frequently at the site of the previous tumour, even after whole brain irradiation. It can, however, also occur following treatment of benign lesions such as AVMs (Kihlstrom and Karlsson 1999). Radiation necrosis appears as a ring enhancing mass on CT and MR scans, and is surrounded by a variable amount of oedema. Clinically, these lesions are associated with focal neurological deficit and may require treatment with surgical resection and/or steroid therapy.

Radiation-induced white matter injury is a demyelinating process, which involves the periventricular region and can extend, usually in more severe cases, peripherally into the juxtacortical region. On MRI it appears as non-enhancing, confluent, usually symmetrical areas of T2 high signal. There is a poor correlation between the severity of the imaging findings and clinical symptoms.

Radiation can also cause atrophy of the cerebrum and cerebellum. In a study of a cohort of bone marrow transplant patients, we have found that subtle changes in brain volume are detectable after only 1 week following irradiation with a relatively small dose of 1440 cGy (Jäger et al. 1996).

Teleangiectasias are due to dilatation of capillary vessels in the cerebral white matter and have been found in patients receiving doses from 1800 to 7800 cGy. Occasionally these can haemorrhage (Poussaint et al. 1995) and the MR appearances can then be confused with cavernomas.

Optic neuropathy is most commonly seen following therapy of sellar and parasellar lesions and represents a late complication, showing a high T2 signal change typically in the intracranial portion of the optic nerve (Fig. 24.8).

Radiation induced large vessel steno-occlusive disease can occur between 4 months and 20 years after irradiation and is caused by intimal proliferation, thrombosis and accelerated arteriosclerotic change (Rabin et al. 1996). It typically affects the extra- or intracranial portions of the internal carotid arteries (see Fig. 24.7).

Meningioma represents the most commonly encountered radiation induced tumour. The latency period for meningiomas depends on the radiation dose and can vary between 19 and 35 years (Rabin et al. 1996).

a

b

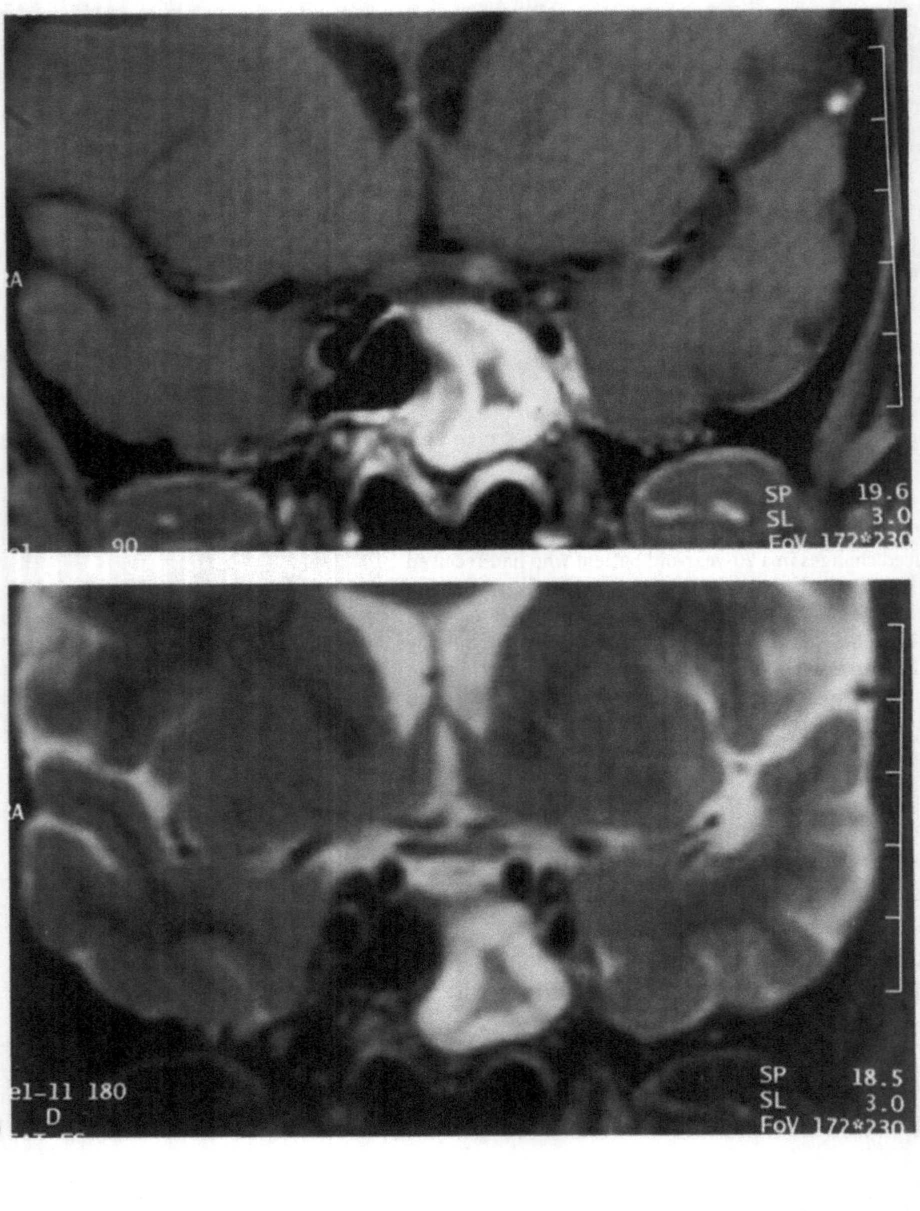

Fig. 24.8a,b. Coronal contrast-enhanced T1-weighted sequence through the intracranial portion of the optic nerves (**a**) and T2-weighted sequence through the optic chiasm (**b**) in a patient who had received radiotherapy for a left-sided orbital lymphoma. There is enhancement of the intracranial potion of the left optic nerve and thickening and T2 hyperintensity of the left side of the chiasm (**b**). The appearances are consistent with radiation damage to the left optic nerve

24.3.1.2
Chemotherapy

A larger number of chemotherapeutic agents are potentially neurotoxic affecting the peripheral or central nervous system. Clinical symptoms of CNS toxicity include acute and chronic encephalopathy, cerebellar syndrome and stroke-like episodes (Keime-Guilbert et al. 1998). The most frequent imaging findings are chronic leukoencephalopathy, which produces bilateral white matter lesions that are of low density on CT and T2-hyerintense on MRI. The changes affect predominantly the periventricular region but may extend into the juxtacortical white matter. Chemotherapeutic agents can be administered by intravenous, intra-arterial, intrathecal and intraventricular (through an Ommaya reservoir) routes. The occurrence and severity of neurotoxic effects depend on route of administration, dose, and combination with radiotherapy (see below). Chronic leukoencephalopathy is most likely to occur after high-dose intravenous or intrathecal methotrexate (Lövblad et al. 1998) (Fig. 24.9) and high-dose intravenous fludarabine. With intra-arterial (intracarotid) BCNU infusion, the white matter changes are confined to the treated vascular territory.

24.3.1.3
Combined treatment with radiotherapy and chemotherapy

Multimodality treatment combining chemotherapy and radiotherapy can result in additive and synergistic effects of neurotoxicity. Although it may be sometimes difficult to identify the offending agent in this context, there is clinical experience of "dangerous liaisons" between radiotherapy and chemotherapy (Keime-Guilbert et al. 1998). The effects do not only depend on the dose but also on the order of administration. Several interactions are possible: chemotherapeutic agents given prior to radiotherapy may act as radiosensitisers, radiotherapy given prior to chemotherapeutic agents may increase the permeability of the blood-brain barrier for the latter and lastly both forms of treatment may have an additive effect by targeting the same cellular structures.

There is experimental and clinical evidence that cisplatin and cytosine arabinoside are radiosensitisers and increase the risk of leukoencephalopathy when given prior to radiotherapy. Combined treatment with methotrexate and cranial irradiation for acute lymphatic leukaemia, or sometimes primary brain tumours, represents the best-known clinical

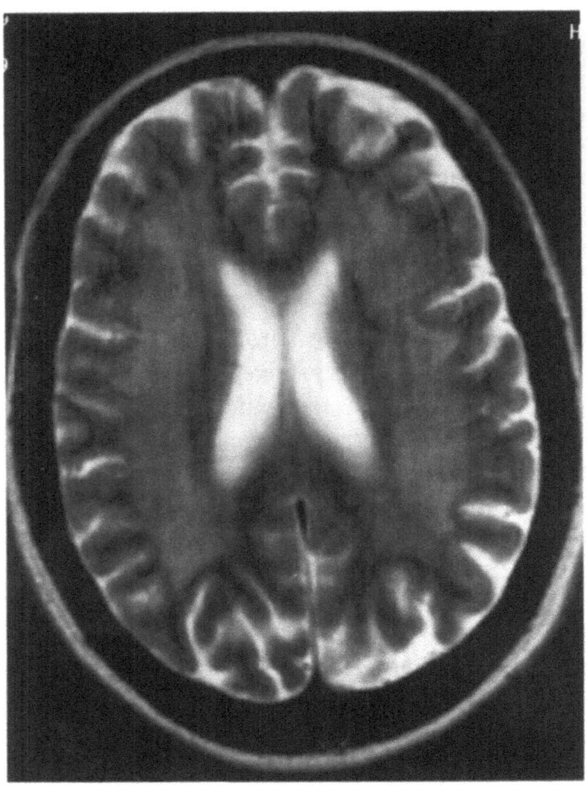

a

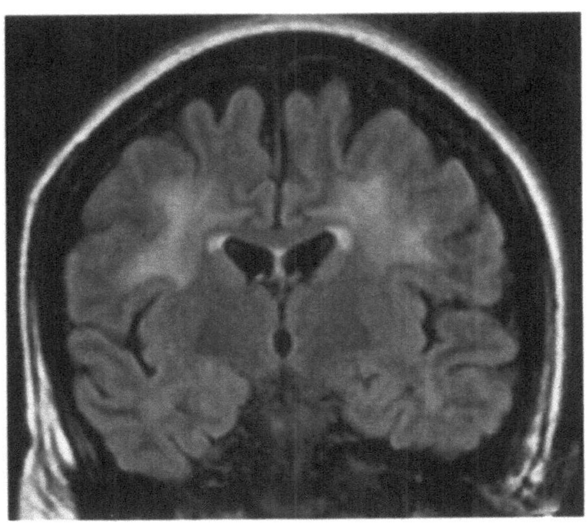

b

Fig. 24.9a,b. Twenty-year-old female patient who had received intrathecal methotrexate for treatment of acute lymphatic leukaemia. Axial T2-weighted MRI (**a**) and the coronal FLAIR sequence (**b**) show confluent symmetrical high signal in the cerebral white matter consistent with leukoencephalopathy example of synergistic toxicity. The dependence of the neurotoxic effects on the sequence of administration is well documented in this case: the risk of developing leukoencephalopathy is lower if methotrexate is given before radiotherapy but is considerably increased when this sequence is reversed or the treatments are given concurrently. Sometimes it is not possible to avoid a reversal of the ideal sequence of administration as in the case of intrathecal treatment with methotrexate for a relapse of acute lymphatic leukaemia after bone marrow transplantation, which will have included cranial irradiation as part of the conditioning procedure.

24.3.2 Malignant Cerebral Tumours

24.3.2.1 Glioma

Surgery and radiotherapy represent currently the mainstay in the treatment of high-grade gliomas (anaplastic astrocytomas and glioblastoma multiforme). Surgery is essential for accurate diagnosis and debulking to relieve intracranial pressure. The effect of radical surgery on survival is debatable but an inverse relationship between the amount of neoplastic tissue left after operation and survival has been described by some authors (Hildebrand et al. 1997). The extent of resection is often difficult to judge during surgery and a contrast-enhanced CT or, preferably, MR scan within 3–4 days of surgery provides a much clearer picture. After this time enhancement of neovascularised tissue may interfere. Long term follow-up scans are used to assess growth of any residual tumour or recurrence of an apparently completely resected tumour.

Survival rates following surgery alone, even after a large resection, are poor but can be substantially increased by radiotherapy. The standard treatment is external beam irradiation with 6000 cGy delivered in 30 fractions over 6 weeks, including a safety margin of 2 cm around the tumour. With this fractionation radiation necrosis is unlikely to occur. Single fraction radiosurgery with a gamma knife can only be used for small tumours and carries a higher risk of radiation necrosis. It may have a role in the treatment of malignant gliomas as a boost after conventional surgery and radiotherapy (Hildebrand et al. 1997).

Imaging following radiotherapy is useful to monitor the tumour response and identify associated side effects (Fig. 24.10). The different types of radiation injury to the brain and their imaging appearances have been discussed above. In the case of treated malignant gliomas, differentiation between tumour recurrence and radiation necrosis can represent a diagnostic challenge on follow-up scans. Both conditions present as an enhancing mass lesion and may be indistinguishable on conventional CT and MRI. A number of additional investigations have been proposed to aid their differentiation. Positron emission tomography (PET) using fluorine-18 fluorodeoxyglucose and single positron emission tomography (SPECT) using thallium-201 show an increased tracer uptake in recurrent high-grade tumours and a decreased tracer uptake in areas of radiation necrosis (Stokkel et al. 1999). Recent studies have cast some doubt on the accuracy of 18-FDG PET in differentiating radiation necrosis from tumour. Ricci et al. (1998) found a considerable number of false positive and false negative results on PET scanning, which would have led to inappropriate treatment of nearly one-third of their patients. These results are corroborated by Stokkel et al. (1999), who performed a systematic comparison of 18-FDG PET and 201 Tl SPECT and found the latter to be much more sensitive for detection of tumour recurrence.

On MR proton spectroscopy recurrence of high-grade tumours is usually associated with an increase in choline and decrease in *N*-acetyl-aspartate levels, whereas radiation necrosis shows a decrease in both metabolites and sometimes also an increase in lactate levels (Taylor et al. 1996). Nelson et al. (1997) underlined the superiority of multivoxel MR spectroscopy (chemical shift imaging) in distinguishing areas of radiation necrosis and tumour recurrence occurring simultaneously and lying close together.

There is preliminary evidence that dynamic contrast-enhanced MR perfusion imaging is able to distinguish radiation necrosis from tumour. Hazle et al. (1997) had previously looked at signal-enhancement-time curves on sequential T1-weighted fast spin echo images and found a much more rapid contrast medium uptake in tumour tissue than in radiation necrosis reflecting increased perfusion in the former. Differences in tissue perfusion can also be investigated with T2*-weighted perfusion imaging, and commercial software programs generating colour perfusion maps from T2*-weighted images are now available. This method appears promising in the distinction of radiation necrosis from recurrent tumour (Fig. 24.11) (Tannenbaum, personal communication 1999).

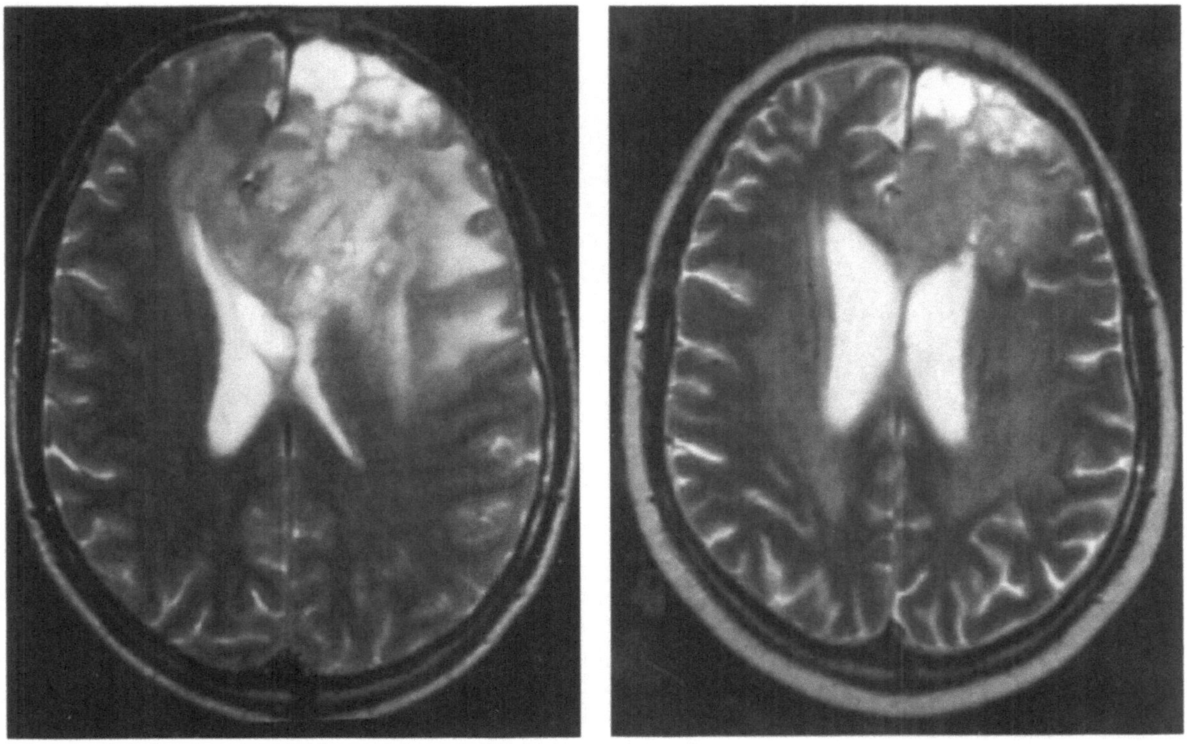

a b

Fig. 24.10a,b. T2-weighted MRI scans of a 31-year-old male patient with an anaplastic glioma before (**a**) and after (**b**) fractionated radiotherapy. The pre-treatment scan (**a**) shows a large heterogeneous mass in the left frontal lobe which extends across the corpus callosum and is surrounded by oedema. There is mass effect with displacement and compression of the lateral ventricles. An MRI scans performed 4 months after radiotherapy (**b**) shows a marked reduction in tumour size, surrounding oedema and mass effect with re-expansion of the lateral ventricles. There is, however, also a more subtle, diffuse signal increase in the white matter of both hemispheres, consistent with radiation-induced leukoencephalopathy

The role of adjuvant chemotherapy in malignant gliomas is not clear at the moment, with a variety of regimens being proposed including intravenous, intrathecal and local intra-arterial delivery (HILDEBRAND et al. 1997).

New methods of treatment such as gene therapy and immunotherapy are in an experimental stage and should be rigorously assessed in randomised trials. These trials should integrate standardised imaging protocols, preferably including state-of-the-art MR perfusion and diffusion imaging as well as volumetric 3D MR sequences with coregistration programs to assess subtle changes in tumour volume and enhancement between serial examinations.

There is less consensus on the treatment of low grade gliomas. It appears that radiotherapy may be of some benefit in delaying the progression to high-grade tumours but it is doubtful that overall survival can be prolonged by this. BAUMAN et al. (1999) used linear, area and segmented volume measurements on CT and MRI scans to quantify the radiological response of low grade gliomas to radiation therapy which they subsequently correlated with symptom control and patient survival. It appeared that only those patients where the tumour mass had been reduced by over 50% had a longer survival. Quantification of tumour volume following radiation treatment may therefore have prognostic implications.

TEDESCHI et al. (1997) used serial proton magnetic resonance spectroscopy in grade 2 and grade 3 gliomas, which had been treated with surgery and radiotherapy, in an attempt to predict malignant degeneration. They found that stable brain tumours showed either a decrease of choline or an increase of less than 35% whereas those progressing to a higher grade showed a choline increase of more than 45%.

24.3.2.2
Other Malignant Tumours

There is an increasing incidence of primary non-Hodgkin's lymphomas (PNHL) of the CNS, not only in immunocompromised but also in immunocompetent patients. At least 50% of these tumours show a

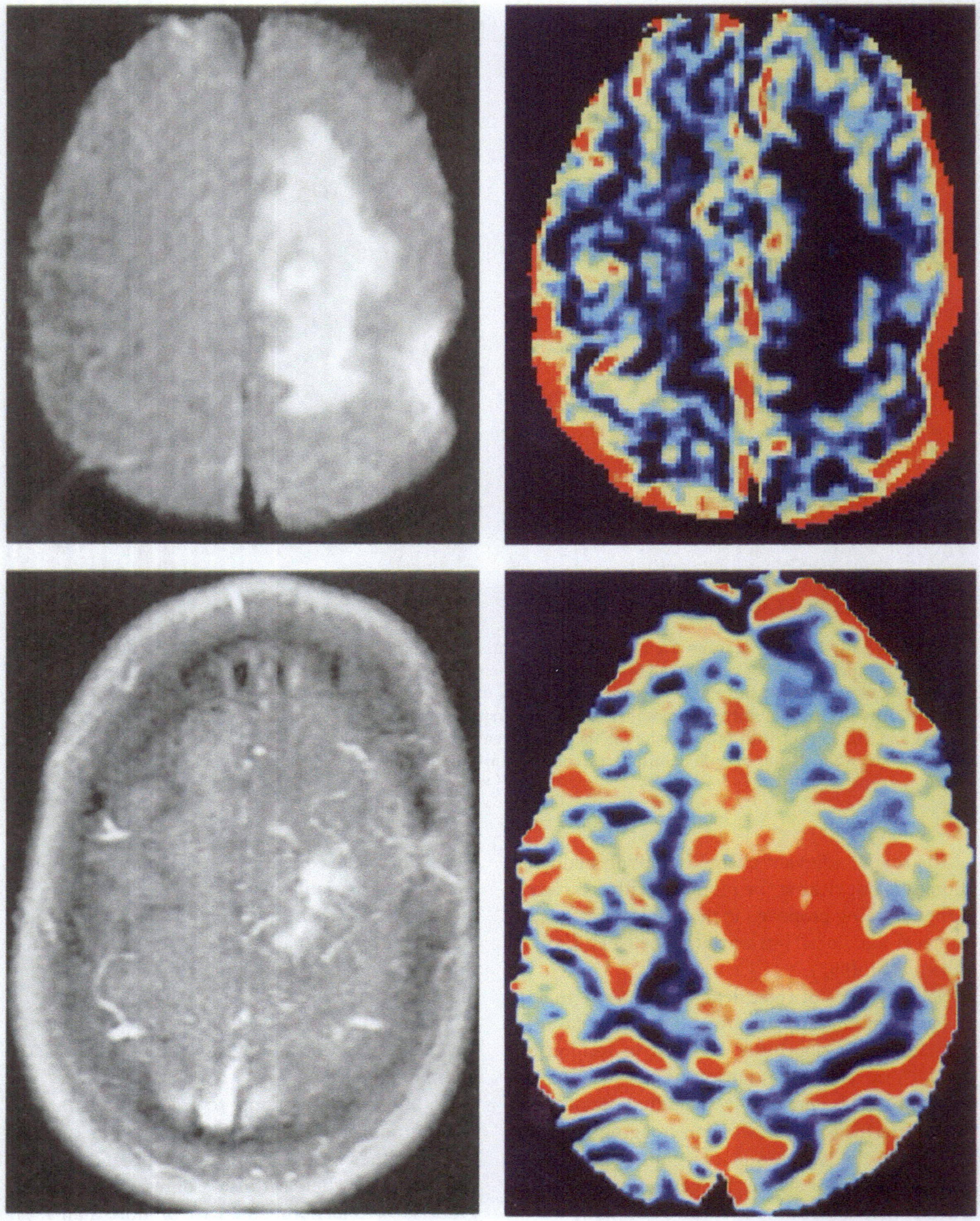

Fig. 24.11a–d. Distinction of radiation necrosis (**a**,**b**) and tumour recurrence (**c**,**d**) using MR perfusion imaging. In the first case, there is a frontoparietal mass lesion with oedema (**a**), which shows a decrease in blood volume on the rCBV map of the MR perfusion scan (**b**). Biopsy of the lesion confirmed radiation necrosis. In the second case, there is an enhancing mass in the left posterior frontal lobe (**c**) with an increased blood volume on the rCBV map (**d**). This proved to be tumour recurrence. Courtesy of Dr. Larry Tannenbaum, JFK Imaging Centre, Edison, New Jersey, USA

rapid response to treatment with glucosteroids, which can take effect in 24 h and has been ascribed to their cytolytic effect. Although a rapid response to steroids on serial neuroimaging may be highly suggestive of the diagnosis of PNHL, it is preferable to perform biopsy before commencing treatment with steroids since their cytolytic effects may compromise the pathological diagnosis.

Most lymphomas recur after a few months of steroid treatment but longer lasting effects with remission up to several years have been documented (PIROTTE et al. 1997). The therapy of PNHL continues to evolve, but there is now sufficient evidence that a combination of high-dose systemic and intrathecal therapy with methotrexate, possibly combined with cytosine arabinoside and irradiation, can increase the median survival to about 40 months (HILDEBRAND et al. 1997). This combination therapy carries, however, a high risk of neurotoxic effects.

Amongst the malignant brain tumours, medulloblastomas and ependymomas have a more favourable course. Surgical resection should be performed and its extent represents an important prognostic feature. The 5-year survival rate for both tumours lies above 80% following complete resection and, in the case of medulloblastoma, additional irradiation. MR imaging plays a key role in determining the extent of resection and detection of recurrence, even after seemingly complete initial resection (Fig. 24.12).

Whole brain radiotherapy has been the mainstay of the treatment of brain metastases, surgical resection being only an option for a single metastasis. Radiosurgery has recently been used in some centres for treatment of cerebral metastases. The survival of these patients is often related to the state of the systemic malignancy and the indication for post-therapeutic neuroimaging remains uncertain. HAWIGHORST et al. (1997) performed serial MR imaging following radiosurgery of intracranial metastases and found the disappearance of central or homogeneous contrast-enhancement to be a good prognostic sign.

24.3.3 Benign Cerebral Tumours

24.3.3.1 Meningiomas

The treatment of choice for meningiomas is surgical resection, which may be complete or partial. Some patients with residual or recurrent disease may subsequently be treated with radiotherapy. At our institution we reviewed postoperative MRI and CT scans in 60 patients who were followed up for an average of 6.5 years (HODGSON et al. 1995). Tumour recurrence was found only in 2 of 34 patients who had had a macroscopic clearance at the initial operation. Both patients had developed new symptoms and signs. Of the patients with residual tumours, patient management was influenced by imaging in 7 of 18 patients who had further surgery or radiotherapy or both. The conclusion of this study was that routine follow-up MRI and CT scans in patients with complete resection is of little use, unless new symptoms or signs become manifest. Imaging has, however, a role in monitoring patients with incompletely resected meningiomas.

24.3.3.2 Pituitary Tumours

The management of pituitary tumours has changed in recent years (BEVAN 1999). Radiotherapy is no longer given routinely following surgery of endocrinologically non-active macroadenomas. This is largely a consequence of modern imaging techniques, mainly high resolution MRI scanning, which enable the assessment of the extent of resection and the detection of tumour regrowth with serial imaging. Prolactinomas are treated medically with bromocriptine or newer dopamine agonists and MRI imaging, along with blood tests, is important for monitoring of the tumour response. Even large tumours compressing the optic pathways can resolve (Fig. 24.13).

24.3.4 Imaging Following Bone Marrow Transplantation

Allogeneic bone marrow transplantation (BMT) is increasingly being used for treatment of haematological and solid malignancies (DUNCOMBE 1997). Prior to transplantation, the bone marrow recipient undergoes a conditioning program, which includes total body irradiation and administration of cytotoxic drugs, most often high dose chemotherapy with cyclophosphamide. Following the bone marrow transplantation, the recipient is treated with immunosuppressive agents to prevent graft-versus-host disease. Both the conditioning treatment and the immunosuppressive therapy can have neurotoxic effects, with abnormal findings on MRI. In a prospective study using co-registered serial MR examinations

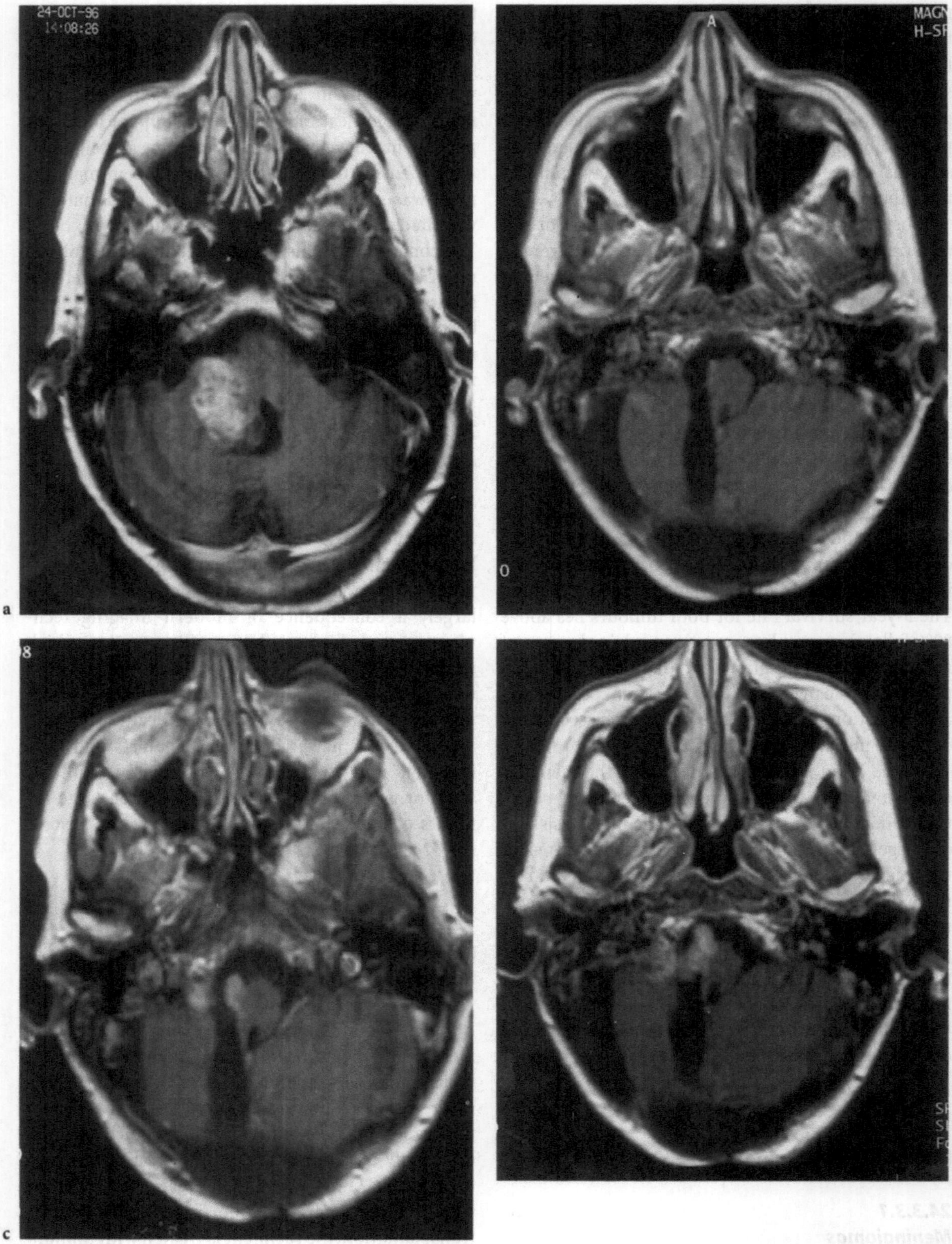

Fig. 24.12a–d. Contrast-enhanced T1-weighted MRI scans in a 53-year-old female with a posterior fossa ependymoma before operation (**a**) and at 6 months (**b**), 2 years (**c**) and 3 years (**d**) after surgery. The scans at 6 months after surgery show a small area of linear enhancement adjacent to the medulla oblongata along the medial resection margin. This could have been postoperative enhancement, but follow-up scans showed progressive enlargement (**c,d**), consistent with tumour recurrence

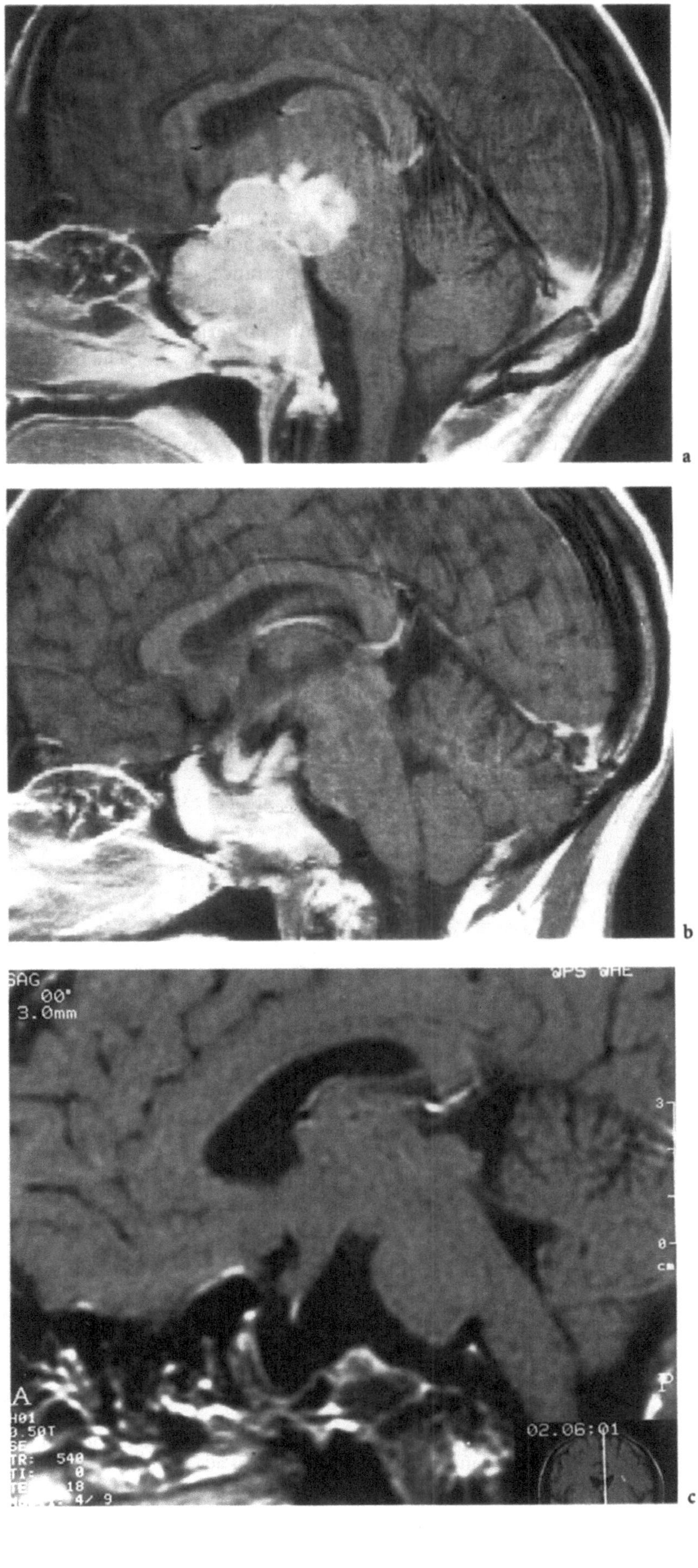

Fig. 24.13a–c. A series of sagittal contrast-enhanced T1-weighted MRI scans in a patient with a prolactin-secreting pituitary macroadenoma. The pre-treatment scan (**a**) shows a large tumour, which compresses the optic chiasm and third ventricle and indents the midbrain and pons. Three months after treatment with bromocriptine (**b**) there has been a marked decrease in tumour size with re-expansion of the third ventricle, the residual tumour remaining mainly in the sella and sphenoid sinus. Six months after bromocriptine treatment (**c**), the tumour has completely resolved and the enlarged sella is empty

(Jäger et al. 1996), we found subtle enlargement of the ventricles as early as 1 week after conditioning and a continued increase of the CSF spaces, including cortical sulci, over a 3–6 month period (Fig. 24.14). Although the precise cause for this remains unclear, it is likely to be due to synergistic effects of cranial radiation and cytotoxic drugs.

Amongst the immunosuppressive drugs used to prevent a graft-versus-host reaction, cyclosporin is the most neurotoxic. Typical imaging appearances of cyclosporin toxicity are high signal change in the white matter of the parietal, occipital and posterior frontal lobes (Shah 1999). The signal abnormality involves usually the juxtacortical matter but may also extend into the cortex (Fig. 24.15). The imaging abnormalities resolve after discontinuation of cyclosporin. The mechanism of cyclosporin toxicity is likely to be a breakdown of the blood-brain barrier, resulting in leakage of fluid into the interstitial space (Shah 1999). This theory has been corroborated in a recent study by Coley et al. (1999), who used quantitative MR diffusion imaging in two patients with cyclosporin-induced neurotoxicity. They showed that the areas of increased T2 signal intensity corresponded to regions of increased diffusion, consistent with extravasation of fluid into the extracellular space and not with cytotoxic oedema, which would restrict the diffusion.

The imaging appearances are indeed very similar to other reversible posterior leukoencephalopathy syndromes, such as hypertensive encephalopathy, eclampsia and interferon alpha toxicity (Hinchey et al. 1996). The predominant involvement of the posterior white matter in these cases has been attributed to a decreased autoregulatory response of the posterior circulation, which has less a-adrenergic receptors than the anterior circulation. Neurotoxicity of cyclosporin is multifactorial and does not depend on cyclosporin levels alone. Coexisting promoting factors are hypertension, hypocholesterolaemia, hypoalbuminaemia and cytochrome p450 activity. There is also evidence of cyclosporin toxicity occurring more frequently in patients with an HLA disparity between the donor and host, which increases

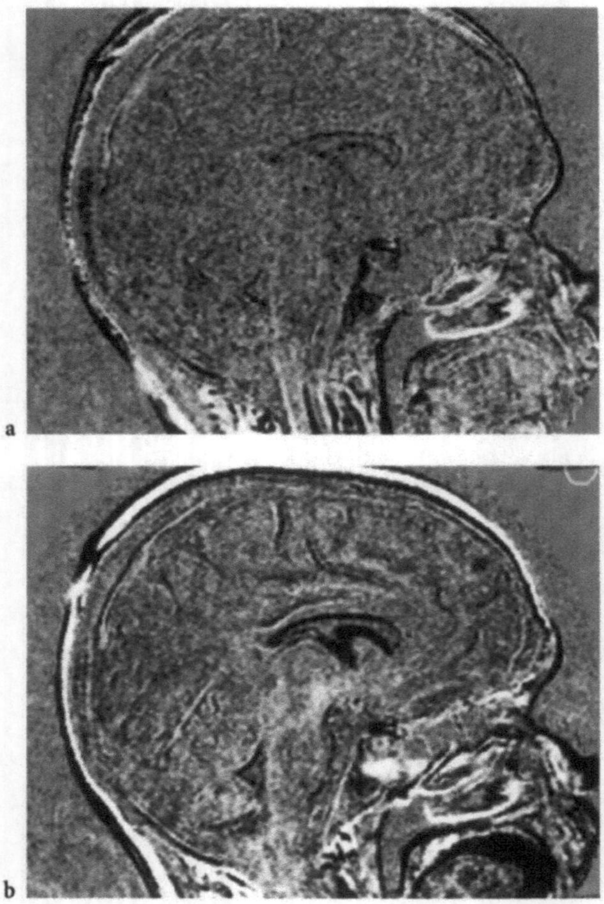

Fig. 24.14a,b. Difference images obtained by subtraction of a baseline MRI from follow-up scans obtained at 6 days (a) and 3 months (b) following bone marrow transplantation. This technique used serial T1-weighted 3D volume scans and a subvoxel registration program. *Dark lines* indicate an increase in size of the lateral ventricles after 6 days (a). This becomes more marked after 3 months (b) and there is additional sulcal enlargement

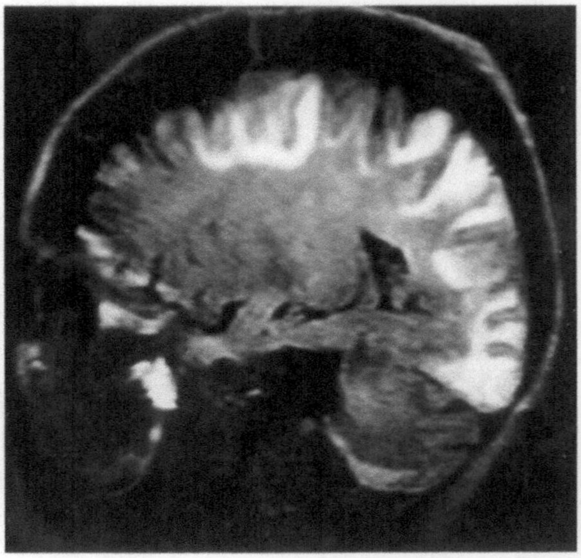

Fig. 24.15. Cyclosporin toxicity in a bone marrow recipient. A sagittal FLAIR sequence shows high signal change in the subcortical white matter of the occipital, parietal and posterior frontal lobes. In some areas the abnormal signal extends into cortex. The changes resolved after discontinuation of the cyclosporin treatment

the chance of developing graft-versus-host disease (ZIMMER et al. 1998), since GVHD represents a risk factor for immune-mediated microangiopathy leading to increased capillary permeability.

Immunosuppression puts patients at risk of developing CNS infections, which occur in approximately 2% of all BMT recipients. Since the clinical signs of infection are often obscured or non-specific during the neutropenic phase, neuroimaging assumes an important role in making the diagnosis. Various types of host defence mechanisms are impaired after BMT. These follow a relatively predictable time course and are paralleled by an increased risk of viral, fungal, bacterial and parasitic infections at specific times post-BMT. This has been described in detail elsewhere (COLEY et al. 1999). It is important to bear in mind that drugs used for treatment and prophylactics of infection can also have neurotoxic effects. BLOHM et al. (1997) described a case of acyclovir neurotoxicity producing reversible enhancing lesions in the cortical and subcortical regions.

Sometimes it is necessary to treat a relapse of acute lymphatic leukaemia following BMT with intrathecal methotrexate. This can be complicated by a particularly devastating leukoencephalopathy since the neurotoxic effects of methotrexate are potentiated by the preceding radiotherapy given for conditioning.

24.4 Imaging Following Therapy for Non-vascular and Non-neoplastic Disease

24.4.1 Epilepsy

In patients with epilepsy, MRI plays a key role in the diagnosis of mesial temporal sclerosis. Imaging following temporal lobe resection in patients with intractable seizures provides an objective measure of the volume of tissue resected. KITCHEN et al. (1995) described a method for the estimation of removed tissue volume in lesional epilepsy. There is emerging evidence that the success of the operation is in some way dependent on the volume of resected tissue. MORAN et al. (1999) have recently described a process of volumetric analysis of temporal lobe resections. With this method, the authors hope to establish a relation between anatomical resection and seizure as well as neuropsychological outcome.

MR imaging in patients developing side effects of medical treatment can be useful to document neurotoxic effects of antiepileptic drugs. Cerebellar atrophy following treatment with phenytoin is well known but other anticonvulsants can also be neurotoxic. A recent report described focal lesions in the corpus callosum of patients receiving dilantin and/or vigabatrim which disappeared after discontinuing the drugs and are likely to represent reversible toxic demyelination (KIM et al. 1999).

24.4.2 Movement Disorders

Although treatment with levadopa represents one of the most significant advances in the treatment of Parkinson's disease, long term treatment can result in levadopa-induced dyskinesias or symptoms unresponsive to dopaminergic therapy. In recent years neurosurgical procedures such as thalamotomy and pallidotomy have been facilitated by imaging guidance (QUINN and BHATIA 1998). There is now an increasing demand for these procedures, which use heat lesioning electrodes into the appropriate nuclei. Unilateral pallidotomy dramatically reduces contralateral levadopa induced dyskinesias but is less effective in alleviating ipsilateral symptoms. Bilateral pallidotomy is on the other hand associated with a much higher complication rate. The search for other ways of altering damaged brain function and the discovery that stimulating electrodes used to guide lesion placement for pallidotomy could abolish tremor at high frequency discharges, has led to the implantation of chronic electronic pulse stimulators, up to now primarily used in pain control. Stimulation of either the thalamic 15 or subthalamic 16 nuclei provides control of parkinsonian tremor and dyskinesias (POWELL 1999). The procedure is less risky than thalamotomy or pallidotomy, its effects are reversible (by switching off) and bilateral stimulation can be applied.

MRI scans following destructive pallidotomy or stimulator placement are useful to document the site and extent of the lesion or position of the electrode (Fig. 24.16), and to rule out procedure-related complications such as haemorrhage.

24.4.3 Inflammatory Disease

In remitting/relapsing multiple sclerosis, treatment with interferon beta-1a has been shown to decrease the number of new and enlarging lesions on T2-weighted MR images, compared to placebo (PRISMS

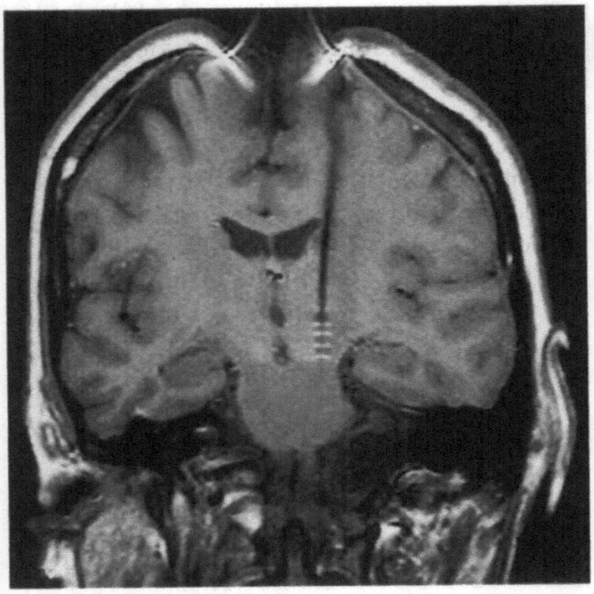

Fig. 24.16. A coronal T1-weighted MRA in a 51-year-old patient following insertion of a right-sided subthalamic electronic stimulator for Parkinson's disease. The position of the stimulator is well shown and there is some susceptibility artefact over the skull vault from metallic connections

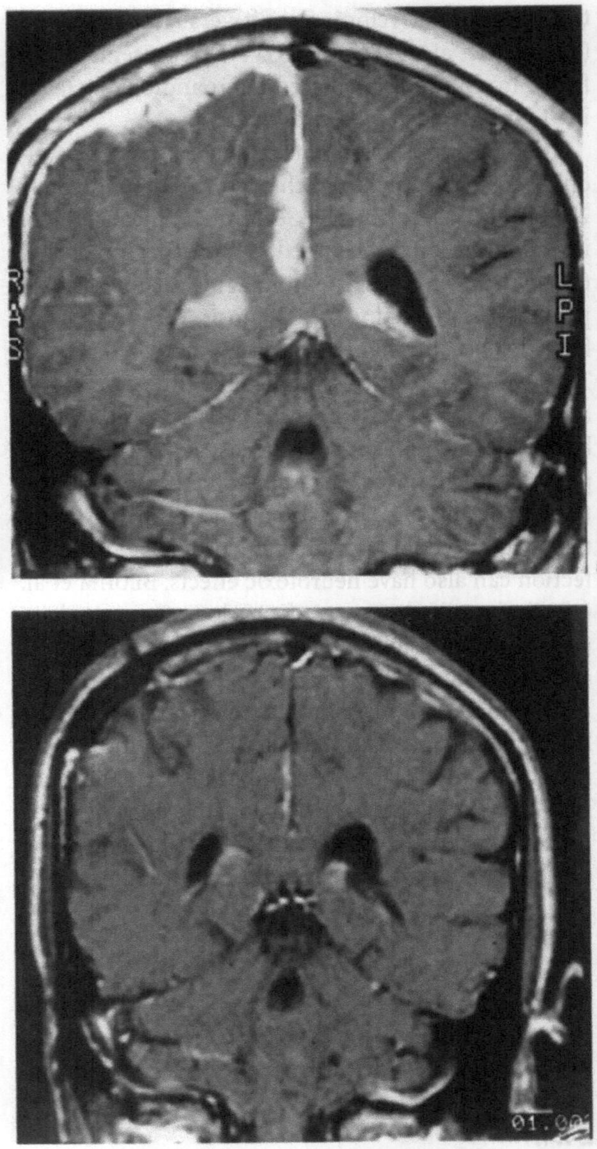

a

b

Fig. 24.17a,b. Contrast-enhanced T1-weighted MRI scans in 32-year-old male patient with a flat-based enhancing dural mass adjacent to the falx and over the right lateral convexity. There is also marked bilateral choroid plexus enhancement (**a**). The diagnosis of neurosarcoidosis was established by a meningeal biopsy. Following treatment with steroids there has been almost complete resolution of the dural masses and a marked reduction in size and enhancement of the choroid plexus (**b**). Note biopsy burr hole over right convexity

Study Group 1998). A more recent placebo controlled trial in patients with secondary progressive multiple sclerosis (Miller et al. 1999) showed that interferon beta-1b significantly decreased the number of new or enlarging T2 lesions, the total lesion volume and number of enhancing lesions. Post-therapeutic imaging in multiple sclerosis is currently only indicated as part of drug trials and has no place in clinical routine.

Serial MRI imaging can sometimes be useful to monitor the treatment response of other inflammatory diseases, such as sarcoidosis or histiocytosis X. Sarcoidosis in particular can occasionally present as a dural mass lesion mimicking a meningioma (Sender et al. 1997). Dural sarcoidosis responds usually well to treatment with steroids (Fig. 24.17).

24.4.4 Infectious Disease

Cross-sectional neuroimaging forms an integral part of the monitoring of treatment response in CNS infections. Some conditions merit special consideration. Serial neuroimaging is crucial in the clinical management of patients suffering from neurological complications of AIDS. Toxoplasmosis represents the commonest CNS infection in this group of patients. It can present as single or multiple enhancing intracerebral mass lesions and its main differential diagnosis is cerebral lymphoma. In clinical practice the diagnosis is often established by the radiological response to empirical antitoxoplasmosis treatment

(Fig. 24.18). Toxoplasmosis will respond to treatment within 14 days in over 90% of patients and a biopsy is indicated if there is lack of response, if new lesions appear and if the patient's condition deteriorates (Chiang et al. 1998). When making a decision on the basis of the radiological response, it is important to ensure that the patient has been compliant in taking the prescribed treatment.

In the past few years a number of antiviral drugs have become available for the treatment of patients with AIDS. Combination therapy with these drugs has resulted in clinical improvement, reduction in disease progression, elevation of the CD 4+ count and decrease in viral load. Treatment with these drugs has also an effect on the T2 high signal change seen on T2-weighted MRI scan. Wilkinson et al. (1997) described a mixed response of white matter changes and spectroscopic data following treatment with zidovudine (AZT) alone. Filippi et al. (1998) compared the signal changes on serial MRI examinations in patients who either received or did not receive a new class of protease inhibitors as part of an antiretroviral combination therapy. They found nearly complete regression of white matter changes in four and stable appearances in another four of nine patients receiving protease inhibitor therapy, which compared favourably with the control group where eight of nine patients showed progression of white matter disease. The radiological improvement in the patients receiving protease inhibitors was paralleled by a cognitive improvement.

Cysticercosis is the commonest parasitic CNS infection worldwide. It may affect the brain parenchyma or meninges and its MR appearances depend on the evolutionary stage of the cysticerci. As long as the parasite is alive, there is little enhancement or surrounding oedema. Degeneration and death of the parasite prompt an inflammatory response of the host. It is therefore not uncommon to see an increase in enhancement and large areas of surrounding oedema during or early after treatment with praziquantel (Chang and Han 1998). It is important to recognise this as a normal response and not to mistake it for treatment failure. An extensive inflammatory reaction should be treated with steroids.

A paradoxical response to treatment with lesion expansion has also been reported in some cases of intracranial tuberculomas (Hejazi and Hassler 1997). Interestingly, intracranial tuberculomas can enlarge at a stage when systemic tuberculosis is regressing. The paradoxical reaction does not require a change in antituberculous therapy, but adjuvant steroid treatment may be helpful. In the presence of intracranial lesions, antituberculous treatment should be given for at least 12 months.

24.4.5 Hydrocephalus

Serial assessment of ventricular size in patients with ventriculoperitoneal shunts has been used since the early days of CT. Fluctuations in size of the ventricles, in particular of the temporal horns, continues to be a useful indicator of shunt function.

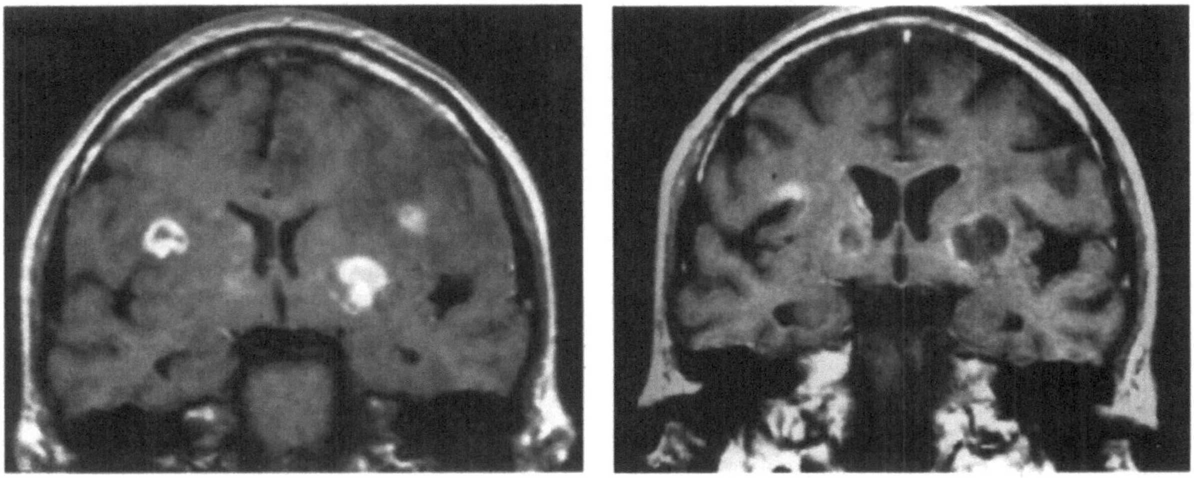

a b

Fig. 24.18a,b. Coronal contrast-enhanced T1-weighted images in a 28-year-old patient with AIDS before (**a**) and 2 weeks after (**b**) treatment for toxoplasmosis. Multiple ring-enhancing lesions with surrounding oedema (**a**) show a favourable response to antitoxoplasmosis treatment (**b**), thereby confirming the diagnosis

Neuroendoscopic third ventriculostomy represents an alternative way of decompressing the ventricular system. This technique consists in opening the floor of the third ventricle under endoscopic control and has proven to be a successful treatment in obstructive, non-communicating hydrocephalus. Treatment failure can be due to closure of the fenestration by membrane formation or malabsorption of CSF. In the case of recurrent or residual symptoms it is important to differentiate closure of the fenestration from malabsorption, since the former requires re-exploration and the latter external shunting.

Cardiac gated multislice spin echo MR imaging has been successfully used to demonstrate patency of third ventriculostomies by MAEDER et al. (1996). More recently, FUKUHARA et al. (1999) performed a comparative study of two-dimensional phase contrast (PC) MR imaging and direct surgical re-exploration of the floor of the third ventricle in 11 patients with recurrent symptoms after third-ventriculostomy, which included headaches, lethargy and confusion. They found cine PC MRI to be a reliable indicator of patency of the ventriculostomy. Complete occlusion of the ventriculostomy by new membranes was correctly diagnosed by cine PC MRI in four of five patients and the presence of minor flow from the pontine cistern to the third ventricle was an early sign of impending closure.

24.5 Conclusion

MRI scanning using conventional sequences has an established role in monitoring the effects and side effects of medical and surgical treatment of CNS disease and is, with a few exceptions, superior to CT scanning.

Non-invasive vascular imaging with MRA and CTA will have a significant impact on the follow-up of patients treated for neurovascular diseases. MR and CT perfusion imaging will give an insight of the haemodynamic repercussions of this treatment.

Serial MR spectroscopy allows detection of changes at molecular level over time which is likely to be useful in the follow-up of neuro-oncological patients. The precision of serial structural imaging of the brain parenchyma and detection of subtle changes is greatly facilitated by the application of registration algorithms and volumetric 3D data acquisitions. With further improvement in processing speed the interpretation of images which result from a subtraction of the baseline from the follow-up scan will play an important role in assessing response to treatment and influence early decision making in clinical management.

References

Atlas S, Sheppard L, Goldberg HI, Hurst RW, Listerud J, Flamm E (1997) Intracranial aneurysms: detection and characterization with MR angiography with use of an advanced postprocessing technique in a blinded-reader study. Radiology 203: 807–814

Bauman G, Pahapill P, Macdonald P, Fisher B, Leighton C, Cairncross G (1999) Low grade glioma: measuring radiographic response to radiotherapy. Can J Neurol Sci 26: 18–22

Bevan J (1999) Management of pituitary tumours. BMJ 318: 1226–1227

Blohm M, Aulich A, Englebrecht V, Burdach S (1997) Reversible brain MRI changes in acyclovir neurotoxicity. Bone Marrow Transplant 19: 1049–1051

Brada M (1999) Radiosurgery for brain tumours. BMJ 318: 411–412

Brown J, Lustrin E, Lev M, Ogilvy C, Taveras J (1999) Reduction of aneurysm clip artifacts on CT angiograms: a technical note. AJNR 20: 694–696

Chang K, Han M (1998) MRI of CNS parasitic diseases. J Magn Reson Imaging 8: 297–307

Chiang F, Walot I, Sinow R, Mehringer C (1998) Diagnostic imaging of the brain in acquired immunodeficiency syndrome (AIDS). Semin Ultrasound CT MR 19: 133–153

Coley S, Jäger H, Szydlo R, Goldman J (1999) CT and MRI manifestations of central nervous system infection following allogenic bone marrow transplantation. Clin Radiol 54: 390–397

Coley S, Porter D, Calamante F, Chong W, Connelly A (1999) Quantitative MR diffusion mapping and cyclosporine-induced neurotoxity. AJNR 20: 1507–1510

Derdeyn CP, Graves VB, Turski PA, Masaryk AM, Strother CM (1997) MR angiography of saccular aneurysms after treatment with Guglielmi detachable coils: preliminary experience. AJNR 18: 279–286

Duncombe A (1997) ABC of clinical haematology: bone marrow and stem cell transplantation. BMJ 314: 1179–1190

Filippi C, Sze G, Farber S, Shahmanesh M, Selwyn P (1998) Regressionof HIV encephalopathy and basal ganglia signal intensity abnormality at MR imaging in patients with AIDS after the initiation of protease inhibitor therapy. Radiology 206: 491–498

Flickinger J, Lunsford L, Konziolka D (1992) Radiosurgery and brain tolerance: an analysis of neurodiagnostic imaging changes after gamma knife radiosurgery for arteriovenous malformations. Int J Radiat Oncol Biol Phys 23: 19–26

Fukuhara T, Vorster S, Ruggieri P, Luciano M (1999) Third ventriculostomy patency: comparison of findings at cine phase-contrast MR imaging and at direct exploration. AJNR 20: 1560–1566

Gillard J, Hardingham C, Kirkpatrick P, Antoun N, Freer C, Griffiths P (1998) Evaluation of carotid endarterectomy with sequential MR perfusion imaging: a preliminary report. AJNR 19: 1747–1752

Grieve J, Stacey R, Moore E, Kitchen ND, Jäger H (1999) Arti-

fact on MRA post aneurysm clipping: a prospective comparative study with DSA. Neuroradiology 41: 680–686
Hartman J, Nguyen T, Larson D, Teitelbaum G (1997) MR artifacts, heat production, and ferromagnetism of Guglielmi detachable coils. AJNR: 497–501
Hawighorst H, Essig M, Debus J et al (1997) Serial MR imaging of intracranial metastases after radiosurgery. Magn Reson Imaging 15: 1121–1132
Hazle J, Jackson E, Schomer D, Leeds N (1997) Dynamic imaging of intracranial lesions using fast spin-echo imaging: differentiation of brain tumors and treatment effects. J Magn Reson Imag 7: 1084–1093
Heiserman JE, Dean BL, Hodak JA, Flom RA, Bird CR, Drayer BP (1994) Neurologic complications of cerebral angiography. AJNR: 1401–1407
Hejazi N, Hassler W (1997) Multiple intracranial tuberculomas with atypical response to tuberculostatic chemotherapy: literature review and a case report. Infection 25: 233–239
Hildebrand J, Dewitte O, Dietrich P, Tribolet ND (1997) Management of malignant brain tumors. Eur Neurol 38: 238–253
Hinchey J, Chaves C, Appignani B et al (1996) A reversible posterior leukoencephalopathy syndrome. N Engl J Med 22: 494–500
Hodgson T, Kingsley D, Moseley I (1995) The role of imaging in the follow up of meningiomas. J Neurol Neurosurg Physchiatr 59: 545–547
Jäger H, Williams E, Savage D, Rule S et al (1996) Assessment of brain changes with registered MR before and after bone marrow transplantation for chronic myeloid leukemia. AJNR 17: 1275–1282
Jäger HR, Grieve J, Moore E, Kitchen N, Taylor W (1999) Comparison of CTA and intra-arterial DSA in patients with cerebral AVMs. Neuroradiology 41: 227
Jäger HR, Moore EA, Grieve JP, Parkers L, Taylor W (1999) MR perfusion imaging in cerebral AVMs using gadolinium bolus tracking and arterial spin tagging methods. Radiology 213(P): 393
Jäger HR, Moore EA, Grieve JP, Taylor W (1999) 3D TOF, contrast-enhanced TOF and 3D FSE sequences in cerebral AVMs. Neuroradiology 41: S100-S101
Kähärä V, Seppänen S, Rymin P, Mattila P, Kuurne T, Laasonen E (1999) MR angiography with three dimensional time-of-flight and targeted maximum-intensity-projection reconstructions in the follow-up of intracranial aneurysms embolized with Guglielmi detachable coils. AJNR 20: 1470–1475
Keime-Guilbert F, Napolitano M, Delattre J (1998) Neurological complications of radiotherapy and chemotherapy. J Neurol 245: 695–708
Kihlstrom L, Karlsson B (1999) Imaging changes after radiosurgery for vascular malformations, functional targets, and tumors. Neurosurg Clin Am 10: 167–180
Kim S, Chang K, Kim S et al (1999) Focal lesion in the splenium of the corpus callosum in epileptic patients: antiepileptic drug toxicity. AJNR 20: 125–129
Kitchen ND, Cook MJ, Shorvon SD, Fish DR, Stevens JM, Thomas DG (1995) Estimation of resection volumes in lesional epilepsy surgery. AJNR 16: 208–210
Lansberg M, Tong D, Norbash A, Yenari M, Moseley I (1999) Intra-arterial rtPA treatment of stroke assessed by diffusion-and perfusion-weighted MRI. Stroke 30: 678–680
Lovblad K, Kellar P, Ozdoba C, Ramelli G, Remonda L, Schroth G (1998) Pure methotrexate encephalopathy presenting seizures: CT and MRI features. Pediatr Radiol 28: 86–91
Maeder PP, Meuli RA, Tribolet Nd (1996) Three-Dimensional volume rendering for magnetic resonance angiography in the screening and preoperative workup of intracranial aneurysms. J Neurosurg 85: 1050–1055
Miller DH, Molyneux PD, Barker GJ, MacManus DG, Moseley IF, Wagner K (1999) Effect of interferon-beta1b on magnetic resonance imaging outcomes in secondary progressive multiple sclerosis: results of a European multicenter, randomized, double-blind, placebo-controlled trial. European Study Group on Interferon-beta1b in Secondary Progressive Multiple Sclerosis. Ann Neurol 46: 850–859
Miyawaki J, Dowd C, Wara W et al (1999) Five year results of LINAC radiosurgery for arteriovenous malformations: outcome for large AVMs. Int J Radiation Oncology Biol Phys 44: 1089–1106
Moran N, Lemieux L, Maudgil D, Kitchen N, Fish D, Shorvon S (1999) Analysis of temporal lobe resections in MR images. Epilepsia 40: 1077–1084
Nelson S, Huhn S, Vigneron D et al (1997) Volume MRI and MRSI techniques for the quantitation of treatment response in brain tumors: presentation of a detailed case study. J Magn Reson Imag 7: 1146–1152
Oelerich M, Lentschig MG, Zunker P, Reimer R, Rummeny EJ, Schuirer G (1998) Intracranial vascular stenosis and occlusion: comparison of 3D time-of-flight and 3D phase-contrast MR angiography. Neuroradiology 40: 567–573
Ohue S, Kohno K, Kusunoki K et al (1998) Magnetic resonance angiography in patients with acute stroke treated by local thrombolysis. Neuroradiology 40: 536–540
Pirotte B, Levivier M, Goldman S, Brucher J, Brotchi J, Hildebrand J (1997) Glucocorticoid-induced long-term remission in primary cerebral lymphoma: case report and review of the literature. J Neurooncol 32: 63–69
Poussaint TY, Siffert J, Barnes PD et al (1995) Hemorrhagic vasculopathy after treatment of central nervous system neoplasia in childhood: diagnosis and follow-up. AJNR 16: 693–699
PRISMS Study Group (1998) Randomised double-blind placebo-controlled study of interferon beta-1a in relapsing/remitting multiple sclerosis. PRISMS (Prevention of Relapses and Disability by Interferon beta-1a Subcutaneously in Multiple Sclerosis) Study Group. Lancet 352: 1498–1504
Powell M (1999) Recent advances Neurosurgery. BMJ 318: 35
Quinn N, Bhatia K (1998) Functional neurosurgery for Parkinson's disease. BMJ 316: 1259–1260
Rabin B, Meyer J, Berlin J, Marymount M, Palka P, Russell E (1996) Radiation-induced changes in the central nervous system and head and neck.Radiographics 16: 1055–1072
Ricci P, Karis J, Heiserman J, Fram R, Bice A, Drayer B (1998) Differentiating recurrent tumor from radiation necrosis: time for re-evaluation of positron emission tomography? AJNR 19: 407–413
Sencer S, Minareci O, Poyanli A (1999) Management of a rare complication of endovascular treatment of direct carotid cavernous fistula. AJNR 20: 1465–1466
Sender P, Jäger H, Hersch M, Chaudri KR, Bajaj N, Frackowiak R (1997) Neurosarcoidosis mimicking meningioma en-plaque: report of two cases and review of the literature. Eur J Neurol 4: 307–314

Shah A (1999) Cyclosporine neurotoxicity among bone marrow transplant recipients. Clin Neuropharmacol 22: 67–73

Sorensen A, Buonanno F, Gonzalez R et al (1996) Hyperacute stroke: evaluaton with combined multisection diffusion-weighted and hemodynamically weighted echo-planar MR imaging. Radiology 199: 391–401

Stokkel M, Stevens H, Taphoorn M, Rijk PV (1999) Differentiation between recurrent brain tumour and post-radiation necrosis: the value of 201TI SPECT versus 18F-FDG PET using a dual-headed coincidence camera – a pilot study. Nucl Med Commun 20: 411–417

Takano K, Carano R, Tatlisumak T et al (1998) Efficacy of intra-arterial and intravenous prourokinase in an embolic stroke model evaluated by diffusion-perfusion magnetic resonance imaging. Neurology 50: 870–875

Taylor J, Langston J, Reddick W et al (1996) Clinical value of proton magnetic resonance spectroscopy for differentiating recurrent or residual brain tumor from delayed cerebral necrosis. Int J Radiat Oncol Biol Phys 36: 1251–1261

Tedeschi G, Lundbom N, Raman R et al (1997) Increased choline signal coinciding with malignant degeneration of cerebral gliomas: a serial proton magnetic resonance spectroscopy imaging study. J Neurosurg 87: 516–524

Velthuis BK, Leeuwen MS, Witkamp TD, Boomstra S, Ramos L, Rinkel GJE (1997) CT angiography: Source images and post-processing techniques in the detection of cerebral aneurysms. AJR 169: 1411–1417

Vieco P, Morin E, Gross C (1996) CT angiography in the examination of patients with aneurysm clips. AJNR 17: 455–457

Wilkinson I, Griffiths P, Gains P, Cleveland T, Venables G (1999) Unilateral leptomeningeal enhancement resulting from carotid angioplasty/stenting. Proc ISMRM 2: 879

Wilkinson ID, Lunn S, Miskiel KA et al (1997) Proton MRS and quantitative MRI assessment of the short term neurological response to antiretroviral therapy in AIDS. J Neurol Neurosurg Psychiatr 63: 477–482

Yamamoto M, Hara M, Ide M, Ono Y, Jimbo M, Saito I (1998) Radiation-related adverse effects observed on neuro-imaging several years after radiosurgery for cerebral arteriovenous malformations. Surg Neurol 49: 385–398

Zimmer W, Hourihane M, Wang H, Schriber J (1998) The effect of human leukocyte antigen disparity on cyclosporine neurotoxicity after allogenic bone marrow transplantation. AJNR 19: 601–610

Spine and Spinal Cord

25 Guidelines for Spinal MR Imaging

PHILIPPE DEMAEREL

CONTENTS

25.1 Introduction

The technical advances in spinal MR imaging have been overshadowed by the advances in brain imaging (ROSS 1999). Although significant progress in sequence design has been achieved, the acquisition of high quality axial images at the cervical level remains an important problem. The major part of this chapter will be devoted to the evaluation of sequences in spinal MR imaging and to the role of spinal MR imaging in healthcare, including the development of guidelines. The latter is not unimportant because of the significant radiation dose associated with plain X-ray, myelography and CT.

25.2 The Problems with Terminology of Degenerative Disease

The terminology of degenerative changes lacks uniformity. Clinicians and radiologists use different terms. This renders the interpretation of CT and MR images particularly difficult. What is the significance of a protrusion, a prolapse, a herniation, bulging or an extrusion?

Disc herniation and annular tears are known to occur in people without low back pain or sciatica (JENSEN et al. 1994; STADNIK et al. 1998). A disc bulge was seen in 52% (JENSEN et al. 1994) and 81% (STADNIK et al. 1998) of asymptomatic volunteers. A disc protrusion was seen in 27% and 33% respectively. Annular tears were observed in 14% and 20% respectively. From these observations, it is clear that MR imaging in the absence of clear clinical signs or symptoms should be interpreted cautiously in order to avoid unnecessary surgery.

Recently the problem of terminology in lumbar vertebral disc disease has been reviewed and a standardized nomenclature has been proposed (MILETTE 1997). Why has it been so difficult to reach a consensus on this topic?

Two factors have influenced this process: the normal age-related disc changes and the physiopathology of disc disease, which remains incompletely understood. When reporting CT scans in the 1980s, the description was limited to: normal disc, disc bulging without nerve root compression and disc herniation with nerve root compression.

Knowing that sciatica can also be caused by chemical changes leading to inflammation of the nerve root, a new simple classification was developed (BRANT-ZAWADZKI et al. 1995). The "disc extension beyond the interspace" (DEBIT) determined the classification. A normal disc, bulging, protruded and extruded disc were distinguished. The latter two terms may be jointly called herniation but it was preferred to retain the two terms because extrusion is extremely rare in people without low back pain as opposed to protrusion. This classification generated only moderate interobserver agreement (BRANT-ZAWADZKI et al. 1995). One of the problems was the difficult interpretation of the images when the bony spinal canal was narrowed. Spinal narrowing is an important factor that may accelerate symptoms of disc herniation.

PH. DEMAEREL, MD, PhD
Consultant Neuroradiologist, Department of Radiology, University Hospitals, Herestraat 49, 3000 Leuven, Belgium

Milette (1997) proposed a classification based on the assessment of the anatomy and pathology of the disc and the adjacent vertebral bodies.

The "normal young disc" still has a central high signal on T2-weighted images. The central high signal decreases in the "normal aging disc" (over 40 years of age and no symptoms) and osteophytes make their appearance. A definite loss of the high signal is accepted as evidence of a major annular tear. The "scarred (or deteriorated) disc" (all ages and frequent symptoms) is characterized by a loss of height of the disc and prominent osteophyte formation. This is considered to be pathological degeneration as opposed to the normal aging disc changes. Finally "herniated discs" need to be further specified taking into account the size of the spinal canal. The division of the spinal canal into three parts on an axial slice is recommended.

To specify the location several possibilities are available. The Nomenclature Committee of the North American Spine Society uses the following terms: for the sagittal plane: discal, suprapedicular, pedicular and infrapedicular; for the axial plane: central, subarticular (at the medial edge of the facets), foraminal, extraforaminal and anterior (part of the vertebral body).

When the herniated disc is separated from the intervertebral disc, the term disc fragment migration is preferred to sequestered disc.

One should be aware that the reliability of this classification has not been tested. The advantage of this classification is that it allows correlation with surgical and postmortem findings which is necessary for the validation of any nomenclature.

This classification does not solve our daily problem of differentiating bulging from herniation. However, this is unimportant because the two terms are not mutually exclusive.

In conclusion, it is clear that the clinical symptomatology will determine every therapeutic decision and imaging alone should never justify a treatment.

25.3 Use of Plain Lumbar Spine X-Ray

Everyone is convinced that too many lumbar spine X-rays are performed. Plain X-rays are indicated whenever there is a suspicion of fracture, tumour, or infection. When they are requested in patients with low back pain and/or sciatica, the purpose is to exclude one of the above mentioned bone abnormalities. However, a delay of 2 or 3 weeks has been recommended before ordering plain X-rays unless the diagnosis of malignant disease, infection or fracture is clinically likely (Suarez-Almazor et al. 1997). Routine oblique views should be discouraged and only performed after review of the anteroposterior and lateral views. Apart from reducing the cost, this would also significantly reduce radiation exposure. The gonadal radiation dose from lumbar spine X-ray is 40 times the dose received during chest X-ray. Lifetime risk analyses have shown that 1 million lumbar spine radiographs can result in 20 excess deaths from leukaemia and 400 excess cases of genetic diseases (Whalen and Balter 1982).

Disc herniation and annular tears are known to occur in people without low back pain (Jensen et al. 1994; Stadnik et al. 1998). What must be guarded against is a decision to operate on a patient solely on the imaging findings and not the clinical features. The relation between symptoms of back pain and findings on plain radiographs has been studied (Van Tulder et al. 1997). These data have been used to estimate the combined proportion of false positives, i.e. the proportion of positive findings among individuals who had no back pain. This number varied from 41% to 48% depending on the severity of imaging abnormalities. At present reports of plain radiographs, and probably MR imaging, too, are relayed in a manner that is unintentionally damaging the patients because they promote wrong guidelines on management of back pain. Even the statistically significant association between degenerative changes and symptoms of low back pain should be interpreted cautiously, since the magnitude of this association was weak and several potential resources of bias were identified (Van Tulder et al. 1997). To emphasize the limited predictive value of plain radiographs and the high prevalence of symptomless abnormalities, insertions have been recommended for radiology reports (Roland and Van Tulder 1998). An example of such a statement is: roughly 40% of patients with advanced disc degeneration do not have back pain and this finding may therefore be unrelated. Other statements concern findings such as slight degeneration or spina bifida or transitional vertebrae which occur in almost half of the patients who do not have back pain. Roughly half of the patients with spondylosis or spondylolisthesis do not have back pain and more than 40% of the patients with Scheuermann's disease do not have back pain. It would certainly be useful to include these comments because it may be of benefit to the patient, by avoiding inappropriate management by the physician and/or inappropriate behaviour by the patient, and it may help reduce the number of plain radiographs carried out. This report relates to plain X-rays, but the same problem exists with MR imaging, as it is well known that the prevalence of abnormal findings is very high and that abnormal findings can frequently be seen in the absence of clinical signs or symptoms (Jensen et al. 1994; Stadnik et al. 1998).

At this moment plain X-ray and CT cannot be replaced by MR imaging. It can reasonably be expected that this may occur in a not too distant future, provided that there is a more widespread availability of MR systems.

There have been trials that compared rapid MR imaging with plain X-ray (Jarvik et al. 1997). The four- to sixfold increase in the throughput, thanks to a rapid imaging protocol, results in a lower cost, close to the cost of plain X-ray. While it seems unrealistic to replace plain X-ray by MR imaging routinely, the first step in that direction has certainly been made. One of the problems that will be encountered is the development of a reliable but rapid examination. Recently the use of a single sagittal T2-weighted sequence has been compared with a routine imaging protocol consisting of sagittal T1- and T2-weighted sequences and T2-weighted axial images (Rankine et al. 1997). The conclusion was that the extra information gained by using all three sequences was considered to be of greater benefit than the time saved by using a single sagittal T2-weighted sequence. Compared to the three sequence examination, the sensitivity to diagnose disc protrusions was only 38%.

25.4 Guidelines for Spinal MR Imaging

Similarly to our discussion in Chap. 7, the development of guidelines depends on the access to MR imaging. One important difference compared to brain imaging is that MR imaging with its multiplanar capability can replace examinations such as conventional myelography, CT and plain X-ray. The latter are associated with a significant radiation dose and their replacement by MR imaging is of even more benefit to the patient than the replacement of brain CT by brain MR imaging.

In examinations of the spine/ spinal cord our recommendation is to perform MR imaging as much as possible thereby replacing CT and conventional myelography. CT may occasionally be useful to depict calcification in an intra- or extraspinal mass. Occasionally a conventional myelogram may be necessary to further investigate the anatomic boundaries of an intraspinal cyst. Recently the therapeutic impact of lumbar spine MR imaging was assessed on patients with low back and leg pain (Rankine et al. 1998). The authors found a poor agreement between the clinical diagnosis and the MR findings. There was a move towards conservative treatment after MR imaging in 47.9% of patients with an initial management plan of surgery. The large variety of clinical features that influence the management is partly due to the variety of possible diagnoses. In this study the presence of abnormal neurological signs only was not a good predictor of surgery because 17 patients without neurological findings were treated by surgery. Because of the not unimportant psychological benefit of undergoing an MR examination it is extremely difficult, if not impossible, to define guidelines for MR imaging. The relative importance of non-biomedical variables in the decision to request MR imaging has been demonstrated (Robling et al. 1998). On the other hand one should never operate on a patient based solely on the imaging findings. The decision to operate should be taken on clinical grounds and MR imaging can be useful in the surgical work-up.

This is certainly true for the lumbar and thoracic spine. As far as the cervical spine is concerned there are a few more limitations. Generally speaking the image quality of axial images is usually good as far as the spinal cord is concerned but they are more prone to swallowing artefacts. The axial images are most helpful in defining the focal nature of a disc protrusion, its relationship to nerve roots and the presence of facet joint disease and central canal stenosis. Because of the sometimes suboptimal image quality at the cervical level, cervical myelography and CT may still be indicated despite the availability of MR imaging.

Our routine imaging protocol for low back pain and sciatica consists of sagittal SE T1, sagittal fast SE T2-weighted, axial fast SE T2-weighted and four (anteroposterior, lateral, left and right oblique MR myelographic) images. Others will prefer axial SE T1-weighted images. Whenever bone abnormalities are suspected, an additional T2-weighted inversion recovery sequence with fat suppression is obtained.

At our institute, contrast enhanced scans are obtained in approximately 20% of all spinal MR examinations. We certainly recommend a contrast enhanced scan whenever there is a suspicious lesion on a pre-contrast image that cannot be specified sufficiently (see Chaps. 27, 28 and 29). Most patients with neurological signs will require a contrast enhanced scan if the cause of the symptoms is not elucidated on the pre-contrast images. We routinely administer intravenous contrast if the patient is known with a primary tumour and when he is referred for the exclusion of metastases. Precontrast T1-weighted images are mandatory in order not to overlook bone marrow metastases. Leptomeningeal enhancement is typically only depicted on contrast enhanced scans and can be due to metastatic disease (see Chap. 27), inflammatory disease (see Chap. 28) or lymphoproliferative disease (see Chap. 29).

The use of intravenous contrast agents in postoperative lumbar spine imaging is discussed in Chap. 31. The first results of intrathecal administration of contrast are being reported (see Chap. 30).

25.5 The Battlefield of Pulse Sequences

Contrary to brain MR imaging, the choice of sequences for spinal MR imaging is more limited. A technical discussion on the different types of sequences can be found in Chap. 3. The priorities of spinal imaging are different from those of brain imaging. The occurrence of intrinsic (e.g. swallowing artefacts) and extrinsic (e.g. cerebrospinal fluid flow artefacts) artefacts are the major challenges.

After T1-weighted and T2-weighted spin-echo (SE) sequences, T2-weighted fast or turbo SE imaging was introduced, dramatically reducing the examination time. The 2D version of fast SE has become the gold standard for spinal sagittal T2-weighted imaging (Fig. 25.1). Axial imaging is more difficult and there is no consensus about the best approach. Axial images are important in assessing the degree of nerve root compression, and routine SE T1- and T2-weighted images cannot confidently differentiate osteophytes from disc material. The image quality is patient dependent and swallowing artefact can cause image

a

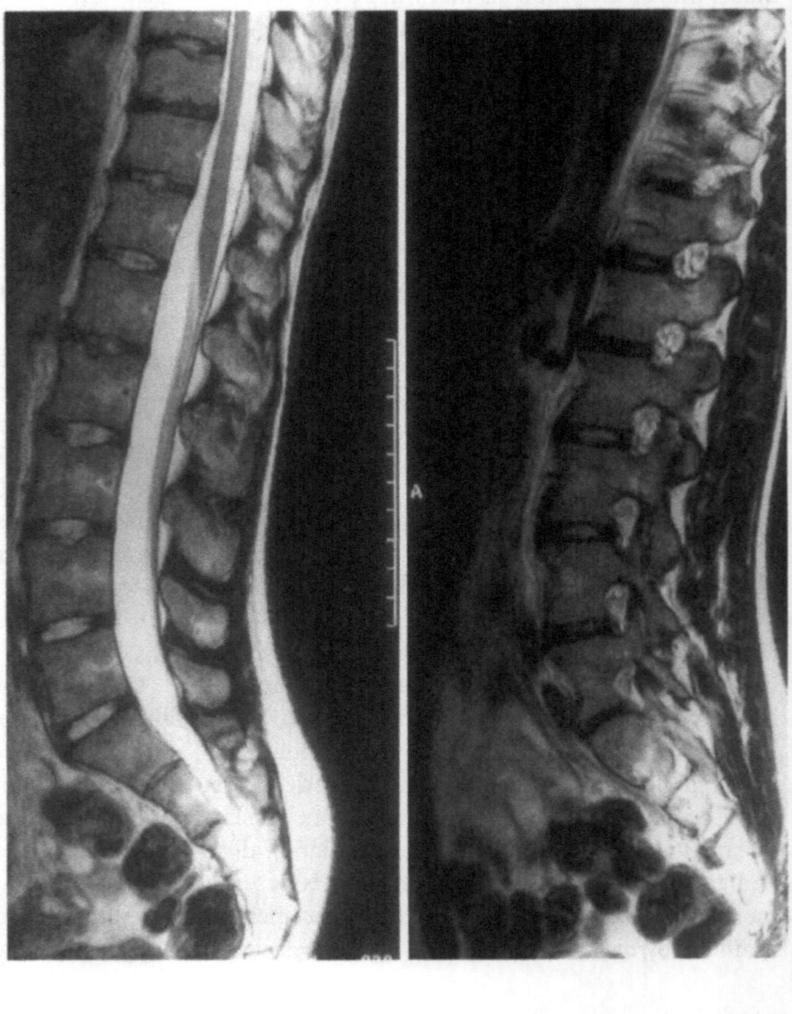

b

Fig. 25.1a,b. Sagittal T2-weighted fast SE images through the midline (**a**) and through the left foramina (**b**) degradation. The discussion on the different types of sequences will now be focused on axial imaging.

T2*-weighted gradient-echo (GE) imaging, using steady-state sequences, relies on a reduced flip angle to enhance signal with short TR and can be obtained in 2D or 3D data sets (Fig. 25.2). The contrast resolution of GE sequences for the assessment of spinal cord abnormalities is not as good as that of (fast)SE sequences but imaging times are shorter. Oblique sagittal reconstructions in the plane of the cervical foramina can display nerve root compression (Fig. 25.3). There are no cerebrospinal fluid flow artefacts. The necessity of using a low flip angle (5–8°) to obtain a high signal of cerebrospinal fluid means a low S/N and a grainy image. The sequence is prone to motion artefacts too. Despite these disadvantages it is often recommended as the sequence of choice for axial imaging of the cervical spine. Magnetization transfer (MT) may be useful in solving these problems (Finelli 1998). The addition of an MT pulse increases the sensitivity to intramedullary disease and improves the cord/cerebrospinal fluid contrast. A shorter TE can be used which minimizes the magnetic susceptibility (Melhem et al. 1996). The less clear visualization of the disc space on the axial images is one drawback.

Using T2-weighted fast SE volume imaging there are more cerebrospinal fluid pulsation artefacts because flow compensation can only be applied in one direction and signal intensity of cerebrospinal fluid is lower (Maldjian et al. 1999). The quality of the axial reconstructed images is less good. The contrast is adequate on a high field magnet contrary to the contrast on a low field magnet (Swainson et al. 1997). The S/N is better than on the axial 3D GE sequence and there are less susceptibility artefacts (Fig. 25.4). The 3D fast SE has been compared with the 2D fast Se in the detection of MS plaques and the former proved superior (Stevenson et al. 1998).

2D GE T2-weighted imaging is the alternative sequence of choice for axial imaging of the cervical spine and is particularly useful when the 3D image data set is degraded by motion artefacts. For axial images of the thoracic spine the same sequences can be recommended with a slight preference for the 2D GE sequence. Axial images of the lumbar spine are best achieved using the fast SE sequence (Fig. 25.5).

Recently T2*-weighted GE steady-state sequences with balanced gradients have been used (Georgy et al. 1998; Duerk et al. 1998). These sequences provide a high signal cerebrospinal fluid with higher flip angles and therefore with a better S/N. The CISS technique has been successfully applied to visualize the intradural cervical nerve roots but is less good in the assessment of the foramina (Georgy et al. 1998).

T1-weighted imaging is usually performed using SE sequences.

Short tau inversion recovery (STIR) and fast STIR, using the adequate field-strength dependent inversion time (usually 100–150 ms), suppresses the signal from fat while being very sensitive to changes in water content. The SE pulse sequence is applied at the time when only water protons have longitudinal magnetization because of their faster recovery after the 180° radiofrequency pulse. Using fastSE techniques the acquisition times are relative-

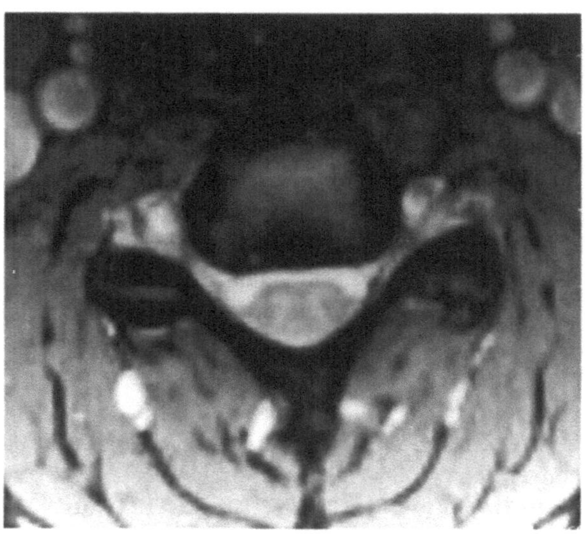

a

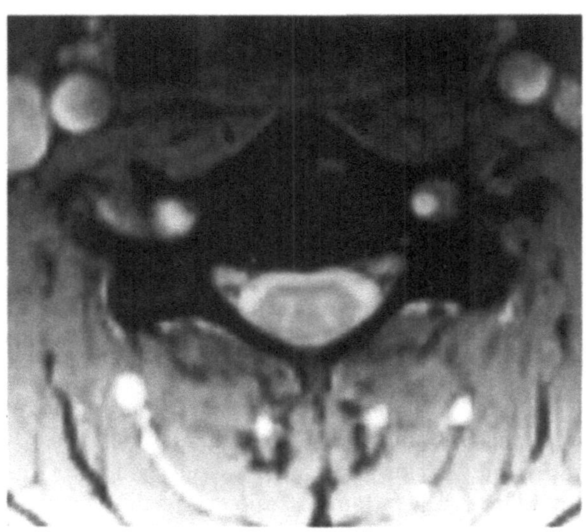

b

Fig. 25.2a,b. Axial GE T2-weighted images at the level of the C5C6 disc (**a**) and through the body of C6 (**b**)

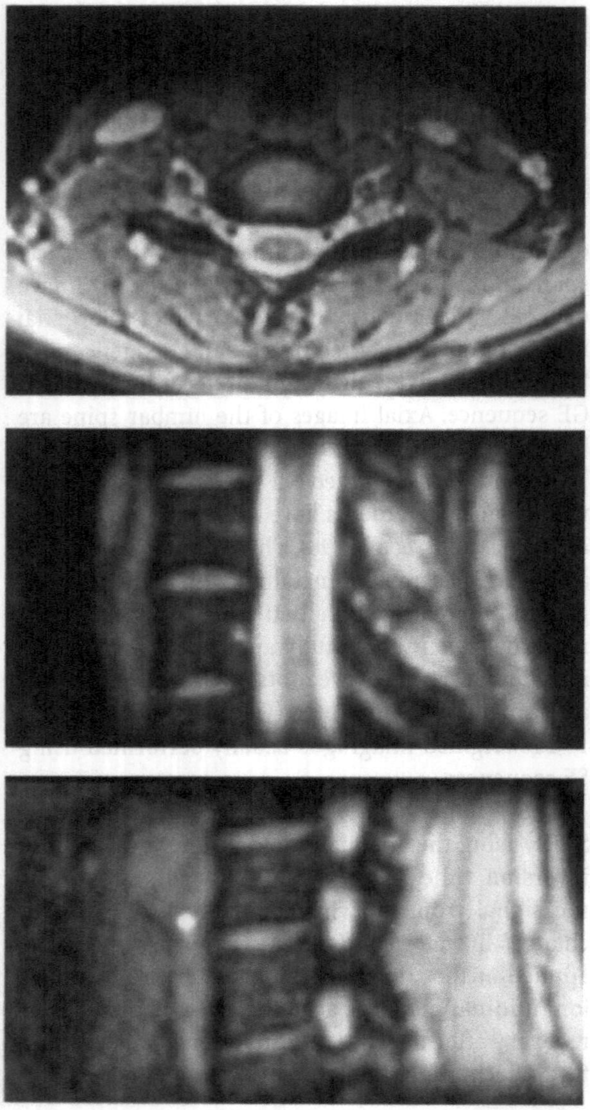

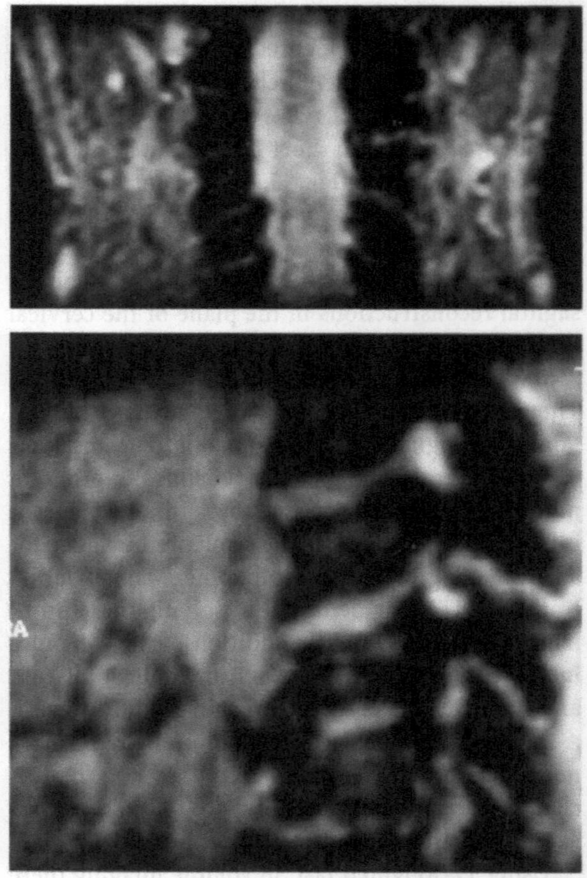

Fig. 25.3a–e. 3D GE sequence at C5C6. Native axial 1-mm slice (**a**). Reformatted midline sagittal (**b**) and oblique (**c**) image through the foramina in a volunteer. Coronal (**d**) and oblique (**e**) images in a patient with osteophytoses and uncarthrosis causing narrowing of the foramina

ly short (Hittmair et al. 1996; Lycklama à Nijeholt et al. 1998). The disadvantages are the moderate spatial resolution and the motion/flow artefacts. The use of this sequence has been recommended in the assessment of the cervical spinal cord to depict MS plaques (Hittmair et al. 1996). The fast STIR sequence has been compared with the fast SE and MT-GE sequence in terms of lesion detection and the former proved to be superior (Rocca et al. 1999).

Another technique achieves fat suppression by applying a frequency selective (chemical shift) saturation pulse prior to the imaging pulses. This is followed by a conventional SE pulse sequence to generate signal from other tissues than fat. The FATSAT sequence can be used in combination with any imaging technique and can be used in conjunction with intravenous gadolinium chelates.

STIR and FATSAT sequences are routinely used when bone marrow disorders are suspected. Bone marrow imaging is discussed in Chap. 29.

The application of fluid attenuated inversion recovery (FLAIR) sequences for spinal cord imaging has not been as straightforward as for brain imaging (Hittmair et al. 1996). More recently a T1-weighted hybrid-RARE FLAIR technique was compared to a conventional T1-weighted SE sequence in 20 patients (Melhem et al. 1997). Using a TR/TI of 2000/

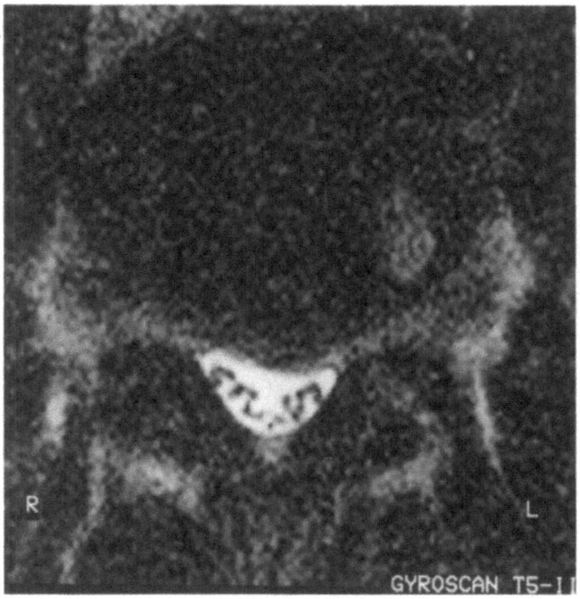

Fig. 25.4. Axial fast SE 3D dataset, 3-mm-thick partition, 0.5 T. Protrusion at L4–L5 without root compression. (Courtesy of Jan Wilmink, MD, PhD, Department of Radiology, Academic Hospital Maastricht)

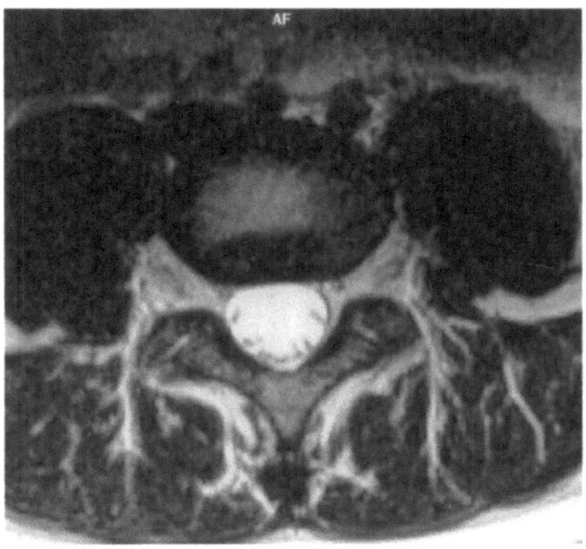

Fig. 25.5. Axial T2-weighted fast SE image at the L3–L4 level

862, an optimal contrast could be obtained between abnormal tissues and spinal cord/bone marrow.

Although it is accepted that MR imaging has superseded CT myelography for the diagnosis of most disorders, there has been interest in the so-called MR myelography. There are two techniques that are used to produce MR myelographic images. The first is based on 3D GE or fastSE pulse sequences and the examination time varies between 5 and 13 min. This method requires postprocessing with a maximum-intensity-projection algorithm visualization (El Gammal et al. 1995; Hofman and Wilmink 1996) (Fig. 25.6). The second technique is based on the rapid acquisition with relaxation enhancement technique. The advantages of this method are the extremely fast imaging time and the absence of postprocessing techniques since each image is acquired in approximately 2 s. One slice encompasses the entire thecal sac and its contents, making a projective image. One of the possible sequences is the single-shot turbo SE (Demaerel et al. 1997). We use this method routinely as part of the imaging protocol for patients presenting with low back pain and/or sciatica. Although the contribution of these MR myelographic to the diagnosis is limited to approximately 10% of the cases, the images increase the confidence of the radiologist. Nerve root compression is seen extremely well at a glance and the technique is very useful when there is a moderate or severe scoliosis (Fig. 25.7). The technique successfully demonstrates arteriovenous fistulae and postoperative changes such as arachnoiditis. The disadvantage of the MR myelographic techniques is that only the thecal sac is imaged and all surrounding structures are dark. This can cause problems of localizing an abnormality, but can be solved by demonstrating the chosen axial T2-weighted images on the MR myelogram (Fig. 25.8). At the cervical level this technique is less successful because the amount of cerebrospinal fluid around the cord and roots provides an insufficient MR signal and the image is further degraded by accelerated pulsatile cerebrospinal fluid movements.

Three-dimensional MR myelography, using a constructive interference in steady state (CISS) technique or turboSE 3D, has been used in patients with traumatic lesions of the brachial plexus (Gasparotti et al. 1997). Compared to CT myelography the authors found 89% sensitivity, 95% specificity and 92% diagnostic accuracy.

The CISS technique has been successfully applied to visualize the intradural cervical nerve roots but is less good in the assessment of the foramina (Georgy et al. 1998).

Diffusion-weighted sequences have been used in differentiating benign from malignant vertebral compression but at this stage more experience is needed to determine the potential of this technique in spine imaging (Baur et al. 1998; Ross 1999).

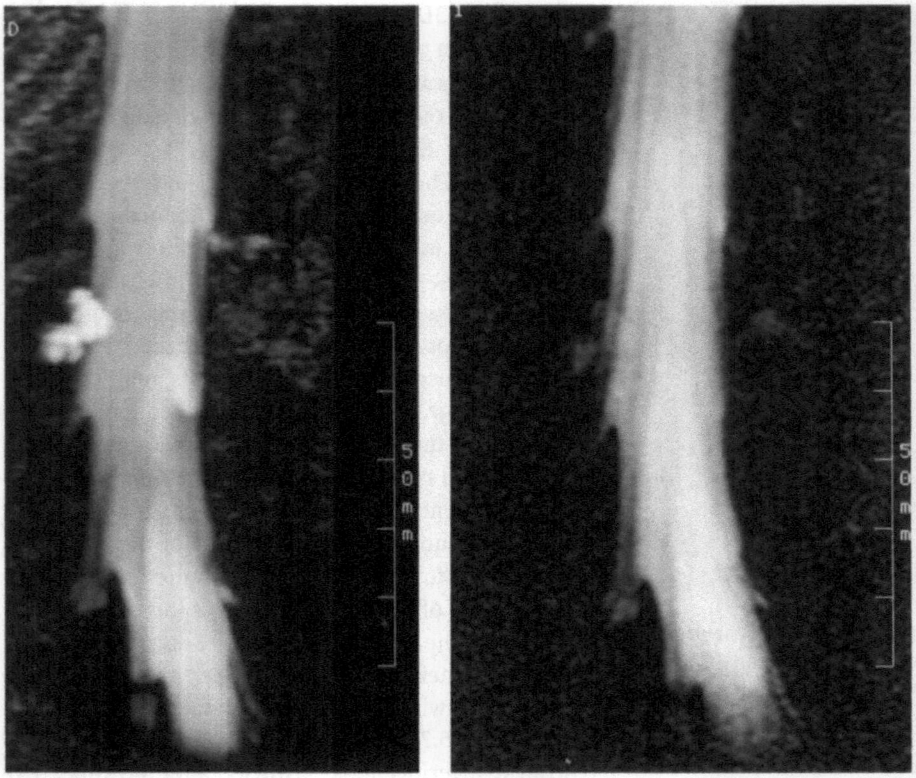

a b

Fig. 25.6a,b. Fast SE myelogram, multislice MIP (scantime 6:36 min) (a). Single slice, single-shot multi-acquisition MR myelogram (scan time 0:36 min) (b). (Courtesy of Jan Wilmink, MD, PhD, Department of Radiology, Academic Hospital Maastricht)

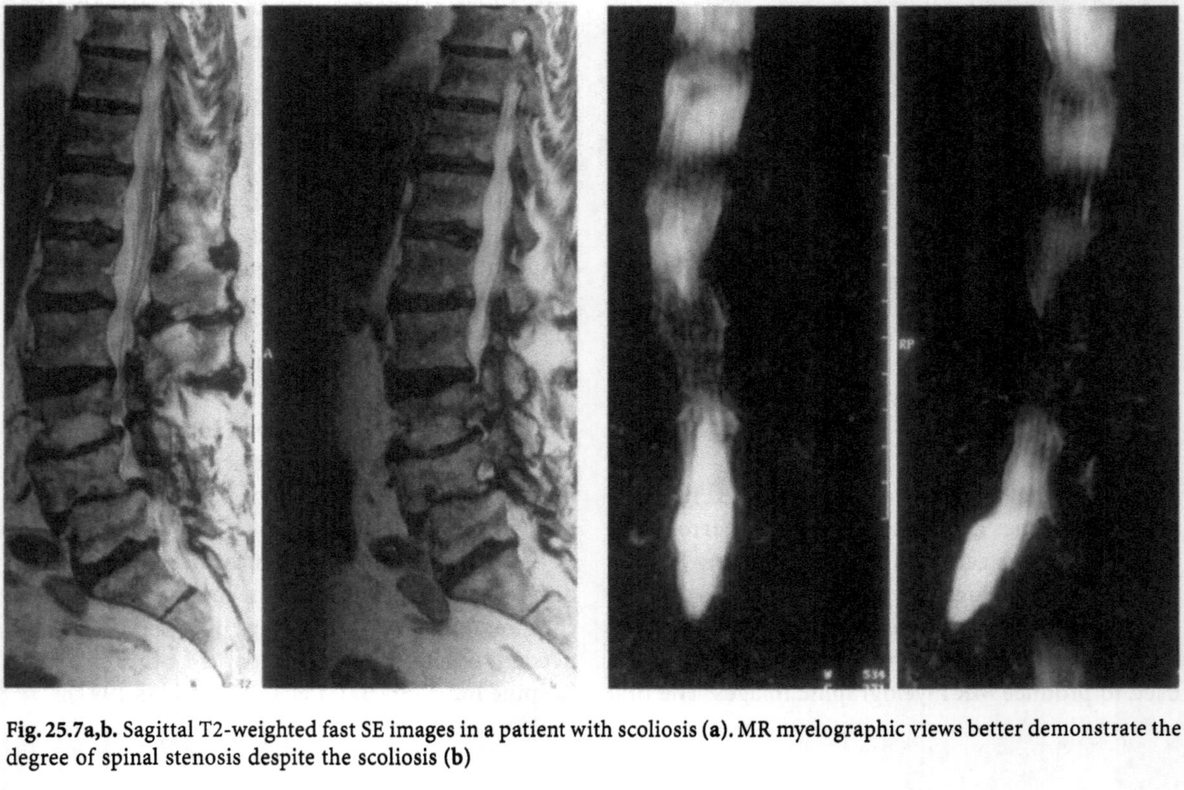

a b

Fig. 25.7a,b. Sagittal T2-weighted fast SE images in a patient with scoliosis (**a**). MR myelographic views better demonstrate the degree of spinal stenosis despite the scoliosis (**b**)

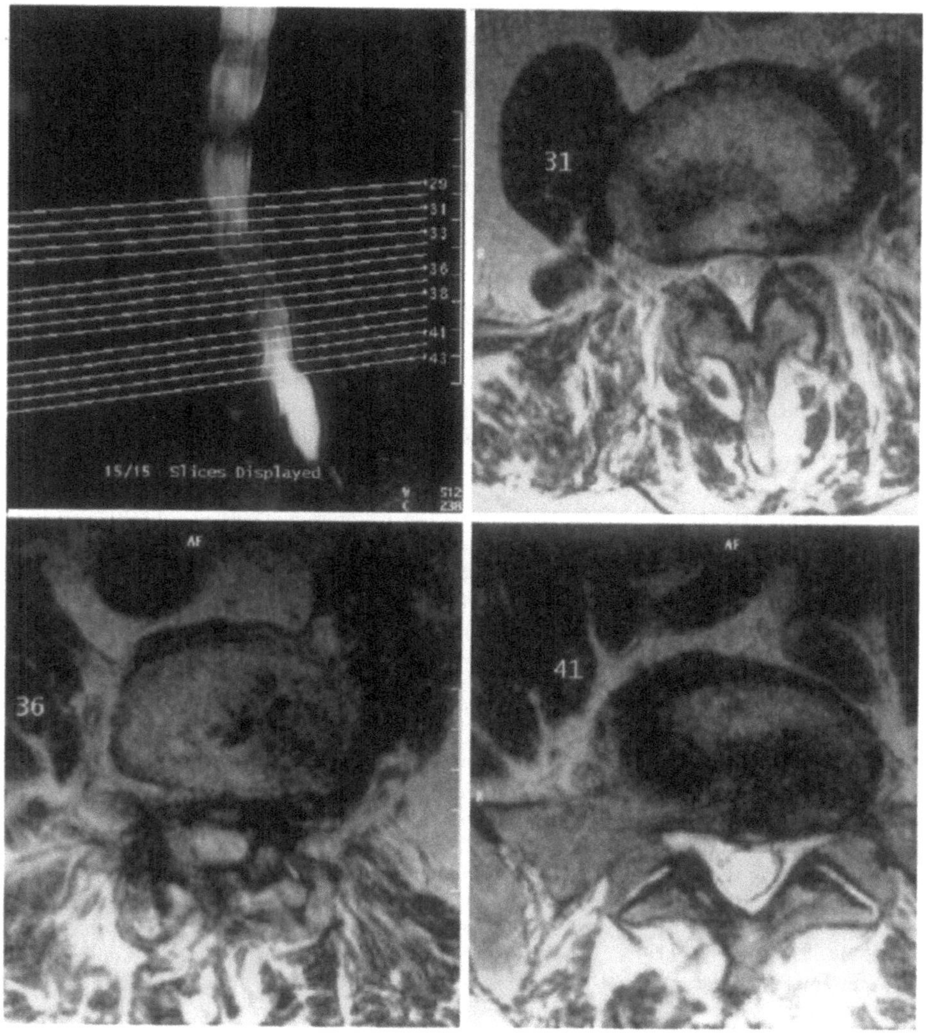

Fig. 25.8. The chosen axial T2-weighted fast SE images are displayed on the MR myelographic image, taking away the uncertainty of locating any abnormality on the myelographic image

25.6 Conclusion

Compared with plain X-ray, myelography and CT myelography, thoracic and lumbar spine MR imaging have dramatically changed our approach to spine and spinal cord disease. The advantages of spinal MR imaging are even greater than those of brain MR imaging because techniques such as myelography are invasive and are associated with a significant radiation exposure. With the further development of rapid MR imaging, it is to be expected that plain X-ray, myelography and CT myelography may no longer play a significant role in the diagnostic work-up of spine and spinal cord diseases, except perhaps when a fracture is suspected.

Although there are significant advantages of cervical spine MR imaging in degenerative disease compared to the other imaging techniques, MR imaging cannot replace these techniques at present. Although several MR sequences have been recommended, many are system dependent and most do not systematically deliver optimal image quality. Partly this is due to the limited amount of cerebrospinal fluid at the cervical level and partly it is due to the occurrence of swallowing artefacts. The development of new surface coils may be the solution for further improving the image quality. This means that plain X-ray, CT and myelography still play an important role in the diagnostic work-up of degenerative cervical spine disease.

Acknowledgements. I am very grateful to Jan Wilmink, MD, PhD, for his advice in the preparation of this chapter.

References

Baur A, Stabler A, Bruning R et al (1998) Diffusion-weighted MR imaging of bone marrow: differentiation of benign versus pathological compression fractures. Radiology 207: 349–356

Brant-Zawadzki MN, Jensen MC, Obuchowski N, Ross JS, Modic MT (1995) Interoberver and intraobserver variability in interpretation of lumbar disc abnormalities. Spine 20: 1257–1264

Demaerel Ph, Bosmans H, Wilms G et al (1997) Rapid lumbar spine MR myelography using rapid acquisition with relaxation enhancement. AJR 168: 377–378

Duerk JL, Lewin JS, Wendt M, Petersilge C (1998) Remember true FISP? A high SNR, near 1-second imaging method for T2-like contrast in interventional MRI at .2 T. J Magn Reson Imaging 8: 203–208

El Gammal T, Brooks BS, Freedy RM, Crews CE (1995) MR myelography: imaging findings. AJR 164: 173–177

Finelli DA (1998) Magnetization transfer in neuroimaging. Magn Reson Imaging Clin N Am 6: 31–52

Gasparotti R, Ferraresi S, Pinelli L et al (1997) Three-dimensional MR myelography of traumatic injuries of the brachial plexus. AJNR Am J Neuroradiol 18: 1733–1742

Georgy BA, Hesselink JR, Joseph PH (1998) 3D CISS in MR imaging of the cervical spine. 36th Annual Meeting of the ASNR, 1998

Hittmair K, Mallek R, Prayer D, Schindler EG, Kollegger H (1996) Spinal cord lesions in patients with multiple sclerosis: comparison of MR pulse sequences. AJNR Am J Neuroradiol 17: 1555–1565

Hofman PAM, Wilmink JT (1996) Optimizing the image of the intradural nerve root: the value of MR radiculography. Neuroradiology 38: 654–657

Jarvik JG, Maravilla KR, Haynor DR, Levitz M, Deyo RA (1997) Rapid MR imaging versus plain radiography in patients with low back pain: initial results of a randomized study. Radiology 204: 447–454

Jensen MC, Brant-Zawadski MN, Obuchowski N et al (1994) MR imaging of the lumbar spine in people without back pain. New Eng J Med 331: 69–73

Lycklama à Nijeholt GJ, Castelijns JA, Weerts J et al (1998) Sagittal MR of multiple sclerosis in the spinal cord: fast versus conventional spin-echo imaging. AJNR Am J Neuroradiol 19: 355–360

Maldjian C, Adam RJ, Akhtar N, Bonakdarpour A, Boyko OB (1999) Volume fast spin-echo imaging of the cervical spine. Acad Radiol 6: 84–88

Melhem ER, Benson ML, Beauchamp NJ, Lee RR (1996) Cervical spondylosis: three-dimensional gradient-echo MR with magnetization transfer. AJNR Am J Neuroradiol 17: 705–711

Melhem ER, Israel DA, Eustace S, Jara H (1997) MR of the spine with a fast T1-weighted fluid-attenuated inversion recovery sequence. AJNR Am J Neuroradiol 18: 447–454

Milette PC (1997) The proper terminology for reporting lumbar intervertebral disk disorders. AJNR Am J Neuroradiol 18: 1859–1866

Mühle C, Metzner J, Weinert D et al (1998) Classification system based on kinematic MR imaging in cervical spondylitic myelopathy. AJNR Am J Neuroradiol 19: 1763–1771

Rankine JJ, Hutchinson CE, Hughes DG (1997) MRI of lumbar spondylosis: a comparison of sagittal T2 weighted and three sequence examinations. Br J Radiol 70: 1112–1121

Rankine JJ, Gill KP, Hutchinson CE, Ross ERS, Williamson JB (1998) The therapeutic impact of lumbar spine MRI on patients with low back and leg pain. Clin Radiol 53: 688–693

Robling M, Kinnersley P, Houston H, Hourihan M, Cohen D, Hale J (1998) An exploration of GP's use of MRI: a critical incident study. Fam Pract 15: 236–243

Rocca MA, Mastronardo G, Horsfield MA, et al (1999) Comparison of three MR sequences for the detection of cervical cord lesions in patients with multiple sclerosis. AJNR Am J Neuroradiology 20: 1710–1716

Roland M, Van Tulder M (1998) Should radiologists change the way they report plain radiography of the spine? Lancet 352: 229–230

Ross JS (1999) Newer sequences for spinal MR imaging: smorgasbord or succotash or acronyms. AJNR Am J Neuroradiol 20: 361–373

Stadnik TW, Lee RR, Coen HL et al (1998) Annular tears and disk herniation: prevalence and contrast enhancement on MRI in the absence of low back pain and sciatica. Radiology 206: 49–55

Stevenson VL, Moseley IF, Phatouros CC, MacManus D, Thompson AJ, Miller DH (1998) Improved imaging of the spinal cord in multiple sclerosis using three dimensional fast spin echo. Neuroradiology 40: 416–419

Suarez-Almazor ME, Belseck E, Russell AS, Mackel JV (1997) Use of lumbar radiographs for the early diagnosis of low back pain. JAMA 277: 1782–1786

Swainson CJ, Hutchinson CE, Watson Y (1997) A comparison of 2-D and 3-D FSE imaging in MR of the cervical spine. Clin Radiol 52: 194–197

Van Tulder MW, Assendelft WJJ, Koes BW, Bouter LM (1997) Spinal radiographic findings and nonspecific low back pain. Spine 22: 427–434

Vroomen PCAJ, van Hapert SJM, van Acker REH et al (1998) The clinical significance of gadolinium enhancement of lumbar disc herniations and nerve roots on preoperative MRI. Neuroradiology 40: 800–806

Whalen JP, Balter S (1982) Radiation risks associated with diagnostic radiology. Dis Mon 28: 73

26 Emergencies in Spine and Spinal Cord Imaging

Luc van den Hauwe, Johan W. Van Goethem

CONTENTS

26.1 Introduction

"Emergency" is defined as a sudden, unforeseen occurrence needing immediate action. The ultimate goal in emergency situations is to preserve the function of the spinal cord and column whenever possible. According to the clinical presentation, the neuroradiologist together with the neurologist, neurosurgeon or orthopedic surgeon should decide to perform the most appropriate imaging modality to obtain the maximum of information without delay and at the minimum of expense.

26.2 Imaging Techniques

A wide range of imaging modalities is at our disposal to examine patients presenting in an emergency situation. The choice of just one imaging technique or the combination of different imaging modalities will largely depend on the clinical questions to be solved. Technical advances have shifted medical imaging from plain film radiography towards (helical) computed tomography (CT) and magnetic resonance (MR) imaging. Conventional polydirectional tomography and myelography can be used occasionally to solve specific puzzling cases or when patients cannot be examined otherwise (e.g. contraindications for MR examinations).

26.2.1 Plain Film

In spinal imaging, plain film radiography remains the initial imaging technique of choice, especially in the traumatic patient. Also in the non-trauma patient, plain film radiography often gives some clues towards the diagnosis. Therefore, specialized imaging techniques such as CT and MRI should usually not be performed without using plain films for guidance (Fig. 26.1) (Daffner 1996).

Differing opinions exist of how many and which views should be obtained routinely in emergency situations. It is general practice that plain film radiography of the cervical spine should include at least 3 views: cross table lateral (CTL), anteroposterior (AP) and open mouth (OM) odontoid views. Additional imaging can be used, such as oblique views to evaluate the neuroforamina, a swimmer's view for the cervicothoracic junction can be added and if the patient is sufficiently stable flexion-extension views can be obtained.

For the initial evaluation of the thoracico-lumbar spine (TLS), AP and CTL views may be sufficient.

Analysis of emergency department admissions and imaging studies in a level I trauma center demonstrated the high number of patients that presented with traumatic lesions of the spine (Lee and Chew 1998). Among all bone radiographs, the most commonly performed was the cervical spine (19% of bone studies). Plain film studies of the thoracic spine and the lumbar spine were performed in 4.1% and 9% respectively. Studies of the cervical spine yielded the highest percentage of normal findings (88.7%).

L. van den Hauwe, MD; J.W. Van Goethem, MD, PhD
Department of Radiology, University Hospital Antwerp, Wilrijkstraat 10, 2650 Antwerp (Edegem), Belgium

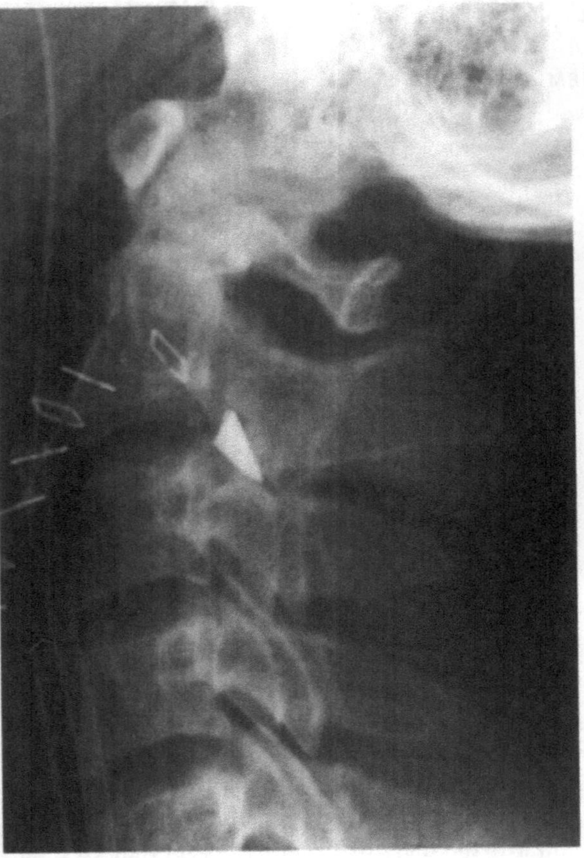

a

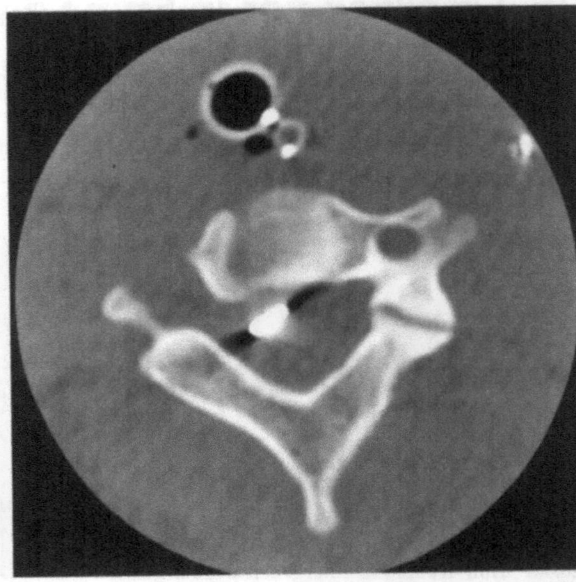

b

Fig. 26.1a,b. Stabbing lesion: The lateral plain film in the young male with a stabbing lesion shows the broken tip of a knife projected intraspinally at the C2–C3 level. Emergency CT shows the metal fragment intraspinally but extramedullary (**b**). CT is unable to demonstrate intrinsic medullary changes. MR was not performed since the presence of a large superparamagnetic or even ferromagnetic fragment in the spinal canal is an absolute contraindication

Radiographs of the thoracic spine and lumbar spine were negative in 86.3% and 82.4% of cases. Other studies demonstrated a low sensitivity for identifying traumatic cervical spine lesions. In a large series of patients with cervical injuries the combination of CTL, AP and OM views missed 61% of all fractures, 36% of subluxations and dislocations and falsely identified 23% of the patients, half of whom had unstable cervical injuries, as having normal cervical spines (Fig. 26.2) (Woodring and Lee 1993).

Reasons for this high number of negative studies need to be analyzed. Clinical examination of the cervical spine is often unreliable since movement of this area in patients with possible spinal injury is prohibited. Therefore, emergency physicians have to rely on imaging studies instead. Mirvis et al. demonstrated that 96% of hospitals that treat trauma in North America follow the guidelines of the American College of Surgeons, which include that radiographs of the cervical spine are obtained in all patients with major trauma (Mirvis et al. 1989). These factors have compelled emergency physicians to make these studies a routine part of the evaluation of trauma patients. Imaging studies are also ordered because of medicolegal aspects; to document a normal condition. In a study of 333 patients, no positive cervical spine radiographs were reported in alert patients with no clinical signs of cervical trauma (Fischer 1984). Others concluded that in the absence of specific clinical findings cervical spine radiographs can be omitted (Cadoux et al. 1987). On the other hand, plain film abnormalities can be found in patients without symptoms of cervical injury (Walter et al. 1984). In a recent publication by Blackmore et al., severe head injury, high-energy cause, focal neurologic deficit and patient's age were used as predictors of cervical spine fractures (Blackmore et al. 1999). Frequently, radiographs taken in the emergency room are of suboptimal quality because of an uncooperative patient or the necessity of taking of cross-table lateral (CTL) views and portable views. Other causes of negative plain radiographs can be low quality radiographs (especially the craniocervical junction and the cervicothoracic junction) and misinterpretation of the findings due to lack of experience (Blacksin and Lee 1995). To increase the sensitivity of imaging, trauma victims with plain films positive for cervical injury, or negative for cervical injury but with a high clinical suspicion of injury, should undergo helical CT or MR for a more definitive evaluation of the cervical spine (Nunez and Quencer 1998).

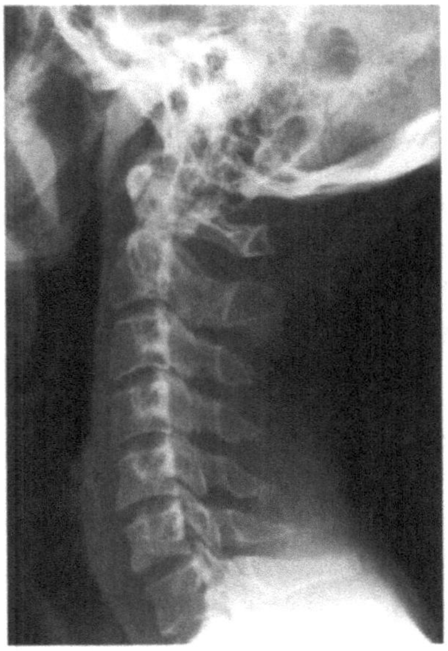

a

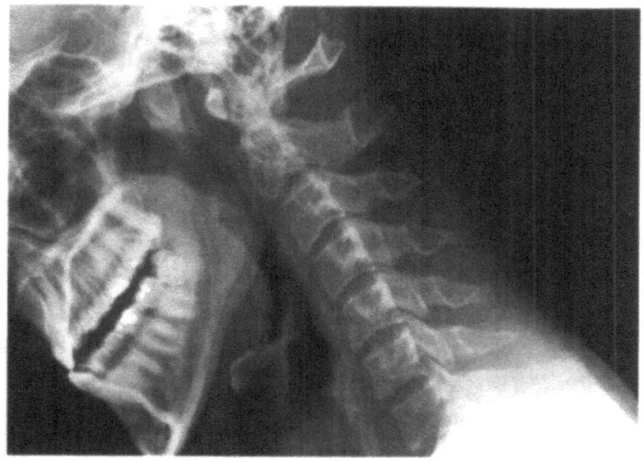

b

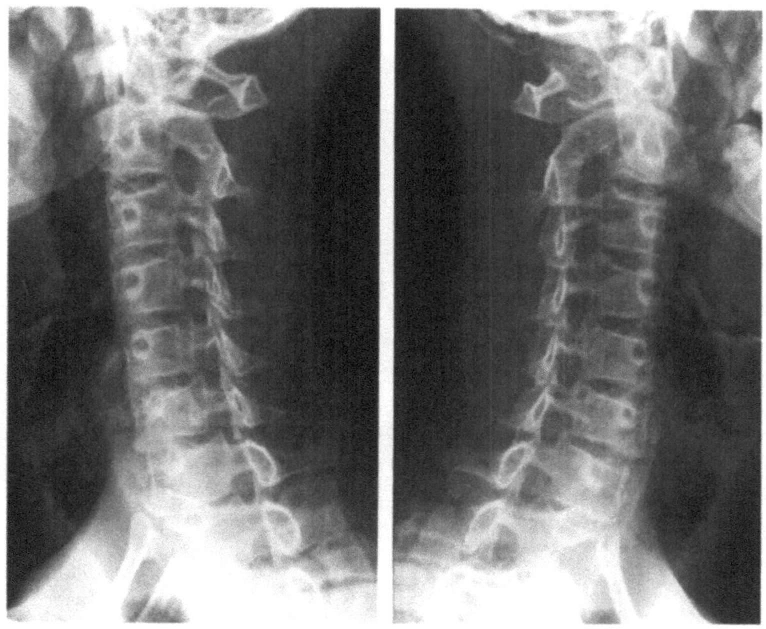

c

Fig. 26.2a–c. Fracture/luxation C6–C7: Plain films of a 28-year-old man after a motor vehicle accident. He complained of neck and irradiating pain immediately after the trauma. The lateral flexion/extension films show a minimal anterolisthesis at the C6–C7 level on the dorsiflexion film (extension), but this could be paranormal (**a,b**). Also the superior facets of C7 are less clearly delineated. For further examination oblique films were made (**c**). These show an obvious fracture of the superior articular process of C7 with secondary subluxation and foraminal narrowing

26.2.2
Computed Tomography

Spiral or helical CT (Johnson and Tanenbaum 1998) is performed in the axial plane and then reformatted in the sagittal and coronal plane. Also 3D-surface rendered reconstructions may be achieved. Therefore, the thinnest stacked contiguous sections possible need to be achieved. The choice of section thickness depends on the area studied and on the indication of the examination. Whereas 2–3 mm thick axial sections may be sufficient to evaluate the cervical spine for degenerative disease, thinner sections (1–1.5 mm) are required in patients with trauma to the craniocervical junction (CCJ) or when complex lateral mass fractures are suspected (Kaiser and Holland 1998). In the TLS, 4–5 mm axial slices are usually sufficient.

CT has been proposed as a method of screening trauma patients to exclude cervical fractures (Nunez et al 1994; Link et al. 1995). Advantages of CT in the examination of patients with craniocervical trauma include its higher sensitivity when compared to plain radiography (Bachulis et al. 1987; Woodring et al. 1992; Nunez et al 1994) and the lack of valuable time loss when CT of the cervical spine is performed in conjunction with CT scanning of the brain (Nunez et al. 1994). However, availability is variable through the countries in the EC and higher medical costs are involved when screening all patients with cervical trauma. Therefore patients should be classified into various groups according to their level of probability for injury (Blackmore et al. 1999a, 1999b). In high and moderate risk groups for cervical spine fracture, CT screening is cost-effective and prevents cases of paralysis due to spinal cord injury (Blackmore et al.

1999b). Indications for CT of the cervical spine in trauma patients therefore include severe head injury, focal neurologic deficit and high-energy causes (Blackmore et al. 1999a, 1999b). In our institution CT is also performed when visualization of the complete C-spine (C1–C7) on plain film is not complete, when unexplained focal neck pain is present, in cases of unexplained prevertebral soft-tissue swelling or if initial plain films show any abnormality (Fig. 26.3).

CT also has an important role in imaging thoracic or lumbar fractures detected on plain film (Fig. 26.4). Evaluation of the extent of the fracture and the compression of neurologic structures is important in the therapeutic planning.

26.2.3 Magnetic Resonance Imaging

Whenever possible, circular polarized coils should be used to obtain high quality images with high SNR (Van Goethem 1999). Multiple small surface coils, often circularly polarized, can be used together in a so-called array coil (phased-array coils). With this concept, larger regions can be covered with a significant higher SNR when compared to the body coil (Nitz 1999).

For MR imaging of the C-spine in general, sagittal conventional spin echo (SE) T1-W and sagittal turbo spin echo (TSE aka fast spin echo, FSE) T2-W se-

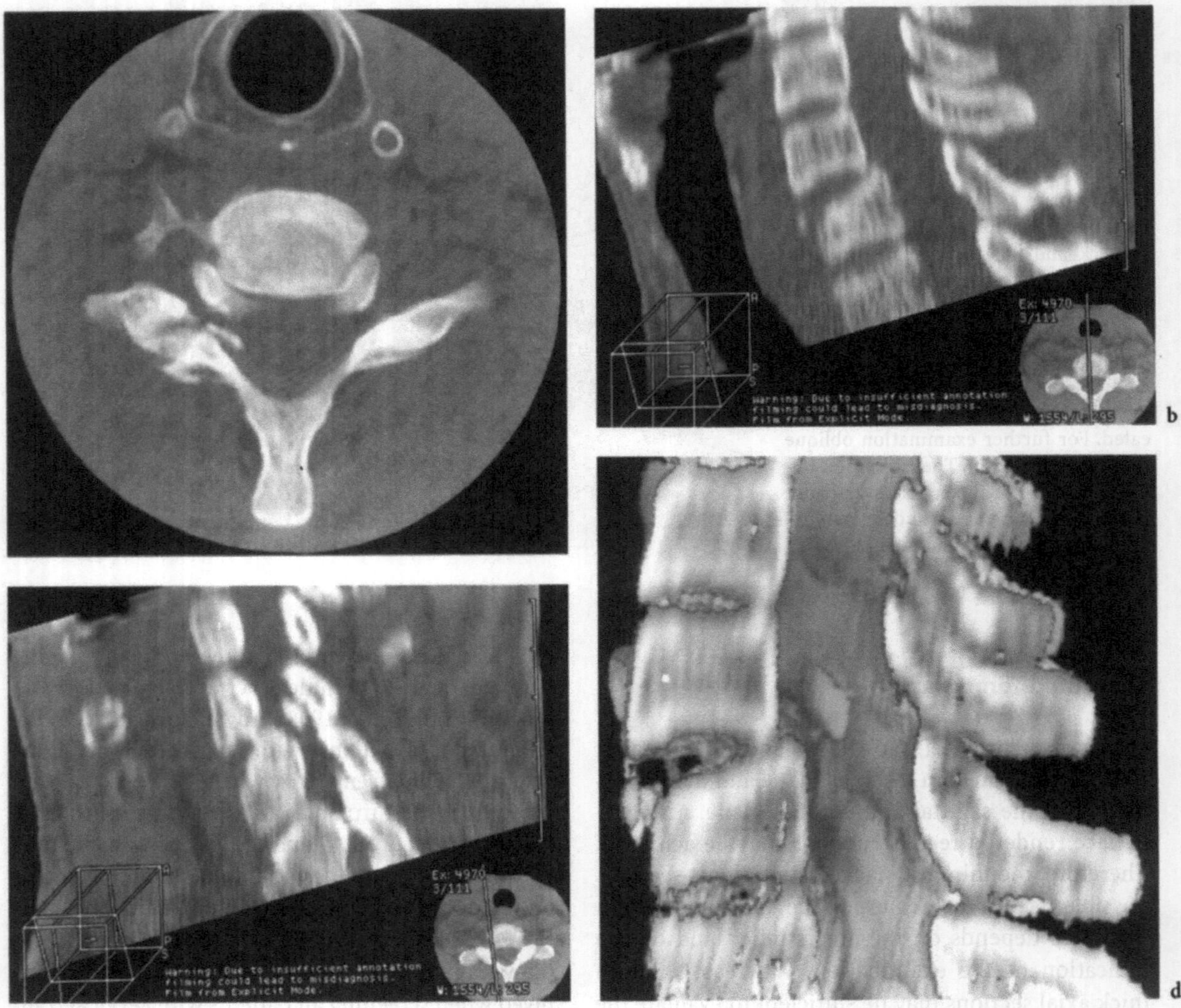

Fig. 26.3a–d. Cervical fracture/luxation, use of reformatted images and 3D reconstructions: A 57-year-old man had a fracture at the right C5–C6 facet joint after an accidental fall. The axial CT image (**a**) shows the fracture at the facet with small bony chips intra- and extraspinally. Due to the secondary subluxation the neuroforamina are narrowed. Since foraminal narrowing is better appreciated on (para-)sagittal images reformatted images were made (**b,c**). These images more clearly depict the anterolisthesis (luxation) of C5 on C6 and the bony fragment at the right C5–C6 neuroforamen. 3D surface renderings (**d**), although spectacular to look at, usually do not yield more information. The quality of reformatted images and the possibility of 3D images is greatly enhanced with the introduction of spiral CT as was used in this case (compare with reformats in classic CT in Fig. 26.1)

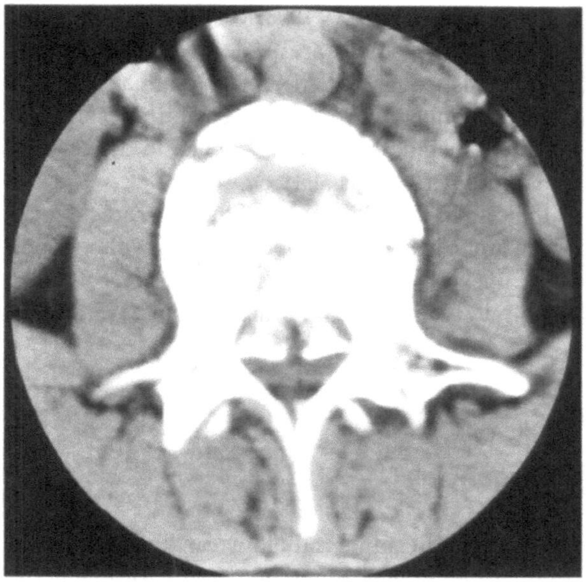
a

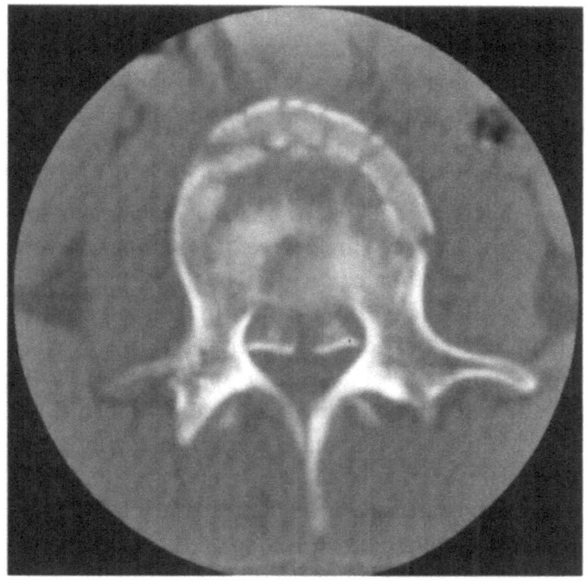
b

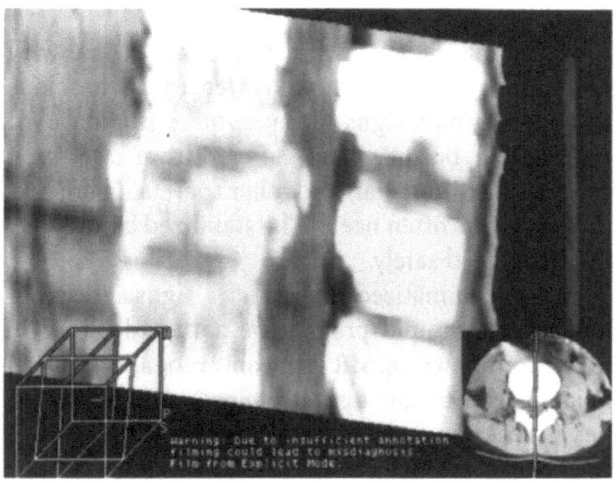
c

Fig. 26.4a–c. Burst fracture L3: This 25-year-old woman sustained a single level lumbar fracture. The axial images at the level of the L3 pedicles (**a,b**) show an important displacement of bone fragments in the spinal canal. The image with a bony window (1800/350, W/C) clearly depicts the fragments which are radially displaced in a typical example of a burst fracture. The soft tissue window (400/30, W/C) is more suited to exclude intraspinal or paraspinal soft tissue pathology, e.g., epidural or paravertebral hematoma. It is therefore always recommended to make two prints of the images, one in bone and one in soft tissue windows. A reformatted parasagittal image (**c**) more clearly demonstrates the sagittal extension of the spinal stenosis due to displaced bone fragments

quences with relatively short echo train lengths are used. When compared to conventional SE, FSE sequences allow us to achieve images with comparable image quality in a considerably shorter imaging time (Van Goethem 1999). Routinely, axial gradient echo (GE) T2*, perpendicular to the intervertebral disk space, is added to examine the cervical spine. It has been published, however, that standard GE T2*-W sequences are inaccurate for evaluating intramedullary cord lesions (Kaiser and Holland 1998). When an intramedullary lesion is suspected clinically, an additional true T2-W axial sequence should be performed.

At the level of the lumbar spine, an axial T2-W TSE sequence is used, when available. The latter sequence should not be used at the cervico-thoracic level since they are more vulnerable to CSF pulsation artifacts. Also axial SE or TSE T1-W sequences can be performed.

If there is suspicion of tumor or infection, then a fat-suppressed sequence should be added. Examples include vertebral metastases, osteomyelitis or diskitis (Kaiser and Holland 1998).

Recently, novel MR imaging techniques have been developed, allowing for sequences with high contrast to noise ratios and short examination times. A lot of these sequences have been described in the literature but still have to prove their real clinical impact on spinal imaging (Ross 1999). Such sequences include three-dimensional (3D) GE, fast fluid-attenuated inversion recovery (FLAIR) and diffusion-weighted (DW) sequences. Also half Fourier techniques such as 3D constructive interference in steady state (3D CISS) and HASTE, which is a half Fourier TSE sequence, have been described. HASTE has the advantage of reducing artifacts from spinal metal implants (Rudisch et al. 1998; Mathews et al. 1998).

An axial T2*-W 3D low-flip angle GE sequence allows for better visualization of the neural foramina of the cervical spine, reserving the 2D GE for uncooperative patients. However, in comparing this 3D GE sequence with thin-section CT, Yousem et al. reported that the findings on MR agreed with CT in only 76% of cases (Yousem et al. 1991). As a result of magnetic susceptibility artifacts, the degree of foraminal narrowing was overestimated on MR. The use of magnetization transfer with 3D GE results in less exaggeration of the degree of foraminal stenosis (Finelli et al. 1994; Melhem et al. 1996). The application of FLAIR for the detection of subtle spinal cord abnormalities (e.g., MS plaques) remains controversial (White et al. 1992; Hittmaier et al.1996; Keiper et al. 1997). Short-inversion-time inversion recovery (STIR) and fast STIR cannot only be used to detect vertebral metastases but appear to be useful to evaluate the cervical spinal cord (Baker et al. 1990; Jones et al. 1994; Hilfiker et al. 1995; Ross 1999). Only few results are available on the application of echo-planar imaging (EPI) in imaging of the spinal cord. Recently, the presence of cord abnormalities has been demonstrated in a small number of traumatic and myelopathic cases, using an SE EPI sequence (Teresi et al. 1997; Holder et al. 1998). Dousset et al. demonstrated areas with increased apparent diffusion coefficient (ADC) in the spinal cord at the level of medullary compression in patients with acquired spinal stenosis, secondary to degenerative disorders (Dousset et al. 1999).

Various investigators have recommended obtaining "MR myelograms" (MRM), thereby simulating conventional myelogram views (VanDyke et al. 1992; El Gammal et al. 1996; Edal et al. 1997). Some claim, however, that this technique is of minimal value since only the deformity of the CSF is displayed and not the structure actually causing the deformity, similar to the limitations of conventional myelography (Kaiser and Holland 1998).

It has been stated that diffusion-weighted imaging of the spine allows the differentiation of benign from pathologic compression fractures (Baur et al. 1998). Benign vertebral compression fractures are hypo- to isointense to normal bone marrow in the adjacent vertebral bodies, whereas pathologic compression fractures are hyperintense to normal vertebral bodies (Baur et al. 1998). When a quantitative approach is applied (using bone marrow contrast ratios) to discriminate these two types of compression fractures, a negative bone marrow contrast ratio is observed in benign compression fractures and a positive marrow contrast ratio in pathologic compression fractures (Baur et al. 1998). Other investigators have criticized the value of this technique (Le Bihan 1998; Ross 1999; Castillo et al. 1999). Further studies are needed to assess the added value of this sequence in MR imaging of patients with vertebral bone marrow abnormalities. Diffusion weighted imaging can also be applied to the cervical spinal cord (Clarck et al. 1999).

Indications for MR imaging of the spine are progressive neurologic deficit, spinal cord injury without bone injury, unexpected level of signs above the level of radiographically seen injury and whiplash injuries (Fig. 26.5).

26.3 Emergencies

Emergencies in spinal radiology can be classified as traumatic emergencies and non-traumatic emergencies.

In trauma patients, we mostly have to deal with polytraumatized patients who often are unconscious and not only have signs and symptoms of spinal cord dysfunction, but may have suffered from associated cranial (maxillo-facial) and other trauma. Therefore, these patients often need to be stabilized before they can be imaged safely.

In non-traumatized emergencies, signs and symptoms indicate rapid progressive abrupt decrease in spinal cord function. MR is the only modality that can reliably demonstrate discrete spinal cord abnormalities as for example in multiple sclerosis (MS).

26.3.1 Traumatic Emergencies

Trauma is the most frequent cause of chronic spinal cord dysfunction. It typically occurs in young adults as a result of motor vehicle accidents, falls, or accidents in recreational activities (diving, riding, skiing). Imaging of spinal trauma is used to detect and assess the extent of osseous, spinal cord and nerve root lesions, ligamentous and other soft tissue injuries and to evaluate instability (An 1998).

26.3.1.1 Spinal Cord Injury

Spinal cord injuries are usually associated with traumatic lesions of the vertebrae, intervertebral disks and/or ligaments which may cause cord compression due to dislocated bone, herniated disk and epidural hematoma. However, notably in newborns and chil-

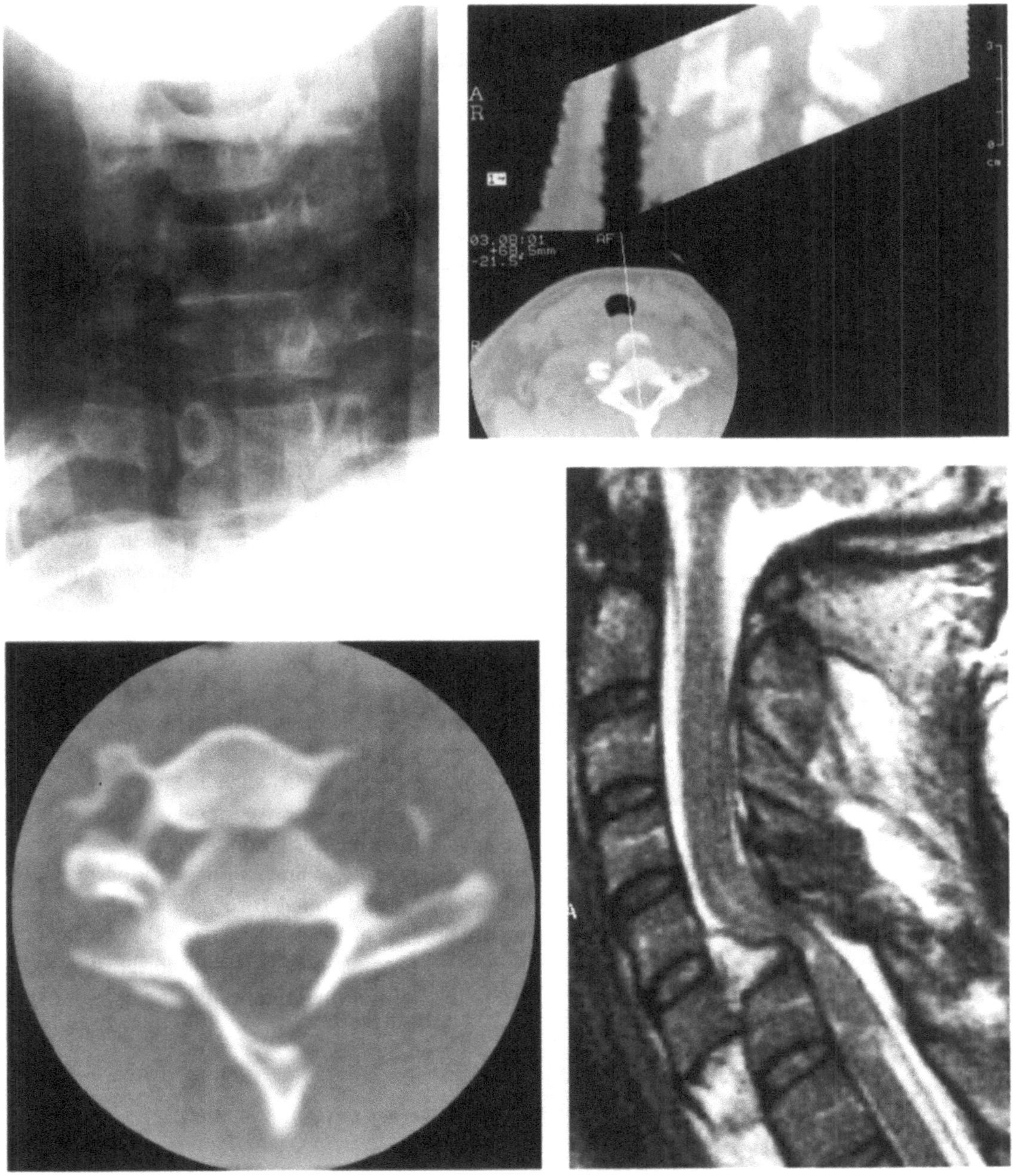

a b c d

Fig. 26.5a–d. Cord section after traumatic vertebral luxation: This 30-year-old woman was paraplegic when she arrived at the hospital after a car accident. Lateral plain films did not adequately image the lower cervical spine, in an obese patient. The frontal plain film (**a**) clearly shows a narrowed C6–C7 disk space which urged for a subsequent CT. The axial CT image (**b**) and the reformatted CT image (**c**) show a complete luxation of C6 on C7 with spinal canal narrowing. Finally MR was performed, confirming a complete cord transection at the level of the luxation (**d**)

dren, severe cord injury may occur without spinal damage as a result of traction and stretching forces (Mascalchi et al. 1993).

26.3.1.1.1
Acute Phase

Findings in the acute phase of spinal cord trauma include edema, hematoma and transection of the spinal cord (Fig. 26.5). Also posttraumatic extradural lesions, such as epidural hematomas, herniated disks (Fig. 26.6) and retropulsed bony fragments, compressing the spinal cord are readily visualized (El Khoury et al. 1995). In patients with acute spinal injury presenting with neurological deficit, MR imaging is an emergency examination. In these cases MR should be performed to establish the cause of

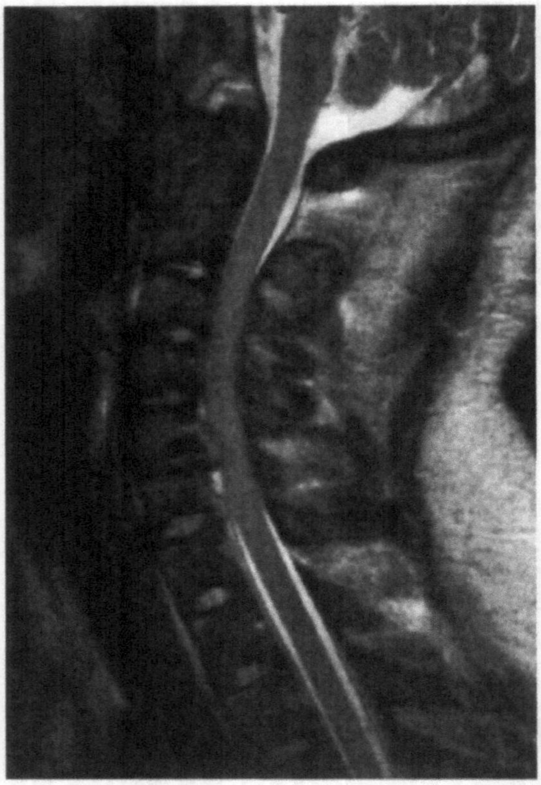

a

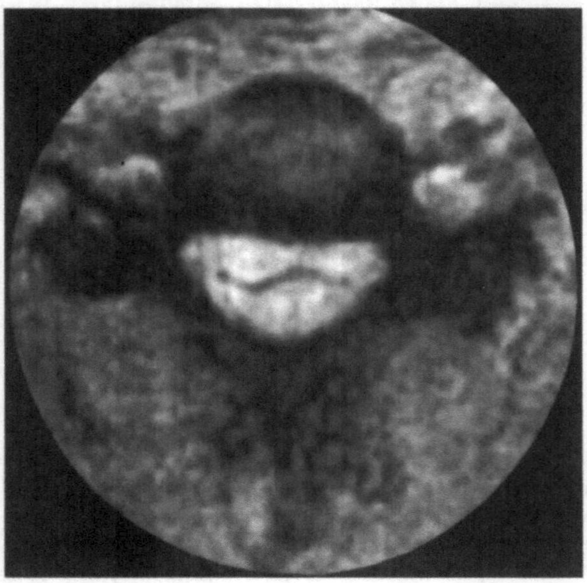

b

Fig. 26.6a,b. Traumatic disk herniation with medullary contusion: This 19-year-old male polytrauma sustained a severe motor vehicle accident. He developed an increasing paraparesis in the hours following the accident. Emergency MR was carried out (**a,b**). The sagittal T2-weighted image (**a**) shows a large C5–C6 disk herniation. A smaller hernia is seen at the level C6–C7. The axial T2*-weighted image at the C5–C6 level (**b**) shows an epidural mass with high signal corresponding to the herniated disk material. The high signal intensity is caused by hemorrhage and edema in the acutely herniated material. A curtain sign is seen in which the disk material protrudes left and right of the posterior ligament on the midline

cord compression requiring surgical decompression after proper reduction and/or to detect and characterize contusions of the spinal cord. Distinction between grossly hemorrhagic and non-hemorrhagic contusions has significant prognostic implications (Flanders et al. 1996). In fact the former lesions usually carry a worse prognosis with incomplete recovery of clinical deficit and more extensive cystic necrosis at follow-up MR imaging. Another application of acute MR imaging of spinal trauma is the evaluation of spinal ligament disruption and tears which may be relevant in planning stabilization procedures (Mascalchi et al. 1994). In the acute phase T2* weighted gradient echo images can be of use for demonstration of hemorrhagic contusions of the cord, especially at low- and mid-field strength. The acutely injured spinal cord may appear either normal, enlarged because of hemorrhagic or non-hemorrhagic contusion, or thinned because of compression or transection.

26.3.1.1.2
Chronic Phase

In the chronic phase, MR imaging is justified when the patient presents with late functional deterioration in order to detect conditions such as syringomyelia or arachnoid cysts amenable to surgical treatment. Other imaging findings include cord atrophy, myelomalacia, wallerian degeneration and meningeal adhesions. The chronically injured spinal cord may appear normal, thinned because of atrophy, or enlarged because of an intramedullary cyst. In addition the cord can be tethered to the walls of the spinal canal due to meningeal adhesions.

26.3.1.2
Vertebral Artery Lesions

A recent report has emphasized the high yield of vertebral artery abnormalities in patients with acute cervical spinal injury examined with MR angiography in addition to MR imaging (Friedman et al. 1995). Since vertebral artery abnormalities do not alter management of these patients, the extra time needed to acquire MR angiography has to be balanced against the often difficult clinical and monitoring conditions of these patients.

26.3.1.3
Nerve Root Lesions

Avulsions of the nerve roots and posttraumatic meningocoeles are the result of hyperextension in-

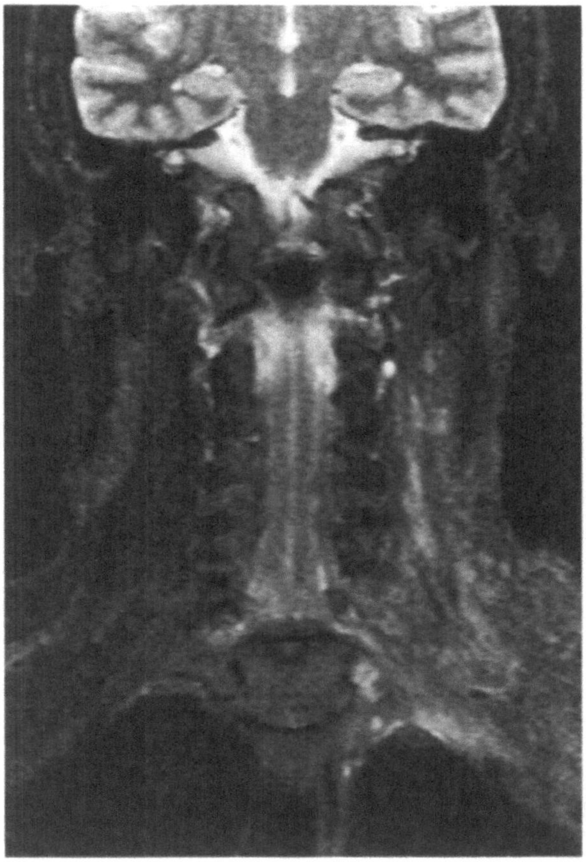

a

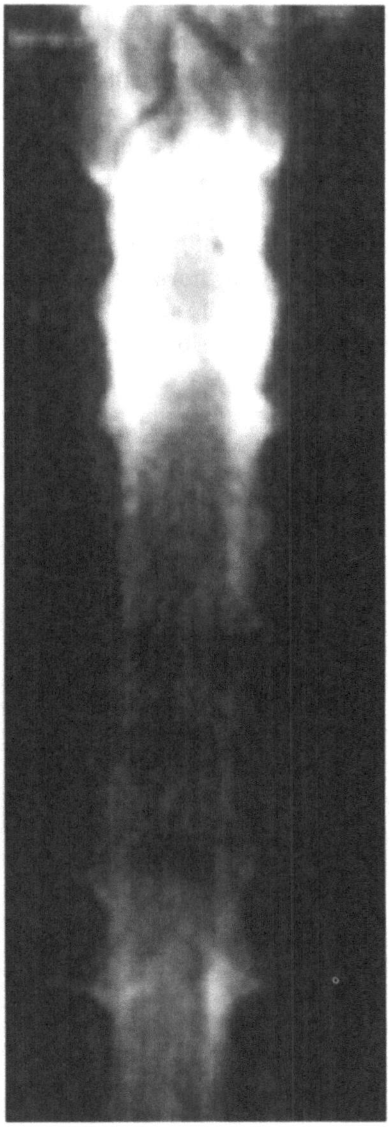

b

Fig. 26.7a,b. Plexus avulsion: This 41-year-old man fell with his motor bike 2 weeks earlier. He had a monoparesis of his right arm since the accident with little or no recuperation. The coronal T2-weighted image shows an area with diffuse high signal paravertebral on the left side, in the region of the brachial plexus (**a**). This probably represents diffuse edema. The MR myelography depicts a normal thecal sac without root avulsion (**b**). This is explained by the fact that the plexus lesion was more lateral

juries of the arm (Fig. 26.7). When located in or near the spinal canal, they can be clearly identified obtaining myelographic images. Nowadays, 3D MR myelography is able to demonstrate plexus avulsions in a non-aggressive manner (Edal et al. 1997; Gasparotti et al. 1997).

26.3.1.4 Whiplash Trauma

Whiplash is one of the most common mechanisms of injury to the cervical spine and cord. The term whiplash is not a diagnosis but only describes the manner in which a head is moved to produce a sprain of the neck (Crowe 1928; Newman 1990). The whiplash injury usually is a non-contact lesion resulting from sudden acceleration of the body and subsequent hyperextension of the neck due to the inertia of the head. It typically occurs after rear-end automobile collisions. "Whiplash" has become an emotional term, common in the popular vocabulary, frequently used by attorneys and sometimes the object of scorn by physicians (Hirsch et al. 1988). Since many cases result in litigation some physicians have considered persistent symptoms to be a form of compensation neurosis (Gotten 1956; Evans et al. 1994;). Evidence however suggests that whiplash injuries are real and are manifested by symptoms consistent with the anatomic lesion sustained and that they are a potential cause of significant impairment.

The anatomy of injury not only includes musculoligamentous sprain, but also musculoligamentous rupture, bone bruising (Fig. 26.8), disk avulsion, disk protrusion/herniation, soft-tissue hemorrhage or hematoma, cervical sympathetic nerve damage, vascular injury and surface hemorrhages, contusions of the brain, brainstem and cervical cord, and any combination of these (HIRSCH et al. 1988; FLANDERS et al. 1990; PEARCE 1993; VAN GOETHEM et al. 1998). Ligamentous injuries particularly include anterior longitudinal ligament (ALL) rupture (Fig. 26.9), sometimes with either avulsion of the involved vertebrae from the adjacent disk or horizontal rupture of the disk (DAVIS et al. 1991). More severe extension may also damage the posterior longitudinal ligament (PLL) and/or interspinous ligament. The role of medical imaging in the evaluation of whiplash injuries remains to be determined. Plain radiographs cannot be relied upon either to definitively determine the true extent and severity of cervical injuries in trauma victims or to exclude cervical injuries in these patients (WOODRING and LEE 1993). The more routine use of complex-motion tomographic studies and/or CT increases the detection of dislocations, subluxations and fractures (WOODRING and LEE 1992) but often fails to determine or visualize the

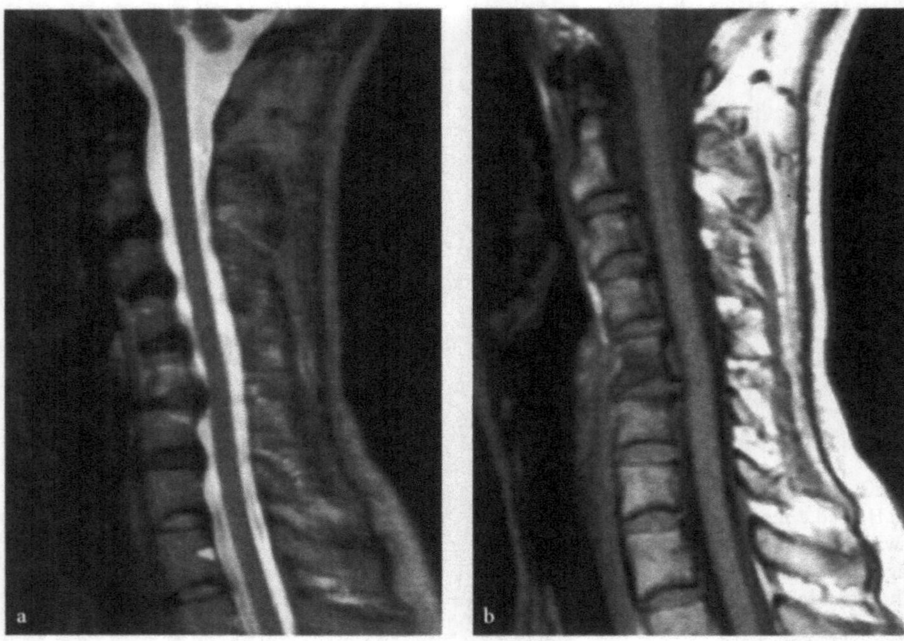

Fig. 26.8a,b. Bone bruising: This 20-year-old woman had a whiplash injury 3 days prior to this MR examination. Plain films showed a cervical kyphosis and narrowing of the C5–C6 disk space. Subsequently an MR was performed (**a,b**). This examination not only shows a large C5–C6 disk herniation, but also signal intensity changes in both vertebrae, especially anteroinferiorly in C5. The changes (low on T1, high on T2) correspond to bone edema in a case of compressive bone bruising without fracture. MR signal intensities returned to normal after 6 months

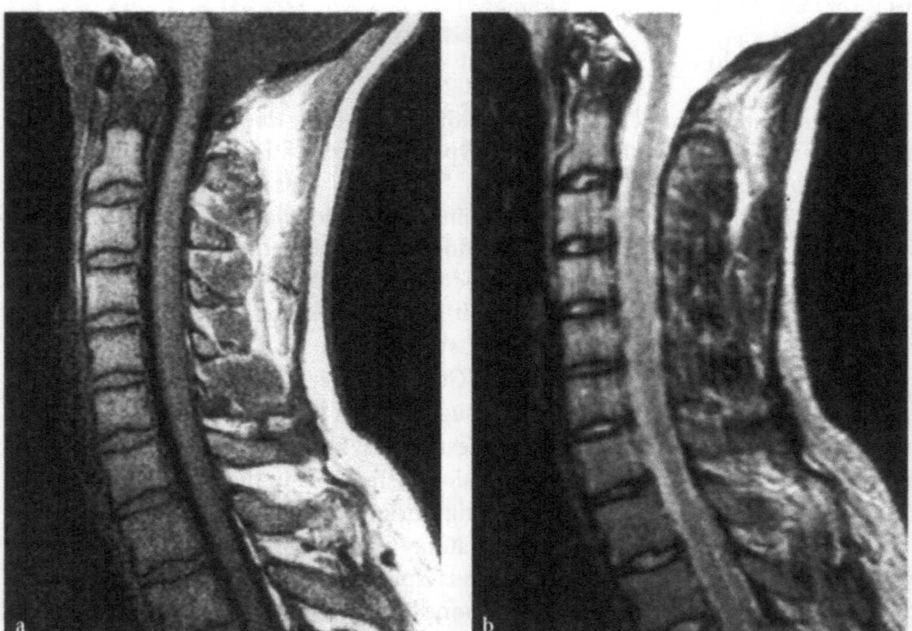

Fig. 26.9a,b. Anterior longitudinal ligamentous lesion: MR examination with sagittal T1-weighted (**a**) and T2-weighted (**b**) images 2 weeks after a whiplash injury in a young woman. The examination reveals no disk or bone abnormalities. The anterior longitudinal ligament (ALL) however is abnormally thick and has a high signal intensity at the C2 level. These changes correspond to an ALL lesion after whiplash trauma with forced dorsiflexion (extension). The posterior ligaments are normal

cause of a whiplash syndrome. Isotope scans fail to play a major role in the evaluation of whiplash injuries (HILDINGSON et al. 1989; BARTON et al. 1993). MR however is able to assess different types of soft-tissue lesions related to whiplash injuries, and is especially useful in the evaluation of intervertebral disks, cervical ligaments and spinal cord (FLANDERS et al. 1990; DAVIS et al. 1991). Finally dynamic imaging, albeit plain radiography, CT or MR, is able to show functional disturbances in patients suffering from whiplash injuries (NAGELE et al. 1992; DVORAK et al. 1993).

Since there are so many different pathological processes that may cause the symptoms and signs in a whiplash injury, it is not surprising that imaging findings are also very diverse. In a large retrospective study of 200 patients who claimed litigation after a whiplash injury the most common abnormalities on imaging findings were functional disturbances (VAN DEN HAUWE et al. 1995). These can be demonstrated on plain radiography, CT and/or MR. The second most common finding is preexisting spondylotic changes which are more frequent among whiplash injured patients than in the general population of the same age group. In addition patients with a narrower sagittal diameter of the spinal canal before the injury have a higher chance of sustaining a permanent spinal cord injury (KANG et al. 1994).

It is important to classify cervical sprains into different categories since each has different clinical and imaging findings, and what is more important a different clinical course (ERDMANN 1983; VAN GOETHEM et al. 1996).

Class I cervical sprains are what most of us call true whiplash injuries. They are also the most common form, comprising more than 95% of all whiplash injuries. There are no pathological roentgenographic findings on the initial imaging studies which can be attributed with certainty to the trauma. However newer techniques such as dynamic or high-resolution MR imaging may soon be able to diagnose abnormalities in these patients. Typically these patients have a symptom-free period between the initial accident and the onset of symptoms. The length of this time interval may vary between a few hours to 1 day and may be correlated to the severity of the sprain. This is similar to other ligamentous injuries elsewhere in the body.

Class III neck sprains are usually seen in severely traumatized patients with acute onset of symptoms immediately after the accident. This class is only a minority of all whiplash injuries (1%). Their initial imaging studies show fractures, dislocations or subluxations of the cervical spine, and therefore it could be advocated not to classify them as whiplash injuries.

Class II neck sprains are somewhere in between and usually show no primary radiological findings. Nevertheless they may exhibit secondary abnormalities later on, such as early onset disk degeneration or functional disturbances. Most physicians classify these lesions also as whiplash injuries.

MR findings in whiplash injuries are very diverse and are different depending on the time of imaging since the accident. In the chronic phase, more than 1 year after the original trauma, findings are mostly non-specific and include degenerative disk disease, disk protrusion and herniations (VAN GOETHEM et al. 1998). Only a minority of patients show bony or ligamentous lesions. In the subacute phase, within 4 months of the whiplash trauma, more characteristic findings such as separation of the disk from the vertebral end plate and ligamentous lesions are reported (DAVIS et al. 1991). The ALL is more often injured than the PLL or interspinous ligament. Aspecific findings such as degenerative disk disease or disk herniations are also reported in this stage. In the acute phase, within 15 days after the original trauma, no specific findings are made. Degenerative changes with osteophytes and disk protrusion or herniation are the most common findings (PETTERSON et al. 1994; FAGERLUND et al. 1995). In this particular study no ligamentous lesions were noted. One-third of all patients had a completely normal MR examination.

Indications for MR imaging after whiplash injury include myelopathy, radiculopathy, progressive neurologic deficit, spinal cord injury and an unexpected level of signs above the level of radiographically seen injury (DAVIS et al. 1991). MR should probably also be used in all patients with whiplash injury who have persistent complaints or significant findings at any other investigation, since these patients have a worse prognosis and may exhibit significant MR findings (VAN GOETHEM et al. 1998)

Open-design low-field MR magnets have some advantages over tunnel-shaped high-field magnets, since they allow easier dynamic extension/flexion or rotation MR examinations to be performed. This way ligamentous injuries can sometimes be detected that were not visible on the static MR examination (DVORAK et al. 1993; IGNELZI 1993). Also abnormal motion and interaction between the different anatomical constituents can be assessed.

Radiological management of patients who sustained a whiplash injury depends on the classification of the injury. Severely traumatized patients should first be examined with CTL, AP and open-mouth plain radiography. Those with positive findings on these films (class III) and those with negative findings but clinical suspicion of severe neck trauma (class II) subsequently should have cervical CT scan. If these examinations are normal cervical MRI sometimes shows soft-tissue lesions and should be performed.

26.3.2 Non-Traumatic Emergencies

Almost all non-traumatic emergencies are related to lesions that interfere with normal function of the spinal cord. "Myelopathy" and "myelitis" are non-specific terms that are often used interchangeably to describe various pathological conditions of the spinal cord. Myelopathy usually indicates a non-inflammatory, degenerative disorder of the spinal cord resulting from compressive, vascular, toxic or metabolic origin. Myelitis results from inflammation, as seen in infections (mainly viral), or presumed autoimmune (e.g., multiple sclerosis) or idiopathic conditions (Balériaux et al. 1992). Clinical presentation of the patient can orientate the diagnosis; an acute or rapidly progressive pathology is usually related to an intrinsic medullary lesion, whereas a slowly progressive onset is more likely due to extrinsic spinal cord compression.

26.3.2.1 Intrinsic Medullary Lesions

MR is the only imaging technique that reliably demonstrates intrinsic abnormalities of the spinal cord, and is therefore the imaging method of choice. In these cases, MR imaging may show an enlarged spinal cord. Focal areas of high signal intensity can be seen on T2-weighted sequences. In the acute phase, these lesions may have breakdown of the blood cord barrier and therefore show enhancement after intravenous injection of gadolinium. Intrinsic medullary lesions include infection (Fig. 26.10), inflammatory/demyelinating disease, ischemic or tumoral lesions. Sometimes, no definite cause can be found. Also radiation therapy may damage the spinal cord, which is frequently seen at the level of the cervical spine, since head and neck tumors frequently are irradiated (Wang et al. 1995). The clinical history and the presence of associated bone marrow changes may help in the differential diagnosis.

Infectious diseases of the spinal cord may be viral, bacterial or parasitic in origin, the latter being a rare cause of myelitis in immune compromised patients (Fig. 26.11) (Cumming 1992).

Inflammatory/demyelinating disease of the spinal cord includes multiple sclerosis (MS), sarcoidosis, autoimmune disorders such as lupus and paraneoplastic effects. Infectious myelitis usually presents with more mass effect and shows more extensive segmental involvement, whereas MS more frequently affects the spinal cord over only one to three segments, usually without significant mass effect (Brant-Zawadski 1999). MS lesions are typically localized within the dorsal bundles of the spinal cord (Tartaglino et al. 1995), whereas infectious lesions show more tendency to involve the centromedullary portions of the spinal cord. Sarcoidosis of the spinal cord may mimic MS on MR imaging (Junger et al. 1993).

Vascular causes of myelopathy include infarction, arteriovenous malformations and dural fistulas. Acute infarction of the spinal cord is caused by occlusion of the anterior spinal artery of Adamkiewicz. Possible underlying causes include abdominal aortic aneurysm surgery (Mawad et al. 1990) and extensive progressive atherosclerosis. Vascular lesions more often involve the anterior and central part of the cord and are more frequently seen in the lower thoracic spine and at the level of the conus.

When extensive spinal cord swelling and gadolinium enhancement is observed, MS, sarcoidosis and myelitis may be difficult to differentiate from medullary tumors. Spinal cord tumors may involve extensive portions of the spinal cord, before clinical symptoms develop, because of the great plasticity of the spinal cord. Most frequently encountered intramedullary tumors include astrocytoma, ependymoma and hemangioblastoma. An extensive tumor will usually be an astrocytoma. Hemorrhagic components are more typical for ependymoma, but may also be found in astrocytoma. Hemangioblastoma frequently has cystic components (Brotchi et al. 1991).

26.3.2.2 Extrinsic Medullary Compression

Causes of extrinsic medullary compression in non-trauma patients include degenerative disease (spondylotic myelopathy) (Fig. 26.12), non-traumatic compression fractures, epidural collections such as hemorrhage or infectious collections and extramedullary tumors (both intra- and extra-durally located) (Fig. 26.13). The spinal cord compression may be associated with focal signal abnormalities on T2-weighted images. When quick and appropriate surgical treatment is performed, these findings may be reversible and the patient may recover. In the

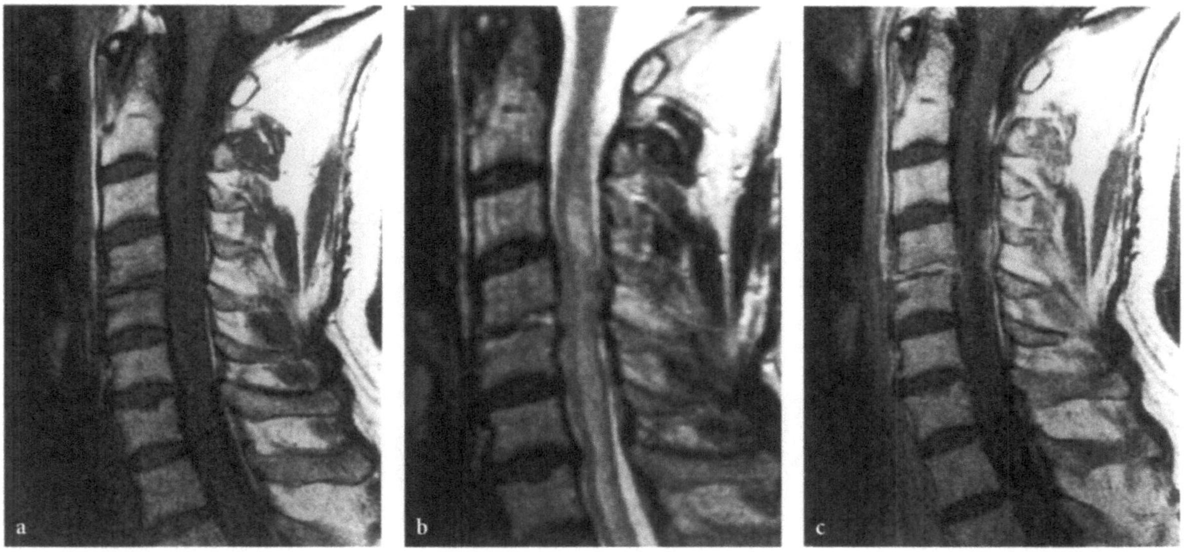

Fig. 26.10a–c. Infectious myelomeningitis after diskectomy: This 55-year-old patient underwent cervical diskectomy at the C4–C5 level. Fourteen days later, while still being hospitalized, he developed severe neck pain, fever and neurologic signs in the arms and legs. An emergency MR with T1- and T2-weighted images before contrast (**a,b**) and T1-weighted images after contrast (**c**) was performed. The operated disk space is narrowed. On the T2-weighted image the disk space partially has a high signal intensity. Also there is an extensive medullary lesion with high signal from C3 downward. After contrast administration (**c**) diffuse meningeal thickening and enhancement is noted. Disk space biopsy revealed a tuberculous infection in this case of tb myelomeningitis

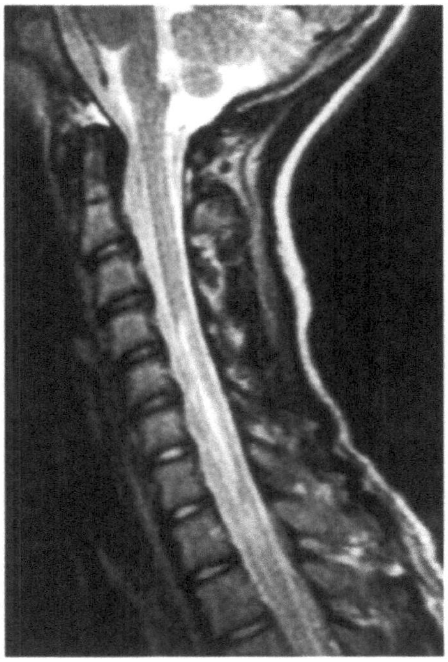

a

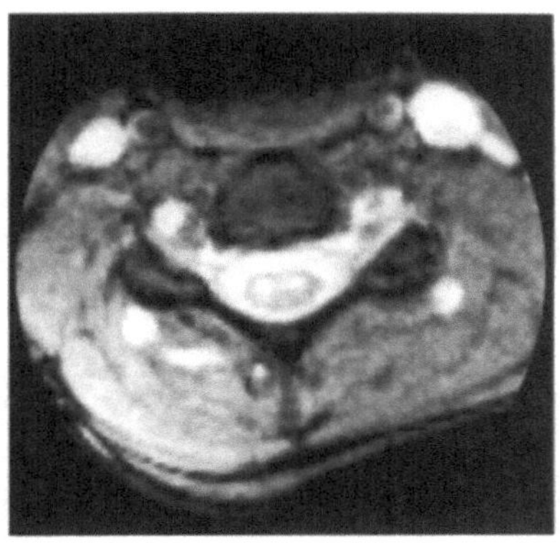

b

Fig. 26.11a,b. Poliomyelitis: A 12-year-old girl with weakness in both arms presented at the emergency department. The loss of strength in both arms had gradually developed over the previous 24 h. Emergency MR was performed and showed a high intensity medullary lesion in the cervical gray matter at the C4–C7 level on the T2-weighted images (**a,b**). There was no enhancement after contrast administration. Further laboratory testing revealed a poliovirus infection. This girl was not vaccinated for poliomyelitis although the vaccination is obligatory in Belgium

presence of intramedullary hemorrhage or cyst formation, prognosis is usually poor with permanent neurological deficit (see also Sect. 26.3.1.1.2).

We will not discuss the imaging findings in degenerative disease of the spine, since this is beyond the scope of this chapter. However it should be clear that although plain film and CT may adequately show the etiology of medullary compression, the possible associated abnormalities of the spinal cord can only be evaluated using MR imaging.

Non-traumatic compression fractures may be of osteoporotic, pathologic or infectious etiology. A

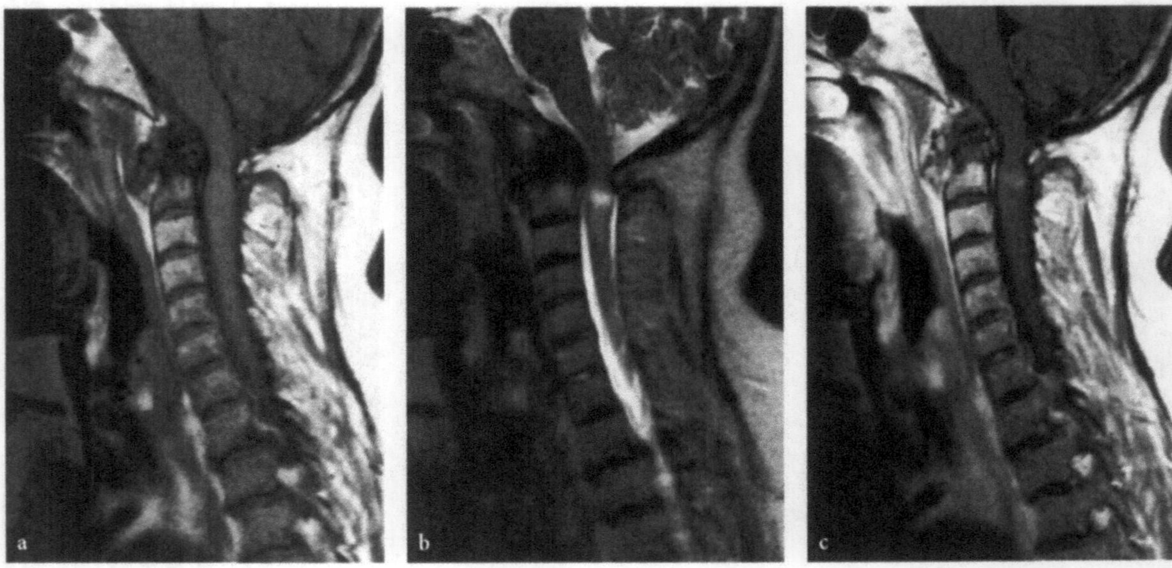

Fig. 26.12a–c. Rheumatoid arthritis with myelopathy: MR examination in an older patient with known rheumatoid arthritis. The images show bony erosion at the C1-C2 level with an inhomogeneous soft tissue swelling at the anterior joint (pannus). Due to the soft tissue swelling anteriorly and the compression of the dural sac posteriorly, secondary to subluxation, the spinal canal is narrowed (**a**). The cervical medulla is compressed and shows a focal area of myelopathy (**b**). After gadolinium administration this area shows enhancement (**c**). Enhancement corresponding to breakdown of the blood-cord barrier is believed to be a sign of (still) reversible myelopathy

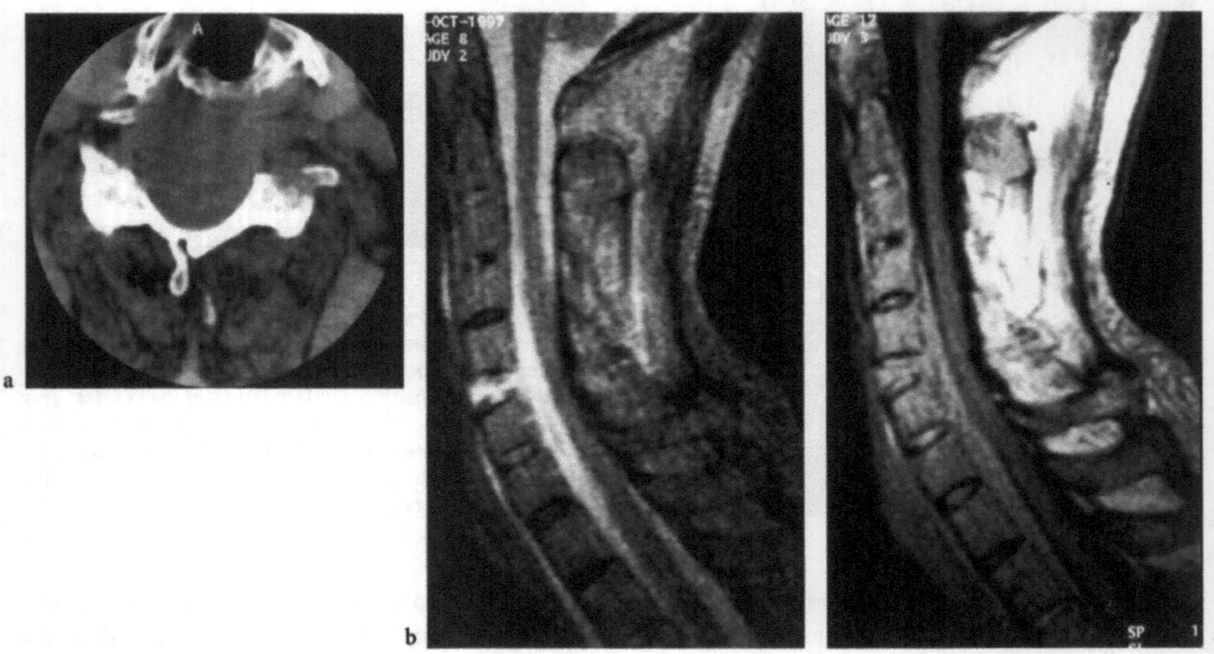

Fig. 26.13a–c. Metastatic disease with vertebral collapse and epidural hematoma: This 55-year-old man with lung cancer and known metastatic disease experienced rapidly evolving cervical pain and paraparesis. The initial CT examination (**a**) shows a complete destruction of the C6 vertebral body. The intraspinal extent is, however, not completely clear. Subsequent MR imaging (**b,c**) confirms a subtotal vertebral collapse, but also shows a large epidural mass. This mass is slightly hyperintense on the T1-weighted image suggestive of a large hematoma. This was confirmed on surgery

STIR sequence may be very helpful to distinguish between old and recent compression fractures, since recent compression fractures are clearly visible with high signal intensity on this sequence (Dousset et al. 1999).

Some MR imaging features may allow us to discriminate between benign and malignant compression fractures (An et al. 1995). In general, traumatic and osteoporotic compression fractures show preservation of some normal marrow signal intensity, especially in the region of the pedicles. Presence of an associated soft tissue mass around the compressed vertebral body may indicate a neoplastic or infectious etiology. Disk space invasion is seen in spondylodiskitis. An associated epidural pus collection may be present, compressing the dural sac and its contents (Friedman et al. 1996). This is also seen in non-bacterial spondylodiskitis (e.g., tuberculosis). Metastatic disease tends to spare the intervertebral disk space (Brant-Zawadski 1999).

Although many case reports have described spontaneous spinal epidural hematoma (SSEH), traumatic spinal epidural hematomas are much more frequently observed (Sklar et al. 1999). SSEH are most frequently found in the anterior epidural space, but may also occur in the posterior epidural space (Holtas et al. 1996). The upper thoracic region is the most common location. Concomitant systemic disease (plasma cell myeloma, hemophilia) or anticoagulant (warfarin) or antithrombotic (e.g., thrombolysis for myocardial infarction) therapy is frequently observed. Spinal arteriovenous malformations are seldom found as the underlying cause of SSEH space (Holtas et al. 1996). The diagnosis and the age of the epidural hematoma can be made on the relative signal intensities on T1- and T2-weighted images.

Extramedullary tumors may compress the dural sac and its contents. They are described in detail in Chap. 27.

26.4 Conclusion

Plain film radiography still remains the imaging method of choice to examine traumatized patients and to depict bony lesions, such as fractures and dislocations. An abundance of CT facilities allows further investigation when necessary. MR imaging is the imaging modality of choice for the evaluation of the spinal cord.

References

An HS, Andreshak TG, Nguyen C, Williams A, Daniels D (1995) Can we distinguish between benign versus malignant compression fractures of the spine by magnetic resonance imaging? Spine 20: 1776–1782

An HS (1999) Cervical spine trauma. Spine 23: 2713–2729

Bachulis BL, Long WB, Hynes GD, Johnson MC (1987) Clinical indications of cervical spine radiographs in the traumatized patient. Am J Surg 153: 473–478

Baker LL, Goodman SB, Perkash I, Lane B, Enzmann DR (1990) Benign versus pathologic compression fractures of vertebral bodies: assessment with conventional spin-echo, chemical-shift, and STIR MR imaging. Radiology 174: 495–502

Balériaux D, Parizel PM, Bank WO (1992) Intraspinal and intramedullary pathology. In: Manelfe C (ed) Imaging of the spine and spinal cord. Raven Press, New York, pp 513–564

Barton D, Allen M, Finlay D, Belton I (1993) Evaluation of whiplash injuries by technetium 99^misotope scanning. Arch Emerg Med 10: 197–202

Baur A, Stabler A, Bruning R, Bartl R, Krodel A, Reiser M, Deimling M (1998) Diffusion-weighted MR imaging of bone marrow: differentiation of benign versus pathologic compression fractures. Radiology 207: 349–356

Blackmore CC, Emerson SS, Mann FA, Koepsell TD (1999) Cervical spine imaging in patients with trauma: determination of fracture risk to optimize use. Radiology 211: 759–765

Blackmore CC, Emerson SS, Mann FA, Koepsell TD (1999) Cervical spine screening with CT in trauma patients: a cost-effectiveness analysis. Radiology 212: 117–125

Blacksin MH, Lee HJ (1995) Frequency and significance of fractures of the upper cervical spine detected by CT in patients with severe neck trauma AJR 165: 1201–1204

Brant-Zawadski M (1999) Acute myelopathy. In: Jeffry RB, Ralls PW, Leung AN, Brant-Zawadski M (eds) Emergency imaging. Lippincott Williams & Wikins, Philadelphia, pp 49–63

Brotchi J, Dewitte O, Levivier M et al. (1991) A survey of 65 tumors within the spinal cord: surgical results and the importance of preoperative magnetic resonance imaging. Neurosurgery 29: 651–657

Cadoux CG, White JD, Hedberg MC et al. (1987) High-yield roentgenographic criteria for cervical spine injuries. Ann Emerg Med 16: 738–742

Castillo M, Arbelaez A, Smith JK, Fisher L (1999) Diffusion-weighted imaging vs conventional MR imaging in spinal metastatic disease. 37th annual meeting of the ASNR, p 198–198 (abstract)

Clarck CA, Barker GJ, Tofts PS (1999) Magnetic resonance diffusion imaging of the human cervical spinal cord in vivo. Magn Reson Med 41: 1269–1273

Crowe H (1964) A new diagnostic sign in neck injuries. Calif Med 100: 12–13

Cumming WJ (1992) Myelitis and toxic, inflammatory and infectious disorders. Curr Opin Neurol Neurosurg 5: 549–553

Daffner RH (1996) Imaging of vertebral trauma, 2nd edn. Lippincott-Raven Publishers, Philadelphia New York

Davis SJ, Teresi LM, Bradley WG Jr, Ziemba MA, Bloze AE (1991) Cervical hyperextension injuries: MR findings. Radiology 180: 245–251

Dousset V (1999) JFR '99, Paris, October 25–29, 1999, personal communication. Accepted for publication in AJNR
Dvorak J, Panjabi MM, Grob D, Novotny JE, Antinnes JA (1993) Clinical validation of functional flexion/extension radiographs of the cervical spine. Spine 18: 120–127
Edal A, Balériaux D, Metens T et al. (1997) Three-dimensional turbo spin echo cervical magnetic resonance myelography. Int J Neuroradiol 3: 130–135
El Gammal TAM, Crews CE (1996) MR myelography of the cervical spine. Radiographics 16: 77–88
El-Khoury GY, Kathol MH, Daniel WH (1995) Imaging of acute injuries of the cervical spine: value of plain radiography, CT and MR imaging. AJR 164: 43–50
Erdmann H (1983) Versicherungsrechtliche Bewertungen des Schleudertraumas. In: Hohmann D, Kügelen B, Liebig K, Schirmer M (eds) Neuroorthopädie 1. Springer, Berlin Heidelberg New York
Evans RW, Evans RI, Sharp MJ (1994) The physician survey on the post-concussion and whiplash syndromes. Headache 34: 268–274
Fagerlund M, Bjornebrink J, Petterson K, Hildingsson C (1995) Magnetic resonance imaging in acute phase of whiplash injury. Eur Radiol 5: 297–301
Finelli DA, Hurst GC, Karaman BA, Simon JE, Duerk JL, Bellon EM (1994) Use of magnetization transfer for improved contrast on gradient-echo MR images of the cervical spine. Radiology 193: 165–171
Fischer RP (1984) Cervical radiographic evaluation of alert patients following blunt trauma. Ann Emerg Med 13: 905–907
Flanders AE, Schaefer DM, Doan HT, Mishkin MM, Gonzalez CF, Northrup BE (1990) Acute cervical spine trauma: correlation of MR imaging findings with degree of neurologic deficit. Radiology 177: 25–33
Flanders AE, Spetell CM, Tartaglino CM, Friedman DP, Herbison GJ (1996) Forecasting motor recovery after spinal cord injury: value of MR imaging. Radiology 201: 649–655
Friedman DP, Hills JR (1994) Cervical epidural spinal infection: MR imaging characteristics. AJR Am J Roentgenol 163: 699–704
Friedman D, Flanders A, Thomas C, Millar W (1995) Vertebral artery injury after acute cervical spine trauma: rate of occurrence as detected by MR angiography and assessment of clinical consequences. AJR Am J Roentgenol 164: 443–447
Gasparotti R, Ferraresi s, Pinelli L et al. (1997) Three-dimensional MR myelography of traumatic injuries of the brachial plexus. AJNR 18: 1733–1742
Gotten N (1956) Survey of one hundred cases of whiplash injury after settlement of litigation. JAMA 162: 865–867
Hildingsson C, Hietala SO, Toolanen G (1989) Scintigraphic findings in acute whiplash injury of the cervical spine. Injury 20: 265–266
Hilfiker P, Zanetti M, Debatin JF, McKinnon G, Hodler J (1995) Fast spin-echo inversion-recovery imaging versus fast T2-weighted spin-echo imaging in bone marrow abnormalities. Invest Radiol 30: 110–114
Hirsch SA, Hirsch PJ, Hiramoto H, Weiss A (1988) Whiplash syndrome: fact or fiction? Orthop Clin North Am 19: 791–795
Hittmair K, Mallek R, Prayer D, Schindler EG, Kollegger H (1996) Spinal cord lesions in patients with multiple sclerosis: comparison of MR pulse sequences. AJNR 17: 1555–1565
Holder CA, Eastwood JD, Muthupillai R, Hudging PA (1998) Diffusion-weighted MR imaging of the normal human spinal cord in vivo. 36th annual meeting of the ASNR; p 190–190 (abstract)
Holtas S, Heiling M, Lonntoft M (1996) Spontaneous spinal epidural hematoma: findings at MR imaging and clinical correlation. Radiology 199: 409–413
Ignelzi R (1993) The potential role of low field MR with open design in assessing ligamentous injury in acute cervical trauma. Surg Neurol 39: 519–529
Johnson BA, Tanenbaum LN (1998) Contempory spinal CT applications. Neuroimag Clin North Am 8: 559–575
Jones KM, Schwartz RB, Mantello MT et al. (1994) Fast spin-echo MR in the detection of vertebral metastases: comparison of three sequences. AJNR 15: 401–407
Junger SS, Stern BJ, Levine SR, Sipos E, Marti-Masso JF (1993) Intramedullary spinal sarcoidosis: clinical and magnetic resonance imaging characteristics. Neurology 43: 333–337
Kaiser JA, Holland BA (1999) Imaging of the cervical spine. Spine 23: 2701–2712
Kaneriya PP, Schweitzer ME, Spettell C, Cohen MJ, Karasick D (1998) The cost-effectiveness of oblique radiography in the exclusion of C7-T1 injury in trauma patients. AJR 171: 959–962
Kang JD, Figgie MP, Bohlman HH (1994) Sagittal measurements of the cervical spine in subaxial fractures and dislocations. An analysis of two hundred and eighty-eight patients with and without neurological deficits. J Bone Joint Surg [Am] 76: 1617–1628
Keiper MD, Grossman RI, Brunson JC, Schnall MD (1997) The low sensitivity of fluid-attenuated inversion-recovery MR in the detection of multiple sclerosis of the spinal cord. AJNR 18: 1035–1039
Le Bihan DJ (1998) Differentiation of benign versus pathologic compression fractures with diffusion-weighted MR imaging: a closer step toward the "holy grail" of tissue characterization? Radiology 207: 305–307
Lee SI, Chew FS (1998) Radiology in the emergency department: technique for quantitative description of use and results AJR 171: 559–564
Link TM, Schuierer G, Hufendiek A, Horch C, Peters PE (1995) Substantial head trauma: value of routine CT examination of the cervicocranium. Radiology 196: 741–745
Mascalchi M, Dal Pozzo G, Dini C et al. (1993) Acute spinal trauma: prognostic value of MRI appearances at 0.5 T. Clin Radiol 48: 100–108
Mathews VP, Greenspan SL, Caldemeyer KS, Patel MR (1998) FLAIR and HASTE imaging in neurologic diseases. Magn Reson Imaging Clin North Am 6: 53–65
Mawad ME, Rivera V, Crawford S, Ramirez A, Breitbach W (1990) Spinal cord ischemia after resection of thoracicoabdominal aortic aneurysms: MR findings in 24 patients. AJNR 11: 987–991
Melhem ER, Benson ML, Beauchamp NJ, Lee RR (1996) Cervical spondylosis: three-dimensional gradient-echo MR with magnetization transfer. AJNR 17: 705–711
Mirvis SE, Diaconis JN, Chirico PA, Reiner BI, Joslyn JN, Militello P (1989) Protocol-driven radiologic evaluation of suspected cervical spine injury: efficacy study Radiology 1989: 831–834
Modic MT, Ross JS (1990) Morphology, symptoms, and causality. Radiology 175: 619–620
Nagele M, Koch W, Woll B, Reiser M (1992) Dynamic function MR of the cervical vertebral column. RoFo 157: 222–228
Newman PK (1990) Whiplash injury: long term prospective studies are needed and, meanwhile, pragmatic treatment. Br Med J 301: 395

Nitz W (1999) Principles of magnetic resonance imaging and magnetic resonance angiography. In: Reimer P, Parzel PM, Stichnoth FA (eds) Clinical MR imaging. A Practical approach. Springer Verlag, Berlin Heidelberg, pp 1-36

Nunez DB Jr, Ahrmad AA, Coin CG et al. (1994) Clearing the cervical spine in multiple trauma victims: a time-effective protocol using helical computed tomography. Emerg Radiol 1: 273-278

Nunez DB Jr, Zululuga A, Fuentes-Bernardo DA, Rivas LA, Becerra JL (1996) Cervical spine trauma: how much more do we learn by routinely using helical CT? Radiographics 16: 1307-1318

Nunez DB Jr, Quencer RM. (1998) The role of helical CT in the assessment of cervical spine injuries. AJR 171: 951-957

Pearce JMS (1993) Subtle cerebral lesions in "chronic whiplash syndrome"? J Neurol Neurosurg Psychiatry 56: 1328-1329

Petterson K, Hildingsson C, Toolanen G, Fagerlund M, Bjornebrink J (1994) Magnetic resonance imaging and neurology in acute whiplash trauma: no correlation in prospective examination of 39 cases. Acta Orthop Scand 65: 525-528

Ross JS (1999) Newer sequences for spinal MR imaging: Smorgasbord or Succotash of acronyms? AJNR 20: 361-373

Rudisch A, Kremser C, Peer S, Kathrein A, Judmaier W, Daniaux H (1998) Metallic artifacts in magnetic resonance imaging of patients with spinal fusion. A comparison of implant materials and imaging sequences. Spine 23: 692-699

Sklar EM, Post JM, Falcone S (1999) MRI of acute spinal epidural hematomas. J Comput Assist Tomogr 23: 238-243

Tartaglino LM, Friedman DP, Flanders AE, Lublin FD, Knobler RL, Liem M (1995) Multiple sclerosis in the spinal cord: MR appearance and correlation with clinical parameters. Radiology 195: 725-732

Teresi L, Atkinson DJ, Chen DY et al. (1997) Diffusion-weighted imaging of the C-spine: a new means of contrast for cord lesions. 35th annual meeting of the ASNR, p 270-270 (abstract)

van den Hauwe L, De Schepper AM, Van Goethem JW, de Deurwaerder R, Parizel PM (1995) Whiplash trauma: a study of 200 litigation claims. Eur Radiol 5: S290

Van Dyke CW, Modic MT, Beale SM, Amartur S, Ross JS (1992) 3D MR myelography. JCAT 16: 497-500

Van Goethem JWM, Biltjes IGGM, van den Hauwe L, Parizel PM, De Schepper AMA (1996) Whiplash injuries: is there a role for imaging. Eur J Radiol 22: 30-37

Van Goethem JWM, Biltjes IGGM, van den Hauwe L, Parizel PM, De Schepper AMA (1998) Imaging of whiplash injuries. Riv di Neurorad 11: 337-346

Van Goethem JWM, Widelec J, de Moor J et al. (1998) Normal imaging of the cervical spine:roentgen anatomy, variants, and pitfalls. In: Gunzburg R and Szpalski M (eds) Whiplash injuries:current concepts in prevention, diagnosis and treatment of the cervical whiplash syndrome. Lippincott-Raven Publishers, Philadelphia, pp 21-30

Van Goethem J (1999) Magnetic Resonance Imaging of the Spine. In: Reimer P, Parzel PM, Stichnoth FA (eds) Clinical MR Imaging. A Practical approach. Springer Verlag, Berlin Heidelberg, pp 127-152

Walter J, Doris PE, Shaffer MA (1984) Clinical presentation of patients with acute cervical spine injury. Ann Emerg Med 13: 512-515

Wang (1995) Serial MRI changes in radiation myelopathy. Neuroradiol. 37: 374-377

White AA III, Panjabi MM (1990) The problem of clinical instability in the human spine: a systematic approach. In: White AA, Panjabi MM (eds) Clinical biomechnics of the spine 2nd ed. JB Lippincott, Philadelphia, pp 277-238

White SJ, Hajnal JV, Young IR, Bydder GM (1992) Use of fluid-attenuated inversion-recovery pulse sequences for imaging the spinal cord. Magn Reson Med 28: 153-162

Woodring JH, Lee C (1992) The role and limitations of computed tomographic scanning in the evaluation of cervical trauma. J Trauma 33: 698-708

Woodring JH, Lee C (1993) Limitations of cervical radiography in the evaluation of acute cervical trauma. J Trauma 34: 32-39

Yousem DM, Atlas SW, Goldberg HI, Grossman RI (1991) Degenerative narrowing of the cervical spine neural foramina: evaluation with high-resolution 3-DFT gradient-echo MR imaging. AJNR 12: 229-236

27 Imaging Tumours of the Spine and Spinal Cord

Daniëlle Balériaux, Fatima Rio, Philippe David

CONTENTS

27.1 Introduction

Spine and spinal cord tumours are rare (Osborn 1994; Sze 1996). Still, these tumours are often found in younger patients or children and should be properly identified. Early diagnosis plays an important role in the management of spinal cord tumours and will interfere with the prognosis and final outcome of the patient (Balériaux 1999). Plain X-ray still has an important role to play providing a first overview of the spine including an easy dynamic approach of the spine. CT remains the imaging modality of choice for the evaluation of the bony vertebral structures but is of limited diagnostic value in the case of intramedullary pathology. MRI should be performed as soon as possible and firstly whenever an intrinsic spinal cord lesion is clinically suspected. Systematic analysis of the MR images together with a basic knowledge of the most common spinal cord tumours encountered eases early recognition of the disease and leads to appropriate treatment (Balériaux et al. 1999; Zileli et al. 1996).

Tumours of the spine may be classified according to their site of origin in primary bony vertebral tumours, epidural tumours, intracanalar extramedullary tumours and, finally, intramedullary tumours.

Primary bony tumours of the spine are rare. Epidural tumours are mostly malignant and often include metastatic spread. On the contrary, intradural extramedullary tumours are mostly benign tumours including meningiomas and neurinomas. Intramedullary tumours are predominantly slow growing low-grade tumours (75%) although fast growing highly malignant intramedullary tumours do exist with metastatic spread to the entire neural axis.

Thanks to the recent advances of imaging procedures and the widespread diffusion of knowledge due to the development of computer based literature on the one hand and to recent advances in the surgical management (Zileli et al. 1996; Brotchi et al. 1992) of spine and spinal cord tumours on the other hand, our knowledge and care of these lesions has improved in the last 10 years. In this review we will summarize the basic knowledge and most recent progress in this field.

27.2 Imaging Techniques

27.2.1 Plain Films

Plain films should still routinely be performed: they provide a first static and dynamic overview of the entire spine. They are useful in detecting primary vertebral bony tumours although complementary CT will be needed. This applies also to epidural or intradural extramedullary tumours. Still, plain film radiographs are often normal in the initial phase of spinal bony tumours: indeed, 50% of the calcium must disappear before the lesion is noticed on plain

D. Balériaux, MD, PhD; F. Rio, MD; P. David, MD
Department of Neuroradiology, Université Libre de Bruxelles, Hôpital Erasme, route de Lennik 808, Brussels, 1070, Belgium

films. Therefore technetium-99 scintigraphy has been advocated but unfortunately this procedure is not specific for tumours and is today less sensitive than MRI for the detection of bone metastases (Algra et al. 1991).

In extramedullary intradural lesions, bony erosions and widening of the canal are frequently observed due to slow growth and chronic erosion.

In the case of intramedullary tumours, the abnormal findings will be often subtle and nonspecific: in adults, the commonest signs include straightening of the spine with disappearance of the normal curvatures. Progressive scoliosis should alert the clinician to an underlying intramedullary lesion. Widening of the spinal canal occurs in children but not in adults except in the case of myxopapillary ependymoma found in young adults and exclusively located in the conus medullaris and filum terminale. These tumours grow very slowly and may become extremely large expanding progressively the spinal canal and neural foramina. If plain films are rarely abnormal in adults with an intramedullary tumour, they are more often positive (58–81%) in children, demonstrating expansion of the canal, straightening of the spine or scoliosis.

27.2.2 Computed Tomography

CT is the optimal imaging technique for the evaluation of the vertebral bony structures including vertebral bodies, pedicles, articular facets and laminae. CT clearly shows widening of the bony canal. High-resolution bone algorithms available today allow superb evaluation of the bony lesions and perivertebral spread of the tumour. Spiral CT provides useful secondary 3D reconstructions. On the contrary, plain CT should not be chosen as a screening modality for intramedullary lesions as visualization of the canalar content remains limited on CT.

27.2.3 Myelography

Myelography has been the preferred imaging modality for the visualization of the spinal cord: this method should be definitely avoided nowadays as patients' symptomatology may occasionally be exacerbated by the procedure. Moreover, only the cord contours are delineated with myelography and no information is obtained concerning the intramedullary appearance.

27.2.4 Magnetic Resonance Imaging

Today MRI is the most sensitive method for the early detection of bone tumours although MRI was initially considered of poor value for the evaluation of bony structures. MRI is moreover definitely the imaging procedure of choice for the demonstration of the spinal cord: any patient in whom intramedullary pathology is clinically suspected should be subjected to an MR examination.

The MR technique must include systematically T1- and T2-weighted images as well as gadolinium enhanced T1 WI (Bydder et al. 1985). The entire spinal cord must be studied with dedicated phased array spinal surface coils. At least two different imaging planes must be used in order to locate the tumour properly and differentiate intra- from extramedullary tumours.

Bearing in mind the need for a systematic image analysis the radiologist may provide useful preoperative information to the surgeon: the histology may be suspected, the tumour borders assessed and surgical planning facilitated.

MR myelography may be a useful complementary technique to better show the nerve roots and spinal cord displacements (Edal et al. 1997).

MR angiography does not yet allow identification of small normal medullary vessels such as Adamkiewicz's artery but may clearly demonstrate enlarged vessels in tumour cases or spinal AVM (Mascalchi et al. 1999).

MR diffusion imaging of the human cervical spine in vivo has recently been demonstrated in the literature but further technical developments are currently in progress and its clinical utility especially in cases of spinal cord tumours is still under clinical evaluation (Clark et al. 1999).

27.2.5 Medullary Angiography

Angiography is rarely performed today for diagnostic purposes. Still, it should be performed whenever the vascularization of the cord has to be known before surgery in order to locate the artery of Adamkiewicz at the lower thoracic level or to demonstrate the vascular feeding of highly vascular tumours like hemangioblastomas. Embolization may be recommended in richly vascular tumours as well (Eskridge et al. 1996; Shi et al. 1999; Bowen and Pattany 1999).

27.3 Spinal Tumours

27.3.1 Vertebral Tumours

Although almost any bone tumour may be found in the vertebral column, primary vertebral bony tumours are uncommon except hemangioma. On the contrary, the spine is a common location for metastases. It is often difficult or even impossible to differentiate benign from malignant tumours, hence the need for biopsy. Still, signal heterogeneity on MRI, ill-defined contours and cortical bone disruptions are often signs of malignancy (Warnock and Yu 1993). Some MRI findings are characteristic and rather specific such as fluid-fluid levels in aneurysmal bone cysts or hyperintensity on both T1- and T2-weighted images of vertebral hemangiomas.

27.3.1.1 Benign Bone Tumours

Benign bone tumours include hemangioma, osteochondroma, osteoid osteoma, osteoblastoma, aneurysmal bone cyst, giant cell tumour, eosinophilic granuloma, and fibroma.

Vertebral hemangiomas are common and usually incidental findings in the vertebral bodies at the thoracolumbar region. They vary from predominantly fatty lesions to true hemangioma with mature thin-walled vessels and large blood-filled endothelial-lined spaces (Laredo et al. 1990). Still, some hemangiomas behave more aggressively and present with fracture and epidural extension with acute cord compression (Fig. 27.1). On plain films the honeycomb appearance is easily recognizable. The MRI presentation is variable according to the tissue components: most frequently hemangiomas are hyperintense on both T1- and T2-weighted images. Fat suppression sequences are useful in order to differentiate fatty components from highly vascular components that do strongly enhance after gadolinium injection.

Osteoid osteoma is relatively common, especially in young male patients, accounting for 12% of benign bony tumours. They affect more often the lumbar spine favoring the posterior arch of the vertebrae. Bone scintigraphy remains an excellent procedure to detect these lesions and complementary CT is the imaging procedure of choice, demonstrating a small lytic lesion surrounded by a dense area of sclerosis. A central calcified nidus is often seen.

Osteoblastomas are rare primary bone tumours but do affect the spine in 40% of cases. They are mostly located in the posterior arch although they may involve the vertebral body as well. Typically they are lytic expansile masses with extension to the perivertebral region, often lucent with a thin bony or sclerotic rim (Osborn 1994). On MRI, osteoblastomas have an intermediate signal in T1 WI and mixed high signal areas on T2 WI.

a 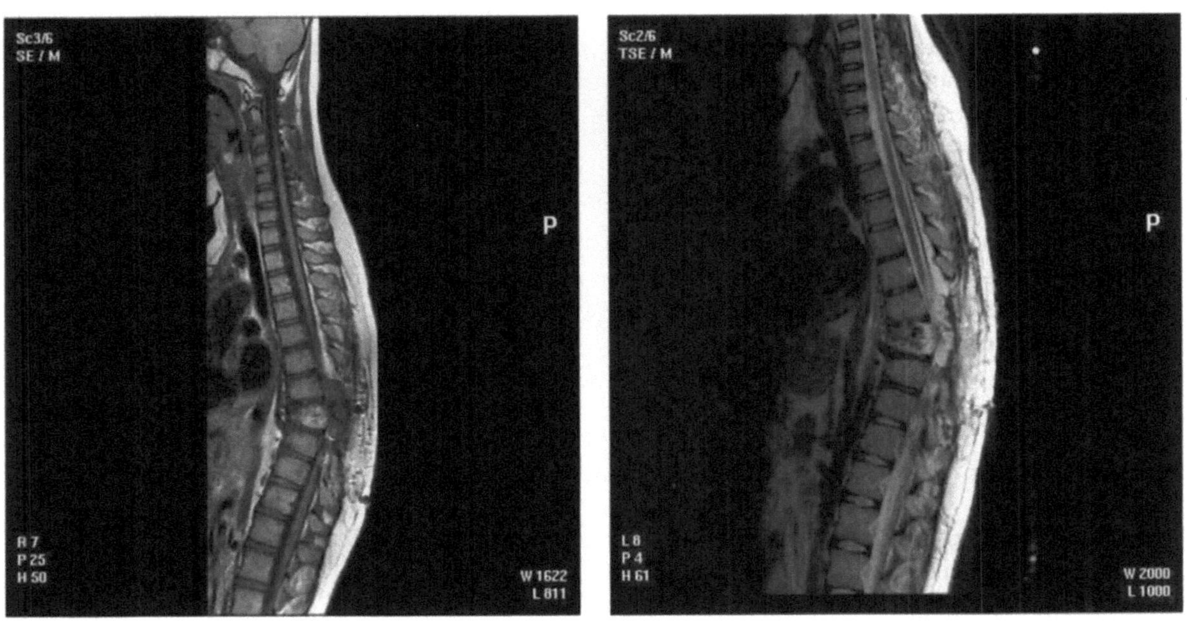 b

Fig. 27.1a,b. Aggressive vertebral hemangioma of Th8 in a 13-year-old girl. Sagittal T1 (**a**) and sagittal T2-weighted image (**b**). Severe secondary cord compression

Giant cell tumours are found in older patients with a peak incidence in the 3rd decade. They rarely affect the spine choosing preferentially the sacrum. Giant cell tumours are mostly lytic, expansile destructive masses of the sacrum with mixed signal, multicompartmented cystic components with a huge amount of blood degradation products (Aoki et al. 1991).

Aneurysmal bone cysts affect preferentially the posterior elements of the cervical and thoracic spine. They occur mostly in young patients (80% are under 20 years) complaining of pain and swelling. The most suggestive element of aneurysmal bone cysts is fluid-fluid levels and blood degradation products best seen on MRI. At angiography those tumours are extremely vascular.

Osteochondromas are frequent at the cervical level (50%) affecting the spinous or transverse processes mainly of C2 and growing as a cauliflower with the cortical bone of the tumour continuing with the normal cortical bone. They show mixed signal intensity on both T1 and T2 WI (Osborn 1994).

Eosinophilic granuloma is a benign, nonneoplastic vertebral lesion typically found in the young child (5–10 years). This lesion is usually hyperintense on T2 WI and of variable intensity on T1 WI. As many bony lesions it tends to extend within the epidural space and may compress the spinal cord secondarily (Fig. 27.2). It enhances strongly after contrast administration.

27.3.1.2
Malignant Bone Tumours

Malignant bone tumours are mostly metastatic lesions. Other malignant tumours are the following: multiple myeloma, lymphoma, leukemia, neuroblastoma, chordoma, chondrosarcoma, osteosarcoma, and Ewing's sarcoma.

They are rare bone tumours and have no characteristic appearance except the chordoma that is the only hyperintense signal tumour on T2 WI. It enhances moderately and inhomogeneously after gadolinium injection.

27.3.2
Epidural Tumours

Extradural metastatic tumours are the most common. Lymphoma, leukemia, multiple myeloma, and angiolipoma are also seen (Klisch et al. 1999). Nerve sheath tumours are extradural in 15% of cases.

27.3.3
Extramedullary Intradural Tumours

Nerve sheath tumours and meningiomas are the most common intradural extramedullary tumours accounting for almost 90% of them. Nerve sheath tumours comprise schwannoma, neurofibroma, ganglioneuroma and rarely neurofibrosarcoma.

Schwannomas commonly enlarge the neural foramina and rarely calcify. On T1 WI, 75% are isointense while 25% are hyperintense. More than 95% are hyperintense on T2 WI. Intramedullary neurinomas are rare but may occur (Innocenzi et al. 1997; Balériaux 1999).

Spinal *meningiomas* typically are found in middle-aged women at the thoracic level. Meningiomas are slow growing, intradural extramedullary tumours in 90% of cases. Associated bony erosion is rare. Calcification may be seen rarely in 1%–5% of cases. On T1 WI and T2 WI, meningiomas are well-delineated tumours, isointense to the cord. A broad-based dural attachment, sometimes calcified, may be seen but is less frequently observed compared to intracranial meningiomas. Homogeneous contrast uptake is usually observed.

In neurofibromatosis type I, primarily intraforaminal spinal tumours are seen extending into the spinal canal while in NF2 they are mostly intraspinal intradural tumours (Thakkar et al. 1999).

Epidermoids are either congenital or acquired tumours in which case they are usually a late complication of a lumbar puncture (ranging from 1 to more than 20 years). Epidermoid cysts are uncommon, typically seen in young patients. Associated spinal malformations are often present such as spina bifida, and hemivertebrae in the case of congenital epidermoids. Epidermoids may be difficult to disclose when small as they do have a signal behavior similar to CSF. The best imaging sequence to pick them up is still proton density images. Contrast injection is unnecessary, as they do not enhance typically.

Spinal *dermoids* are mostly detected during the 1st year of life. They may be both intramedullary or extramedullary. The MR signal behavior is variable, linked to the different nature of their components. Still, a hyperintense appearance is usually found on T1 WI.

27.3.4
Tumours of the Spinal Cord

Tumours of the spinal cord are rare (Fischer and Brotchi 1996). In a general hospital, only 5% of spinal tumours are intramedullary for 40% intradural extramedullary and 55% extradural.

In children, astrocytomas are by far the most frequent while in adults ependymomas represent 60% of the intramedullary tumours. Astrocytomas account for about 30% of spinal cord gliomas. Hemangioblastomas are less frequent and represent 5%.

Clinical presentation is poorly specific with pain being the most common finding and usually the first symptom to be reported. Sensory and motor deficits are variable, occurring in function of tumour localization. Urinary disturbance and impotence are rarer and appear late in the clinical course of the disease: they occur usually coincident with motor paralysis of the legs.

In children, pain is equally the most frequent symptom as reported in 42% of cases. Motor regression is present in 36%, gait abnormality in 27%, tor-

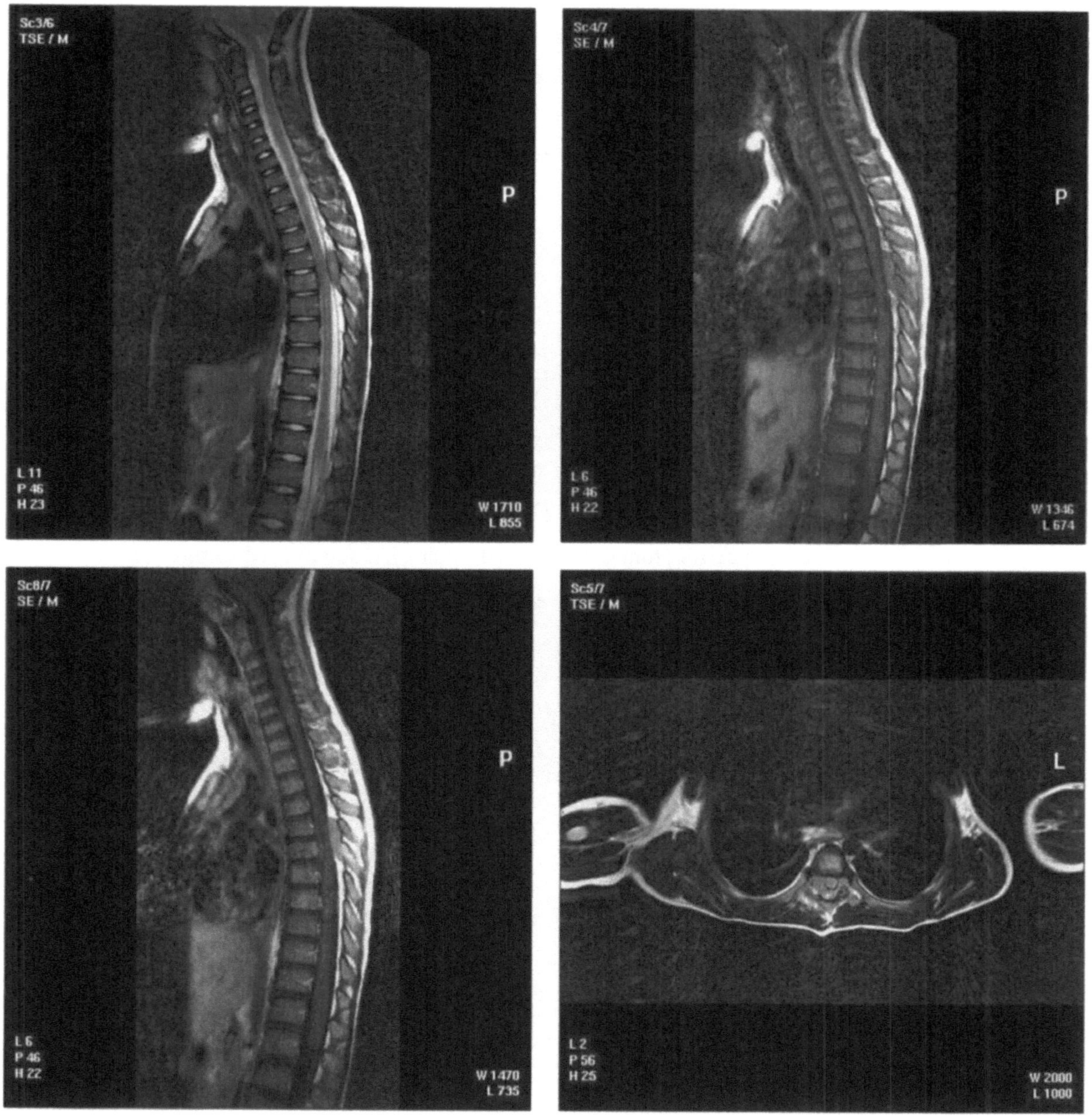

a b c d

Fig. 27.2a–d. Eosinophilic granuloma (bone histiocytosis). A 7-year-old boy with nocturnal dorsal pain. The right vertebral pedicle on Th6 was missing on plain X-ray films. MRI showed a right posterior epidural mass lesion compressing the cord anteriorly. The bony involvement is seen as a hyperintense lesion on T2 WI, isointense on T1 WI while the epidural solid component is isointense to the cord on both T1 and T2 weighted images. It enhances strongly after gadolinium administration. Sagittal T2 WI (**a**), sagittal T1 WI (**b**), sagittal Gd T1 WI (**c**), axial Gd T1 WI (**d**) ticollis in 27% and progressive kyphoscoliosis is 24%; 89% are low-grade lesions (Constantini et al. 1996; Lunardi et al. 1993).

Clinical symptoms of cord tumours are usually of insidious onset: pain may be for a long time the only complaint while motor deficits often appear later (Balériaux 1999). Before the advent of MRI the diagnosis of cord tumour was often delayed. It is important, however, to diagnose these tumours at an early stage as new, efficient, surgical techniques including the use of CUSA may heal the patient or at least stop tumoural evolution (Brotchi et al. 1991, 1992; Chandy and Babu 1999). Adequate management by using the proper diagnostic tools and careful analysis of the MRI images will lead to a description of important features such as solid nodules, cystic components, and associated hydrosyringomyelia, guiding the surgeon in an optimal way (Balériaux and Brotchi 1992).

Systematic analysis of the MRI images must be done and both morphological anomalies as well as signal behavior anomalies described in order to identify the extent of the tumour and separate tumour components (Bourgouin et al. 1998; Balériaux 1999; Del Carpio O'Donovan 1998; Li and Holtas 1991; Parizel et al. 1989; Scotti et al. 1987). It is of the utmost importance to differentiate tumour infiltration from associated edema, and solid nodules from cystic elements. Edema is most extensive in hemangioblastomas. It is seen in 60% of all ependymomas and only in 23% of astrocytomas. Intratumoural cystic components are located entirely within the boundaries of the tumour with contrast enhancement frequently observed in the cyst wall. The signal behavior of these cysts is usually different from CSF, due to the high protein content of the fluid. On the contrary, associated, "satellite" cysts are located cephalad or caudal to the solid nodule and their walls do not enhance after gadolinium injection. They develop as an intramedullary reaction to the presence of the tumour and the liquid has a similar behavior to CSF. They spontaneously collapse after surgery. Finally, extensive associated hydromyelia may develop as well: these cavities will equally disappear spontaneously after total tumour removal.

Solid tumour components have either clear limits as in the case of low-grade tumours such as ependymomas or hemangioblastomas, or ill-defined borders in the case of more infiltrating and more aggressive tumours.

Contrast enhancement patterns should also be carefully described: ependymomas usually enhance more intensely and homogeneously while astrocytomas enhance moderately and in an inhomogeneous way.

It is important to know that not all tumours do enhance while, on the contrary, any enhancing intramedullary mass expanding the cord must not be considered as being a neoplasm.

Hemorrhage may occur within spinal cord tumours (Nemoto et al. 1992) and can be recognized on T1 WI as hyperintense areas, when the hemorrhage is 1 week to approximately 4 months old. Hemosiderin deposits can later be identified as low signal areas on both T1 WI and T2 WI, preferably obtained by gradient echo sequences. When MR imaging shows an intramedullary tumour with hypointensity at the margin, it is suggestive, but not pathognomonic, of an ependymoma (Osborn 1994; Nemoto et al. 1992).

Subarachnoid hemorrhage with a spinal origin is a rare clinical entity and the most common source of SAH is an arteriovenous malformation (Lahanis et al. 1993). Still, a few cases of SAH due to bleeding from a hemangioblastoma have been reported in the literature: this etiology should thus be kept in mind in documented cases of SAH with normal cerebral angiography and MRI of the spine performed in order to rule out this classical although very rare cause of SAH (Minami et al. 1998).

Finally, hydrocephalus associated with spinal cord tumours is a well-documented but infrequent occurrence (Rifkinson-Mann et al. 1990). Especially in the presence of childhood hydrocephalus and increased intracranial pressure without a clearly defined etiology, a spinal cord tumour should always be considered (Caviness et al. 1998).

27.3.4.1 Common Spinal Cord Tumours

Astrocytomas, ependymomas and hemangioblastomas are by far the most frequent intramedullary tumours. Astrocytomas are more often located in the thoracic region. Moreover, a panmedullary-infiltrating tumour is usually an astrocytoma. Ependymomas are more frequently found in the cervical region. Hemangioblastomas may be found at any level.

The radiologist should avoid predicting with too great confidence the resectability of a lesion. According to the literature (Chandy and Babu 1999), indicators of radical excision are good tumour-cord interface, cranially located tumours, presence of syringomyelia and histology of ependymoma. In our experience some lesions with sharp borders and associated cystic components could only partially be removed while ill defined infiltrating tumours turned out to be totally resected on follow-up examinations. For these reasons, we have learned always to biopsy a tumour and attempt cautious total resection (Brotchi et al. 1992). We confirm the better prognosis of ependymoma.

Astrocytoma. Astrocytomas are common tumours and account for 24%–30% of intramedullary tumours in adults (Epstein et al. 1992), while it is by far the most common tumour in children (up to 90%) (Przybylski et al. 1997). Even in adults, they are mostly encountered in younger patients (mean age in our series was 29) with a predominance of males (63%). Congenital spinal cord astrocytomas have rarely been reported but do exist.

The typical astrocytoma is large and located in the thoracic region. If a cystic component is present, it is typically an intratumoural one. However, satellite cysts and secondary hydromyelia can also be observed.

The astrocytoma is usually eccentrically located and exhibits heterogeneous, moderate, and partial contrast

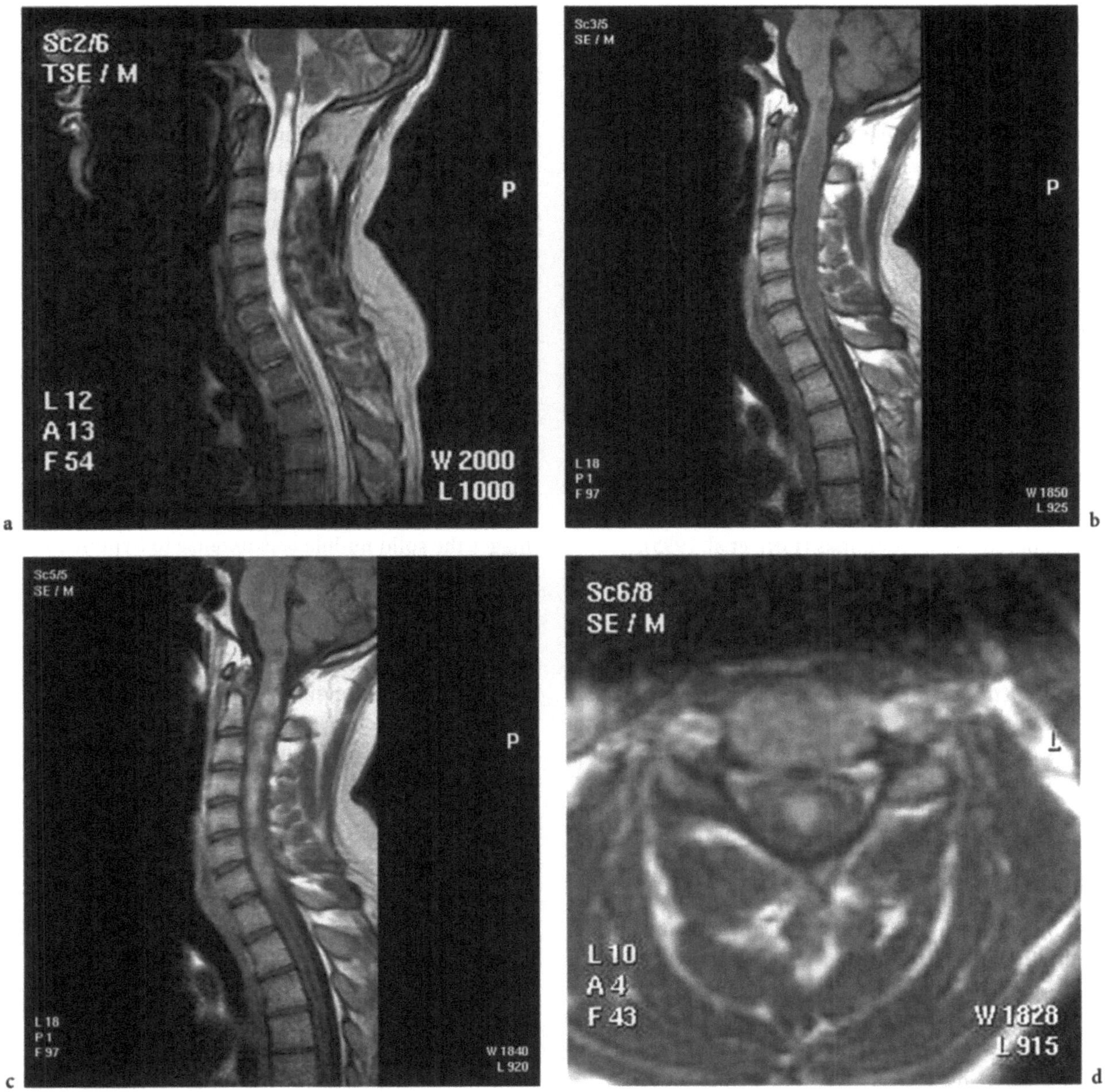

Fig. 27.3a–d. Low grade, pilocytic astrocytoma of the cervical spinal cord. A 22-year-old man with a 2-year history of cervicobrachialgia. Sagittal T2 WI (**a**), sagittal T1 WI (**b**), sagittal (**c**) and axial Gd T1 WI (**d**). The entire cervical spinal cord is enlarged by an ill-defined mass, hypointense on T1 WI, hyperintense on T2 WI and showing patchy, irregular enhancement after gadolinium injection. Biopsy only could be performed due to the infiltrating aspect of the tumour without clear-cut limits

enhancement after gadolinium injection. Astrocytoma borders are frequently ill defined (Fig. 27.3).

Cervicomedullary astrocytomas are a unique subset of brainstem gliomas in childhood that present with a long duration of symptoms and a greater long-term survival than pontine gliomas (Young Poussaint et al. 1999). The majority of these tumours are pilocytic astrocytomas. Our experience concurs with this recent report from Young et al.: we even observed spontaneous regression of the residual tumour in cases of partial resection without adjuvant radiotherapy. For these reasons we recommend radiotherapy only in cases of malignant astrocytomas and would rather operate again later if necessary in cases of slow progression of those low-grade astrocytomas typically encountered in the pediatric population. Nadkarni and Rekate (1999) also share this opinion.

Ependymoma. The typical ependymoma is located in the cervical region and associated large satellite cysts are frequently seen. A so-called "cap sign" is often seen and corresponds to low signal intensity areas capping at both sides the tumour limits: these caps are hemosiderin deposits due to chronic hemorrhage. Ependymomas do enhance vividly and homogeneously, and have well-defined borders (Kahan et al. 1996).

Ependymomas originate from the ependymal walls and as such are more centromedullary located compared to astrocytomas (Fine et al. 1995).

The mean tumour size of the ependymoma corresponds to a mean height of 3 to 4 vertebral bodies (min. 2, max. 13), while astrocytomas are usually more extensive, with a mean height of 5.6 vertebral bodies (min. 2, max. 19). More recently, we were able to diagnose several cases of smaller ependymoma of less than 2 cm thanks to the ever-increasing spatial resolution of MR images (Fig. 27.4).

Ependymoma accounts for most of the tumours arising from the filum terminale (Sevick and Wallace 1999).

Rare cases of spinal cord *subependymoma* are described in the literature and were reviewed by Bret et al. in 1997. It is likely that these rare lesions account for less than 2% of all spinal cord tumours. The majority of the cases involved the cervical cord or cervicothoracic junction. On MRI no specific pattern could help in diagnosing these lesions except the tendency for subependymoma to grow eccentrically within the cord or to show an exophytic component.

Finally, *myxopapillary ependymoma* of the conus medullaris and filum terminale is a relatively common spinal intradural neoplasm found in children (Nagib and O'Fallon 1997) and young adults although they may be seen at older ages. There is a slight male predominance. Tumour location is typical. They are slow growing tumours and may become very large before the diagnosis is finally made in patients with a classical longstanding history of chronic low back pain exacerbated at night when in the horizontal position. On MRI, the lesion is isointense compared to the cord and hyperintense on T2-weighted images. They enhance strongly after gadolinium injection. Hemorrhage often occurs, explaining the sudden worsening of clinical symptoms with occurrence of leg weakness and sphincter disturbances (Friedman and Hollander 1998).

Hemangioblastoma. Hemangioblastomas are benign, usually richly vascular spinal cord tumours, often located superficially, in the subpial region. Hemangioblastomas represent 2–6% of all spinal tumours. These tumours are either solitary (80%) or multiple, when associated with von Hippel-Lindau disease (Baker et al. 1999).

Tumour nodules are usually small and they are typically associated with extensive hydrosyringomyelia. When no cystic component is present, extensive edema is found with diffuse cord enlargement. Hemangioblastomas are therefore often easily identified.

Still, exophytic hemangioblastoma may occur with minimal cord reaction as well as extramedullary hemangioblastoma (Fig. 27.5). On T1-weighted images the solid nodule is isointense to hypointense and isointense to slightly hyperintense on T2-weighted images. After gadolinium injection, intense and homogeneous contrast uptake is seen (Colombo et al. 1986). Contrast administration is especially useful in the case of small, often multiple nodules. Preoperative endovascular embolization of craniospinal hemangioblastomas is recommended (Eskridge et al. 1996).

27.3.4.2 Uncommon Spinal Cord Tumours

Lymphoma. An intramedullary lymphoma may occur as part of a multifocal lymphoma, with cerebral, cerebellar or brain stem lesions associated with the intramedullary lesion (0.9% of primary CNS non-Hodgkin's lymphomas). Primary intramedullary lymphomas are rare especially in immunocompetent patients but are more frequent in AIDS patients. MRI was "nonspecific" in the cases reported in literature (see Chap. 29).

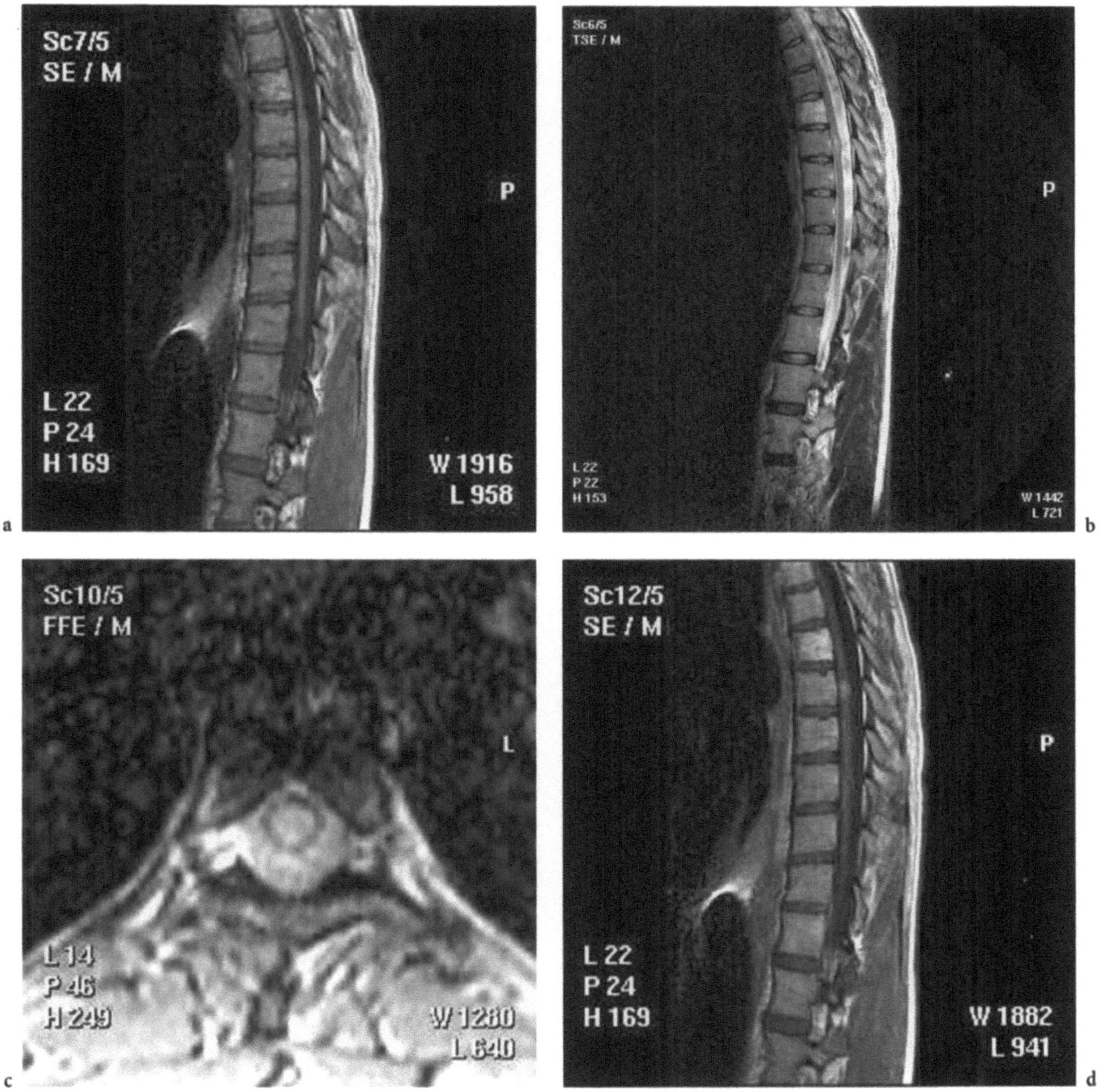

Fig. 27.4a–d. Small thoracic ependymoma. A 32-year-old woman with right lumbosciatalgia and sensory problems. Sagittal T1 WI (**a**), sagittal T2 WI (**b**), axial T2 WI (**c**), sagittal Gd T1 WI (**d**). The spinal cord is focally enlarged at the level of Th8 by a small lesion isointense to the spinal cord on T1 WI (**c**), hyperintense on T2 WI (**b,c**) and enhancing clearly after contrast administration (**d**). Note a hemangioma of the vertebral body of Th7

Metastasis. Four percent of intramedullary tumours are metastases. Still, it is difficult to ascertain the true incidence of spinal cord metastases, as the clinical picture often is atypical and seen in terminally ill patients. Autopsy material is also biased, as the cord is often not systematically examined. On the other hand, 2.4% of metastases removed surgically from the CNS are located in the cord. Clinical symptoms are often nonspecific, but usually involve root pain. The exquisite sensitivity of MRI enables intramedullary metastases to be easily detected. No specific MRI characteristics are seen. Usually they are small, nodular, well-defined lesions, hypointense on T2 WI. The enhancement pattern may be either ring-like or homogeneous and intense (Ijaz and Jones 1997).

Ganglioglioma. Spinal cord gangliogliomas are rare tumours, representing 3.8% of all central nervous system tumours (Hamburger et al. 1997). They involve the upper cervical cord in the great majority of

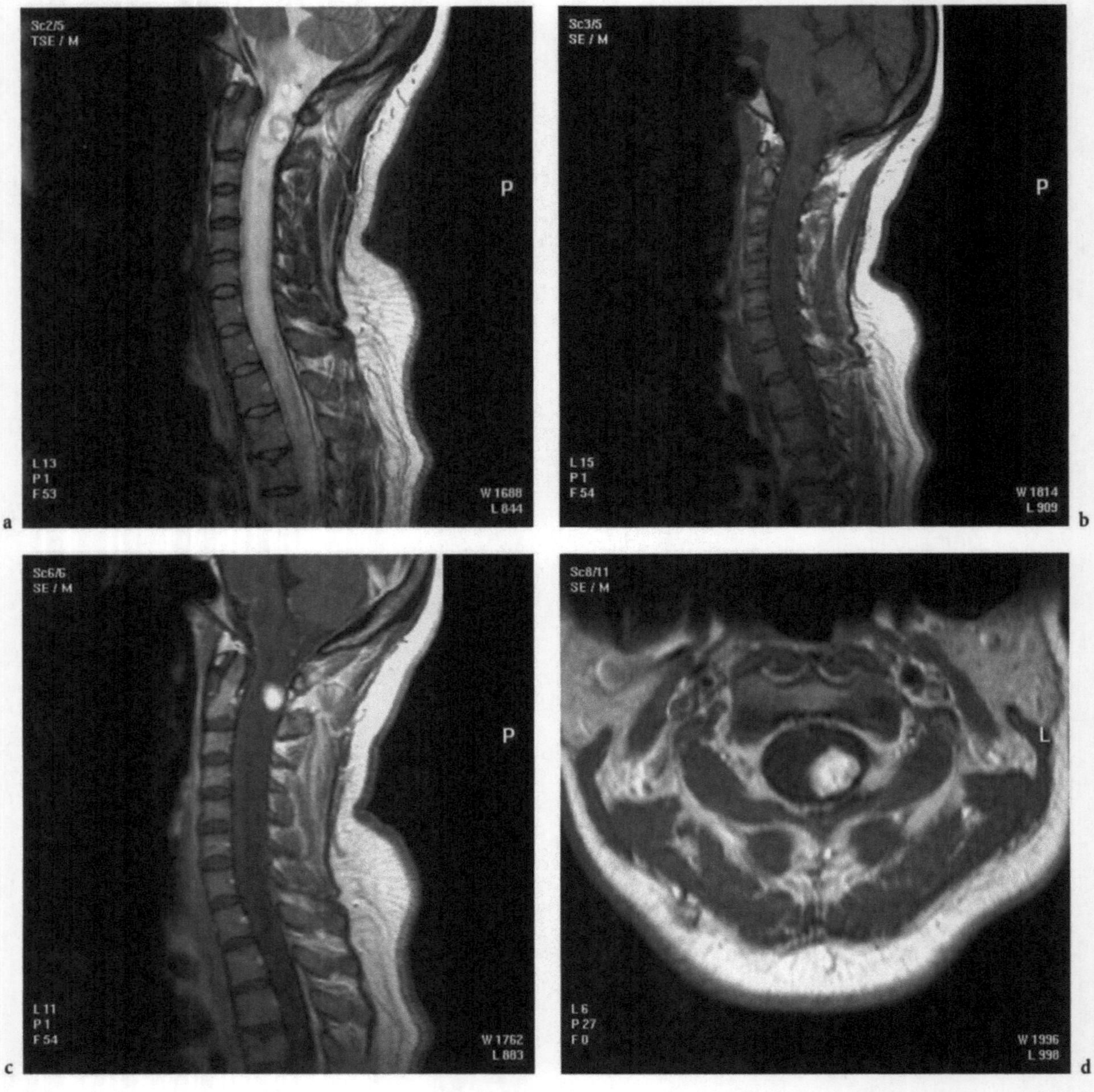

Fig. 27.5a–d. Cervical hemangioblastoma at the level of C1. Chronic left cervicobrachialgia in a middle-aged woman. Sagittal T2 WI (**a**), sagittal T1 WI (**b**), sagittal Gd T1 WI (**c**), axial Gd T1 WI (**d**). Small solid nodular mass lesion, with faint hyperintense rim on T1 WI, isointense to the cord on T2 WI and surrounded by extensive edema. Strong and homogeneous enhancement after gadolinium injection

cases. One-third of the gangliogliomas are seen in children of which spinal cord involvement (1.7%) is greater than cerebral (1.4%) or cerebellar (0.7%) involvement. A large series of 27 patients was recently reported by Patel et al. (1998): the diagnosis can be strongly suspected according to these authors in young patients (mean 12 years) with long tumour length, presence of tumoural cyst, presence of bone erosion and scoliosis, absence of edema, presence of mixed signal intensity on T1-weighted images and presence of patchy enhancement and cord surface enhancement. However, the ultimate diagnosis still depends on histopathologic investigation.

Paragangliomas. Paragangliomas of the spinal canal are more common than previously thought and can be located anywhere along the spine, although the lumbosacral level is the most common. Their appearance on MRI is nonspecific. In general they are benign, slowly growing tumours but some are more aggressive and may give rise to metastatic spread (SUNDGREN et al. 1999).

Oligodendroglioma. Oligodendrogliomas are rare in the spinal cord. They exhibit no specific MRI characteristics. However, the few cases in our experience were relatively small tumours (two vertebral segments), with ill-defined borders and slight hyperintensity on T1 WI. No peritumoural edema or contrast enhancement was observed.

Congenital spinal masses: lipomas, epidermoids, teratomas and midline spinal cord hamartomas.

Lipoma. Lipomas are relatively rare spinal cord tumours, representing 6% of intramedullary tumours. True intramedullary lipoma must be differentiated from cauda equina lipomas or lipomas associated with dysraphism, the clinical, radiological, and surgical problems raised by these lesions being totally different (Timmer et al. 1993).

Although these tumours appear well defined on MRI, often no cleavage plane from the surrounding spinal cord is found at surgery. Therefore, the tumour usually cannot be completely resected without causing severe neurological damage.

The typical hyperintensity of lipomas on T1 WI makes these lesions easy to diagnose with MRI.

Angiolipoma. Angiolipomas of the spine are rare benign tumours containing vascular and mature adipose tissue. In 90% of cases they are located within the epidural space. Only four cases of intramedullary angiolipoma have been reported. The diagnosis may be suggested from the richly vascularized components and lipomatous content (KLISCH et al. 1999).

Teratomas. Intradural spinal teratoma is a rare tumour and its pathogenesis remains unclear. KOEN et al. (1998) present a series of patients in whom an intradural teratoma arose at the same site as a developmental spinal cord abnormality and postulate that these lesions are the result of a dysembryogenic mechanism and are not neoplastic.

Spinal cord hamartomas. Congenital midline spinal hamartomas are rare and a relatively unknown entity (CASTILLO et al. 1998). MRI shows a mass lesion that is isointense with the spinal cord on all sequences. A small dermal sinus tract that tethers the cord at the level of the lesion is often found.

Cavernoma. Cavernomas are vascular malformations that may remain clinically silent for a long period of time. Often they are responsible for an acute or rapidly progressive neurological medullary deficit. Cavernomas represent 2.4% of all intramedullary tumours. All cases presented with hemorrhage. Before the advent of MRI these lesions were extremely difficult to diagnose, especially in the spinal cord, as they usually are small and do not enlarge the spinal cord. On the contrary, on MRI, intramedullary cavernomas (or cavernous hemangiomas) are usually easily recognized. A reticulated appearance with areas of mixed signal intensity in both T1- and T2- or T2*-weighted images is the most common finding. A prominent rim of decreased signal intensity is less commonly seen than in the brain. Contrast enhancement may occur (Fig. 27.6). As cavernomas may be multiple, we recommend cerebral MRI whenever the diagnosis of cavernoma is suspected. If multiple similar lesions are found in the brain, this should support the final diagnosis of cavernoma of the spinal cord.

27.4 Conclusion

It is often not possible to provide a diagnosis of a spinal or spinal cord tumour with absolute certainty, and biopsy should always be performed to establish the final histological diagnosis: still, the radiologist will suggest a histological diagnosis and discuss the differential diagnosis.

It should be stressed that numerous nonneoplastic intramedullary lesions may simulate tumour infiltration and be distinguished properly in order to avoid unnecessary biopsy. Typically, these lesions include MS plaques, inflammatory lesions, granulomas, and abscesses. Sarcoidosis is rare in the spinal cord. Diagnosis of an intramedullary lesion is facilitated when the patient has known systemic sarcoidosis. In two of our cases, the patient had a solitary spinal cord lesion presenting as an intramedullary tumour (LEVIVIER et al. 1991). MRI demonstrated nonspecific findings of a nodular lesion which usually strongly enhances on gadolinium enhanced T1 WI. Sarcoidosis should thus be included in the differential diagnosis of a nodular lesion. Biopsy may be required and should be performed to establish the diagnosis when no systemic signs of sarcoidosis are present.

In a recent paper LEE et al. (1998) stressed the fact that even with MRI it may be difficult or impossible to differentiate spinal tumours from intramedullary

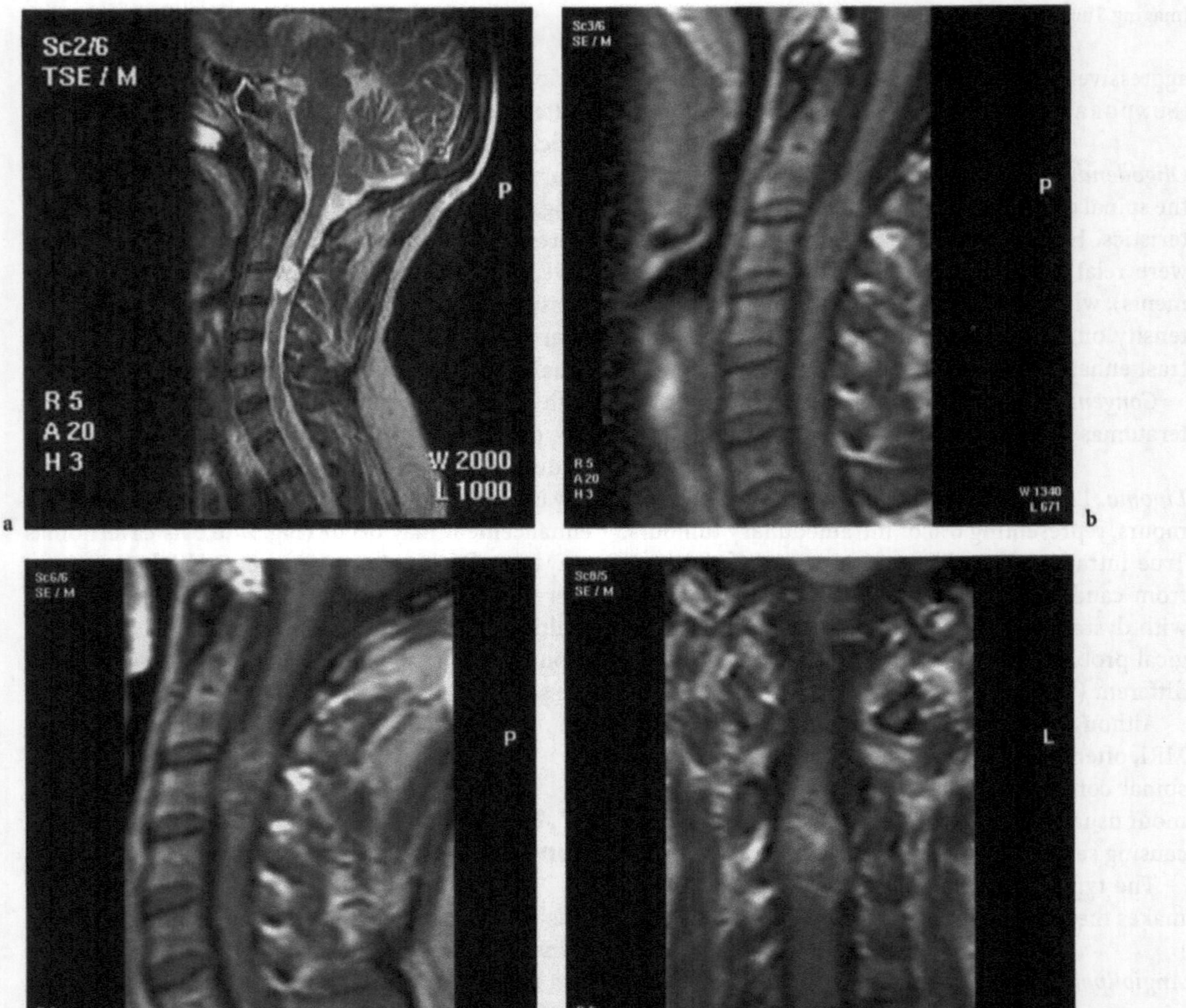

Fig. 27.6a–f. Cervical cavernoma. This 43-year-old woman complained of progressive loss of strength in the superior and inferior left limbs occurring over a period of 3 years. Lhermitte's sign is also reported on clinical examination. Sagittal T2 WI (**a**), sagittal T1 WI (**b**), sagittal Gd T1 WI (**c**), coronal T1 WI (**d**). Focal enlargement at the cervical cord by an almost isointense lesion with patchy areas of hyperintensities on T1 WI. The lesion is hyperintense on T2 WI and better delineated on this pulse sequence. There is only moderate contrast uptake. Sagittal T1 WI (**e**) and sagittal T2 WI (**f**) obtained after total removal of a C4 cavernoma

nonneoplastic lesions: they reported 4% of nonneoplastic lesions in a series of 212 patients undergoing surgery for intramedullary spinal cord tumours: histology showed demyelinating disease, sarcoidosis, amyloid angiopathy and a mass of nonneoplastic inflammatory cells of unknown origin!

Let us stress the fact that the radiologist has an important role to play but must know the limits of imaging procedures: in particular, he or she will be unable to predict the resectability of a tumour. In particular, in spinal cord tumours, although no clear-cut separation between tumour and normal spinal cord is found on MRI, the surgeon will discover a cleavage plane at surgery. Alternatively, a clearly definable tumour on MRI may not be easily resectable, as in the case of spinal lipoma, where MRI shows sharp tumour margins, while the surgeon finds diffuse infiltration with no separation between cord and fatty tissue (Balériaux 1999).

In the case of diagnostic uncertainty it may be useful to perform a baseline study and then follow-up MR examinations of the spinal cord rather than a biopsy. Spinal cord tumours are usually slow growing lesions and have a relatively stable appearance on MRI.

References

Algra PR, Bloem JL, Tissing H, Falke TH, Arndt JW, Verboom LJ (1991) Detection of vertebral metastases: comparison between MR imaging and bone scintigraphy. Radiographics 11: 219–232

Aoki J, Moriya K, Yamashita K et al. (1991) Giant cell tumours of bone containing large amounts of hemosiderin: MR-pathologic correlation. J Comput Assist Tomogr 15: 1024–1027

Baker KB, Moran CJ, Wippold FJ2nd et al. (2000) MR imaging of spinal hemangioblastoma. AJR 174: 377–382

Balériaux DL (1999) Spinal cord tumours. Eur Radiol 9: 1252–1258

Balériaux D et al. (1999) MRI of spinal cord diseases. CD ROM. Lasion (ed) 2nd edition

Balériaux D, Brotchi J (1992) Spinal cord tumours. Neuroradiological and surgical considerations. Riv Neuroradiol 5: 29–41

Balériaux D, Parizel P, Bank WO (1992) Intraspinal and Intramedullary Pathology. In: Manelfe C (ed) Imaging of the Spine and Spinal Cord. Raven Press, New York, pp 513–564

Bourgouin PM, Lesage J, Fontaine S et al. (1998) A pattern approach to the differential diagnosis of intramedullary spinal cord lesions on MR imaging. AJR Am J Roentgenol 170: 1645–1649

Bowen BC, Pattany PM (1999) Vascular anatomy and disorders of the lumbar spine and spinal cord. Magn Reson Imaging Clin North Am 7: 555–571

Bret P, Bougeard R, Saint-Pierre G, Guyotat J, Rricci AC, Confavreux C (1997) Intramedullary subependymoma of the cervical spinal cord. Review of the literature a propos of a case. Neurochirurgie 43: 158–163

Brotchi J, Dewitte O, Levivier M et al. (1991) A survey of 65 tumours within the spinal cord: surgical results and the importance of preoperative magnetic resonance imaging. Neurosurgery 29: 651–657

Brotchi J, Noterman J, Balériaux D (1992) Surgery of intramedullary spinal cord tumours. Acta Neurochir (Wien) 116: 176–178

Bydder GM, Brown J, Niendorf HP, Young IR (1985) Enhancement of cervical intraspinal tumours in MR imaging with intravenous gadolinium-DTPA. J Comput Assist Tomogr 9: 847–851

Castillo M, Smith MM, Armao D (1999) Midline spinal cord hamartomas: MR imaging features of two patients. AJNR 20: 1169–1171

Caviness JA, Tucker MH, Pia SK, Tam DA (1998) Hydrocephalus as a possible early symptom in a child with a spinal cord tumour. Pediatr Neurol 18: 169–171

Chandy MJ, Babu S (1999) Management of intramedullary spinal cord tumours: review of 68 patients. Neurol India 47: 224–228

Clark CA, Barker GJ, Tofts PS (1999) Magnetic resonance diffusion imaging of the human cervical spinal cord in vivo. Magn Reson Med 41: 1269–1273

Colombo N, Kucharczyk W, Brant-Zawadzki M, Norman D, Scotti G, Newton TH (1986) Magnetic resonance imaging of spinal cord hemangioblastoma. Acta Radiol (Diagn) 769: S734-S737

Constantini S, Houten J, Miller DC et al. (1996) Intramedullary spinal cord tumours in children under the age of 3 years. J Neurosurg 85: 1036–1043

Del Carpio O'Donovan R (1998) A pattern approach to the differential diagnosis of intramedullary spinal cord lesions on MR imaging. AJR Am J Roentgenol 170: 1645–1649

Edal E, Balériaux D, Metens T et al. (1997) Three-dimensional turbo spin echo cervical magnetic resonance myelography. Int J Neuroradiol 3: 130–135

Epstein FJ, Farmer JP, Freed D (1992) Adult intramedullary astrocytomas of the spinal cord. J Neurosurg 77: 355–359

Eskridge JM, McAuliffe W, Harris B, Kim DK, Scott J, Winn HR (1996) Preoperative endovascular embolization of craniospinal hemangioblastomas. AJNR 17: 525–531

Fischer G, Brotchi J (1996) Intramedullary Spinal Cord Tumours. Thieme, Stuttgart New York

Fine MJ, Kricheff II, Freed D, Espstein FJ (1995) Spinal cord ependymomas: MR imaging features. Radiology 197: 655–658

Friedman DP, Hollander MD (1998) Myxopapillary ependymoma of the conus medullaris or filum terminale resulting in superficial siderosis and dissemination of tumour along CSF pathways. Radiographics 18: 794–798

Hamburger C, Buttner A, Weis S (1997) Ganglioglioma of the spinal cord: report of two rare cases and review of the literature. Neurosurgery 41: 1410–1415

Innocenzi G, Cervoni L, Caruso R (1997) Intramedullary cervical neurinoma. A case report and review of the literature. Minerva Chir 52: 679–682

Ijaz T, Jones K (1997) Images in clinical medicine. Intramedullary spinal cord metastases. N Engl J Med 13; 336(11): 768

Kahan H, Sklar EML, Donovan Post MJ, Bruce JH (1996) MR characteristics of histopathologic subtypes of spinal ependymoma. AJNR 17: 143–150
Klisch J, Spreer J, Bloss HG, Baborie A, Hubbe U (1999) Radiological and histological findings in spinal intramedullary angiolipoma. Neuroradiology 41: 584–587
Koen JL, McLendon RE, George TM (1998) Intradural spinal teratoma: evidence for a dysembryogenic origin. Report of four cases. J Neurosurg 89: 844–851
Lahanis S, Vlahos L, Gouliamos A, Papavasiliou C (1993) Arteriovenous malformation of the spinal cord mimicking a tumour. Neuroradiology 35: 598–599
Laredo JL, Assouline E, Gelbert F et al. (1990) Vertebral hemangiomas: fat content as a sign of aggressiveness. Radiology 177: 467–472
Lee M, Epstein FJ, Rezai AR, Zagzag DD (1998) Nonneoplastic intramedullary spinal cord lesions mimicking tumours. Neurosurgery 43: 788–794
Levivier M, Brotchi J, Balériaux D, Pirotte B, Flament-Durand J (1991) Sarcoidosis presenting as an isolated intramedullary tumour. Neurosurgery 25: 271–276
Li MH, Holtas S (1991) MR imaging of spinal intramedullary tumours. Acta Radiol 32: 505–513
Lunardi P, Licastro G, Missori P, Ferrante L, Fortuna A (1993) Management of intramedullary tumours in children. Acta Neurochir (Wien) 120: 59–65
Manelfe C (1992) Imaging of the Spine and Spinal Cord. Raven Press, New York
Mascalchi M, Cosottini M, Ferrito G, Quilici N, Bartolozzi C, Villari N (1999)
Contrast-enhanced time-resolved MR angiography of spinal vascular malformations. J Comput Assist Tomogr 23: 341–345
Minami M, Hanakita J, Suwa H, Suzui H, Fujita K, Nakamura T (1998) Cervical hemangioblastoma with a past history of subarachnoid hemorrhage. Surg Neurol 49: 278–281
Nagib MG, O'Fallon MT (1997) Myxopapillary ependymoma of the conus medullaris and filum terminale in the pediatric age group. Pediatr Neurosurg 26: 2–7
Nadkarni TD, Rekate KL (1999) Pediatric intramedullary spinal cord tumours. Critical review of the literature. Childs Nerv Syst 15: 17–28
Nemoto Y, Inoue Y, Tashiro T et al. (1992) Intramedullary spinal cord tumours: significance of associated hemorrhage at MR imaging. Radiology 182: 793–796
Ng TH, Fung CF, Goh W, Wong VC (1991) Ganglioneuroma of the spinal cord. Surg Neurol 35: 147–151
Osborn AG (1994) Chapter 21: Tumours, Cysts and Tumour-like Lesions of the Spine and Spinal Cord. In: Anne G (ed) Diagnostic Neuroradiology. Mosby, pp 876–918
Papadatos D, Albrecht S, Mohr G, del Carpio-O'Donovan R (1998) Exophytic primitive neuroectodermal tumour of the spinal cord. AJNR 19: 787–789
Parizel P, Balériaux D, Rodesch G et al. (1989) Gd-enhanced MR imaging of spinal tumours. AJNR 10: 249–258
Przybylski GJ, Albright AL, Martinez AJ (1997) Spinal cord astrocytomas: long-term results comparing treatments in children. Childs Nerv Syst 13: 375–382
Patel U, Pinto RS, Miller DC et al. (1998) MR of spinal cord ganglioglioma. AJNR 19: 879–887
Rifkinson-Mann S, Wishoff JH, Epstein F (1990) The association of hydrocephalus with intramedullary spinal cord tumours: a series of 25 patients. Neurosurgery 27: 749–754
Russo CP, Katz DS, Corona RJ Jr, Winfield JA (1995) Gangliocytoma of the cervicothoracic spinal cord. AJNR 16: 889–891
Scotti G, Scialfa G, Colombo N, Landoni L (1987) Magnetic resonance diagnosis of intramedullary tumours of the spinal cord. Neuroradiology 29: 130–135
Sevick RJ, Wallace CJ (1999) MR imaging of neoplasms of the lumbar spine Magn Reson Imaging Clin North Am 7: 539–553
Shi HB, Suh DC, Lee HK et al. (1999) Preoperative transarterial embolization of spinal tumour: embolization techniques and results. AJNR 20: 2009–2015
Sibilla L, Martelli A, Farina L et al. (1995) Ganglioneuroblastoma of the spinal cord. AJNR 16: 875–877
Sundgren P, Annertz M, Englund E, Stromblad LG, Holtas S (1999) Paragangliomas of the spinal canal. Neuroradiology 41: 788–794
Sze G (1996) Chapter 27: Neoplastic disease of the spine and spinal cord. In: Atlas SW (ed) Magnetic Resonance Imaging of the Brain and Spine, 2nd edition, Lippincott-Raven, pp 1339–1385
Thakkar SD, Feigen U, Mautner VF (1999) Spinal tumours in neurofibromatosis type 1: an MRI study of frequency, multiplicity and variety. Neuroradiology 41: 625–629
Timmer FA, van Rooij WJ, Beute GN, Teepen JL (1993) Intramedullary lipoma. Neuroradiology 38: 159–160
Warnock NG, Yuh, WTC (1993) Magnetic resonance imaging in the discrimination of benign from malignant disease of the lumbosacral vertebral column. Neuroimaging Clin North Am 3: 609–623
Young Poussaint T, Yousuf N, Barnes PD et al. (1999) Cervicomedullary astrocytomas of childhood: clinical and imaging follow-up. Pediatr Radiol 29: 662–668
Zileli M, Coskun E, Ozdamar N et al. (1996) Surgery of intramedullary spinal cord tumours. Eur Spine J 5: 243–250

28 Infectious Diseases of the Spine and Spinal Cord

Alan J. Holz, Evelyn Sklar, Judith M. Donovan Post, J. Randy Jinkins

CONTENTS

28.1 Introduction

The wide variety of presentations together with improvements in imaging techniques make this area one of the most exciting topics in neuroimaging.

The incidence of spinal infections has increased in recent years for which several factors are believed to be responsible. The first and most obvious is the increasingly large population of immunocompromised patients. This includes chronically debilitated patients, such as diabetics, alcoholics, intravenous drug abusers, transplant and chemotherapy patients, as well as those with acquired immunodeficiency syndrome (AIDS). In 1993 there were an estimated 14 million individuals infected by the human immunodeficiency virus (HIV) worldwide. That number is expected to rise to 30–40 million by the year 2000. Diseases such as tuberculosis (TB), which had been on the decline in the United States for decades, are now on the rise. Between 1985 and 1991 an estimated 40,000 new cases of TB occurred as a direct result of the AIDS epidemic (Sharif et al. 1995). At present, approximately 30% of patients with TB are believed to be HIV positive (Thurnher et al. 1997).

Spinal infections have also increased, in part due to the emergence of medically resistant strains of organisms, including TB and other bacterial infections. These organisms may disseminate widely both systemically and throughout the neuraxis with devastating consequences. In the spine sequelae include destruction of the vertebral bodies and intervening intervertebral disc space with resultant deformity and neural compromise. Infection may also primarily or secondarily involve the perispinal tissues, spinal cord and nerves potentially producing permanent neurologic deficits.

This chapter includes an overview of recent developments in MR imaging of spinal infections. Advances in pulse sequences and coil design with improved detection of epidural, paraspinal, marrow, subarachnoid space and spinal cord pathology are reviewed (Ross 1999). Specific pathogens will be discussed as they relate to infection of the vertebral body, intervertebral disc, paraspinal soft tissues, epidural and subarachnoid spaces, spinal cord and nerve roots.

28.2 Technical Aspects

Magnetic resonance (MR) imaging, because of its noninvasive nature, multiplanar capabilities and superb soft tissue characterization, is the study of choice for the diagnostic evaluation of spinal infections. Pathological changes in the spine are not only best imaged with MR, but also seen earlier with MR than any other imaging modality (Thurnher et al. 1997). Recent advances in pulse sequences and coil design have led to even greater detection of spinal cord, subarachnoid, epidural, paraspinal and marrow pathology.

The spine is routinely imaged in at least two planes, typically sagittal and axial. Sagittal views are

A.J. Holz, MD; E. Sklar, MD; J.M. Donovan Post, MD
Department of Radiology, Section of Neuroradiology (R-308), University of Miami School of Medicine, 1115 NW 14th Street, Miami, FL 33136, USA
J.R. Jinkins, MD, FACR
Professor and Director of Neuroimaging Research, Department of Radiology, 981045 Nebraska Medical Center, Omaha, NE 68198-1045, USA

useful to assess the vertebral bodies, intervertebral disc, epidural and subarachnoid spaces, as well as the spinal cord. Axial images are complementary and help to evaluate the paraspinal soft tissues, epidural and subarachnoid spaces. Occasionally supplemental coronal images are added for improved visualization of the foramina and paraspinal soft tissues.

Different techniques are available to obtain suppression of fat signal. The frequency selective (chemical shift) fat suppression technique in conjunction with intravenous contrast increases the conspicuity of contrast enhancement by suppressing the hyperintense signal of fat in marrow, the epidural space, foramina and paraspinal soft tissues. Studies have shown that images obtained with contrast and fat suppression detect more abnormalities than do images obtained with contrast alone (GEORGY and HESSELINK 1994). Unfortunately, magnetic susceptibility artifacts may arise in regions of varying morphology, such as the craniocervical and cervicothoracic junctions.

Gradient echo fat suppression technique is based on chemical shift phenomenon. Using different echo times (TE) results in fat and water being in-phase and out-of-phase. This data can be combined to produce either fat-selective or water-selective images. While this method may produce more homogeneous fat suppression than frequency-selective sequences it is seldom used because it requires greater imaging time and is therefore more susceptible to patient motion (PETERFY et al. 1994).

Short-inversion-time inversion recovery (STIR) is an alternate method of fat suppression in which fat is suppressed on the basis of its T1 relaxation. Inflammatory infiltration of vertebral body marrow produces patchy areas of increased signal, which are even more hyperintense than on T2-weighted images (Fig. 28.1). The synergistic effect of prolonged T1 and T2 relaxation times characteristic of myelitis results in greater lesion conspicuity on STIR images than on conventional T2-weighted images in the cervical region

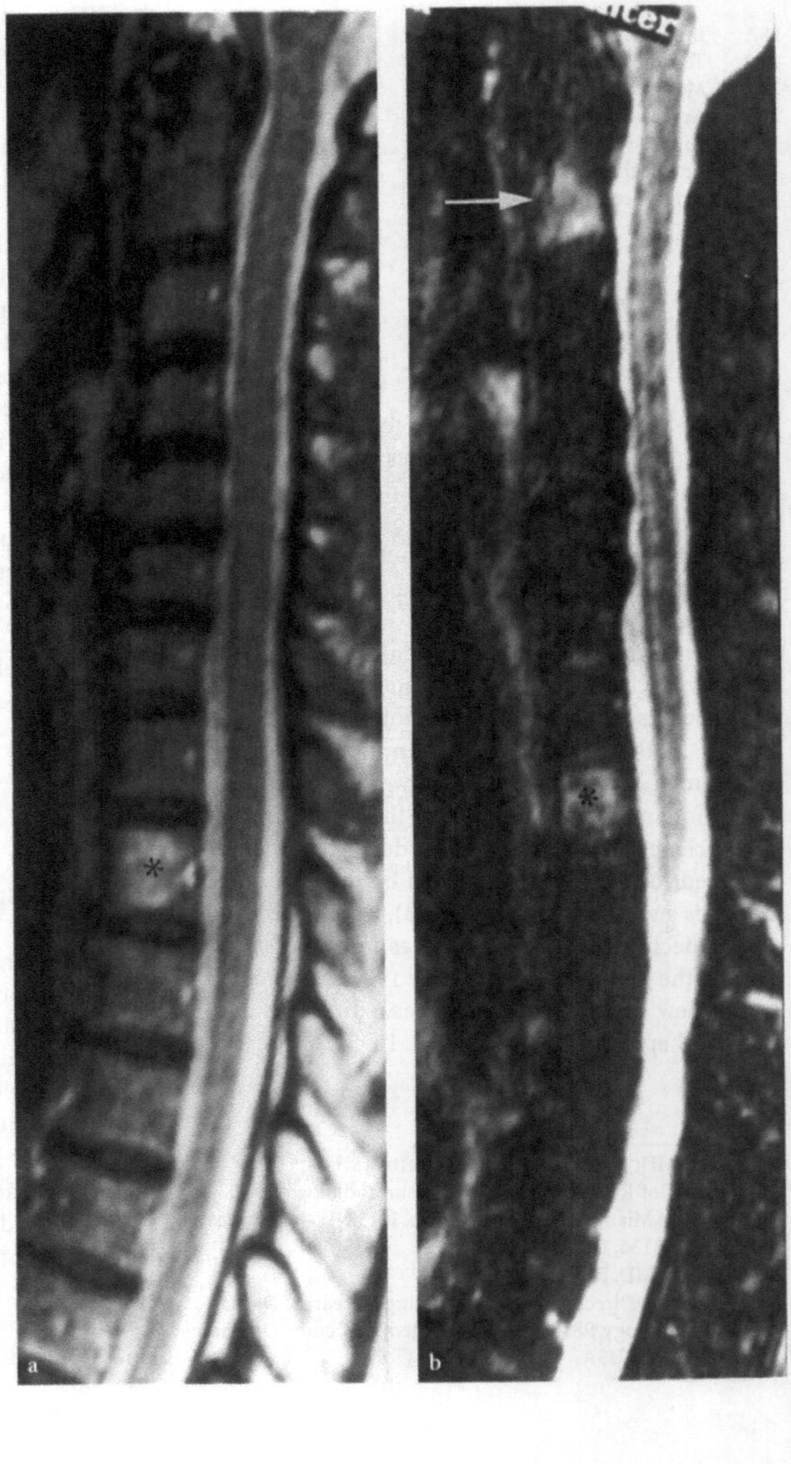

Fig. 28.1a,b. Osseous metastasis. Sagittal T2 weighted (**a**) and STIR (**b**) large FOV MR images acquired with a phased array coil. The lesion in the T2 vertebral body (*asterisk*) is well seen on both pulse sequences. However, the lesion in the C2 vertebral body (*arrow*) is only identified on the STIR sequence

(HITTMAR et al. 1996; ROSS 1999). Disadvantages of the STIR technique include longer imaging time, decreased spatial resolution and incompatibility with gadolinium (GEORGY and HESSELINK 1994; PETERFY et al. 1994).

28.3 Myelitis

Myelitis is a nonspecific inflammation of the spinal cord that may be seen with infectious, inflammatory and neoplastic processes. Unlike spinal cord tumors, which present insidiously, infectious or inflammatory myelitis usually presents acutely. Clinical signs include rapidly progressive weakness, hyporeflexia, urinary bladder and anal sphincter disturbances. Disease predominates in immunocompromised patients and includes bacterial, fungal, viral and parasitic pathogens.

Bacterial infections of the spinal cord are postulated to occur only in the setting of systemic bacteremia. A respiratory infection, usually staphylococcus or streptococcus, is the most common source. Other possible etiologies include a congenital dermal sinus or bacterial endocarditis. Sequential imaging studies suggest the progression from infectious myelitis to frank cord abscess parallels the evolution from cerebritis to abscess formation in the brain (MURPHY et al. 1998). Early findings in infectious myelitis include an increase in cord diameter with diffuse, ill-defined hyperintensity on T2-weighted images and poorly defined enhancement on postcontrast T1-weighted images. In later stages findings include decreased signal abnormalities on T2-weighted images with well-defined ring-enhancement following contrast administration corresponding to intramedullary abscess formation. Following antibiotic therapy, serial scans may show a progressive decrease in the size of the enhancing lesion and associated edema (MURPHY et al. 1998).

TB is estimated to be up to 500 times more common in AIDS patients than in HIV-negative individuals. Of those with AIDS-related TB approximately 10% have CNS involvement (THURNHER et al. 1997; WHITEMAN 1997). As with TB elsewhere in the spine, infection is usually the result of hematogenous spread from a primary pulmonary site. Pathologically, mature tuberculomas have a central area of solid caseous necrosis and a capsule of collagenous tissue, epitheloid cells, multinucleated giant cells and mononuclear inflammatory cells. MR imaging features of intramedullary tuberculomas vary depending on whether the granuloma is noncaseating, caseating with a solid center or caseating with a liquid center. Noncaseating granulomas are usually hypointense on T1-weighted images, hyperintense on T2-weighted images and enhance homogeneously (Fig. 28.2). Caseating granulomas with a solid center are hypointense to isointense on T1-weighted images, isointense to hypointense on T2-weighted images and demonstrate peripheral enhancement following contrast administration. Caseating granulomas with a liquid center are generally hypointense on T1-weighted images, hyperintense on T2-weighted images and enhance peripherally (JINKINS et al. 1995; WHITEMAN 1997). The variable appearance of intramedullary tuberculomas means these lesions are often indistinguishable from pyogenic infections, noninfectious granulomatous diseases such as spinal sarcoidosis or even some intramedullary tumors (GERO et al. 1991).

Other granulomatous infections include fungal agents that affect immunocompromised hosts, as well as those agents endemic to particular geographic regions. Typically, immunosuppressed patients may be infected with aspergillus, cryptococcus and candida. Aspergillus is reported to involve the CNS in approximately 10–25% of AIDS patients and cryptococcus in approximately 5–10% of AIDS patients. As with TB, CNS involvement is almost always due to hematogenous spread of a primary pulmonary site of infection (THURNHER et al. 1997). Coccidiomycosis is endemic in the southwest, blastomycosis in the southeast and histoplasmosis in the midwest United States and may be seen in AIDS subpopulations in these regions (Fig. 28.3). Infection usually involves the vertebral bodies; intraspinal involvement is rare.

Viral infections of the cord are seen exclusively or with increased incidence and severity in AIDS patients. In fact, the incidence of myelopathy in AIDS patients may be as high as 20% (QUENCER and POST 1997). Most have associated brain lesions. Cord pathology includes vacuolar myelopathy, tract pallor, myelitis, opportunistic infections and neoplasms. A recent study by PETITO et al. found vacuolar myelopathy to be the most common cord pathology in AIDS patients (PETITO 1997; QUENCER and POST 1997). Vacuolar myelopathy is defined microscopically as vacuolation in the white matter of the spinal cord, in association with lipid-laden macrophages. It may occur with or without tract pallor in which a loss of myelin staining occurs without vacuolation or the presence of numerous macrophages (QUENCER and POST 1997; SANTOSH et al. 1995). Both conditions

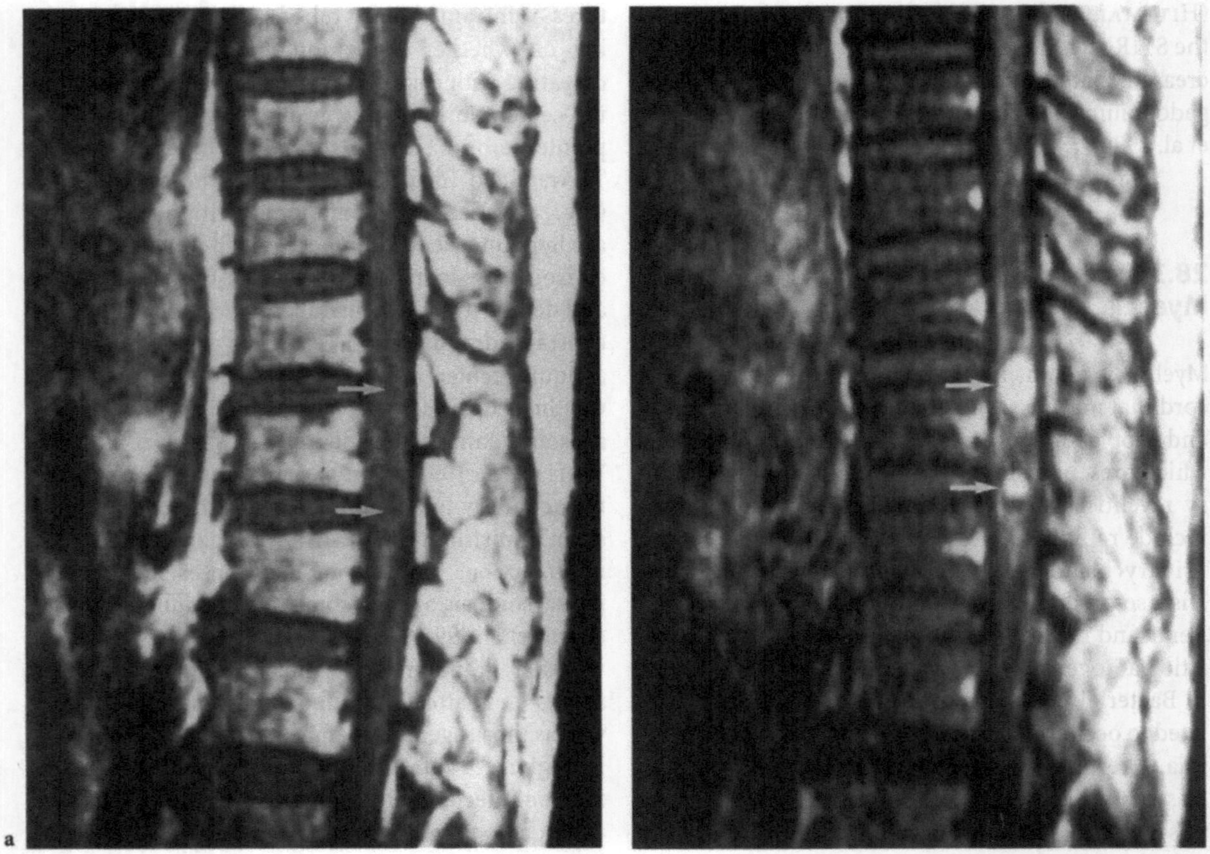

Fig. 28.2a,b. Noncaseating TB granulomata of the thoracic spinal cord. T1-weighted sagittal MR precontrast (**a**) and postcontrast (**b**) images. Moderate swelling of the distal thoracic cord (*arrows*), with solid nodular enhancement (*arrows*) representing noncaseating TB granulomata. TB bacilli were isolated from pulmonary sputum. The spinal cord lesions resolved completely following antituberculous medical therapy

typically involve the dorsal columns and lateral corticospinal tracts of the cervical and thoracic segments of the spinal cord. On gradient echo (T2*-weighted) MR images intramedullary hyperintensity may be detected in approximately two-thirds of patients (SANTOSH et al. 1995), without associated cord enlargement or contrast enhancement on T1-weighted sequences (Fig. 28.4). Patients with vacuolar myelopathy generally have a steadily progressive spastic-ataxic paraparesis and urinary incontinence, while those with tract pallor primarily have a sensory neuropathy (QUENCER and POST 1997). In HIV myelitis discrete microglial nodules with multinucleated giant cells involve either the gray or white matter. HIV myelitis is most often seen in patients with severe HIV encephalitis. It occurs much more frequently in pediatric AIDS patients than either vacuolar myelopathy or opportunistic infections (QUENCER and POST 1997). Opportunistic infections of the cord are typically those of the herpes family including cytomegalovirus (CMV) and herpes simplex virus (HSV) 1 and 2. CMV has been shown pathologically to infect endothelial cells in the periphery of the lumbar and thoracic cord, including the posterior columns and dorsal roots (QUENCER and POST 1997; THURNHER et al. 1997). It may produce tract pallor, myeloradiculitis or polyradiculopathy. Unenhanced MR images are often unremarkable, but may display subtle thickening of the conus and cauda equina. Postcontrast images may demonstrate enhancement of the conus medullaris, nerve roots and leptomeninges over the cord (Fig. 28.5). HSV may pathologically affect the same regions of the spine and present similar clinically to CMV; however, it has not been described as having clearly visible imaging characteristics (THURNHER et al. 1997). Unfortunately, identification of the causative agent producing myelitis is often difficult.

Parasitic infections include toxoplasmosis, schistosomiasis and cysticercosis. *Toxoplasma gondii* is an obligate intracellular organism, which may produce a self-limited subclinical infection in immuno-

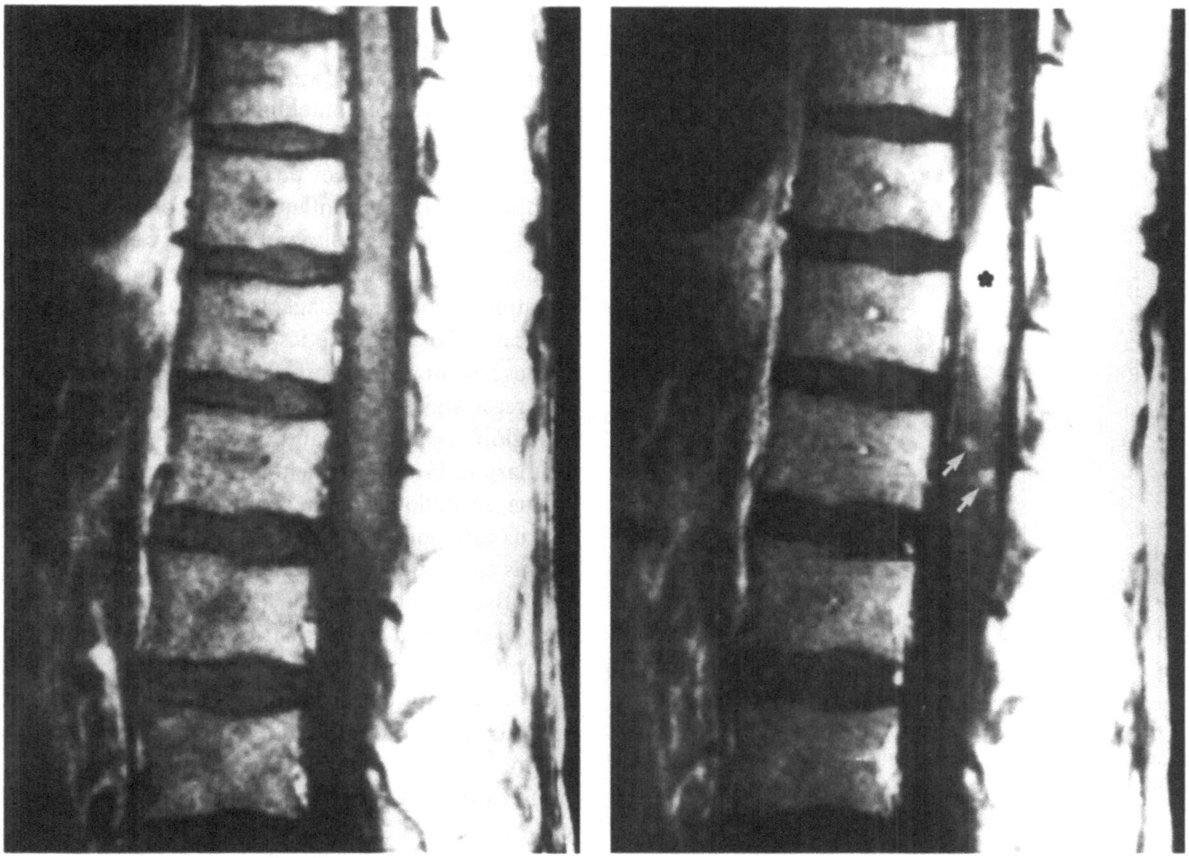

Fig. 28.3a,b. Histoplasma myelitis. T1-weighted sagittal MR precontrast (**a**) and postcontrast (**b**) images show a large enhancing lesion at the T11 level (*star*) with two satellite enhancing lesions in the conus (*arrows*)

competent individuals (Reddy et al. 1995). In AIDS patients, toxoplasmosis is the most common opportunistic brain infection. It is rarely found in the spine, but when present often coexists with brain lesions. In one autopsy study of 138 AIDS patients, toxoplasmosis was found in the brain in 32 patients, in the cord in only 1 patient (Henin et al. 1992; Thurnher et al. 1997). MR imaging findings include hypointensity to isointensity on T1-weighted images, hyperintensity on T2-weighted images with homogeneous enhancement following contrast administration (Fig. 28.6). In the cord, as in the brain, distinguishing toxoplasmosis from lymphoma on the basis of imaging alone is difficult. To date, radionuclide scanning with thallium-201 SPECT has not been successful in imaging the cord. However, one may suggest *Toxoplasma* myelitis in a patient with coexisting spinal cord and brain lesions and a negative brain thallium-201 SPECT examination. Schistosomiasis is a disease of developing countries; more than 200 million people are believed to be systemically infected worldwide (Murphy et al. 1998; Reddy et al. 1995). Rarely schistosome eggs may infect the spinal cord either antegrade through the systemic circulation or retrograde through valveless vertebral/paravertebral veins. The result may be an acute transverse myelitis or a chronic focal granulomatous response (Reddy et al. 1995). Cysticercosis is the most common CNS parasitic infection in Latin America, southern Asia and Africa. Spinal involvement is uncommon and is almost always accompanied by intracranial disease. Intramedullary cysticercosis is believed to result from hematogenous dissemination. The thoracic cord is most commonly affected because it receives the greatest blood flow of all spinal segments. As expected, the cystic component of the lesion is generally isointense to CSF on all sequences. The scolex is isointense to cord parenchyma and best seen on T1-weighted images (Fig. 28.7). It may not be visualized on T2-weighted images because it is often isointense to cyst fluid (Leite et al. 1997). As with cerebral lesions, when the scolex begins to break down, ring enhancement will be observed following contrast administration.

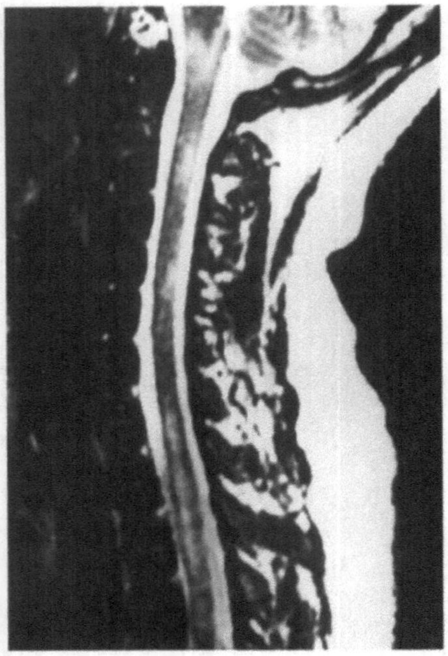

Fig. 28.4. Nonspecific AIDS myelitis. Sagittal T2-weighted MR image in a patient with CSF cultures positive for HTLV III. Patchy areas of hyperintensity are seen within an atrophic (i.e., absent normal cervical enlargement) cervical and upper thoracic spinal cord

28.4 Arachnoiditis

Arachnoiditis or leptomeningitis is a broad term denoting inflammation of the meninges and subarachnoid space. A variety of possible etiologies exist, including infectious, inflammatory and neoplastic processes. Noninfectious, inflammatory etiologies include surgery, intrathecal hemorrhage and the administration of intrathecal agents, such as myelographic contrast media, anesthetics or steroids. Neoplasia includes hematogenous spread of systemic tumors, such as breast and lung carcinoma, melanoma and non-Hodgkin's lymphoma, and direct CSF seeding from primary CNS tumors including glioblastoma multiforme, medulloblastoma, ependymoma and choroid plexus carcinoma. These topics are beyond the scope of this chapter and the reader is referred to Chap. 27.

With regard to infection, etiologies include bacterial, viral, fungal and parasitic agents. TB is the most common cause of spinal meningitis, usually secondary to dissemination through the subarachnoid space of an intracranial tuberculous meningitis. Infection may also spread to the meninges hematogenously from a source outside the CNS or by intraspinal extension of a discitis/osteomyelitis (GUPTA et al. 1994; WHITEMAN 1997). Pathologically, subarach-

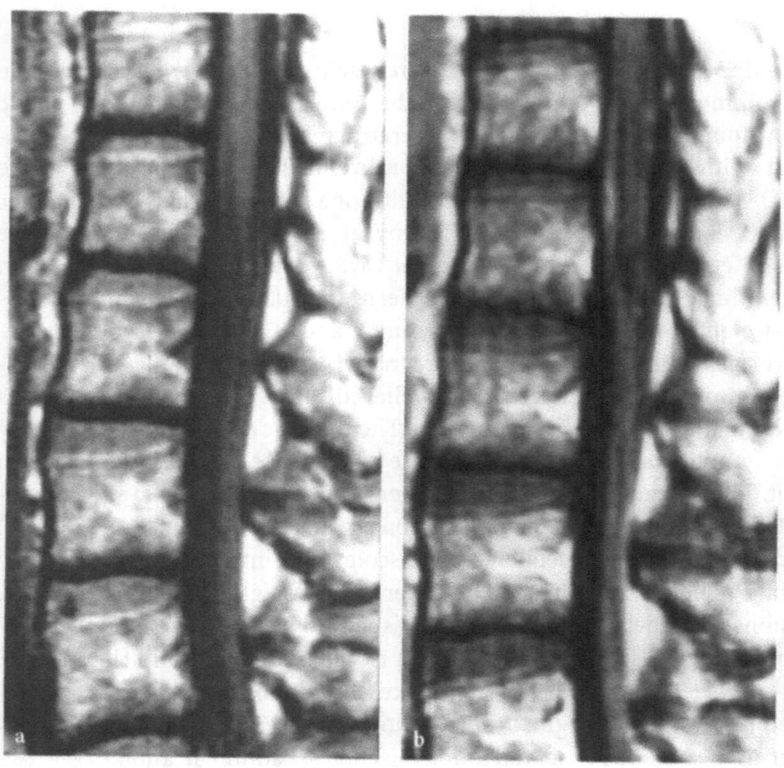

Fig. 28.5a,b. CMV Radiculitis. T1-weighted sagittal MR precontrast (**a**) and postcontrast (**b**) images show mild thickening and enhancement of the conus medullaris and cauda equina

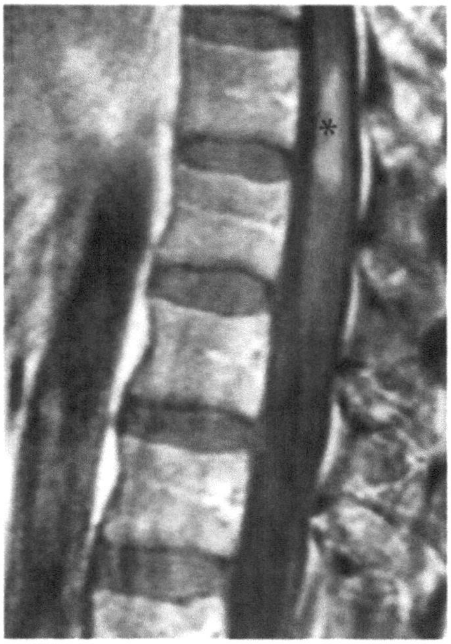

Fig. 28.6. *Toxoplasma* myelitis. T1-weighted sagittal postcontrast MR image shows an enhancing lesion in the lower thoracic cord (*asterisk*)

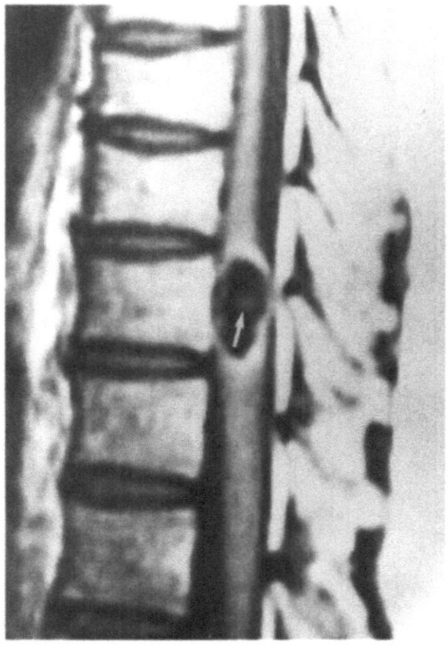

Fig. 28.7. Intramedullary spinal cysticercosis. Unenhanced T1-weighted sagittal MR image with a hypointense intramedullary lesion at the T11 level. Note the scolex (*arrow*) within the cyst cavity

noid infection produces meningeal inflammation leading to congestion and inflammatory exudate. Adhesions form between fibrin-coated nerve roots and meninges causing them to adhere to one another. Subsequently, collagenized adhesions are formed by proliferating fibroblasts producing root tethering, blockage of CSF flow and the formation of CSF loculations. The spinal cord may also be affected as a complication of arachnoiditis. Vascular involvement due to inflammation or compression by fibrous tissue or CSF loculations may produce spinal cord ischemia, infarction, myelomalacia and late cavitation (Sharma et al. 1997).

In cases of arachnoiditis, T1-weighted MR images reveal an indistinct or absent cord outline due to an increase in signal intensity of the surrounding CSF. This may be due to an elevation in CSF protein content, the presence of inflammatory exudate and/or the formation of adhesions along the surface of the cord. T2-weighted images, particularly those acquired with an MR myelographic technique (heavily T2-weighted FSE with fat suppression), best demonstrate the "classic" appearance of arachnoiditis. In the cervical and thoracic region images demonstrate CSF loculation and obliteration of the subarachnoid space. In the lumbar region nerve root matting may produce irregularly thickened, clumped nerve roots which may occasionally be misinterpreted as a tethered cord or a thickened filum terminale. With more severe arachnoiditis, progression of nerve root clumping and leptomeningeal adhesions may lead to angular defects in the dural sac. Peripheral adherence of the nerve roots to the thecal walls leads to the so-called "featureless" or "empty" sac (Johnson and Sze 1990).

Contrast enhancement in lumbar arachnoiditis is an inconstant finding. Enhancement, when it does occur, may be due to development of a vascular network within the fibrous stroma proliferating in the subarachnoid space. Three patterns of enhancement have been described. The most common is a smooth, linear layer of enhancement outlining the surface of the cord and nerve roots. Next is a nodular pattern with discrete foci of enhancement seen along the surface of the cord and nerve roots. The least common pattern consists of diffuse, thick intradural enhancement completely filling the subarachnoid space (Fig. 28.8). Unfortunately, no enhancement pattern is characteristic of any specific infectious agent or any specific pathologic process. For example, smooth, linear enhancement of the cord and nerve roots may be seen in bacterial, viral or fungal arachnoiditis, as well as in leptomeningeal carcinomatosis (Gero et al. 1991; Gupta et al. 1994). In general, benign arachnoiditis enhances less avidly than does carcinomatous meningitis. However, MR find-

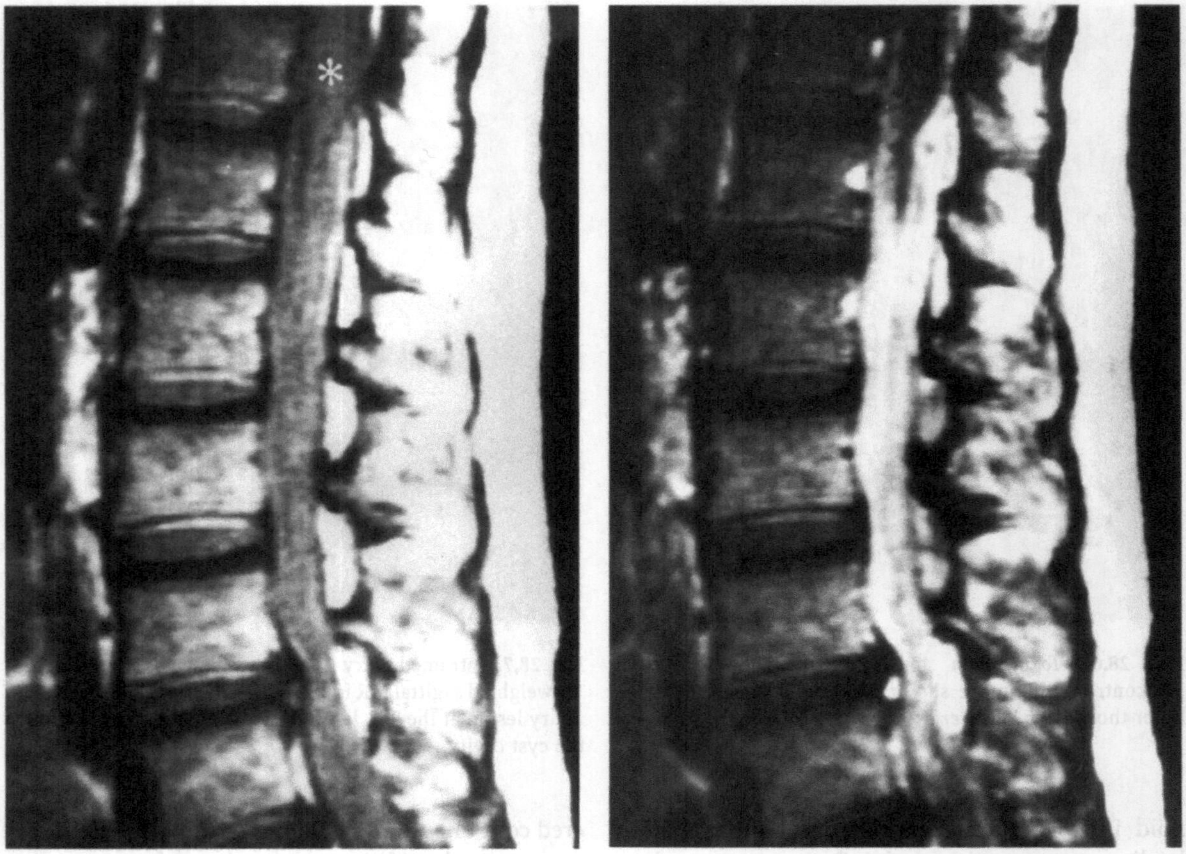

Fig. 28.8a,b. Tuberculous arachnoiditis. Sagittal T1-weighted MR precontrast (a) and postcontrast (b) images. Diffuse hyperintensity of the subarachnoid space relative to the cord (*asterisk*) with intense enhancement indicative of arachnoiditis. TB bacilli were isolated from the CSF

ings alone cannot differentiate infection from neoplasm.

With regard to the signs and symptoms associated with arachnoiditis, paresis may result from compression of the spinal cord and cauda equina, polyradiculopathy from compression or involvement of the cauda equina alone. Patients may complain of low back or radicular pain, leg weakness, gait disorder and incontinence. However, the pattern of contrast enhancement does not correlate with the severity or chronicity of neurologic symptoms (GERO et al. 1991).

28.5 Discitis and Vertebral Osteomyelitis

Infectious spondylitis involves both the vertebral body and the adjacent intervertebral disc. The initial focus of spinal infection is usually by vascular dissemination from a primary source to the most richly vascularized structure in the spine. In infants and children this is the intervertebral disc into which organisms may enter hematogenously and spread across to involve the adjacent vertebral bodies. The disease process typically takes a more benign course in children than it does in adults.

Vertebral osteomyelitis usually affects otherwise healthy adults in the 6th and 7th decades of life. In adults, the cancellous bone adjacent to the cartilaginous end plate retains its rich vascularization, especially in the peripheral metaphyseal region, and is thus the first and most common site of spinal infection in this age group. At the time of diagnosis, spread has almost always occurred to the adjacent intervertebral disc, and often across the disc to the next contiguous vertebral end plate. In a surgical review by MALAWSKI (1977), approximately 66% of patients have infection limited to the intervertebral disc and the two adjacent vertebral bodies. Another 25% show contiguous involvement at more than one segmental level. However, multiple separate spinal foci can rarely be seen without contiguous involvement statistically; the sites of involvement in descending order are the lumbar, thoracic and cervical spine. Men are affected twice as often as women. With regard to therapy, adult patients with vertebral osteomyelitis are routinely treated with parenteral antibiotics for 6 weeks. Surgical treatment becomes necessary when progressive neurologic symptoms supervene or if antibiotic treatment fails and bony destruction causes spinal canal malalignment or instability.

The most common organism responsible for spondylitis is *Staphylococcus aureas*. Conventional radiographic findings are typically subtle and not detectable until later in the course of the disease. The hallmark is disc space narrowing, which is minor at first. Findings become more evident as the adjacent vertebral bodies are eroded. The end stage is characterized by vertebral sclerosis with partial or complete bony fusion across the disc space. On MR, findings often reflect both the replacement of bone by inflammatory tissue and associated structural changes such as disc space narrowing (Modic et al. 1985). A finding highly suggestive of infectious spondylitis is that of vertebral body MR signal abnormality in the vertebrae adjacent to the intervertebral disc. Initially the disc space is markedly hyperintense on T2-weighted images due to increased water content. Later marrow signal intensity changes are noted. The replacement of marrow by inflammatory tissue is seen as abnormally low signal intensity on T1-weighted images and increased signal intensity on T2-weighted images (Fig. 28.9).

Non-enhanced MR has been reported to be as sensitive and specific as radionuclide scans in detecting infectious spondylitis. Modic et al. (1985) found non-enhanced MR to have a sensitivity of 96%, specificity of 92%, and an accuracy of 94% in detecting vertebral osteomyelitis. The changes of osteomyelitis on MR appeared at approximately the same time as abnormalities were detected on gallium and technetium-99m hydroxydiphosphonate bone scans.

In almost all patients, bone and disc abnormalities are accompanied by adjacent inflammatory tissue anteriorly and laterally in the paraspinal region and/or posteriorly in the epidural space. With extensive disc space involvement the cortical vertebral margins may become difficult or impossible to de-

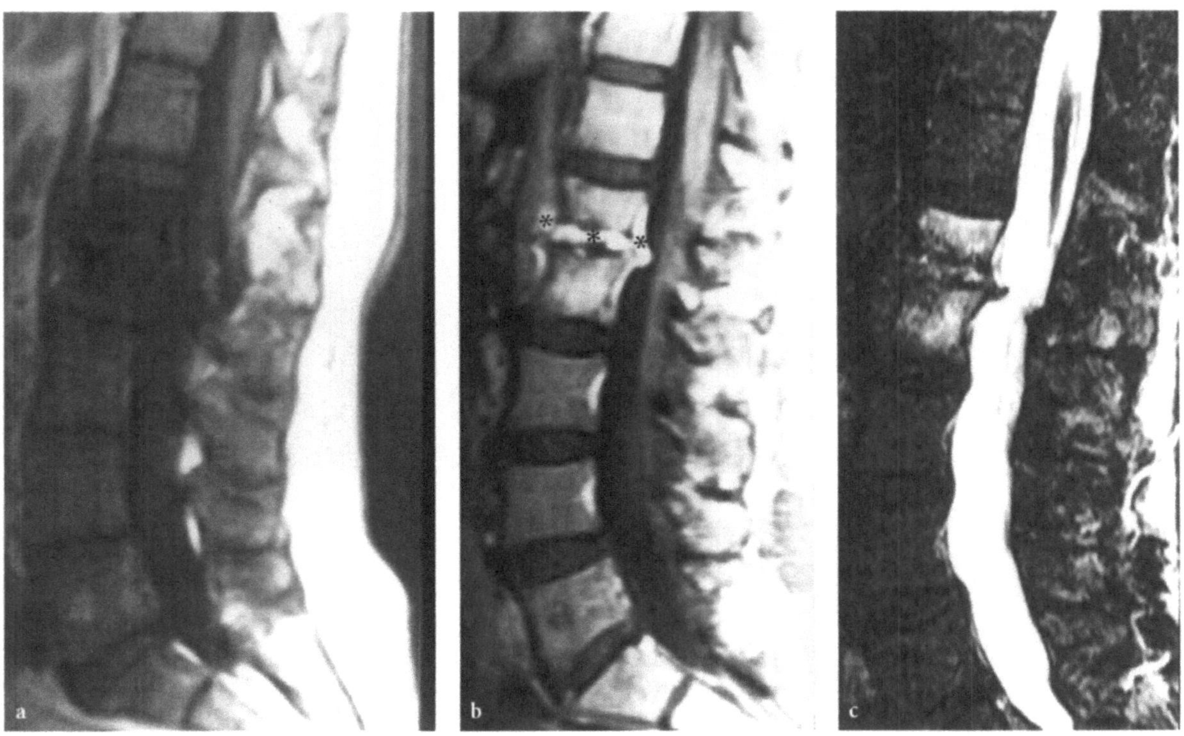

Fig. 28.9a–c. Disc space infection. Sagittal T1-weighted MR precontrast (**a**) and postcontrast (**b**) images, and sagittal STIR (**c**) image. The L1 and L2 vertebral bodies have ill-defined cortical bone and abnormally decreased marrow signal on T1-weighted image and increased signal on STIR image. Postcontrast T1-weighted image shows enhancement of the disc space, prevertebral and epidural soft tissues (*asterisks*)

lineate due to bony destruction. Often the marrow fat involved in the infection is not restored after the infection is cured.

Following the intravenous injection of gadolinium, contrast enhancement is seen in the substance of periphery of the infected disc and adjacent vertebral marrow (Fig. 29.10). Enhancement of the disc and adjacent bone increases observer confidence in the diagnosis of intravertebral disc infection and may be helpful in those patients whose clinical situations are complicated by a history of malignancy or trauma. POST et al. (1990) found that the diagnosis of discitis and osteomyelitis could not be confidently made in 6 of 26 patients on the basis of non-enhanced MR, whereas with gadolinium-enhanced MR, the correct diagnosis was usually clearly established.

In an attempt to determine the MR imaging appearance of spinal infection in patients who have been receiving antibiotic therapy, the factors that best correlated with clinical improvement were resolution of the epidural collections and perispinal soft tissue inflammatory changes. Over time the vertebral bodies maintained MR signal abnormalities and underwent a progressive decrease in height, while the disc spaces showed some prolonged enhancement and had abnormal signal despite evidence of clinical improvement.

Postoperative disc space infections follow 0.2–3.0% of spinal surgical procedures (ENZMANN 1990). In this setting, infection usually begins within the disc space. One to 4 weeks after surgery patients may develop severe back pain that radiates to the legs, testes, perineum and abdomen (ENZMANN 1990).

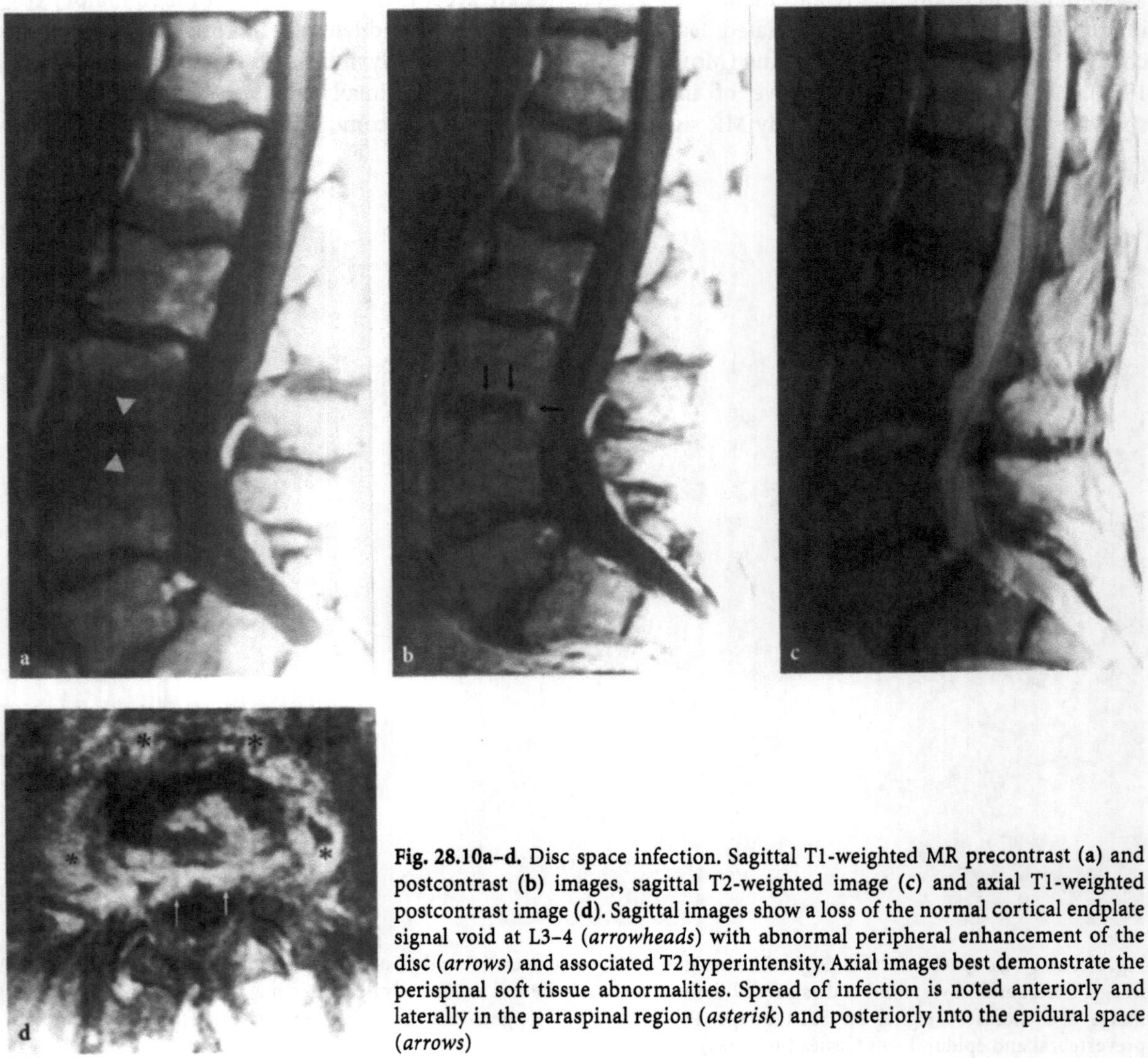

Fig. 28.10a–d. Disc space infection. Sagittal T1-weighted MR precontrast (**a**) and postcontrast (**b**) images, sagittal T2-weighted image (**c**) and axial T1-weighted postcontrast image (**d**). Sagittal images show a loss of the normal cortical endplate signal void at L3–4 (*arrowheads*) with abnormal peripheral enhancement of the disc (*arrows*) and associated T2 hyperintensity. Axial images best demonstrate the perispinal soft tissue abnormalities. Spread of infection is noted anteriorly and laterally in the paraspinal region (*asterisk*) and posteriorly into the epidural space (*arrows*)

Typically there is an elevated erythrocyte sedimentation rate and a mild increase in the white blood cell count. DINA et al. (1995) found that the most reliable finding of postoperative discitis was contrast enhancement of the vertebral bone marrow adjacent to the involved disc space. This together with enhancement of the posterior annulus fibrosus (which may be seen in some normal post-operative discectomy patients) and within the intervertebral disc space (which is seen in the minority of normal post-operative discs) is highly indicative of post-operative discitis.

In North America, tuberculous spondylitis is most prevalent in adults with a mean age of 41–44 years (SMITH et al. 1989). TB infections are usually more insidious and may have a better prognosis than pyogenic infections. TB spondylitis occurs by the hematogenous spread of infectious organisms from a remote primary site in the pulmonary, gastrointestinal or genitourinary systems.

The most common site of infection of TB spondylitis is usually L-1. Classically, spinal TB is thought to begin in the anterior-inferior portion of the vertebral body. Spread of infection can occur beneath the longitudinal ligaments directly to involve multiple vertebral bodies (Fig. 28.11). Disc space narrowing occurs secondarily and is limited relative to the degree of bone destruction, which is typically more extensive than that seen in pyogenic infection. Contiguous vertebral body involvement with destruction of the intervening disc occurs in approximately half the cases (DAGIRMANIAN et al. 1996). On the other hand, preservation of intervertebral discs is often seen (DIGIORGIO et al. 19??). A lack of proteolytic enzymes associated with mycobacteria has been proposed as one of the causes of this relative preservation as compared with pyogenic infection of the intervertebral disc. Involvement of the posterior bony elements appears to be more common with tuberculosis than with other infectious agents (ENZMANN 1990; SMITH et al. 1989). Recognition of posterior element involvement is important because successful treatment requires laminectomy and de-

a 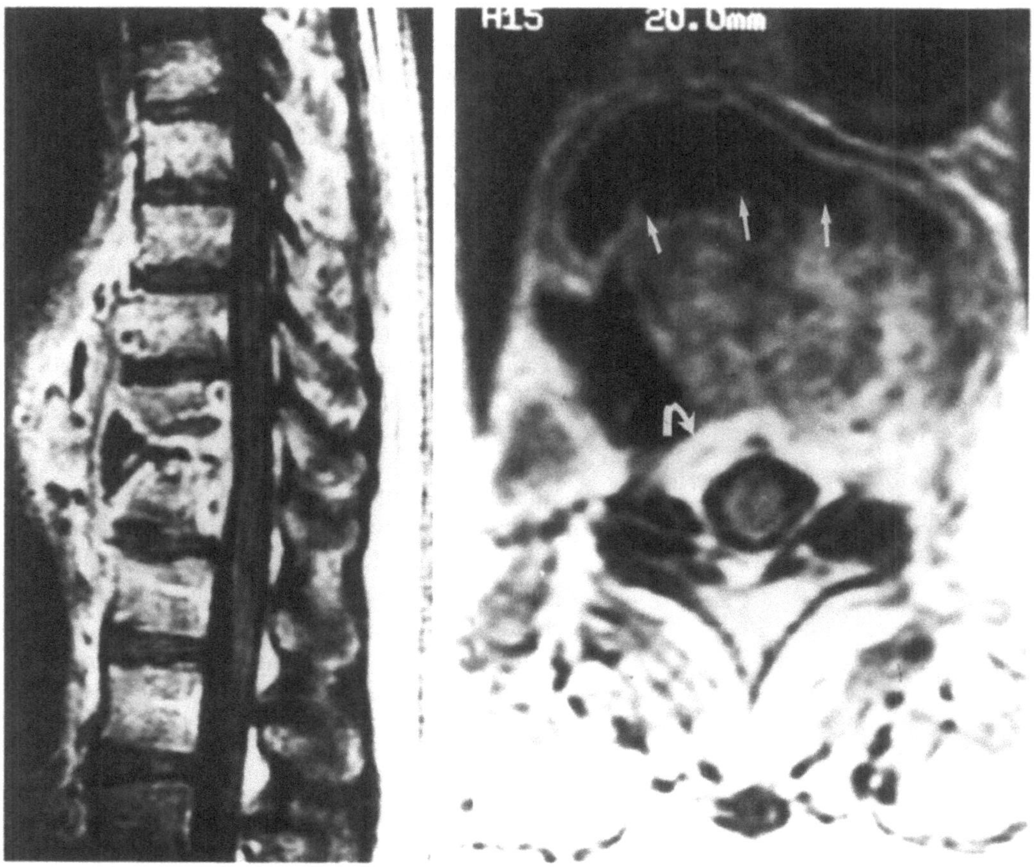 b

Fig. 28.11a,b. Tuberculous spondylitis. Sagittal (**a**) and axial (**b**) T1-weighted MR postcontrast images. Extensive bony destruction of adjacent vertebral bodies is noted with spread of infection beneath the anterior (*arrows*) and posterior (*curved arrow*) longitudinal ligaments bridement in addition to medical therapy. The multiplicity of vertebral body involvement in tuberculous spondylitis makes differentiation from metastatic neoplastic disease difficult. If involvement of the disc space is present, MR can often distinguish infection from tumor by showing abnormal signal and enhancement of the intervertebral disc and adjacent vertebral bodies. In addition, the middle column of the spine has been shown to be destroyed more often than the anterior column. This may be caused by the difference in the blood supply to each column of the spine (Kim et al. 1994). Because mycobacterium need a high concentration of oxygen to survive, it is hypothesized that the micro-organisms require the high blood flow supplied by the posterior equatorial artery located in the posterior aspect of the vertebral body.

Paraspinal infection and a gibbus deformity are common in tuberculous spondylitis. The size of the paraspinal lesions has been noted to be generally larger and more longitudinally extensive in TB than in pyogenic infections. The reported incidence of paraspinal lesions that are out of proportion to the amount of bony destruction varies from 55% to 96% (Smith et al. 1989). The inflammatory masses extend into the psoas muscles and may result in paravertebral abscesses, which have a tendency to calcify (Fig. 28.12).

Granulomatous infections are a frequent cause of infectious spondylitis in many parts of the underdeveloped world. The granulomatous reaction is a nonspecific response of tissues to an antigenic stimulus. This type of reaction has been identified in infectious, neoplastic, and autoimmune diseases. Organisms infecting the spine associated with a granulomatous reaction include brucellosis, tuberculosis and various types of fungi.

Brucellosis is a small gram-negative coccobacillus. The predominant species in the United States is *Brucella abortus*, most commonly found in cattle, or *Brucella suis*, found in swine. This infection typically involves the lower lumbar spine. The vertebral body is usually morphologically intact despite evidence of osteomyelitis. The degree of fibrosis is more marked than in either TB or in non-granulomatous infections. Extension into the epidural space may be mild or moderate. The paraspinal soft tissues are only infrequently affected by such inflammatory reactions.

In some parts of the world, there is relatively frequent involvement of the spine in certain disseminated fungal infections, including coccidiomycosis, blastomycosis, and actinomycosis. Coccidiomycosis involves multiple spinal foci with preservation of the disc space. Sclerotic margins surrounding lytic foci are typical of the spinal lesions. Inflammatory soft tissue paraspinal masses may also occur. Blastomycosis commonly produces paravertebral masses and lytic lesions with surrounding sclerosis (Dagirmanian et al. 1996).

Candida and aspergillus usually cause infections in immunocompromised hosts. Intervertebral disc and vertebral body changes are similar to those seen in pyogenic infections. In candidiasis, micro-abscess in the brain and meningitis have been reported. This gives rise to the possibility of both epidural and intradural foci of infection with systemic candidiasis. In aspergillosis, the radiographic appearance of spinal infection is similar to that of TB. Cryptococcosis can also affect the spine of an immunocompromised host. Involvement is due to hematogenous spread and

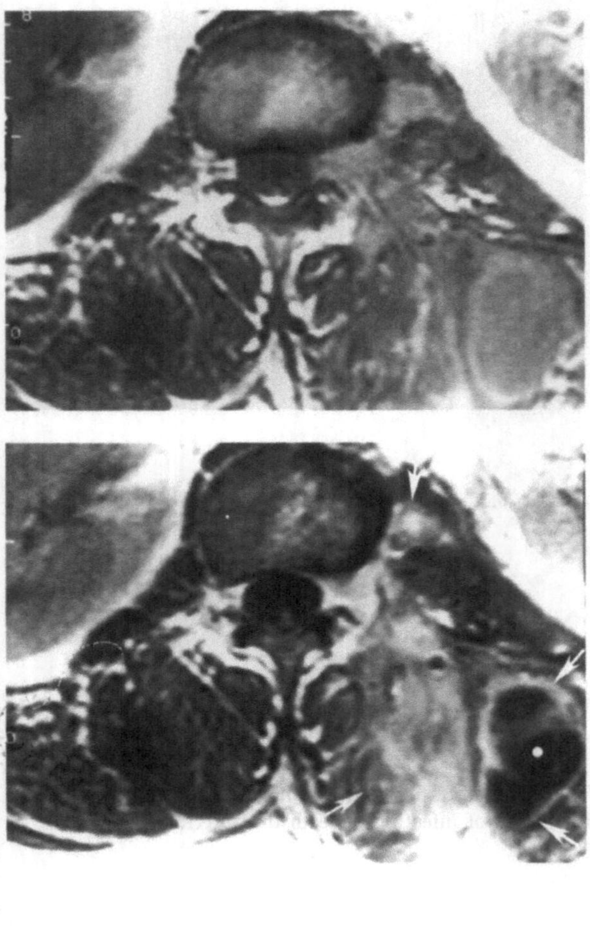

Fig. 28.12a,b. Tuberculous abscess. Axial T1-weighted MR precontrast (**a**) and postcontrast (**b**) images. Inflammatory changes are noted on the left, involving the neural foramen and paraspinal musculature (*arrows*), including a large psoas muscle abscess (*dot*) with ring enhancement and capsule formation

is characterized by sharply marginated lytic lesions in the vertebral bodies and posterior elements. Paravertebral inflammatory masses may also be seen.

Nocardia is a gram-positive bacteria that resembles a fungus. Radiographic findings are similar to those of TB. Involvement of several vertebral bodies with sparing of the disc space is seen together with inflammatory paraspinal masses.

28.6 Epidural Abscess

Epidural abscess is commonly associated with discitis/osteomyelitis. MR greatly facilitates early diagnosis and may improve patient outcome as timely decompression may save neurologic function.

Symptoms of lumbar spinal epidural abscess primarily include back and radicular pain followed by paresthesias. Weakness and paralysis appear later and may be irreversible if prompt treatment by evacuation is not initiated. While epidural abscesses may progress rapidly over a period of 24 h to a few days, some abscesses may have a more chronic course, progressing over weeks to months. An experimental model of epidural abscesses has shown direct compression of neural tissue as the cause of neurologic injury (Kim et al. 1994). White matter is usually more affected than gray matter. Vascular thrombosis or direct inflammation is not a prominent pathologic feature.

MR is as sensitive (91%) as CT myelography (92%) (Modic et al. 1985) in detecting epidural abscesses. MR advantages include its non-invasive nature, thus eliminating the potential for spread of infection to other portions of the spine, and its greater ability to distinguish epidural abscesses from other extradural processes, such as disc herniations, hematomas or neoplasms. On non-contrast MR, an epidural abscess appears as a clearly defined mass that is usually isointense as compared to spinal cord on T1-weighted images and relatively hyperintense on T2-weighted images. In cases of both epidural abscess and meningitis, the epidural collection may be difficult to distinguish from the adjacent infected subarachnoid space. In patients with an epidural abscess but no concomitant disc space infection, the epidural abscess also may go unrecognized if its signal is similar to that of adjacent cerebrospinal fluid (CSF) (Modic et al. 1985). Contrast enhancement can help clearly delineate epidural abscesses (Fig. 28.13). Homogeneous enhancement is seen with phlegmon (i.e., solid soft tissue inflammation), while peripheral rim enhancement is seen with frank liquid abscesses. The majority of epidural abscesses occur adjacent to an infected disc space and typically extend from two to four spinal segments. In extraordinary cases, spread is more extensive and may progress throughout the entire length of the spine.

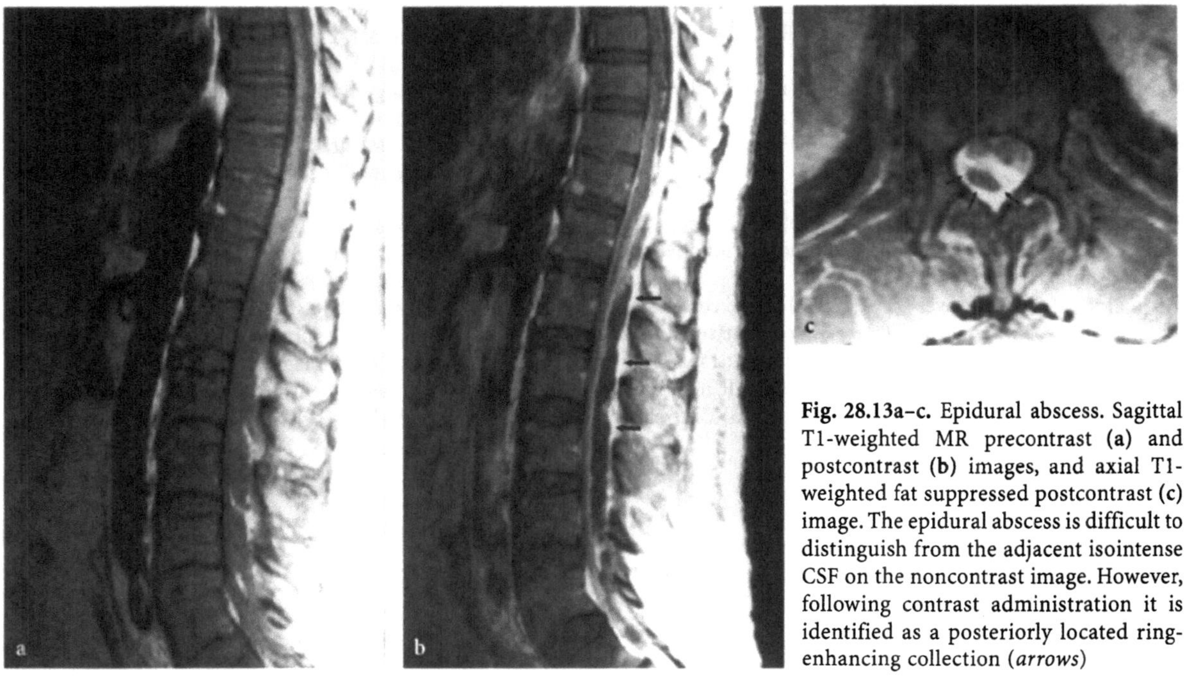

Fig. 28.13a–c. Epidural abscess. Sagittal T1-weighted MR precontrast (**a**) and postcontrast (**b**) images, and axial T1-weighted fat suppressed postcontrast (**c**) image. The epidural abscess is difficult to distinguish from the adjacent isointense CSF on the noncontrast image. However, following contrast administration it is identified as a posteriorly located ring-enhancing collection (*arrows*)

Staphylococcus aureus is the organism most commonly responsible for epidural abscesses in both immunocompetent and immunocompromised patients. Other agents encountered include gram-negative organisms, TB and fungal infections, such as coccidiomycosis, blastomycosis, actinomycosis, candidiasis, and aspergillus.

Treatment consists of a combination of antibiotics and surgical decompression/debridement. MR may help determine the mode of treatment. A small epidural collection in a patient without motor weakness may be treated with antibiotics alone followed by close interval MR follow-up (Enzmann 1990). In contrast, MR evidence of epidural abscess causing severe cord or cauda equina compression will likely be treated by emergency decompressive surgery.

References

Dagirmanian A, Schils J, McHenry M et al. (1997) MR imaging of vertebral osteomyelitis revisited. AJR Am J Roentgenol 169: 1459

Dina TS, Boden SD, Davis DOC (1995) Lumbar spine after surgery for herniated disc: imaging findings in the early postoperative period. AJNR Am J Neuroradiol 164: 665–671

El Gammal T, Brooks BS, Freedy MR et al (1995) MR myelography: imaging findings. AJR Am J Roentgenol 164: 173–177

Enzmann DR (1990) Infection and Inflammation In: Enzmann DR, dela Paz RL, Ruben J (eds) Magnetic Resonance of the Spine. St. Louis, CV Mosby, p 260

Friedman DP, Hills JR (1994) Cervical epidural spinal infection: MR imaging characteristics. AJNR Am J Neuroradiol 163: 699

Gero B, Sze G, Sharif H (1991) MR imaging of intradural inflammatory diseases of the spine. AJNR Am J Neuroradiol 12: 1009–1019

Georgy BA, Hesselink JR (1994) MR imaging of the spine: recent advances in pulse sequences and special techniques. AJR Am J Roentgenol 162: 923–934

Gupta RK, Gupta S, Kumar S et al. (1994) MRI in intraspinal tuberculosis. Neuroradiology 36: 39–43

Henin D, Smith TW, De Girolami U et al. (1992) Neuropathology of the spinal cord in the acquired immunodefiency syndrome. Hum Pathol 23: 1106–1114

Hittmair K, Mallek R, Prayer D et al (1996) Spinal cord lesions in patients with multiple sclerosis: comparison of MR pulse sequences. AJNR Am J Neuroradiol 17: 1555–1565

Jinkins RJ, Gupta R, Chang KH et al (1995) MR imaging of central nervous system tuberculosis. Radiol Clin North Am 33: 771–785

Johnson CE, Sze G (1990) Benign lumbar arachnoiditis: MR imaging with gadopentetate dimeglumine. AJNR Am J Neuroradiol 11: 763–770

Kim, N, Lee H, Suh J (1994) Magnetic resonance imaging for the diagnosis of tuberculous spondylitis. Spine 19: 2451–2455

Leite CC, Jinkins RJ, Escobar BE et al. (1997) MR imaging of intramedullary and intradural-extramedullary spinal cysticercosis. AJR Am J Roentgenol 169: 1713–1717

Malawski SK (1977) Pyogenic infection of the spine. Int Orthop (SICOT) 1: 125

Modic MT, Feiglin DH, Piraino DW et al. (1985) Vertebral osteomyelitis: assessment using MR. Radiology 151: 157

Murphy KJ, Brunberg JA, Quint DJ et al. (1998) Spinal cord infection: myelitis and abscess formation. AJNR Am J Neuroradiol 19: 341–348

Peterfy CG, Linares R, Steinbach LS (1994) Recent advances in magnetic resonance imaging of the musculoskeletal system. Radiol Clin North Am 32: 291–310

Petito CK (1997) The neuropathology of human immunodeficiency virus infection of the spinal cord. In: Berger JR, Levy RM (eds) AIDS and the Nervous System, 2nd ed. Lippincott-Raven Publishers, Philadelphia, pp 451–459

Post MJD, Sze G, Quencer RM et al. (1990) Gadolinium-enhanced MR in spinal infection. J Comput Assist Tomogr 14: 721–729

Quencer RM, Post MJD (1997) Spinal cord lesions in patients with AIDS. Neuroimag Clin North Am 7: 359–373

Reddy S, Leite CC, Jinkins JR (1995) Imaging of infectious disease of the spine. Spine: state of the art reviews 9: 119–139

Roemer PB, Edelstein WA, Hayes CE et al. (1990) The NMR phased array. Magn Reson Med 16: 192–225

Ross JS (1999) Newer sequences for spinal MR imaging: smorgasbord or succotash of acronyms? AJNR Am J Neuroradiol 20: 361–373

Santosh CG, Bell JE, Best JJK (1995) Spinal tract pathology in AIDS: postmortem MRI correlation with neuropathology. Neuroradiology 37: 134–138

Sharif HS, Clark DC, Aabed MY et al. (1990) Granulomatous spinal infections: MR imaging. Radiology 177: 101–107

Sharif HS, Morgan JL, Al Shahed MS et al. (1995) Role of CT and MR imaging in the management of tuberculous spondylitis. Radiol Clin North Am 33: 787–803

Sharma A, Goyal M, Mishra NK (1997) MR imaging of tubercular spinal arachnoiditis. AJR Am J Roentgenol 168: 807–812

Smith AS, Weinstein MA, Mizushima A et al. (1989) MR imaging characteristics of tuberculous spondylitis vs. vertebral osteomyelitis. AJR 153: 399–405

Thurnher MM, Jinkins RJ, Post MJD (1997) Diagnostic imaging of infections and neoplasms affecting the spine in patients with AIDS. Neuroimaging Clin North Am 7: 341–357

Whiteman MLH (1997) Neuroimaging of central nervous system tuberculosis in HIV-infected patients. Neuroimaging Clin North Am 7: 199–214

29 Lymphoproliferative Disorders

MIRIAM DROESSAERT, PETER BRYS

CONTENTS

29.1 Introduction

MR has become the noninvasive imaging modality of choice for diagnosing many bone marrow disorders.

Despite its lack of specificity, MR imaging has the potential to play a role in the management of patients with primary neoplastic disorders of the hematopoietic system, including lymphomas, leukemias and multiple myeloma. In addition to its use in the assessment of spinal cord compression, bone marrow MR imaging could be used as a prognostic method or as a technique to assess the response to treatment.

M. DROESSAERT, MD; P. BRYS, MD
Department of Radiology, University Hospitals, Herestraat 49, 3000 Leuven, Belgium

29.2 Normal MR Appearance of Bone Marrow

At birth, bone marrow is predominantly hematopoietically red marrow, involved in the production of red cells, white cells and platelets. With aging, there is a gradual and progressive conversion to hematopoietically inactive fatty, yellow marrow. This process generally occurs from the periphery to the center but at different rates and different sites within each bone. It is normally completed by the age of 25 years, when the adult marrow distribution is reached. At that time, red marrow predominates in the axial skeleton and the proximal portions of the femora and humeri. With aging, there is continued involution of hematopoietic tissue (WEINREB 1990).

There is no direct correlation between the MR appearance and the histologic pattern of red and yellow distribution, because MR imaging is more sensitive to the presence of microscopic fat in bone marrow (MOORE and DAWSON 1990). The MR appearance, however, can serve as a guide to marrow distribution. Although red marrow is hematopoietically active, in the adult it has a large adipose component. It consists of approximately 40% water, 40% fat and 20% protein. Yellow marrow contains about 80% fat. On routine spin echo MR images, water protons and fat protons both contribute to the signal intensity of tissue. In bone marrow, the signal from the fat component is averaged with that of the water component to produce a summed marrow signal intensity. The higher signal of yellow marrow on the T1-weighted images reflects primarily the preponderance of fat. The lesser signal of red marrow reflects a weighted average of relatively short T1 fat and long T1 water (DAFFNER et al. 1986).

In the axial skeleton of the adult, considerable marrow inhomogeneity is a normal finding, due to an irregular admixture of red and yellow marrow, as well as larger areas of fatty infiltration superimposed on regions of uniform hematopoietic marrow.

On T1-weighted images, four main patterns of marrow distribution are identified throughout the spine and correlated with the age of the patients (Ricci et al. 1990).

Under the age of 30, a uniform low intensity pattern, except for linear areas of high intensity superior and inferior to the basivertebral vein, was recognized throughout the whole spine.

With increasing age, in the lumbar and the cervical spine, areas of bandlike or triangular hyperintensity near the end plates and at the corners of the vertebral body, were noted. This pattern may also relate to mechanical stress and/or degenerative disk disease (Fig. 29.1).

The remaining two patterns showed diffusely distributed areas of high signal intensity, either numerous indistinct dots, measuring a few millimeters or less, or well circumscribed areas, ranging in size from 0.5 to 1.5 cm (Fig. 29.1).

29.3 Reconversion of Bone Marrow

At times at which the body's demand for hematopoiesis increases, a reconversion of yellow to red marrow occurs. Numerous factors play a role in the reconversion: oxygen tension, alterations in vascularity, erythropoietin, elevations in temperature, stress situations and marrow replacement diseases. However, it is certain that other factors may affect the appearance of bone marrow, such as prolonged immobilization, drugs, other systemic diseases, and obesity (Weinreb 1990).

The extent of reconversion depends on the severity and the duration of the stimulus. The order of reconversion is the reverse of the sequence of normal conversion, progressing centripetally from the axial to the appendicular skeleton. Thus the axial skeleton is first affected.

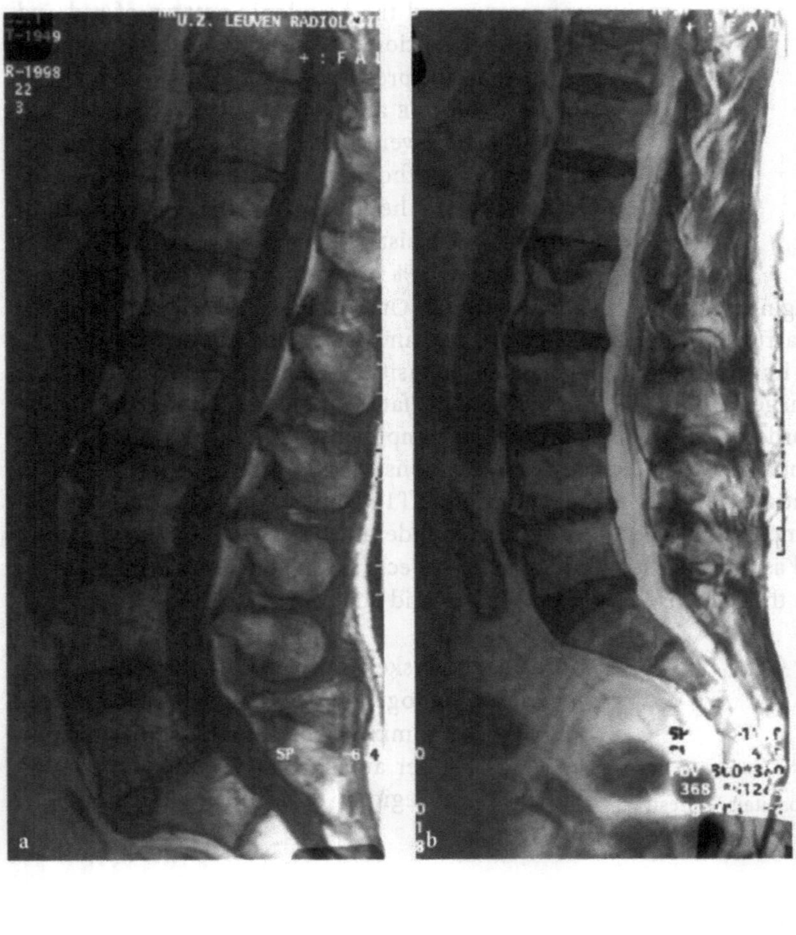

Fig. 29.1a,b. Sagittal T1-weighted SE image (a) shows uniform low intensity pattern, except for a bandlike area near the basivertebral vein, and at the corners of the vertebral bodies. Remarkable signal inhomogeneity on a sagittal T2-weighted SE image (b) in a 65 year old patient

When the disorder affecting hematopoietic demands occurs in childhood, there is a failure or arrest in normal conversion.

On MR images, reconverted marrow has the same signal intensity characteristics as normal hematopoietic marrow, but the distribution is more extensive and more heterogeneous.

29.4 Replacement of Bone Marrow in Lymphoproliferative Disorders

Any process that alters or displaces marrow fat will decrease the T1 signal. The T2 strength will depend on the type of tissue that replaces the normal marrow. Necrotic tissue, hemorrhagic or inflammatory tissue return a higher T2 signal than neoplastic tissue, while sclerotic or fibrotic tissue returns a low signal (DAFFNER et al. 1986).

The distribution of marrow lesions parallels that of hematopoietic marrow either because they originate from red marrow or because of the rich vascularity of red marrow is more favorable to their development than the sparse vascularity of fatty marrow.

Different types of bone marrow involvement are described. These patterns are not specific and can also be seen in non-neoplastic marrow disorders such as inflammatory conditions or metabolic disorders. They can also vary from one anatomical region to another in the same patient. Sometimes it is even difficult to differentiate between red marrow hyperplasia or reconversion and marrow infiltration (VANDE BERG et al. 1998).

The focal pattern of bone marrow involvement is characterized by the presence of an area of marrow replacement with low signal intensity on T1-weighted images, and variable signal intensity on T2-weighted sequences. The margins appear well circumscribed on T1-weighted images, but on T2-weighted images adjacent marrow edema can produce a halo sign. The focal pattern can be observed in multiple myeloma, and high grade non-Hodgkin's and Hodgkin's lymphoma (Fig. 29.2).

A diffuse pattern of marrow involvement is characterized by a diffuse and homogeneous decrease in signal intensity lower than that of discs or adjacent muscles on T1-weighted images (Fig. 29.3). This involvement pattern can cause the intervertebral discs

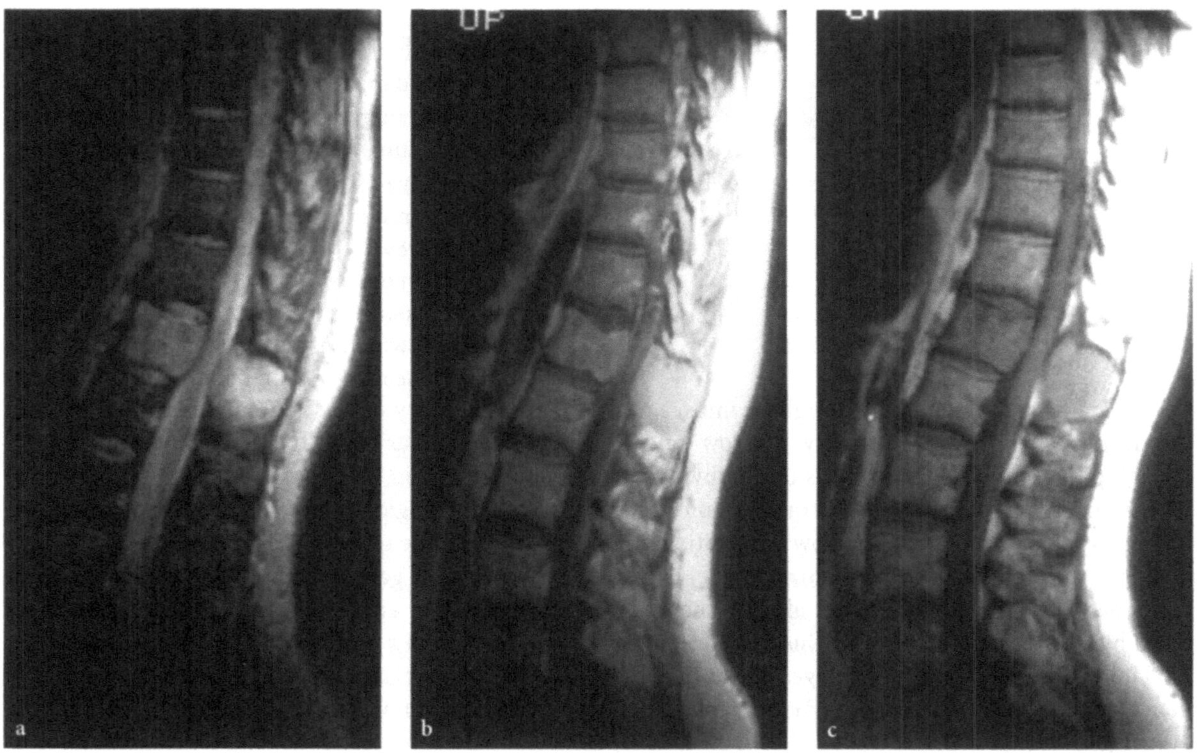

Fig. 29.2a–c. Sagittal T2-weighted turbo inversion recovery (**a**), T1-weighted SE (**b**) and Gd-enhanced T1-weighted SE (**c**) images of a plasmocytoma in vertebra Th12. Note the involvement of the posterior part of the vertebra and the spinal cord compression

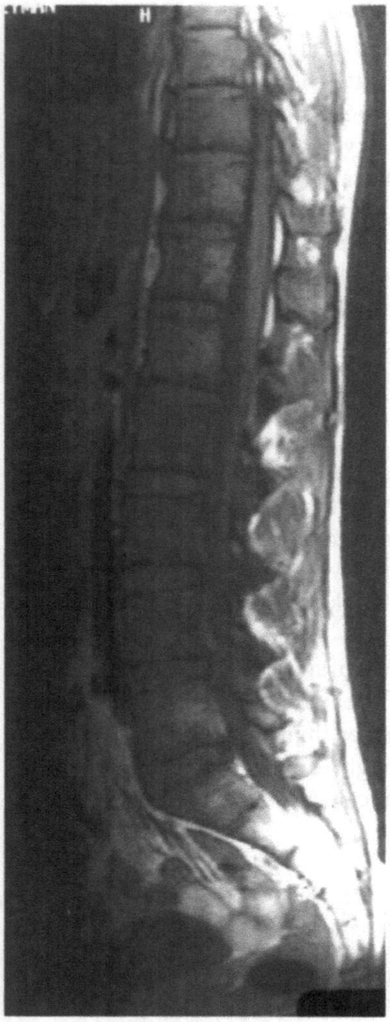

Fig. 29.3. Sagittal T1-weighted SE image showing diffuse bone marrow involvement in a patient with NHL

to have a bright signal on T1-weighted images. The finding of high signal intensity marrow on T2-weighted or equivalent sequences or an obvious increase in signal intensity on contrast-enhanced MR images helps to confirm marrow infiltration and helps to differentiate this from normal hypercellular marrow. The diffuse pattern can also be characterized by a diffuse and heterogeneous decrease in signal intensity on T1-weighted images due to the presence of multiple tiny areas of marrow replacement (variegated or pepper and salt pattern) (Fig. 29.4). The diffuse pattern is observed in multiple myeloma, leukemia and low-grade non-Hodgkin's lymphoma (Vande Berg et al. 1998).

29.5 Multiple Myeloma

29.5.1 Clinical Presentation

Multiple myeloma (MM) is due to malignant proliferation of plasma cells and classically produces marrow plasmocytosis, a monoclonal protein band on urine or serum electrophoresis, and bone lesions affecting the axial skeleton. MM is detected at variable stages of disease development, and patients with advanced disease have bone pain and fractures, anemia and hypercalcemia at initial examination (Vande Berg et al. 1996).

A clinical staging system is proposed (Durie and Salmon 1975). It is based on serum concentrations of hemoglobin, calcium and paraprotein, urinary Bence-Jones protein excretion and the number of skeletal lesions seen on radiographs. Serum beta-2 microglobulins levels are thought to be the single most powerful determinant of outcome (Libshitz et al. 1992).

However, some variants of MM pose diagnostic problems:

Non-secretory myeloma is characterized by involvement of the bone marrow, but no evidence of abnormal protein in the blood or urine. The atypical plasma cells cannot excrete paraproteins or have lost the capability to produce them. So, assessment of the clinical course depends on repeated marrow aspirations because there is no detectable monoclonal peak in the serum. An iliac aspirate may not always be representative of the marrow involvement due to both nodular and interstitial tumor growth patterns (Barti et al. 1989).

In light chain deposition disease, a variant of MM, the atypical plasma cells produce immunoglobulins (light chains), which are deposited in the interstitium of the bone marrow and in other organs. Due to a strong affinity of the light chains with tissue, the light chains clear out of the blood, and no immunoglobulin peak in electrophoresis is seen. Masses of light chain conglomerates are the predominant feature in the bone marrow (Baur et al. 1998).

Monoclonal gammopathies of unknown significance (MGUS) are a relatively frequent laboratory finding. In a few cases, such as a mild increase of bone marrow plasmocytosis or slight morphologic plasma-cell abnormalities, differentiation between MGUS and MM may be difficult. Another point is that 11–24% of MGUS cases turn into MM or other malignant hemopathy, sometimes after a very long delay of up to 35 years (Bellaiche et al. 1997).

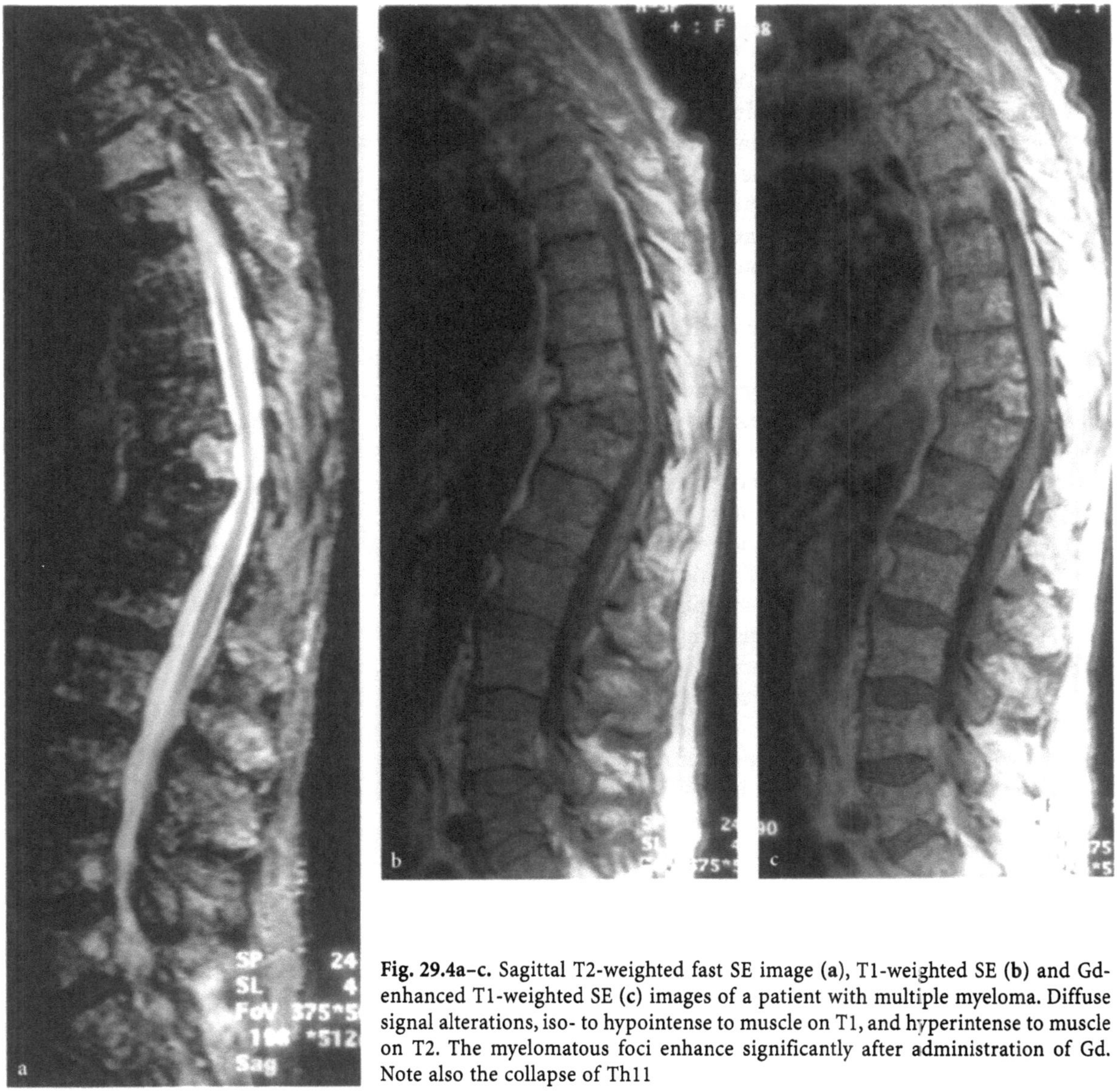

Fig. 29.4a–c. Sagittal T2-weighted fast SE image (**a**), T1-weighted SE (**b**) and Gd-enhanced T1-weighted SE (**c**) images of a patient with multiple myeloma. Diffuse signal alterations, iso- to hypointense to muscle on T1, and hyperintense to muscle on T2. The myelomatous foci enhance significantly after administration of Gd. Note also the collapse of Th11

29.5.2 Role of Bone Marrow Biopsy

Marrow biopsy is essential for diagnosis of multiple myeloma and gives direct proof for atypical plasma cells. Because the biopsy sample is small, however, the result does not always represent the whole marrow, especially in cases of nodular involvement. In contrast to diffuse myeloma infiltration, no correlation was found in nodular involvement between MR imaging and marrow biopsy. False-negative results were seen when the biopsy was taken beside a nodule, and false positive results of a high grade tumor involvement were seen when the biopsy was taken from a solitary nodule (Staebler et al. 1996). Therefore, biopsy may be false negative in 26% of cases.

29.5.3 Imaging

The presence and the extent of osteolytic bone lesions in patients with MM are important factors in the staging of the disease. MR imaging is more sensitive than conventional radiography for MM (Ludwig et al. 1987; Fruewald et al. 1988). Spinal MR imaging depicted marrow abnormalities in half of the patients with asymptomatic myeloma and normal skeletal radiographs (Moulopoulos et al. 1995). In patients with newly diagnosed disease, spinal MR revealed marrow involvement in 69% of the patients (Moulopoulos et al. 1992).

When minimal plasma cell infiltration is present, usually it is accompanied by a normal or increased amount of marrow fat cells. Apparently, monoclonal plasma cells produce factors that inhibit normal hematopoiesis, thus increasing the relative fat component. Therefore, despite tumor infiltration and replacement of hematopoietic cells, marrow fat may be normal or even increased. As long as no critical shift is seen in the fat-water ratio of the marrow, myeloma remains undetected. No signal abnormalities were found when biopsy showed that marrow contained less than 20% plasma cells (Staebler et al. 1996).

It is recognized that bone marrow infiltration in MM takes three forms: either focal, variegated (with innumerable tiny foci on a background of uninvolved marrow), or diffuse (with total replacement of fatty marrow) (Moulopoulos et al. 1992).

Myelomateous tumor nodules show signal intensities similar to or lower than that of muscle on T1-weighted images (Fig. 29.4). One study reported hyperintense nodules on T1-weighted imaging on the initial study, but on follow-up MR-imaging they resolved to become hypo-intense, suggesting the presence of hemorrhage within the focus of myelomatous involvement at the time of the initial study (Moulopoulos et al. 1992).

Before treatment, all myelomatous tumor nodules have homogeneous T2 high signal intensity and all homogeneously after bolus injection of a contrast agent (Rahmouni et al. 1993) (Fig. 29.4).

There is also a greater sensitivity of T2-weighted imaging for myelomatous nodules, as in 9 of the 32 patients focal abnormalities were only seen on the T2-weighted images, and in no patient were they only seen on the T1-weighted imaging (Rahmouni et al. 1993) (Fig. 29.5).

Interestingly, different signal alterations were described in patients with light chain deposition disease. They found focal areas of low signal intensity on both T1- and T2-weighted images. As specific laboratory parameters for light chain deposition disease are lacking, MR can be helpful in monitoring light chain deposition disease (Baur et al. 1998).

In MGUS, all findings on MR imaging were normal. It seems reasonable, therefore, to propose MR imaging of the spine as a valuable diagnostic tool in the long term follow-up study of MGUS, when a new biological or clinical event suggests the diagnosis of a malignant disorder (Bellaiche et al. 1997).

Most vertebral compression fractures in patients with MM appear benign at MR imaging, and their distribution is similar to that observed in osteoporotic fractures; 67% of fractures had MR features suggestive of benign osteoporotic vertebral compression fracture, and 87% were observed between T6 and L4. Only 33% of fractures showed MR features suggestive of malignant fractures (Lecouvet et al. 1998).

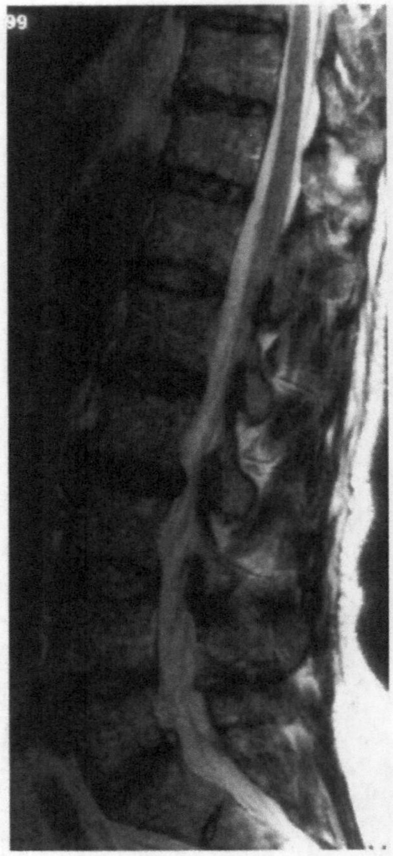

Fig. 29.5. Sagittal T2-fast SE image of a patient with multiple myeloma. The variegated pattern is well depicted

Inability to identify MM in all cases with MR imaging makes it difficult to distinguish benign from malignant causes of vertebral compression fractures. This problem is completed by the significant osteoporosis present in MM.

In MM, a vertebral compression fracture may occur without the MR imaging observation of marrow being totally replaced by tumor cells, possibly because, in addition to tumorous marrow infiltration, osteoclast activating factors also contribute to the development of vertebral compression fractures (Moulopoulos et al. 1992).

The presence and the size of focal marrow lesions are not major or sufficient determinants of fracture occurrence in patients with MM. Actually, a diffuse myeloma induced bone resorption rather than focal osteolysis could be the major cause of bone weakening and of fractures. Increased osteoclastic resorption is observed in association with the widespread dissemination of myeloma cells, due to the synthesis of various osteoclast-activating factors. The demonstration in several studies that a high percentage of myelomatous compression fractures represents an MR appearance of benign osteoporotic fracture, rather than that of malignant fractures, points in the same direction (LECOUVET et al. 1998).

Other series demonstrated that pretreatment MR imaging of the bone marrow in patients with stage III MM had prognostic relevance to detect patients at risk for subsequent development of vertebral compression fractures. Patients with either diffuse or more than ten focal lesions at initial MR imaging had statistically shorter fracture free survivals before the occurrence of the first three fractures than patients with either fewer than ten focal lesions or normal appearing bone marrow (MOULOPOULOS et al. 1995).

29.5.4 Clinicoradiological Correlation

In a group of patients with untreated newly diagnosed disease, 66% had no bone pain, 33% reported bone pain. A significant relationship between MR patterns and serum B_2 microglobulin, monoclonal protein, and serum creatinine was not observed with either test. All patients with normal MR imaging study were free of bone pain (MOULOPOULOS et al. 1992).

The stage of the disease could not be related to the absence of definite evidence of bone marrow involvement (BAUR et al. 1998).

All patients with normal appearing marrow and variegated pattern were in stage I, whereas five of the seven patients with a diffuse pattern were in stage III. All but two of the patients with focal and diffuse or focal tumor infiltration were in stage II or III (STAEBLER et al. 1996).

The abnormal signal intensity of bone marrow in patients with MM results from an increase in bone marrow cellularity. Although there is no histologic correlation, MOULOPOULOS believed that focal plasma cell aggregates accounted for focal lesions and that a generalized infiltration accounted for the diffuse patterns. In the variegated pattern, they believed that small clusters are dispersed on a background of normal bone marrow. In normal patients, either no tumor cells are present or a low number of tumor cells are dispersed in such a way that they do not alter cellularity to a degree that is evident on MR images (MOULOPOULOS et al. 1995).

29.5.5 Treatment and Prognosis

No chemotherapy is justified for patients with no or minimal harmful features in whom the likelihood for prolonged stability is high. By contrast, therapy soon after diagnosis could be useful for patients at high risk for early progression (DIMOPOULOS et al. 1993; ALEXANIAN and DIMOPOULOS 1995) and should not be delayed for symptomatic patients (ALEXANIAN and DIMOPOULOS 1995).

Radiation therapy, in association with chemotherapy, has a major place in the management of focal complicated myeloma lesions, which account for major discomfort, morbidity and even mortality in MM patients. Its rapid and highly effective therapeutic effect on epidural involvement and neurologic compression is well demonstrated. Local irradiation reduces the incidence of new fractures and local lesions in irradiated vertebrae (LECOUVET et al. 1997).

Surgery, and more recently cement vertebroplasty, have been proposed as alternative therapeutic approaches in the urgent management of impending lytic lesions and cord compression, alone or in association with radiation therapy (WEILL et al. 1996).

The presence of bone marrow involvement at MR imaging had a high predictive value for developing aggressive disease. It is clear, however, that normal MR imaging findings do not enable prediction of a stable clinical course with a high level of confidence, although patients with normal MR findings demonstrated a statistically significantly longer progression-free interval than patients with abnormal MR imaging findings. In patients with bone marrow abnormalities demonstrated by MR, the progression-free interval was a median of 10 months, compared with a median of 32 months for patients in whom MR imaging findings were normal (VANDE BERG et al. 1996).

In patients with a diffuse pattern, the disease progressed earlier than in patients with a variegated or focal pattern (MOULOPOULOS et al. 1995, 1994). Conversion of a diffuse to a focal or variegated pattern in patients who responded suggested that diffuse myeloma is associated with more advanced disease (MOULOPOULOS et al. 1994).

After a sequence of standard and intensive therapies, approximately 70% of patients with MM achieve a remission of good quality and many months duration, approximately 2 years. Yet the disease remains incurable (ALEXANIAN and DIMOPOULOS 1995).

29.5.6 Response to Treatment

The effect of successful treatment in diseased marrow was associated with different changes in the three patterns. The marrow often returned to normal when the pattern was diffuse or variegated, but residual abnormalities persisted in patients with a focal pattern. In focal myeloma, dense, nodular plasma cell aggregates may destroy normal bone substrate and cause permanent fibrotic change. In patients with variegated or diffuse patterns, abnormal cells are interspersed in normal marrow, so focal aggregates may not be large enough to produce changes on radiographs. In such cases, the tumor may resolve without any evidence of residual abnormality on MR images.

Most persistent focal abnormalities in patients who had a complete response either did not show enhancement or showed a peripheral rim enhancement on Gd-enhanced images. Rim enhancement may represent a peripheral reparative process and may suggest treated, inactive disease. In complete responders with focal lesions, persistent homogeneous enhancement of focal lesions within irradiated vertebrae was observed in both partial and complete responders. The effect of treatment on focal lesions in irradiated or collapsed vertebrae was difficult to assess with MR imaging because persistent enhancement in such cases may not necessarily indicate resistant disease (Moulopoulos et al. 1994).

After treatment, on T2-weighted images, lesions remained hyperintense, even in good and partial responders, probably related to necrosis within the lesion.

On T1-weighted enhanced images, three patterns could be distinguished:

- Rim enhancement or no enhancement, representing a good response to treatment
- Arterial and complete enhancement and no arterial enhancement, with or without peripheral delayed enhancement, correlates with good or partial response
- No changes in signal intensity, usually represents evidence of progressive disease (Rahmouni et al. 1992)

MR imaging may help clarify the cause of the fracture and guide selection of treatment (Moulopoulos et al. 1994). T1-weighted MR images before and after administration of contrast material best demonstrate the effect of treatment (Moulopoulos et al. 1994; Rahmouni et al. 1992).

29.6 Lymphoma

29.6.1 Clinical Presentation

The malignant lymphomas, which encompass Hodgkin's disease (HD) and a heterogeneous group of tumors termed non-Hodgkin lymphomas (NHL), are primary neoplasms of the lymphatic system. They differ in modes of presentation, treatment and prognosis.

For HD, the Ann Arbor clinical staging was introduced and takes account of the extent of nodal disease and the presence of extranodal extension (Sandrasegaran et al. 1994).

In NHL, the histologic subtype (based on the cell of origin, i.e., Working Formulation, which divides NHL into low, intermediate and high grade types) and other parameters such as tumor bulk and specific organ involvement are more important than the anatomical extent in determining initial therapy and prognosis (Sandrasegaran et al. 1994).

Knowledge of the bone marrow status is essential for the staging and treatment of patients with lymphoma (Tardivon et al. 1995).

In HD, it contributes to the classification, which is critical for the therapeutic strategy: localized disease without bone marrow involvement is mainly treated with radiotherapy (Tardivon et al. 1995).

In NHL, bone marrow involvement indicates advanced disease, and worse prognosis than involvement of liver, lung or osseous bone (Sandrasegaran et al. 1994).

The bone marrow status is of further importance in patients who relapse since most of them will be treated with therapy including autologous hematopoietic cell transplantation (Tardivon et al. 1995).

Patients with lymphoma and with bone marrow involvement seen on MR appear to have an overall lower survival rate than those with normal marrow on MR, whatever the results of the marrow biopsy (Tsunoda et al. 1997).

In HD, bone marrow involvement is uncommon at diagnosis. However, during the course of the illness, 5–15% of patients will develop bone marrow involvement. In NHL, abnormal findings at bone marrow aspiration are found in 20–25% of patients at presentation (Vande Berg et al. 1998; Tardivon et al. 1995; Sandrasegaran et al. 1994).

There is still controversy about the existence of lymphoid tissue in the spinal epidural space. Epidural spinal cord disease occurs in 1–6.5% of patients with systemic NHL (Salvati et al. 1996). Primary spinal epidural NHL, i.e., in the absence of any detectable extraspinal lymphoproliferative disorder, should be considered in the older patient who presents with symptoms of spinal cord compression manifested by a prodrome of back pain followed by a paid neurological deterioration. Plain X-ray is typically normal.

The treatment consists of systemic chemotherapy with possibly additional intrathecal chemotherapy. Radiotherapy is used when complications may occur in later stages of the disease. In emergency situations, high dose steroids and radiotherapy are used.

29.6.2 Role of Bone Marrow Biopsy

Bone marrow biopsy (BB) is recommended in all cases of NHL, but its value in HD is controversial and only a small proportion of patients with early HD have positive bone marrow aspirates (Sandrasegaran et al. 1994).

There is a significant association of abnormal MR imaging with constitutional symptoms or bone pain or elevated alkaline phosphatase level (Tardivon et al. 1995).

MRI is also recommended for patients with negative BB, who would otherwise be candidates for radiotherapy, e.g., stage I high grade NHL (Sandrasegaran et al. 1994).

MR imaging has not replaced BB, but it is used as a complementary tool.

Unilateral blind biopsy is subject to frequent sampling errors compared to bilateral biopsies.

Studies comparing uni- to bilateral BB confirm this by demonstration tumor infiltration at only one site in NHL in 17–23% of patients with proven BM infiltration (Hoane et al. 1991). Moreover, because the infiltrated bone marrow frequently exhibits a focal pattern of distribution in most cases of HD, and in high grade NHL, bone marrow involvement is also likely to be missed at bilateral biopsy, due to the small volume of the sample, and, again, sampling errors exist (Brunning et al. 1975).

Discordant results were found in 48% of cases between MR results and BB findings and follow-up data reinforced the value of MR abnormalities as predictive of bone marrow infiltration (Tardivon et al. 1995).

29.6.3 Imaging

Typically, regions involved with lymphoma are hypo-intense compared with fat on T1-weighted images. On T2-weighted images, abnormal areas are hyperintense compared with muscle and iso- to hyperintense compared with fat. Of special interest are regions of bright signal intensity on T2-weighted images within areas of tumor replacement. This pattern is most often found in nodular sclerosing HD and may represent immature fibrosis within the tumor foci. Early fibrosis is characterized by rich vascularity and relatively few reticulin fibers, so that areas of bright signal intensity may represent early fibrosis, edema, or inflammation surrounded by mature fibrosis or tumor (Steiner et al. 1993; Hermann et al. 1997).

The patterns in abnormalities range from discrete, small (3–5 mm) marrow lesions to diffusely abnormal marrow representing near-complete marrow replacement (Hoane et al. 1991) (Figs. 29.6, 29.7).

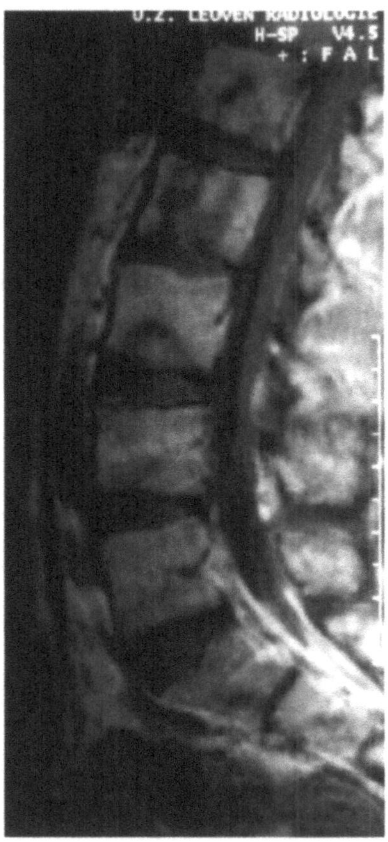

Fig. 29.6. Sagittal T1-weighted SE image of a patient with non-Hodgkin lymphoma, nodular pattern

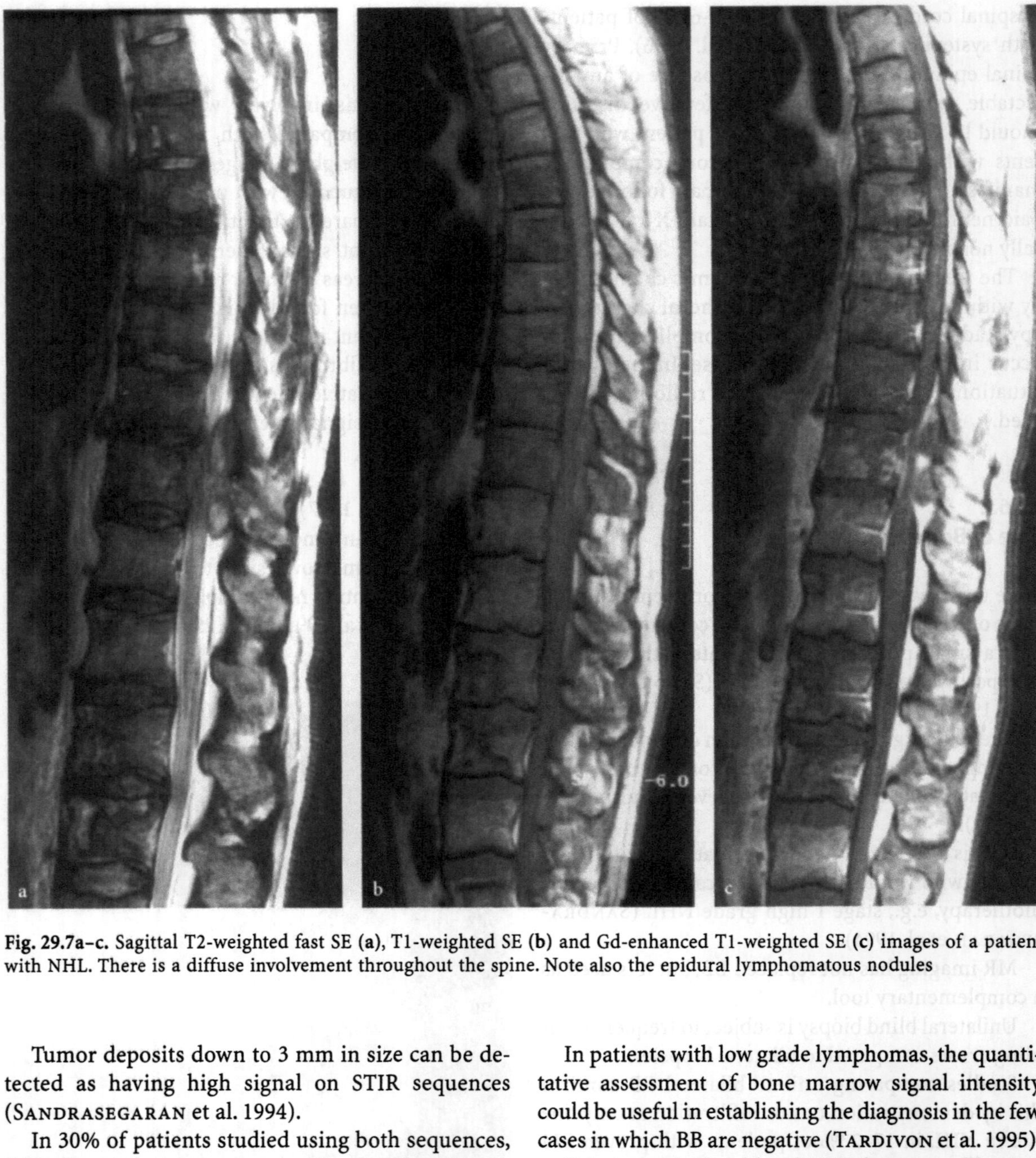

Fig. 29.7a–c. Sagittal T2-weighted fast SE (**a**), T1-weighted SE (**b**) and Gd-enhanced T1-weighted SE (**c**) images of a patient with NHL. There is a diffuse involvement throughout the spine. Note also the epidural lymphomatous nodules

Tumor deposits down to 3 mm in size can be detected as having high signal on STIR sequences (Sandrasegaran et al. 1994).

In 30% of patients studied using both sequences, STIR detected marrow tumor missed by the conventional T1 sequence (Hoane et al. 1991).

Bone marrow involvement was nodular in 65% of patients with HD, and in 85% of high grade NHL (Tardivon et al. 1995).

Bone marrow involvement in low grade NHL is typically diffuse but in intermediate to high grade NHL, and in HD, marrow disease is likely to be focal (Sandrasegaran et al. 1994).

Analysis showed biopsy somewhat better at finding low grade disease; however, MR better depicted intermediate – and high grade NHL and Hodgkin's disease (Hoane et al. 1991; Doehner et al. 1989).

In patients with low grade lymphomas, the quantitative assessment of bone marrow signal intensity could be useful in establishing the diagnosis in the few cases in which BB are negative (Tardivon et al. 1995).

Primary spinal epidural NHL has a predilection for the thoracic spine and is often located posteriorly to the spinal cord (Boukobza et al. 1996) (Fig. 29.7). Histologically these lesions are often low or intermediate grade NHL. A potentially favorable outcome has been postulated for the primary epidural NHL compared to secondary disease of the spine. Intradural NHL may also occur along the cauda equina (Figs. 29.8, 29.9). Intravenous administration of gadolinium is mandatory to assess the spinal canal and to follow-up treatment (Fig. 29.9).

Quantitative MR of bone marrow signal intensities may improve the detection of bone marrow in-

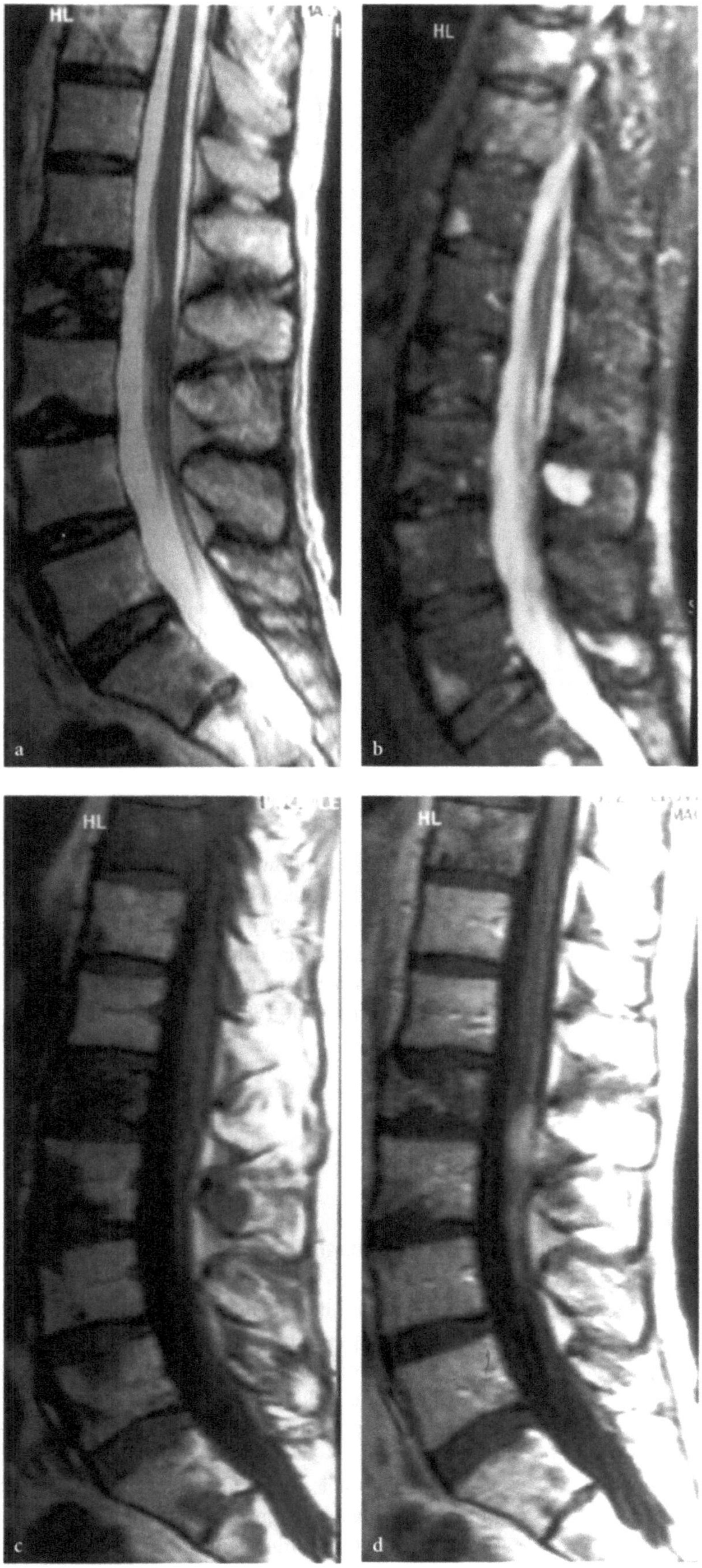

Fig. 29.8a–d. Sagittal T2-weighted fast SE (**a**), turbo inversion recovery (**b**), T1-weighted SE (**c**) and Gd-enhanced T1-weighted SE (**d**) images showing variable involvement of most vertebral bodies and involvement of the cauda equina

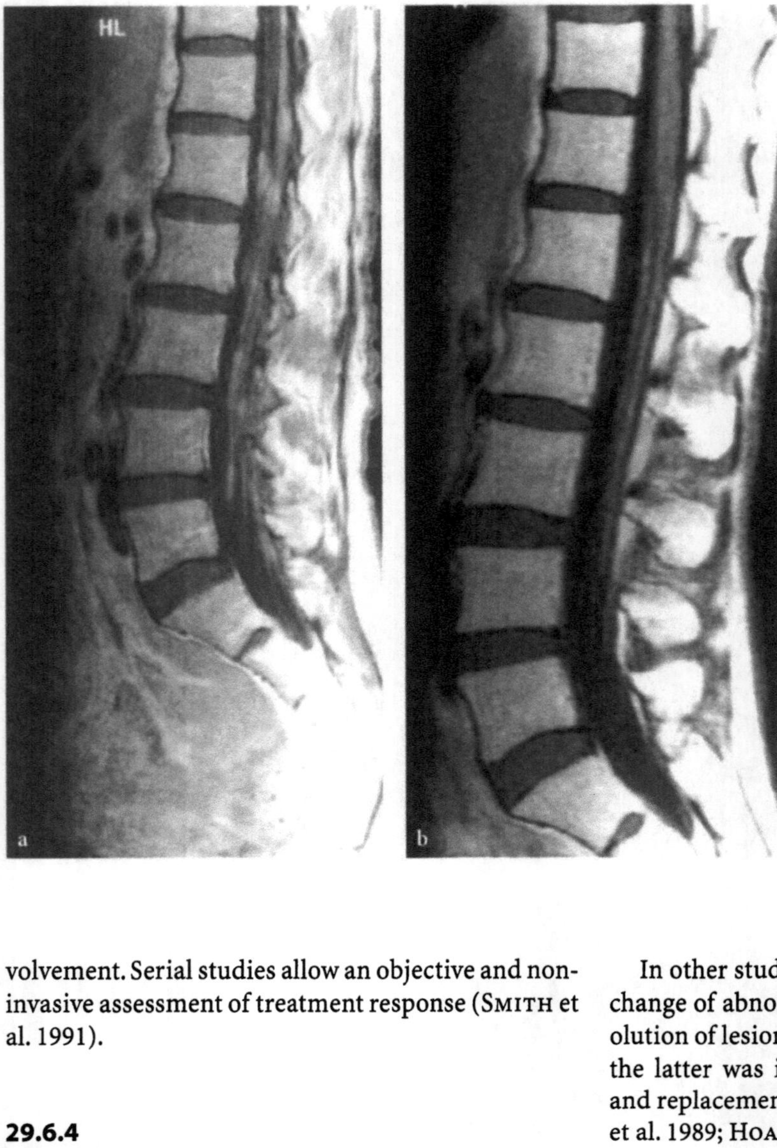

Fig. 29.9a,b. Sagittal Gd-enhanced T1-weighted SE images of a patient with intradural NHL during treatment. Note the significant decrease of the involvement of the cauda equina and the homogeneous high signal of the vertebral bodies due to the treatment

volvement. Serial studies allow an objective and non-invasive assessment of treatment response (Smith et al. 1991).

29.6.4 Response to Treatment

During treatment, follow-up MR studies may demonstrate no change, resolution of focal or diffuse marrow abnormalities, and appearance of necrotic tissue or of marrow fat (Vande Berg et al. 1998).

After chemotherapy, the signal intensities of the bone marrow lesions were the opposite of those seen before treatment. The high signal on T1 and the low signal on STIR images on the post-treatment studies indicated that the tumor tissue had been replaced by fat. Fat saturated images confirmed the fatty nature of the lesions (Lien and Holte 1996). This has been described for the nodular sclerosing subtype of HD. This subtype has a marked reactive fibrous tissue compartment, which may destroy the normal hematopoietic and stromal supportive tissue to a greater extent than most other malignancies.

In other studies, follow-up studies have shown no change of abnormalities (Linden et al. 1989) or resolution of lesions approaching a normal appearance; the latter was interpreted as elimination of tumor and replacement with normocellular tissue (Linden et al. 1989; Hoane et al. 1991).

29.7 Leukemia

29.7.1 Clinical Presentation

Leukemias are a heterogeneous group of malignant neoplasms composed of clonal expansions and marrow accumulations of mature and immature cells of the white blood cell lineage (i.e., granulocytes in myeloid and lymphocytes in lymphocytic leukemia).

Acute leukemia is characterized by a proliferation of immature, blast cells, chronic leukemia by a proliferation of cells that underwent differentiation.

Acute lymphocytic leukemia (ALL) is a disease of the young (peak incidence 5 years), whereas acute myeloid leukemia (AML) accounts for only 10% of the malignancies in childhood. The incidence of AML increases with age.

Chronic leukemia is a disease of the middle aged (CML 30–60 years, CLL 45–75 years).

Acute leukemia can be preceded by a myelodysplastic syndrome. MDS are disorders that are characterized by peripheral cytopenia, a cellular or hypercellular bone marrow, frequent cytogenic abnormalities and a risk of evolution to acute leukemia (Jacobs 1985). The frequency of evolution to acute leukemia occurs in as many as 66% of MDS patients (Bain 1990).

29.7.2 Imaging

On T1-weighted images, leukemic infiltration is characterized by a diffuse decrease in signal intensity, compared with normal marrow (Steiner et al. 1993). The pattern is usually diffuse (scattered or uniform) (Takagi et al. 1995), although others report that this diffuse pattern is found mostly in ALL, and that focal patterns may also be noted, especially in AML (Steiner et al. 1993).

The critical role of MR in patients with chronic leukemia is barely studied. In one series of 21 patients with early chronic lymphocytic leukemia, two-thirds of the patients showed normal MR findings (Lecouvet et al. 1997). When MR abnormalities occurred, the pattern was homogeneous (Lewis et al. 1994).

In AML, MR findings may lack prognostic value (Vande Berg et al. 1996).

In the study of Lecouvet of 21 patients with early chronic lymphocytic leukemia, the treatment free survival rate was shorter in patients with abnormal MR findings. Quantitative MR imaging could be a useful tool to assess the presence of disease progression.

In patients with MDS, the MR pattern of the femoral marrow changes from a fatty, nodular or faint pattern to a uniform pattern in association with disease progression (Takagi et al. 1995). Evolution to AML is associated with high signal intensities on STIR and with extension of the involved areas. Different types of MDS were noted: fatty, nodular, faint and diffuse. Different stages of disease can be reflected. The fatty, nodular or faint patterns were not seen in patients with advanced disease states (Takagi et al. 1995).

In a series of 80 adult patients with acute leukemia, signal intensity of the vertebral bone was lower than that of discs in 73 patients with AML and in all patients with ALL (Vande Berg et al. 1995). Several methods, including bulk T1-relation time measurement, chemical shift imaging techniques and spectroscopy, may more consistently demonstrate marrow involvement (Vande Berg et al. 1998). However, 10% of patients with AML have normal quantitative MR imaging findings (Bongers et al. 1992).

29.7.3 Response to Treatment

Islam noted three different stages of human bone marrow regeneration after chemotherapy for acute leukemia at histologic examination. Initially, there is an acute edematous stage, when the marrow becomes hypocellular and has widely dilated sinuses. In the second stage, precursors of multiloculated fat cells are seen. By the third stage, islands of regenerating hematopoietic cells are seen almost exclusively in areas of close proximity to relatively uniform aggregates of fat cells (Islam 1980). These observations suggest that fat cells may play an essential role in regenerating human hematopoietic marrow in acute leukemia. Vande Berg showed that sequential quantitative MR imaging (bulk T1 values) are valuable for prediction of response in patients with ALL, but not in those with AML (Vande Berg et al. 1995, 1996). In ALL, bulk T1 relaxation time measurements were statistically different among responder and non-responder patients after 2 weeks of treatment, as the mean bulk T1 values decreased in patients with ALL, who responded well (Vande Berg et al. 1996).

In patients with AML, neither the early increase in bulk T1, nor the rate or magnitude of the subsequent decrease in bulk T1 were predictive of a positive response to treatment (Vande Berg et al. 1995).

In chronic leukemia, regenerating hematopoietic marrow may be less dependent on precursor fat cells (Gerard et al. 1992).

References

Alexanian R, Dimopoulos MA (1995) Management in multiple myeloma. Semin Hematol 32: 20–30

Bain BJ (1990) The myeloysplastic syndromes in leukemia diagnosis. A guide to the FAB classification. Gower, London, p 44

Barti R, Frisch B, Diem H et al. (1989) Bone marrow histology and serum beta 2 microglobulin in multiple myeloma: a prognostic strategy. Eur J Haematol 43 (suppl 51): 88–98

Baur A, Stabler A, Lamerz R, Bartl R, Reiser M (1998) Light chain deposition disease in multiple myeloma: MR imaging features correlated with histopathological findings. Skelet Radiol 27: 173–176

Bellaiche L, Laredo JD, Liote F et al. (1997) Magnetic resonance appearance of monoclonal gammopathies of unknown significance and multiple myeloma. Spine 22: 2551–2557

Bongers H, Schick F, Skalej M, Jung WI, Einsele H (1992) Localized in vivo 1H spectroscopy and chemical shift imaging of the bone marrow in leukemic patients. Eur Radiol 2: 350–356

Boukobza M, Mazel C, Touboul E (1996) Primary vertebral and spinal epidural non-Hodgkin's lymphoma with spinal cord compression. Neuroradiology 38: 333–337

Brunning RD, Bloomfield CD, McKenna RW et al.(1975) Bilateral trephine bone marrow biopsies in lymphoma and other neoplastic diseases. Ann Intern Med 83: 365–366

Daffner RH, Lupetin AR, Dash N, Deeb ZL, Sefczek RJ, Schapiro RL (1986) MRI in the detection of malignant infiltration of bone marrow. AJR 146: 353–358

Dimopoulos MA, Moulopoulos A, Smith T, Delasalle KB, Alexanian R (1993) Risk of disease progression in asymptomatic multiple myeloma. Am J Med 94: 57–61

Döhner H, Gückel, Knauf W, Semmler W, van Kaik G, Ho AD, Hunsein W (1989) Magnetic resonance imaging of bone marrow in lymphoproliferative disorders: correlation with bone marrow biopsy. Br J Haematol 73: 12–17

Durie BGM, Salmon SE (1975) A clinical staging system for multiple myeloma. Cancer 36: 842–854

Fruehwald FXJ, Tscholakoff D, Schwaighfer B et al. (1988) Magnetic resonance imaging of the lower vertebral column in patients with multiple myeloma. Invest Radiol 23: 193–199

Gerard EL, Ferry JA, Amrein PC et al (1992) Compositional changes in vertebral bone marrow during treatment for acute leukemia: assessment with quantitative chemical shift imaging. Radiology 183: 39–46

Hermann G, Klein MG, Abdelwahab IF, Kenan S (1997) MRI appearance of primary non-Hodgkin's lymphoma of bone. Skeletal radiology 26: 629–632

Hoane BR, Shields AF, Porter BA, Shulman HM (1991) Detection of lymphomateous bone marrow involvement with magnetic resonance imaging. Blood 78: 728–738

Islam A, Catovsy D, Galton D (1980) Histological study of bone marrow regeneration following chemotherapy for acute myeloid leukemia and chronic granulocytic leukemia in blast transformation. Br J Haematol 45: 535–540

Jacobs A (1985) Myelodysplastic syndromes: pathogenesis, functional abnormalities, and clinical implications. J Clin Path 38: 1201–1217

Lecouvet F, Richard F, Vande Berg B, Malghem J, Maldague B, Jamart J (1996) Long-terms effects of localized spinal radiation therapy on vertebral fractures and focal lesions appearance in patients with multiple myeloma. Br J Haematol 96: 743–745

Lecouvet FE, Vande Berg BC, Michaux L, Jamart J, Maldague BE, Malghem J (1998) Development of vertebral fractures in patients with multiple myeloma: does MRI enable recognition of vertebrae that will collapse? J Comput Assist Tomogr 22: 430–436

Lecouvet FE, Vande Berg BC, Michaux L et al. (1997) Early chronic lymphocytic leukemia: prognostic value of quantitative bone marrow MR imaging findings and correlation with hematologic variables. Radiology 204: 813–818

Lewis S, Wainscoat JS, Moore NR, Golding SJ (1994) Magnetic resonance imaging in myelodysplastic syndromes. Br J Radiol 68: 121–127

Libshitz HI, Malthouse SR, Cunningham D, MacVicar AD, Husband JE (1992) Multiple myeloma: appearance at MR imaging. Radiology 182: 833–837

Lien HH, Holte H (1996) Fat replacement of Hodgkin disease of bone marrow after chemotherapy: report of three cases. Skelet Radiol 25: 671–674

Linden A, Zankovich R, Theissen P, Diehl V, Schica H (1989) Malignant lymphoma: bone marrow imaging versus biopsy. Radiology 28: 199–205

Ludwig H, Tscholakoff D, Neuhold A et al (1987) Magnetic resonance imaging of the spine in multiple myeloma. Lancet ??: 364–366

Moore SG, Dawson KL (1990) Red and yellow marrow in the femur: age related changes in appearance at MR imaging. Radiology 177: 219–223

Moulopoulos LA, Dimopoulos MA, Smith TL et al. (1995) Prognostic significance of magnetic resonance imaging in patients with asymptomatic multiple myeloma. J Clin Oncol 13: 251–256

Moulopoulos LA, Varma DGK, Dimopoulos MA et al. (1992) Multiple myeloma: spinal MR imaging in patients with untreated newly diagnosed disease. Radiology 185: 833–840

Rahmouni A, Divine M, Mathieu D et al. (1993) Detection of multiple myeloma involving the spine: efficacy of fat-suppression and contrast-enhanced MR imaging. AJR 160: 1049–1052

Rahmouni A, Divine M, Mathieu D et al. (1993) MR appearance of multiple myeloma of the spine before and after treatment. AJR 160: 1053–1057

Ricci C, Cova M, Kang YS et al. (1990) Normal age related patterns of cellular and fatty bone marrow distribution in the axial skeleton: MR imaging study. Radiology 177: 83–88

Salvati M, Cervoni L, Artico M, Raco A, Ciapretta P, Delfini R (1996) Primary spinal epidural non-Hodgkin's lymphomas: a clinical study. Surg Neurol 46: 339–344

Sandrasegaran K, Robinson PJ, Selby P (1994) Review: Staging of lymphoma in adults. Clin Radiol 49: 149–161

Smith SR, Williams CE, Edwards RHT, Davies JM (1991) Quantitative magnetic resonance studies of lumbar vertebral marrow in patients with refractory or relapsed Hodgkin's disease. Ann Oncol 2: 39–42

Stabler A, Baur A, Bartl R, Munker R, Lamerz R, Reiser MF (1996) Contrast enhancement in quantitative signal analysis in MR imaging of multiple myeloma: assessment of focal and diffuse growth patterns in marrow correlated with biopsies and survival rates. AJR 167: 1029–1036

Steiner RM, Mitchell DG, Rao VM, Schweitzer ME (1993) Magnetic resonance imaging of diffuse bone marrow disease. Radiol Clin North Am 31: 383–409

Takagi S, Tanaka O, Miura Y (1995) Magnetic resonance imaging of femoral marrow in patients with myelodysplastic syndromes or leukemia. Blood 86: 316–322

Tardivon AA, Munck JN, Shapeero LG et al. (1995) Can clinical data help to screen patients with lymphoma for MR imaging of the bone marrow? Ann Oncol 6: 795–800

Tsunoda S, Takagi S, Tanaka O, Miura Y (1997) Clinical and prognostic significance of femoral marrow magnetic resonance imaging of bone marrow in patients with malignant lymphoma. Blood 89: 286–290

Vande Berg BC, Lecouvet FE, Michaux L, Ferrant A, Maldague B, Malghem J (1998) Magnetic resonance imaging if the bone marrow in hematological malignancies. Eur Radiol 8: 1335–1344

Vande Berg BC, Lecouvet FE, Michaux L et al. (1996) Stage I multiple myeloma: value of MR imaging of the bone marrow in the determination of prognosis. Radiology 201: 243–246

Vande Berg BC, Malghem J, Lecouvet FE, Ferrant A, Scheiff JM, Maldague B (1995) Leucémies et IRM. In: Scintzoff S, Laredo JD, Caroit M (eds) Imagerie de l'os et la moelle osseuse. Sauramps Medical, Montpellier, pp 173–184

Vande Berg BC, Michaux L, Scheiff JM et al. (1996) Sequential quantitative MR analysis of bone marrow: differences during treatment of lymphoid versus myeloid leukemia. Radiology 201: 519–523

Vande Berg BC, Schmitz PJ, Scheiff M et al. (1995) Acute myeloid leukemia: lack of predictive value of sequential quantitative MR imaging during treatment. Radiology 197: 301–305

Weil A, Chiras J, Simon JM, Rose M, Sola-Martinez T, Enkaoua E (1996) Spinal metastases: indications for and results of percutaneous injection of acryl surgical cement. Radiology 199: 241–247

Weinreb JC (1990) MR imaging of bone marrow: a map could help. Radiology 177: 23–24

30 Intrathecal Gadolinium-Enhanced MR Myelography/Cisternography

J. Randy Jinkins, Qingyu Zeng, Lin Xiong, Zhanming Fan, Zhongsheng Liu

CONTENTS

30.1 Introduction

The high level of safety and tolerance of IV administrated gadolinium has been proved through extensive clinical use (Goldstein et al. 1990; Niendorf et al. 1991a, 1991b). However, only a limited number of laboratory studies have been performed focusing on the possible usage and neurotoxic or inflammatory reactions of paramagnetic contrast agents injected into the subarachnoid space (DiChiro et al. 1985; Allard et al. 1987; Ray et al. 1996; Skalpe and Tang 1997; Ray et al. 1998; Skalpe 1998; Jinkins et al. 1999). Only one study on two human patients with meningeal carcinomatosis who underwent intraventricular gadolinium injection has been published (Siebner et al. 1997). The present chapter details the results of a controlled pilot medical experiment (Zeng et al. 1999). It should be noted that the intrathecal gadolinium is not presently an approved route of administration of gadolinium worldwide.

J. R. Jinkins, MD, FACR
Professor and Director of Neuroimaging Research, Department of Radiology, 981045 Nebraska Medical Center, Omaha, NE 68198-1045, USA
Q. Zeng, MD; L. Xiong, MD; Z. Fan, MD; Z. Liu, MD
Department of Radiology, General Coal Hospital, Xi Ba He Nan Li 29, Beijing 100028, P.R. China

30.2 The Pilot Study

No patient demonstrated gross behavioral change, neurologic alteration or seizure activity following the intrathecal gadolinium administration. The intrathecal gadolinium enhanced MR myelography demonstrated: intervertebral disc herniations (n=4) (Fig. 30.1a), a spinal vascular malformation with related spinal cord infarction (intradural arteriovenous fistula: n=1) (Fig. 30.2), a post-surgical non-communicating cyst (n=1) (Fig. 30.3), posttraumatic/postoperative spinal stenosis (n=3) (Fig. 30.4), a case of transverse myelitis (n=1), and a solitary intradural-extramedullary mass (n=1).

Two cases demonstrated complete obstruction of CSF flow following intrathecal gadolinium administration on both immediate and delayed MR imaging studies (Fig. 30.4). This phenomenon (i.e., complete CSF obstruction) could not be reliably assessed on the preceding unenhanced conventional spin-echo MR studies. The third patient revealed apparent complete obstruction of CSF flow on the immediate exam after intrathecal gadolinium injection; however, partial obstruction was confirmed on the delayed examination by visual evidence of the passage of the CSF gadolinium enhancement above the obstruction site. One patient presented with a post-operative paraspinal focal fluid collection (i.e., cyst) at the surgical site. The non-communication of the cystic fluid collection at the surgical site was clearly demonstrated on both immediate and delayed intrathecal post-gadolinium injection examinations. The intramedullary spinal cord lesions were expectedly better visualized on the unenhanced T2-weighted imaging than on the gadolinium enhanced T1-weighted MR myelogram in two patients (one with transverse myelitis, and one with spinal cord infarction secondary to an intradural arteriovenous fistula).

Fat saturated, T1-weighted gadolinium enhanced MR myelography demonstrated a focal hyperintense CSF leak (i.e., gadolinium enhancement) along the needle track between two adjacent lumbar spinous

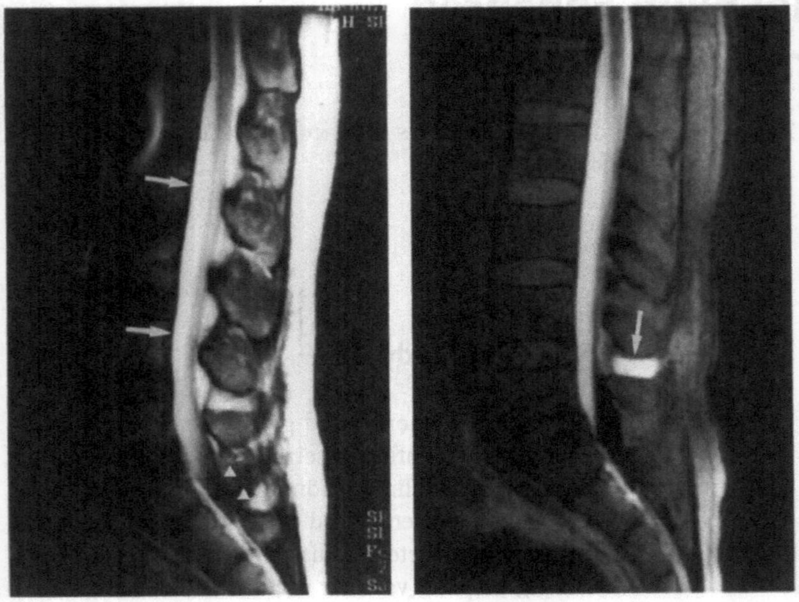

Fig. 30.1a,b. Forty-four-year-old male presenting with a 3 year history of low back pain. Diagnosis: L5/S1 disc herniation with CSF leak along lumbar spinal needle track. **a** Sagittal T1-weighted (640/12/1: TR/TE/excitations) MR myelogram obtained immediately after 1.0 ml intrathecal gadolinium administration shows the CSF to be hyperintense cranially (*white arrows*) and hypointense (*arrowheads*) at the level of the dependent terminal thecal sac. The latter hypointensity resulted from highly concentrated gadolinium. **b** Sagittal fat suppressed T1-weighted (375/15/1) MR myelogram immediately following the intrathecal gadolinium administration shows enhancement of the L4/L5 interspinous space (*arrow*) indicating CSF leakage along the needle track at the level of the lumbar puncture

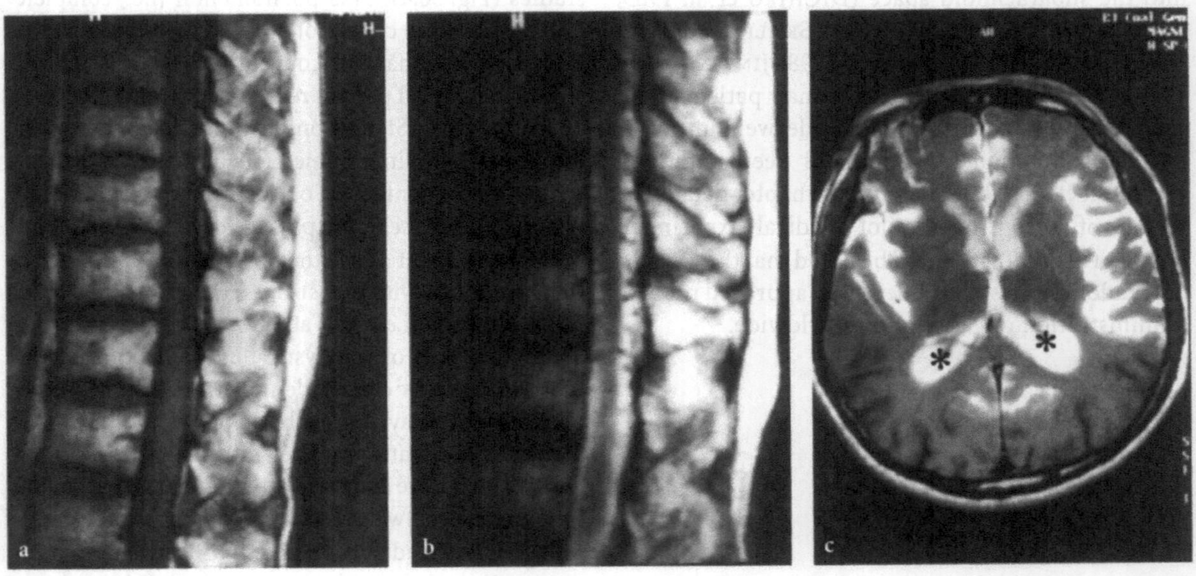

Fig. 30.2a–c. Sixty-six-year-old male presenting with a 7 year history of back pain and bilateral lower extremity weakness. Diagnosis: dural arteriovenous malformation and associated communicating hydrocephalus. **a** Unenhanced sagittal T1-weighted (640/12/1) conventional spin-echo MR image at the level of the thoracolumbar junction reveals no discrete abnormality. **b** Sagittal T1-weighted (640/12/1) MR myelogram immediately following 0.5 ml intrathecal gadolinium administration reveals serpentine filling defects/flow voids within the subarachnoid space. This appears similar to image **b**. **c** Eight hour delay axial TI-weighted (640/12/1) MR myelogram/cisternogram following intrathecal gadolinium administration demonstrates the progressive enhancement of the subarachnoid space and the lateral ventricles (*asterisks*). The latter indicates abnormal ventricular reflux associated with the communicating hydrocephalus

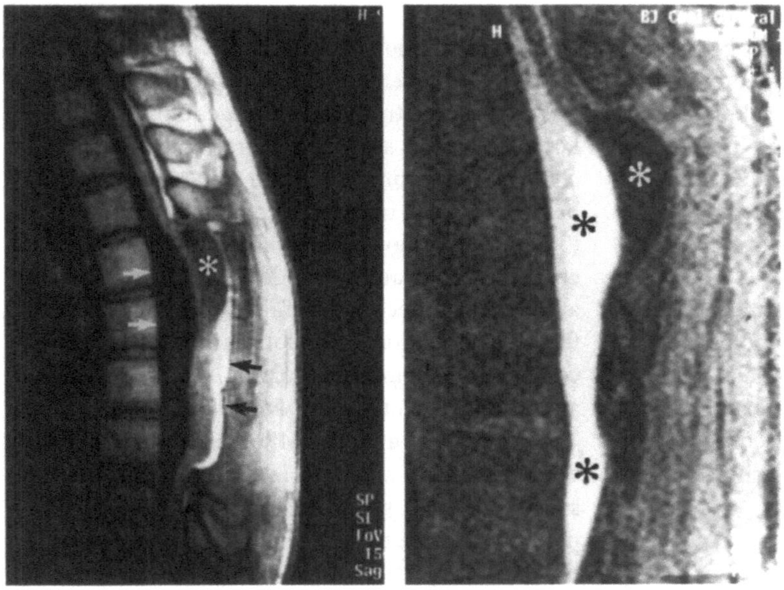

a b

Fig. 30.3a,b. Twenty-three-year-old male presenting with a 2 year history of bilateral lower extremity weakness. Diagnosis: noncommunicating post-surgical paraspinal subarachnoid space fluid collection (i.e., cyst) with residual congenital lipoma. The patient was status-post partial resection of a developmental spinal lipoma at the thoracolumbar junction. **a** Unenhanced sagittal T1-weighted (640/12/1) conventional spin-echo MR image reveals post-surgical changes which include: focal dilatation of the subarachnoid space (*white arrows*), soft tissue and bony defects at the thoracolumbar junction and a crescenteric fluid collection (*asterisk*) posterior to the dilated subarachnoid space. An irregular, thin band-like area of hyperintensity (*black arrows*) represents the residual congenital lipoma. **b** Six hour delay sagittal fat-suppressed T1-weighted (640/12/1) MR myelogram following 0.5 ml intrathecal gadolinium administration shows enhancement of the CSF in the spinal subarachnoid space (*black asterisks*). There is no enhancement of the focal fluid collection (*white asterisk*) indicating no communication with the subarachnoid space

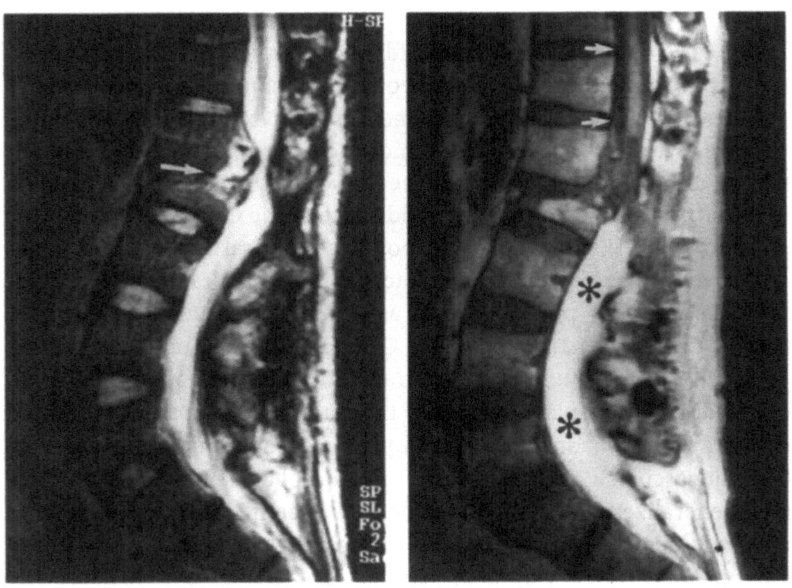

a b

Fig. 30.4a,b. Twenty-eight-year-old male presenting with bilateral lower extremity paralysis secondary to L1 burst fracture. Diagnosis: post-traumatic spinal canal stenosis with complete CSF pathway obstruction. **a** Sagittal T2-weighted (4500/112/1) MR image shows a burst type fracture of L1–2 (*arrows*) with retropulsion of bony fragments and encroachment on the central spinal canal. **b** Time-delayed sagittal T1-weighted (640/12/1) MR myelogram obtained 6 h after intrathecal gadolinium injection shows gadolinium CSF enhancement (*asterisks*) below the fracture site and no gadolinium CSF enhancement (*arrows*) above the fracture site. This finding is consistent with complete obstruction of CSF flow at the fracture site due to extreme posttraumatic spinal stenosis processes at the level of the subarachnoid space puncture in one patient with a surgically proven disc herniation (Fig. 30.1c). One case with communicating hydrocephalus (Fig. 30.2d,e) showed progressive reflux of gadolinium enhanced CSF into the cerebral ventricular system. No other patient sequentially followed over time by MR imaging showed such ventricular reflux following the lumbar intrathecal gadolinium injection.

One year follow up MR imaging studies in three patients demonstrated no gross morphologic or MR signal changes as compared to the initial baseline or intrathecal gadolinium enhanced MR examinations. No gross neurologic sequelae were recorded in any of the 11 cases during the 9–15 month clinical follow up period.

30.3 Discussion

Generally speaking, MR imaging provides excellent anatomic depiction of the CSF spaces and surrounding tissues. However, in certain clinical situations, such as possible CSF flow obstruction, possibly communicating or noncommunicating cystic lesions bordering on the CSF pathways, and in cases of suspected CSF leakage, further imaging evaluation may be required.

Gadolinium has been widely used via the IV route of administration. Its safety and tolerance have been established based upon preclinical studies and extensive clinical trials. However, reports have revealed some potential adverse systemic effects, although they are seen at a very low incidence (Niendorf et al. 1991a, 1991b; Tardy et al. 1992; Harbury 1991; Tishler and Hoffman 1991). Nausea or vomiting, and headache are most common side effects, having a frequency ranging from 0.26% to 0.42% (Tardy et al. 1992). Other very rare reactions reported following IV administration of gadolinium include: paresthesias, dizziness, focal convulsions, urticaria, mucosal reactions, generalized flush, cardiovascular reactions (e.g., tachycardia, arrhythmia), generalized seizures, laryngospasm, and anaphylactic shock (Niendorf et al. 1991a, 1991b; Tardy et al. 1992; Harbury 1991; Tishler and Hoffman 1991).

In one published report, the effects of intraventricular gadolinium (Magnevist: gadopentetate dimeglumine) injection in an animal model included behavioral and neurologic alteration (focal seizure activity, ataxia, delayed tremor) and histologic changes (loss of oligodendroglia, hypertrophy of astrocytes, formation of eosinophilic granules) (Ray et al. 1996). However, these pathologic alterations were only seen at relatively high dosages of intraventricular gadolinium; such behavioral and morphologic changes were not seen in the same reported study below 15 µl total intraventricular gadolinium dosage (3.3 µmol/g brain) (Ray et al. 1996). Similarly, a recent study in an animal model which was carried out at lower intrathecally administered dosages of a different formulation of gadolinium (Omniscan; Nycomed Amersham, Oslo, Norway) did not reveal CNS alterations (Skalpe and Tang 1997).

Although unenhanced MR imaging generally provides excellent anatomic delineation of the CSF spaces, certain *functional* derangements of CSF pathways may be better seen following the subarachnoid space injection of gadolinium. In this pilot human trial, the benefits found in the gadolinium enhanced MR myelogram were in detecting complete CSF flow obstruction (n=2) (Fig. 30.4), and in visualizing the lack of communication between the subarachnoid space and a paraspinal fluid collection (n=1) (Fig. 30.3).

Unexpectedly, abnormal gadolinium reflux into the cerebral ventricular system was observed on delayed cranial imaging in one patient with communicating hydrocephalus (Figs. 30.2d,e); this may provide an avenue of further research in the future in patients with suspected normal pressure hydrocephalus under consideration for ventricular shunt placement. Spontaneous, posttraumatic or postsurgical CSF leakage is another good example of the potential use of this technique to determine the exact anatomic location of the leakage anywhere bordering upon the subarachnoid space of the CNS (Fig. 30.1c).

Overall, the possible practical applications for gadolinium enhanced MR myelography/cisternography include: the assessment of communication or obstruction of the CSF pathways (e.g., arachnoid cysts; inflammatory, traumatic, posttherapeutic and neoplastic stenosis), the evaluation of gross subarachnoid space CSF flow dynamics (e.g., communicating "normal pressure" hydrocephalus, postinflammatory arachnoidal adhesions), the investigation of spontaneous/acquired craniospinal CSF fistulae, and possibly the analysis of extracellular space CNS parenchymal extracellular space gadolinium perfusion in various pathologic conditions (DiChiro et al. 1986; Rosen et al. 1987).

Additional animal and human studies need to be carried out in order to evaluate the long term safety and prove the potential clinical applications of this technique, and how these observations relate to other currently approved imaging methods. Furthermore, this article describes the intrathecal usage of only one gadolinium agent: Magnevist (gadopentetate dimeglumine). No inferences should be made regarding the intrathecal use of other gadolinium preparations, as differing results may obtain from the use of other agents.

References

Allard M, Kien P, Caille JM, Bonnemain B, Simonnet G (1987) Brain distribution of MRI contrast media in rats after intracisternal injection. J Neuroradiol 14: 383–387

DiChiro G, Knop RH, Girton MR et al. (1985) MR cisternography and myelography with GD GTPA in monkeys. Radiology 157: 373–377

DiChiro G, Girton ME, Frank JA et al. (1986) Cerebrospinal fluid rhinorrhea: depiction with MR cisternography in dogs. Radiology 160: 221–222

Goldstein HA, Kashanian FK, Blumetti RF, Holyoak WL, Hugo FP, Blumenfield DM (1990) Safety assessment of gadopentetate dimeglumine in U.S. clinical trials. Radiology 174: 17–23

Harbury OL (1991) Generalized seizure after IV administration of gadopentetate dimeglumine. Am J Neuroradiol 12: 666

Jinkins JR, Williams RF, Xiong L (1999) Evaluation of gadopentetate dimeglumine magnetic resonance cisternography in an animal model: preliminary report. Invest Radiol 34: 156–159

Niendorf HP, Haustein J, Cornelius I, Alhassan A, Claub W (1991a) Safety of gadolinium-DTPA: extended clinical experience. Mag Reson Med 22: 222–228

Niendorf HP, Haustein J, Louton T, Beck W, Laniado M (1991b) Safety and tolerance after intravenous administration of 0.3 mmol/kg Gd-DTPA: results of a randomized, controlled clinical trial. Invest Radiol 26: S221-S223

Ray DE, Cavanagh JB, Nolan CC, Williams SCR (1996) Neurotoxic effects of gadopentetate dimeglumine: behavioral disturbance and morphology after intracerebroventricular injection in rats. Am J Neuroradiol 17: 365–373

Ray DE, Holton JL, Nolan CC, Cavanagh JB, Harpur ES (1998) Neurotoxic potential of gadodiamide after injection into the lateral cerebral ventricle of rats. Am J Neuroradiol 19: 1455–1462

Rosen GM, Griffeth LK, Brown MA, Drayer BP (1987) Intrathecal administration of nitroxides as potential contrast agents for MR imaging. Radiology 163: 239–243

Siebner HR, Grafin von Einsiedel H, Conrad B (1997) Magnetic resonance ventriculography with gadolinium DTPA: report of two cases. Neuroradiology 39: 418–422

Skalpe IO, Tang GJ (1997) Magnetic resonance imaging contrast media in the subarachnoid space: a comparison between gadodiamide injection and gadopentetate dimeglumine in an experimental study in pigs. Invest Radiol 32: 140–148

Skalpe IO (1998) Is it dangerous to inject MR contrast media into the subarachnoid space? Acta Radiol 39: 100

Tardy B, Guy C, Barral G, Page Y, Ollagnier M, Bertrand JC (1992) Anaphylactic shock induced by intravenous gadopentetate dimeglumine. Lancet 339: 494

Tishler S, Hoffman JC (1990) Anaphylactoid reactions to IV gadopentetate dimeglumine. Am J Neuroradiol 11: 1167

Zeng Q, Xiong L, Jinkins JR, Fan Z, Liu Z (1999) Intrathecal gadolinium (gadopentetate dimeglumine)-enhanced MR myelography/cisternography: A pilot study in human patients. Am J Roentgenol (in press)

31 Posttherapeutic Spine Imaging

J. Randy Jinkins, Francesco Calabro

CONTENTS

J. R. Jinkins, MD, FACR
Professor and Director of Neuroimaging Research, Department of Radiology, 981045 Nebraska Medical Center, Omaha, NE 68198-1045, USA
F. Calabro, MD
TMA-Clinica Villa Salus, Via Montallegro 48, 16145 Genoa, Italy

31.1 Introduction

One of the most challenging areas of diagnosis is to be found in acquiring and interpreting medical images in the patient who has undergone one or more forms of therapy for spinal disease. This may have involved conservative treatment, surgery, radiation therapy, antibiotic therapy, chemotherapy, or other forms of medical treatment. The imaging findings may be either of an expected or unexpected nature. In some instances, the treated tissues may be left with benign scarring; in other cases, there may be a recurrence of disease or spread of the disease beyond the original site. In still other situations, the observation may represent a true complication of the therapy. All of these possibilities complicate medical image analysis.

In order to critically evaluate the posttherapeutic patient, it is imperative to understand several factors in reasonably specific detail. These include: (a) the primary diagnosis, (b) the treatment(s) undergone by the patient, (c) the elapsed time since the various therapies, and (d) the current clinical syndrome. The answers to these questions will in large part determine which imaging modality or modalities are chosen for the patient work-up, how the images are acquired, and whether or not an enhancing agent is used.

The sections of this chapter illustrate the features of expected and abnormal posttherapeutic spinal imaging. The discussions provide the background, practical information, and graphic examples necessary to enable the medical imaging physician to better approach the clinicoradiologic evaluation of the posttherapeutic patient (Jinkins 1997).

31.2 Lumbosacral Spine Imaging Following Intervertebral Disc Surgery

It has been estimated by some authors that up to 80% of certain populations will have back pain at some time in their life. In patients between 20 and 50 years old, the evaluation and treatment of low back and radicular pain is one of the highest overall costs of health care. The many mechanisms responsible for back and lower extremity pain include the nonspecific mechanical or chemical irritation of: (a) afferent somatic and sympathetic neural branches, (b) spinal nerves in the spinal canal or neural foramen, and (c) medial neural branches of the posterior primary spinal nerve rami (Jinkins 1993a). Complicating the diagnosis and treatment of these conditions is the fact that different types of pathology can produce similar clinical syndromes. In addition, the same abnormality may present in typical as well as atypical ways.

The likelihood of pain relief through surgical correction has been correlated with several factors. One prospective study showed that such diverse factors as female gender, psychological problems, sick leave from work of more than 3 months' duration coupled with degenerative radiographic spinal alterations were generally associated with an unsatisfactory surgical outcome.

31.2.1 The Failed Back Surgery Syndrome

Despite the loose application of criteria for judging operative success, lumbosacral spinal surgery has been so often unsuccessful (10–40%) that failed back surgery is now labeled as a syndrome: *the failed back surgery syndrome* (FBSS) (Shafaie et al. 1997).

The FBSS is characterized by postsurgical intractable pain in the low back and lower extremity(ies) combined with varying degrees of functional incapacitation. The major identifiable causes of the FBSS include "clinically" relevant epidural fibrosis, recurrent or residual disk herniation, postoperative spinal infection, sterile arachnoiditis, postsurgical pseudomeningocele formation and lateral recess, and foraminal or central spinal stenosis that may preexist or follow the spinal surgery. Other less common causes of the FBSS include surgery inadvertently performed on the wrong side or at the incorrect segmental level, direct nerve injury at the time of surgery, spinal pain of mechanical origin (e.g., facet joint disease), and attempted surgical fusion failure. Still further causes of the FBSS are recurrent or residual clinical symptoms related to anterior spinal disc protrusion, spinal nerve root radiculitis (i.e., neuritis), disc herniation at a spinal level other than that operated on, facet joint fracture, and progressive spinal instability with spondylolisthesis. These conditions should be distinguished from acceptable and expected postoperative findings found after successful lumbar surgery (i.e., that surgery associated with clinical sign and symptom relief).

31.2.2 Technical Considerations

Progressive improvements in magnetic resonance imaging have substantially improved the ability of the medical imaging physician to critically analyze the postoperative lumbosacral spine following discectomy. Compared to other imaging methods, MR images acquired in multiple planes have superior diagnostic potential, in part because of their greater spatial and contrast resolution characteristics. Nevertheless, the similarity of some postsurgical pathologic processes in regard to MR signal intensity often makes even this imaging technique somewhat difficult to interpret. The development of intravenously (IV) administered paramagnetic MR contrast agents (e.g., gadolinium) has materially assisted the diagnostic sensitivity and specificity of MR in the evaluation of the FBSS because of the differential improvement in contrast resolution afforded by these agents.

In general, T2-weighted fast spin-echo images are superior to conventional spin-echo images of the lumbosacral spine in part because of improved image quality resulting from better spatial resolution and reduced motion artifact. Sagittal (with fat suppression) and axial (without fat suppression) fast spin-echo T2-weighted images are helpful in assessing neural foramen narrowing, central and lateral recess spinal stenosis, hydration status of the intervertebral disc, abnormal signal intensity of the disc and cancellous bone, and signal intensity of abnormal intra- or perispinal soft tissue masses (e.g., disc herniation, epidural scar, epidural abscess, epidural phlegmon). Sagittal and axial T1-weighted spin-echo images obtained before and immediately after the bolus IV injection of a gadolinium product are almost imperative in the evaluation of the postoperative lumbar spine. Fat-suppression techniques can also often be used after IV gadolinium administration because they improve the relative intensity and homogeneity of contrast enhancement of epidural fibrosis, thereby distinguishing it from centrally nonenhancing recurrent disc herniation. However, it makes the critical interpretation of possible abnormal postoperative intrathecal nerve root enhancement (i.e., sterile radiculitis) impossible because small degrees of apparently normal nerve root enhancement are not infrequently observed when fat suppression MR imaging techniques are used.

The initiation of MR imaging within approximately 2 min of the IV gadolinium injection is important because some disc herniations can be somewhat vascularized and therefore may enhance relatively early. The basis for this imaging strategy is that the vessels in the scar tissue are relatively homogeneously distributed, whereas in disc herniation the vessels are quite heterogeneous or are centrally absent. Therefore, a markedly heterogeneously or centrally nonenhancing epidural mass would be labeled a partially vascularized disc herniation, but homogeneous enhancement of an epidural process would be termed epidural fibrosis. It should be noted that imaging after 20–30 min of the IV contrast agent administration is not helpful because many recurrent disc herniations enhance centrally within this delayed time frame as the gadolinium progressively seeps into the disc.

Intravenously administered gadolinium compounds are also an important adjunct to the MR evaluation of the postoperative lumbosacral spine in the elucidation and differentiation of spinal, leptomeningeal, and/or neural inflammation (infectious or aseptic). The proper differentiation of these varied pathologic phenomena on MR imaging should allow improved patient triage toward appropriate medical-surgical therapy.

If the patient cannot undergo an MR imaging examination for medical reasons or because of spinal metallic surgical implants, a "high" dose (40–60 g of iodine equivalent) IV iodinated contrast-enhanced CT study is recommended after a precontrast survey examination is performed in order to search for the same problems in much the same manner outlined in the foregoing paragraphs. Myelography is helpful for documenting arachnoiditis and its sequelae such as loculations, adhesions and obstructions but is otherwise not very informative. Computed tomography continues to be the mainstay in evaluating ossific or calcific pathologic changes (e.g., spinal neural foramen, lateral recess or central canal stenosis) of the postoperative lumbosacral spine. Kinetic or dynamic (i.e., flexion-extension) MR imaging and flexion-extension conventional radiography both have the potential of depicting postoperative bony instability in the spine (Shafaie et al. 1997).

31.2.3 Normal Postoperative Changes

The interpretation of images of the lumbosacral spine acquired in the immediate postoperative period (i.e., initial 6–8 postsurgical weeks) should be undertaken with caution. Normal postoperative changes occur in the bony structures as well as the soft tissues, that vary depending on the time lapsed since the surgical procedure.

The most common surgical approach is a posterior midline incision that allows access to the posterior elements, spinal canal, and disc space. The term laminotomy refers to removal of only the inferior margin of the lamina and is often used in cases of microdiscectomy. In unilateral laminectomy, the lamina on one side of the spine is removed. A total or bilateral laminectomy involves removal of both laminae and the spinous process. Laminotomies and laminectomies are often performed to improve access for discectomies and for decompression in cases of trauma and symptomatic stenosis of the central spinal canal. An overzealous laminectomy/facetectomy may contribute to postoperative spinal instability.

On MR, the surgical absence of bone can be best demonstrated on axial T1-weighted images. There is often an associated asymmetry in the muscle-fat planes posteriorly. The paraspinal musculature may also be temporarily indistinct secondary to edema in the subacute phase after surgery. The posterior border of the dural tube margin may expand posteriorly toward the surgical site and laminectomy defect, reflecting this relative bony insufficiency. This is an expected, clinically irrelevant finding and does not represent a pseudomeningocele.

In discectomy, often performed in association with the postsurgical changes outlined in the foregoing, a partial or complete resection of the degenerated or herniated disc is undertaken. On unenhanced images acquired immediately after surgery, postdiscectomy changes can mimic the preoperative appearance of disc herniation because of annular disc disruption and epidural tissue edema. This renders the outline of the dural sac and intervertebral disc indistinct and may efface the thecal sac. Homogeneous enhancement of this epidural process on MR after IV gadolinium administration may be observed. This is caused by granulation tissue and/or fibrosis, and it explains the mild regional epidural mass effect seen commonly in postoperative imaging of successful lumbar discectomy patients.

In one recent study of asymptomatic postoperative patients following intervertebral disc surgery, 100% of subjects showed evidence of epidural fibrosis (Fig. 31.1) (Jinkins et al. 1993). In addition, enhancing lumbosacral vertebral end plates have been observed between 6 and 18 months after surgery in 19% of patients, and enhancement of the posterior anulus fibrosis has been reported in the majority of asymptomatic postoperative patients (Shafaie et al. 1997).

One reason anterior epidural and lateral recess scar almost always enhances on IV gadolinium enhanced

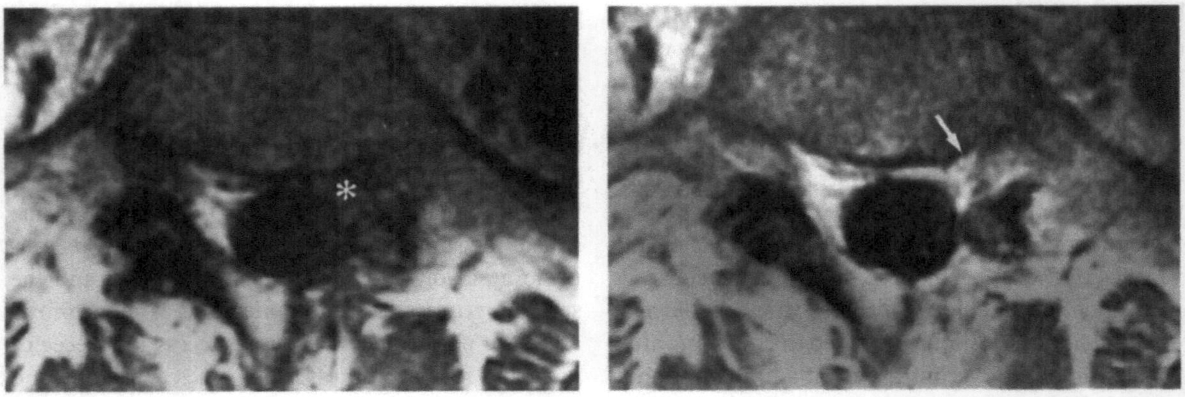

Fig. 31.1a,b. Asymptomatic postdiscectomy epidural fibrosis. a Axial T1-weighted (TR/TE: 500/15) MR image shows obliteration/replacement of the epidural fat on the left side anteriorly (*asterisk*). b IV gadolinium enhanced (0.1 mmol/kg) axial T1-weighted (500/15) MR shows uniform enhancement of the epidural space (*arrow*) indicating postoperative epidural fibrosis. [From Jinkins JR, Leite C da C (1998) Neurodiagnostic imaging. Lippincott-Williams & Wilkins, Philadelphia, with permission]

MR imaging is that fibrosis maintains a fairly large extracellular space. Another major determinant of enhancement grade in epidural scar older than 2 months is the capillary endothelial gap-junction status. If these endothelial junctions are open, the degree of enhancement after IV gadolinium administration will be greater. In general, the vascular density of scars does not correlate with enhancement grade and, regardless of scar site, appears to remain stable after 2 months of inception (Shafaie et al. 1997).

31.2.4 Postoperative Complications

31.2.4.1 Recurrent Disc Herniation

As noted above, the lack of early central contrast enhancement associated with disc herniations after IV gadolinium administration is claimed to be the major criterion by which recurrent disc herniation can be distinguished from isolated epidural scar (Fig. 31.2). The accuracy of contrast-enhanced MR imaging in the differentiation of herniated disc and epidural scar is estimated to be 95–100% (Shafaie et al. 1997).

31.2.4.2 Postoperative Infection

The onset of progressively severe back pain occurring soon after surgery, especially when accompanied by a persistently elevated erythrocyte sedimentation rate, is suggestive of postoperative infection. T2-weighted MR imaging is more sensitive early on in the pathologic process than are combined bone and gallium radionuclide scanning in the diagnosis of postoperative spondylitis and discitis. However, the specificity of the radionuclide studies is greater than that of MR imaging

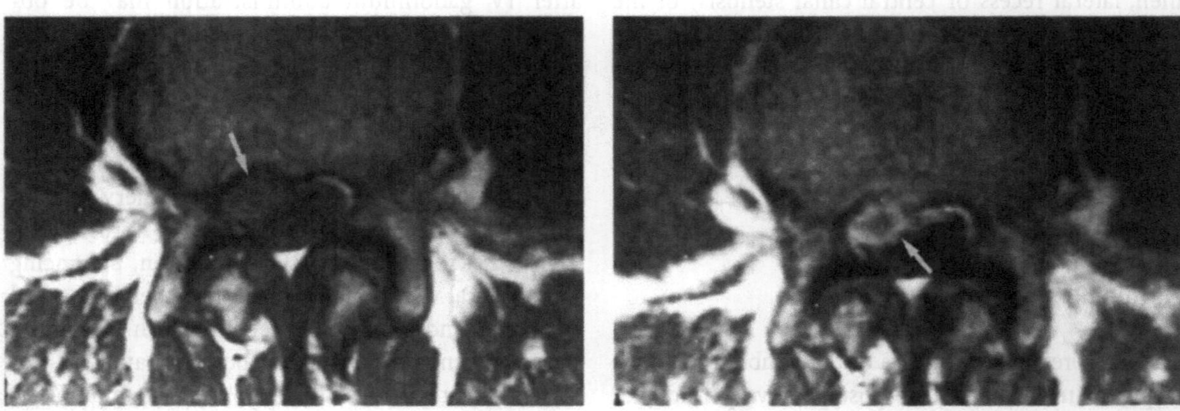

Fig. 31.2a,b. Recurrent postoperative intervertebral disc extrusion. a Axial T1-weighted (500/15) MR image shows subtle obliteration/replacement of the epidural fat on the right side (*arrow*). b IV gadolinium enhanced axial T1-weighted (500/15) MR image shows peripheral enhancement (*arrow*) surrounding a nonenhancing central area indicating recurrent disc herniation. [From Jinkins JR, Leite C da C (1998) Neurodiagnostic imaging. Lippincott-Williams & Wilkins, Philadelphia, with permission]

(100% versus 92%, respectively) (SHAFAIE et al. 1997). The MR manifestations of discitis include loss of the outline of the vertebral end plates, relatively low signal on T1-weighted images within the peridiscal vertebral bony marrow, and consonant high signal intensity on T2-weighted acquisitions within the abnormal vertebral marrow. The combination of extensive disc intervertebral enhancement, posterior anulus fibrosus enhancement, and enhancement of the adjacent vertebral marrow after IV gadolinium administration is not typically seen on MR images of asymptomatic postoperative patients in the immediate period after surgery. However, as noted in the foregoing, limited posterior anulus and peridiscal enhancement is commonly seen in asymptomatic postoperative discs.

Epidural or paravertebral infection may be present postoperatively with or without findings of spondylitis or discitis. Epidural infection can appear either as a homogeneously or slightly heterogeneously enhancing phlegmonous mass within the spinal canal on IV gadolinium enhanced T1-weighted MR images, or it may present as a peripherally enhancing mass with a hypointense nonenhancing center representing liquefactive abscess formation (Fig. 31.3).

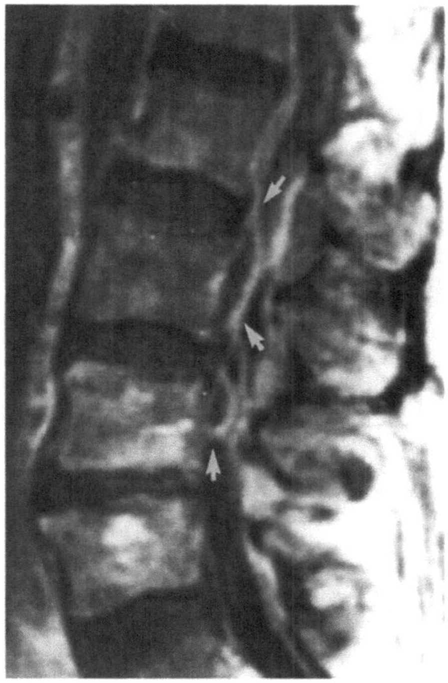

Fig. 31.3. Postoperative spinal infection (staphylococcus). IV gadolinium enhanced sagittal T1-weighted (500/15) MR image shows irregular rim enhancement over extensive areas within the lumbosacral spinal canal (*arrows*) indicating postoperative epidural abscess formation following discectomy. [From Jinkins JR, Leite C da C (1998) Neurodiagnostic imaging. Lippincott-Williams & Wilkins, Philadelphia, with permission]

Because of the nonspecific appearance of the postoperative spine with regard to spinal infection, correlation of both clinical (e.g., blood or cerebrospinal fluid cultures) and the imaging studies is mandatory in such circumstances. The overall appearance on MR of the spinal tissues with or without contrast enhancement after surgical intervention may be somewhat indeterminate, and percutaneous needle aspiration may be necessary in such cases in order to establish or exclude the presence of active postoperative infection (SHAFAIE et al. 1997).

31.2.4.3
Chronic Sterile Arachnoiditis

The factors inciting chronic sterile spinal arachnoiditis are much debated but include the surgical procedure itself, the presence of intradural blood, following surgery or preceding myelography lumbar puncture treated perioperative spinal infection, the previous use of myelographic contrast media (especially oil-based), and the prior intraspinal injection of anesthetic or anti-inflammatory agents (e.g., steroids). Chronically persistent lumbosacral signs and symptoms in 6–16% of postsurgical patients may be caused by sterile arachnoiditis.

The degrees of severity of the imaging findings in a patient with chronic sterile arachnoiditis do not appear to correlate well with one another. The symptoms when present are usually polyradicular, with pain and paresthesias extending into both lower extremities. Despite the presence of arachnoiditis, coexisting bony lateral stenosis or recurrent or residual disc herniation should be sought because they may imply a favorable chance of pain relief or diminution with repeat surgery.

Myelography and CT myelography usually clearly depict the changes indicative of arachnoiditis. However, subtle changes of focal arachnoiditis (i.e., absence of nerve-root sheath filling) may mimic the presence of a herniated disc. The three MR imaging patterns that have been described in adhesive arachnoiditis include: (a) matted or clumped nerve roots, (b) an "empty" thecal sac caused by adhesions of the nerve roots to the walls of the thecal sac, and (c) an intrathecal soft tissue mass with a broad dural base that may obstruct the CSF pathways (Fig. 31.4) (SHAFAIE et al. 1997). These alterations may be either focal or diffuse. Enhancement of the thickened meningeal scarring and involved underlying intrathecal nerve roots on IV gadolinium enhanced MR imaging, when present, does not seem to correlate well with the clinical severity of the arachnoidi-

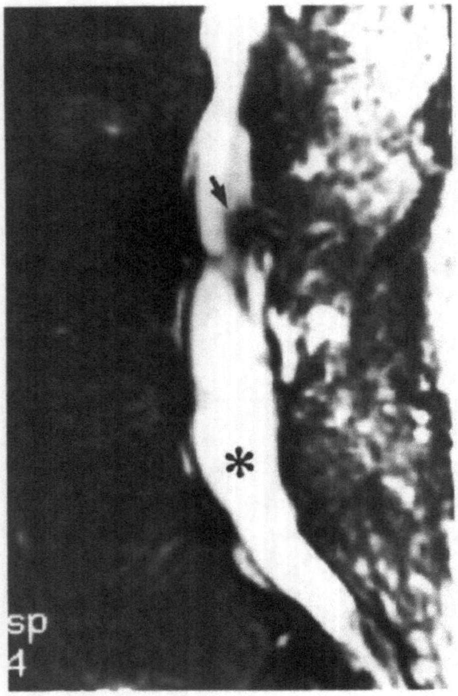

Fig. 31.4. Sterile postoperative adhesive arachnoiditis. Axial T2-weighted (4000/90) fast spin echo MR image shows matting of the intrathecal nerve roots (*arrow*) and a distal "empty" thecal sac (*asterisk*) indicating sterile adhesive postoperative arachnoiditis. [From Jinkins JR, Leite C da C (1998) Neurodiagnostic imaging. Lippincott-Williams & Wilkins, Philadelphia, with permission]

tis. Because pathologic enhancement is not always present in such cases, IV gadolinium administration does not invariably aid in visualization of arachnoiditis. On the other hand, gadolinium may on occasion demonstrate abnormal enhancement of the thickened leptomeninges and matted nerve roots on enhanced MR imaging. At present, the most reliable method of demonstrating the advanced findings of arachnoiditis on MR is the use of unenhanced axial T2-weighted fast spin-echo acquisitions. The classic findings of arachnoiditis identified on MR correlate well with identical findings seen on myelography and postmyelographic CT. A 92% sensitivity, 100% specificity and 99% accuracy have been reported in the diagnosis of moderate to severe arachnoiditis by MR imaging alone (Shafaie et al. 1997).

31.2.4.4
Postoperative Radiculitis

On MR imaging, enhancement of the intrathecal spinal nerve roots of the cauda equina following IV gadolinium administration at a conventional dosage of 0.1 mmol/kg (0.2 cc/kg) is not a normal observation. In other words, spinal nerve roots have a visually intact blood-nerve barrier (BNB) on IV gadolinium enhanced spin-echo MR. On the other hand, the distinction should be noted that there is little or no BNB within the spinal dorsal root ganglia, which explains their intense enhancement pattern after IV gadolinium administration. With frank compression injury to spinal nerves and nerve roots, however, this otherwise relatively intact BNB may break down. The complex and as yet poorly understood sequelae of chronic neural trauma/ischemia are believed to be the cause of the abnormal neurophysiologic changes resulting in clinical radiculopathy that may continue long after the initially offending influence (e.g., disc herniation) has been surgically removed (Jinkins 1993b).

In a recent study of symptomatic postoperative patients, enhancement of spinal nerve roots after IV gadolinium administration was demonstrated at, and extending away from, the surgical site in the chronic postoperative period (i.e., more than 6–8 months after surgery) (Fig. 31.5) (Jinkins 1993b). It has been shown in laboratory models that mechanical injury alone is sufficient to cause focal BNB disruption and nerve root enhancement on MR. It has also been proven in laboratory models of neural crush that wallerian axon degeneration and regener-

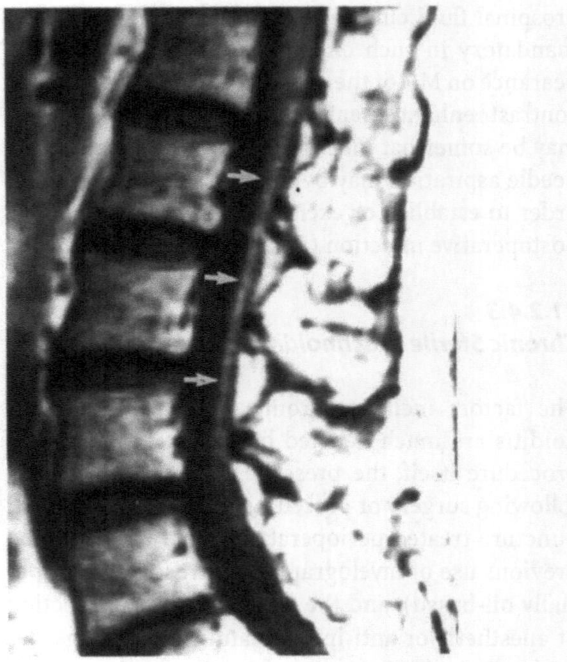

Fig. 31.5. Postoperative sterile lumbosacral radiculitis. IV gadolinium enhanced sagittal T1-weighted (500/15) MR image shows enhancement of an intrathecal lumbosacral nerve root (*arrows*) indicating sterile postoperative radiculitis. [From Jinkins JR, Leite C da C (1998) Neurodiagnostic imaging. Lippincott-Williams & Wilkins, Philadelphia, with permission]

ation are associated with and may even induce and prolong the BNB breakdown; in fact, BNB disruption is believed to serve as an indicator of such degenerative activity. Almost certainly, the instances of nerveroot enhancement on MR remote to the site of injury (i.e., distant from disc herniation and surgery) are associated with ongoing degenerative and regenerative phenomena within injured nerves.

From a practical standpoint, chronic postoperative nerve root enhancement on MR correlates well with the radicular clinical presentation. However, a caveat should be noted in that, during the first 6–8 months after intervertebral disc surgery, nerve root enhancement can be seen in the asymptomatic patient; this enhancement apparently reflects the nerve root under repair. Nevertheless, in the proper clinical setting of the chronic FBSS, nerve root enhancement may be used to confirm the presence of clinically relevant imaging findings in etiologically uncertain cases of postoperative radiculopathy (Jinkins 1993b).

31.2.4.5 Spinal Stenosis

Stenosis of the central spinal canal, the lateral recess of the spinal canal, and the neural foramen may be a cause of the FBSS. These forms of spinal stenosis may preexist or follow the spinal surgery. When the stenosis follows surgery, it may be the result of accelerated degeneration of spinal segments above or below a level of bony spinal fusion. Although published studies have methodologic biases and small sample sizes, it appears that the sensitivity and specificity of MR imaging and CT for depicting spinal stenosis are similar to one another (i.e., true-positive rate of approximately 90%, false-positive rate of approximately 10%) (Shafaie et al. 1997). The appearance of central spinal canal lateral recess spinal stenosis on MR is best depicted utilizing T2-weighted fast spin-echo axial acquisitions. Spinal neural foramen narrowing is best imaged with direct sagittal T1-weighted MR imaging (Fig. 31.6).

31.2.4.6 Postoperative Pseudomeningocele

Postsurgical pseudomeningocele formation results either from an inadvertent intraoperative dural tear or from a persistent opening in the dura following intradural surgery. The term pseudomeningocele is used because it is not a true arachnoid-lined sac. This potential cause of the FBSS usually presents as a recur-

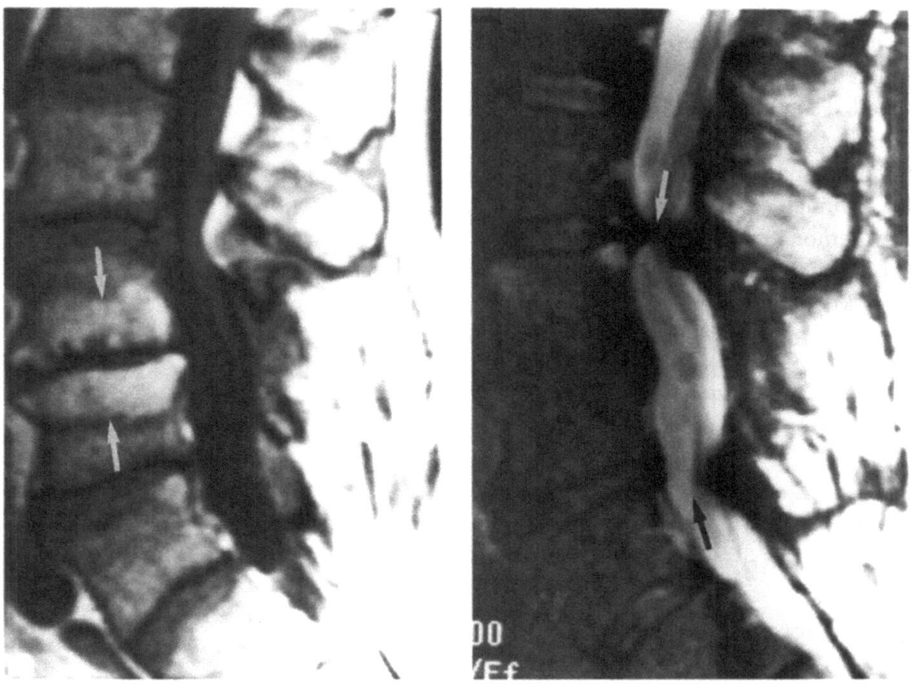

a b

Fig. 31.6a,b. Acquired postoperative central spinal stenosis secondary to accelerated fusion adjacent to fused segment. **a** Sagittal T1-weighted (500/10) MR image shows laminectomy at L4 and intervertebral fusion at the L4–5 level. Note the paradiscal fatty conversion (*arrows*) at L4–5 indicating probable stable fusion at that level. **b** Sagittal T2-weighted (4500/) MR image showing central stenosis supra- (*upper arrow*, L3–4) and subjacent (*lower arrow*, L5–S1) to the L4–5 fusion. [From Jinkins JR, Leite C da C (1998) Neurodiagnostic imaging. Lippincott-Williams & Wilkins, Philadelphia, with permission]

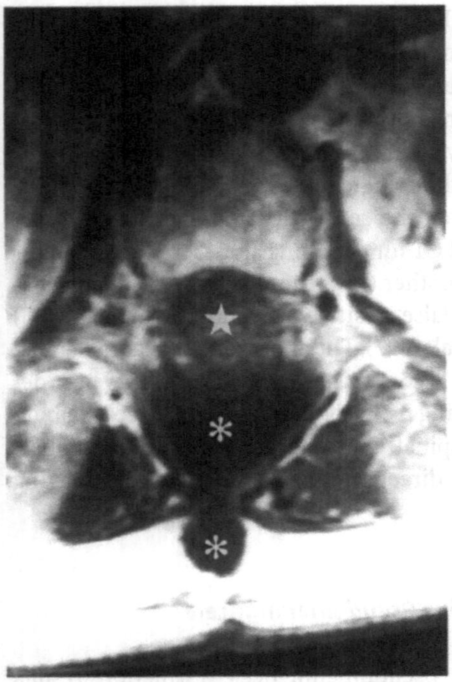

Fig. 31.7. Postoperative pseudomeningocele. Axial T1-weighted (500/15) MR image shows the thecal sac (*c*) and a postoperative pseudomeningocele extending posteriorly (*asterisks*). [From Jinkins JR, Leite C da C (1998) Neurodiagnostic imaging. Lippincott-Williams & Wilkins, Philadelphia, with permission]

rence of low back pain following an asymptomatic interval of several weeks. There may also be radicular signs and symptoms as well. Pseudomeningoceles appear as well-defined fluid collections abutting upon the surgical site and extending into the posterior paraspinal soft tissues. Although postoperative pseudomeningoceles usually demonstrate CSF signal intensity on all MR sequences, sometimes fluid-fluid levels or relative differences in MR signal intensity are seen secondary to blood products, high protein content or gross internal debris (Fig. 31.7) (Shafaie et al. 1997).

31.3 Cervicothoracic Spine Following Intervertebral Disc Surgery and Decompressive Laminectomy

31.3.1 Intervertebral Disc Surgery

Unlike the lumbosacral spine, the cervical and thoracic regions of the spine operated previously for disc disease and spinal stenosis do not require IV contrast agents when imaged by CT or MR, unless postoperative infection is suspected. Without repeating what has previously been stated for the lumbosacral spine, generally speaking, MR is superior when evaluating soft tissue abnormalities (e.g., recurrent disc herniation, progressive myelomalacia) whereas high resolution CT with reconstructions is better for analyzing bony postoperative abnormalities (e.g., spinal stenosis, postoperative spondylolisthesis). Even in these two areas, the two modalities are often complimentary or confirmatory to variable degrees with regard to the information yielded. Otherwise, many of the complications that may be seen on medical imaging in the lumbosacral spine may also be observed in the cervicothoracic region. Two exceptions to this observation include: the possibility of direct surgical injury to the cervical or thoracic spinal cord (i.e., the spinal cord is not normally present in the lumbosacral spine below the L1 level) and the general absence of visible cervicothoracic sterile radiculitis as evidenced by postoperative nonenhancement of cervical or thoracic spinal nerve roots in cases of clinical radiculopathy.

31.3.2 Decompressive Surgery for Chiari I and II Malformations

One specific area that deserves further specific discussion is the treatment and follow-up of syringohydromyelia associated with Chiari I and II malformations. Depending upon the individual case, simply opening up the foramen magnum (occipital bone) posteriorly in the midline together with posterior surgical unroofing (i.e., bilateral laminectomy) of C1 and perhaps C2 may take the constrictive pressure off the cervicomedullary junction sufficiently to allow spontaneous drainage of the syringohydromyelic cavity through the obex (Fig. 31.8). Not infrequently a fibrous band simultaneously constricts the cervicomedullary junction posteriorly as well, and requires surgical section to enable full decompression.

31.3.3 Decompressive surgery for Spinal Canal Stenosis

Stenosis of the central canal of the spine in the cervicothoracic region will result in varying degrees of spinal cord compression. This may in turn lead to

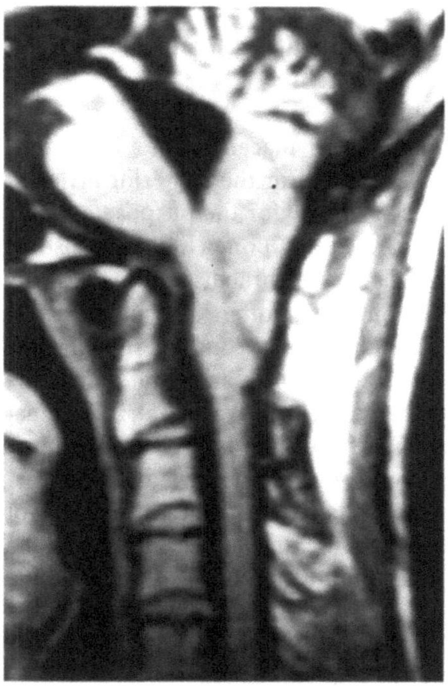

Fig. 31.8. Chiari malformation following posterior cervico-occipital surgical decompression for related syringohydromyelia. Sagittal T1-weighted (800/15) MR image following posterior surgical decompression of the cervicomedullary junction shows spontaneous drainage of the syringohydromyelic cavity observed in the cervical spinal cord on preoperative MR examination (not shown). Note the continued tonsillar and medullary ectopia. [From Jinkins JR, Leite C da C (1998) Neurodiagnostic imaging. Lippincott-Williams & Wilkins, Philadelphia, with permission]

clinical myelopathy. While there may be an element of preexistent developmental/congenital central canal stenosis (i.e., "short vertebral pedicles"), the major cause is usually acquired: posttraumatic stenosis, postinfectious stenosis, degenerative ossification of the posterior longitudinal ligament and/or the ligamentum flavum leading to spinal stenosis, and stenosis associated with generalized spondylosis.

On imaging, delayed conventional (i.e., water soluble iodinated contrast media) CT myelography may show uptake of the contrast agent into the spinal cord (Jinkins 1986), and MR imaging will reveal spinal cord compression, atrophy and hyperintensity of the most severely affected areas of the spinal cord on T2WI. Pathologically these alterations correspond to myelomalacia which may be microcystic; some degree of cord edema may or may not be present.

Following surgical decompression, these MR signal changes in the spinal cord may only partially resolve or not resolve at all (Fig. 31.9). This indicates the largely permanent nature of the pathologic change of the spinal cord underlying the imaging findings, and therefore the serious clinical implications of this disease process.

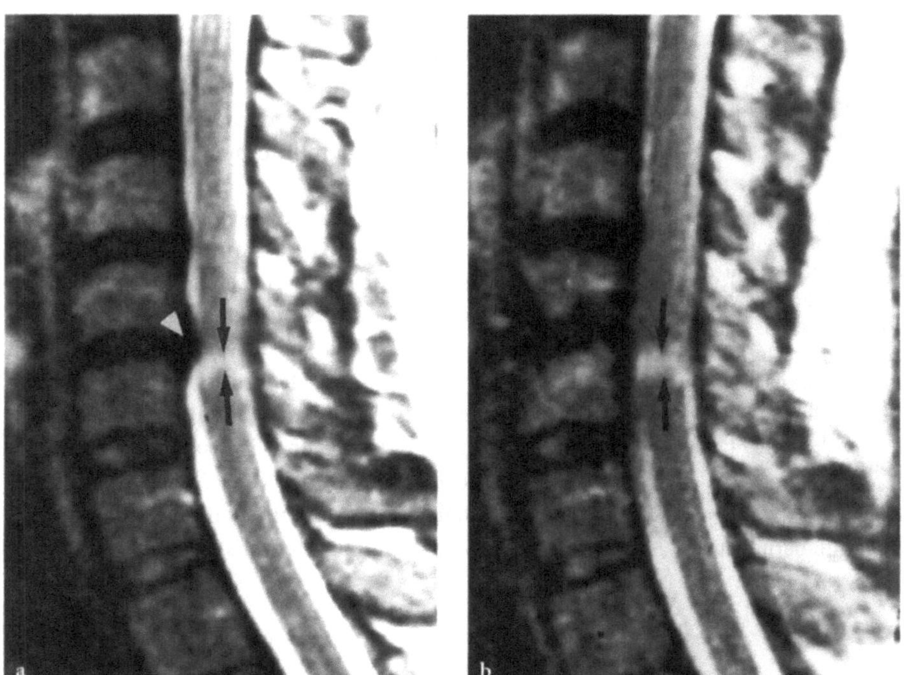

Fig. 31.9a,b. Compressive myelomalacia secondary to spinal stenosis. **a** Sagittal T2-weighted (2500/80) MR image shows hyper-intense spondylotic/stenotic (*arrowhead,* disc herniation) myelomalacia (*arrows*) of the cervical spinal cord. **b** Sagittal T2-weighted (2500/80) MR image following surgical decompression (discectomy) of the cervical spinal canal shows residual postoperative hyperintense myelomalacia (*arrows*). [From Jinkins JR, Leite C da C (1998) Neuro-diagnostic imaging. Lippin-cott-Williams & Wilkins, Philadelphia, with permission]

31.4 Imaging of Postoperative Segmental Spinal Instability: Spondylolisthesis

Failed operative fusion with resultant spinal instability may reveal a change in bony spinal relationships on MR imaging. Spondylolisthesis secondary to spinal instability from excessive posterior element surgical resection or postoperative facet fracture in the absence of a surgical fusion produces similar findings. It is important to note that this spondylolisthesis may be associated with stenosis of the central spinal canal and spinal neural foramina with symptomatic spinal cord compression and/or entrapment of nerve roots, respectively (Fig. 31.10) (Shafaie et al. 1997).

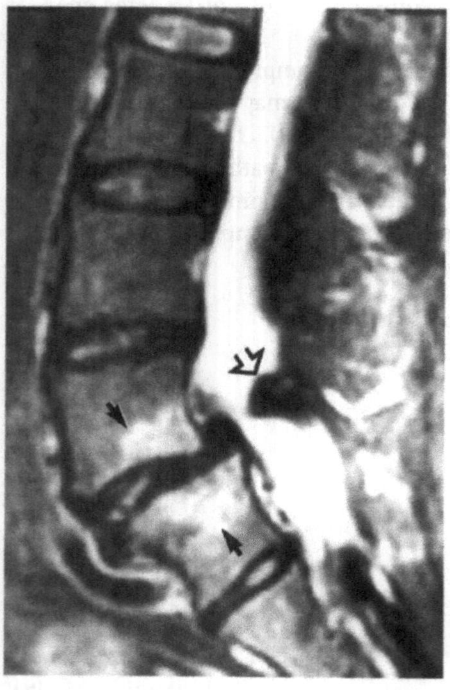

Fig. 31.10. Postoperative spinal instability with spondylolisthesis. Sagittal T2-weighted (4000/90) MR image following bilateral laminectomy, partial facetectomy and discectomy shows grade I anterolisthesis of L5 on S1 with resultant stenosis of the central spinal canal. This is caused by encroachment of the bony elements of the posterior neural arch (*open arrow*) as a result of spondylolisthesis occurring in the face of incomplete resection of the spinal laminae. The abnormal L5–S1 paradiscal marrow is hyperintense (*solid arrows*) on this acquisition indicating marrow edema consistent with spinal instability at this level. [From Jinkins JR, Leite C da C (1998) Neurodiagnostic imaging. Lippincott-Williams & Wilkins, Philadelphia, with permission]

31.5 Imaging of Postoperative Bony Intervertebral Fusion

In surgical spinal fusion, placement of a bone graft across the transverse and/or the posterior articular processes of the vertebrae for the purpose of spine stabilization is carried out. Bone chips may also be placed within the intervertebral disc space following discectomy. Although it is often difficult to determine by MR imaging alone, complete fusion may demonstrate a contiguity of marrow fat across the fused bony elements (i.e., intervertebral, intertransverse, interarticular fusion) on T1-weighted acquisitions. The bone graft itself has a varied MR appearance depending on its site of origin, the extent of trauma to the graft at the time of harvesting, and the degree of vascular infiltration of the graft. On axial CT with multiplanar reconstructions a similar vertebral element to vertebral element bony continuity is sought in order to confirm fusion.

In the absence on MR imaging of transdiscal marrow continuity, stable fusions cause a conversion of paradiscal vertebral red marrow to yellow (fatty) marrow secondary to a decrease in biomechanical stresses. On MR imaging this is manifested as a subchondral region paralleling the vertebral end plates demonstrating relative high signal intensity on T1-weighted images and isotensity on T2-weighted acquisition (Fig. 31.11). On the other hand, persistent segmental instability may show paradiscal vertebral marrow hypointensity on T1-weighted images and relative hyperintensity on T2-weighted acquisitions, perhaps representing cancellous marrow bony microfractures and resultant vertebral bone marrow edema (Fig. 31.12). These edematous marrow areas may enhance on IV gadolinium enhanced MR imaging. It should be noted that a time interval of 1 year or more is usually needed between the attempted surgical fusion and the MR examination in order to fully appreciate and judge these changes with some significance. Kinetic flexion-extension MR imaging utilized to judge spinal stability, accomplished with the patient in the lateral decubitus position, may be of use when using MR units that allow such studies to be performed. However, it is probably more practical to perform dynamic (i.e., flexion-extension) conventional radiographs in such patients to evaluate for physical intersegmental spinal instability.

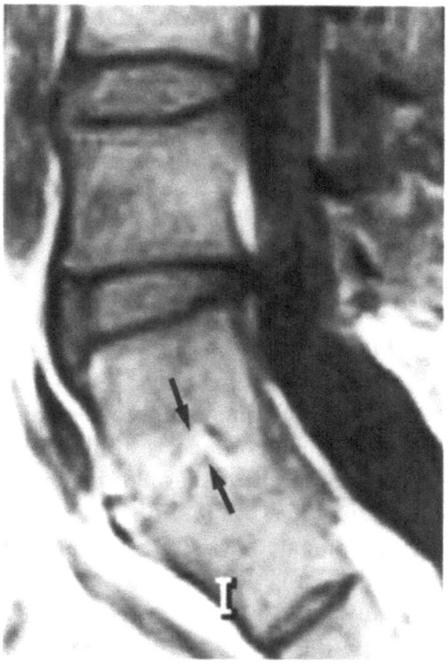

Fig. 31.11. Complete stable spinal fusion. Sagittal T1-weighted (500/15) MR image shows continuity of hyperintense marrow fat across the L5–S1 intervertebral disc space (*arrows*) indicating complete, stable bony intersegmental spinal fusion

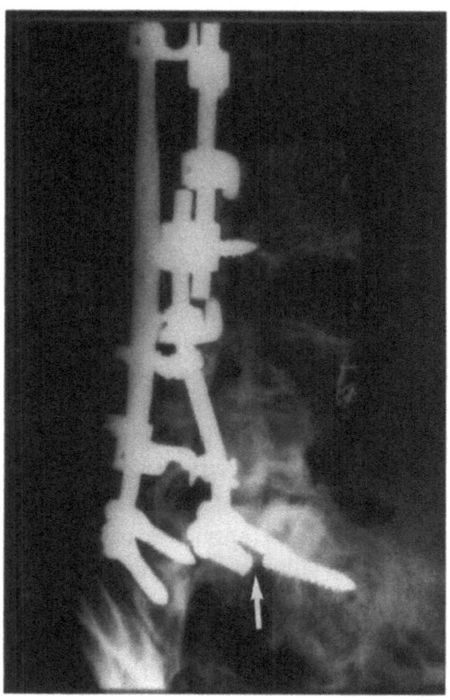

Fig. 31.12. Spinal surgical instrument failure. Conventional radiograph in the lateral projection shows a fracture of one of the pedicle screws (*arrow*) attaching the intersegmental surgical appliance to the spinal column. [From Jinkins JR (1997) Posttherapeutic neurodiagnostic imaging. Lippincott-Raven, Philadelphia, with permission]

31.6 Principles, Imaging, and Complications of Surgical Spinal Instrumentation

Spinal fusion is often required for the purpose of successful correction or repair of spinal instability or deformity. For certain selected problems, a single-level fusion can be accomplished without the aid of surgically implanted fixation devices. For other types of pathology it is difficult or impossible to adequately fuse the spine without surgical instrumentation. The likelihood of a successful solid arthrodesis (i.e., intersegmental bony fusion) increases when instrumentation is used to span multiple segments.

Metal wires, plates, screws, and rod instrumentation systems are the most common materials that have been used in the treatment of spinal abnormalities resulting from fractures, degenerative disease, and congenital anomalies. The instrumentation is used to provide stability, restore and maintain anatomic alignment, and limit motion as the spine undergoes osseous fusion in the cases commonly treated with concomitant bone graft placement. Although metal instrumentation provides immediate stability, it is subject to fatigue failure, with eventual loosening or metallic fracture from repeated stress. The success of spinal fusion greatly increases with bone grafting placed in conjunction with the surgical instrumentation. Exceptions to this rule include patients who have a decreased life expectancy, such as those with metastatic neoplastic spinal disease, who require stabilization but not arthrodesis (Slone and McEnery 1997).

The primary purpose of instrumentation is to provide purchase to an individual level and rigid linkage to other levels. Different instrumentation systems use varying specific approaches to accomplish these two goals. In general, spinal instrumentation using internal surgical stabilization is superior to external immobilization, such as braces and casts, for stabilizing and immobilizing the spine during the bony fusion process.

Bony spinal elements that are infected, crushed, or involved with tumor often must be removed (i.e., corpectomy), leaving a large bony defect and a mechanically unstable spine. Replacement materials such as structural bone grafts, methylmethacrylate, and titanium cages are used to maintain height in such cases and to restore alignment. Methylmethacrylate is typically used only for the treatment of metastatic tumors to replace vertebral body content if the life expectancy of the patient is short; it is contraindicated in the treatment of osteomyelitis.

Significant recent changes in spinal fixation have occurred with the development of biocompatible materials that can be left in place permanently and that can withstand the repeated stresses of weight bearing, flexion and extension until arthrodesis occurs. The instrumentation is no longer needed once osseous fusion has occurred, but it is nevertheless generally left in place indefinitely because of the potential risks associated with repeated surgery. Infection and intractable pain are two indications for removal of the instrumentation following fusion. Fractured and dislodged implants are typical signs of failed fusion and pseudoarthrosis formation across the construct; the instrumentation in such cases is usually removed for the purpose of revision of the fusion (Sloan and McEnery 1997).

31.6.1 Specific Types of Spinal Instrumentation

Spinal instrumentation includes longitudinal members such as plates and rods attached directly to vertebral bodies or posterior elements using wires, cables, screws or hooks. Wires and screws can also be used independently as a primary means of fixation. The techniques of fixation differ with their site of attachment to the spine (e.g., lamina, pedicles or vertebral body), and means of attachment (e.g., screws, wires, or hooks). In addition, instrumentation used variously at the cervico-occipital junction, the mid- to lower cervical spine, the thoracic and lumbar spines, and the lumbosacral spine differs significantly. Generally speaking, spinal instrumentation fixation techniques may be classified as anterior, posterior, or combined (Sloan and McEnery 1997).

31.6.2 Imaging Techniques

Conventional radiographs remain the mainstay of surgical implant evaluation. Radiographs demonstrate the position of the spinal elements, the instrumentation itself, the graft material, and often evidence of gross complications if present. Orthogonal views of the appliance and spine are necessary because complications are often visible in only one projection. Spinal fusion evaluation usually begins with conventional radiographs acquired in the anteroposterior, lateral and occasionally the oblique projections. Serial radiographs obtained over time may show subtle changes that become more evident on dynamic lateral flexion-extension films obtained in the erect position. Such dynamic radiographs can be helpful in establishing the presence or absence of motion and therefore integrity of the fusion.

31.6.3 Complications of Spinal Fusion Utilizing Spinal Instrumentation

31.6.3.1 Soft Tissue Complications

Operative complications of spinal surgery generally include injury to the spinal cord, nerve roots, dura, vessels and other regional soft tissues. Postoperative neurologic injury can be the result of direct surgical neural trauma, instrumentation failure or surgical appliance migration. Neurologic injury is an uncommon complication of spinal surgery, occurring in only about 1% of patients (Sloan and McEnery 1997). Malpositioned instrumentation and overdistraction of bony elements are common causes of surgical fusion failure. Other postoperative complications include hematoma formation, infection, superficial pressure sores developing over spinal instruments and spinal instability as a result of a failure of spinal element purchase or a failure of accomplishment of rigid linkage. When spinal instrumentation is incorrectly selected or placed, it may contribute to fixation failure. Careful patient technique and instrument selection are important factors in determining the success of a particular procedure.

31.6.3.2 Spinal Instrument Failure

Spinal fusion instrumentation may fail at the site of attachment to the spine (e.g., dislodged hooks, loose screws, broken wires or cables) at the junction of the instrument components (e.g., pedicle screw coming loose from the rod), or along the rigid linkage (e.g., fracture along the midportion of a plate or rod). A dislodged or fractured surgical appliance usually indicates instability, clinical failure of the fusion, or both. Fracture of the instrumentation may occur as a result of metal fatigue from the repeated stresses of flexion, extension and lateral bending (Fig. 31.13). As a result of the loss of stability, these problems can lead to failure of bony fusion (i.e., pseudoarthrosis). Resulting displacement of the spine can result in associated neurologic injury (Sloan and McEnery 1997).

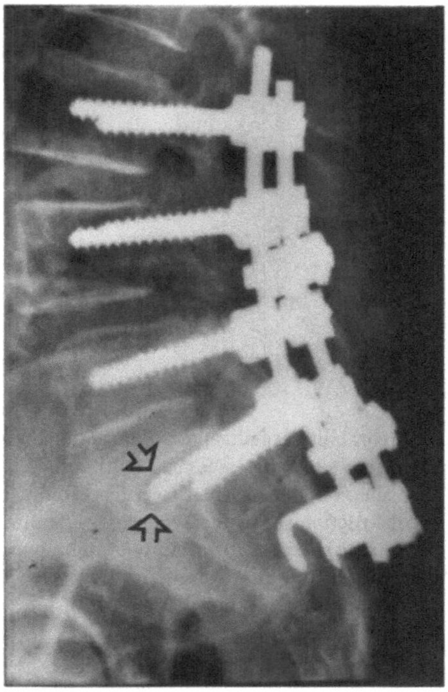

Fig. 31.13. Postsurgical peri-instrumental bone resorption. Conventional radiograph in the lateral projection shows a radiolucent halo within the vertebra (*arrows*) surrounding the surgical appliance indicating loosening of the bolt/screw within the bone. [From Jinkins JR (1997) Posttherapeutic neurodiagnostic imaging. Lippincott-Raven, Philadelphia, with permission]

31.6.3.3 Failed Spinal Fusion (Pseudoarthrosis) Following Instrument Placement

Typically 6–9 months is required for the development of a solid radiographic bony fusion, and 2 years for a solid fusion to completely remodel.

Pseudoarthrosis or fibrous union is a potential complication of spinal fusion. Early recognition and repair of this complication helps prevent surgical implant failure, loss of correction and clinical pain. An increasing risk of pseudoarthrosis is seen with increasing complexity and extent of the spinal surgery and with patient age. Any motion at the intended level of fusion during the healing phase increases the risk of pseudoarthrosis development, and therefore external braces (i.e., orthoses) are not uncommonly worn by the patient in order to minimize motion and maintain stability during attempted bony fusion.

Although perfect surgical technique does not guarantee a successful bony fusion, the rate of pseudoarthrosis occurrence is reduced by utilizing meticulous surgical technique. Nevertheless, a fibrous union can still sufficiently limit motion to enable a reduction of pain; conversely, a solid bone union does not necessarily ensure a good clinical outcome. Reoperation for surgical repair is necessary only if the patient presents with gross implant failure or pain. In the asymptomatic patient, intervention may be deferred while the patient's condition is followed. However, a pseudoarthrosis allows continued stress on the implant, and therefore instrumentation fracture may eventually follow. Failure of bony fusion may also result from bone graft fracture or infection occurring in the bony graft site (Sloan and McEnery 1997).

31.6.3.4 Peri-instrumental Bone Resorption

Bone resorption can occur around surgical screws/bolts and under implants that are in direct contact with bone (Fig. 31.14). Such resorption usually is associated with motion of the implanted instrument. It may lead to fracture of the weakened bone or to detachment of the surgical component with a resultant loss of fixation. The pattern of bone resorption occasionally indicates a mechanical etiology such as the arc-like motion of a loose screw about a pivot point. Infection must also be considered when a radiolucency is seen surrounding an implant (Sloan and McEnery 1997).

31.7 Imaging Following Intervertebral Fusion Cage Surgery

The first intervertebral fusion cages (also called "disc cages" or simply "cages") were implanted to stabilize lumbar motion segments in patients independently by a neurosurgeon (C.D. Ray) and by an orthopedic surgeon (J.W. Brantigan) in May 1989 (Kaech and Jinkins 1999). Since that time an increasing number of different cages have appeared on the market. For the radiologist it is important to distinguish between the radiolucent carbon cages and the radiopaque titanium cages. In addition, these disc cages may be implanted alone or in association with pedicle screws, plates or rods.

Irrespective of their composition and shape, intervertebral disc cages have a dual function: (1) mechanical – cages act as a spacer, restoring intervertebral disc space height, and stabilizing potential motion between adjacent vertebrae, and (2) biological – most cages are implanted together with autologous bone which will ideally eventually achieve bony

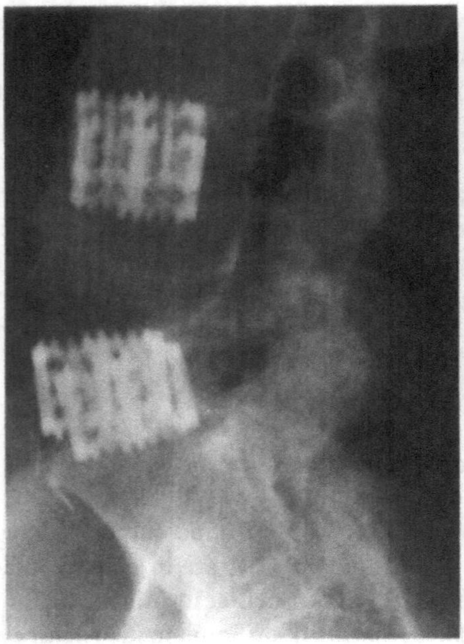
a

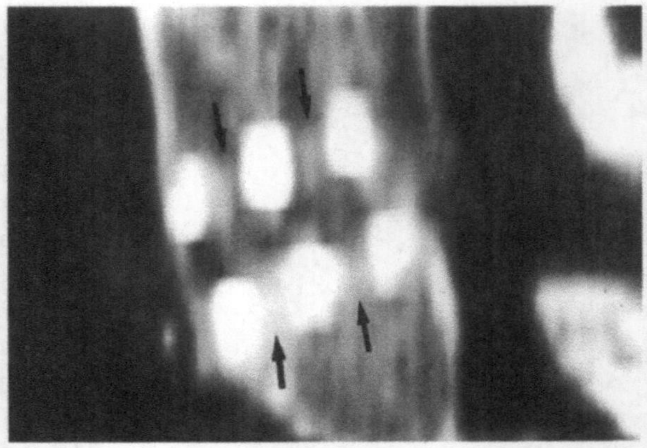
b

Fig. 31.14a,b. Successful intervertebral disc cage fusion. **a** Conventional radiograph in the lateral projection shows two disc cages each within the L4–5 and L5–S1 intervertebral disc spaces following dual level discectomy. **b** High resolution sagittal CT reconstruction shows the hyperdense titanium intervertebral disc cage within the disc space, and continuity of radiodense bone (*arrows*) traversing the disc space and the cage interior between the adjacent vertebral marrow, indicating successful transdiscal bony fusion

fusion between the two adjacent vertebrae (Kaech and Jinkins 1999).

Disc cages allow the treatment of problems related to degenerative instability of the lumbar spine at vertebral segments where it is common. The problem of deficient load sharing capacity in the anterior column is also solved by disc cage implantation, thereby allowing restoration of appropriate weight bearing to the anterior aspect of the spinal column.

31.7.1 Indications for Fusion Cage Surgery

The indications for disc cage implantation are primary segmental instability of the spine and secondary segmental spinal instability after decompressive surgery. Practically speaking, spinal fusion with disc cages is currently recommended for treatment of disc herniation subsequent to discectomy associated with instability (including spondylolisthesis up to grade 1), for isolated postoperative spinal instability and when extensive decompressive surgery is planned and signs of associated instability are present preoperatively. Chronic disabling low back pain (i.e., at least 6 months duration and not responding to conservative treatment) is another relative indication, if the pain can be proved to be of spondylodiscogenic origin. Disc cage surgery is primarily considered for symptomatic degenerative disc disease involving one or at most two segments (Kaech and Jinkins 1999).

The contraindications to a cage implantation are active regional infection, extreme osteopenia, symptomatic peripheral vascular disease, active malignancy, gross obesity, pregnancy and the presence of a spondylolisthesis at the anticipated operative level of greater than grade I (Kaech and Jinkins 1999).

31.7.2 Imaging

Standard non-stress conventional radiographs are generally performed before the patient leaves the hospital. These images are typically repeated after 6 weeks. Dynamic (i.e., flexion-extension) radiographic studies are obtained at 3, 6, 12 and 24 months, according to the surgeon's particular follow-up protocol or to the clinical presentation of the patient postoperatively.

Thin section CT scanning with bone window filming and sagittal/coronal reconstructions is best for proving that fusion has occurred by documenting bony bridge formation traversing the cages and between the vertebrae across the intervertebral disc spaces. In the case of postoperative complications, more detailed imaging investigations will be required (Kaech and Jinkins 1999).

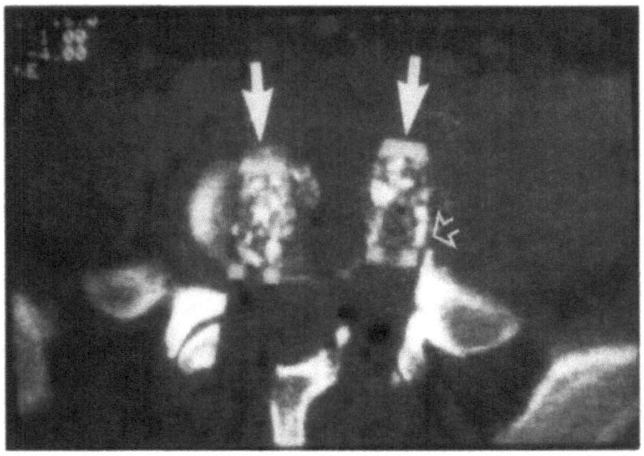

Fig. 31.15. Postoperative intervertebral disc cage displacement. Axial CT scan shows two intervertebral disc cages (*arrows*) in place. Note the slippage of the intervertebral disc cage on the left into the left L5–S1 intervertebral neural foramen. (Case courtesy of D.L. Kaech, MD)

31.7.3 Indications of Successful Fusion Following Cage Surgery

Specific postoperative criteria of successful fusion for radiopaque intervertebral disc cages packed with morsellized bone include: (1) absence of any discernible movement (less than 2 degrees of angular change) at the intervertebral segment as visualized on dynamic flexion-extension filming, (2) absence of either a radiolucent halo surrounding the disc cage or marked new sclerosis of the endplates as seen on lateral conventional radiographic images, (3) bone visible inside and surrounding the cages on Ferguson projection radiograph(s) (i.e., anteroposterior radiograph acquired parallel to the plane of the intervertebral disc space(s)), and (4) normal or reduced radionuclide uptake at the fused level on bone scintigraphy (Fig. 31.15). With good patient selection and with optimal surgical technique, successful fusion rates of 91–98% after 2 years should be possible, as reported in the literature (Kaech and Jinkins 1999).

31.7.4 Indications of Failed Fusion Following Cage Surgery

Radiologic criteria of failed fusion of radiopaque intervertebral disc cages packed with morsellized bone (with or without posterior instrumentation) include: (1) collapse of the construct (i.e., subcage subsidence into adjacent vertebrae), (2) progressive postoperative spondylolisthesis, (3) broken instrumentation (i.e., transpedicular screws), (4) resorption of the bone graft, and (5) radiolucency (i.e., "halo") visible surrounding the fusion area (e.g., 2 mm diameter or more around the entire periphery of the intervertebral fusion cage) (Fig. 31.16) (Kaech and Jinkins 1999).

31.8 Imaging Following Medical Therapy of Spinal Infection

In some circumstances, infections of the spine may be followed on medical therapy once the specific diagnosis of organism type and antibiotic sensitivity have been determined by tissue culture (e.g., blood, CSF, needle biopsy tissue). This is true in cases of infectious arachnoiditis, myelitis, spinal cord abscess/granuloma, and in some instances of spondylitis. However, because infectious spondylitis may result in spinal instability, segmental spinal collapse and/or infectious disc extrusion, careful clinicoradi-

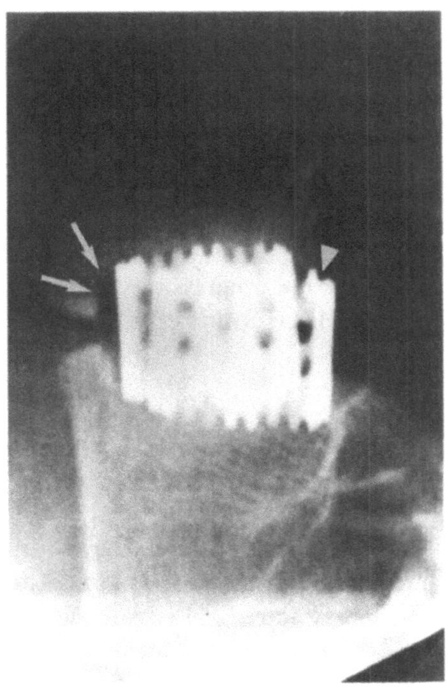

Fig. 31.16. Intervertebral disc cage displacement/failure of fusion. Conventional radiograph in the lateral projection shows a radiolucent halo (*arrow*) surrounding the intervertebral disc cage indicating posterior slippage (*arrowhead*) and possibly failure of bony fusion (i.e., vertebral subsidence of cage, loosening of cage). In the absence of recurrent patient signs and symptoms, repeat surgery may not be indicated in such a case. (Case courtesy of D.L. Kaech, MD)

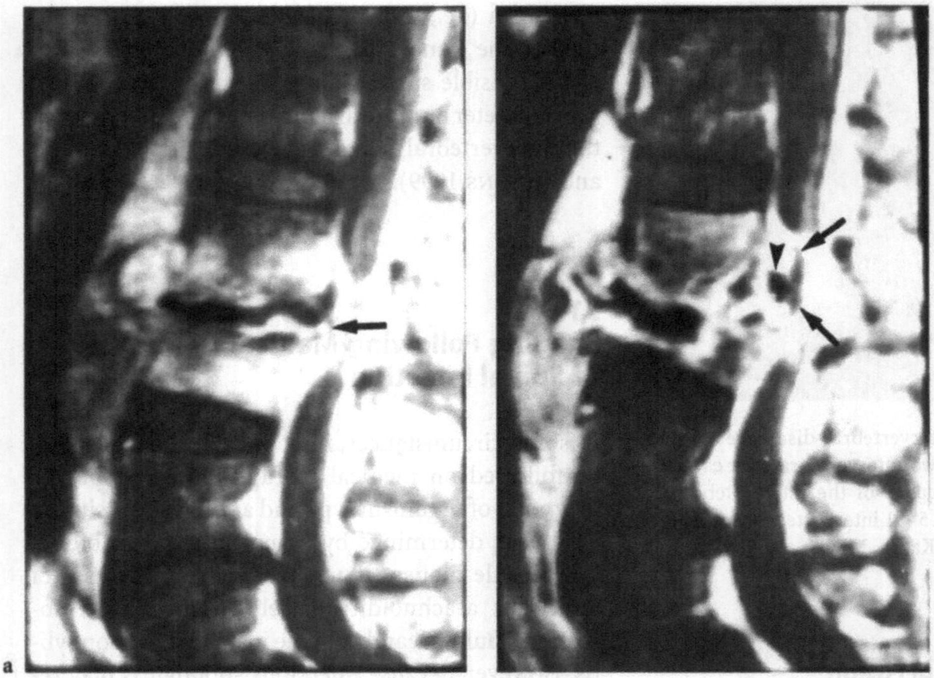

Fig. 31.17a,b. Progression of infectious disc extrusion on medical therapy (staphylococcus). **a** Initial IV gadolinium enhanced T1-weighted (500/15) MR image shows L2–3 disc collapse, peridiscal enhancement and epidural enhancement (*arrow*) surrounding a surgically proved infectious disc extrusion. **b** Repeat IV gadolinium enhanced T1-weighted (500/15) MR image acquired following 4 weeks of specific antibiotic therapy shows further collapse of the segmental spondylitis, persistence and enlargement of the epidural infectious process (*arrows*) and increased severity of the resulting central spinal stenosis. The patient subsequently underwent surgical debridement that revealed an infectious disc extrusion (*arrowhead*). [From Jinkins JR, Bazan C III, Xiong L (1996) MR of disc protrusion engendered by infectious spondylitis. J Comput Assist Tomogr 20(5):715–718, with permission]

ologic follow-up must be undertaken in order to sequentially evaluate the spine for satisfactory resolution or alternatively for progressive deleterious complications (Fig. 31.17) (Jinkins et al. 1996).

31.9 Imaging Following Surgery for Neoplasia

A number of neoplasms can affect this region, including: intramedullary tumors such as astrocytomas and ependymomas; intradural extramedullary tumors such as schwannomas and meningiomas; and epidural tumors such as neoplastic vertebral/epidural metastases and primary bone neoplasms. MR imaging is the modality of choice for postsurgical evaluation of spinal tumors. MR imaging before and after IV gadolinium administration can reveal residual or recurrent neoplasia, secondary effects on the spinal cord by the tumor mass, pseudomeningocele formation, and other complications of surgery. Recurrent neoplasia is simply judged by residual enhancement and/or progressive mass formation on segmental imaging studies following attempted surgical resection (Fig. 31.18). Seeding of the subarachnoid space from primary spinal cord tumors should also be sought on IV gadolinium enhanced MR imaging (Fig. 31.19) (Leite et al. 1996).

31.10 Imaging Following Radiation Therapy for Neoplasia

External spinal radiation leads to progressive changes in the hematopoietic bone marrow included in the radiation port. Immediately after completion of treatment, the vertebral marrow may show decreased MR signal on T1-weighted imaging and contrast enhancement after IV gadolinium administration, particularly if fat suppression techniques are used. This is believed to be related to edema, which typically resolves approximately 14 days after the completion of the therapy.

Further postradiation bone marrow alterations may begin to appear as early as 2 weeks after cessation of the radiation therapy. Some investigators have suggested that the findings are more time- than dose-dependent. After irradiation it has been shown histologically that initially there is a reduction in the cellular marrow. Subsequently the cellular marrow (i.e., "red" marrow) is progressively replaced by fatty marrow (i.e., "yellow" marrow). The typical MR appearance of postradiation fatty marrow conversion is one of diffusely increased intensity on T1-weighted images (Fig. 31.18). As expected, this fatty marrow will undergo fat suppression on appropriate fat-suppressed MR acquisition sequences. There are no known clear clinical implications of this phenomenon when the region of fatty marrow conversion is limited to small areas of the skeleton (Jinkins and Leite 1998).

Radiation-induced myelitis is a rare but serious complication of radiation therapy. There is no precise tolerance threshold of the spinal cord to radiation therapy. Histologically, radiation induced chronic progressive myelitis is characterized by demyelination, erythrodiapedesis, perineuronal edema and obliterative endoarteritis in the acute stage, and by perivascular and interstitial fibrosis and cord atrophy in the subacute and chronic stages. The clinical diagnosis of radiation induced myelitis is made on the basis of two main criteria: the spinal cord must have been included in the radiation field, and the symptomatology must correspond to the medullary segment involved. The differential diagnosis must include primary or recurrent intramedullary neoplastic lesions, necrotizing carcinomatous myelitis and myelopathy due to other intra- or extramedullary pathology. The latency period between the end of radiation therapy and the onset of radiation induced chronic progressive myelitis ranges from a few months up to 6 years. Typically this latent period is from 6 to 24 months.

The MRI findings most commonly described in radiation myelitis include: (a) spinal cord swelling of varied extent, (b) intramedullary hypointensity on the T1- and hyperintensity on the T2-weighted images; and (c) intramedullary contrast enhancement following IV gadolinium administration of varying extent both in the longitudinal and in the transverse planes (Fig. 31.20). The natural evolution on MRI of postradiation myelopathy progresses slowly and is characterized by eventual stabilization of the clinical picture and by gross spinal cord atrophy or, more rarely, intramedullary cavitation (Alfonso et al. 1991).

31.11 Imaging Progressive Posttraumatic Syringomyelia

Even in the face of adequate surgical spinal stabilization, in the chronic stages of severe trauma to the spinal cord, the cord itself may cavitate. Termed posttraumatic syringomyelia, this alteration can be seen within months of the traumatic episode. In some instances the syringomyelic cavity may be static and remain localized to the area of involvement of the actual spinal cord trauma. This is mirrored in the stabilization of the clinical syndrome shortly after the injury. However, in other cases there is an advancement in the signs and symptoms related to the spinal cord after an initial period of clinical stabilization. This is seen clinically as a progressively ascending sensory level of involvement and a deterioration of remaining spinal cord function. If followed on MR, these cases show a progressively enlarging syringomyelic cavity. While the cyst may potentially enlarge in both of the caudal and cranial directions within the spinal cord, for unknown reasons there is a strong tendency for the enlargement to extend superiorly. This results in an expansion of the syrinx into relatively more normal areas of the spinal cord cranial to the injury and accounts for the temporally progressive signs and symptoms in these cases.

On MR, posttraumatic syringomyelia is seen as an intramedullary cavity that is hypointense on T1-weighted imaging and variably hyperintense on T2-weighted acquisitions. Some variation in intensity may be seen if chronic blood products (e.g., hemosiderin) are present in the area of the initial cord trauma. If progressive, some posttraumatic syringomyelic cavities may have an area of parenchymal hyperintensity within the spinal cord adjacent to the leading edge of the cyst. This spinal cord hyperintensity on T2-weighted images is usually seen in the cord adjacent to the cranial extent of the syringomyelic cavity and probably represents an escape of cyst fluid into the spinal cord in the direction of syringomyelic cavity growth. In cases where the cyst cavity is followed on MR after surgical stenting/shunting with successful collapse of the cavity, the leading edge of parenchymal edema may disappear with resolution of the progressive signs and symptoms or even a return of some recently lost spinal cord function (Fig. 31.20). Therefore, hyperintensity within the spinal cord adjacent to a posttraumatic spinal cord cavity on T2-weighted imaging may be a sign on MR imaging of advancing syringomyelia (Jinkins et al. 1998).

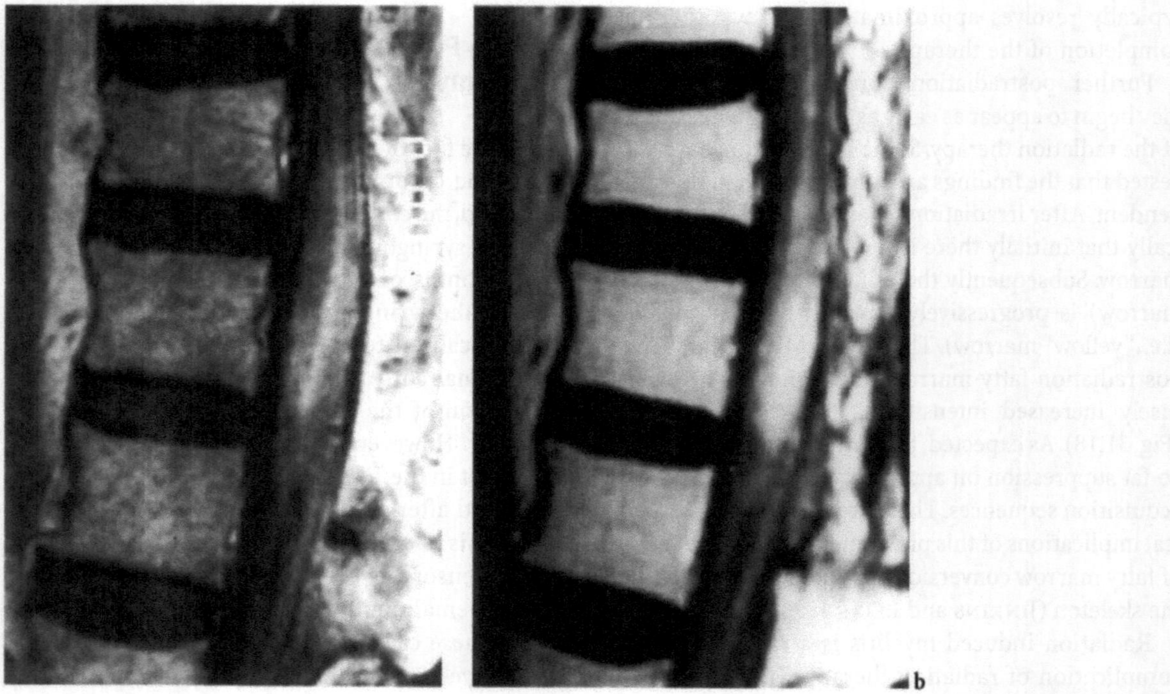

Fig. 31.18a,b. Postradiation vertebral marrow alteration and recurrent spinal cord ependymoma (15 year old patient). **a** Initial IV gadolinium enhanced sagittal T1-weighted (500/15) MR image showing normally mixed intensity vertebral bone marrow and irregular enhancement of a conus medullaris ependymoma. **b** IV gadolinium enhanced sagittal T1-weighted (500/15) MR image 2 months following regional external beam radiation therapy shows interim conversion of the vertebral marrow to uniform, marked hyperintensity (i.e., fatty marrow). Note the increased enhancement of the conus medullaris indicating residual/recurrent ependymoma (surgically proven)

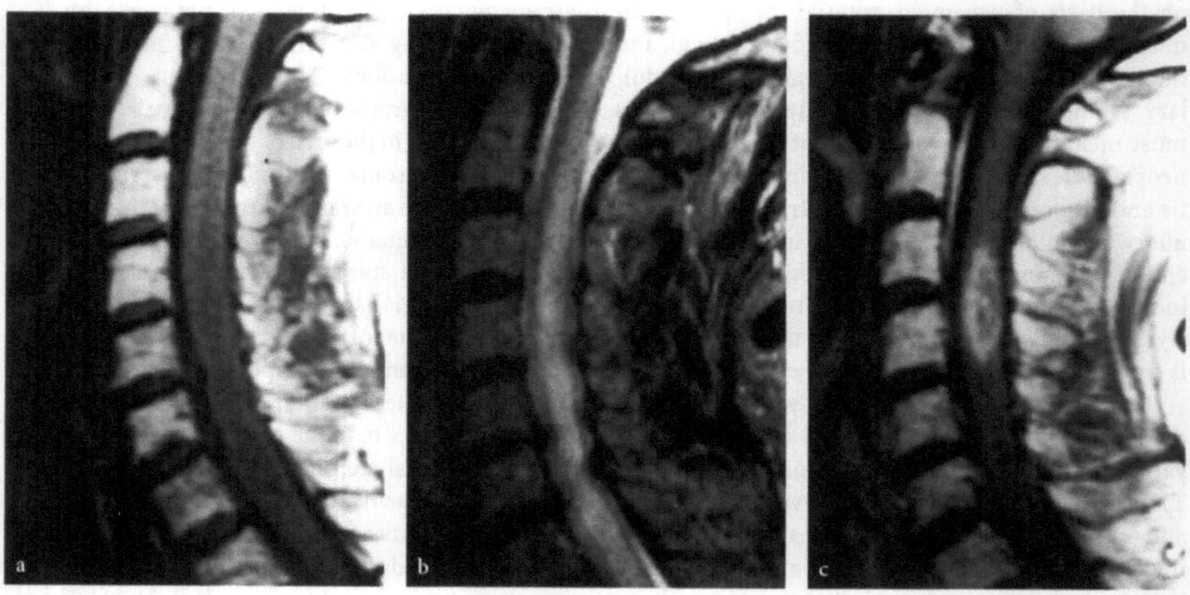

Fig. 31.19a–c. Radiation induced myelitis (prior radiation therapy for cervical extraspinal soft tissue neoplasm: tonsillar squamous cell carcinoma). **a** Sagittal T1-weighted (500/15) MR image shows swelling of the cervical spinal cord 12 months following radiation of a cervical extraspinal soft tissue neoplasm. **b** Sagittal T2-weighted (2000/80) MR image shows hyperintensity of the involved spinal cord. **c** IV gadolinium enhanced T1-weighted (500/15) MR image shows irregular enhancement of the cervical spinal cord indicating radiation myelitis. These changes resolved to spinal cord atrophy over a period of months with conservative therapy (not shown)

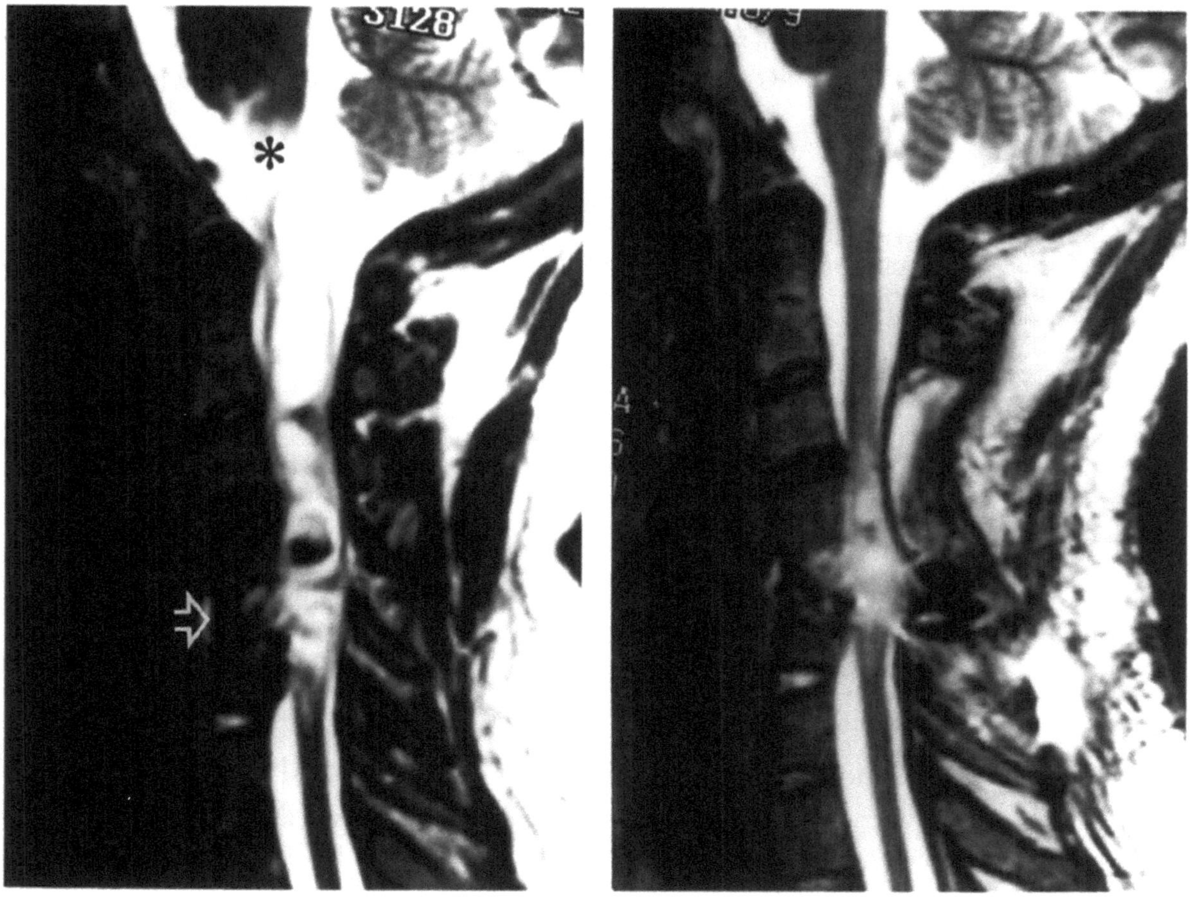

Fig. 31.20a,b. Progressive posttraumatic syringomyelia before and after shunt placement. **a** Sagittal T2-weighted (4000/120) MR fast spin echo image shows a mixed intensity syringomyelic cavity of the cervical spinal cord 12 months following cord trauma. Note the cervical spinal fusion (*arrow*) and the cranial leading edge of parenchymal edema (*asterisk*) within the lower brainstem. The latter is an indicator of active advancement of the syrinx. **b** Sagittal T2-weighted (4000/120) fast spin echo MR image following cystoperitoneal shunt placement shows collapse of the cyst and resolution of the lending edge of edema within the lower brainstem (compare with **a**). [From Jinkins JR, Reddy S, Leite C da C, Bazan III, Xiong L (199) MR of parenchymal spinal cord signal change as a sign of active advancement in clinically progressive posttraumatic syringomylia. Am J Neuroradiol 19:177–182, with permission]

31.12 Conclusion

It should be clear to those who perform and interpret medical images of the spine following one or more forms of surgical or nonsurgical therapy that the images are often difficult to interpret in part because of the superimposition of pathology engendered by the therapy per se, and/or because of a complication of the therapeutic procedure. Although long-term experience in this area is without doubt helpful in regard to improving interpretive skills, nevertheless, certain sequelae can be predicted regardless of the interpreter's background.

Once the normal or expected posttherapeutic findings are understood, the subtle and gross changes that depart from these observations can be better analyzed. The importance of a high level of competence in the domain of posttherapeutic neurodiagnostic imaging is in the knowledge that the patient returning for restudy may be acutely in distress or even in medical danger (e.g., postoperative spondylitis). In fact, the clinical presentation posttherapeutically may well be more severe or dire than was observed pretherapeutically. Thus, an in-depth appreciation of the broad range of clinicoradiologic possibilities as presented here should place the medical imaging physician in an excellent position to provide an experienced diagnostic evaluation in the patient presenting with recurrent or new signs and symptoms following spinal treatment (Tables 31.1, 31.2).

Table 31.1. Possible modes of spinal therapy

- Intervertebral disc surgery for disc disease
- Segmental intervertebral bony fusion for spinal instability
- Laminectomy for central spinal stenosis (developmental, acquired)
- Foraminotomy for lateral recess and spinal neural foramen stenosis
- Spinal instrumentation [intervertebral, interlaminar, interspinous, transpedicular instrumentation; vertebral replacement (vertebroplasty)]
- Syringomyelia shunting (posttraumatic, postinfectious, related to Chiari malformations, idiopathic)
- Medical therapy for spinal infection
- Radiation therapy for primary or secondary spinal neoplasia

Table 31.2. Potential complications of therapeutic spinal procedures

- Infection (e.g., bone, disc, peri-intraspinal tissues)
- Pseudomeningocele formation
- Recurrent/residual disease (e.g., recurrent disc disease/neoplasia, spinal stenosis)
- Sterile radiculitis
- Sterile adhesive arachnoiditis
- Pseudoarthrosis (i.e., failed intervertebral bony fusion)
- Progressive spinal instability (spondylolisthesis: antero-/retro-)
- Accelerated degenerative alteration (e.g., disc disease, spinal stenosis) supra- and subjacent to fused spinal segment(s)
- Direct neural injury (e.g., spinal cord, spinal nerve roots/nerves)
- Bone graft migration
- Spinal instrument failure/migration
- Syringomyelia shunt failure
- Radiation neuritis/myelitis/necrosis

References

Alfonso ER, De Gregorio MA, Mateo P et al. (1997) Radiation myelopathy in over-irradiated patients: MR imaging findings. Eur Radiol 7: 400–404

Jinkins JR, Bashir R, Al-Mefty O, Al-Kawi MZ, Fox JL (1986) Cystic necrosis of the spinal cord in compressive cervical myelopathy: Demonstration by iopamidol CT-myelography. AJNR 7: 693–701

Jinkins JR (1993a) The pathoanatomic basis of somatic and autonomic syndromes originating in the lumbosacral spine. Neuroimaging Clin North Am 3: 443–463

Jinkins JR (1993b) Magnetic resonance imaging of benign nerve root enhancement in the unoperated and postoperative lumbosacral spine. Neuroimaging Clin North Am 3: 525–541

Jinkins JR (1997) Posttherapeutic neurodiagnostic imaging. Jinkins JR (ed) Lippincott-Raven, Philadelphia

Jinkins JR, Bazan C, Xiong L (1996) MR of disc protrusion engendered by infectious spondylitis. J Comput Assist Tomogr 20: 715–718

Jinkins JR, Osborn AG, Garrett D Jr, Hunt S (1993) Spinal nerve enhancement with Gd-DTPA: MR correlation with the postoperative lumbosacral spine. AJNR 14: 383–394

Jinkins JR, Leite da Costa C (1998) Neurodiagnostic imaging: pattern analysis and differential diagnosis in the posttherapeutic spine. In: Jinkins JR and Leite da Costa Leite C (eds) Neurodiagnostic imaging. Lippincott-Raven, Philadelphia, pp 932–953

Jinkins JR, Reddy S, Leite CC, Bazan C, Xiong L (1998) MR of clinically progressive posttraumatic syringomyelic cysts: reversible perilesional parenchymal spinal cord signal change as a sign of active advancement. AJNR 19: 177–182

Kaech DL, Jinkins JR (1999) Clinicoradiologic assessment after disc cage implantation. Riv Neuroradiol 12(S): 129–140

Leite CC, Jinkins R, Bazan C et al. (1996) MR of subarachnoid seeding from CNS glial tumors. Int J Neuroradiol 2: 561–569

Shafaie FF, Bundschuh C, Jinkins JR (1997) The posttherapeutic lumbosacral spine. In: Jinkins JR (ed) Posttherapeutic neurodiagnostic imaging. Lippincott-Raven, Philadelphia, pp 223–243.

Slone RM, McEnery KW (1997) Principles, imaging, and complications of spinal instrumentation: radiologist's perspective. In: Jinkins JR (ed) Posttherapeutic neurodiagnostic imaging. Lippincott-Raven, Philadelphia, pp 245–266

Subject Index

List of Contributors

ABDELOUHAB ABANOU, MD
Centre Hospitalier National d'Ophthalmologie
des Quinze-Vingts
Service de Neuro-imagerie et radiologie
Rue de Charenton 28
75571 Paris Cedex 12
France

ERIC ACHTEN, MD, PhD
Professor, MR Department
University Hospital Gent
De Pintelaan 185
9000 Gent
Belgium

DANIËLLE BALÉRIAUX, MD, PhD
Professor, Hôpital ERASME
Service de Neuroradiologie
Route de Lennik 808
1070 Brussels
Belgium

FREDERIK BARKHOF, MD, PhD
Department of Radiology
MR Centre for MS Research
Academic Hospital "Vrije Universiteit"
PO Box 7057
1007-MB Amsterdam
The Netherlands

LUC BELLINGER, MD
Centre Hospitalier National d'Ophthalmologie
des Quinze-Vingts
Service de Neuro-imagerie et radiologie
Rue de Charenton 28
75571 Paris Cedex 12
France

ELISABETH BERGERS, MD, PhD
Department of Radiology
MR Centre for MS Research
Academic Hospital "Vrije Universiteit"
PO Box 7057
1007-MB Amsterdam
The Netherlands

PETER BRYS, MD
Department of Radiology
University Hospitals K.U.L.
Herestraat 49
3000 Leuven
Belgium

JAMES BYRNE, MD
Consultant Neuroradiologist
Department of Neuroradiology
The Radcliffe Infirmary
Woodstock Road
Oxford, OX2 6HE
UK

EMMANUEL A. CABANIS, MD
Professor
Centre Hospitalier National d'Ophtalmologie
des Quinze-Vingts
Service de Neuroradiologie, 28
Rue de Charenton
75571 Paris
France

FRANCESCO CALABRO, MD
TMA-Clinica Villa Salus
Via Montallegro 48
16145 Genoa
Italy

ANDREW G. CLIFTON, MD
Consultant Neuroradiologist, Department of Neuroradiology
Atkinson Morley's Hospital
Copse Hill
Wimbledon
London SW20 0NE
UK

PHILIPPE DAVID, MD
Professor, Hôpital ERASME
Service de Neuroradiologie
Route de Lennik 808
1070 Brussels
Belgium

PHILIPPE DEMAEREL, MD, PhD
Professor, Department of Radiology
University Hospitals K.U.L.
Herestraat 49
3000 Leuven
Belgium

JUDITH M. DONOVAN POST, MD
Department of Radiology, Section of Neuroradiology (R-308)
University of Miami School of Medicine
Neuroradiology
1115 NW 14th Street
Miami, FL 33136
USA

VINCENT DOUSSET, MD, PhD
Professor, Service de Neuroradiologie
CHU Pellegrin
Place Amélie Raba-Léon
33076 Bordeaux Cédex
France

MIRIAM DROESSAERT, MD
Department of Radiology
University Hospitals K.U.L.
Herestraat 49
3000 Leuven
Belgium

ZHANMING FAN, MD
Department of Radiology
General Coal Hospital
Xi Ba He Nan Li 29
Beijing 100028
P.R. China

PATRICK FLAMEN, MD
Department of Nuclear Medicine
University Hospitals
Herestraat 49
3000 Leuven
Belgium

DANIELLE GAMBARELLI, MD, MCU-PH
Department of Neuropathology
Hôpital Timone
Université de la Méditerranée
13915 Marseille Cédex 20
France

NADINE GIRARD, MD
Professor, Department of Radiology
Hôpital Nord, Université de la Méditerranée
Chemin des Bourrellys
13915 Marseille Cédex 20
France

PAUL D. GRIFFITHS, MD
Professor of Radiology
Section of Academic Radiology
The University of Sheffield
Royal Hallamshire Hospital, Floor C
Glossop Road, Sheffield
South Yorkshire, S10 2JF
UK

MARINA GRISOLI, MD
Department of Neuroradiology
Istituto Nazionale Neurologico "C. Besta"
Via Celoria 11
20133 Milan
Italy

SHAWN HALPIN, MRCP, FRCR
Department of Radiology
University Hospital of Wales
Heath Park
Cardiff, CF4 4XW
UK

ALAN J. HOLZ, MD
Department of Radiology
Section of Neuroradiology (R-308)
University of Miami School of Medicine
Neuroradiology
1115 NW 14th Street
Miami, FL 33136
USA

MARGARET D. HOURIHAN, MD
Consultant Neuroradiologist
Radiology Directorate
University Hospital of Wales
Heath Park
Cardiff, CF4 4XW
UK

MARIE-THÉRÈSE IBA-ZIZEN, MD
Centre Hospitalier National d'Ophthalmologie
des Quinze-Vingts
Service de Neuro-imagerie et radiologie
Rue de Charenton 28
75571 Paris Cedex 12
France

ALAN JACKSON, PhD, MB, ChB, MRCP, FRCR
Imaging Science and Biomedical Engineering
Medical School, Professor of Neurology
Department of Diagnostic Radiology
The University of Manchester
Stopford Building
Oxford Road
Manchester, M13 9PT,
UK

ROLF H. JÄGER, MD
Senior Lecturer in Neuroradiology and Consultant
Neuroradiologist, Institute of Neurology
University College London
University Department of Neurosurgery
The National Hospital for Neurology
and Neurosurgery
Queen Square
London, WC1N 3BG
UK

OLAV JANSEN, MD
Department of Neuroradiology
University of Heidelberg Medical School
Im Neuenheimer Feld 400
69120 Heidelberg
Germany

MOHAMMED JIDAL, MD
Centre Hospitalier National d'Ophthalmologie
des Quinze-Vingts
Service de Neuro-imagerie et radiologie
Rue de Charenton 28
75571 Paris Cedex 12
France

J. Randy Jinkins, MD, FACR
Professor and Director of Neuroimaging Research
Department of Radiology
981045 Nebraska Medical Center
Omaha, NE 68198-1045
USA

Zhongsheng Liu, MD
Department of Radiology
General Coal Hospital
Xi Ba He Nan Li 29
Beijing 100028
P.R. China

Frederik Maes, PhD
Medical Image Computing
ESAT-PSI and Radiology
Faculties of Engineering and Medicine
Kardinaal Mercierlaan 94
Heverlee
3001 Leuven
Belgium

Katherine Miszkiel, MRCP, FRCR
Consultant Neuroradiologist
Lysholm Department of Radiology
The National Hospital for Neuroradiology and Neurosurgery
Queen Square
London, WC1N 3BG
UK

William Mukonoweshuro
Specialist Registrar in Radiology
Radiology Department
The University of Sheffield
Royal Hallamshire Hospital, Floor C
Glossop Road
Sheffield
South Yorkshire, S10 2JF
UK

Thomas P. Naidich, MD, FACR
Professor of Radiology
Director of Neuroradiology
The Mount Sinai Medical Center
One Gustave L. Levy Place
Department of Radiology
Box 1234
New York, NY 10029-6574
USA

Paul M. Parizel, MD, PhD
Department of Radiology, University of Antwerp
Wilrijkstraat 10
2650 Edegem
Belgium

Zoltán Patay, MD, PhD
Consultant Neuroradiologist
Department of Radiology, MBC 28
King Faisal Specialist Hospital and Research Centre
PO Box 3354
11211 Riyadh
Kingdom of Saudi Arabia

Charles Raybaud, MD
Department of Neuroradiology
Hôpital Timone
Université de la Méditerranée
13915 Marseille Cédex 20
France

Fatima Rio, MD
Professor, Hôpital ERASME
Service de Neuroradiologie
Route de Lennik 808
1070 Brussels
Belgium

Max Ryan, FFR RCSI, FRCR
Department of Radiology
University Hospital of Wales
Heath Park
Cardiff, CF4 4XW
UK

Mario Savoiardo, MD
Department of Neuroradiology
Istituto Nazionale Neurologico "C. Besta"
Via Celoria 11
20133 Milan
Italy

Peter D. Schellinger, MD
Department of Neuroradiology
University of Heidelberg, Medical School
Im Neuenheimer Feld 400
69120 Heidelberg
Germany

Evelyn Sklar, MD
Department of Radiology
Section of Neuroradiology (R-308)
University of Miami School of Medicine
Neuroradiology
1115 NW 14th Street
Miami, FL 33136
USA

Stefan Sunaert, MD
Department of Radiology, University Hospitals
Herestraat 49
3000 Leuven
Belgium

Wendy Taylor, MD
Consultant Neuroradiologist
Lysholm Department of Radiology
The National Hospital for Neurology and Neurosurgery
Queen Square
London, WC1N 3BG
UK

Luc van den Hauwe, MD
Department of Radiology
University Hospital Antwerp
Wilrijkstraat 10
2650 Antwerp (Edegem)
Belgium

DIRK VANDERMEULEN, PhD
Professor, Medical Image Computing
ESAT-PSI and Radiology
Faculties of Engineering and Medicine
Kardinaal Mercierlaan 94
Heverlee
3001 Leuven
Belgium

JOHAN VAN GOETHEM, MD, PhD
Department of Radiology
University Hospital Antwerp
Wilrijkstraat 10
2650 Antwerp (Edegem)
Belgium

PAUL VAN HECKE, MD, PhD
Professor, Department of Radiology
University Hospitals K.U. Leuven
Herestraat 49
3000 Leuven
Belgium

KOEN VAN LEEMPUT, MSc
Medical Image Computing
ESAT-PSI and Radiology
Faculties of Engineering and Medicine
Kardinaal Mercierlaan 94
Heverlee
3001 Leuven
Belgium

ADAM D. WALDMAN, MA, PhD, MRCP, FRCR
Lysholm Department of Radiology
The National Hospital for Neurology and Neurosurgery
Queen Square
London, WC1 3BG
UK

GUY WILMS, MD, PhD
Professor, Department of Radiology
University Hospitals K.U.L.
Herestraat 49
3000 Leuven
Belgium

LIN XIONG, MD
Department of Radiology
General Coal Hospital
Xi Ba He Nan Li 29
Beijing 100028
P.R. China

INDRA YOUSRY, MD
Medizinische Abteilung für Neuroradiologie
am Institut für Radiologische Diagnostik
Klinikum Großhadern
Ludwig Maximilians Universität München
Marchioninistrasse 15
81377 München
Germany

TAREK A. YOUSRY, MD
Medizinische Abteilung für Neuroradiologie
am Institut für Radiologische Diagnostik
Klinikum Großhadern
Ludwig Maximilians Universität München
Marchioninistrasse 15
81377 München
Germany

QINGYU ZENG, MD
Department of Radiology
General Coal Hospital
Xi Ba He Nan Li 29
Beijing 100028
P.R. China

MEDICAL RADIOLOGY
Diagnostic Imaging and Radiation Oncology

Titles in the series already published

DIAGNOSTIC IMAGING

Innovations in Diagnostic Imaging
Edited by J.H. Anderson

Radiology of the Upper Urinary Tract
Edited by E.K. Lang

The Thymus - Diagnostic Imaging, Functions, and Pathologic Anatomy
Edited by E. Walter, E. Willich, and W.R. Webb

Interventional Neuroradiology
Edited by A. Valavanis

Radiology of the Pancreas
Edited by A.L. Baert, co-edited by G. Delorme

Radiology of the Lower Urinary Tract
Edited by E.K. Lang

Magnetic Resonance Angiography
Edited by I.P. Arlart, G.M. Bongartz, and G. Marchal

Contrast-Enhanced MRI of the Breast
S. Heywang-Köbrunner and R. Beck

Spiral CT of the Chest
Edited by M. Rémy-Jardin and J. Rémy

Radiological Diagnosis of Breast Diseases
Edited by M. Friedrich and E.A. Sickles

Radiology of the Trauma
Edited by M. Heller and A. Fink

Biliary Tract Radiology
Edited by P. Rossi

Radiological Imaging of Sports Injuries
Edited by C. Masciocchi

Modern Imaging of the Alimentary Tube
Edited by A. R. Margulis

Diagnosis and Therapy of Spinal Tumors
Edited by P. R. Algra, J. Valk, and J. J. Heimans

Interventional Magnetic Resonance Imaging
Edited by J. F. Debatin and G. Adam

Abdominal and Pelvic MRI
Edited by A. Heuck and M. Reiser

Orthopedic Imaging
Techniques and Applications
Edited by A.M. Davies and H. Pettersson

Radiology of the Female Pelvic Organs
Edited by E.K.Lang

Magnetic Resonance of the Heart and Great Vessels
Clinical Applications
Edited by J. Bogaert, A. J. Duerinckx, and F. E. Rademakers

Modern Head and Neck Imaging
Edited by S. K. Mukherji and J. A. Castelijns

Radiological Imaging of Endocrine Diseases
Edited by J. N. Bruneton in collaboration with B. Padovani and M.-Y. Mourou

Trends in Contrast Media
Edited by H. S. Thomsen, R. N. Muller, and R. F. Mattrey

Functional MRI
Edited by C. T. W. Moonen and P. A. Bandettini

Radiology of the Pancreas
2nd Revised Edition
Edited by A. L. Baert
Co-edited by G. Delorme and L. Van Hoe

Emergency Pediatric Radiology
Edited by H. Carty

Spiral CT of the Abdomen
Edited by F. Terrier, M. Grossholz, and C. D. Becker

Liver Malignancies
Diagnostic and Interventional Radiology
Edited by C. Bartolozzi and R. Lencioni

Medical Imaging of the Spleen
Edited by A. M. De Schepper and F. Vanhoenacker

Radiology of Peripheral Vascular Diseases
Edited by E. Zeitler

Diagnostic Nuclear Medicine
Edited by C. Schiepers

Radiology of Blunt Trauma of the Chest
P. Schnyder and M. Wintermark

Portal Hypertension
Diagnostic Imaging-Guided Therapy
Edited by P. Rossi
Co-edited by P. Ricci and L. Broglia

Virtual Endoscopy and Related 3D Techniques
Edited by P. Rogalla, J. Terwisscha Van Scheltinga, and B. Hamm

Recent Advances in Diagnostic Neuroradiology
Edited by Ph. Demaerel

Transfontanellar Doppler Imaging in Neonates
A. Couture and C. Veyrac

Springer

MEDICAL RADIOLOGY
Diagnostic Imaging and Radiation Oncology

Titles in the series already published

RADIATION ONCOLOGY

Lung Cancer
Edited by C.W. Scarantino

Innovations in Radiation Oncology
Edited by H.R. Withers and L.J. Peters

Radiation Therapy of Head and Neck Cancer
Edited by G.E. Laramore

Gastrointestinal Cancer – Radiation Therapy
Edited by R.R. Dobelbower, Jr.

Radiation Exposure and Occupational Risks
Edited by E. Scherer, C. Streffer, and K.-R. Trott

Radiation Therapy of Benign Diseases - A Clinical Guide
S.E. Order and S.S. Donaldson

Interventional Radiation Therapy Techniques - Brachytherapy
Edited by R. Sauer

Radiopathology of Organs and Tissues
Edited by E. Scherer, C. Streffer, and K.-R. Trott

Concomitant Continuous Infusion Chemotherapy and Radiation
Edited by M. Rotman and C.J. Rosenthal

Intraoperative Radiotherapy – Clinical Experiences and Results
Edited by F.A. Calvo, M. Santos, and L.W. Brady

Radiotherapy of Intraocular and Orbital Tumors
Edited by W.E. Alberti and R.H. Sagerman

Interstitial and Intracavitary Thermoradiotherapy
Edited by M.H. Seegenschmiedt and R. Sauer

Non-Disseminated Breast Cancer Controversial Issues in Management
Edited by G.H. Fletcher and S.H. Levitt

Current Topics in Clinical Radiobiology of Tumors
Edited by H.-P. Beck-Bornholdt

Practical Approaches to Cancer Invasion and Metastases
A Compendium of Radiation Oncologists' Responses to 40 Histories
Edited by A.R. Kagan with the Assistance of R.J. Steckel

Radiation Therapy in Pediatric Oncology
Edited by J.R. Cassady

Radiation Therapy Physics
Edited by A.R. Smith

Late Sequelae in Oncology
Edited by J. Dunst and R. Sauer

Mediastinal Tumors. Update 1995
Edited by D.E. Wood and C.R. Thomas, Jr.

Thermoradiotherapy and Thermochemotherapy

Volume 1:
Biology, Physiology, and Physics

Volume 2:
Clinical Applications
Edited by M.H. Seegenschmiedt, P. Fessenden, and C.C. Vernon

Carcinoma of the Prostate
Innovations in Management
Edited by Z. Petrovich, L. Baert, and L.W. Brady

Radiation Oncology of Gynecological Cancers
Edited by H.W. Vahrson

Carcinoma of the Bladder
Innovations in Management
Edited by Z. Petrovich, L. Baert, and L.W. Brady

Blood Perfusion and Microenvironment of Human Tumors
Implications for Clinical Radiooncology
Edited by M. Molls and P. Vaupel

Radiation Therapy of Benign Diseases. A Clinical Guide
2nd Revised Edition
S.E. Order and S.S. Donaldson

Carcinoma of the Kidney and Testis, and Rare Urologic Malignancies
Innovations in Management
Edited by Z. Petrovich, L. Baert, and L.W. Brady

Progress and Perspectives in the Treatment of Lung Cancer
Edited by P. Van Houtte, J. Klastersky, and P. Rocmans

Combined Modality Therapy of Central Nervous System Tumors
Edited by Z. Petrovich, L. W. Brady, M. L. Apuzzo, and M. Bamberg

Age-Related Macular Degeneration
Current Treatment Concepts
Edited by W. A. Alberti, G. Richard, and R. H. Sagerman

Springer

MIX
Papier aus verantwortungsvollen Quellen
Paper from responsible sources
FSC® C105338

If you have any concerns about our products,
you can contact us on
ProductSafety@springernature.com

In case Publisher is established outside the EU,
the EU authorized representative is:
Springer Nature Customer Service Center GmbH
Europaplatz 3, 69115 Heidelberg, Germany

Printed by Libri Plureos GmbH
in Hamburg, Germany